Stedman's
MEDICAL ABBREVIATIONS,
ACRONYMS & SYMBOLS

FOURTH EDITION

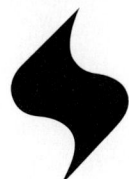

Stedman's
MEDICAL ABBREVIATIONS,
ACRONYMS & SYMBOLS

FOURTH EDITION

Wolters Kluwer Health | Lippincott
Williams & Wilkins

Publisher: Julie K. Stegman
Senior Product Manager: Eric Branger
Managing Editor: Amy Millholen
Typesetter: Josephine Bergin
Printer & Binder: RR Donnelley Crawfordsville

Copyright © 2008 Wolters Kluwer Health|Lippincott Williams & Wilkins
351 West Camden Street
Baltimore, Maryland 21201-2436

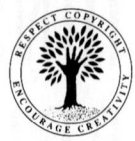

Printed in the United States of America

2008

Library of Congress Cataloging-in-Publication Data
Stedman's medical abbreviations, acronyms & symbols. -- 4th ed.
    p. ; cm.
Rev. ed. of: Stedman's ABBREV abbreviations, acronyms & symbols. 3rd ed. 2003.
Includes bibliographical references.
ISBN-13: 978-0-7817-7261-7 (alk. paper)
ISBN-10: 0-7817-7261-3 (alk. paper)
    1. Medicine--Abbreviations--Dictionaries. 2. Medicine--Acronyms--Dictionaries. I.
Stedman's ABBREV abbreviations, acronyms & symbols. II. Title: Medical abbreviations,
acronyms & symbols. III. Title: Stedman's medical abbreviations, acronyms, and symbols.
    [DNLM: 1. Medicine--Abbreviations. W 13 S811903 2008]
    R123.S69 2008
    610.1'48--dc22

2007042790

08
1 2 3 4 5 6 7 8 9 10

Contents

Acknowledgements

An essential part of our editorial process is the involvement of medical transcriptionists — as advisors, reviewers, and/or editors.

We extend special thanks to Ellen Atwood for diligently editing the manuscript and for her commitment to making this edition even better than the previous. We are grateful to May Updegrove for her assistance with the manuscript review. Thanks also to Pati Howard for her help on this project.

We thank editorial advisory board members Lucinda Allshouse, Barb Blank, Robin Koza, and Suzanne Kusar for their valuable input. Our appreciation goes to Marty Cantu, Robin Koza, and Helen Littrell for helping to enhance the A-to-Z content of this edition. We extend thanks to Jeanne Bock for conducting research for this reference, and to Angela Kelly for helping to revise and expand the appendices. Additional thanks to Helen Littrell for performing the final prepublication review.

As with all our *Stedman's* word references, this resource incorporates the suggestions and expertise of our many contacts in the medical transcriptionist community. Thanks to all of our advisory board participants, reviewers, editors, and others who have written us with requests and comments — keep talking, and we'll keep listening.

Editor's Preface

Abbreviations are the rogues, the rebels, of the tidy medical language world. Despite our best efforts to stomp them out, abbreviations, acronyms, and symbols continue to proliferate like some mad scientist's project gone horribly wrong. There is no cure! They have interesting life spans, some coming to stay, others slinking off into obscurity. Scientists of one specialty may create and use an abbreviation as a one-time thing, for a journal article. That term may be spotted, join the lists of word-watching people, and assume a life of importance beyond its true usefulness. Conversely, it may become as coddled as a beloved pet, used as though it were the "real" word. As if to balance these, there are those occupying the *Do Not Use* and *Dangerous Abbreviations* lists.

Abbreviations, along with their relatives, acronyms, initialisms, and short forms, are very nearly a formal language, with complicated rules of style, usage, and meaning dependent on context. Other than for a handful of technical terms, the world of short forms is a jumble of styles and combinations of letters that nimbly avoid being rounded up into a general, unified, cohesive order. But, medicine and science cannot get along without them and the world in general seems bent on producing and using abbreviations at an alarming rate, as evidenced by terms generated by text messaging, another jargon on the fast track to becoming its own language.

Delving into the mystery of life via proteins and genes has contributed vast numbers of new abbreviations, some of which bear absolutely no resemblance to the expanded meaning, or are purely whimsical. Now that the genome is catalogued, there is a shift away from irregular capitalization and italics to more regular, all upper case capitalization in standard font. However, as genes and protein identification proliferate, new forms of abbreviations have emerged, built on abbreviations within abbreviations, on the order of those Russian nesting dolls. Perhaps tracking down all those genes was the easier task than updating and translating these changes.

Some abbreviations or acronyms, such as *laser* and *radar*, slip so easily into mainstream usage that we are unaware that they are not really a word, but a compilation of letters derived from the original expansion. Newly promoted terms in this category include *faber* and *fabere*, now sporting their stylish lower-case configurations. Others are sure to follow in time.

Other sources of terms include research activities richly productive of new techniques, medications, understanding of disease—and abbreviations. In this 4th edition of *Stedman's Medical Abbreviations, Acronyms, & Symbols*, a generous chunk of new abbreviations arrived by way of the science and practice of war: IED, WMD, TBI, WIA, along with the reawakening of NATO codes used for chemical weapons.

Organizations active in overseeing safe medical practices have identified a group of abbreviations that are considered *DANGEROUS* to use in patient medications and handwritten documentation, now expanded to include all patient documentation. Given the concept's massive impact, the list itself is quite short. Medical transcriptionists and others on the documentation side of medical language are super-cautious about using any abbreviation, or scrutinize each for correctness, while the clinicians and practitioners continue to dictate in the usual jargon. Patient-care providers are charged with compiling in-house lists of abbreviations that are either acceptable for use or are those not to be used, in addition to the lists provided by ISMP and JCAHO. Those responsible for such lists want to nail down "the" correct abbreviation. Sadly, most of the world of abbreviations precludes there being "only one" in the bewildering varieties and spellings generated.

To make life more challenging for medical transcriptionists, many brand name medical equipment terms are variations of commonly used words or phrases. Or vice versa. For example, dictators routinely refer to a Band-Aid, which can only be literally applied to Johnson & Johnson products. A lab test dictated "MONO rapid test," could be the brand name or the slang version for mononucleosis, or some strange amalgam of the two.

We've gone to great lengths to put these seemingly disparate parts together into a comprehensive reference. This gargantuan task was additionally challenged by changing technology. At no time in the 10-plus years that I have edited for Stedman's has the importance of teamwork been more clear.

Huge thanks to Amy Millholen for her professionalism and steadiness. May Updegrove jumped in feet first with great attention to detail. The entire Stedman's staff, as usual, provided support, direction, and belief that this book would emerge.

Ellen Atwood

Publisher's Preface

Stedman's Medical Abbreviations, Acronyms & Symbols, Fourth Edition, offers an authoritative assurance of quality and exactness to the healthcare community including practitioners, educators, students, and the wordsmiths of the healthcare professions—medical transcriptionists, medical editors and copyeditors, health information management personnel, and court reporters. In addition, this reference offers valuable abbreviations, acronyms, symbols, and their meanings to many other areas such as insurance companies, law firms, and others who work or are exposed to medical terminology and medical documentation.

Stedman's Medical Abbreviations, Acronyms & Symbols, Fourth Edition, a compilation of more than 60,000 clinically relevant abbreviations, acronyms, and symbols, is the product of reviews of medical and allied health professional literature since the publication of the third edition in 2003. Our intention with this reference is to present sought-after information in a format that facilitates efficient searching, easy reading, and quick comprehension. New for this edition, we have included a special icon next to error-prone and "dangerous" abbreviations so that they can easily be identified. We encourage you to read the Explanatory Notes section that follows for descriptions of the organization, format, and style, to make the most of the book's features.

The creation of new abbreviations and usage changes outpace compilation of them. Thousands of new abbreviations appear monthly, many of them simply reworking of existing material to the individual specifications of untold numbers of medical specialty journals. We have carefully culled these specialty abbreviations, focusing on quality and usability. We at Lippincott Williams & Wilkins strive to provide you with the most up-to-date and accurate word references available. Your use of this reference will prompt new editions, which we will publish as often as updates and revisions justify. We welcome your suggestions for improvements, changes, corrections, and additions—whatever will make this Stedman's product more useful to you.

Explanatory Notes

Organization

All terms listed within the A-Z portion of this book are referred to and treated as abbreviations, regardless of any formal designations such as initialisms, acronyms, symbols, short form, or other such terms, adhering to the same sequence, style, and format throughout. Abbreviations are represented as singular. To form a plural, add a lower case s.

AVM
arteriovenous malformation
AVMs
arteriovenous malformations

Expansions, too, are singular, except when plural is needed for sense, or if there is an irregular plural:

mm
millimeter
muscles [plural]
NS
no sequela [singular] (sequelae [plural])

Most abbreviations are formed by the first letter of each word in the expansion, frequently ignoring articles (a, an, the). Words containing "of" frequently have two abbreviations, one with an O and one without.

DB
date of birth
DOB
date of birth

Gene and protein names do not always adhere to this pattern, and in future editions may not be considered short forms at all.

SPCA
    coagulation factor VII (serum prothrombin conversion accelerator) [gene F7]

CROSS REFERENCES: Terms having more than one abbreviation are cross-referenced, with the reference appearing in parentheses, following italicized *See also*.

O
    obese (obesity) (*See also* OB)
    obstetrics (*See also* OB, OBS)

OB
    obese (obesity) (*See also* O)
    obstetric(s) (*See also* O, OBS, obstet)

OBS
    obsolete
    obstetric(s) (*See also* O, OB, obstet)

obstet
    obstetric(s) (*See also* O, OB, OBS)

Alphabetical Order

Entries in the A-Z portion of the book are alphabetized letter by letter, then numeric (Arabic or Roman) order, without consideration for superscript, subscript, leading or trailing. Uppercase precedes lower case. Mixed case relies upon first letter of the abbreviation. Standard punctuation and spaces are ignored in the alphabetization. Greek characters require special treatment, as described. Some special characters, such as # or ° (degree sign) are considered part of the abbreviation, and will be separate from a solely alphabetic or alphanumeric term.

OSAS
    obstructive sleep apnea syndrome

O2 sat.
oxygen saturation
OSBCL
Ottawa School Behavior Checklist

R0
no residual tumor [TNM classification]
R1
longitudinal relaxivity
microscopic residual tumor [TNM classification]
R2
macroscopic residual tumor [TNM classification]
transverse relaxivity
∘R
[degree] Rankine [obsolete temperature scale]
[degree] Réaumur [obsolete temperature scale]
+R
Rinne test positive
R#1
good risk [for anesthesia]

Exceptions

A few exceptions to the strict order have been made for ease of use. One such is the varieties of the radiopharmaceutical technetium, listed immediately following the main entry Tc, regardless of isotope designation.
T&C
type and crossmatch
Tc
technetium
temporal complex
^{99}Tc
technetium-99

99mTc
 technetium-99m
99mTc-DMSA
 technetium-99m dimercaptosuccinic acid

VARIANT ABBREVIATIONS: If an abbreviation has more than one form, the varieties are separated by commas, with alphanumeric sequence considering only the first term in the series.
 CN 1–12, CN I–XII
  cranial nerves 1–12 (I–XII)

 CN 1, CN I
  first cranial nerve [olfactory]

ABBREVIATIONS CONTAINING RANGES: Many otherwise identical abbreviations have numerical or alphabetical designators. Rather than listing each one independently, we use the range format, as shown above. Unlike the example above, some abbreviations a designator attached, directly or with a hyphen. The format will then be:
 NRG1–NRG4
  neuregulin 1–4 [protein]

 TIMP-1–TIMP-3
  tissue inhibitor of metalloproteinase 1–3

Again, only the letters and numerals of the first term are considered in sequencing.

GREEK CHARACTERS: Greek characters are alphabetized as pronounced in English, except for those characters that look the same as English characters.
 B
  bel [sound intensity]
  Benoist scale [physics]
  beta [second letter of Greek alphabet uppercase]

β, beta
    probability of type II error
    β [second letter of Greek alphabet lowercase]
    second in series or group

Another exception is the Greek character μ, which is pronounced "mu" but symbolizes "micro." Therefore, all the units of measure using μ will be found in the alphabetical sequence following "micro."

micro
    microscopic [findings]

μ
    mu [12th letter of Greek alphabet lowercase]
    population mean [statistics]

μA
    microampere

micro-AVM
    cerebral microarteriovenous malformation

Format and Style

Each entry consists of a boldface abbreviation, below which is listed its expansions, which are the meanings or, in some instances, interpretations of the individual letters of the abbreviation. Expansions are in alphanumeric order as above, indented, and in lightface. Italics denote genus and/or species.

ABG
    air-bone gap
    aortoiliac bypass graft
    arterial blood gas
    axiobuccogingival

CAPITAL LETTERS, LOWER CASE LETTERS, MIXED CASE: Correctness does not depend upon case for the majority of abbreviations. It is perfectly acceptable to have all capital letters, all lower case letters, and/or mixed case letters denoting the same expansion.

EX

example

ex

example

Ex

example

For this reason, to avoid repetition or confusion, Stedman's has selected a representative term, wherever possible, to consolidate the multiplicity of upper, lower, and mixed case into a single upper case abbreviation.

EX

example

If your institution prefers lower case or mixed case, those are acceptable formats, with the following exceptions:

TECHNICAL AND STANDARDIZED ABBREVIATIONS: Specific abbreviations, case-dependent, are required in technical fields. See below for specific information. However, you will see entries that cannot be merged.

KW

Kruskal-Wallis [test, statistics]

Kw

dissociation constant of water

kW

kilowatt

KWAV

Kwatta virus

kWh, kW-hr

kilowatt-hour

GENUS/SPECIES: Formal representation is initial capital letter and italic font to represent genus, with species in lower case italic. General reference to a microorganism is in normal lower case roman font.

MOTT
mycobacteria other than tubercle (*Mycobacterium tuberculosis*)

RATIO: Abbreviations involving ratios have two formats. One is a standard letter-for-letter abbreviation including "r" for ratio.

RAR
renal to aortic ratio

In the other format, a colon (:) represents the words "to" and "ratio"

S:N
sample to negative control ratio
signal to noise ratio
speech to noise ratio

LATIN TERMS: Upper case Latin abbreviations require no periods; lower case do. These are represented as separate main entries in this edition.

TID
three times a day
t.i.d.
three times a day

ETYMOLOGY: Terms derived from foreign languages are accompanied by etymology information, enclosed in square brackets.

ODT
right occiput transverse (occipitotransverse) [fetal position] [L. *occipitodextra transversa*]

Special Features

MULTIPLE EXPANSIONS: Many terms have multiple expansions with usage a matter of preference, not correctness. Such expansions have been combined, in the manner of variants, with subsequent terms in parentheses. Your institution may have specific rules regarding preferred usage of these terms.

ASCUS
   atypical squamous cells of uncertain (undetermined) significance
ASCVD
   arteriosclerotic (atherosclerotic) cardiovascular disease

Other terms have multiple similar meanings. These too are enclosed in parentheses, for ease of choice.

UAL
   ultrasonic-assisted lipoplasty (liposuction) (lipectomy)

Some terms are too long, cumbersome, or dissimilar for effective combination. In such cases, they are left as separate subentries.

SDB
   seated diastolic blood pressure
   standing diastolic blood pressure
   supine diastolic blood pressure

STT
   scaphoid, trapezium, trapezoid [joint]
   scaphotrapeziotrapezoid [joint]
   scaphotrapezoid-trapezial [joint]

INFLECTED FORMS: Terms that are used in a variety of inflections are shown with base word, then inflected forms in parentheses, for ease of choice:

EEG
   electroencephalograph(y) (electroencephalogram)

OGTT
oral glucose tolerance test(ing)

EXPANDED OR EXPLANATORY INFORMATION: For terms that may be unclear out of context, or need extra information to point towards specialty or application, we have put such explanatory information in brackets, usually at the end of the expansion.

SAF
self-articulating femoral [hip prosthesis]
standard error [statistics]

DANGEROUS ABBREVIATIONS: In keeping with the Institute for Safe Medication Practices (ISMP) and The Joint Commission (JCAHO) directives regarding *Do Not Use* and *Dangerous* abbreviations, such terms are designated with ⚠

SLANG: An abbreviation in red font indicates a slang term, or one in such common usage that there is a specific meaning to its use. The corresponding expansion is also indicated in red font. In some instances, several different expansions will be red. Context will decide the appropriate expansion. Danger symbols are added as appropriate.

⚠ **OD**
occipital dysplasia
occupational dermatitis
occupational disease
oculus dexter [right eye] [L. oculus dexter] (*See also* o.d., RE) ⚠
once daily (*See also* od)⚠
overdose (overdosage)

DRUG ABBREVIATIONS: For additional precaution in medication safety, most drug abbreviations, other than those marked as dangerous or as slang, have been removed from this edition.

ACCEPTED-USE ABBREVIATIONS: Stedman's has gathered terms from across the globe, from a wide variety of scientific and medical sources, and consolidated them into this comprehensive reference. JCAHO's directive indicates each institution is to provide employees with instructions on proper use of abbreviations. An abbreviation included in this edition may be acceptable to one hospital, but not permissible in another setting. The vast numbers of abbreviations (with more coined daily) limits the effectiveness of creating a one-size-fits-all approved abbreviation list.

SCIENTIFIC NOTATION: Standardized terms requiring specific-case abbreviations.

UNITS OF MEASURE

ampere	A
becquerel	Bq
celsius	C
coulomb	C
curie	Ci
Fahrenheit	F
farad	F
joule	J
liter	L [SI formal unit is l, but upper case is preferred because of confusion with numeral 1 or I, and the letter I]
gray	Gy
henry	Hz
newton	N
pascal	Pa
siemens	S
tesla	T
volt	V
watt	W

AMINO ACID ABBREVIATIONS: Each amino acid has 2 recognized abbreviations: a trivial name and a letter symbol. The essential amino acids are:

Amino Acid	Trivial Name	Symbol
alanine	Ala	A
asparagine	Asn	N
cysteine	Cys	C
glutamic acid	Glu	E
histidine	His	H
arginine	Arg	R
aspartic acid	Asp	D
glutamine	Gln	Q
glycine	Gly	G
isoleucine	Ile	I
leucine	Leu	L
lysine	Lys	K
methionine	Met	M
phenylalanine	Phe	K
proline	Pro	P
serine	Ser	S
threonine	Thr	T
tryptophan	Trp	W
tyrosine	Tyr	Y
valine	Val	V

References

The AAMT Book of Style, 2nd Edition. Modesto, CA: AAMT, 2002.

The Charles Press Handbook of Current Medical Abbreviations, Fifth Edition. Philadelphia: The Charles Press, 1997

Davis NM. Medical Abbreviations: 26,000 Conveniences at the Expense of Communication and Safety, 12th Edition. Warminster, PA: Neil M Davis Associates, 2005.

Drake E. Sloane's Medical Word Book, 4th Edition. Philadelphia: Saunders, 2001.

Jablonski S. Cardiology Acronyms and Abbreviations. Baltimore: Lippincott Williams & Wilkins, 2001.

Jablonski S. Dictionary of Medical Acronyms & Abbreviations, 5th Edition. Philadelphia: Elsevier, 2005.

Lance LL. Quick Look Drug Book. Baltimore: Lippincott Williams & Wilkins, 2007.

Marcucci L. Marcucci's Handbook of Medical Eponyms. Baltimore: Lippincott Williams & Wilkins, 2001.

Mitchell-Hatton SL. Davis Book of Medical Abbreviations. Philadelphia: F.A. Davis Company, 1991.

Sloane SB. Medical Abbreviations & Eponyms. Philadelphia: Saunders, 1997.

Stedman's Abbreviations, Acronyms & Symbols, 3rd Edition. Baltimore: Lippincott Williams & Wilkins, 2003.

Stedman's Alternative Medicine Words, 2nd Edition. Baltimore: Lippincott Williams & Wilkins, 2005.

Stedman's Anatomy & Physiology Words, 2nd Edition. Baltimore: Lippincott Williams & Wilkins, 2002.

Stedman's Cardiovascular & Pulmonary Words, 5th Edition. Baltimore: Lippincott Williams & Wilkins, 2007.

Stedman's Dermatology & Immunology Words, 3rd Edition. Baltimore: Lippincott Williams & Wilkins, 2005.

Stedman's Endocrinology Words, 2nd Edition. Baltimore: Lippincott Williams & Wilkins, 2005.

Stedman's GI & GU Words, 4th Edition. Baltimore: Lippincott Williams & Wilkins, 2005.

Stedman's Internal Medicine & Geriatric Words. Baltimore: Lippincott Williams & Wilkins, 2002.

Stedman's Medical Dictionary, 28th Edition. Baltimore: Lippincott Williams & Wilkins, 2005.

Stedman's Medical & Surgical Equipment Words, 5th Edition. Baltimore: Lippincott Williams & Wilkins, 2007.

Stedman's Neurology & Neurosurgery Words, 4th Edition. Baltimore: Lippincott Williams & Wilkins, 2006.

Stedman's OB-GYN & Pediatric Words, 4th Edition. Baltimore: Lippincott Williams & Wilkins, 2005.

Stedman's Oncology Words, 5th Edition. Baltimore: Lippincott Williams & Wilkins, 2006.

Stedman's Ophthalmology Words, 4th Edition. Baltimore: Lippincott Williams & Wilkins, 2006.

Stedman's Organisms & Infectious Disease Words. Baltimore: Lippincott Williams & Wilkins, 2001.

Stedman's Orthopaedic & Rehab Words, 5th Edition. Baltimore: Lippincott Williams & Wilkins, 2005.

Stedman's Pathology & Lab Medicine Words, 4th Edition. Baltimore: Lippincott Williams & Wilkins, 2005.

Stedman's Plastic Surgery, ENT & Dentistry Words, 4th Edition. Baltimore: Lippincott Williams & Wilkins, 2005.

Stedman's Psychiatry Words, 4th Edition. Baltimore: Lippincott Williams & Wilkins, 2007.

Stedman's Radiology Words, 5th Edition. Baltimore: Lippincott Williams & Wilkins, 2006.

Stedman's Surgery Words, 3rd Edition. Baltimore: Lippincott Williams & Wilkins, 2006.

Vera Pyle's Current Medical Terminology, 8th Edition. Modesto, CA: Health Professions Institute, 2000.

A

abortus
absorbance [spectroscopy]
acceptor
accommodation (*See also* ACC)
acetone
acetum [vinegar]
acid (*See also* a, AC)
acidophil (acidophile) (acidophilic)
Acinetobacter
Actinomyces
adenine (*See also* Ade)
adenoma
adrenaline (*See also* Adr)
adult
aesthetic
age
akinetic
alanine (*See also* Ala)
alive
allergy (allergic) (*See also* ALL)
alpha [first letter of Greek alphabet uppercase]
alveolar gas [subscript]
amalgam
ampere
amyloid
anaphylaxis
androsterone
anesthesia (anesthetic) (*See also* AA, AN, ANA, anes, anesth)
anisotropic [band in striated muscle]
annum [year] (*See also* a)
anode (anodal) (*See also* a, AN)
ante [before]
apex [singular] (apices [plural])
aqueous (water) [L. *aqua*] (*See also* aq.)
assessment
asymmetric (*See also* AS)
atomic mass number
atrium (atrial) (*See also* At)
auricle (auricular) [obsolete in reference to heart] (*See also* aur)
auris [ear] (*See also* a, aur)
auscultation
average
axial (*See also* a, ax.)
axilla (axillary) (*See also* ax.)
axillary [temperature] (*See also* (a))
blood group in the ABO system
Helmholtz free energy
[start of] anesthesia (anesthetic)
subspinale [craniometric point A]

A₁

aortic first sound
first auditory area

A₂

aortic second sound
second auditory area

A₄

androstenedione

AI–AIII, A1–A3

angiotensin I–III (*See also* ATI–ATIII, AT1–AT3, ANGI–ANGIII, ANG1–ANG3)

A1–A5

anterior cerebral artery segments 1–5

A250

5% albumin, 250 mL

A1000

5% albumin, 1000 mL

Å

angstrom [non-SI unit of length]

A+

blood type A positive

A-

blood type A negative

(a)

axillary temperature (*See also* A)

a

acceleration (*See also* accel)
accommodation (*See also* A, ACC)
acid (*See also* A, AC)
acidity (*See also* AC)
after
agar
annum [year] (*See also* A)
anode (*See also* AN)
anterior (*See also* AN, ANT, ant.)
area (*See also* S)
arterial blood [subscript]
atto-
auris [ear] (*See also* A, aur)
axial (*See also* A, ax.)

ā

before [L. *ante*] (*See also* bef)
of each

a.

artery (arteria) [singular] [L. *arteria*] (*See also* ART)
before [L. *ante*] (*See also* bef)

a

absorptivity

AA

Academic Alertness
accommodative amplitude
acetabular anteversion
acetic acid

AA *(continued)*
achievement age
active alcoholic
active assistance
active-assisted (active-assistive) [range
   of motion] *(See also* AAROM)
active avoidance
acupuncture analgesia
acute appendicitis
acute asthma
adjuvant arthritis
adrenal androgen
adrenocortical autoantibody
affected area
aggregated albumin
aggregative adherence
agranulocytic angina
alcohol abuse
Alcoholics Anonymous
allergic alveolitis
alopecia areata
alveoloarterial
aminoacetone
amino acid
aminoacyl
amplitude of accommodation
amyloid A
amyloid-associated
anaplastic astrocytoma
androgenetic alopecia
anesthesia (anesthetic) *(See also* A, AN,
   ANA, anes, anesth)
anterior apical
antiarrhythmic agent
anticipatory avoidance
antigen aerosol
aortic amplitude
aortic aneurysm
aortic arch
aplastic anemia
arachidonic acid
Ascaris antigen
ascending aorta *(See also*
   ASCAo)
atlantoaxial
atomic absorption [spectroscopy]
atrial activity
atypical angiomyolipoma
audiologic assessment
authorized absence
autoanalyzer
automobile accident
axonal arborization
A:A
arm to ankle [pulse ratio]
A&A
aid and attendance
arthroscopy and arthrotomy
awake and aware

A-a
alveolar-arterial [gradient]
aortic artery
A-a 0$_2$
alveolar-arterial oxygen tension
aA
abampere
azure A [stain]
aa.
⎯⎯ arteria (arteries) [plural] [L. *arteriae*]
a͞a
of each
AAA
abdominal aortic aneurysm(ectomy)
achalasia-addisonism-alacrimia
acne-associated arthritis
acquired aplastic anemia
acute anxiety attack
addiction, autoimmune diseases, aging
amalgam *(See also* aaa)
amino acid analysis
androgenic anabolic agent
aneurysm of ascending aorta
angiography of abdominal aorta
antigen-extracted allogenic [bone]
aromatic amino acid
arrest after arrival
autolyzed, antigen-extracted, allogenic
   [bone]
[cardiac] arrest after arrival
[diagnostic] arthroscopy, [operative]
   arthroscopy, [possible operative]
   arthrotomy
aaa
amalgam *(See also* AAA)
AAAAA
aphasia, agnosia, apraxia, agraphia,
   alexia
AAAD
aromatic amino acid decarboxylase
AA/AD
alcohol abuse [and] alcohol dependence
AAAE
amino acid activating enzyme
AAAF
albumin autoagglutinating factor
AAAP
autologous blood [selective] aortic arch
   perfusion
AAAV
avian adenoassociated virus
AAB
action against burns
aminoazobenzene
AABCC
alertness [consciousness] airway,
   breathing, circulation, cervical spine
AABR
automated auditory brainstem response

AAC
    acute acalculous cholecystitis
    advanced adrenocortical cancer
    antibiotic-associated colitis
    antigen-antibody crossed
        [electrophoresis]
    antimicrobial agent-induced colitis
    antimicrobial agents and chemotherapy
    augmentative and alternative
        communication
A1AC
    alpha-1 (α1) antichymotrypsin
AACD
    abdominal aortic counterpulsation
        device
    age-associated cognitive decline
AACE
    antigen-antibody crossed electrophoresis
AACG
    acute angle-closure glaucoma
AACI
    arachidonic acid cascade inhibitor
AACLR
    arthroscopic anterior cruciate ligament
        reconstruction
AACSH
    adrenal androgen corticotropic
        stimulating hormone
AAD
    acid-ash diet
    acroangiodermatitis
    acute agitated delirium
    acute aortic dissection
    alcohol abuse or dependence
    alloxazine adenine dinucleotide
    alpha (α) antitrypsin deficiency
    antiarrhythmic drug
    antibiotic-associated diarrhea
    aromatic acid decarboxylase
    atlantoaxial dislocation
A1AD
    alpha (α)1-antitrypsin deficiency
Aad
    alpha (α) aminoadipic acid
AADA
    Abbreviated Antibiotic Drug Application
        [FDA]
AADC
    amino acid decarboxylase
    aromatic L-amino acid decarboxylase
AAdC
    anterior adductor of coxa
AADI
    anterior atlantodental interval
(A-a)D$_{N2}$
    alveolar gas and arterial blood nitrogen
        tension difference

(A-a)DO$_2$
    alveolar gas and arterial blood oxygen
        tension difference
AADP
    amyloid A-degrading protease
AADPPO
    alveolar-arterial difference in partial
        pressure of oxygen
AADR
    age-adjusted death rate
AAE
    acquired angioedema
    active assistive exercise (*See also*
        A/AEX)
    acute allergic encephalitis
    annuloaortic ectasia
AAECS
    amino acid-enriched cardioplegic
        solution
AAEV
    Aedes aegypti entomopoxvirus
A/AEX
    active assistive exercise (*See also* AAE)
AAF
    acetamidofluorene
    acetic acid-alcohol-formalin [fixative]
    2-acetylaminofluorene
    aggregative adherence fimbria [adhesin]
    altered auditory feedback
    aortic arch flush
    ascorbic acid factor
AAFB
    alcohol- [and] acid-fast bacilli
AAFO
    active ankle-foot orthosis
AAG
    allergic angiitis and granulomatosis
    alpha (α)1-acid glycoprotein (*See also*
        AGP)
    alveolar-arterial gradient
    antral atrophic gastritis
    autoantigen
aAg
    autoantigen
AAGS
    adult adrenogenital syndrome
AAH
    acute alcoholic hepatitis
    aortic arch hypoplasia
    atypical adenomatous hyperplasia
AAI
    activating adjusting instrument
    acute adrenal insufficiency
    acute alcohol intoxication
    acute alveolar injury
    Adolescent Alienation Index
    arm-ankle indices

AAI *(continued)*
 atlantoaxial instability
 atrial demand-inhibited
  [pacemaker]
 axial acetabular index
AAIB
 alpha (α)1-aminoisobutyrate
AAIN
 acute allergic interstitial nephritis
AAK
 allo activated killer [cell]
 atlantoaxial kyphosis
AAL
 anterior axillary line
AAM
 acute aseptic meningitis
 aggressive angiomyxoma
 amino acid mixture
AAMD
 age-associated memory disorder
 atrophic age-related macular
  degeneration
AAME
 acetyl arginine methyl ester
AAMI
 age-associated memory impairment
AAML
 atypical angiomyolipoma
AAMRS
 automated ambulatory medical record
  system
AAMS
 acute aseptic meningitis syndrome
AAN
 AIDS-associated nephropathy
 alpha (α)-amino nitrogen
 amino acid nitrogen
 analgesic-associated nephropathy
AA-NAT
 arylalkylamine *N*-acetyltransferase
AAO
 amino acid oxidase
 automated assay optimization
 awake, alert, oriented
(A-a)O$_2$
 alveolar-arterial oxygen gradient
AAOC
 antacid of choice
AAOx3
 alert, awake, oriented to time, place,
  person
AAP
 achromatic automated perimetry
 acute abdominal pain
 acute anterior poliomyelitis
 acute apical periodontitis
 acute appendicitis
 air at atmospheric pressure
 alpha (α)1-antiprotease

 assessment adjustment pass
 attenuated adenomatous polyposis
A-aP$_{CO2}$
 alveolar-arterial carbon dioxide
  difference
a2AP
 a2-antiplasmin
AAPBDS
 anomalous arrangement of
  pancreaticobiliary ductal system
AAPC
 antibiotic-associated pseudomembranous
  colitis
AAPF
 antiarteriosclerosis polysaccharide
  factor
AAPMC
 antibiotic-associated pseudomembranous
  colitis
AaPO$_2$
 arterial to alveolar oxygen pressure
  [tension] ratio
AAPSA
 age-adjusted prostate-specific antigen
AAR
 active avoidance reaction
 acute articular rheumatism
 antigen-antibody reaction
 antigen-antiglobulin reaction
 Australia antigen radioimmunoassay
 automated anesthesia record
AARE
 automobile accident, rear end
AARF
 acute alveolar respiratory failure
 atlantoaxial rotatory fixation
AAROM
 active ankle [joint complex] range of
  motion
 active-assisted (active-assistive) range of
  motion (*See also* AA)
AAS
 acid aspiration syndrome
 acute abdominal series
 alcoholic abstinence syndrome
 allergic *Aspergillus* sinusitis
 amino-alkylsilane
 anabolic-androgenic steroid
 aneurysm of atrial septum
 anthrax antiserum
 aortic arch syndrome
 atlantoaxial subluxation
 atomic absorption spectrophotometry
  (spectrophotometer)
 atypical absence seizure
AASA
 acetabular sector angle
aa seq
 amino acid sequence

AASH
adrenal androgen-stimulating hormone
AASP
acute atrophic spinal paralysis
ascending aorta synchronized pulsation
AASV
antibody-associated systemic vasculitis
AAT
Aachen aphasie test
academic aptitude test
- activity as tolerated
acute abdominal tympany
alanine aminotransferase
alkylating agent therapy
alpha (α)1 antitrypsin (*See also* A1AT)
aminoazotoluene
androgen ablation therapy
animal-assisted therapy
atrial-demand triggered [pacemaker]
atypical antibody titer
auditory apperception test
automatic atrial tachycardia
A1AT
alpha (α)1-antitrypsin (*See also* AAT)
A2AT
alpha (α)2-antitrypsin
AATD
alpha (α)1-antitrypsin disease
AAT-R
Academic Aptitude Test-Revised
AAU
acute anterior uveitis
AAV
(antineutrophil cytoplasmic antibody)
ANCA-associated vasculitis
AAV 1–5
adenoassociated virus 1–5
AAV-CF
adenoassociated virus cystic fibrosis
AAVNRT
atypical atrioventricular nodal reentrant
tachycardia
AAVT
acral arteriovenous tumor
AAVV
accumulated alveolar ventilatory volume
AAW
anterior aortic wall
AAWD
antiandrogen withdrawal
AB
abdominal
abnormal (abnormality) (*See also* ABN,
abn, abnor, abnorm)
abortion
abortus
Ace bandage

active bilaterally
aid to the blind
air bleed
air-bone [conduction]
Alcian blue
ankle-brachial [index]
anterior basal
antibiotic (*See also* ATB, anti bx, ABx,
abx)
antibody (*See also* Ab)
antigen binding
apex (apical) beat
apnea and bradycardia (*See also* A&B)
armboard
asbestos body
asthmatic bronchitis
attentional blink
axiobuccal
blood group in ABO system
3AB
3-aminobenzamide
⚠ **A>B**
air greater than bone [conduction] ⚠
A:B
acid to base ratio
A&B
apnea and bradycardia (*See also* AB)
Ab
antibody (*See also* AB)
aB
azure B [stain]
ABA
abscissic acid
allergic bronchopulmonary aspergillosis
antibacterial activity
applied behavioral analysis
Apraxia Battery for Adults
[cardiac] arrest before arrival
ABA-2
Apraxia Battery for Adults Second
Edition
ABAb
antibeta (β)1 adrenoreceptor antibody
AB/AD
abduction [and] adduction
abductor [and] adductor
ABAER
automated brainstem auditory evoked
response
A band
dark-staining zone of striated muscle
AbAP
antibody-against-panel
ABAV
Abandina virus
ABB
acute bronchitis (bronchiolitis)

A

ABBI
> advanced breast biopsy instrumentation

ABBQ
> Acquired Immunodeficiency Syndrome Beliefs and Behavior Questionnaire

abbr, abbrev
> abbreviate(d) (abbreviation)

ABC
> abbreviated blood count
> Aberrant Behavior Checklist
> absolute band count
> absolute basophil count
> absolute bone conduction
> acalculous biliary colic
> acid balance control
> Activities-Specific Balance Confidence Scale
> adenosine triphosphate (ATP) binding cassette
> advanced breast cancer
> airway, breathing, circulation
> all but code [resuscitation order]
> alternative birth center
> aneurysmal bone cyst
> antigen-binding capacity
> antigen-binding cell
> aortic-brachiocephalic [vein, trauma]
> apnea, bradycardia, cyanosis
> applesauce, bananas, cereal [diet]
> argon beam coagulator
> artificial beta cells
> aspiration biopsy cytology
> assessment of basic competency
> Assessment Battery for Children
> atomic, biological, chemical [warfare, weapon]
> autism behavior checklist
> automated blood count
> avidin-biotin [horseradish peroxidase] complex [method]
> axiobuccocervical

A&BC
> air and bone conduction

ABC and C&C
> airway, breathing, circulation and cervical spine, and consciousness level

ABCD
> airway, breathing, circulation, defibrillate
> airway, breathing, circulation, differential
> airway, breathing, circulation, disability [trauma evaluation]
> Arizona Battery for Communication Disorders of Dementia
> asymmetry, border irregularity, color variegation, and diameter greater than 6 mm [melanoma evaluation]
> avidin-biotin complex assay

ABCDE
> airway, breathing, circulation, disability, exposure
> pentavalent botulism toxoid

ABCDES
> alignment, bone mineralization, calcifications, distribution [of lesions], erosion, soft tissue/nails [x-ray features in arthritis]

ABCIC
> airway, breathing, circulation, intravenous crystalloid

ABCIL
> antibody-mediated cell-dependent immunolympholysis

ABCs
> affect, behavior, cognition [geriatric psychiatry]

ABCT
> (adenosine triphosphate) ATP-binding cassette transporter [gene]

ABD
> abdomen (abdominal) (*See also* abd, abdom)
> adynamic bone disease
> after bronchodilator
> aged, blind, disabled
> aggressive behavioral disturbance
> autologous blood donation
> automatic (automated) boundary (border) detection
> average body dose

abd
> abdomen (abdominal) (*See also* ABD, abdom)
> abduction (*See also* abduc)
> abductor [muscle] (*See also* abduc)

ABDCT
> atrial bolus dynamic computed tomography

abd hyst
> abdominal hysterectomy (*See also* AH)

abdom
> abdomen (abdominal) (*See also* ABD, abd)

abd poll
> abductor pollicis [muscle]

abduc
> abductor [muscle] (*See also* abd)
> abduction (*See also* abd)

ABE
> acute bacterial endocarditis
> adult basic education
> anatomy-based extraction [computed tomography]
> average bioequivalence
> botulism equine trivalent antitoxin

ABECB
  acute bacterial exacerbation of chronic bronchitis
ABEP
  auditory brainstem-evoked potential
ABER
  abducted and externally rotated
  abduction and external rotation
  auditory brainstem evoked response
aber
  aberrant
ABES
  Adaptive Behavior Evaluation Scale
ABES-R
  Adaptive Behavior Evaluation Scale-Revised
ABF
  aortic blood flow
  aortobifemoral [bypass]
  attempted breastfeed
ABG
  air-bone gap
  aortoiliac bypass graft
  arterial blood gas
  axiobuccogingival
ABG PCT
  arterial blood gas point-of-care test
ABH
  angina bullosa haemorrhagica
AbH
  abdominal hysterectomy
ABI
  acquired brain injury
  ankle-brachial index
  atherosclerotic (arteriosclerotic) brain infarction
  atherothrombotic brain infarction
  auditory brainstem implant
ABIC
  Adaptive Behavior Inventory for Children
  antibody excess immune complex
ABID
  antibody identification
ABIT
  assertive behavior inventory tool
ABK
  aphakic bullous keratopathy
ABL
  Abelson protooncogene
  abetalipoproteinemia
  acceptable blood loss
  acute basophilic leukemia
  African Burkitt lymphoma
  allograft-bound lymphocyte
  angioblastic lymphadenopathy
  antigen-binding lymphocyte

  automated biological laboratory
  axiobuccolingual
ABLB
  alternate binaural loudness balance
ABLE
  Adult Basic Learning Examination
ABLV
  Australian bat lyssavirus
ABM
  adjusted body mass
  adult bone marrow
  alveolar basement membrane
  autologous bone marrow
ABMA
  antibasement membrane antibody
ABMD
  anterior basement membrane dystrophy
ABMI
  autologous bone marrow infusion
AbMLV
  Abelson murine leukemia virus
ABMR
  autologous bone marrow rescue
ABMS
  autologous bone marrow support
A/B MS
  apnea [and] bradycardia mild stimulation
ABMT, ABMTx
  allogeneic bone marrow transplant(ation)
  autologous blood and marrow transplantat(ion)
  autologous bone marrow transplant(ation)
ABMV
  Abu Mina virus
ABN, abn
  abnormal (abnormality) (*See also* AB, abnor, abnorm)
  advance beneficiary notice
AbN
  antibody nitrogen [content]
ABNC
  abnormal curve
ABN F%
  abnormal forms percent [sperm count]
ABNG
  AB negative [blood type]
abnor, abnorm
  abnormal (abnormality) (*See also* AB, ABN, abn)
ABO
  absent bed occupant
  blood group system [groups A, AB, B, and O]
ABO-HD
  ABO hemolytic disease

ABP
actin-binding protein
acute biliary pancreatitis
ambulatory blood pressure
androgen-binding protein
antigen-binding protein
arterial blood pressure
automated boundary protection
automatic [systolic] blood pressure
avidin-biotin peroxidase

aBP
arterial blood pressure

ABPA
acute bronchopulmonary asthma
allergic bronchopulmonary aspergillosis

AB/PAS
Alcian blue [and] periodic acid-Schiff [stain]

ABPB
axillary brachial plexus block

ABPC
antibody-producing cell
argon beam plasma coagulation

ABPE
acute bovine pulmonary edema

ABPI
ankle-brachial pressure index

ABPM
allergic bronchopulmonary mycosis
ambulatory blood pressure monitor(ing)

ABR
abortus-Bang-ring [test]
abrasion
absolute bedrest
anterior band remover
arterial baroreflex
artery to bronchus ratio
auditory (audiometric) brainstem response

ABr
agglutination test for brucellosis

abr, abras
abrasion

ABRS
acute bacterial rhinosinusitis

ABRV
Abras virus
Arbroath virus

ABS
abdominal surgery
abnormal brainstem
absent
absolute
absorbed
absorption (*See also* absorb.)
Accu-Chek blood sugar
acrylonitrile-butadiene-styrene [polymer]
acute brain syndrome
Adaptive Behavior Scale

admitting blood sugar
adult bovine serum
Affect Balance Scale
aging brain syndrome
alkylbenzene sulfonate
amniotic band sequence
antibody screen
anti-B serum
arterial blood sample
arterial blood supply
artificial bowel sphincter
at bedside

AB-SAAP
autologous blood selective aortic arch perfusion

absc
abscess
abscissa

AbSD
abductor spasmodic dysphonia

ABSe
ascending bladder septum

ABSEG
atlas-based segmentation [MRI image]

abs feb
fever absent

absorb.
absorption (*See also* ABS)

ABSR
auditory brainstem response

AbSR
abnormal skin reflex

A/B SS
apnea [and] bradycardia self-stimulation

abst, abstr
abstract

ABSV
Absettarov virus

ABT
abstract behavioral type
alcohol breath tester
aminopyrine breath test
antibiotic therapy
autologous blood therapy
autologous blood transfusion
autologous bone marrow transplant(ation)

abt
about

ABTX
alpha (α)-bungarotoxin

ABU
aminobutyrate
asymptomatic bacteriuria

ABV
Agaricus bisporus virus
Aglaonema bacilliform virus
Aransas Bay virus
arthropod-borne virus

AbV
　Agaricus bisporus virus
ABW
　actual body weight
　average body weight
ABx, abx
　antibiotic (*See also* ATB, AB, anti bx)
ABY
　acid bismuth yeast [medium]
aby
　antibody
AbYV
　Abutilon yellow virus
AC
　abdominal circumference
　abdominal compression
　ablation catheter
　abrupt closure
　absorption coefficient
　absorptive cell
　abuse case
　accommodative convergence
　acetate
　acid (*See also* A, a)
　acidified complement
　acidity (*See also* a)
　Acinetobacter calcoaceticus
　aconitine
　acromioclavicular [joint]
　activated charcoal
　acupuncture clinic
　acute
　acute cholecystitis
　adenocarcinoma (*See also* ACA)
　adenylate cyclase
　adenylyl cyclase
　adherent cell
　adrenal cortex
　adrenocorticoid
　aftercoming [placenta]
　air chamber
　air changes
　air conduction
　alcoholic cirrhosis
　alcoholic coma
　all culture [broth]
　alternating current
　alveolar crest
　ambulatory care
　ambulatory controls
　anchored catheter
　anesthesia circuit
　angiocellular
　antecubital
　anterior chamber [of eye]
　anterior circulation
　anterior colporrhaphy

　anterior column
　anterior commissure
　anterior cruciate [ligament]
　antibiotic concentrate
　anticholinergic
　anticoagulant
　anticomplement
　anticomplementary
　anticonvulsant
　antiinflammatory corticoid
　antiphlogistic corticoid
　aortic closure
　aortic compliance
　aortocoronary
　arm circumference
　arterial capillary
　ascending colon
　assist control [ventilation]
　atrial contraction
　atriocarotid
　autoclave
　autologous cell
　axiocervical
　before meals [L. *ante cibum*] (*See also* a.c.)
　NATO code for HCN [hydrogen cyanide]
A2C
　apical two-chamber [view TEE]
A4C
　apical four-chamber [view TEE]
A-C
　adult-versus-child
　aortocoronary [bypass]
A&C
　alert and controlled
A:C
　albumin to coagulin ratio
　albumin to creatinine ratio
　amylase to creatinine clearance ratio
Ac
　acetyl
　actinium
aC
　abcoulomb
　azure C [stain]
a.c.
　before meals [L. *ante cibum*] (*See also* AC)
ACA
　abnormal coronary artery
　accessory conduction ablation
　achylic chloroanemia
　acrodermatitis chronica atrophicans
　acute cerebellar ataxia
　adenine-cytosine-adenine [nucleotide]
　adenocarcinoma (*See also* AC)

ACA *(continued)*
  adenylate cyclase activity
  against clinical advice
  ammoniacal copper arsenate
  amyotrophic choreoacanthocytosis
  anomalous coronary artery
  anterior cerebral artery
  anterior choroidal artery
  anterior communicating aneurysm
  anterior communicating artery (*See also*
    ACoA, AComA, A-comm)
  anticanalicular antibody
  anticardiolipin antibody (*See also*
    ACLA, ACLAb)
  anticentromere antibody (autoantibody)
  anticollagen autoantibody
  anticomplement activity
  anticytoplasmic antibody
  arrhythmic cardiac arrest
  asthma care algorithm
  augmentative communication aid
  automatic chemical agent alarm
  automatic clinical analyzer
7-ACA
  aminocephalosporanic acid
AC:A
  accommodative convergence to
    accommodation ratio
ACAD
  allograft coronary artery disease
  anterior circulation arterial dissection
  asymptomatic coronary artery disease
  arteriosclerotic (atherosclerotic) carotid
    artery disease
  arteriosclerotic (atherosclerotic) coronary
    artery disease
A-CAH
  autoimmune chronic active hepatitis
ACAID
  anterior chamber-associated immune
    deviation
ACAN, ACANTH
  acanthocyte
  acanthrocyte [obsolete]
ACAO
  acylcoenzyme A oxidase
ACAPI
  anterior cerebral artery pulsatility index
ACAS
  asymptomatic carotid artery stenosis
ACASH
  Automated Child/Adolescent Social
    History
ACAT
  acyl coenzyme A cholesterol
    acyltransferase
  aged care assessment team
  automated computed axial
    tomography

ACAV
  Acara virus
ACB
  albumin cobalt binding
  alveolar-capillary block
  antibody-coated bacteria
  aortocoronary bypass
  arterialized capillary blood
  asymptomatic carotid bruit
AC&BC
  air conduction and bone conduction
ACBE
  air contrast barium enema
ACBG
  aortocoronary bypass graft
ACBGS
  aortocoronary bypass graft surgery
ACBS
  aortocoronary bypass surgery
ACC
  acalculous cholecystitis
  acceleration
  accelerator
  accident (*See also* accid)
  accommodation (*See also* A, accom)
  according
  acetylcoenzyme A carboxylase
  acinar cell (acinic-cell) carcinoma
  adenoid cystic carcinoma
  adrenocortical carcinoma
  advanced colorectal cancer
  agenesis of corpus callosum
  alveolar cell carcinoma
  amylase to creatinine clearance [ratio]
  anterior central curve
  anterior cingulate cortex
  antitoxin-containing cell
  aplasia cutis congenita
  articular chondrocalcinosis
  automated cell count
accel
  acceleration (*See also* a)
  accelerations [labor]
ACCHN
  adenoid cystic carcinoma of head and
    neck
ACCI
  Adult Career Concerns Inventory
accid
  accident (*See also* ACC)
ACCLA
  anticardiolipin lupus anticoagulant
accom
  accommodation (*See also* A, ACC)
AcCPV
  Arctia caja cypovirus
ACCR
  amylase to creatinine clearance
    ratio

ACCS
    acute change clinical score
ACCSCI
    acute central cervical spinal cord injury
accum
    accumulate(d) (accumulation)
accur.
    accurate(ly) [L. *accuratissime*]
ACD
    absolute cardiac dullness
    absolute claudication distance
    absorbent cover dressing
    acid-citrate-dextrose [blood collection
      tube]
    active compression-decompression
    adult celiac disease
    advanced care directive
    allergic contact dermatitis
    alopecia, contracture, dwarfism
    alpha-chain disease
    alternative communication device
    anemia of chronic disease
    angiokeratoma corporis diffusum
    annihilation coincidence detection
    anterior capsular distance
    anterior cervical discectomy
    anterior chamber depth [eye]
    anterior chamber diameter
    anterior chest diameter
    anticonvulsant (antiepileptic) drug
      (*See also* AED)
    area [of] cardiac dullness
    arrhythmia control device
    Assessment of Career Development
AcD
    alive with disease
AC-DC
    alternating current [and] direct current
ACD-CPR
    active compression-decompression
      cardiopulmonary resuscitation
ACDF
    adult child of dysfunctional family
    anterior cervical discectomy and fusion
ACDK
    acquired cystic disease of kidney
ACDM
    Assessment of Career Decision Making
ACDV
    Acado virus
ACE
    acetonitrile
    actinium emanation
    acute care for elderly
    acute cerebral encephalopathy
    acute coronary event
    adrenocortical extract

    advanced combined encoder
    adverse clinical event
    aerobic chair exercise
    aerosol cloud enhancer
    alcohol, chloroform, ether (mixture)
    angiotensin-converting enzyme
    antegrade colonic enema
    antegrade continence enema
    autologous-cultured epithelium
ace
    accessory cholera enterotoxin
ace.
    acentric
ACE I–II
    angiotensin-converting enzyme I–II
ACED
    anhidrotic congenital ectodermal
      dysplasia
ACE-DD
    angiotensin-converting enzyme DD
      [genotype]
ACEDS
    angiotensin-converting enzyme
      dysfunction syndrome
ACEH
    acid cholesterol ester hydrolase
ACEI
    angiotensin-converting enzyme inhibitor
ACE IT
    AsthmaCare Education: Intensive
      Training
AcEst
    acetyl esterase
ACET
    aquatic cardiac evaluation and testing
acetyl-CoA
    acetylcoenzyme A
ACEV
    Anomala cuprea entomopoxvirus
ACF
    aberrant crypt focus
    accessory clinical findings
    active case finding [for tuberculosis]
    advanced communications function
    anterior cervical fusion
    anterior cranial fossa
    area correction factor
    asymmetric crying facies
ACFM
    automated cardiac flow measurement
ACFn
    additional cost of false negatives
ACFp
    additional cost of false positives
ACFS
    anterior cervical plate fixation
      system

ACG
angiocardiograph(y) (angiocardiogram)
angle-closure glaucoma
aortocoronary graft
apexcardiograph(y) (apexcardiogram)
Assessment of Core Goals

AcG
accelerator globulin [factor V]

aCGH
array-based comparative genomic
hybridization

ACH
acetaldehyde
achalasia
active chronic hepatitis
adrenal cortical (adrenocortical) hormone
aftercoming head
air change per hour
amyotrophic cerebellar hypoplasia
arm girth, chest depth, and hip width
[nutritional index]

ACh
acetylcholine

ACHA
air-conduction hearing aid

AChA
anterior choroidal artery

AChE
acetylcholinesterase

AChEI
acetylcholinesterase inhibitor

ACHES
abdominal pain, chest pain, headache,
eye problems, severe leg pain

ACHOO
autosomal dominant compelling
helioophthalmic outburst [syndrome]

AChR
acetylcholine receptor

AChRAb
acetylcholine receptor antibody

AC&HS
before meals and at bedtime [L. *ante
cibum* + *hora somni*]

AcHV
Acciptrid herpesvirus

ACI
acceleration index
acoustic comfort index
acute cardiac ischemia
acute coronary infarct(ion)
acute coronary insufficiency
adenylate cyclase inhibitor
adrenocortical insufficiency
aftercare instructions
anabolic-catabolic index
anemia of chronic illness
anticlonus index
asymptomatic cardiac ischemia

autologous chondrocyte implantation
average cost of illness

ACID
Arithmetic, Coding, Information, and
Digit Span

ACIDS
acquired cellular immunodeficiency
syndrome

ACIF
acute care index of functions
anterior cervical interbody fusion
anticomplement immunofluorescence

AC IOL, ACIOL
anterior chamber intraocular lens

ACIP
acute canine idiopathic polyneuropathy
Advisory Committee on Immunization
Practices

ACIS
ambulatory care information system
Assessment of Communication and
Interaction Skills
automated cellular imaging system

ACIT
allogeneic cellular immune therapy

ACJ
acromioclavicular joint

ACKD
acquired cystic kidney disease

ACL
accessory collateral ligament
Achievement Checklist
acromegaloid features, cutis verticis
gyrata, corneal leukoma
Adjective CheckList
Allen Cognitive Level
anal canal length
anterior cruciate ligament

aCL
anticardiolipin

ACLA, ACLAb
anticardiolipin antibody (*See also* ACA)

ACLC
Assessment of Children's Language
Comprehension

AcLDL
acetylated low-density lipoprotein

ACLE
acute cutaneous lupus erythematosus

ACLF
adult congregate living facility

ACLR
anterior capsulolabral reconstruction
anterior cruciate ligament reconstruction
(repair)

ACLS
acrocallosal syndrome
advanced cardiac life support
Allen Cognitive Level Screen

AcLV
> avian acute leukemia virus

ACM
> acute cerebrospinal meningitis
> acute confusional migraine
> albumin, calcium, magnesium
> [containing saline]
> alcoholic cardiomyopathy
> alternative/complementary medicine
> alveolar capillary membrane
> anterior chamber maintainer
> anticardiac myosin
> Arnold-Chiari malformation
> asbestos-containing material
> automated cardiac flow measurement

ACME
> aphakic cystoid macular edema

ACMF
> arachnoid cyst of middle fossa

ACMI
> age-consistent memory impairment

ACML, aCML
> atypical chronic myeloid leukemia

AcMNPV
> *Autographa californica* multicapsid
> nucleopolyhedrovirus

ACMP
> alveolar-capillary membrane permeability

ACMS
> acute quadriplegic myopathy syndrome

ACMT
> advanced combined modality therapy
> artificial circus-movement tachycardia

ACMV
> assist-controlled (assist-control)
> mechanical ventilation

ACN
> accessory cuneate nucleus [Monakow
> nucleus]
> acute conditioned neurosis

ACO
> acute coronary occlusion
> alert, cooperative, oriented
> anterior capsular opacification
> Assessment of Conceptual Organization

ACOA
> adult child of alcoholic

ACoA
> anterior communicating artery (*See also*
> ACA, AComA, A-comm)

ACOM
> automated cardiac output measurement

AComA
> anterior communicating artery (*See also*
> ACoA, ACA, A-comm)

A-comm
> anterior communicating artery (*See also*
> ACA, ACoA, AComA)

acor
> apex cornea

acous
> acoustic (acoustics)

ACP
> absorbable collagen paste
> accessory conduction pathway
> acid phosphatase (*See also* AcP, AC-PH,
> ac phos, AP)
> acyl carrier protein
> adamantinomatous craniopharyngioma
> adenocarcinoma of prostate
> anterior cervical plate
> antrochoanal polyp

AcP
> acid phosphatase (*See also* ACP,
> AC-PH, ac phos, AP)

ACPA
> anticytoplasmic antibody
> (autoantibody)

AC-PC
> anterior commissure-posterior
> commissure

ACPE
> acute cardiogenic pulmonary edema

AC-PH
> acid phosphatase (*See also* ACP, AcP,
> AP, ac-phos)

ac-phos
> acid phosphatase (*See also* ACP, AcP,
> AC-PH, AP)

ACPL
> antibody-conjugated paramagnetic
> liposome

ACPO
> acute colonic pseudoobstruction

ACPP
> adrenocorticopolypeptide (adrenocortical
> polypeptide)

ACPR30
> adipocyte complement related protein of
> 30 kilodalton

ACPS
> acrocephalopolysyndactyly
> (acrocephalosyndactyly)
> anterior cervical plate stabilization

ACQ
> Achenbach-Conners-Quay [Behavior]
> Checklist

acq
> acquired
> acquisition

ACR
> abnormally contracting regions
> absolute catabolic rate
> adenomatosis of colon and rectum
> albumin to creatinine ratio
> anterior chamber reformation

ACR *(continued)*
anticonstipation regimen
axillary count rate

Acr
acrylic

ACRC
advanced colorectal cancer

ACRF
acute-on-chronic respiratory failure

ACS
abdominal compartment syndrome
acetyl strophanthidin
acrocallosal syndrome
acrocephalosyndactyly [type I–V]
acute chest syndrome
acute confusional state
acute coronary syndrome
acute mountain sickness
Advanced Cardiovascular Systems
Advanced Catheter System
Alcon Closure System
anterior compartment syndrome
anterior cricoid split
antireticular cytotoxic serum
aperture current setting
arterial cannulation support
automated corneal shaper

ACSF
abdominal computed tomography
artificial cerebrospinal fluid

ACSL
automatic computerized solvent
litholysis

ACSV
aortocoronary-saphenous vein [bypass,
graft]

ACSVBG
aortocoronary-saphenous vein bypass
graft

ACT
ablation catheter tip
Achievement Through Counseling and
Treatment
acid clearance test
activated clotting time
activated coagulation time
adaptive control of thought
adaptive current tomography
adenylate cyclase toxin
adoptive cellular therapy
advanced coronary treatment
aggressive comfort treatment
allergen challenge test
alpha (α) antichymotrypsin
alternate cover test
antichymotrypsin
anticoagulant therapy
antrocolic transposition
anxiety control training

asthma care training
atropine coma therapy
axial computed tomography

act.
active (activity) *(See also* α)

ACTA
automatic computed transverse axial
[scan(ning) scanner]

ACTeRS
ADD-H: Comprehensive Teacher's
Rating Scale, Second Edition

Act Ex
active exercise

ACTH
adrenocorticotropic hormone
(corticotropin)

ACTH-LI
adrenocorticotropin-like immunoreactivity

ACTHR
adrenocorticotropic hormone receptor

ACTH-RF
adrenocorticotropic hormone-releasing
factor

ACTHR/MC-2
adrenocorticotropin receptor/melanocortin
receptor 2

ACTN
adrenocorticotropin

ACTP
adrenocorticotropic polypeptide

ActR
activin receptor

ACTRS
Abbreviated Conners Teacher Rating
Scale

ACTS
acute cervical traumatic sprain
(syndrome)
Auditory Comprehension Test for
Sentences

ACTV
Acatinga virus

ACU
acquired cold urticaria

ACUP
adenocarcinoma of unknown
primary

ACUTENS
acupuncture and transcutaneous
electrical nerve stimulation

ACUV
air-contrast ultrasound venography

A-C-V
A wave, C wave, V wave

ACV
acute cardiovascular [disease]
adaptive cardio volume [reconstructive
approach]
assist/control ventilation

atrial/carotid/ventricular
autonomic conduction velocity
ACVB
aortocoronary venous bypass
ACVD
acute cardiovascular disease
arteriosclerotic (atherosclerotic)
cardiovascular disease
autoimmune collagen vascular disease
ACVRD
arteriosclerotic (atherosclerotic)
cardiovascular renal disease
ACW
anterior chest wall
AC/W
acetone in water
ACx
anomalous circumflex [coronary artery]
acyl-CoA
acylcoenzyme A
⚠ **AD**
abdominal diameter
above diaphragm
absorbed dose
accidental death
accident dispensary
acetate dialysis
achievement drive
active disease
acute dermatomyositis
addict(ion) (addictive) (*See also*
addict.)
adductor
adenoid degeneration [agent]
adenovirus
adherent
adipocyte
adjuvant disease
admitting diagnosis
adnexa
adrenal
adrenodoxin [protein]
adult disease
advance directive
aerodynamic mass diameter
aerosol deposition
affective disorder
after discharge
air dyne
alcohol dehydrogenase
Aleutian disease [of mink] (*See also*
AMD)
alternating days
alveolar diffusion
alveolar duct
Alzheimer dementia (disease)
analgesic dose

analog device
androgen deprivation
androstenedione
anisotropic disc
anterior displacement
anterior division
antidepressant
antidiarrheal
antigenic determinant
aortic diameter
aortic dissection
appropriate disability
arthritic dose
assistive device
atopic dermatitis
attentional disturbance
autistic disorder
autogenic drainage
autonomic dysreflexia
autosomal dominant
average day
average deviation
average difference
axillary dissection
axiodistal
axis deviation
right ear [L. *auris dexter*] (*See also*
a.d., RE) ⚠
A&D
admission and discharge
alcohol and drugs
ascending and descending
vitamins A and D
A/D
analog-to-digital [converter]
⚠ **a.d.**
alternating days (every other day) [L.
alternis dies]
as desired
right ear [L. *auris dextra*] (*See also*
AD, RE) ⚠
ad.
let there be added [L. *addetur*]
(*See also* add.)
ADA
adenosine deaminase
alternated delay acquisition
Americans with Disabilities Act
anterior descending artery
antideoxyribonucleic acid antibody
approved dietary allowance
ADA #
American Diabetes Association diet
number
ADACS
automatic data acquisition and control
system

ADAD
  Adolescent Drug and Alcohol
  Diagnostic Assessment
ADAM
  adjustment disorder with anxious mood
  aerosol-derived airway morphometry
  amniotic deformity, adhesion, mutilation
  [syndrome]
  androgen deficiency in aging males
  [syndrome, questionnaire]
  arrestee drug abuse monitoring
  a disintegrin and metalloprotease
  (metalloproteinase)
ADAMHA
  Alcohol, Drug Abuse, and Mental
  Health Administration [local level]
ADAMTS 13
  a disintegrin and metalloprotease
  (metalloproteinase) with
  thrombospondin domain 13
ADAP
  AIDS Drug Assistance Program
ADAPC
  alcohol and drug abuse prevention and
  control
ADAPTS
  acute directional atherectomy prior to
  stenting
ADAS
  Alzheimer Disease Assessment Scale
ADAS-Cog, ADAS-cog
  Alzheimer Disease Assessment Scale,
  cognitive subscale
ADase
  adenosine deaminase
ADASI
  Atopic Dermatitis Area and Severity
  Index
ADAT
  advance diet as tolerated
ADAU
  adolescent drug abuse unit
ADB
  anti-DNase B
ADC
  adult day care
  Aid to Dependent Children
  AIDS dementia complex
  albumin, dextrose, catalase [medium]
  ambulance design criteria
  analog-to-digital converter
  antibody-directed catalysis
  antral diverticulum of colon
  apparent diffusion coefficient
  average daily census
  axiodistocervical
AdC
  adenylate cyclase
  adrenal cortex

ADCA
  autosomal dominant cerebellar ataxia
ADCC
  acute disorder of cerebral circulation
  antibody-dependent cell(ular) cytotoxicity
ADCD
  antibody complement-dependent
  cytolysis
ADCHF
  acutely decompensated congestive heart
  failure
ADCMC
  antibody-dependent complement-mediated
  cytotoxicity
AD-CPEO
  autosomal dominant chronic progressive
  external ophthalmoplegia
ADD
  acceptable daily dose
  adduction
  adenosine deaminase
  alcohol and drug dependency
  angled delivery device
  attention deficit disorder
  auditory discrimination
  average daily dose
ADD1
  adipocyte determination and
  differentiation factor 1
add.
  addition
  let there be added [L. *addetur*]
  (*See also* ad.)
ADDBD
  attention deficit and disruptive behavior
  disorder
ADDBRS
  Attention Deficit Disorder Behavior
  Rating Scale
addend.
  to be added [L. *addendus*]
ADDES
  Attention Deficit Disorders Evaluation
  Scale
ADD-HA
  attention deficit disorder with
  hyperactivity (*See also* ADHD,
  ADD-H)
addict.
  addict(ion) (addictive) (*See also* AD)
ADDM
  adjustment disorder with depressed
  mood
AdDNV
  Acheta domestica densovirus
ADE
  acute disseminated encephalitis
  (encephalomyelitis) (*See also* ADEM)
  adverse drug effect

adverse drug event
antibody-dependent enhancement
apparent digestible energy
apparent digestive efficiency
Ade
adenine (*See also* A)
ADEAR
Alzheimer's Disease Education and
Referral
AdeCbl
adenosyl cobalamin
ADEE
age-dependent epileptic encephalopathy
ADEM
acute disseminated encephalitis
(encephalomyelitis) (*See also* ADE)
ADEPT
antibody-directed enzyme prodrug
therapy
adeq
adequate
A-DES
Adolescent Dissociative Experiences
Scale
ADF
aortoduodenal fistula
AD:FHD
acetabular depth to femoral head
diameter ratio
ADFN
albinism-deafness [syndrome]
AD-FSP
autosomal dominant familial spastic
paraplegia
ADFT
atrial defibrillation threshold
ADFU
agar diffusion for fungus
ADG
adjustable-depth gauge [needle]
atrial diastolic gallop
axiodistogingival
ADH
adhesion (adhesive)
alcohol dehydrogenase
antidiuretic hormone
atypical ductal hyperplasia
AdHCC
advanced hepatocellular carcinoma
ADHD, ADD-H
attention deficit hyperactivity disorder
(*See also* ADD-HA)
ADHD-PI
attention deficit hyperactivity
disorder-predominantly inattentive
ADHF
acute decompensated heart failure

ad hoc
for this [purpose] (temporary) [L. *ad
hoc*]
ADI
absolute dose intensity
acceptable (allowable) daily intake
Adolescent Diagnostic Interview
Adolescent Drinking Index (Inventory)
antral (artificial) diverticulum of ileum
atlantodens interval
Autism Diagnostic Interview
autosomal-dominant ichthyosis
axiodistoincisal
ADI-R
Autism Diagnostic Interview Revised
ADJ
adjustable dynamic joint
adj
adjacent
adjoining
adjunct
adjust(ment)
adjuvant
ADK
adenosine kinase [gene]
automated disposable keratome
ADKC
atopic dermatitis with
keratoconjunctivitis
ADL
activities of daily living
adolescent medicine [pediatrics]
adrenoleukodystrophy
Amsterdam Depression List
ADL-AMN
adrenoleukodystrophy-
adrenomyeloneuropathy
ADLC
antibody-dependent lymphocyte-mediated
cytotoxicity
ad lib.
ad libitum [as desired, freely] [L. *ad
libitum*]
ADLR
advanced design LINAC radiosurgery
ADM
abductor digiti minimi [muscle]
administration (*See also* admin)
administrative medicine
admission
admit
Allen Diagnostic Module
amyopathic dermatomyositis
apparent distribution mass
atypical diabetes mellitus
AdM
adrenal medulla

ADMA
asymmetric dimethylarginine

ADMCKD
autosomal dominant medullary cystic kidney disease

Adm Dr
admitting doctor

ADME
absorption, distribution, metabolism, excretion

admin
administer
administration (*See also* ADM)

ADMLX
adhesion moleculelike X-linked [gene]

Adm Ph
admitting physician

ADMR
average daily metabolic rate

ADMX
adrenal medullectomy

ADN
aortic depressor nerve

adn
adenoid(ectomy)

ADNase
antideoxyribonuclease

ADNase-B
antideoxyribonuclease B (*See also* anti-DNase B)

ad naus.
to the point of producing nausea [L. *ad nauseam*]

ADNR
anterior displacement no reduction [fracture]

ADO
adolescent medicine
axiodistoocclusal

ADO2
autosomal dominant osteopetrosis type 2

Ado
adenosine

ADOA
autosomal dominant ocular albinism

ADOD
arthrodentoosteodysplasia

ADODM
adult-onset diabetes mellitus

AdoHcy
S-adenosyl-L-homocysteine (*See also* SAH)

AdoHcyase
S-adenosyl-L-homocysteine hydrolase

adol
adolescent

AdoMet
S-adenosyl-L-methionine (*See also* SAM)

ADOS
Autism Diagnostic Observation Schedule
autosomal dominant Opitz syndrome

Adox
oxidized adenosine

ADP
adenopathy
adenosine diphosphate (adenosine 5'-diphosphate)
adenovirus death protein
ammonium dihydrogen phosphate
approved drug product
area diastolic pressure
artrial demand pacing
automatic data processing

ADPA
aggressive digital papillary adenoma

ADPase
adenosine diphosphatase (adenosine 5'-diphosphatase)

ADP/ATP
adenosine 5'-diphosphate [and] adenosine triphosphate

ADPKD
autosomal dominant polycystic kidney disease

ADPL
average daily patient load

ADPR
adenosine diphosphate ribose

ADPRT
adenosine diphosphoribosyl transferase

ADPV
anomaly of drainage of pulmonary vein

ADQ
abductor digiti quinti [muscle]
adequate
adolescent drinking questionnaire

ADR
absence of deep reflexes
acceptable dental remedies
activation, depression, repetition [bone remodeling]
actual death rate
acute dystonic reaction
adrenergic receptor
adrenodoxin reductase
adverse drug[-induced] reaction
airways dilation reflex
allergic drug reaction
arrested development of righting response
ataxia-deafness-retardation [syndrome]

Adr
adrenaline (*See also* A)

adr
adrenal(ectomy)

ADRA
alpha (α) adrenergic receptor

ADRA2
alpha (α)2 adrenergic receptor
ADRA1A
alpha (α)1A adrenergic receptor
ADRA1B
beta (α)1B adrenergic receptor
ADRA2C
alpha (α)2C adrenergic receptor
ADRBR
adrenergic beta (β)-receptor
ADRD
Alzheimer disease and related disorders
ADRF
adiabatic demagnetization in rotating
frame
ADROM
ankle dorsiflexion range of motion
ADRP
adipocyte differentiation-related protein
adRP
autosomal-dominant retinitis pigmentosa
ADRS
Alzheimer Disease Rating Scale
ADRV
adult diarrhea rotavirus
ADS
acute death syndrome
acute diarrheal syndrome
Alcohol Dependence Scale
alternative delivery system
anatomical dead space
anonymous donor sperm
anterior drawer sign
antibody deficiency (antibody-deficient)
syndrome
antidiuretic substance
autonomous detection system
AdSD
adductor spasmodic dysphonia
ADSI
Atopic Dermatitis Severity Index
ADSQC
adenosquamous cell carcinoma
ADSU
ambulatory diagnostic surgery unit
ADSV
Arboledas virus
Arborea virus
ADT
accepted dental therapeutics
adenosine triphosphate
admission, discharge, transfer
agar (agar-gel) diffusion test
alternate day therapy
androgen deprivation therapy
anterior drawer test
anticipate discharge tomorrow

any desired thing
Auditory Discrimination Test
automated dithionite test
ADTP
adolescent day treatment program
alcohol dependence treatment program
ADU
acute duodenal ulcer
ADV
adventitia
A/DV
arterial [and] deep venous
AdV
adenovirus
adv
advance(d)
advice
advise
ADVIRC
autosomal-dominant
vitreoretinochoroidopathy
ADVS
Activities of Daily Vision Scale
ADW
assault with deadly weapon
A5D5W
5% alcohol and 5% dextrose in water
ADWOR
anterior disc displacement without
reduction
ADWR
anterior displacement with reduction
ADX
adrenalectomy (adrenalectomized)
AE
above-elbow [amputation]
accident and emergency [British for
emergency room] (*See also* A&E)
accurate empathy
acrodermatitis enteropathica
activation energy
acute exacerbation
adaptive equipment
adrenal epinephrine
adult erythrocyte
adverse event
aftereffect
agarose electrophoresis
air embolism
air entry
airplane ear
alcoholic embryopathy
androstanediol
anion exchange
anoxic encephalopathy
antiembolitic
antiepileptic

AE *(continued)*
  Antitoxineinheit [German for antitoxin unit]
  apoenzyme
  arm ergometer
  aryepiglottic [fold]
  arteriosclerotic (atherosclerotic) encephalopathy
  atrial ectopic
  avian encephalomyelitis
AE1
  anion exchanger 1
  antikeratin
A&E
  accident and emergency [British for emergency room] (*See also* AE)
A/E
  assess and evaluate
  assessment and evaluation
AEA
  above-elbow amputation (*See also* AE)
  adrenal epithelioid angiosarcoma
  alcohol, ether, acetone [solution]
  allergic extrinsic alveolitis
  antiendomysium antibody
  autoerotic asphyxiation
AEB
  acute erythroblastopenia
  as evidenced by
  atrial ectopic beat
  avian erythroblastosis
AEC
  absolute [blood] eosinophil count
  3-amino-9-ethylcarbazole [solution]
  ankyloblepharon, ectodermal defect, cleft lip and/or palate [syndrome]
  aortic ejection click
  at earliest convenience
  Atomic Energy Commission
  automatic exposure control
AECA
  antiendothelial cell antibody (autoantibody)
AECB
  acute exacerbation of chronic bronchitis
AECD
  allergic eczematous contact dermatitis
  automatic external cardioverter-defibrillator
AECG
  ambulatory echocardiogram
  ambulatory electrocardiograph(y) (electrocardiogram)
AECGM
  ambulatory electrocardiography monitoring
AECOPD
  acute exacerbation of chronic obstructive pulmonary disease

AECP
  antiepiligrin cicatricial pemphigoid
AECS
  acute exacerbation of chronic sinusitis
  acute exertional compartment syndrome
AECUS
  atypical endocervical cells of undetermined (unknown) significance
AED
  aerodynamic equivalent diameter
  antiepileptic (anticonvulsant) drug (*See also* ACD)
  antihidrotic ectodermal dysplasia
  anxious ego dissolution
  automatic (automated) external defibrillator
AEDF
  absent end-diastolic blood flow [umbilical artery Doppler]
AEDP
  assisted end-diastolic pressure
  automated external defibrillator pacemaker
aEEG
  amplitude-integrated electroencephalogram
AEF
  allogenic effect factor
  amyloid-enhancing factor
  aortoenteric fistula
  aryepiglottic fold
  auditory-evoked magnetic field
AEFB
  aerobic endospore-forming bacterium
AEFI
  acute esophageal food impaction
  Adverse Event Following Immunization [WHO]
AEFV
  acceleration of early flow velocity
AEG
  acute erosive gastritis
  air encephalograph(y) (encephalogram)
  atrial electrogram
Ae-H interval
  anterograde conduction
AEI
  atrial emptying index
AEIOU TIPS
  alcohol, epilepsy, insulin, overdose, uremia, trauma, infection, psychiatric, stroke [causes of decreased level of consciousness]
AEL
  acute erythroleukemia
AELBM
  after each loose bowel movement
AELT
  ascites euglobulin lysis time

AELV
avian enterolike virus
AEM
active electrode monitoring
ambulatory electrocardiographic
(electrogram) monitoring
analytical electron microscopy
(microscope)
antiepileptic medication
avian encephalomyelitis
AEMB
abdominal electromyography
AEMK
ataxia episodica with myokymia
AEN
anal epithelial neoplasia
aseptic epiphyseal necrosis
AENNS
Albert Einstein Neonatal Developmental
Scale
AEO
apraxia of eyelid opening
AEP
acute edematous pancreatitis
admission evaluation protocol
appropriateness evaluation protocol
artificial endocrine pancreas
auditory evoked potential
average evoked potential
AEq
age equivalent
AER
abduction-external rotation
acoustic evoked response
acute exertional rhabdomyolysis
agranular endoplasmic reticulum
aided equalization response
albumin excretion rate
alcohol elimination rate
aldosterone excretion rate
apical ectodermal ridge
auditory evoked response
automatic endoscopic reprocessor
average electroencephalic response
average evoked response
aer
aerosol
AERA
average evoked response audiometry
AERD
aspirin-exacerbated respiratory
disease
atheroembolic renal disease
AerM
aerosol mask
Aero
Aerobacter

AERP
antegrade effective refractory period
atrial effective refractory period
auditory event related potential
AERPAP
antegrade effective refractory period
accessory pathway
AerT
aerosol tent
AES
acetone-extracted serum
Alzheimer euphoria state
anal endosonography
anterior esophageal sensor
antielevation syndrome
antiembolic stockings
antieosinophilic serum
antral ethmoidal sphenoidectomy
aortic ejection sound
Auger electron spectroscope
AESOP
automated endoscopic system for
optimal positioning
AESP
applied extrasensory projection
AEST
aeromedical evacuation support team
AET
absorption-equivalent thickness
alternating esotropia
aminoethylisothiouronium bromide
atrial ectopic tachycardia
AEU
[Allercoat] enzyme allergosorbent unit
AEV
avian encephalomyelitis-like virus
avian erythroblastosis virus
AeV
Antheraea eucalypti virus
AEVS
automated eligibility verification system
AEX, AEx
aerobic exercise
AEZ
acrodermatitis enteropathica, zinc
deficient
AF
abnormal frequency
acid fast
adult female
afebrile (*See also* AFEB)
aflatoxin (*See also* AFT)
aggressive fibromatosis
albumose-free [tuberculin]
alcoholic female
aldehyde fuchsin
alleged father

AF *(continued)*
    amaurosis fugax
    ameloblastic fibroma
    amniotic fluid
    anchoring fibril
    angiogenesis factor
    anteflex(ed) (anteflexion)
    anterior fontanelle
    anterior frontal (anterofrontal)
    antibody forming
    antifibrinogen
    antifungal
    aortic flow
    aortofemoral
    apical foramen
    arcuate fasciculus
    artificial feeding
    artificially fed
    ascitic fluid (*See also* ascit fl)
    atrial fibrillation (*See also* AFib, At Fib, at.fib., ATR FIB, atr fib)
    atrial flutter (*See also* AFL)
    atrial fusion
    attenuation factor
    attributable fraction
    audiofrequency

AF-1
    antifertility factor-1

A-F
    air-fluid [level]
    ankle-foot [orthosis]

aF
    abfarad

AFA
    acromegaloid facial appearance
    advanced first aid
    alcohol-formaldehyde-acetic acid [fixative, solution]

AFAFP
    amniotic fluid alpha fetoprotein

A-FAIR
    arrhythmia-insensitive flow-sensitive alternating inversion recovery

AFAP
    attenuated familial adenomatous polyposis

AFB
    acid-fast bacillus
    aflatoxin B
    aflatoxin biomarker
    air-fluidized bed
    aortofemoral bypass
    aspirated foreign body

AFB1
    aflatoxin B1

AFBG
    aortofemoral bypass graft

AFBN
    acute focal bacterial nephritis

AFC
    acid-fast culture
    adult foster care
    air-filled cushion
    allergic fungal sinusitis
    alveolar fluid clearance
    antibody-forming cell
    antral follicle count

AFCI
    acute focal cerebral ischemia

AFCL
    atrial fibrillation cycle length

AFD
    accelerated freeze-drying
    acrofacial dysostosis
    assessment of fat distribution

AFDC
    Aid to Families with Dependent Children

AFE
    5-aminolevulinic acid-induced fluorescence endoscopy
    amniotic (amnionic) fluid embolism (embolization)

AFEB
    afebrile (*See also* AF)

AFF
    atrial fibrillation-flutter
    atrial filling fraction

AF/F
    atrial fibrillation and/or flutter

aff
    afferent

AF/FL
    atrial fibrillation [and] atrial flutter

AFFN
    acrofrontofacionasal

AFG
    aflatoxin G
    alpha (α)-fetoglobulin
    amniotic fluid glucose
    auditory figure-ground

aFGF, a-FGF
    acidic fibroblast growth factor (*See also* FGFa)

AFH
    adenofibromatous hyperplasia
    angiofollicular hyperplasia
    angiomatoid fibrous histiocytoma
    anterior facial height

AFI
    acute febrile illness
    amaurotic familial idiocy
    amniotic (amnionic) fluid index

AFib
    atrial fibrillation (*See also* AF, At Fib, at.fib., ATR FIB, atr fib)

AFIP
    Armed Forces Institute of Pathology

AFIS
    amniotic fluid infection syndrome
AFKO
    ankle-foot-knee orthosis
AFL
    air-fluid level
    antifatty liver [factor]
    antifibrinolysin
    atrial flutter (*See also* AF)
AFLH, AFLNH
    angiofollicular lymphoid (lymph node)
    hyperplasia
AFLP
    acute fatty liver of pregnancy
    amplified fragment length polymorphism
    [PCR]
AFM
    aerosol face mask
    aflatoxin M
    atomic force microscopy
AFN
    afunctional neutrophil
    antegrade femoral nail
AFND
    acute febrile neutrophilic dermatosis
AFO
    ankle-foot orthosis (orthotic)
AFP
    acute flaccid paralysis
    adiabatic fast passage
    alpha (α)-fetoprotein (*See also* aFP)
    anterior faucial pillar
    ascending frontal parietal
    atrial filling pressure
    atypical facial pain
aFP
    alpha (α)-fetoprotein (*See also*
    AFP)
AFP-EIA
    alpha (α)-fetoprotein enzyme
    immunoassay
AFPP
    acute fibropurulent pneumonia
AFQ
    aflatoxin Q
AFQT
    Armed Forces Qualification Test
AFR
    aqueous flare response
    ascorbic free radical
    atrial flutter response
AFRAX
    autism-fragile X [syndrome]
AFRD
    acute febrile respiratory disease
AFRI
    acute febrile respiratory illness

AFROC
    alternative-free response receiver
    operating characteristic
AFRT
    altered fractionation radiotherapy
AFS
    acid-fast smear
    acquired (adult) Fanconi syndrome
    acromegaloid facial syndrome
    aldehyde-fuchsin stain
    allergic fungal sinusitis
    Alzheimer fugue state
    antifibroblast serum
    atomic fluorescence spectrometry
AFSLQ
    adolescent family and social life
    questionnaire
AFSP
    acute fibrinoserous pneumonia
AFT
    adaptive focusing technology
    aflatoxin (*See also* AF)
    agglutination-flocculation test
    autologous fat transfer
AFT$_3$
    absolute free triiodothyronine
AFT$_4$
    absolute free thyroxine
AFTC
    apparent free testosterone concentration
AFTN
    autonomously functioning thyroid nodule
AFTP
    ascitic fluid total protein
AFV
    amniotic fluid volume
    aortic flow velocity
AFV, AFV-F, AVF-S
    Aspergillus foetidus virus, F, S
AFVSS
    afebrile, vital signs stable
AFX
    air-fluid exchange
    atypical fibroxanthoma
AG
    abdominal girth
    acidophilic granulocyte
    agarose
    aminoglutethimide (*See also* AGL)
    aminoglycoside
    Amsler grid [vision test]
    analytical grade
    angular gyrus
    anion gap
    antigen (*See also* AGN)
    antiglobulin
    antigravity

AG *(continued)*
    atrial gallop
    attached gingiva
    autograft
    axiogingival
    azurophilic granule
A:G
    albumin to globulin ratio
Ag
    silver [L. *argentum*]
AGA
    accelerated growth area
    acetylglutamate
    acute gonococcal arthritis
    allergic granulomatosis and angiitis
    androgenetic alopecia
    antigliadin antibody
    antiglomerular antibody
    anti-immunoglobulin A autoantibody
    appropriate for gestational age
    average gestational age
Ag-Ab
    antigen-antibody [complex]
AGAG
    acidic glycosaminoglycans
AGAS
    accelerated graft atherosclerosis
    acetylglutamate synthetase
Ag-AS
    silver-acidified serum
AG/BL
    aminoglycoside [and] beta-lactam
        [combination antibiotic therapy]
AGC
    absolute granulocyte count
    advanced gastric cancer
    anatomic graduated component
    atypical glandular cells
    automatic gain control
AgCl
    silver chloride
AgCPV
    Autographa gamma cypovirus
AGCT
    adult granulosa cell tumor
    antiglobulin consumption test
    Army General Classification
        Test
AGCUS
    atypical glandular cells of uncertain
        (undetermined) (unknown) significance
        (*See also* AGUS)
AGD
    agar/agarose-gel diffusion [method]
    agar gel diffusion
    antigonadotropic decapeptide
AGDD
    agar and agarose-gel double diffusion
        (method)

AGE
    acrylamide gel electrophoresis
    acute gastroenteritis
    advanced glycation (glycosylation)
        end-product (*See also* AGEP)
    angle of greatest extension
    anterior gastroenterostomy
    arterial gas embolism
AGECAT
    automatic geriatric examination for
        computer-assisted taxonomy
AGED
    automated general experimental
        device
AGENT
    angiogenic gene therapy agent
AGEP
    acute generalized exanthematous
        pustulosis
    advanced glycosylation end product
        (*See also* AGE)
AGEPC
    acetyl glyceryl ether phosphorylcholine
AGF
    adrenal growth factor
    angle of greatest flexion
    autologous growth factor
AGG
    agammaglobulinemia
agg
    agglutinate (agglutination) (*See also*
        aggl, agglut, AGL)
    aggregation
aggl, agglut
    agglutinate (agglutination) (*See also* agg,
        AGL)
AGGS
    antigas-gangrene serum
AGH
    amenorrhea, galactorrhea,
        hypothyroidism
AGI
    alpha (α)-glucosidase inhibitor
agit.
    shake [L. *agita*]
AGL
    acute granulocytic leukemia
    agglutinate (agglutination) (*See also* agg,
        aggl, agglut)
    aminoglutethimide (*See also* AG)
    anterior glenoid labrum
A-GLACTO-LK
    alpha (α)-galactoside leukocyte
AGLMe
    N-alpha (α)-acetylglycyl-L-lysine
AGM
    absorbent gelling material
AGMK, AGMk
    African green monkey kidney [cell]

AGML
acute gastric mucosal lesion

AgMNPV
Anticarisia gemmatalis multiple nucleopolyhedrovirus

AGN
acute glomerulonephritis
agnosia (*See also* agn)
antigen (*See also* AG, ag)

AGNB
aerobic gram-negative bacillus

AgNO₃
silver nitrate

AgNOR
argyrophilic nucleolar organizer region [method]

AgNO₃ sol
silver nitrate solution

AGP
acute gallstone pancreatitis
agar-gel precipitation [test] (*See also* AGPT)

AGPNHL
aggressive good prognosis non-Hodgkin lymphoma

AGPT
agar-gel precipitation test (*See also* AGP)

AGR
aniridia, ambiguous genitalia, mental retardation
anticipatory goal response

AGRP
agouti-related peptide (protein)

AGS
adrenogenital syndrome
antiglucagon
audiogenic seizures

AGT
abnormal glucose tolerance
activity group therapy
acute generalized tuberculosis
adrenoglomerulotropin
angiotensinogen test
antiglobulin test

AGTH
adrenoglomerulotropin hormone

AGTT
abnormal glucose tolerance test

AGU
aspartylglycosaminuria (aspartylglucosaminuria)

AGUS
atypical glandular cells of uncertain (undetermined) (unknown) significance (*See also* AGCUS)

AGUV
Aguacate virus

AGV
Ahmed glaucoma valve
aniline gentian violet

AGVHD
acute graft-versus-host disease

A-H
atrium (atrio)-His [bundle]

AH
abdominal hysterectomy (*See also* abd hyst)
absorptive hypercalciuria
accidental hypothermia
acid hydrolysis
acute hepatitis
adenomatous hyperplasia
adrenal hypoplasia
affected hemisphere
afterhyperpolarization (*See also* AHP)
agnathia holoprosencephaly
alcoholic hepatitis
amenorrhea and hirsutism
amenorrhea and hyperprolactinemia
anterior heel
anterior hypothalamus
antihyaluronidase
aqueous humor
Arachis hypogaea
arcuate hypothalamus
arterial hypertension
artificial heart
ascites hepatoma
assisted hatching
astigmatic hypermetropia
ataxic hemiparesis
atrium (atrio)-His [bundle]
atypical hyperplasia
auditory hallucination
autoimmune hepatitis
autonomic hyperreflexia
axillary hair

A&H
accident and health [policy]

Ah
ampere-hour
hyperopic (hypermetropic) astigmatism

aH
abhenry

AHA
abortive hereditary ataxia
acquired hemolytic anemia
acute hemolytic anemia
alpha hydroxy acid
anterior hypothalamic area
antiheart antibody
antihistone antibody

AHA *(continued)*
arthritis-hives-angioedema [syndrome]
aspartylhydroxamic acid
Australian hepatitis antigen
autoimmune hemolytic anemia
AHase
antihyaluronidase [titer]
AHA.SOC
American Heart Association Stroke
Outcome Classification
AHB
alpha (α)-hydroxybutyric dehydrogenase
AHBC
hepatitis B core antibody
AHC
academic health care
acute hemorrhagic conjunctivitis
acute hemorrhagic cystitis
adrenal hypoplasia congenita
alternating hemiplegia of childhood
antihemophilic factor C
AHCD
acquired hepatocellular degeneration
AHC/HHG
adrenal hypoplasia congenita [and]
hypogonadotropic hypogonadism
[syndrome]
AHCPR
Agency for Healthcare Policy and
Research
AhCPV
Agrochola helvolva cypovirus
AHCY, ACHY
S-adenosylhomocysteine hydrolase [gene]
AHD
acquired hepatocerebral degeneration
acute heart disease
antihypertensive drug
arteriohepatic dysplasia
arteriosclerotic (atherosclerotic) heart
disease
autoimmune hemolytic disease
AHDMS
automated hospital data management
system
AHDP
azacycloheptane diphosphonate
AHE
acute hemorrhagic edema
acute hemorrhagic encephalomyelitis
AHEI
acute hemorrhagic edema of infancy
AHES
artificial heart energy system
AHF
accelerated hyperfractionation
acute heart failure
antihemophilic factor [factor VIII]
Argentinian hemorrhagic fever

AHFS
American Hospital Formulary
Service
AHFTRT
accelerated hyperfractionated thoracic
radiotherapy
AHG
aggregated human globulin
antihemophilic globulin
antihuman globulin
AHG-CDC
antiglobulin-enhanced
complement-dependent cytotoxicity
AHGG
aggregated human gamma globulin
AHGS
acute herpetic gingival stomatitis
AHGXM
antihuman globulin crossmatch
AHH
alpha (α)-hydrazinohistidine
anosmia and hypogonadotropic
hypogonadism [syndrome]
arylhydrocarbon hydroxylase
AHHD
arteriosclerotic (atherosclerotic)
hypertensive heart disease
AHI
acetabular head index
acromiohumeral interval
active hostility index
acute HIV1 infection
anterior horn index
apnea-hypopnea index
Arthritis Helplessness Index
AHJ
artificial hip joint
AHL
aggressive histology lymphoma
apparent half-life
AHLE
acute hemorrhagic leukoencephalitis
AHLG
antihuman lymphocyte globulin
AHLS
antihuman lymphocyte serum
AHLT
auxiliary heterotopic liver
transplant(ation)
AHLV
American hop latent virus
AHM
ambulatory Holter monitor(ing)
anterior hyaloid membrane
apical holosystolic murmur
AHMA
antiheart muscle autoantibody
AHMD
alcoholic heart muscle disease

AHMO
anterior horizontal mandibular osteotomy
AHN
adenomatous hyperplastic nodule
AHNS
arteriolar hyperplastic nephrosclerosis
AHO
acute hematogenous osteomyelitis
Albright hereditary osteodystrophy
AHP
acute hemorrhagic pancreatitis
afterhyperpolarization (*See also* AH)
afterspike hyperpolarization
air at high pressure
American Hand Prosthetics
AHPCT
autologous hematopoietic progenitor cell
transplant(ation)
AHPO
anterior hypothalamic preoptic [area]
AHR
acute humoral rejection
airways hyperreactivity
(hyperresponsiveness)
antihyaluronidase reaction
aryl hydrocarbon receptor
atrial heart rate
autonomic hyperreflexia
AHRE
atrial high-rate event
AHRF
acute hypoxemic respiratory failure
AHRQ
Agency for Healthcare Research and
Quality
AHS
adaptive hand skills
African horse sickness
alien hand syndrome
allopurinol hypersensitivity syndrome
alveolar hypoventilation syndrome
antiepileptic [drug] hypersensitivity
AHSCT
autologous hematopoietic stem cell
transplant(ation)
AHSDF
area health service development fund
AHSV 1–9
African horse sickness virus 1–9
AHT
aggregation half-time
alternating hypertropia
amiodarone [and] iodine-induced
thyrotoxicosis
antihyaluronidase titer
augmented histamine test
autoantibodies to human thyroglobulin

AHTG
antihuman thymocyte globulin
AHTP
antihuman thymocyte plasma
AHTS
antihuman thymus serum
AHU
acute hemolytic uremic [syndrome]
arginine, hypoxanthine, uracil [auxotype]
AHuG
aggregated human immunoglobulin G
AHV
Abu Hammad virus
avian herpesvirus
AhV
Atkinsonella hypoxylon virus
aHyl
allohydroxylysine
AHYS
acquired hyperostosis syndrome
AI
acceleration index
acceptable intake
accidental injury
accidentally incurred
accommodative insufficiency
acetabular index
acute inflammation
adiposity index
aggregation index
allergy and immunology (*See also* A&I)
allergy index
amylogenesis imperfecta
anal index
anaphylatoxin inactivator
anaphylatoxin inhibitor
angiogenesis inhibitor
angiotensin inhibitor
anxiety index
aortic incompetence
aortic insufficiency
apical impulse
apnea index
apoptotic index
aromatase inhibitor
articulation index
artificial insemination
artificial intelligence
atherogenic index
atrial insufficiency
autoimmune (autoimmunity)
avidity index
axioincisal
A-I
aortoiliac
A&I
allergy and immunology (*See also* AI)

AIA
adjuvant-induced arthritis
allergen-induced asthma
allyl isopropyl acetamide
amylase inhibitor activity
antigen-induced arthritis
antiimmunoglobulin antibody
antiinsulin antibody (*See also* AI-Ab)
aortoiliac aneurysm
aspirin-induced (intolerant) asthma
automated image analysis
AI-Ab
antiinsulin antibody (*See also* AIA)
AIB
aminoisobutyric acid (*See also* AIBA)
avian infectious bronchitis
AIBA
aminoisobutyric acid (*See also* AIB)
AIBF
anterior interbody fusion
AIBH
ACTH-independent bilateral
macronodular hyperplasia
AICA
anterior inferior communicating artery
anterior internal cerebellar artery
AI-CAH
autoimmune-type chronic active hepatitis
AICB
anterior interbody cervical bone graft
AICC
antiinhibitor coagulant complex
AICD
activation-induced cell death
automatic implantable (implanted)
cardioverter-defibrillator
AICE
angiotensin I converting enzyme
AICF
autoimmune complement fixation
AICP, AIPC, AI-PCa
androgen-independent prostate carcinoma
AICS
acute ischemic coronary syndrome
artery of inferior cavernous sinus
AID
absolute iron deficiency
activation-induced cytidine deaminase
acute infectious disease
acute ionization detector
aggressive insulin-dependent diabetes
antiinflammatory drug
aortoiliac disease
argon ionization detector
artificial insemination by donor
autoimmune deficiency
autoimmune disease
automatic implantable defibrillator
average interocular difference

AIDA
automatic interpretation for diagnostic
assistance
AIDCI
angle independent Doppler color
imaging
AIDH
artificial insemination donor,
husband
atypical intraductal hyperplasia
AIDNV
Aedes albopictus densovirus
AIDP
acute inflammatory demyelinating
polyneuropathy
(polyradiculoneuropathy)
(polyradiculopathy)
AIDS
acquired immune deficiency
(immunodeficiency) syndrome
Assessment of Intelligibility of
Dysarthric Speech
AIDS-HAQ
acquired immunodeficiency syndrome
health assessment questionnaire
AIDS-KS
acquired immunodeficiency syndrome
with Kaposi sarcoma
AIDS-related Kaposi sarcoma
AIDSLINE
online information on acquired
immunodeficiency syndrome
AIE
acute inclusion-body encephalitis
acute infective endocarditis
autoimmune enteropathy
AIED
autoimmune inner ear disease
AIEP
amount of insulin extractable from
pancreas
AIF
anemia-inducing factor
antiinflammatory
antiinvasion factor
apoptosis-inducing factor
arterial input function
AIF-1
anemia-inducing factor 1
AIFD
acute intrapartum fetal distress
AIG
antiimmunoglobulin
AIgA
absence of immunoglobulin A
AIgE
antiimmunoglobulin E antibody
AIGF
androgen-induced growth factor

AIgM
absence of immunoglobulin M
A-IGP
activity-interview group psychotherapy
AIH
amelogenesis imperfecta, hypomaturation
type
anterior interhemispheric approach
aortic intramural hemorrhage
(hematoma)
artificial insemination, homologous
(husband)
autoimmune hepatitis
AIHA
autoimmune hemolytic anemia
AIHD
acquired immune hemolytic disease
AIHQ
Ambiguous Intentions Hostility
Questionnaire
AII
acute intestinal infection
AIIS
anterior inferior iliac spine
AIIT
amiodarone-iodine induced thyrotoxicosis
AIL
acute infectious lymphocytosis
angiocentric immunoproliferative lesion
angioimmunoblastic lymphadenopathy
angioimmunoblastic lymphoma
angioimmunoproliferative lesion
AILA
angioimmunoblastic lymphadenopathy
AILC
adult independent living center
AILD
alveolar-interstitial lung disease
angioimmunoblastic lymphadenopathy
with dysproteinemia
aIle
alloisoleucine
AILT
amiloride-inhibitable lithium transport
angioimmunoblastic T-cell lymphoma
AIM
Ace intramedullary [nail]
aerosol inhalation monitor
antiinflammatory medication
area of interest magnification
artificial intelligence in medicine
atypical immature squamous metaplasia
AIMD
abnormal involuntary movement disorder
active implantable medical device
A-IMF
areola to inframammary fold [distance]

AIMO
anterior inferior mandibular osteotomy
AIMS
Abnormal Involuntary Movements Scale
Alberta Infant Motor Scale
Arthritis Impact Measurement Scale
AIN
acute interstitial nephritis
allergic interstitial nephritis
anal intraepithelial neoplasia
anterior interosseous nerve
autoimmune neutropenia
AINA
automated immunonephelometric assay
AINS
antiinflammatory nonsteroidal [agent]
A Insuf
aortic insufficiency
AIO
activity, interest, option
all-in-one
amyloid of immunoglobulin origin
AIOD
aortoiliac occlusive (obstructive) disease
AION
anterior ischemic optic neuropathy
AIP
acute idiopathic pericarditis
acute infectious polyneuritis
acute inflammatory polyneuropathy
acute intermittent porphyria
acute interstitial pneumonia
(pneumonitis)
aldosterone-induced protein
asymptomatic inflammatory prostatitis
autoimmune pancreatitis
automated immunoprecipitation
average intravascular pressure
A/I-PACG
acute intermittent primary angle-closure
glaucoma
AIPC
androgen-independent prostate cancer
AIPE
acute interstitial pulmonary emphysema
AIPFP
acute idiopathic peripheral facial nerve
palsy
AIPH
attenuation in phantom method
AIR
accelerated idioventricular rhythm
(*See also* AIVR)
acetylcholine-induced relaxation
acute insulin response
airways responsiveness
aminoimidazole ribonucleotide (ribotide)

AIR *(continued)*
5-aminoimidazole ribose 5′-phosphate
aortoiliac reconstruction
automatic image registration
average impairment rating
AIRA
antiinsulin receptor antibody
AIRE
autoimmune regulator [gene]
AIRF
alteration in respiratory function
AIROM
active integral range of motion
AIRR
acute infusion-related reaction
AIRS
Amphetamine Interview Rating Scale
AIS
Abbreviated Injury Scale (Score)
acute ischemic stroke
adenocarcinoma in situ
adolescent idiopathic scoliosis
Advanced Interventional Systems
aggregate injury score
amniotic infection syndrome
amputation index score
analyzer of interrater sequences
androgen insensitivity syndrome
anterior interosseous [nerve] syndrome
antiinsulin serum
automotive injury score
AISA
acquired idiopathic sideroblastic anemia
AIS/ISS
Abbreviated Injury Score [and] Injury
Severity Score
AIS/MR
Alternative Intermediate Services for the
Mentally Retarded
AIT
acute intensive treatment
adoptive immunotherapy
auditory integration training
AITD
autoimmune thyroid disease
AITN
acute interstitial tubular nephritis
AITP
autoimmune thrombocytopenia
autoimmune thrombocytopenic
purpura
AITT
arginine/insulin tolerance test
augmented insulin tolerance test
AIU
absolute iodine uptake
antigen-inducing unit
AIVC
absence of vena cava

AIVR
accelerated idioventricular rhythm
(*See also* AIR)
AIVV
anterior internal vertebral vein
AJ
adherens junction
ankle jerk
AJC
ankle joint complex
AJPBD
anomalous junction of pancreatobiliary
duct
AJR
abdominojugular reflux maneuver
abnormal jugular reflex
AJS
acute joint syndrome
AJT
automatic junctional tachycardia
AK
above knee [amputation] (*See also*
AKA)
acne keloidalis
actinic keratosis
adenosine kinase
adenylate kinase
amebic keratitis
applied kinesiology
artificial kidney
astigmatic keratotomy
AKA
above-knee amputation (*See also* AK)
alcoholic ketoacidosis
all known allergies
alpha (α)-allokainic acid
also known as
antikeratin antibody
AKAP
protein kinase A-anchoring protein
AKAV
Akabane virus
AKBR
arterial ketone body ratio
AKD
atypical Kawasaki disease
AKE
acrokeratoelastoidosis
active knee extension
A/kg
ampere per kilogram
AKR
aldo-keto reductase
AKRMLV
AKR endogenous murine leukemia virus
AKS
alcoholic Korsakoff syndrome
arthroscopic knee surgery
auditory and kinesthetic sensation

Akt1
akt/protein kinase B [gene]
AKU
alkaptonuria
artificial kidney unit
AKV
acrokeratosis verruciformis
⚠ **AL**
absolute latency
acinar lumina
acute leukemia
adaptation level
albumin [5%, followed by amount in mL] (*See also* ALB)
alcoholism (*See also* ALC)
alignment mark
allantoic
allergic
amyloidosis
angiographic [area of] lateral [projection]
annoyance level
anterior leaflet
anterolateral
antihuman lymphocytic [globulin]
argininosuccinate lysate
argon laser
arterial line (*See also* A-line, art. line)
avian leukosis
axial length
axiolingual
left ear [L. *auris laeva*] (*See also* a.l., AS, a.s.) ⚠
lethal antigen
primary amyloidosis
Al
aluminum
⚠ **a.l.**
left ear [L. *auris laeva*] (*See also* AL, AS, a.s.) ⚠
ALA
Activity Loss Assessment
alpha (α) lactalbumin
alpha (α) linolenic acid (*See also* LNA)
alpha (α) lipoic acid
amebic liver abscess
aminolevulinic acid
anterior lip of acetabulum
antileukotriene agent
antilymphocyte antibody
axiolabial (*See also* ALa)
delta (δ)-aminolevulinic acid
5-ALA
5-aminolevulinic acid
ALa
axiolabial (*See also* ALA)

Ala
alanine (*See also* A)
AL-Ab
antilymphocyte antibody
ALAC
antibiotic-loaded acrylic cement
ALAD
abnormal left axis deviation
aminolevulinic acid dehydrase (*See also* ALA-D)
ALA-D
aminolevulinic acid dehydrase (*See also* ALAD)
ALADP
aminolevulinic acid dehydrogenase deficiency porphyria
ALaG
axiolabiogingival
ALaL
axiolabiolingual
ALAO
angiographic [area of] left anterior oblique [projection]
ALA-PDT
5-aminolevulinic acid photodynamic therapy
ALARA
as low as reasonably achievable [radiation exposure]
ALARM
adjustable leg and ankle repositioning mechanism
ALARP
as low as readily practicable [amount of radiation]
ALAS
aminolevulinic acid synthetase
ALAT
alanine aminotransferase
ALAX
apical long axis
ALB
albumin [5%, followed by amount in mL] (*See also* AL)
Assessment of Ludic Behaviors
avian lymphoblastosis
alb.
white [L. *albus*]
ALB:GLOB
albumin to globulin ratio (*See also* A:G)
ALBPSQ
Acute Low Back Pain Screening Questionnaire
ALBUMS
aldehyde-linker based ultrasensitive mismatch scanning [molecular analysis]

ALC
absolute lymphocyte count
acetyl-L-carnitine
acute lethal catatonia
alcohol
alcoholic liver cirrhosis
alcoholism (*See also* AL)
allogeneic lymphocyte cytotoxicity
alternate level of care
Alternative Lifestyle Checklist
amyotrophic lateral sclerosis
approximate lethal concentration
avian leukosis complex
axiolinguocervical

ALCA
anomalous left coronary artery

ALCAPA
anomalous [origin of] left coronary
artery from pulmonary artery

ALCAT
antigen leukocyte cellular antibody test

ALCEQ
Adolescent Life Change Event
Questionnaire

ALCL
anaplastic large cell lymphoma

AlCPV
Agrochola lychnidis cypovirus

AlCPV-10
Aporophyla lutulenta cypovirus

ALCR
alcohol rub

AL:CR
axial length to corneal radius ratio

AlCr
aluminum crown

ALD
adrenoleukodystrophy
alcoholic liver disease
aldolase (*See also* Ald)
aldosterone
anterior latissimus dorsi
appraisal of language disturbances
approximate lethal dose
assistive listening device
average lens density

Ald
aldolase (*See also* ALD)

ALD-AMN
adrenoleukodystrophy [and]
adrenomyeloneuropathy

ALDH
aldehyde dehydrogenase

Aldo
aldosterone

ALDP
adrenoleukodystrophy protein

ALDS
albinism-deafness syndrome

ALE
active life expectancy
allowable limits of error
amputated lower extremity

ALEC
artificial lung-expanding compound

ALEP
atypical lymphoepithelioid cell
proliferation

ALERT
antibody-based lateral flow economical
recognition ticket [system]

ALEV
Alenquer virus

ALF
acute liver failure
anterior long fiber
arterial line filter
automated laser fluorescence

ALFT
abnormal liver function test

ALG
Annapolis lymphoblast globulin
antilymphocyte globulin
axiolinguogingival

ALH
angiolymphoid hyperplasia
anterior lobe hormone
anterior lobe of hypophysis
atypical lobular hyperplasia

ALHE
angiolymphoid hyperplasia with
eosinophilia

ALHV
Alcelaphine herpesvirus

ALI
acute limb ischemia
acute lung injury
argon laser iridotomy
average lobe index

ALIF
anterior lumbar interbody fusion

A-line
arterial line (*See also* AL, art. line,
ART)

ALIP
abnormal localization of immature
precursors

ALJV
Alajuela virus

ALK, alk
alkaline
alkylating [agent]
anaplastic lymphoma kinase
automated lamellar keratoplasty
automated laser keratomileusis

ALK-E
automated lamellar keratoplasty-
excimer

alk phos, alk p'tase
  alkaline phosphatase (*See also* ALP, AP, P'ase)
ALL
  acute lymphoblastic (lymphocytic) leukemia
  allergy (allergic) (*See also* A)
  anterior longitudinal ligament
  antihypertensive and lipid lowering
ALLA
  acute lymphocytic leukemia antigen
ALLD
  arthroscopic lumbar laser discectomy
ALLO
  atypical *Legionella*-like (legionellalike) organism
allo-BMT
  allogeneic (allogenic) bone marrow transplantation
allo-HSCT
  allogeneic (allogenic) hematopoietic stem cell transplantation
ALM
  acral lentiginous melanoma
  adhesive leptomeningitis
  alveolar lining material
ALMCA
  anomalous left main coronary artery
ALME
  acetyl-lysine methyl ester
ALMI
  anterior lateral myocardial infarct(ion)
ALMN
  adrenoleukomyeloneuropathy
ALMV
  Almpiwar virus
  anterior leaflet of mitral valve
ALN
  anterior lymph node
  axillary lymph node
ALND
  axillary lymph node dissection
ALNM
  axillary lymph node metastasis
ALO
  acute laryngeal obstruction
  Aerococcus-like organism
  average lymphocyte output
  axiolinguoocclusal
Al₂O₃
  aluminum oxide
ALOC
  altered level of consciousness
ALOH
  average length of hospitalization
ALOS
  average length of stay

ALP
  actinic lichen planus
  acute leukemia protocol
  acute lupus pericarditis
  acute lupus pneumonitis
  alkaline phosphatase (*See also* alk phos, alk p'tase, AP, P'ase)
  ankle ligament protector
  anterior lobe of pituitary
  antileukoproteinase
  antilymphocyte (antilymphocytic) plasma
  argon laser photocoagulation
α
  active (activity) (*See also* act.)
  alpha [first letter of Greek alphabet lowercase]
  alpha (α) particle
  angular acceleration [rate of change of angular velocity over time SI unit is radiax]
  Bunsen solubility coefficient
  constituent of alpha protein plasma fraction
  first in alpha series or group
  heavy chain of immunoglobulin A
  probability of type I error [statistics]
[α]
  specific optical rotation
alpha (α)2-AP
  alpha (α)2-antiplasmin
alpha (α)-APA
  alpha (α)-anilinophenyl-acetamide
alpha (α)1-AT
  alpha (α)1-antitrypsin
alpha (α)2-B(β)1
  alpha (α)2-beta (β)1 integrin cell-surface collagen
alpha (α)-BSM
  alpha (α)-bone substitute material
alpha (α)-cat
  alpha (α)-catenin
alpha (α)-GST
  alpha (α)-glutathione S-transferase
alpha (α)-HCD
  alpha (α)-heavy-chain disease
alpha (α)-hCG
  alpha (α)-human chorionic gonadotropin
3-alpha (α)-HSD
  3-alpha (α)-hydroxysteroid dehydrogenase
alpha (α)-IFN
  alpha (α)-interferon
alpha (α)-KG
  alpha (α)-ketoglutarate
alpha (α)-KIC
  alpha (α)-ketoisocaproic acid

alpha (α)-LP
alpha (α)-lipoprotein
alpha (α)2-M
alpha (α)2-macroglobulin
alpha (α)-MHC
alpha (α)-myosin heavy chain
alpha (α)-MSH
alpha (α)-melanocyte-stimulating
hormone
alpha (α)-NREM
alpha (α)-nonrapid eye movement
[sleep]
1-alpha (α)-OHase
25-hydroxy-vitamin D 1alpha
(α)-hydroxylase
alpha (α)1-PI
alpha (α)-protease inhibitor
5-alpha (α)R
5-alpha (α)-reductase
5-alpha (α)RA
5-alpha (α)-reductase activity
alpha (α)-T
alpha (α)-tocopherol
ALPI
alkaline phosphatase isoenzyme
argon laser peripheral iridoplasty
ALPL
alkaline phosphatase liver
ALPP
abdominal leak-point pressure
alkaline phosphatase placental
ALPPL
alkaline phosphataselike placental
ALPS
alcoholism, leukopenia, pneumococcal
sepsis
anterior locking plate system
Aphasia Language Performance Scale
autoimmune lymphoproliferative
syndrome
autologous leukapheresis, processing,
and storage [container]
ALPSA
anterior labroligamentous periosteal
sleeve avulsion
anterior labrum periosteal sleeve avulsion
ALPV
aphid lethal paralysis virus
ALQTS
acquired long QT syndrome
ALR
adductor leg raise
ALRI
acute lower respiratory infection
anterolateral rotary (rotational) instability
ALRTI
acute lower respiratory tract infection
ALS
acid-labile subunit

acute lateral sclerosis
advanced life support [protocol]
afferent loop syndrome
amyotrophic lateral sclerosis
angiotensin-like substance
anterolateral sclerosis
anticipated lifespan
antilymphocyte serum
antiviral lymphocyte serum
atypical lichenoid stomatitis
ALSAR
Assessment of Living Skills and
Resources
ALSD
Alzheimer-like senile dementia
ALS-PD
amyotrophic lateral sclerosis-
parkinsonism dementia [complex]
AlStV
Alstromeria streak virus
ALT
alanine aminotransferase
anterolateral tract
antibiotic lock technique
argon laser trabeculoplasty
(trabeculopexy)
autolymphocyte therapy [adoptive
cellular therapy]
avian laryngotracheitis
alt
alternate
altitude
ALT:AST
alanine aminotransferase to aspartate
aminotransferase ratio
ALTB
acute laryngotracheobronchitis
ALTE
apparent life-threatening event
ALTEE
acetyl-L-tyrosine ethyl ester
ALTK
automated lamellar therapeutic
keratoplasty
ALTP
argon laser trabeculoplasty
(trabeculopexy) (*See also* ALT)
ALT-RCC
autolymphocyte-based treatment for
renal cell carcinoma
ALTS
acute lumbar trauma syndrome
ALTV
Altamira virus
ALV
Abelson leukemia virus
adenolike virus
ascending lumbar vein
avian leukosis virus

alv
  alveolar
  alveolus [singular] (alveoli [plural])
ALV-A
  avian leukosis virus RSA
ALVAD
  abdominal left ventricular assist device
ALVF
  acute left ventricular failure
ALV-J
  avian leukosis virus-subgroup J
ALVM
  alveolar mucosa
ALVT
  aortic and left ventricular tunnel
alv vent
  alveolar ventilation (*See also* VA, V_A)
alvx
  alveolectomy
ALW
  arch-loop-whorl [fingerprint system]
ALWMI
  anterolateral wall myocardial infarct(ion)
A-LYM
  atypical lymphocyte
AM
  acrylamide
  actomyosin
  acute myelofibrosis
  adrenomedullin
  adult male
  adult monocyte
  aerosol mask
  aerospace medicine
  akinetic mutism
  alternative medicine
  alveolar macrophage
  alveolar mucosa
  amacrine cell
  amalgam (*See also* AMAL)
  ametropia (*See also* am.)
  ammeter
  amnion
  amplitude modulation (*See also* A-mod)
  amyl
  anovular menstruation
  anterior midpapillary
  anteromeatal
  antimycotic
  arabinomannan
  arithmetic mean
  arousal mechanism
  arterial malformation
  arterial mean
  articulation manipulation
  atrial myxoma
  attitude to medication

  Austin Moore [prosthesis]
  aviation medicine (*See also* AV, AVM)
  axiomesial
  before noon [L. *ante meridiem*] (*See also* a.m.)
  mixed astigmatism
  myopic astigmatism (*See also* ASM, AsM, am.)
A/m
  ampere per meter
A/m²
  ampere per square meter
Am
  americium
²⁴¹Am
  americium-241
a.m.
  before noon [L. *ante meridiem*] (*See also* AM)
am
  ammeter
am.
  ametropia (*See also* AM)
  amplitude
  meter angle [unit of ocular convergence]
  myopic astigmatism (*See also* ASM, AsM, AM)
AMA
  actual mechanical advantage
  advanced maternal age
  against medical advice
  alkaline membrane assay
  antimitochondrial antibody
  antimyosin antibody
  antithyroid microsomal antibody
  apocrine membrane antigen
  arm muscle area
  augmentation of mandibular angle
  autoregressive moving average [statistics]
AMAC
  adults molested as children
AMAD
  Assessment Measure for Atopic Dermatitis
  morning admission
AMA-Fab
  antimyosin monoclonal antibody with Fab [fragment]
AMAG
  adrenal medullary autograft
  autoimmune metaplastic atrophic gastritis
AMAL
  amalgam (*See also* AM)

AMAN
    acute motor axonal neuropathy
AMAP
    as much as possible
AMAS
    antimalignin antibody screen
AMAT
    antimalignin antibody test
    Arm Motor Ability Test
A-MAT
    amorphous material
AMATC
    Amplatz maceration aspiration
        thrombectomy catheter
AMAV
    Amapari virus
AMB
    ambulate (ambulation) (ambulatory)
        (*See also* ambul)
    anomalous muscle bundle
    avian myeloblastosis
amb
    ambient
    ambiguous (*See also* ambig)
    ambulance
AMBER
    advanced multiple-beam equalization
        radiography
AMBI
    acute multiple brain infarcts
ambig
    ambiguous (*See also* amb)
AMBRI
    atraumatic, multidirectional, bilateral
        radial instability [multidirectional
        glenohumeral instability shoulder
        dislocation]
AMBU
    air mask bag unit
ambul
    ambulate (ambulation) (ambulatory)
        (*See also* AMB)
AMBV
    Anhembi virus
AMC
    antibody-mediated cytotoxicity
    antimalaria campaign
    arm muscle circumference
    arthrogryposis multiplex congenita
    ataxia-microcephaly-cataract [syndrome]
    automated mixture control
    automatic mode conversion
    axiomesiocervical
AMCHA
    aminomethylcyclohexane-carboxylic acid
AMCN
    anteromedial caudate nucleus
AmCPV
    Antheraea mylitta cypovirus

AM:CR
    amylase to creatinine ratio
AMCV
    avian myelocytomatosis virus
AMD
    acid maltase deficiency
    acromandibular dysplasia
    adrenomyelodystrophy
    age-related macular degeneration
    Aleutian mink disease (*See also* AD)
    alpha (α) methyldopa
    arthroscopic microdiscectomy
    articular motion device
    axiomesiodistal
AMDGF
    alveolar macrophage-derived growth
        factor
AMDR
    acceptable macronutrient distribution
        range
AMDV
    Aleutian mink disease virus
AME
    anthrax meningoencephalitis
    apparent mineralocorticoid excess
        [syndrome]
    aseptic meningoencephalitis
    Austin Medical Equipment
AMEAE
    acute monophasic experimental
        autoimmune encephalomyelitis
AMegL
    acute megakaryoblastic leukemia [FAB
        M7]
AMERIND
    American Indian Sign Language
AMES
    age, [distant] metastases, extent, size
Ameslan
    American Sign Language (*See also*
        ASL)
AMeX
    acetone, methylbenzoate, xylene [tissue
        processing method]
AMF
    aerobic metabolism facilitator
    antimuscle factor
    autocrine motility factor
AMFH
    angiomatoid malignant fibrous
        histiocytoma
AM/FM
    alopecia mucinosa [and] follicular
        mucinosis
AMFR
    autocrine motility factor receptor
AMG
    acoustic myography
    aminoglycoside

A

amyloglucosidase
antimacrophage globulin
arterial migraine grinder
autometallography
axiomesiogingival

A₂MG
alpha₂ (α₂)-macroglobulin

AMH
antimüllerian hormone
automated medical history

Amh
mixed astigmatism with myopia
predominating [over hyperopia]

AMHT
automated multiphasic health testing

AMI
acquired monosaccharide intolerance
acute mesenteric ischemia
acute myocardial infarct(ion)
adolescent medicine, internal
anterior myocardial infarction
antibody-mediated immunity
Athletic Motivation Inventory
axiomesioincisal

AMIS
anterior minimally invasive surgery
antibody-mediated immune
suppression

AMK
anatomic modular knee

AMKL
acute megakaryoblastic leukemia

AML
acute monoblastic leukemia
acute monocytic leukemia (*See also*
AMOL)
acute mucosal lesion
acute myeloblastic leukemia
acute myelocytic leukemia
acute myelogenous (myeloid) leukemia
[acute granulocytic, acute
nonlymphocytic]
anatomic medullary locking
angiomyolipoma
anterior mitral leaflet
automated multitest laboratory

AMLA
antimyolemmal antibody

AMLB
alternate monaural loudness balance
[test]

AMLC
adherent macrophagelike cell
autologous mixed lymphocyte culture

AMLR
auditory middle latency response
autologous mixed lymphocyte reaction

AMLS
antimouse lymphocyte serum

AMLSGA
acute myeloblastic leukemia surface
glycoprotein antigen

AMLV-RT
avian myeloblastosis leukemia virus
reverse transcriptase

AMM
agnogenic myeloid metaplasia
ammonia (*See also* ammon.)
antibody to murine cardiac
myosin

AMML, AMMOL, AMMoL
acute myelomonocytic
(myelomonoblastic) leukemia

ammon.
ammonia (*See also* AMM)

AMN
acquired melanocytic nevus
adrenomyeloneuropathy
alloxazine mononucleotide
angiomyoneuroma
anterior median nucleus
atypical melanocytic nevus

AMNGT
atypical melanocytic nevus of genital
type

amnio
amniocentesis

AMN SC
amniotic fluid scan

AMO
Allergan Medical Optics
axiomesioocclusal

A-mod
amplitude modulation

AMOL
acute monocytic (monoblastic) leukemia
(*See also* AML)

AMOR, AMORP
amorphous [sediment]

AMOVA
analysis of molecular variance
[statistics]

AMP
accelerated mental processes
acid mucopolysaccharide
adenosine monophosphate (adenosine
5′-monophosphate)
amphetamine
amplification
ampule (*See also* ampul.)
amputation
amputee
assisted medical procreation
average mean pressure

AMPA
    alpha (α)-amino-3-hydroxy-5-
    methylisoxazole-4-propionic acid
    [receptor]
AMP-c
    cyclic adenosine monophosphate
    (*See also* cAMP)
AMPD1
    adenosine monophosphate deaminase 1
AMPH
    amphetamine
amph
    amphoric [respiratory sound]
amp-hr
    ampere-hour
AMP-HSA
    ampicillin-human serum albumin
AMPK
    adenosine monophosphate-activated
    protein kinase
AMPLE
    allergies, medications, past medical
    history, last meal, events preceding
    present condition [mnemonic for
    history taking]
AMPPE
    acute multifocal placoid pigment
    epitheliopathy
AMPPPE
    acute multifocal posterior placoid
    pigment epitheliopathy
A-M pr
    Austin Moore prosthesis
AMP-S
    adenylosuccinic acid
AMPS
    acid mucopolysaccharide
    Assessment of Motor and Process
    Skills
AMPT
    alpha-methyl-para-tyrosine
ampul.
    ampule [L. *ampulla*] (*See also* AMP)
AMR
    abnormal muscle response
    acoustic muscle reflex
    activity metabolic rate
    acute mitral regurgitation
    alopecia mental retardation [syndrome]
    alternating motion rate
    ambulatory medical record
    ataxia, microcephaly, retardation
    [syndrome]
AMRI
    anteromedial rotatory instability
AMRS
    automated medical record system
AMRV
    Almeirim virus

AMS
    ablepharon macrostomia syndrome
    accelerator mass spectrometry
    Access Management Survey
    acute maxillary sinusitis
    acute mitral stenosis
    acute mountain sickness
    admission multiphasic screening
    aggravated in military service
    altered mental status
    amylase
    antimacrophage serum
    antimigration system
    aseptic meningitis syndrome
    atypical measles syndrome
    auditory memory span
    automated multiphasic screening
    automatic mode switching
AMSA
    anterior middle superior alveolar
AMSAN
    acute motor-sensory axonal neuropathy
AMSIT
    appearance, mood, sensorium,
    intelligence, thought process [portion
    of mental status examination]
AMT
    active motion testing
    acute miliary tuberculosis
    air medical transportation
    allogeneic [bone] marrow
    transplant(ation)
    alpha (α)-methyltyrosine
    amniotic (amnionic) membrane
    transplant(ation)
    Anxiety Management Training
    area of maximum thinning
    atherogenic metabolic triad
amt
    amount
AMTDT
    amplified *Mycobacterium tuberculosis*
    direct test
AMTP
    alpha (α)-methyltryptophan
AMTR
    anteromedial temporal lobe resection
AMTV
    Arumowot virus
amu
    atomic mass unit
AMuLV
    Abelson murine leukemia virus
    amphotropic murine leukemia virus
AMV
    alveolar minute ventilation
    apex to mitral valve [axis]
    assisted mechanical ventilation
    avian myeloblastosis virus

AMVI
  acute mesenteric vascular insufficiency
AMVL, aMVL
  anterior mitral valve leaflet
AMY
  amylase
AmyA
  antimyocardial antibody
AMY-SP
  amylase urine spot [test]
AN
  acanthosis nigricans
  acne neonatorum
  acoustic neuroma
  adult normal
  ala nasi [singular] (alae nasi [plural])
  aminonucleoside
  amyl nitrate
  anabiosis
  anesthesia (anesthetic) (*See also* A, AA,
    ANA, anes, anesth)
  aneurysm
  anisometropia (*See also* An)
  anode (anodal) (*See also* A, a)
  anorexia nervosa
  antenatal
  anterior (*See also* a, ANT, ant.)
  anticipatory nausea
  antineuraminidase
  aseptic necrosis
  atrionodal
  autonomic neuropathy
  avascular necrosis
A/N
  artery and/or nerve
  as needed
A:N
  adenoidal to nasopharyngeal ratio
A$_n$
  normal atmosphere
An
  actinon [isotope of radon]
  anatomic
  aniridia
  anisometropia (*See also* AN)
  Aspergillus niger
ANA
  acetylneuraminic acid
  anesthesia (anesthetic) (*See also* A, AA,
    AN, anes, anesth)
  antinuclear antibody
  articular/nonarticular
  aspartyl naphthylamide
ANAD
  anorexia nervosa and associated
    disorders
ANAE
  alpha-naphthyl acetate esterase

ANA-FL
  antinuclear antibody fluid
ANAG
  acute narrow angle glaucoma
anal.
  analgesia (analgesic)
  analysis (analytic)
ANAP
  agglutination negative, absorption
    positive [reaction]
  anionic neutrophil-activating peptide
ANAS
  anastomosis
  auditory nerve activating substance
anat
  anatomic(al)
  anatomy
ANB
  atrioventricular nodal block
  avascular necrosis of bone
ANBV
  Anopheles B virus
ANC
  absolute neutrophil count
  acid neutralization (acid-neutralizing)
    capacity
  adult neuronal ceroid [lipofuscinosis]
ANCA
  antineutrophil cytoplasmic antibody
    (autoantibody)
ANCA-SVV
  antineutrophil cytoplasmic autoantibody
    [and] small vessel vasculitis
anch
  anchor(ed)
ANCL
  adult neuronal ceroid lipofuscinosis
ANCOVA
  analysis of covariance [statistics]
AND
  administratively necessary days
  algoneurodystrophy
  anorexia, nausea, diarrhea
  anterior nasal discharge
  axillary node dissection
and.
  androgen
ANDA
  Abbreviated New Drug Application
andro, andros
  androsterone
ANDV
  Andasibe virus
  Andes virus
anes, anesth
  anesthesia (anesthetic) (*See also* A, AA,
    AN, ANA)
  anesthesiology

ANESR
    apparent norepinephrine secretion rate
ANF
    alpha-naphthoflavone
    antineuritic factor
    antinuclear factor
    atrial natriuretic factor
ANG
    angiogenin
    angiograph(y) (angiogram)
    angiopoietin
    angiotensin
ang
    angle (*See also* A)
    angular
ANGEL
    angiolipoma, posttraumatic neuroma,
      glomus tumor, eccrine spiradenoma,
      leiomyoma cutis [syndrome]
ANGFA
    antinerve growth factor antibody
Ang GR
    angiotensin generation rate
AngHV
    anguillid herpesvirus
ANG I–III, ANG 1–3
    angiotensin I–III (*See also* AI–AIII,
      A1–A3, ATI–ATIII, AT1–AT3)
angio
    angiograph(y) (angiographic)
      (angiogram)
ang pect
    angina pectoris
ANH
    acute normovolemic hemodilution
    artificial nutrition and hydration
    atrial natriuretic hormone
anh
    anhydrous
ANHV
    Anhanga virus
ANI
    acute nerve irritation
    autoimmune neutropenia of infancy
ANIA
    automated nephelometric immunoassay
ANIS
    Anorexia Nervosa Inventory for
      Self-Rating
ANISO
    anisocyte (anisocytosis)
ANIT
    alpha-naphthyl-isothiocyanate
ANK
    appointment not kept
ank
    ankle
ANKENT
    ankylosis and ankylosing enthesopathy

ANLI
    antibody-negative with latent infection
ANLL
    acute nonlymphocytic (nonlymphoid)
      (nonlymphoblastic) leukemia
ANM
    auxiliary nurse midwife
ANN
    alloimmune neonatal neutropenia
    artificial neural network
    axillary node negative
ann.
    annual
ANNA
    antineuronal nuclear antibody
    artificial neural network analysis
ann fib
    annulus fibrosus
annot.
    annotation
ANoA
    antinucleolar antibody
ANOTHER
    alopecia, nail [dystrophy], ophthalmic
      [complication], thyroid [dysfunction],
      hypohidrosis, ephelides, enteropathy,
      respiratory [tract infection] [syndrome]
ANOVA
    analysis of variance [statistics]
ANP
    acute necrotizing pancreatitis
    A-norprogesterone
    atrial natriuretic peptide (polypeptide)
    autonomic nerve preservation
    axillary node positive
ANP-A–ANP-C
    atrial natriuretic peptide (polypeptide)
      A–C
A-NPP
    absorbed normal pooled plasma
ANQ
    Adult Neuropsychological Questionnaire
ANRBC
    absolute nucleated red blood cell
ANRL
    antihypertensive neural renomedullary
      lipids
ANS
    acute nephritic syndrome
    antenatal corticosteroid treatment
    anterior nasal spine [craniometric]
    antineutrophilic serum
    arteriolonephrosclerosis
    arterionephrosclerosis
    autonomic nervous system
ANSD
    autonomic nervous system dysfunction
ANSI
    American National Standards Institute

ANSIE
    Adult Nowicki Strickland Internal
    External Control Scale
AN-SIR
    advice nurse structured implicit review
    [telemedicine]
ANT
    acoustic noise test
    adenosine nucleotide translocator
    aminoglycoside nucleotidyl transferase
    anterior (*See also* a, AN, ant.)
    antimycin (*See also* ant.)
ant.
    anterior (*See also* a, AN, ANT)
antag
    antagonist
ant. ax
    anterior axillary
ant. ax line
    anterior axillary line
anti.
    antidote
ANTI A:AGT
    antiblood group A antiglobulin
    [test]
anti-BrDU
    antibromodeoxyuridine
anti-BSA
    antibovine serum albumin
anti bx
    antibiotic (*See also* ATB, AB, ABx,
    abx)
anti-C100
    antibody to C100 [protein]
anti-CEA
    anticarcinoembryonic antigen
anti-CMV
    anticytomegalovirus
anticoag
    anticoagulant
anti-CP9
    antibody to core peptide 9
anti-CP10
    antibody to core peptide 10
anti-D
    anti-D immune globulin
    (immunoglobulin)
anti-DNA
    antideoxyribonucleic acid
anti-DNase B
    antideoxyribonuclease B (*See also*
    ADN-B, ADNase-B)
anti-dsDNA
    antidouble-stranded deoxyribonucleic
    acid
anti-E2
    envelope 2 antigen

anti-EBV
    anti-Epstein-Barr virus
anti-EMA
    antiendomysial antibody
anti-ENA
    antiextractable nuclear antibody
anti-GAD
    antiglutamic acid decarboxylase
anti-GBM
    antiglomerular basement membrane
anti-GOR
    antibody to GOR [epitope]
anti-HA
    antihepatitis antigen
anti-HAA
    antibody to hepatitis-associated
    antigen
anti-HAV
    antibody to hepatitis A virus
anti-HBc
    antibody to hepatitis B core antigen
anti-HBs
    antibody to hepatitis B surface antigen
anti-HCV
    antibody to hepatitis C virus
anti-HDV
    antibody to hepatitis D virus
anti-HEV
    antibody to hepatitis E virus
anti-HTLV-I
    antibody to human T-cell lymphotropic
    virus type 1
anti-IFN-gamma (γ)
    anti-interferon gamma (γ)
anti-IgE
    antiimmunoglobulin E
anti-IL-2R Ab
    antiinterleukin 2R antibody
anti-log
    antilogarithm
anti-MPO
    antimyeloperoxidase
anti-MPO Ab
    antimyeloperoxidase antibody
anti-NADase
    antinicotinamide adenine dinucleotidase
anti-PCAM
    antiplatelet endothelial cell adhesion
    molecule
anti-PCNA
    antiproliferating cell nuclear antigen
anti-PNM Ab
    antiperipheral nerve myelin antibody
anti-RNP
    antiribonucleoprotein
anti-RSV
    antirespiratory syncytial virus

anti-S
  antisulfanilic acid
anti-Scl-70
  antiscleroderma-70 antibody
anti-Sm
  anti-Smith [antibody]
anti-SMA
  antismooth muscle actin
anti-Sm/RNP
  anti-Smith ribonucleoprotein
anti-SRP
  antisignal recognition particle
anti-SSA
  anti-Sjögren syndrome A [antibody]
anti-SSAA(x)
  silicone surface-associated antigen
    antibody
anti-SSB
  anti-Sjögren syndrome B [antibody]
anti-Tac
  humanized antihuman IL-2 receptor
    antibody
anti-Tg
  antithyroglobulin
anti-TPO
  antithyroperoxidase
anti-TSH
  antithyroid-stimulating hormone
anti-vWF
  anti-von Willebrand factor
ANTR
  apparent net transfer rate
ant. sag D
  anterior sagittal diameter
ant. sup. spine
  anterior-superior spine
ANTU
  alpha (α)-naphthylthiourea
ANTV
  Antequera virus
ANUG
  acute necrotizing ulcerative
    gingivitis
ANUV
  Ananindeua virus
ANV
  acute nausea and vomiting
  anorexia, nausea, vomiting
  avian nephritis virus
ANX, anx
  anxiety
  anxious
anx neur
  anxiety neurosis
anx react
  anxiety reaction
A-O
  acoustic-optic
  atlantooccipital [joint] (See also AO)

AO
  abdominal aorta
  abdominally obese
  abdominal obesity
  academic orientation
  achievement orientation
  acid output
  acridine orange [dye or test]
  Agent Orange
  age of onset
  airway obstruction
  American Optical
  anaplastic oligodendroglioma
  ankle orthosis
  anodal opening
  anterior oblique
  aorta (See also Ao)
  aortic opening
  Arbeitsgemeinschaft für
    Osteosynthesefragen [internal
    fixation]
  arthroophthalmopathy
  atlantooccipital [joint] (See also A-O)
  atomic orbital
  atrioventricular valve opening
  auriculoventricular valve opening
    [obsolete]
  average optical density
  avoidance of others
  axioocclusal
A&O
  alert and oriented
Ao
  aorta (See also AO)
AOA
  abnormal oxygen affinity
  anaplastic oligoastrocytoma
  average orifice area
AOAA
  aminooxyacetic acid
AO:AC
  aortic valve opening to aortic valve
    closing ratio
AoAD
  acute aortic dissection
AoAF
  aortic arch flush
AOA-MCA
  alternative occipital artery middle
    cerebral artery
AOAP
  as often as possible
AoArE
  aortic arch epinephrine
AOB
  accessory olfactory bulb
  alcohol on breath
AOBC
  aortic occlusion balloon catheter

AoBP
aortic blood pressure
AOBS
acute organic brain syndrome
AOC
abridged ocular chart
advanced ovarian cancer
amyloxycarbonyl
antacid of choice
aortic opening click
area of concern
AOCD
anemia of chronic disease
AOCLD
acute on chronic liver disease
AOCS
anatomy-oriented colon segmentation
AOD
adult-onset diabetes [mellitus] (*See also* AODM)
airflow obstruction disease
alcohol and other drugs
alleged onset date
aortic occlusive disease
arterial occlusive disease
arterial oxygen desaturation
arteriosclerotic (atherosclerotic) occlusive disease
auriculoosteodysplasia
azotemic osteodystrophy
AODA
alcohol and other drug abuse
AODM
adult-onset diabetes mellitus (*See also* AOD)
AODP
alcohol and other drug problems
AODT
Animal and Opposite Drawing Technique
AOE
[injury, condition] arising out of employment
AoE
aortic epinephrine
AOF
Assessment of Occupational Functioning
AOFMD
adult-onset foveomacular dystrophy
AoG
androsterone glucuronide
AOI
apnea of infancy
area of induration
Ao-il
aorta-iliac (aortoiliac)

AOIVM
angiographically occult intracranial vascular malformation
AOL
acroosteolysis
anterior oblique ligament
augmentation of labor
AOLD
automated open lumbar discectomy
AOM
acute otitis media
alternatives of management
ambulatory oximetry monitoring
arthroophthalmopathy
AOMM
amelanotic oral malignant melanoma
AoMP
aortic mean pressure
AON
anterior olfactory nucleus
A-ONE
Arnadottir Occupational Therapy Activities of Daily Living Neurobehavioral Evaluation
AOO
atrial asynchronous [pacing]
AOP
aminooxypentane
anemia of pregnancy
aortic pressure
apnea of prematurity
AoP
left ventricle to aorta pressure gradient
AOPP
advanced oxidation protein product
AOP-RANTES
aminooxypentane regulated-on-activation normal T-expressed and secreted
AoPW
aortic posterior wall
AOR
adjusted odds ratio
auditory oculogyric reflex
Ao regurg
aortic regurgitation (*See also* AR)
AOS
acridine orange staining
Agent Orange syndrome
ambulatory outpatient surgery
anterior oesophageal sensor [British]
aortic ostial stenosis
A2-OS
aortic second sound opening snap
AOSC
acute obstructive suppurative cholangitis
AOSD
adult-onset Still disease

Ao sten
    aortic stenosis (*See also* AS)
AOT
    accessory optic tract
    acute occlusive thrombus (thrombosis)
    adenomatoid odontogenic tumor
    antiovotransferrin
AOU
    amount of use
    apparent oxygen utilization
AoV
    aortic valve
AOVM
    angiographically occult vascular
      malformation
A&Ox3
    alert and oriented to person, place, time
A&Ox4
    alert and oriented to person, place,
      time, date
AOZ
    anterior optical zone
A-P
    abdominoperineal [resection] (*See also*
      AP)
    analytic-psychologic
    anterior-posterior
AP
    abdominal pain
    abdominoperineal [resection] (*See also*
      A-P)
    accelerated phase
    accessory pathway
    acid phosphatase (*See also* ACP, AcP,
      AC-PH, ac phos)
    acinar parenchyma
    action potential
    activator protein
    active pepsin
    active pressure
    acute pancreatitis
    acute phase
    acute pneumonia
    acute proliferative
    adductor pollicis
    adenomatous polyp(osis)
    adolescent psychiatry
    after parturition
    after polarization
    alkaline phosphatase (*See also* alk phos,
      alk p'tase, ALP, KA, P'ase)
    alum-precipitated [vaccine]
    alveolar permeability
    aminopeptidase
    amyloid P-component
    amyloid peptide
    anatomic profile
    angina pectoris
    antepartum [L. *ante partum*]

    anterior pituitary
    anterior and posterior (anteroposterior)
      (*See also* A&P)
    antidromic potential
    antiparkinsonian (*See also* APK)
    antiplasmin
    antiviral protein
    antral peristalsis
    aortic pressure
    aortic pulmonary (aortopulmonary)
    apical pulse
    apothecary (*See also* ap, apoth)
    appendectomy (*See also* appy)
    appendiceal perforation
    appendicitis
    appendix
    area postrema
    arithmetic progression
    arterial pressure
    artificial pneumothorax
    aspiration pneumonitis
    assessment and plan (*See also* A&P)
    association period
    arteriosclerotic (atherosclerotic) plaque
    atrial pacing
    atrioventricular pathway
    atrium pace
    attending physician
    axiopulpal
    [intra]abdominal [voiding] pressure
AP1
    activator protein 1
8AP
    eighth nerve action potential
A:P
    ascites to plasma ratio
A&P
    abdominal and perineal
    active and present
    anatomy and physiology
    anterior and posterior (anteroposterior)
      (*See also* AP)
    assessment and plan (*See also* AP)
    auscultation and palpation
    auscultation and percussion
A_2P_2
    aortic second sound, pulmonary second
      sound
⚠ **$A_2 < P_2$**
    second aortic sound less than second
      pulmonic sound ⚠
$A_2 = P_2$
    second aortic sound equals second
      pulmonic sound
⚠ **$A_2 > P_2$**
    second aortic sound greater than second
      pulmonic sound ⚠
Ap
    apex

ap
  apothecary (*See also* apoth, AP)
APA
  acute pain attack
  air pollution adaptation
  aldosterone-producing adenoma
  antiparietal antibody
  antipernicious anemia [factor]
  antiphospholipid antibody
  atypical polypoid adenomyofibroma
  atypical polypoid adenomyoma
6-APA
  6-aminopenicillanic acid
APAA
  anterior parietal artery aneurysm
APAAP
  alkaline phosphatase antialkaline
    phosphatase
APAb
  antiphospholipid antibody
APACG
  acute primary angle-closure glaucoma
APACHE
  Acute Physiology and Chronic Health
    Evaluation [score, system]
APACHE II
  Acute Physiology and Chronic Health
    Evaluation II [score, system]
APAD
  anterior-posterior abdominal diameter
APAF
  antipernicious anemia factor
  apoptosis activating factor
APA-LMP
  atypical polypoid adenomyofibroma of
    low malignant potential
APAP
  autotitrating [self-adjusting] nasal
    [continuous] positive airway pressure
APAS
  annular phased array system
APAT
  Accounting Program Admission Test
APB
  abductor pollicis brevis [muscle]
  atrial premature beat
  auricular premature beat [obsolete]
APBD
  adult polyglucosan body disease
  anomalous pancreaticobiliary duct
APBDJ
  anomalous pancreaticobiliary
    (pancreatobiliary) duct junction
APBDU
  anomalous pancreaticobiliary
    (pancreatobiliary) ductal union
APBF
  accessory pulmonary blood flow

APBI
  accelerated partial breast irradiation
APBSCT
  autologous peripheral blood stem cell
    transplant(ation)
APBU
  anomalous pancreaticobiliary
    (pancreatobiliary) union
A-P-C
  adenoidal-pharyngeal-conjunctival [agent
    or virus]
APC
  absolute phagocyte count
  absolute plasma concentration
  activated protein C
  acute pharyngoconjunctival (fever)
  adenomatous polyp(osis) of colon
    (adenomatous polyposis coli)
  advanced pancreatic cancer
  advanced prostate cancer
  allophycocyanin
  all-purpose capsule
  alternative patterns of complement
  ambulatory payment classification
    group
  angiotensin presenting cell
  anterior-posterior compression
  antigen-presenting cell
  antiphlogistic corticoid
  aortopulmonary collateral [artery]
  aperture current
  apneustic center [of brain]
  argon plasma coagulation (coagulator)
  atrial premature complex (contraction)
  autologous packed cells
aPC
  activated protein C
APCA
  antiparietal cell antibody
APCD
  acquired prothrombin complex
    deficiency (syndrome)
APCE
  affinity probe capillary electrophoresis
APCF
  acute pharyngoconjunctival fever
APCG
  apex cardiogram (apexcardiogram)
Ap4CH
  apical four-chamber plane
    [echocardiogram]
APCI
  atrial peptide clearance inhibitor
APCKD
  adult-type polycystic kidney disease
    (*See also* APRD)
ApCPV
  Antheraea pernyi cypovirus

A-PCR
allele-specific polymerase chain reaction

APCR
activated protein C resistance

AP-CT
abdominal and pelvic computed tomography

APD
abdominal postoperative dehiscence
acid peptic disease
acquired perforating dermatosis
action potential duration
acute polycystic disease
adult polycystic disease
afferent pupillary defect
airway pressure disconnect
ambulatory peritoneal dialysis
anteroposterior diameter
antipsychotic drug
arteriopathic dementia
atrial premature depolarization
auditory processing disorder
autoimmune progesterone dermatitis
automated percutaneous discectomy
automated peritoneal dialysis
avoidant personality disorder

APDC
anxiety and panic disorder clinic

APDCC
antropyloroduodenal common chamber

APDER
anterior-posterior dual energy radiography

APDI
Adult Personal Data Inventory

ApDNV
Aedes pseudoscutellaris densovirus

APDT
acellular pertussis vaccine with diphtheria and tetanus toxoid

APE
acetone powder extract
acute polioencephalitis
acute psychotic episode
acute pulmonary edema
Advanced Placement Examination
airway pressure excursion
anterior pituitary extract
aqueous pollen extract
asthma of physical effort
avian pneumoencephalitis

APEC
asymmetric periflexural exanthem of childhood

APECED
autoimmune polyendocrinopathy, candidiasis, ectodermal dystrophy

APELL
Assessment Program of Early Learning Levels

ApEn
approximate entropy

APER
abdominoperitoneal excision of rectum

APERP
accessory pathway effective refractory period

APES
aminopropyltriethoxysilane

APEUV
Apeu virus

A&P ex
active and passive exercise

APEX-PH
Assessment Protocol of Excellence in Public Health

APF
acidulated phosphate fluoride (phosphofluoride)
anabolism-promoting factor
animal protein factor
antiperinuclear factor
aortopulmonary fistula

APG
acid-precipitated globulin
air plethysmography
animal pituitary gonadotropin
antegrade pyelography
Apgar [score]

APGAR
adaptability, partnership, growth, affection, and resolve [family screening, not Apgar score of newborn physical status]
American Pediatric Gross Assessment Record [Not Apgar Score]
appearance [color], pulse [heart rate], grimace [reflex irritability], activity [muscle tone] [mnemonic built on eponym Apgar for newborn screen, but not Apgar score]

APGL
alkaline phosphatase activity of granular leukocytes

APGN
acute postinfectious glomerulonephritis

APH
adult psychiatric hospital
alcohol-positive history
alternative pathway hemolysis
antepartum hemorrhage
anterior pituitary hormone

aph
aphasia

AP/HC
accreditation program [for] hospice care

AP/HHC
  accreditation program [for] home health
    care
APHLT
  auxiliary partial heterotopic liver
    transplant(ation)
APHP
  anti-*Pseudomonas* human plasma
APHSCS
  autologous peripheral hematopoietic
    stem cell support
API
  active pharmaceutical ingredients
  Activity Pattern Indicator
  Adult Personality Inventory
  alkaline protease inhibitor
  analytical profile index
  ankle-arm pressure index
  arterial pressure index
  Autonomy Preference Index
A1PI
  alpha (α)1 proteinase inhibitor
APIB
  Assessment of Preterm Infants Behavior
APIE
  assessment, plan, implementation,
    evaluation
APIP
  additional personal injury protection
APIVR
  artificial pacemaker-induced ventricular
    rhythm
APK
  antiparkinsonian (*See also* AP)
aPKC
  atypical protein kinase C
APKD
  adult polycystic kidney disease (*See also*
    APCKD)
APKG
  acute primary keratotic gingivostomatitis
APKH
  acquired progressive kinking of hair
APL
  abductor pollicis longus [muscle]
  accelerated painless labor
  acquired progressive lymphangioma
  acute promyelocytic leukemia (*See also*
    FAB M3, AProL)
  animal placenta lactogen
  anterior pituitarylike [hormone]
  anterior pulmonary leaflet
  antiphospholipid antibody (*See also* aPL,
    APLA)
AP&L, AP&Lat
  anteroposterior and lateral [radiologic
    view]

aPL, APLA
  antiphospholipid antibody (*See also*
    APL)
APLD
  adult polycystic liver disease
  automated percutaneous lumbar
    discectomy
APLP
  amyloid precursor-like protein
APLS
  Adult Performance Level Survey
  advanced pediatric life support
aPLS
  antiphospholipid antibody syndrome
AP/LTC
  accreditation program [for] long-term
    care
APM
  acid-precipitable material
  alternating pressure mattress
  antepartum monitor
  anterior papillary muscle
  anterior and posterior medialization
  anteroposterior movement
  aspartame
APME
  acute postinfectious measles
    encephalitis
APMET
  aggressive papillary middle ear tumor
APML
  acute promyelocytic leukemia
APMPPE
  acute posterior multifocal placoid
    pigment epitheliopathy
APMV
  avian paramyxovirus
APN
  acute panautonomic neuropathy
  acute pyelonephritis
  arsenic polyneuropathy
  average peak noise
APO
  adductor pollicis obliquus [muscle]
  adverse patient occurrences
  airway peroxidase
  aphoxide
  apoprotein (apolipoprotein)
ApoA–ApoZ
  apoprotein (apolipoprotein) A–Z
apo
  apoenzyme
apobec-1
  apolipoprotein B mRNA-editing catalytic
    polypeptide 1
ApoDCIS
  apocrine ductal carcinoma in situ

ApoHyp
apocrine hyperplasia
APOIV
Apoi virus
APOLT
auxiliary partial orthotopic liver
transplant(ation)
APOPPS
adjustable postoperative protective
prosthetic socket
APORF
acute postoperative renal failure
apoth
apothecary (*See also* ap, AP)
APP
acute-phase protein
addiction-prone personality
alternating pressure pad
alum-precipitated protein
alum-precipitated pyridine
aminopyrazolopyrimidine
amyloid precursor protein
antiplatelet plasma
appendix (*See also* app, appx)
automated physiologic profile
average pixel projection
avian pancreatic polypeptide
app
appendix (*See also* APP, appx)
applied
approximate(ly) (approximation)
(*See also* appr, approx)
AP/PA
anteroposterior [and] posteroanterior
appar
apparatus
apparent
AP-PCR
arbitrary-primed polymerase chain
reaction
APPG
aorticopulmonary paraganglioma
appl
appliance
applicable
application
applied
applan.
flattened [L. *applanatus*]
APPM
antegrade perfusion pressure
measurement
appoint.
appointment (*See also* appt)
appr, approx
approximate(ly) (approximation)
APPT
Adolescent and Pediatric Pain
Tool

appt
appointment (*See also* appoint.)
appx
appendix (*See also* APP, app)
appy
appendectomy (*See also* AP)
APQ
average perturbation quotient
APR
abdominoperineal resection
absolute proximal reabsorption
accelerator-produced radiopharmaceutical
acute pain reaction
acute phase reactant
acute phase reaction
acute phase response
air-purifying respirator
amebic prevalence rate
anatomic porous replacement
anatomic porous revision
anterior pituitary resection
apolipoprotein regulatory protein
auropalpebral reflex
A-PR
anterior-posterior repair
aprax
apraxia
APRE
acute phase response element
APRIL
A proliferation-inducing ligand
APRL
Army Prosthetics Research Laboratory
AProL
acute promyelocytic (progranulocytic)
leukemia (*See also* APL, FAB M3)
APRP
acidic proline-rich protein
acute-phase reactant protein
APRT
abdominopelvic radiotherapy
adenine phosphoribosyltransferase
APRV
airway pressure release ventilation
APS
acute physiology score
adenosine phosphosulfate (adenosine
5′-phosphosulfate)
Adult Protective Services
air plasma spray
air pollution syndrome
anterior pararenal space
anterior plate system
antiphospholipid antibody syndrome
antiphospholipid syndrome
arterioportal vein shunting
attending physician's statement
autoimmune polyglandular syndrome
automated patient system

APS1–3
autoimmune polyendocrine
(polyendocrinopathy) syndrome 1–3
APSAC
anisoylated plasminogen streptokinase
activator complex
APSD
Alzheimer presenile dementia
aortopulmonary (aorticopulmonary)
septal defect
APSGN
acute poststreptococcal
glomerulonephritis
APSP
assisted peak systolic pressure
APSQ
Abbreviated Parent Symptom
Questionnaire
APSR
acute paranoid schizophrenic reaction
APSS
anterior pull skin stretch
APT
Age Projection Test
alum-precipitated toxoid
anomaloscope plate test
antiplatelet trial
antropyloric muscle thickness
arsenic pseudotabes
atopy patch test
attached proton test
automatic peak tracking
AP-T
apical transverse
APTA
aneurysm of persistent trigeminal artery
APTC
anteroposterior talocalcaneal angle
APTD
Aid to Permanently and Totally
Disabled
APTI
airway pressure time index
AP-TNAP
alkaline phosphatase, tissue-nonspecific
isozyme protein precursor
APTT, aPTT
activated partial thromboplastin time
APTX
acute parathyroidectomy
APUD
amine precursor uptake and
decarboxylation [cell]
APV
abnormal posterior vector
Acyrthosiphon pisum virus
amprenavir

ANCA (antineutrophil cytoplasmic
antibody) positive vasculitis
average peak velocity
aPV
acellular pertussis vaccine
APVC
anomalous pulmonary venous connection
APVD
anomalous pulmonary venous drainage
APVM
acute perivascular myelinoclasis
APVR
anomalous pulmonary venous return
anterior proliferative vitreoretinopathy
APW
aortopulmonary window
AQ
accomplishment quotient
achievement quotient
acoustic quantification
anxiety quotient
any quantity
aphasia quotient
aq.
aqueous [water] [L. *aqua*] (*See also* A)
AQAB
acquired abnormality
aq. dist
distilled water
AQLQ
Asthma Quality of Life Questionnaire
AQMS
acute quadriplegic myopathy
syndrome
AQP
aquaporin
AQP1–2
aquaporin 1–2
AQS
additional qualifying symptom
A-R
apical-radial [pulse] (*See also* AR, A/R)
AR
abnormal record
absolute risk
acceptable risk
achievement ratio
Achilles reflex
acoustic reflex
acoustic rhinometry
actinic reticuloid [syndrome]
active resistance
acute rejection
adherence ratio
admitting room
adrenergic receptor
adverse reaction

AR *(continued)*
  airways resistance (*See also* R$_A$, RAW, R$_{AW}$, R(AW))
  alarm reaction
  alcohol related
  aldose reductase
  allergic rhinitis
  allowance region [radiotherapy]
  alloy restoration
  amphiregulin
  amplitude ratio
  analytical reagent
  androgen receptor
  ankle reflex
  anterior root
  aortic regurgitation (*See also* Ao regurg)
  apical-radial [pulse] (*See also* A-R, A/R)
  apical rate
  apoptotic rate
  applied relaxation
  Argyll Robertson [pupil]
  artificially ruptured
  artificial respiration
  assisted respiration
  atrial rate
  atrial regurgitation
  atrial reversal
  at risk
  atrophic rhinitis
  attack rate
  aural rehabilitation
  autoradiography
  autorefraction (autorefractor)
  autoregressive
  autosomal recessive
A&R
  advised and released
A/R
  accounts receivable
  apical/radial [pulse] (*See also* AR, A-R)
Ar
  argon
  articulare [craniometric]
ARA
  acetylene reduction activity
  adenosine regulating agent
  Adolescent Role Assessment
  anorectal angle
  antireticulin antibody
  aortic root angiogram
  Axenfeld-Reiger anomaly
ARAD
  abnormal right axis deviation
ARAL
  adjustment reaction to adult life
ARAM
  antigen recognition activation motif

ARAO
  angiographic [area of] right anterior oblique projection
ARAS
  ascending reticular activating system
ARB
  adrenergic receptor binder
  angiotensin (angiotensin II) receptor blocker
  antibiotic-resistant bacteria
  any reliable brand
arb
  arbitrary [unit]
ARBD
  alcohol-related birth defect
ARBOR
  arthropod-borne [virus]
ARBOW
  artificial rupture of bag of waters
ARBV
  Arbia virus
ARC
  abnormal retinal correspondence
  absolute reticulocyte count
  accelerating rate calorimetry
  active renin concentration
  AIDS-related complex
  alcohol rehabilitation center
  anomalous retinal correspondence
  antigen-reactive cell
  antirotation cable
  anxiety rating for children
  arcuate nucleus [of hypothalamus]
  arthrogryposis-renal dysfunction cholestasis [syndrome]
  atypical reparative changes
  autologous red [blood] cells
  automatic exposure control
  average response computer
ARCA
  acquired red [blood] cell aplasia
ARCD
  acquired renal cystic disease
arch.
  archives
ARCO
  antigen-reactive cell opsonization
ARCON
  accelerated radiotherapy with carbogen and nicotinamide
ARCP
  alcohol-related chronic pancreatitis
ARCS
  azoospermia, renal anomaly, cervicothoracic spine dysplasia
ARD
  absolute reaction of degeneration
  acid-related disorder
  acute radiation disease

acute respiratory disease
acute respiratory distress
allergic respiratory disease
anisotropically rotational diffusion
anorectal dressing
antibiotic removal device
antimicrobial removal device
aortic root diameter
aphakic retinal detachment
arthritis and rheumatic diseases
atopic respiratory disease

ARDS
acute respiratory distress syndrome

ARE
active-resistive exercise
acute red eye
AIDS-related encephalitis

AREDYLD
acrorenal field defect, ectodermal
dysplasia, lipoatrophic diabetes
[syndrome]

ARF
acute renal failure
acute respiratory failure
acute rheumatic fever
Adjective Rating Form
amylase-rich food
area resource file

ArF
argon fluoride

ARFC
active rosette-forming T cell

ARF/CRF
acute renal failure and chronic renal
failure

ARG
alkaline reflux gastritis

Arg
arginine (*See also* R)

arg-gly-asp
arginine-glycine-aspartic acid

ARGNB
antibiotic-resistant gram-negative bacillus

ARGNO
antibiotic-resistant gram-negative
organism

ARGO
Adjustable Advanced Reciprocating Gait
Orthosis

ARH
autosomal recessive hypercholesterolemia

ARHL
age-related hearing loss

ARHNC
advanced resected head and neck cancer

ARHS
acute right heart syndrome

ARI
acute renal insufficiency
acute respiratory infection
airways reactivity index
aldose reductase inhibitor
anxiety reaction, intense
arousal index
arthroscopic reduction and internal
fixation

ARIA
acetylcholine receptor-inducing activity
automated radioimmunoassay

ARIC
acrosome reaction with ionophore
challenge

ARIF
assisted reduction and internal
fixation

ARJ
anorectal junction

ARK
adrenergic receptor kinase

ARK-1
adrenergic receptor kinase 1

ARKD
autosomal recessive kidney disease

ArKr
argon-krypton [laser]

ARKV
Arkonam virus

ARL
AIDS-related lymphoma
average remaining lifetime

ARLD
alcohol-related liver disease

AR-LGMD
autosomal recessive limb muscular
dystrophy

ARLL
AIDS-related lymphoma of lung

ARM
adrenergic receptor material
advanced respiratory mechanics
aerosol rebreathing method
age-related maculopathy
allergy relief medicine
alternating range of motion
anorectal manometry
anxiety reaction, mild
arteriovenous malformation
artificial rupture of membranes
atomic resolution microscopy

ARMD
age-related macular degeneration

ARMS
access [by] radial artery multilink stent
acoustic respiratory motion sensor

ARMS *(continued)*
Adverse Reaction Monitoring System
[FDA]
alveolar rhabdomyosarcoma
amplification refractory mutation system
ARMS-PCR
amplification refractory mutation
system-polymerase chain reaction
ARN
acute renal necrosis
acute retinal necrosis [syndrome]
arcuate nucleus
ARND
alcohol-related neurodevelopmental
disorder
ARNSHL
autosomal recessive nonsyndromic
hearing loss
ARNT
aryl hydrocarbon receptor nuclear
translocator
AROA
autosomal recessive ocular albinism
AROAV
Aroa virus
AROM
active range of motion
artificial rupture of membranes
ARP
abbreviated rapid processing
absolute refractory period
acute radiation proctitis
acute recurrent pancreatitis
adiabatic rapid passage
alcohol rehabilitation program
anticipated recovery path
apolipoprotein regulatory protein
Aptitude Research Project
Argyll Robertson pupil
assay reference plasma
assimilation regulatory protein
atrial refractory period
at-risk period
automaticity recovery phase
ARPD
autosomal recessive polycystic disease
ARPES
angular resolved photoelectron
spectroscopy
ARPF
anterior release posterior fusion
ARPKD, AR-PKD
autosomal recessive polycystic kidney
disease
ARPTH
autosomal recessive renal proximal
tubulopathy and hypercalciuria
ARR
absolute risk reduction

aldosterone to renin ratio
aortic root replacement
arr
arrest(ed)
arrive(d)
ARROM
active resistive range of motion
ARRON
autoimmune-related retinopathy and
optic neuropathy
ARRP
autosomal recessive retinitis
pigmentosa
arry
arrhythmia
ARS
Academic Readiness Scale
acquiescent response scale
acute radiation syndrome (sickness)
acute repetitive seizure
acute retroviral syndrome
adult recovery services
adult Reye syndrome
AIDS-related syndrome
alizarin red S [dye]
amylase-resistant starch
angiographic reference system
antirabies serum
arylsulfatase
ARSA
arylsulfatase A
aberrant right subclavian artery
ARSAC
Administration of Radioactive
Substances Advisory Committee
ARSACS
autosomal recessive spastic ataxia of
Charlevoix-Saguenay
ARSB
arylsulfatase B
ARSC
arylsulfatase C
ARSD
arylsulfatase D
ARSM
acute respiratory system malfunction
ART
absolute retention time
accelerated recovery technique
Achilles [tendon] reflex test
acoustic reflex test
acoustic reflex threshold
acoustic response technology
active-release technique
algebraic reconstruction technique
androgen replacement therapy
antiretroviral therapy (treatment)
arrest-and-reversal treatment
arrhythmia research technology

arterial [line] (*See also* AL, A-line, art. line)

artery (arteria) [singular] [L. *arteria*] (*See also* a.)

articulation

artifact

artificial (*See also* artif)

assessment, review, treatment

assisted reproductive technique (technology)

asymmetry, range [of motion abnormality], tissue [texture abnormality]

atraumatic restorative technique

attention restoration therapy

autologous reactive T cell

automated reagin test

automaticity recovery time

arth.

arthritis

arthrotomy

arthro

arthroscopy

ARTI

acute respiratory tract illness

artif

artificial (*See also* art.)

art. line

arterial line (*See also* AL, A-line, ART)

ARTMA

advanced real-time motion analysis

Art T

art therapy

ARUV

Aruac virus

ARV

acquired immunodeficiency syndrome (AIDS) related virus

Adelaide River virus

AIDS-associated retrovirus

anterior right ventricular [wall]

antiretroviral

ARV-A–ARV-F

Aquareovirus A–F

ARVC

arrhythmogenic right ventricular cardiomyopathy

ARVD

arrhythmogenic right ventricular dysplasia

arteriosclerotic (atherosclerotic) renovascular disease

ARVDD-1

autosomal recessive vitamin D dependency type 1

ARWY

airway

⚠ **AS**

above scale

absence of seizure

acidified serum

acoustic schwannoma

acoustic stimulation

activated sleep

active sarcoidosis

active sleep

acute salpingitis

Adams-Stokes [attack, breathing, disease]

additive solution

adolescent suicide

aerosol sensitivity (sensitization)

aerosol steroid

affective style

alimentary sleep

alveolar sac

alveolar space

amyloid substance

anabolic steroid

anal sphincter

androgen suppression

androsterone sulfate

angiosarcoma

ankylosing spondylitis (*See also* ASP)

annulospiral [ending]

anovulatory syndrome

anterior synechia

anterosuperior

antiserum

antisocial

antistreptolysin [antibody]

antral spasm

anxiety sensitivity

anxiety state

aortic sac

aortic sound

aortic stenosis (*See also* Ao sten)

aqueous solution (suspension)

area of stenosis

arteriosclerosis (atherosclerosis) (*See also* asc, ASCL, ATS)

artificial sweetener

aseptic meningitis

asthma astrocyte

astigmatism (*See also* As, AST, Ast)

asymmetric (*See also* A)

asymptomatic

atrial sense

atrial septum

atrial stenosis

audiogenic seizure

autologous stem

left ear [L. *auris sinistra*] (*See also* AL, a.l., a.s.) ⚠

sickle cell trait [heterozygous genotype]

A-S
ascendance-submission
A(s)
asplenia syndrome
As
arsenic
astigmatism (*See also* AS, AST, Ast)
A·s
ampere-second
aS
absiemens
⚠ **a.s.**
left ear [L. *auris sinistra*] (*See also* AL, a.l., AS) ⚠
ASA
acetylsalicylic acid (aspirin)
active systemic anaphylaxis
acute severe asthma
Adams-Stokes attack
Adaptive Speech Alignment
American Society of Anesthesiologists [classification]
anterior spinal artery
antibody to surface antigen ratio
anticoagulation regimen of aspirin
argininosuccinate
argininosuccinic acid
aspirin-sensitive asthma
asthma, nasal polyps, aspirin intolerance [triad]
atrial septal aneurysm
Asa
arsenate
ASA I–V
American Society of Anesthesiologists patient classifications I to V, followed by "E" for emergency operations
ASAA
acquired severe aplastic anemia
ASAC
acidified serum, acidified complement
ASAD
arthroscopic subacromial decompression
ASA-G
guaiacolic acid ester of acetylsalicylic acid
ASAH
aneurysmal subarachnoid hemorrhage
antibiotic-sterilized aortic valve homograft
ASAI
aortic stenosis and aortic insufficiency
ASAL
argininosuccinic acid lyase
ASAM
adipocyte-specific adhesion molecule
ASAP
as soon as possible

atypical small acinar proliferation of prostate
[Vanderbilt University] Asthma, Sinus and Allergy Program
ASAS
argininosuccinate synthetase
ASB
anencephaly-spina bifida [syndrome]
anesthesia standby
Anxiety Scale for Blind
Aptitude Tests for School Beginners
asymptomatic bacteriuria
ASBESTOS
agent, state, body site, effects, severity, time course, other (diagnoses), synergism
A-SBFM
Andresen Six-Basic-Factors-Model [Questionnaire]
ASBO
adhesive small-bowel obstruction
ASBS
arteriosclerotic brain syndrome
ASC
acetylsulfanilyl chloride
acute suppurative cholangitis
adenosine-coupled spleen cell
altered state of consciousness
ambulatory surgery center
Ancell-Spiegler cylindroma
anterior subcapsular cataract
antibody-secreting cell
antigen-sensitive cell
antimony-sulfur colloid
apical systolic click
apocrine skin cancer
ascorbic acid
asthma symptom checklist
asc
anterior subcapsular
arteriosclerosis (atherosclerosis) (*See also* AS, ASCL, ATS)
arteriosclerotic (atherosclerotic)
ascending
ASCA
anti-Saccharomyces cerevisiae antibody
Anxiety Scales for Children and Adults
ASCAD
arteriosclerotic (atherosclerotic) coronary artery disease
ASCAo
ascending aorta (*See also* Asc-A, AO, AA, Aa)
ASCCC
advanced squamous cell cervical carcinoma
ASCCHN
advanced squamous cell carcinoma of head and neck

ASC-H
> high-grade squamous intraepithelial
> lesion

ASCI
> acute spinal cord injury

ASCII
> American Standard Code for
> Information Interchange

ascit fl
> ascitic fluid (*See also* AF)

ASCL
> arteriosclerosis (atherosclerosis) (*See also*
> AS, asc, ATS)

ASCM
> asymmetrical chest movement

ASCR
> autologous stem cell rescue

ASCS
> acute sickle chest syndrome
> autologous stem cell support

ASCT
> allogeneic stem cell transplant(ation)
> autologous stem cell transplant(ation)

ASCURD
> arteriosclerotic (atherosclerotic)
> cardiovascular renal disease

ASCUS
> atypical squamous cells of uncertain
> (undetermined) significance

ASCVD
> arteriosclerotic (atherosclerotic)
> cardiovascular disease

ASD
> acute stress disorder
> adaptive seating device
> adult/adolescent spectrum of [HIV]
> disease
> air-space disease
> aldosterone secretion defect
> Alzheimer senile dementia
> anterior sagittal diameter
> antisiphon device
> argininosuccinic acid synthetase
> deficiency
> arthritis syphilitica deformans
> atrial septal defect
> autism (autistic) spectrum disorder

ASD1
> primum atrial septal defect

ASD2
> secundum atrial septal defect

A-SDC
> anomaly-symptomatic deformity complex

ASDH
> acute subdural hemorrhage (hematoma)

ASDO
> anterior segmental dentoalveolar
> osteotomy

ASDOS
> atrial septum (septal) defect occluder
> (occlusion) system

ASDP
> anal sphincter dysplasia

ASE
> abstinence symptom evaluation
> acute stress erosion
> axilla, shoulder, elbow [bandage]

A/SE
> action/side effects

ASES
> Adult Self-Expression Scale
> American shoulder and elbow system

ASEx
> anterosuperior external ilium movement

ASF
> African swine fever
> aniline-sulfur-formaldehyde [resin]
> anterior spine (spinal) fusion
> asialofetuin
> asymmetric screen film [x-ray system]

ASFA
> anterior segment fluorescein angiography

ASFP
> ascending frontoparietal

ASFR
> age-specific fertility rate

ASFV
> African swine fever virus

ASG
> advanced stage group

ASGB
> adjustable silicone gastric banding

AS/GP
> antiserum, guinea pig

ASGPR
> antiasialoglycoprotein receptor

ASH
> aldosterone-stimulating hormone
> ankylosing spinal hyperostosis
> antistreptococcal hyaluronidase
> asymmetric septal hypertrophy

A&Sh
> arm and shoulder

AsH
> astigmatism, hypermetropic (hyperopic)

ASHCVD
> arteriosclerotic (atherosclerotic)
> hypertensive cardiovascular disease

ASHD
> arteriosclerotic (atherosclerotic) heart
> disease
> atrioseptal (atrial septal) heart disease

ASHN
> acute sclerosing hyaline necrosis

AS/Ho
> antiserum, horse

ASI
   acromial spur index
   active specific immunotherapy
   addiction severity index
   adrenal stress index
   Anxiety Sensitivity Index
   Anxiety Status Inventory
   arthroscopic screw installation

a-Si
   amorphous silicon

ASIA
   American Spinal Injury Association
   [score]
   angiosclerotic intermittent akinesis

ASIA-A
   American Spinal Injury Association
   complete spinal injury

ASIA-B
   American Spinal Injury Association
   incomplete spinal injury, preserved
   sensation

ASIA-C
   American Spinal Injury Association
   incomplete spinal injury, preserved
   motor [nonfunctional]

ASIA-D
   American Spinal Injury Association
   incomplete spinal injury, preserved
   motor [functional]

ASIA-E
   American Spinal Injury Association
   complete recovery from spinal injury

asialo-galacto-Tg
   asialo-galacto-thyroglobulin

asialo-hCG
   asialo-human chorionic gonadotropin

A-SICD
   Adapted Sequenced Inventory of
   Communication Development

a-SiC:H
   amorphous hydrogenated silicon carbide

ASICT
   amplitude-summation interferential
   current therapy

ASID
   angiosclerotic intermittent dyskinesia

ASIL
   anal squamous intraepithelial lesion

ASIn
   anterosuperior internal ilium
   movement

ASIP
   atypical protein kinase C
   isotype-specific interacting protein

ASIQ
   Adult Suicidal Ideation Questionnaire

ASIS
   anterior superior iliac spine
   aromatic solvent-induced shift

ASK
   antistreptokinase

ASKA
   antiskeletal antibody

ASL
   American Sign Language (*See also*
   Ameslan)
   angiosarcoma of liver
   ankylosing spondylitis, lung
   anterolateral sclerosis
   antistreptolysin

ASLC
   acute self-limited colitis

ASLD
   adenylosuccinate lyase deficiency

ASLN
   axillary sentinel lymph node

ASLO, ASL-O
   antistreptolysin-O (*See also* ASO,
   ASTO)

ASLT
   antistreptolysin test

ASLV
   avian sarcoma and leukosis virus [Rous
   virus]

ASM
   age-specific mortality
   airways smooth muscle
   anterior scalenus muscle
   appendicular skeletal muscle
   atypical squamous metaplasia
   myopic astigmatism (*See also* AsM,
   AM, am.)

AsM
   myopic astigmatism (*See also* ASM,
   AM, am.)

ASMA
   alpha smooth muscle actin
   antismooth muscle antibody

ASMC
   arterial smooth muscle cell

ASMD
   atonic sclerotic muscle dystrophy

ASMI
   anteroseptal myocardial infarct(ion)

As/Mk
   antiserum, monkey

ASMR
   age-standardized mortality ratio

asmt
   assessment

ASN
   acquired splenic neutropenia
   alkali-soluble nitrogen
   arteriosclerotic (atherosclerotic)
   nephritis
   automatic single-needle monitor

Asn
   asparagine (*See also* N)

ASO
adenocarcinoma of uterus with
sarcomatous overgrowth
AIDS service organization
aldicarb sulfoxide
allele-specific oligonucleotide
ankle stabilizing orthosis
antisense oligonucleotides
antistreptolysin-O (*See also* ASLO,
ASL-O, ASTO)
arterial switch operation
arteriosclerosis (atherosclerosis)
obliterans
automatic stop order

As₂O₃
arsenic trioxide

ASOD
anterior segment ocular dysgenesis

ASOR
asialoorosomucoid

ASO-RAD
arteriosclerotic (atherosclerotic) renal
artery disease

ASOT
antistreptolysin-O titer

ASP
abnormal spinal posture
acute suppurative parotitis
acute symmetric polyarthritis
affected sibling pair
African swine pox
aged substrate plasma
alkaline serum phosphatase
alkali-stable pepsin
amnesic shellfish poisoning
ankylosing spondylitis (*See also* AS)
antibody specificity prediction
antisocial personality
aortic systolic pressure
area systolic pressure
asparate
aspartic acid
aspiration
automatic signal processing

asp.
aspirate

ASPAC
anisolated streptokinase-plasminogen
activator complex

ASPAT
antistreptococcal polysaccharide A test

AS-PCR
allele-specific polymerase chain reaction

ASPD
anterior superior pancreaticoduodenal
[artery]
antisocial personality disorder

ASPECT
Ackerman-Schoendorf Scales for Parent
Evaluation of Custody

ASPED
angel-shaped phalangoepiphysial
(phangoepiphyseal) dysplasia

asper
aspergillosis

ASPG
antispleen globulin

Asp-Glu-Tyr
aspartic acid-glutamic acid-tyrosine

ASPI
Adolescent Problem Severity Index

ASPM
angiosclerotic paroxysmal myasthenia

ASPS
advanced sleep phase syndrome
alveolar soft part sarcoma

ASPVD
arteriosclerotic (atherosclerotic)
peripheral vascular disease
arteriosclerotic (atherosclerotic)
pulmonary vascular disease

ASQ
abbreviated symptom questionnaire
Ages and Stages Questionnaire
anxiety scale questionnaire
Attitude to School Questionnaire
Attributional Style Questionnaire

ASR
adrenal to spleen ratio
age/sex rate
aldosterone secretion (secretory) rate
analyte-specific reagent
Arias-Stella reaction
atrial septal resection
automatic speech recognition

AS/Rab
antiserum, rabbit

ASRD
aspirin-sensitive respiratory disease

ASS
acute serum sickness
acute spinal stenosis
anterior-superior (anterosuperior) spine
argininosuccinate synthetase
Asthma Severity Score

ASSAS
aminopterin syndrome sine
aminopterin

ASSC
acute splenic sequestration crisis

AS-SCORE
assessing severity: age of patient,
systems involved, stage of disease,
complications, response to therapy

ASSET
array spatial sensitivity encoding technique
ASSI
Accurate Surgical and Scientific Instruments (Corporation)
Assn, assn
association (*See also* Assoc, assoc)
Assoc, assoc
associate(d)
association (*See also* Assn, assn)
ASSQ
autism spectrum screening questionnaire
ASSR
adult situational (situation) stress reaction
asst
assistant
AST
above selected threshold
acid suppression therapy
acoustic stimulation test
alcohol sniff test
androgen suppression therapy
angiotensin sensitivity test
anterior spinothalamic tract
antistreptolysin titer
antistreptozyme
Aphasia Screening Test
aspartate aminotransferase
astigmatism (*See also* AS, As, Ast)
atrial overdrive stimulation rate
audiometry sweep test
Ast
astigmatism (*See also* AS, As, AST)
ASTA
anti alpha (α)-staphylolysin
Asth
asthenopia
ASTI
acute soft tissue injury
antispasticity index
ASTM
augmented soft tissue mobilization
ASTO
antistreptolysin-O (*See also* ASLO, ASL-O, ASO)
AS TOL, as tol
as tolerated
ASTRA
Advanced Shape Technology Refractive Algorithm
ASTZ
antistreptozyme [test]
ASU
Asthma Symptom Utility
ASV
adaptive support ventilation
anodic stripping voltametry

antisiphon valve
antisnake venom
arteriosuperficial venous (difference)
autologous saphenous vein [graft]
avian sarcoma virus
As/V
ampere-second per volt
ASVAB
Armed Services Vocational Aptitude Battery
ASVD
arterial-superficial venous difference
arteriosclerotic (atherosclerotic) vascular disease
ASVIP
atrial-synchronous ventricular-inhibited pacemaker
ASVS
arterial stimulation and venous sampling
ASW
artificial seawater
asw
artificially sweetened
ASWC
average spike and wave complex [EEG]
Asx
aspartic acid (ASP) or asparagine (Asn) or mono- or diradical
asymptomatic
ASYM, asym
asymmetry (asymmetric)
AT
abdominal thrust
abdominal tympany
abdominothoracic
acceleration time
achievement test
Achilles tendon
activity therapy
activity training
acute thrombosis
adaptive thermogenesis
adipose tissue
adjuvant (adjunctive) therapy
adnexal torsion
air temperature
air trapping
allergy treatment
amegakaryocytic thrombocytopenia
aminotransferase
aminotriazole
anaerobic threshold
anaphylatoxin
anionic trypsinogen
anterior tibia
antithrombin
antitrypsin
antral transplant(ation)
apoptotic index

applanation tonometry (tension)
(*See also* TAP, T APPL)
artificial tears
assistive technology
ataxia-telangiectasia (*See also* A-T)
atraumatic
atresia, tricuspid
atrial tachycardia
atrial tumor
attenuate (attenuation)
autoimmune thrombocytopenia
autologous transplant(ation)
axonal terminal
old tuberculin [Ger. *alt Tuberkulin*]

ATI–ATIII, AT1–AT3
angiotensin 1–3 (*See also* AI–AIII,
A1–A3, ANG1–ANG3,
ANGI–ANGIII)

At
ampere-turn [magnetomotive force]
(*See also* Gi)
astatine
atrium (atrial)

²¹¹At
astatine-211

a.t.
air tight

at.
atom(ic)

A-T
ataxia-telangiectasia (*See also* AT)

ATA
acquired tufted angioma
alimentary toxic aleukia
aminotriazole
anterior temporal artery
antithymic activity
antithyroglobulin antibody
antithyroid antibody
anti-*Toxoplasma* antibody
aspirin-tolerant asthma
atmosphere absolute
aurin tricarboxylic acid

ATAI
acute traumatic aortic injury

ATB
All-Terrain Balloon [catheter]
antibiotic (*See also* AB, anti bx, ABx,
abx)
atrial tachycardia with block
atypical tuberculosis

ATBC
alpha (α) tocopherol beta (β) carotene

ATBF
African tick bite fever

ATC
activated thymus cell

aerosol treatment chamber
aggressive thyroid carcinoma
alcoholism therapy classes
anaplastic thyroid carcinoma
antituberculous chemoprophylaxis
around the clock

ATCC
American Type Culture Collection

ATCL
adult T-cell leukemia (lymphoma)
angioimmunoblastic T-cell lymphoma

ATCS
active trabecular calcification surface
anterior tibial compartment syndrome

ATD
Alzheimer-type dementia
Amplatz thrombectomy device
anterior tonsillar pillar
anthropomorphic test dummy
antithyroid drug
aqueous tear deficiency
asphyxiating thoracic dystrophy
assistive technology device
autoimmune thyroid disease

ATDLG
antithoracic duct lymphocytic
globulin

ATDP
Attitudes Toward Disabled Persons

ATDR
atrial tachycardia detection rate

ATE
acute toxic encephalopathy
acute toxicity end point
adipose tissue extract(ion)
autologous tumor extract

ATEE
N-acetyl-L-tyrosine ethyl ester

ATEM
analytic transmission electron
microscope (microscopy)

A tetra P
adenosine tetraphosphate

ATF
absence of typical findings
activating transcription factor
anterior talofibular ligament
ascites (ascitic) tumor fluid

ATFC
alternative temporal forced choice

At Fib, at. fib.
atrial fibrillation (*See also* AF, AFib,
ATR FIB, atr fib)

ATFL
anterior talofibular ligament

AT III FUN
antithrombin III functional [defect]

ATG
adenine-thymine-guanine [stop codon]
antihuman thymocyte globulin
antithymocyte globulin (*See also* ATGAM)
antithyroglobulin
ATGAM
antithymocyte globulin (*See also* ATG)
AT:GC
adenine-thymine to guanine-cytosine ratio
ATH
acetyltyrosine hydrazide
anthropometric total hip
ATHC
allotetrahydrocortisol
ATHR
angina threshold heart rate
aThr
allothreonine
Athsc
atherosclerosis (*See also* AS, ATS)
ATI
abdominal trauma index
acute traumatic ischemia
AT I–VI
antithrombin I VI
ATIS
HIV/AIDS Treatment Information Service
ATL
Achilles tendon lengthening
acute T-cell leukemia
acute tumor lysis
adult T-cell leukemia (lymphoma) (*See also* ATLL)
anterior temporal lobectomy
anterior tricuspid leaflet
antitension line
argon laser trabeculectomy
atypical lymphocytes
ATLA
adult T-cell leukemia antigen
ATLL
adult T-cell leukemia (lymphoma) (*See also* ATL)
ATLP
anterior titanium thoracolumbar locking plate
ATLS
acute tumor lysis syndrome
advanced trauma life support
ATLV
adult T-cell leukemia virus
ATM
abnormal tubular myelin
acute transverse myelitis (myelopathy)
antithrombin [AT] mutation
asynchronous transfer mode
ataxia telangiectasia mutated
Awareness Through Movement
atm
[standard] atmosphere [unit of pressure]
ATMA
antithyroid plasma membrane antibody
At mA
atrial milliampere
atmos
atmospheric
ATMS
Attitudes Toward Mainstreaming Scale
ATN
acute tubular necrosis
augmented transition network
autonomous thyroid nodule
tyrosinase-negative oculocutaneous albinism
ATNC
atraumatic normocephalic
aTNM
[at autopsy] tumor, nodes, metastases [staging of cancer]
at. no.
atomic number
ATNR
asymmetric tonic neck reflex
ATO
arsenic trioxide
ATOD
alcohol, tobacco, other drugs
ATODC
atraumatic osteolysis of distal clavicle
ATON
adductor tenotomy and obturator neurectomy
A-TP
absorbed test plasma
ATP
addiction treatment program
adenosine triphosphate (adenosine 5′-triphosphate)
ambient temperature and pressure
anatomic pathology
antitachycardia pacemaker (pacing)
autoimmune thrombocytopenic purpura
AT-P
alpha 1 (α) antitrypsin-Pittsburgh
AtP
attending physician
AT-PAS
aldehyde-thionine periodic acid-Schiff [test]
ATPase
adenosine triphosphatase
ATPD
ambient temperature and pressure, dry
ATP-2Na
adenosine triphosphate disodium

ATPS
 ambient temperature and pressure,
  saturated [with water vapor]
ATP-SPECT
 adenosine triphosphate single-photon
  emission computed tomography
ATPTX
 acute thyroparathyroidectomy
ATR
 Achilles tendon reflex
 Achilles tendon repair
 Achilles tendon rupture
 against-the-rule
 alpha-thalassemia mental retardation
 atrium (atrial) (*See also* A, At)
 atrial tachycardia response
 attenuated total reflection
atr
 atrophy
ATRA1
 autoimmune thyroid-related antigen 1
ATR FIB, atr fib
 atrial fibrillation (*See also* AF, AFib,
  At Fib, at. fib.)
AT/RT
 atypical teratoid/rhabdoid tumor
  (*See also* ATT/RhT)
ATRT-CNS
 atypical teratoid/rhabdoid tumor of
  central nervous system
ATRX
 acute transfusion reaction
 X-linked alpha-thalassemia mental
  retardation
ATS
 acid test solution
 adjustable thigh antiembolism stockings
 amphetamine-type stimulant
 antirat thymocyte serum
 antitetanus serum
 antithymocyte serum
 anxiety tension state
 apathetic thyrotoxic storm
 arteriosclerosis (atherosclerosis) (*See also*
  AS, asc, ASCL)
 autologous (autotransfusion) transfusion
  [system]
ATSB
 Aptitude Tests for School Beginners
ATSDR
 Agency for Toxic Substances & Disease
  Registry
ATSMI-AV
 Attitude Toward Serious Mental Illness
  Scale Adolescent Version
ATT
 alternating triple therapy [antibiotic]

 anterior talar translation
 antitetanus toxoid
 arginine tolerance test
 aspirin tolerance time
 atypical teratoid tumor
att
 attending
ATTC
 automated test target calibration
ATTF
 anterior tibiotalar fascicle
ATTR
 amyloidogenic transthyretin
 attached report
ATT/RhT
 atypical teratoid/rhabdoid tumor
  (*See also* AT/RT)
ATU
 alcohol treatment unit
 allylthiourea
ATV
 all-terrain vehicle
 Ambystoma tigrinum stebbinsi virus
 anterior terminal vein
 atrioventricular
 avian tumor virus
AtV
 assisted ventilation (*See also* AV)
at. vol.
 atomic volume
ATW
 all track wire
at. wt.
 atomic weight (*See also* AW)
ATX
 autotoxin [extracellular
  phosphodiesterase]
atyp
 atypical
ATZ
 anal transitional zone
 atypical transformation zone
⚠ **AU**
 absorbance unit [optical density]
 according to custom [L. *ad usum*]
 advanced ultrasonography
 allergy unit
 antitoxin unit
 arbitrary unit
 atomic unit
 Australia antigen (*See also* Au Ag)
 both ears together [L. *aures unitas*]
  (*See also* a.u.) ⚠
 each ear [L. *auris uterque*] (*See also*
  a.u.) ⚠
AU4
 area under pH4

Au
 gold [L. *aurum*]
¹⁹⁸Au
 gold-198
⚠ **a.u.**
 both ears together [L. *aures unitas*]
 (*See also* AU) ⚠
 each ear [L. *auris uterque*] (*See also*
 AU) ⚠
AUA
 asymptomatic urinary abnormality
 [blood concentration] area under curve
Au Ag
 Australia antigen (*See also* AU)
AUB
 abnormal uterine bleeding
AuBMT
 autologous bone marrow
 transplant(ation)
AUC
 area under curve
AuCN
 gold cyanide
AuCPV
 Aglais urticae cypovirus
AUD, aud
 amplifiable units of deoxyribonucleic
 acid (DNA)
 arthritis of unknown diagnosis
 auditory
aud comp
 auditory compensation
AUDEX
 automated urologic diagnostic expert
 [ultrasonographic imaging]
AUDIT
 Alcohol Use Disorders Identification
 Test
aud-vis
 audiovisual (*See also* AV)
AUFS
 absorbance units, full scale
AUG
 acute ulcerative gingivitis
 adenine, uracil, guanine [sequences
 codon]
AUGH
 acute upper gastrointestinal
 hemorrhage
AUGIB
 acute upper gastrointestinal bleeding
AUHAA
 Australia hepatitis-associated antigen
AUI
 alcohol use inventory
AUL
 acute undifferentiated leukemia
AUM
 asymmetric unit membrane

AUMC
 area under first moment curve
AUO
 amyloid of unknown origin
AuP
 Australia antigen protein
AUQ
 Alcohol Usage Questionnaire
AUR
 acute urinary retention
aur
 auricle (auricular) [obsolete reference to
 atrium] (*See also* A)
 auris (*See also* A, a)
AURAV
 Aura virus
AUS
 acute urethral syndrome
 artificial urethral (urinary) sphincter
 auscultation (*See also* ausc, auscul)
ausc, auscul
 auscultation (*See also* AUS)
AuSH
 Australia serum hepatitis [antigen]
AUSR
 acute undifferentiated schizophrenic
 reaction
AUTI
 asymptomatic urinary tract infection
autoAb
 autoantibody
autoMACS
 automated magnetic cell sorting
Auto-PBSC
 autologous peripheral blood stem
 cell
Auto-PBSC BMT
 autologous peripheral blood stem cell
 bone marrow transplant(ation)
autoPEEP
 auto [self-triggered or unintended]
 positive end-expiratory pressure
aux
 auxiliary
AV
 adenoassociated virus
 allergic vasculitis
 alveolar duct
 anteroventral
 anteverted (anteversion)
 anticipatory vomiting
 aortic valve
 arteriovenous
 artificial ventilation
 assisted ventilation (*See also* AtV)
 atrioventricular
 audiovisual (*See also* aud-vis)
 auditory-visual
 augmented vector

aviation medicine (*See also* AM, AVM)
avoirdupois (*See also* AVDP, avdp)
A/V
  alanine [and] valine
  ampere/volt [method]
  arterial [and] venous
  atrial [and] ventricular
A:V
  artery to vein ratio
  arterial to venous ratio [in fundi]
aV
  abvolt
AVA
  advanced vessel analysis
  anthrax vaccine, adsorbed
  antiviral antibody
  aortic valve anulus (annulus)
  aortic valve area
  aortic valve atresia
  Arracacha A virus
  arteriovenous anastomosis
  availability
AvaCPV
  Agraulis vanillae cypovirus
AVAD
  acute ventricular assist device
AV/AF
  anteverted and anteflexed
AVAV
  Avalon virus
AVB
  abnormal vaginal bleeding
  Arracacha B virus
  atrioventricular block
AVBR
  automated ventricular brain ratio
AVC
  aberrant ventricular conduction
  acrylic veneer crown
  aortic valve classification
  aortic valve closure
  arteriovenous communication
  associative visual cortex
  atrioventricular canal
  atrioventricular conduction
  automatic volume control
AVCD
  atrioventricular canal defect
AvCDO$_2$
  arteriovenous oxygen content difference
  (*See also* AVDO$_2$)
AVCN
  anteroventral cochlear nucleus
AVCS
  atrioventricular conduction system
AVCx
  atrioventricular circumflex [branch]

AVD
  aortic valve (valvular) disease
  apparent volume of distribution
  arteriovenous difference
  arteriosclerotic (atherosclerotic) vascular
    disease
  atrioventricular delay
  atrioventricular dissociation
AvDNV
  Agraulis vanillae densovirus
AVDO$_2$
  arteriovenous oxygen [content]
  difference (*See also* AvCDO$_2$)
AVDO$_2$B
  arteriovenous oxygen [content]
  difference, basal
AVDP, avdp
  average diastolic pressure
  avoirdupois (*See also* AV)
AVE
  aortic valve echocardiogram
  atrioventricular extrasystole
AVED
  ataxia with vitamin D deficiency
AVEEG
  audiovisual electroencephalogram
aver
  average (*See also* avg)
AVF
  antiviral factor
  arteriovenous fistula
aVF
  augmented voltage [unipolar limb lead
  on] left leg [in electrocardiography]
AVFM
  arteriovenous fistulous malformation
AVG
  ambulatory visit group [patient
    classification]
  aortic valve gradient
avg
  average (*See also* aver)
AVGC
  autogenous vein graft conduit
AVGCS
  autologous vein graft coated
  stent
AVGS
  autologous vein graft stent
AVH
  acute viral hepatitis
AVHB
  atrioventricular heart block
AVHD
  acquired valvular heart disease
AVHS
  acquired valvular heart syndrome

AVI
air velocity index
atrioventricular interval
AV-ICD
atrial and ventricular implantable
cardioverter-defibrillator
AviCPV
Arctia villica cypovirus
A-V IMA
arteriovenous internal mammary [fistula]
AVIR
aortic valve replacement
AVJ
atrioventricular junction
AVJA
atrioventricular junction ablation
AVJR
atrioventricular junctional rhythm
AVJRe
atrioventricular junctional reentrant
AVJT
atrioventricular junctional tachycardia
AVL
American visceral leishmaniasis
anterior vein of leg
aVL
augmented voltage [unipolar limb lead
on] left arm [in electrocardiography]
AVLINE
audiovisuals on-line
AVM
arteriovenous malformation
atrioventricular malformation
aviation medicine (*See also* AM)
AVN
acute vasomotor nephropathy
arbitrary valve unit
arteriovenous nicking
atrioventricular node (nodal)
avascular necrosis
AVNA
atrioventricular node artery
AVNB
atrioventricular nodal block
AVND
atrioventricular node (nodal) dysfunction
AVNFH
avascular necrosis of the femoral head
AVNFRP
atrioventricular node functional
refractory period
AVNR
atrioventricular nodal reentry
AVNRT
atrioventricular nodal reentrant (reentry)
tachycardia
atrioventricular node recovery time
AVNT
atrioventricular nodal tachycardia

AVO
aortic valve opening (orifice)
atrioventricular opening
A-VO₂
arteriovenous oxygen [difference]
AVOA
amorphous vascular occluding agent
AVOC
avocation
AVP
ambulatory venous pressure
antiviral protein
aortoventriculoplasty
arginine vasopressin
arteriovenous passage [time]
ARTMA virtual patient
AVPR2
antidiuretic arginine vasopressin V2
receptor
AVPU
alert, verbal stimulus response, painful
stimulus response, unresponsive
AVR
accelerated ventricular rhythm
aortic valve replacement
AVr
antiviral regulator
aVR
augmented voltage [unipolar limb lead
on] right arm [in electrocardiography]
AVRB
added viscous resistance to breathing
AVREO
avian reovirus
AVRI
acute viral respiratory infection
AVRP
atrioventricular refractory period
AVRT
atrioventricular reciprocating tachycardia
atrioventricular reentrant tachycardia
AVS
adrenal venous sampling
aneurysm of membranous ventricular
septum
aortic valve stenosis
arteriovenous shunt
auditory vocal sequencing
AVSC
aortic valve cusp separation
AVSD
acquired ventricular septal defect
atrioventricular septal defect
AVSS
afebrile, vital signs stable
AVSV
aortic valve stroke volume
AVT
Allen vision test

area ventralis of Tsai
arginine oxytocin
arginine vasotocin
atrioventricular tachycardia
atypical ventricular tachycardia

AVTB
absolute volume of trabecular bone

AVV
atrioventricular valve

AV3V
anteroventral third ventricle

AvV
Agraulis vanillae virus

AVVM
angiographically visualized vascular
malformation

AvWD
acquired von Willebrand disease

AVWS
anterior vaginal wall sling

AVXR
acute vascular xenograft rejection

AVY
Arracacha virus Y

AVZ
avascular zone

AW
abdominal wall
abnormal wave
above waist
abrupt withdrawal
actual weight
airway
alcohol withdrawal
aluminum wafer
alveolar wall
alveolar wash
Anderson-Wilkins [EKG acuteness
score]
anterior wall
atomic warfare

A3W
crystalline amino acid solution

A/W
able to work

A&W
alive and well

aw
airway

AWA
alcohol withdrawal assessment
as well as
away without authorization

AWAR
anterior wall of aortic root

AWB
autologous whole blood

AWBM
alveolar wall basement membrane

AWD
alcohol withdrawal delirium
alive with disease

AWDW
assault with deadly weapon

AWE
acetowhite epithelium
advancing wavelike epitheliopathy

AWF
adrenal weight factor

AWG
American wire gauge

AWI
anterior wall infarction
authorized walk-in [patient]

AWM
abnormal wall motion

AWMI
anterior wall myocardial infarction

AWMV
amplitude-weighted mean velocity

AWO
airway obstruction

AWOD, AWD
alive without disease

AWOL
absent without leave

AWP
airway pressure

AWR
airway restriction

AWRU
active wrist rotation unit

AWS
AIDS wasting syndrome
alcohol withdrawal syndrome

AWTA
aniridia-Wilms tumor association

awu
atomic weight unit

AX
alloxan

ax.
axial (*See also* A, a)
axilla (axillary) (*See also* A)
axis
axon

AXB
axillary block

AXBF
axillobifemoral [graft, bypass]

AXC
aortic crossclamp

AXF
advanced x-ray facility

AXG
  adult-type xanthogranuloma
ax. grad
  axial gradient
AX-HSA
  amoxicilloyl-human serum albumin
AXL
  axillary lymphoscintigraphy
AXM
  acetoxycycloheximide
AXND
  axillary node dissection
AXP
  total adenine ribonucleotide
AXR
  abdominal x-ray
AXT
  alternating exotropia
  axoplasmic transport
AXUF
  axillounifemoral [graft, bypass]
AYA
  acute yellow atrophy
AYF
  antiyeast factor
AYP
  autolyzed yeast protein
AYV
  Anthriscus yellows virus
AZ
  acquisition zoom
  Aschheim-Zondek [test]
Az
  nitrogen [Fr. *azote*] (*See also* Azo)

AZA
  azelaic acid
AZF
  azoospermia factor
AZH
  assisted zonal hatching
AZM
  acquisition zoom magnification
  [imaging]
AZO, azo
  indicates presence of the group -N:N-
  (*See also* Az)
AZOOR
  acute zonal occult outer retinopathy
AZR
  alizarin [dye, stain]
AZS
  automatic zero set
⚠ **AZT**
  Aschheim-Zondek test
  3′-azido-3′deoxythymidine zidovudine
    (azidothymidine) ⚠
  azidothymidine (zidovudine) ⚠
AZTEC
  amplitude zone time epoch coding
  [electrocardiogram adjunct]
AZTMP
  azidothymidine monophosphate
AZT-R
  azidothymidine-resistant
AZT-S
  azidothymidine-susceptible or sensitive
AZTTP
  azidothymidine triphosphate

B

bacillus (*See also* Bac, bac.)
band
barometric (*See also* BAR)
base [chemistry] (*See also* b)
baseline
bath [L. *balneum*]
Baumé scale [specific gravity of liquids]
behavior
bel [sound intensity]
Benoist scale [physics]
beta [second letter of Greek alphabet uppercase]
bicuspid
black
bloody
blue (*See also* bl)
body
bolus
bone
bone [marrow-derived cell or lymphocyte]
born (*See also* b, n.)
boron
both
bound (*See also* BD)
bovine
bregma [craniometric]
bronchial
bronchus
brother (*See also* BRO)
Brucella
bruit
buccal
Bucky [film in cassette in Potter-Bucky diaphragm]
bursa [cell]
corticosterone [compound B]
supramentale [craniometric point B]
twice [L. *bis*] (*See also* b., bis.)
whole blood (*See also* QB, WB, W Bld)

B̄

magnetic induction

B_0

constant external magnetic field [nuclear magnetic resonance]

B_1

field in nuclear magnetic resonance
thiamin [vitamin B_1]

BI

Billroth I [operation]

B_2

riboflavin [vitamin B_2]

BII

Billroth II [operation]

B_3

niacin (niacinamide, nicotinic acid) [vitamin B_3]

B_5

pantothenic acid [vitamin B_5]

B_6

pyridoxine [vitamin B_6]

B_7

biotin [vitamin B_7]

B_8

adenosine phosphate [vitamin B_8]

B_{12}

cyanocobalamin [vitamin B_{12}]

B19

parvovirus B19

b

barn [unit of area, nuclear physics]
base [of prism]
born (*See also* B, n.)
branch(ed)

b.

twice [L. *bis*] (*See also* B, bis.)

BA

bacillary angiomatosis
backache
bacterial agglutination
bactericidal activity
balloon angioplasty
barbituric acid
basilar artery
benzyladenine
benzyl alcohol (*See also* BnOH)
best amplitude
bilateral asymmetric
bile acid
biliary atony
biliary atresia
bioactive
bioavailability
biologic activity
blocking antibody
blood agar
blood alcohol
bone age
boric acid
bovine albumin
brachial artery
breathing apparatus
bronchial asthma
bronchoalveolar
buccoaxial
buffered acetone
butyric acid

⚠ **B<A**
    bone conduction less than air
        conduction ⚠

⚠ **B>A**
    bone conduction greater than air
        conduction ⚠

B&A
    before and after
    brisk and active

Ba
    barium
    basion [craniometric]

BAA
    benzoylarginine amide
    beta (β) adrenergic agonist

BAAD
    blunt abdominal aortic disruption

BAAP
    bone-anchored auricular prosthesis

BAAV
    bovine adenoassociated virus

BAB
    beta (β) adrenoceptor blocking
    blood agar base
    blood-aqueous barrier

Bab
    Babinski [reflex, sign]

BabK
    baboon kidney

BABV
    Babahoya virus

BAC
    Bacillus amyloliquefaciens
    bacterial adherent colony
    bacterial antigen complex
    bacterial artificial chromosome
    benzalkonium chloride
    blood alcohol concentration
    blood alcohol content
    bronchioloalveolar carcinoma
    bronchoalveolar carcinoma
    bronchoalveolar cell
    buccoaxiocervical

Bac, bac.
    bacillary [L. *Bacillus*]
    bacillus (*See also* B)

BACA
    bronchioalveolar carcinoma

BA:CA
    bone age to chronologic age ratio

BACE
    beta (β) amyloid converting enzyme
    beta (β) site APP (amyloid precursor
        protein) cleaving enzyme

BACI
    bovine anticryptosporidium
        immunoglobulin

BaClr
    barium chloride

BACM
    best available control measures

BACS
    Barriers to Care Scale

BACT
    base-activated clotting time

bact
    bacterial
    bacteriology
    bacterium [singular] (bacteria [plural])

BAD
    benign anorectal disease
    biologic aerosol detection
    biologically active dose
    bipolar affective disorder
    brachial artery diameter

BADF
    bile acid dependent flow

BADGE
    Békésy Ascending-Descending Gap
        Evaluation

BADL
    basic activities of daily living

BADS
    Behavioral Assessment of the
        Dysexecutive Syndrome
    black locks-albinism-deafness syndrome

BadV A–C
    bovine adenovirus A–C

BAE
    basilar artery ectasia
    bone-anchored epithesis
    bone-anchored prosthesis
    bovine aortic endothelium
    bronchial artery embolization

BaE, BaEn
    barium enema (*See also* BE)

BAEC
    bovine aortic endothelial cell

BAEDP
    balloon aortic end-diastolic pressure

BAEE
    benzoyl arginine ethyl ester

BAEF
    brainstem auditory evoked field

BAEP
    brainstem auditory evoked potential

BAER, BSAER
    brainstem auditory evoked response

BAF
    barrier to autointegration factor
        [protein]
    biological aerated filter
    breast adenofibroma
    bronchoalveolar fluid

BAFA
    biologically active food additive

BAFF
    B-cell activating factor

BaFPE
  Bay Area Functional Performance
    Evaluation
BAFS
  biologically active food supplement
BAFT, BaFT
  barium follow-through (followthrough)
BAG
  buccoaxiogingival
BAGF
  brachioaxillary bridge graft fistula
BAGG
  buffered azide glucose glycerol [broth]
BAGP
  bacteria aggregating glycoprotein
BAGV
  Bagaza virus
BAH
  bilateral adrenal hyperplasia
  borderline arterial hypertension
BAHA
  bone-anchored hearing aid
BAHV
  Bahig virus
BAI
  basilar artery insufficiency
  basion-axial interval
  blunt abdominal injury
  blunt aortic injury
  Brain Atrophy Index
  breath-actuated inhaler
  bronchial arterial infusion
BAIB
  beta (β)-aminoisobutyric [acid]
BAIBF
  bile acid-independent bile formation
BAIF
  bile acid-independent flow
BAIP
  bone alkaline phosphatase
BAIQ
  below average intelligence quotient
BAIT
  bacterial automated identification
    technique
BAK
  benzalkonium chloride
BAKUV
  Baku virus
BAKV
  Bakau virus
  Bakelvirus
BAL
  balance (*See also* bal)
  bioartificial liver
  blood alcohol level
  British anti-Lewisite
  bronchoalveolar lavage

bal
  balance (*See also* BAL)
  balsam (*See also* bals)
BALA
  beta (β) alanine
BALB
  binaural alternate loudness balance
BALC
  bronchoalveolar carcinoma
  bronchoalveolar cell
BALF
  bronchoalveolar lavage fluid
B ALL, B-ALL
  B-cell acute lymphoblastic leukemia
BALP
  bone-specific alkaline phosphatase
bals
  balsam (*See also* bal)
BALT
  bronchus-associated lymphoid tissue
BAM
  benzamide
  bilateral augmentation mammoplasty
  bile acid malabsorption
  bioabsorbable membrane
BaM
  brachial artery mean [pressure]
  barium meal
BAME
  benzoylarginine methyl ester
BAMO
  behavioral, anxiety, mood, other [types
    of disorders]
BAMP
  bronchoalveolar mononuclear phagocyte
BAMT
  benefit of allogeneic (allogenic) bone
    marrow transplant(ation)
BAN
  basolateral amygdaloid nucleus
  blood ammonium nitrogen
  British Approved Name [generic drugs,
    British Pharmacopoeia]
  bulimic anorexia nervosa
Ba-N
  basion-nasion [craniometric]
band, stab
  neutrophil
BANF
  bilateral acoustic neurofibromatosis
BANS
  back, arm, neck, scalp
BANV
  Banzi virus
BAO
  basal acid output
  basilar artery occlusion
  brachial artery output

BAO:MAO
  basal acid output to maximal acid
    output ratio
BAP
  bacterial alkaline phosphatase
  basic adaptive process
  Behavior Activity Profile
  Behavioral Assessment of Pain
  beta (β)-amyloid peptide
  blood agar plate
  body adiposity percentage
  bone alkaline phosphatase
  bovine albumin in phosphate buffer
  brachial artery pressure
  brightness area product
BaP
  benzoapyrene
BAPE
  benign asbestos pleural effusion
BAPI
  barley alkaline protease inhibitor
BAPN
  beta (β)-aminopropionitrile fumarate
BAPP
  bacteremia-associated pneumococcal
    pneumonia
  beta (β) amyloid precursor protein
BAPS
  balance activation [of] proprioceptive
    system
  biomechanical ankle platform system
  bovine albumin phosphate saline
BAPV
  basal (baseline) average peak velocity
BAQ
  brain-age quotient
BAR
  bariatrics
  barometer (barometric)
  biofragmentable anastomosis
    (anastomotic) ring
  bronchial artery revascularization
βAR
  beta (β) adrenergic receptor
barb.
  barbiturate
BARE
  bile acid response element
βARK
  beta (β) adrenergic receptor kinase
BARN
  bilateral acute retinal necrosis
  Body Awareness Resource Network
BARS
  Barnes Akathisia Rating Scale
  Behavioral Activity Rating Scale
BARSIT
  Barranquilla Rapid Survey Intelligence
    Test

BART
  biofeedback-assisted relaxation training
BARV
  Barur virus
BAS
  Ballard Assessment Score
  balloon atrial septostomy
  Barnes Akathisia Scale
  behavioral activation system
  benzyl antiserotonin
  beta (β) adrenergic stimulation
  biologically active substance
  boric acid solution
  British Ability Scale
  bronchial asthma status
BaS, Ba swal
  barium swallow (*See also* BS)
bas
  basilar
  basophil (basophilic leukocyte) (*See also*
    baso)
BASA
  Boston Assessment of Severe Aphasia
BASC
  Behavioral Assessment Scale for
    Children
BASE
  B27-arthritis-sacroiliitis-extraarticular
    features [syndrome]
  Brief Aphasia Screening Examination
BASH
  body acceleration synchronous with
    heartbeat (heart rate)
baso
  basophil (basophilic leukocyte) (*See also*
    bas)
BaSO4
  barium sulfate
BASO STIP
  basophilic stippling
BAT
  Basic Aid Training
  basic assurance test
  best available technology
  bilateral advancement transposition
  biliary acid transporter
  blunt abdominal trauma
  B-mode acquisition and targeting
    [radiotherapy]
  bolus arrival time
  brain adjacent tumor
  Brightness Acuity Test
  brown adipose tissue
BATA
  brain-associated thymus antigen
batt
  battery
BATV
  Batai virus

BAU
  bedside abdominal ultrasonograph(y)
    (ultrasonogram)
  bioequivalent allergy unit
  biological allergic unit
  business as usual
BAUP
  Bovie-assisted uvulopalatoplasty
BAUV
  Bauline virus
BAV
  balloon aortic valvotomy (valvuloplasty)
    (*See also* BAVP)
  Banna virus
  BeAr 328208 virus
  bicommissural (bicuspid) aortic valve
  bovine adenovirus
BAVCP
  bilateral abductor vocal cord paralysis
BAVFO
  bradycardia after arteriovenous fistula
    occlusion
BAVM
  brain arteriovenous malformation
BAVP
  balloon aortic valvuloplasty
BAW
  bronchoalveolar washing
BAYV
  Bayou virus
BB
  baby boy
  backboard
  bad breath
  Bandrowski base
  bath blanket
  bed bath
  bed board
  beta blocker (blockade)
  BioBreeding [rat]
  blanket bath
  blood bank (*See also* BLBK, bld bk)
  blood buffer (base)
  blue bloater [emphysema]
  body belt
  Bortfeld/Boyer [radiotherapy]
  both bones [fractures]
  bowel and bladder (*See also* B&B)
  breakthrough bleeding (*See also* BTB)
  breast biopsy (*See also* B Bx, br bx)
  bronchial blocker [tube]
  brush biopsy
  brush border
  buffer base
  bundle branch
  creatine kinase brain band [isoenzyme]
    (*See also* CK-BB, CPK-BB)

B&B
  bismuth and bourbon
  bowel and bladder (*See also* BB)
B/B
  backward bending
Bb
  Borrelia burgdorferi
BBA
  born before arrival
BBB
  baseball bat beating
  blood-brain barrier
  blood buffer base
  bundle branch block
BBBB
  bilateral bundle branch block
BBBM
  bundle branch block morphology
BBBP
  blood-brain barrier permeability
BBC
  biceps, brachialis, coracobrachialis
  bilateral breast cancer (carcinoma)
  bromobenzylcyanide [riot control agent]
  Brown-Buerger cytoscope
  buccal bifurcation cyst
BbCPV
  Biston betularia cypovirus
BBD
  baby born dead
  benign breast disease
  Brief Battery for Dementia
  brittle bone disease
  bronchoscopic balloon dilatation
    (dilatation)
  [heart] beat-to-beat difference
BB3DI
  broad beam three-dimensional
    irradiation
BBDS
  benign bile duct stricture
  bioadhesive drug delivery system
BBE
  Bacteroides bile esculin (agar)
  Bickerstaff brainstem encephalitis
  blood (body fluid) exposure
BBF
  bronchial blood flow
BBFP
  blood and body fluid precautions
BBI
  Bowman-Birk inhibitor
BBM
  banked breast milk
  brush border membrane
BBMI
  baseline body mass index

BB to MM
   belly button to medial malleolus
BBMV
   brush border membrane vesicle
BBN
   broadband noise
BBO
   benign biliary obstruction
BBOV
   Bimbo virus
BBOW
   bulging bag of waters
BBP
   bloodborne (blood-borne) pathogen
   butylbenzyl phthalate
BBPRL
   big big prolactin
BBR
   bacterial breakdown rate
   bibasilar rale
   blood-brain ratio
   bundle branch reentry
BBRS
   Burks Behavior Rating Scale
BBR-VT
   bundle branch reentry ventricular
      tachycardia
BBS
   bashful bladder syndrome
   benign biliary stricture
   benign breast syndrome
   BES buffered saline
   bilateral breath sounds
   bombesin
   brown bowel syndrome
BBSH
   biceps brachii [muscle] short head
BBT
   basal body temperature
   Berg balance test
   Bingham Button Test
   Buteyko breathing technique [for
      asthma]
BBTB
   blood-brain-tumor barrier
BBTD
   baby bottle tooth decay
BBTL
   bilateral basal ganglia thalamic lesion
BBTOP
   Bankson-Bernthal Test of Phonology
BBV
   black beetle virus
   blood-borne virus
   bone [marrow] blood volume
   border membrane vesicle
BBVT
   branch-to-branch ventricular
      tachycardia

BB/W
   BioBreeding/Worcester [rat]
B Bx
   breast biopsy (*See also* BB, br bx)
BC
   back care
   backcross
   background count [radioactivity]
   bactericidal concentration
   basal cell
   base curve
   basket catheter
   basket cell
   battered child
   battle casualty
   bed and chair (*See also* B&C)
   behavior control
   beta (β) carotene
   bicarbonate
   Bilhaut-Cloquet [thumb procedure]
   biliary colic
   biotin carboxylase
   bipolar cell
   birth control
   black carbon
   bladder cancer
   blast crisis
   blastic crisis
   blood cardioplegia
   blood center
   blood count
   blood culture (*See also* BlC, blc, BL
      CuLT, bl cult)
   board certified
   bone conduction
   Bowman capsule
   brachiocephalic
   breast cancer
   bronchial carcinoma
   buccal cartilage
   buccal cusp
   buccocervical
   buffy coat
   bulbus cordis
B/C
   because
B:C
   blood urea nitrogen to creatinine ratio
   benefit to cost ratio
B&C
   bed and chair (*See also* BC)
   biopsy and curettage
   board and care
   breathed and cried
BCA
   balloon catheter angioplasty
   Barrett adenocarcinoma
   basal cell atypia
   bell-clapper anomaly

bichloracetic acid
bicinchoninic acid
bidirectional cavopulmonary anastomosis
blood color analyzer
body composition analysis
brachiocephalic artery
branchial cleft anomaly
breast cancer antigen
BCAA
branched-chain amino acid
BCAF
B-cell activating factor
BCAO
bilateral carotid artery occlusion
BCAP
breast cancer with associated
pregnancy
BCAT
brachiocephalic arterial trunk
breast changes and tenderness
BCAVD
bilateral congenital absence of vas
deferens
BCB
blood-cerebrospinal [fluid] barrier
brilliant cresyl blue [stain]
BCBC
bulbar conjunctival blood column
BCBL
body cavity-based lymphoma
BCBR
bilateral carotid body resection
BCC
basal cell carcinoma (*See also* BCCa)
benign cellular changes
biliary cholesterol concentration
birth control clinic
bcc
body centered cubic [crystal lattice]
BCCA
bifurcation of common carotid artery
BCCa
basal cell carcinoma (*See also* BCC)
branchial cleft carcinoma
BC-CFC
blast cell colony-forming cell
BCCI
Barclay Classroom Climate Inventory
BCCO
bilateral common carotid occlusion
BCCP
biotin carboxyl carrier protein
BCCR
balanced complex chromosomal
rearrangement
BCCV
Black Creek Canal virus

BCD
bad conduct discharge
basal cell dysplasia
binary-coded decimal
blepharocheilodontic
borderline of cardiac dullness
BCDDP
Breast Cancer Detection Demonstration
Project
BCDF
B-cell differentiation factor
BCDH
bilateral congenital dislocated hip
BCDP
balloon catheter dilation of prostate
BCDR
blood capillary density ratio
BCE
barium contrast enema
basal cell epithelioma
B-cell enriched
benign childhood epilepsy
bubble chamber equipment
BCEC
brain capillary endothelial cell
BCECT
benign childhood epilepsy with
centrotemporal [spike]
BCEDP
breast cancer early detection program
BCEI
breast cancer estrogen-inducible [trefoil
factor, gene]
B-cell CLL/SLL
B-cell chronic lymphocytic
leukemia/small lymphocytic lymphoma
BCEOP
benign partial epilepsy with occipital
paroxysm
BCF
basic conditioning factor
basophil chemotactic factor
bioconcentration factor
breast cyst fluid
BCFA
branched-chain fatty acid
BCFP
bacteria colony forming particle
breast cyst fluid protein
BCFU
bacteria colony forming units
BCG
Bacille (Bacillus) Calmette-Guérin
[vaccine]
ballistocardiograph(y)
(ballistocardiogram)
bicolor guaiac [test]

BCG *(continued)*
    bilateral cystogram
    bromcresol green
    bronchocentric granulomatosis
bCgA
    bovine chromogranin A
BCGD
    breast cancer gene database
BCGF
    B-cell growth factor
BCH
    basal cell hyperplasia
    benign cephalic histiocytosis
    benign coital headache
BCHA
    bone conduction hearing aid
BchE
    butylcholinesterase [gene]
BCHL
    bone conduction hearing loss
bChl, Bchl
    bacterial chlorophyll
BCI
    bicaudate index
    blunt cardiac injury
    blunt carotid injury
BCIS
    breast carcinoma in situ
BCKA
    branched chain keto acid
BCKD
    branched chain alpha (α) ketoacid
        dehydrogenase
BCL
    basic cycle length
    B-cell lymphoma
    Békésy comfortable loudness
    biochemiluminescence
BCLD
    B-cell lymphoproliferative disease
        (disorder)
BCLL, B-CLL
    B-cell chronic lymphocytic leukemia
BCLP
    bilateral cleft lip and palate
BCLPD
    B-cell chronic lymphoproliferative
        disorder
BCLS
    basic cardiac life support [system]
BCM
    B-cell maturation
    birth control medication
    birth control method
    blood-clotting mechanism
    body cell mass
    body control and movement
BCMA
    B-cell maturation antigen

BCMD
    benign congenital muscular dystrophy
BCME
    bischloromethyl ether
BCMF
    B-cell maturation factor
BCMI
    B-cell mediated immunity
    body cell mass index
BCMM
    balloon-cell malignant melanoma
BCN
    basal cell nevus
    bilateral cortical necrosis
BCNS
    basal cell nevus syndrome
BCO
    balloon coronary occlusion
    biliary cholesterol output
BCOC
    bowel care of choice
BCOT
    benign cystic ovarian teratoma
BCP
    basic calcium phosphate
    biochemical profile
    birth control pill
    blood cell profile
    bromcresol purple
BCP-D
    bromocresol purple desoxycholate
BCPF
    B-cell proliferation factor
BCP-LBL
    B-cell precursor lymphoblastic
        leukemia
BCPM
    benign cystic peritoneal mesothelioma
BCPR
    basic cardiopulmonary resuscitation
    bystander cardiopulmonary resuscitation
BCPS
    battery-charging power supply
BCPV
    bovine cutaneous papillomavirus
BCQ
    breast central quadrantectomy
BCR
    B-cell antigen receptor
    B-cell reactivity
    behavior control room
    bicaudate ratio
    birth control regimen
    breakpoint cluster region
    buccal cervical ridge
    bulbocavernosus reflex
BCR-ABL
    breakpoint cluster region-Abelson
        murine leukemia [virus]

BCRL
breast cancer-related lymphedema
BCR-negative
breakpoint cluster region negative
BCRP
breast cancer resistance protein
BCR-positive
breakpoint cluster region positive
BCRS
Brief Cognitive Rating Scale
BCRT
Breast Cancer Risk tool
breast conservation [surgery followed
by] radiation therapy
BCRx
birth control drug
BCS
battered child syndrome
blood cell separator
breast conservation (breast-conserving)
surgery
BCSA
bone cross-sectional area
BCSB
bacterial contamination of small
bowel
BCSD
basal cell carcinoma with sebaceous
differentiation
BCSF
B-cell stimulating factor
bloody cerebrospinal fluid
bone cell stimulating factor
BCSI
breast cancer screening indicator
BCSP
breast cystosarcoma phyllodes
Brucella cell surface protein
BCSR
bone-contacting surface ratio
BCSS
Basic Clinical Scoring System
bone cell stimulating substance
breast cancer-specific survival
BCT
benign cystic teratoma
blunt cardiac trauma
brachiocephalic trunk
breast conservation (breast-conserving)
therapy
broad complex tachycardia
BCTC
body coordination test for children
BCU
burn care unit
BCV
Batu Cave virus

blue crab virus
Bunyip Creek virus
BCVA
best-corrected visual acuity
BCVI
blunt cardiovascular injury
BCW
biologic and chemical warfare
BCYE
buffered charcoal yeast extract
BD
band neutrophil
barbital dependent
barbiturate dependence
base deficit
base [of prism] down
basophilic degeneration
Becton Dickinson [catheter, guidewire,
spinal needle]
behavioral disorder
behavior disorder
below diaphragm
Bessel distribution [statistics]
bicarbonate dialysis
bile duct
binocular deprivation
bipolar disorder
birth date
birth defect
black death
bladder drainage
block design [test]
blood donor
blue diaper [syndrome]
board (*See also* Bd)
borderline dull
bottle drainage
bound (*See also* B)
brain dead (death)
brain dysfunction
bronchial drainage
bronchodilation
bronchodilator
buccodistal
band
bundle
butanediol [drug of abuse]
B&D
bondage and discipline
Bd
board (*See also* BD)
buoyant density
BDA
balloon dilation angioplasty
bile duct adenoma
BDAE
Boston Diagnostic Aphasia Examination

BDAS
balloon dilation and septostomy
balloon dilation atrial septostomy
beam data acquisition system [nuclear medicine]

BDAT
best demonstrated available technology

BDAV
Bandia virus

BDB
bis-diazotized-benzidine

BD:BA
bone density to bone age ratio

BDBP
baseline (deoxyribonucleic acid) DNA-binding protein
baseline diastolic blood pressure

BD:PS
bile duct to portal space ratio

BDC
burn dressing change

BDCA
bone density chronological age

BDCC
bile duct cystadenocarcinoma

BDCD
brain-dead cardiac donor

BDCL
basic drive cycle length

BDCM
bromodichloromethane [toxin]

BDCS
Behavioral Dyscontrol Scale

BDD
blistering distal dactylitis
body dysmorphic disorder

BDDE-SR
Body Dysmorphic Disorder Examination-Self Report

BDDQ-DV
Body Dysmorphic Disorder Questionnaire-Dermatology Version

BDDS
biodegradable drug delivery system

BDE
bile duct epithelium
bile duct epithelial [cells]
bile duct exploration

BDF
bilateral distal femoral

BDG
bidirectional Glenn [procedure]
bilirubin diglucuronide
buccal developmental groove
buffered desoxycholate glucose

BDGF
bile duct growth factor
bone-derived growth factor
brain-derived growth factor

BDGR
binding domain of glucocorticoid receptor

BDH
biologically designed hip

BDHI
Buss-Durkee Hostility Inventory

BDI
Baseline Dyspnea Index
basion-dens interval [craniometric]
Battelle Developmental Inventory
Beck Depression Inventory
bile duct injury
burn depth indicator

BDIBS
Boston Diagnostic Inventory of Basic Skills

BDID
bystander dominates initial dominant

BDIP
biomedical digital image processing (processor)

BDIS
Behavior Disorders Identification Scale

BDI SF
Beck Depression Index Short Form

BDL
behaviors of daily living
below detectable levels (limits)
bile duct ligation

BDM
beer-drinkers' myocardiopathy
benzphetamine demethylase
border detection method

BDMP
Birth Defects Monitoring Program

bDNA, b-DNA
branched deoxyribonucleic acid

BDNF
brain-derived neurotrophic factor [avoid using neurotropic]

BDOD
brain-dead organ donor

BDOH
broad determination of health

BDP
bilateral diaphragm paralysis
bronchopulmonary dysplasia

BDR
background diabetic retinopathy
black dot ringworm [syndrome]
bronchodilator response

BDRS
Blessed Dementia Rating Scale

BDS
bile duct stone
biochemical defense system
biohazard (biologic) detection system

Blessed Dementia Scale
botanical dietary supplement
BDSM
bondage and sadomasochism
BDT
binary distance transformation [imaging]
bronchodilator [test]
BDTVMI
Beery Developmental Test of
Visual-Motor Integration
BDV
balloon dilation valvuloplasty
border disease virus
Borna disease virus
BDW
biphasic defibrillation waveform
buffered distilled water
BE
bacillary emulsion [tuberculin]
bacterial endocarditis (*See also* BEC)
barium enema (*See also* BaE, BaEn)
Barrett epithelium
Barrett esophagus
base excess
below-elbow [amputation] (*See also*
BEA, BELB, B/E, B-E)
bile esculin [test]
biological effect
biologically effective
biologically equivalent
board eligible
bovine enteritis
brain edema
bread equivalent
breast examination
bronchiectasis
bronchoesophagology
B↓E
both lower extremities (*See also* BLE)
B&E
brisk and equal
B/E, B-E
below-elbow [amputation] (*See also* BE,
BEA, BELB)
B↑E
both upper extremities (*See also* BUE)
Be
beryllium
BEA
bacillary epithelioid angiomatosis
below-elbow [amputation] (*See also* BE,
B/E, B-E, BELB)
bioelectrical activity
bromoethylamine
bronchitis, emphysema, asthma
BEAC
Barrett esophagus-associated
adenocarcinoma

BEAM
brain electrical activity map(ping)
BeAnV-157575
BeAn 157575 virus
BEAP
bronchiectasis, eosinophilia, asthma,
pneumonia
BEAR
biological effects of atomic radiation
brainstem evoked auditory response
BEB
benign essential blepharospasm
blind esophageal brushing
BEBV
B-cell transformed Epstein-Barr virus
Bebaru virus
BEC
bacterial endocarditis (*See also* BE)
biliary epithelial cell
blood ethanol (ethyl alcohol) content
bronchial epithelial cell
buccal epithelial cell
BECF
blood extracellular fluid
BeCoMo
Bernse Coping Modes
BECT
benign epilepsy of childhood with
centrotemporal spikes
BED
binge-eating disorder
bioeffect dose (biologic effective dose)
biologically equivalent dose
BEE
basal energy expenditure
BEEL
biological equivalent exposure level
(limit) [microorganism or chemical]
BEEP
both end-expiratory pressures
BEER
blood ethanol elimination rate
BEF
bronchoesophageal fistula
Byrne and Euler formula
bef
before [L. *ante*] (*See also* a., ā)
BEFE
bioelectric field enhancement
BEFV
bovine ephemeral fever
beg.
begin(ning)
BEH
benign essential hypertension
benign exertional headache
Beh
behavior(al)

bFGF
basic fibroblast growth factor

BFH
benign familial hematuria

BFHD
Beukes familial hip dysplasia

BFHR
basal fetal heart rate

BFI
Bear-Fedio Inventory
bifrontal index

BFIC
benign familial infantile convulsion

BFL
bird fancier's lung
breast firm and lactating

BFM
benign familial megalocephaly
  (macrocephaly)
bright field microscope
Brunnstrom-Fugl-Meyer [motor test]

BFNC
benign familial neonatal convulsions

BFO
balanced forearm orthosis
ball-bearing forearm orthosis
blood-forming organ
buccofacial obturator

BFP
biologic false-positive

BFPR
biologic false-positive reaction

BFQ
Big Five Questionnaire

BFR
biologic false-positive reactor
blood filtration rate
blood flow rate
bone formation rate
buffered Ringer [solution]

BFS
blood fasting sugar

BFST
behavioral family systems therapy

BF-STS, BFPSTS
biological false-positive serologic test
  for syphilis

BFT
bentonite flocculation test
biofeedback training
bladder flap tube
blunt force trauma
Brooke-Fordyce trichoepithelioma

BFU
burst-forming unit

BFU-E
burst-forming unit erythroid

BFU-MK
burst-forming unit, megakaryocyte

BFV
Barmah Forest virus
blood flow velocity
bovine feces virus
bovine foamy virus

BFVW
blood flow velocity waveform

BG
baby girl
background (*See also* BKG, BKg)
basal ganglion [singular] (basal ganglia
  [plural])
basic gastrin
basophilic granulocyte
Bender-Gestalt [Bender Visual-Motor
  Gestalt test] (*See also* BGT,
  BVMG)
beta (β)-galactosidase
beta (β)-glucuronidase
bicolor guaiac [test]
big gastrin
Birbeck granule
blood glucose (*See also* BGlu)
blood group [system]
bone graft
Bordet-Gengou [agar, bacillus,
  phenomenon]
brilliant green
buccal groove
buccogingival

BGA
blood group antigen
blue-green algae

BGAg
blood group antigen

BGC
basal ganglion calcification
blood glucose concentration
blood group class

BGCA
bronchogenic carcinoma

BGCF
buccal groove of central fossa

BG-corr
background corrected

BGCT
benign glandular cell tumor

BGD
blood group degrading [enzyme]

BGDC
Bartholin gland duct cyst

BGDR
background diabetic retinopathy

BGE
butyl glycidyl ether

BGG
bovine gamma globulin

BGH, bGH
bovine growth hormone

BGIV
Bangui virus
BGL
blood glucose level
BGLB
brilliant green lactose broth
BGlu
blood glucose (*See also* BG)
BGM
bedside glucose monitoring
blood glucose monitoring
BGMR
basal ganglion disorder-mental
retardation
BGMV
bean golden mosaic virus
BGNV
Bangoran virus
BGO
bismuth germanium oxide (bismuth
germanate) ($Bi_{12}GeO_{20}$) [crystal,
optics]
BGP
beta (β)-glycerophosphatase
biliary glycoprotein
bone Gla protein
brain-type glycogen phosphorylase
BGRS
blood glucose reagent strip
BGS
balance, gait, station
blood group substance
bone graft substitute
BGSA
blood granulocyte-specific activity
BGT
basophil granulation test
Bender-Gestalt test (*See also* BG,
BVMG, BVMOT)
blood glucose testing
bungarotoxin
BGTT
borderline glucose tolerance test
BGV
Bahia Grande virus
bleeding gastric varix
BH
base hospital
bill of health
birth history
Bishop-Harman [instrument]
board of health
Bolton-Hunter [reagent]
borderline hypertensive
both hands
bowel habits
brain hormone

Braxton-Hicks [contraction]
breath holding
bronchial hyperreactivity
Bryan high titer [strain of Rous
sarcoma virus]
bundle of His (*See also* BOH)
BH₄
tetrahydrobiopterin [cofactor]
BHA
bilateral hilar adenopathy
bound hepatitis antibody
brain-hair follicle axis
butylated hydroxyanisole
BHAGL
bony humeral avulsion of glenohumeral
ligament
BHAV
Bhanja virus
BHB
beta (β)-hydroxybutyrate (*See also*
BHBA)
bHb
bovine hemoglobin
BHBA
beta (β)-hydroxybutyrate (*See also*
BHB)
beta (β)-hydroxybutyric acid
BHC
benzene hexachloride
Braxton Hicks contractions
bHCG, bhCG, β-hCG
beta (β) human chorionic
gonadotropin
BHD
bilateral hemisphere damage
BHF
Bolivian hemorrhagic fever
BHI
Battery for Health Improvement
beef heart infusion [broth]
biosynthetic human insulin
bone healing index
brain-heart infusion [broth]
breath-holding index
BHIA
brain-heart infusion agar
BHIBA
brain-heart infusion blood agar
BHIRS
brain-heart infusion and rabbit serum
[medium]
BHK
baby hamster kidney [cells]
type-B Hong Kong [influenza virus]
BHL
bilateral hilar lymphadenopathy
biologic half-life

bHLH
    basic helix-loop-helix [transcription factor]

BHN
    Brinell hardness number

BHP
    basic health profile

BHR
    basal heart rate
    borderline hypertensive rat
    bronchial hyperreactivity
    bronchial hyperresponsiveness

BHS
    Beck Hopelessness Scale
    Behavioral Health Systems
    beta (β) hemolytic streptococcus
    breath-holding spell

BHT
    borderline hypertension
    breath hydrogen test
    bronchial hygiene therapy
    butylated hydroxytoluene [food preservative]

BHU
    basic health unit

BHV
    bovine herpesvirus

BH:VH
    [whole] body hematocrit to venous hematocrit ratio

BI
    background interval
    bacterial index
    bactericidal index
    bacteriologic index
    Barthel index
    base [of prism] in
    basilar impression
    bifocal (See also BIF, bif)
    biologic indicator
    bladder insufficiency
    bodily injury
    bone injury
    bowel impaction
    brain infarct
    brain injured
    brain injury
    burn index

Bi
    bismuth

bi
    bilateral (See also BIL, bil, bilat)

BIA
    bicarbonate ingestion alkalosis
    bioelectrical impedance analysis
    bioimmunoassay
    bioimpedance
    biospecific interaction analysis

BIAD
    blind insertion airway device

BIAV
    Bobia virus

BIB, bib
    biliointestinal bypass
    brought in by

bib.
    drink [L. bibe]

BIBA
    brought in by ambulance

biblio
    bibliography

BIBPD
    brought in by police department

B-IBS
    B-immunoblastic sarcoma

BIC
    blood isotope clearance
    bovine immunoglobulin concentrate
    brain injury center

Bic
    biceps

BICAO
    bilateral internal carotid artery occlusion

BICAP
    bipolar circumactive probe

bicarb
    bicarbonate (See also HCO₃)

BiCAT
    bilateral carotid artery traction

BICROS, BiCROS
    bilateral contralateral routing of signals

⚠ **BID**
    bibliographic information and documentation
    bilateral interfacetal dislocation
    body image disturbance
    brought in dead
    twice a day [L. bis in die] (See also b.i.d.) ⚠

⚠ **b.i.d.**
    twice a day [L. bis in die] (See also BID) ⚠

BIDA
    butyl iminodiacetic acid

BIDLB
    block in posteroinferior division of left branch [bundle branch]

BIDS
    bedtime insulin, daytime sulfonylurea (therapy)
    biological integrated detection system
    brittle hair, intellectual impairment, decreased fertility, short stature [syndrome]

BIE
    bayesian image estimation
    bullous ichthyosiform erythroderma

BIEF
bilateral inferior epigastric [artery] flap

BIF, bif
bifocal (*See also* BI)

BIFC
benign infantile familial convulsions

BIG
botulism immune globulin

BIGGY
bismuth glycine glucose yeast [agar]

BIH
basal interhemispheric approach
benign intracranial hypertension
bilateral inguinal hernia

BII
beat inclusion index
benign prostatic hypertrophy (BPH) impact index

bi isch
between ischial tuberosities

BIL, bil
basal insulin level
biceps interval lesion
bilateral (*See also* bilat, bi)
biliary
bilirubin (*See also* bili, bilirub, BR)
brother-in-law

BILAG
British Isles Lupus Assessment Group [index]

BIL:ALB
bilirubin to albumin ratio

bilat
bilateral (*See also* bi, BIL, bil)

BILAT SLC
bilateral short leg cane

BILAT SXO, bilat sxo
bilateral salpingo-oophorectomy

bili
bilirubin (*See also* BIL, bil, bilirub, BR)

BILI:ALB
bilirubin to albumin ratio

bili-c
conjugated bilirubin

bili-D/I
direct and indirect bilirubin

bilirub
bilirubin (*See also* BIL, bil, bili, BR)

bili-T
total bilirubin (*See also* T-bili)

BIMA
bilateral internal mammary arteries

BiMAB
bispecific monoclonal antibody

BIMC
Blessed Information, Memory, Concentration Test

BIMV
Bimiti virus

BIN
benign intradermal nevus

BIND
bilirubin-induced neurologic dysfunction

BINO
binocular internuclear ophthalmoplegia

BINS
Bayley Infant Neurodevelopmental Screener

biochem
biochemical
biochemistry

BIOD
bony interorbital distance

BIOETHICSLINE
Bioethical Information On-Line

biof
biofeedback

Bi(OH)₃
bismuth hydroxide

biol
biologic
biology

bioLH
bioassay of luteinizing hormone

BIOM
binocular indirect ophthalmomicroscope
binocular indirect ophthalmoscope

biophys
biophysical
biophysics

BIOSIS
BioScience Information Service

BIP
Background Interference Procedure
bacterial intravenous protein
biparietal [diameter]
bismuth iodoform paraffin [paste dressing]
brain injury program
brief infertile period
bronchiolitis with interstitial pneumonitis

BiPAP, BIPAP
bilevel (biphasic) positive airway pressure

BiPD
biparietal diameter [fetal skull]

BIPLED
bilateral independent periodic lateralizing epileptiform discharge

BIPP
bismuth iodoform paraffin paste

B

BIR
  backward internal rotation
  basic incidence rate
BI-RADS
  Breast Imaging Reporting and Data
  System
BIRD
  bilinear rotation decoupling
BIRV
  Birao virus
BIS
  behavioral inhibition system
  bioenergy imbalance syndrome
  bioimpedance spectroscopy
  Bispectral Index Sensor
  bone cement implantation
  syndrome
  Brain Information Service
  Brief Impairment Scale
  building illness syndrome
bis.
  twice [L. *bis*] (*See also* B, b.)
BISCC
  basaloid invasive squamous cell
  carcinoma
BISF-W
  Brief Index of Sexual Functioning for
  Women
bis-Gd-MP
  bis-gadolinium-mesoporphyrine
bis-GMA
  bisphenol A-glycidyl methacrylate
BISP, bisp
  between ischial spines
  bispinous [interspinous diameter]
bisp diam
  bispinous diameter
BIT
  Behavioral Inattention Test
BITE
  Bulimic Investigatory Test
BITU
  benzylthiourea
BIU
  billion international units
BIV
  Bohle iridovirus
  bovine immunodeficiency virus
BIVAD
  bilateral ventricular assist device
BIW, biw, bi wk
  biweekly
  twice weekly
  two times per week
BIZ-PLT
  bizarre platelets
BJ
  Bence Jones
  biceps jerk

  body jacket
  bones and joints (*See also* B&J)
B&J
  bones and joints (*See also* BJ)
BJE
  bone and joint examination
  bones, joints, extremities
BJHS
  benign joint hypermobility syndrome
BJI
  bone and joint infection
BJM
  bones, joints, muscles
BJP
  Bence Jones protein(uria)
BJT
  bilateral juxtafoveal telangiectasis
BK
  below knee [amputation] (*See also*
  BKA, BK amp)
  bovine kidney [cells]
  bradykinin
  bullous keratopathy
Bk
  berkelium
bk
  back
BKA, BK amp
  below-knee amputation (*See also* BK)
BK-A
  basophil kallikrein of anaphylaxis
BKC
  blepharokeratoconjunctivitis
BKD
  bacterial kidney disease
bkf, bkfst, bkft
  breakfast (*See also* brkf)
BKG, BKg
  background (*See also* BG)
bkly
  back lying
BKO
  below-knee orthosis
BKS
  Barraquer-Krumeich-Swinger
  [microtome]
  beekeeper serum
BKTT
  below-knee-to-toe [cast]
BKWC
  below-knee walking cast
BKWP
  below-knee walking plaster
BL
  bacterial levan
  basal lamina
  baseline
  Bessey-Lowry [unit] (*See also* BLU,
  B.L. unit)

bifurcation lesion
bioluminescence
black light
bladder channel [acupuncture]
bland
blast [cell]
bleed(ing) (*See also* bldg)
blind loop
blood (*See also* bld)
blood lactate
blood level
blood loss
bone [marrow] lymphocyte
borderline (*See also* BOD, BORD)
borderline lepromatous
bronchial lavage
buccolingual
Bullard laryngoscope
Burkitt lymphoma
butyrolactone [dangerous substance]

B-L
    bursa-equivalent lymphocyte

bl
    black (*See also* blk)
    blood (*See also* b, BL, bld)
    blue (*See also* B)

BL=BS
    bilateral equal breath sounds

BLa
    buccolabial

BLAD
    borderline left axis deviation

blad
    bladder (*See also* ves.)

BLADES
    Bristol Language Development
    Scale

BLAST
    broad-use linear acquisition speed-up
    technique

BLAT
    Blind Learning Aptitude Test

BLB
    Baker-Lima-Baker [mask]
    Bessey-Lowry-Brock [method or unit]
    black light bulb
    blood bank
    Boothby, Lovelace, Bulbulian [mask]
    bronchoscopic lung biopsy
    bulb [syringe]

BLBK
    blood bank (*See also* BB, bld bk)

BLC
    beef liver catalase

BlC, blc
    blood culture (*See also* BC, Bl cult, bl
    cult)

BLCL
    Burkitt lymphoma cell line

BL CULT, bl cult
    blood culture (*See also* BC, BIC, blc)

BLD
    basal-cell liquefactive degeneration
    basal laminar deposit
    benign lymphoepithelial disease
    beryllium lung disease
    bilateral deafness

bld
    blood (*See also* BL, bl)

bld bk
    blood bank (*See also* BB, BLBK)

bld chem
    blood chemistry

bldg
    bleed(ing) (*See also* BL)

bld tm
    bleeding time (*See also* BT, BLEED,
    BLT)

BLDY
    grossly bloody

BLE
    both lower extremities (*See also* B↓E)

BLEED
    bleeding time (*See also* bld tm, BT,
    BLT)
    [ongoing] bleeding, low [blood
    pressure], elevated [prothrombin time],
    erratic [mental status], [unstable
    comorbid] disease [risk factors for
    continued gastrointestinal bleeding]

BLEL
    benign lymphoepithelial lesion

bleph
    blepharoplasty

BLES
    bovine lipid extract surfactant

BLESS
    bath, laxative, enema, shampoo, shower

BLFD
    buccolinguofacial dyskinesia

BLFG
    bilateral firm [hand] grips

BL-FST
    blood fasting [glucose tolerance test]

BLG
    beta (β) lactoglobulin

blH
    biologically active luteinizing hormone

BLHI
    Brief Life History Inventory

BLIC
    beta (β) lactamase inhibitor combination

BLIP
    beta (β) lactamase inhibiting protein

BLIS
breast leakage inhibitor system
BLJ
black liver jaundice
blk
black (*See also* bl)
BLL
below lower limit
benign lymphoepithelial lesion
bilateral lower lobe
blood lead level
brows, lids, lashes
Burkitt-like lymphoma
BLLS
bilateral leg strength
BLLV
Bloodland Lake virus
BLM
basolateral membrane
bilayer lipid membrane
bimolecular liquid membrane
black lipid membrane
borderline malignancy
buccal-lingual-masticatory
BLMV
Belem virus
BLN
bronchial lymph node
BLNAI
Barclay Learning Needs Assessment
Inventory
BlObs
bladder obstruction
BLOC
body location
brief loss of consciousness
BLOT
Bimodality Lung Oncology Team
BLP
beta (β) lipoprotein
bilateral papilledema
BLPB
beta (β) lactamase-producing
bacteria
BLPD
B-cell lymphoproliferative disorder
B-LPH
beta (β)-lipoprotein hormone
B-LPN
beta (β)-lipoprotein
BLPO
beta (β) lactamase-producing
organism
BL PR, bl pr
blood pressure (*See also* BP)
BLQ
both lower quadrants
BLR
baseline record

BLRA
beta (β) lactamase-resistant
antimicrobial
BLS
bare lymphocyte syndrome
basic life support
B-cell lymphoproliferative syndrome
blind loop syndrome
blood and lymphatic system
BlS
blood sugar (*See also* BS)
BLSD
bovine lumpy skin disease
BLS-D
basic life support-defibrillation
BLST
Bankson Language Screening Test
BLT
balanced ligamentous tension [treatment]
bilateral lung transplant(ation)
bladder tumor
bleeding time (*See also* bld tm, BT,
BLEED)
blood-clot lysis time
blood test
blood type (typing)
bright light therapy
brow left transverse
BLT-2
Bankson Language Test 2
BL/T
bilateral tubal ligation
BLU, B.L. unit
Bessey-Lowry unit (*See also* BL)
BLUV 1–24
bluetongue virus 1–24
BLV
blood viscosity
blood volume (*See also* BV)
bovine leukemia virus
BLVR
biliverdin reductase
Blx, blx
bleeding time
BLyS
B lymphocyte stimulator
BM
bacterial meningitis
basal medium
basal membrane
basal metabolism
basement membrane
basilar membrane
Bergersen medium
biomedical
blind matching
blood monitoring
blood monocyte
body mass

Bohr magneton (*See also* γ$_B$)
bone marrow
bone metastasis
bowel movement
breast milk
buccal mass
buccomesial
bullous myringitis

B/M
breath per min

BMA
basaloid monomorphic adenoma
biological movement artifact
bone marrow arrest
bone marrow aspirate
bone mineral area

BmA
Brugia malayi adult antigen

BMAB
bone marrow aspirate and biopsy

BMAL1
brain/muscle ARNT-like protein 1

BMAP
bone marrow acid phosphatase

BMAV
Batama virus

BMB
biomedical belt
bone marrow biopsy

BMBL
benign monoclonal B-cell lymphocytosis

BMC
balloon mitral commissurotomy
blood mononuclear cell (*See also* BMNC)
bone marrow cell
bone marrow culture
bone mineral content

BMCL
blastoid variant of mantle cell lymphoma
blastoma mantle cell lymphoma

BMCMC
bone marrow-derived cultured mast cell

BMD
Becker muscular dystrophy
benchmark dose
bone marrow depression
bone mineral densitometry
bone mineral density
bovine mucosal disease

BMDC
Biomedical Documentation Center

BME
basal medium, Eagle
biomedical engineering

biundulant meningoencephalitis
brief maximal effort

BMEI
benign myoclonic epilepsy in infants

BMET
basic metabolic panel

BMF
bone marrow failure

BMFDS
Burke-Marsden-Fahn dystonia rating scale

BMG
benign monoclonal gammopathy

BMH
biomechanical heart
bone marrow hypoplasia

BMI
bicuculline methiodide
biomedical informatics
body mass index

BMIPP
betamethyliodophenyl pentadecanoic acid

BMJ
bones, muscles, joints
breast milk jaundice

BMK, bmk
birthmark

BML
benign metastasizing leiomyoma (leiomyomatosis)
bone marrow lymphocytosis

BMLM
basement membranelike material

BMLS
billowing mitral leaflet syndrome

BMM
bone marrow-derived macrophage
bone marrow micrometastasis (*See also* BMMM)
bone mineral mass

BMMM
bone marrow micrometastasis (*See also* BMM)

BMMP
benign mucous membrane pemphigoid
bone marrow myeloid precursor

BMN
bone marrow necrosis

BMNC
blood mononuclear cell (*See also* BMC)

BMNR
bone marrow neutrophil reserve

BMOC
Brinster medium for ovum culture

Bmod, B-mod
behavior modification

B-mode
brightness modulation [ultrasonography]
BMP
basic metabolic profile
behavior management plan
bone marrow pressure
bone morphogenetic (morphogenic) protein
BMPC
bone marrow plasmacytosis
BMPI
bronchial mucous proteinase inhibitor
BMPR
bone morphogenetic protein receptor
BMR
basal metabolic rate
best motor response
biologic response modifier
BMRM
bilateral modified radical mastectomy
BMS
bare metal stent
biomedical monitoring system
biometal surface
bronchoscopic microsampling
bulk magnetic susceptibility
burning mouth syndrome
BMST
Bruce maximum (maximal) stress test
BMT
basement membrane thickening (thickness)
behavioral marital therapy
benign mesenchymal tumor
bilateral myringotomy [and] tubes
bone marrow transplant(ation)
Buschke Memory Test
BMT-GVHD
bone marrow transplant(ation) graft-versus-host disease
BMTN
bone marrow transplant(ation) neutropenia
BMU
basic multicellular unit
BMV
balloon mitral valvotomy (valvuloplasty)
billowing mitral valve
BMZ
basement membrane zone
BN
bladder neck
brachial neuritis
bronchial node
brown Norway [rat]
bucconasal
bulimia nervosa
BNA
Basle Nomina Anatomica

bronchoscopic needle aspiration
BNAS
Brazelton Neonatal Assessment Scale
BNBAS
Brazelton Neonatal Behavioral Assessment Scale
BNB
blood-nerve barrier
BNC
binasal cannula
bladder neck closure
bladder neck contracture
BNCT
boron neutron capture therapy
BND
barely noticeable difference
BNDD
Bureau of Narcotics and Dangerous Drugs [Department of Health and Human Services]
bne
but not exceeding
BNEG
B negative [blood type]
BNF
British National Formulary
BNGD
biopsy-negative graft dysfunction
BNGF
beta-nerve growth factor
B-NHL
B-cell non-Hodgkin lymphoma
BNL
breast needle location
BNMSE
Brief Neuropsychological Mental Status Examination
BNO
bladder neck obstruction
bowels not open(ed)
BNOE
benign necrotizing otitis externa
BnOH
benzyl alcohol (*See also* BA)
BNP
beta (β)-natriuretic peptide (B-type natriuretic peptide) (brain natriuretic peptide)
BNPA
binasal pharyngeal airway
BNR
beam nonuniformity ratio [ultrasound]
bladder neck resection
BNS
benign nephrosclerosis
bladder neck suspension
BNT
Boston Naming Test
brain neurotransmitter

BO
  bacterial overgrowth
  base [of prism] out
  behavior objective
  body odor
  bowel
  bowel obstruction
  bowels open(ed)
  bronchiolitis obliterans
  buccoocclusal

B/O
  because of

BOA
  behavioral observation audiometry
  born on arrival
  born out of asepsis

BOB
  ball on back

BOBA
  beta (β)-oxybutyric acid

BOBV
  Bobaya virus

BOC
  beat of clonus
  blood oxygen capacity
  butyloxycarbonyl

BoCV
  bovine enteric calicivirus

BOD
  bilateral orbital decompression
  biochemical oxygen demand
  biologic oxygen demand
  borderline (*See also* BL, BORD)
  brachymorphism, onychodysplasia,
    dysphalangism
  braided occlusion device
  burden of disease

Bod
  Bodansky [unit]

BOE
  benign occipital epilepsy
  bilateral otitis externa

BOEC
  blood outgrowth epithelial cell

BOF
  branchiooculofacial

BOFA
  beta (β)-oncofetal antigen

BOFS
  branchiooculofacial syndrome

BOH
  bundle of His (*See also* BH)

BoHV
  bovine herpesvirus

BOL
  beginning of life [pacemaker battery]
  blood oxygen level

bol
  bolus

BOLD
  blood oxygenation level-dependent

BOLD-fMRI
  blood oxygenation level-dependent
    functional magnetic resonance imaging

BOLD MRI
  blood oxygenation-level dependent
    magnetic resonance imaging

BOLT
  Basic Occupational Literacy Test

BolVX
  Boletus virus X

BOM
  benign ovarian mass
  bilateral otitis media

BOMA
  bilateral otitis media, acute

BOME
  bilateral otitis media with effusion

BONG
  body oscillation neuromuscular gain

BoNT A–E
  botulinum neurotoxin A–E

BOO
  bladder outlet obstruction
  buccinator-orbicularis oris [muscles]

BOOP
  bronchiolitis obliterans-organizing
    pneumonia

BOP
  bilateral occipitoparietal
  bleeding on probe [dental]

BOPP
  boronated porphyrin

BOR
  basal optic root
  before time of operation
  bowels open regularly
  branchiootorenal [syndrome]

BORD
  borderline (*See also* BL, BOD)

BORR
  blood oxygen release rate

BORSA
  borderline resistant *Staphylococcus
    aureus*

BORV
  Boraceia virus

BoRV
  Buthus occitanus reovirus

BOS
  base of skull
  base of support
  Boix-Ochoa score
  bronchiolitis obliterans syndrome

B

bos 1–10
Bos adenovirus 1–10
BOSS
Becker orthopaedic spinal system
bimodal slice select
BOT
base of tongue
benign ovarian tumor
botulinum toxin
bot
botany
bottle
BOTV
Botambi virus
BOU
branchiootoureteral [syndrome]
burning on urination
BOUV
Bouboui virus
BoV
Boolarra virus
BOW
bag of waters
bowel prep
bowel preparation
BOWI
bag of waters intact
BOWR
bag of waters ruptured
BOZOV
Bozo virus
BOZR
back optic zone radius
BP
bacillary peliosis
back pressure
barometric pressure
basic protein
bathroom privileges (*See also* BRP)
bed pan
before polarization
before present
behavior pattern
Bell palsy
benzoyl peroxide
benzpyrene
beta (β)-protein
binding protein
bioequivalence problem
biotic potential
biparietal
biphenyl
bipolar
birthplace
bladder pressure
blood pressure (*See also* BL PR, bl pr)
bodily pain
body part
body plethysmography

boiling point
Bolton point [craniometric]
borderline personality
bowenoid papulosis
breech presentation
bronchopleural
bronchopulmonary
buccopulpal
bullous pemphigus (pemphigoid)
bypass
Pharmacopoeia Britannica (*British Pharmacopoeia*)
bp
base pair
BPA
Bauhinia purpura agglutinin
birch pollen allergy
blood pressure assembly
boronophenylalanine
bovine plasma albumin
bronchopulmonary aspergillosis
bullous pemphigoid antigen
burst-promoting activity
BPAD
bipolar affective disorder
BPAEC
bovine pulmonary artery endothelial cell
BPAQ
Buss-Perry Aggression Questionnaire
BPB
biliopancreatic bypass
black-pigmented bacteria
bone-patella-bone [graft, ACL repair]
bone-patellar ligament-bone (*See also* BPLB)
bone-patellar tendon-bone (*See also* BPTB)
brachial plexus block
bromphenol blue
BPC
Behavior Problem Checklist
benign pheochromocytoma
bile phospholipid concentration
blood pressure cuff
British Pharmaceutical Codex
bronchial provocation challenge
BPCC
bilateral percutaneous cervical cordotomy
BPCF
bronchopleurocutaneous fistula
BPCHI
benign pheochromocytoma with histological invasion
BPCS
back pain classification scale
BPD
biliopancreatic diversion
biparietal diameter

B

bipolar disorder [type 1, 2]
blood pressure decreased
borderline personality disorder
bronchopulmonary dysplasia

BPd
blood pressure diastolic

BPE
bacterial phosphatidylethanolamine
basal promoter element
benign prostatic enlargement

BPEAS
benign partial epilepsy [of childhood]
with affective symptoms

BPEC
benign partial epilepsy with
centrotemporal spike
bipolar electrocoagulation
bipolar electrocardiogram

BPEI
blepharophimosis, ptosis, epicanthus
inversus

BPEIS, BPES
blepharophimosis, ptosis, epicanthus
inversus syndrome

BPF
bradykinin potentiating factor
Brazilian purpuric fever
bronchopleural fistula
bronchopulmonary fistula
burst-promoting factor

BPFM
bronchopulmonary foregut
malformation

BPG
benign paraganglioma
blood pressure gauge
bypass graft

BPH
benign prostatic hyperplasia
(hypertrophy)

BPh
buccopharyngeal

Bph
bacteriopheophytin

BPI
bactericidal/permeability-increasing
[protein]
Basic Personality Inventory
bipolar illness
Bipolar Psychological Inventory
blood pressure increased
blood pressure index
brachial plexus injury
Brief Pain Inventory

BPIG
bacterial polysaccharide immune
globulin

BPIV
bovine parainfluenza virus

BPL
benign proliferative lesion
beta (β) propiolactone
bone phosphate of lime

BPLA, BP lar
blood pressure, left arm

BPLB
bone-patellar ligament-bone (*See also*
BPB)

B-PLL
B-cell prolymphocytic leukemia

BPLN
bilateral pelvic lymph node

BPLND
bilateral pelvic lymph node
dissection

BPM
beat per minute
best partial match
birth per minute
block perfusion monitor
blood perfusion monitor
blood pressure monitor
body protein monitor
breath per minute

BPMS
blood plasma measuring system

BPN
brachial plexus neuropathy

BPO
basal pepsin output
benign prostatic obstruction
benzoyl peroxide
bilateral partial oophorectomy
bile phospholipid output

BPOL
bilateral parietooccipital lesion

BPOP
bizarre parosteal osteochondromatous
proliferation

BPP
binding protein protease
biophysical profile
Bloembergen, Purcell, Pound [theory]
bovine pancreatic polypeptide
brachial plexus paralysis
bradykinin potentiating peptide
breast parenchymal pattern

BP&P
blood pressure and pulse

BPPN
benign paroxysmal positioning
nystagmus

BPPP
bilateral pedal pulses present

BP,P,R,T
blood pressure, pulse, respiration, temperature
BPPV
benign paroxysmal positional vertigo
BPQ
Berne pain questionnaire
BPR
blood per rectum
blood pressure recorder
blood production rate
BPRA, BP rar
blood pressure, right arm
BPRS
Brief Psychiatric Rating Scale
BPRS-C
Brief Psychiatric Rating Scale for Children
BPRS-E
Brief Psychiatric Rating Scale Expanded
BPS
beat per second
bilateral partial salpingectomy
biophysical profile score (scoring)
bovine papular stomatitis
brain protein solvent
breath per second
bronchopulmonary sequestration
BPs
blood pressure systolic
BPSA
bronchopulmonary segmental artery
BPSD
behavioral and psychological symptoms of dementia
bronchopulmonary segmental drainage
BPSV
bovine papular stomatitis virus
BPT
benign paroxysmal torticollis
bronchial provocation test
BPTB
bone-patellar tendon-bone (*See also* BPB)
bPTH
bovine parathyroid hormone
BPTI
basic (bovine) pancreatic trypsin inhibitor
brachial plexus traction injury
BPTT
brachial plexus tension test
BPV
balloon pulmonary valvuloplasty
bat paramyxovirus
bee paralysis virus
benign paroxysmal vertigo
benign positional vertigo
bioprosthetic valve
bovine papillomavirus
bovine parvovirus
BP(VET)
British Pharmacopoeia (Veterinary)
BPXY
buffalopox virus
Bq
becquerel [SI unit of radionuclide activity]
BQC
2,6-dibromoquinone-4-chlorimide solution [reagent]
BQCT
bone quantitative computed tomography
BQL
below quantifiable levels
BQSV
Barranqueras virus
BR
baroreflex
barrier-reared [experimental animals]
baseline recovery
bathroom
bedrest
bedside rounds
benzodiazepine receptor
bilirubin (*See also* BIL, bil, bili, bilirub)
biologic response
birthing room
blink reflex
boiling range
bowel rest
brachial (*See also* brach)
brachialis
brachioradialis
branch
branchial
breast [anatomy]
breath (*See also* brth)
breathing rate
breathing reserve
breech
bridge
broiled
bronchial
bronchial responsiveness
bronchitis
bronchus
brother (*See also* B, BRO)
brown
brucellosis
buccal root
Br
bregma [craniometric]
bromine
BRA
banana, rice, applesauce [diet]
beta (β) resorcylic acid
bilateral renal agenesis

bone-resorbing activity
brain-reactive antibody
branch retinal artery
bra
brassiere
BRAC
basic rest-activity cycle
brach
brachial (*See also* BR)
brady
bradycardia
brady-tachy
bradycardia-tachycardia [syndrome]
(*See also* BTS)
BRAFE
brachial, radial, femoral
BRMS
Bech-Rafaelson Melancholia Scale
BRAO
branch retinal artery occlusion
BRAP
burst of rapid atrial pacing
BrAP
brachial artery pressure
BRAS
bilateral renal artery stenosis
BRAT
bananas, rice, applesauce, toast
[diet]
Baylor rapid autologous transfusion
[system]
BRATT
bananas, rice, applesauce, tea, toast
[diet]
BRB
blood-retinal barrier
bright red blood
BRBC
bovine red blood cell
BRBN
blue rubber bleb nevus
BRBNS
blue rubber bleb nevus syndrome
BRBPR, BRBR
bright red blood per rectum
B1R
bradykinin B1 receptor
B2R
B2 receptor
br bx
breast biopsy (*See also* BB, B Bx)
BRC
brain reserve capacity
BRCA
breast cancer antigen
BRCA1
breast cancer 1 gene

BRCA2
breast cancer 2 gene
BRCD
breast cancer, ductal
BRCM
below right costal margin
BRD
baroreflex dysfunction
bladder retraining drill
BRDS
Blessed-Roth Dementia Scale
BrDu
bromodeoxyuridine
(5-bromodeoxyuridine)
BRE
benign rolandic epilepsy
BRESEK, BRESHECK
brain anomalies, retardation, ectodermal
dysplasia, skeletal malformations,
Hirschprung disease, ear/eye
anomalies, cleft palate/cryptorchidism,
kidney dysplasia/hypoplasia
BRETH
breath releasing energy for
transformation and happiness
BRF
bone-resorbing factor
BRFS
biochemical relapse-free survival
BRFSS
Behavioral Risk Factor Surveillance
System
BRH
benign recurrent hematuria
BRI
Basic Reading Inventory
Bioresearch Index
BRIC
benign recurrent intrahepatic
cholestasis
BRIME
brief repetitive isometric maximal
exercise
Brit
British
BRJ
brachioradialis jerk
brkf
breakfast (*See also* bkf, bkfst, bkft)
BRM
biologic response modifier
biuret-reactive material
BrM
breast milk
BRMP
Biological Response Modification
Program

BRMV
    Berrimah virus
BRO
    bronchoscopy (*See also* bronch)
    brother (*See also* B)
BRO LAC
    bromothymol blue lactose
BROM
    back range of motion
brom
    bromide
bron
    bronchial
    bronchus [singular] (bronchi [plural])
bronch
    bronchoscopy (bronchoscope) (*See also*
        BRO)
BRP
    bathroom privileges (*See also* BP)
    bilirubin production
BRP-2
    Behavior Rating Profile, Second
        Edition
Brph
    bronchophony
BRR
    baroreceptor reflex response
    breathing reserve ratio
BR RVO
    branch retinal vein occlusion
BR S
    breath sounds (*See also* BS)
BRS
    baroreceptor reflex (baroreflex)
        sensitivity
    battered root syndrome
    behavior rating scale
BRSA
    borderline-resistant *Staphylococcus
        aureus*
BRSV
    bovine respiratory syncytial virus
BRT
    Brook reaction test
BrT
    breast tumor
brth
    breath (*See also* br)
B-RTO
    balloon-occluded retrograde transvenous
        obliteration
BRU
    bone remodeling unit
BrU
    bromouracil
BRUV
    Bruconha virus
BRV
    branch retinal vein

BRW
    Brown-Roberts-Wells [stereotactic frame]
BRW-PB
    Brown-Roberts-Wells phantom base
BS
    Babinski sign
    Bacillus subtilis
    barium swallow (*See also* BaS, Ba
        swal)
    bedside
    before sleep
    Bennett seal
    bilateral(ly) symmetric (symmetrical)
    bile salt
    Binet-Simon [test]
    Björk-Shiley [valve]
    blind spot
    blood sugar (*See also* BlS)
    bone scan
    borderline schizophrenia
    bowel sounds
    breaking strength
    breath sounds (*See also* BR S)
    British Standard
    buffered saline
B&S
    Bartholin and Skene [glands]
    bending and stooping
    Brown and Sharp [suture]
BSA
    beef serum albumin
    benzenesulfonic acid
    bismuth-sulfite agar
    bis-trimethylsilylacetamide
    body surface area
    both sexes affected
    bovine serum albumin
    bowel sounds active
    broad-spectrum antibiotic
BSAB
    Balthazar Scales of Adaptive Behavior
BSABS
    Bonn Scale for Assessment of Basic
        Symptoms
BSAG
    Bristol Social Adjustment Guides
BSAP
    bone-specific alkaline phosphatase
    brief short-action potential
    brief, small, abundant [motor-unit
        action] potential
BSAPP
    brief, small, abundant, polyphasic
        potential
BSB
    bedside bag
    body surface burned
BSBC
    buffer-soluble binding component

BS=BL
breath sounds equal bilaterally
BSBV
Bushbush virus
BSC
basosquamous carcinoma
bedside care
bedside commode
bench scale calorimeter
best supportive care
bile salt concentrate (concentration)
biological safety (biosafety) cabinet
Biological Stain Commission
burn scar contracture
BSCA
bidirectional superior cavopulmonary
anastomosis
BSCB
blood-spinal cord barrier
BSCC
basaloid squamous cell carcinoma
bedside commode chair
Björk-Shiley convexoconcave [valve]
BSCP
bovine spinal cord protein
BSCT
breast stimulation contraction test
BSCVA
best spectacle-corrected visual acuity
BSD
baby soft diet
back surface debris
bedside drainage
BSDLB
block in superior division of left branch
[bundle branch]
BSDT
Bryant-Schwan Design Test
BSE
bacillus species enzyme
behavior summarized evaluation
bilateral, symmetrical, equal
bovine spongiform encephalopathy
brain surface extractor
breast self-examination
bystander effect
BSEP
bile salt export pump
brainstem evoked potential
BSER, BSERA
brainstem evoked response [audiometry]
BSF
backscatter factor
basal skull fracture
B-cell stimulatory factor
benign senescent forgetfulness
B-lymphocyte stimulatory factor

BSFR
basal secretory flow rate
BSG
Bagolini striated glasses [eye test]
brachioskeletogenital [syndrome]
BSGA
beta (β) hemolytic streptococcus
group A
BSGF
brachiosubclavian bridge graft fistula
BSH
benign sexual headache
boron sulfhydryl
broad-spectrum heater
BSI
Behavior Status Inventory
bloodstream infection
body substance isolation
borderline syndrome index
bound serum iron
brainstem injury
Brief Symptom Inventory
BSID
Bayley Scales of Infant Development
BSID-II
Bayley Scales of Infant Development II
BSK
Barbour-Stoenner-Kelly [culture]
BSL
benign symmetric lipomatosis
biosafety level 1–4
blood sugar level
brainstem lesion
BSLE
bullous systemic lupus erythematosus
BSLM
body surface laplacian mapping
BSM
bile salt metabolism
Bilingual Syntax Measure [Test]
Björk-Shiley monostrut [prosthetic heart
valve]
bone substitute material
BSMC
bronchial smooth muscle cell
BSM II
Bilingual Syntax Measure II [Test]
BSN
bowel sounds normal
BSNA
bowel sounds normal and active
BSNT
breasts soft and nontender
BSO
behavior, speech, other syndromes
bilateral sagittal osteotomy
bilateral salpingo-oophorectomy

B

BSO *(continued)*
bilateral serous otitis
bile salt output
BSOM
bilateral serous otitis media
BSP
body segment parameter
bone sialoprotein
bromsulphalein [test dye for liver function]
BSp
bronchospasm
BSPA
bowel sounds present and active
BSPM
body surface potential mapping
BSPS
Brief Social Phobia Scale
BSQ
Behavior Style Questionnaire
Biliary Symptoms Questionnaire
BSQV
Bussuquara virus
BSR
basal skin resistance
blood sedimentation rate
body stereotactic radiosurgery
bowel sounds regular
brain stimulation reinforcement
burst suppression ratio
Buschke selective reminding [test]
BSRI
Bem Sex Role Inventory
BSS
balanced saline (salt) solution
Basic Screening Survey
bedside scale
Bernard-Soulier syndrome
bilayered skin substitute
biphasic synovial sarcoma
black silk suture
buffered saline solution
buffered single substrate
BSSE
bile salt-stimulated esterase
BSSI
Basic School Skills Inventory
BSSL
bile salt-stimulated lipase
BSSO
bilateral sagittal split osteotomy
BSSRO
bilateral sagittal split ramus osteotomy
BSSS
benign sporadic sleep spindles [EEG]
BS/ST
brain scan [and] spinal tap
BST
bacteriuria screening test

bedside testing
blood serologic test
bovine somatotropin
breast stimulation test
brief stimulus therapy
BSTFA
bis-trimethylsilyltrifluoroacetamide [reagent]
BSU
Bartholin, Skene, urethral [glands] (*See also* BUS)
basic structural unit
British Standard Unit
BSV
binocular single vision
BSW
bedscale weight
BT
Bacillus thuringiensis
base of tongue
bedtime
behavioral therapy
bitemporal
bitrochanteric
bituberous
bladder tumor
Blalock-Taussig [shunt]
bleeding time (*See also* bld tm, BLEED, BLT)
blood transfusion
blood type (typing)
blue tetrazolium
blue tongue
blunt trauma
body temperature
body type
borderline tuberculoid
bovine turbinate [cells]
bowel tones
brain tumor
breast tumor
bulbotruncal
Bt
Bacillus thuringiensis
BTA
below the ankle
biological terrain assessment
bladder tumor antigen
botulinum toxin A
brief tone audiometry
N-benzoyl-L-tyrosine amide
BTB
back to bed
beat-to-beat
blood-tumor barrier
breakthrough bleeding (*See also* BB)
bromothymol blue
BTBC
Boehm Test of Basic Concepts

BTBV
  beat-to-beat variability
BTC
  body temperature chart
  basal temperature chart
  betacellulin [gene]
  bilateral tubal coagulation
  bladder tumor check
  blood temperature chart
  by the clock
BTD
  biliary tract disease
  bolus thermodilution
BTDS
  benzoylthiamine disulfide
BTE
  Baltimore Therapeutic Equipment [work
    simulator]
  behind-the-ear [hearing aid]
  bovine thymus extract
BTEA
  Boston Test for Examining
    Aphasia
BTF
  blenderized tube feeding
BTFS
  breast tumor frozen section
BTG
  beta (β) thromboglobulin
BTg
  bovine trypsinogen
BTHI
  Brief Test of Head Injury
BTI
  biliary tract infection
  bitubal interruption
BTK
  Bruton tyrosine kinase
BTKA
  bilateral total knee
    arthroplasty
BTKV
  Boteke virus
BTL
  bilateral tubal ligation
btl
  bottle [feeding]
BTLS
  basic trauma life support
BTM
  benign tertian malaria
  bilateral tympanic membranes
BTMSA
  bis-trimethylsilacetylene
BTO
  balloon test occlusion
  bilateral tubal occlusion

BTP
  biliary tract pain
  breakthrough pain
  broad terminal phalanx [singular]
    (phalanges [plural])
BT-PABA
  benzoyl-tyrosyl-paraaminobenzoic acid
  N-benzoyl L-tyrosyl-*P*-aminobenzoic
    acid
BTPD
  body temperature, pressure, dry
BTPS
  body temperature, pressure, saturated
    [with water vapor]
BTR
  Bezold-type reflex
  biceps tendon reflex
  biotoxic reduction
  bladder tumor recheck
  bovine trypsin
  buccal triangular ridge
BTS
  bioptic telescopic spectacle
  bithionol sulfoxide
  Blalock-Taussig shunt
  blood transfusion service
  blue toe syndrome
  bradycardia-tachycardia syndrome
    (*See also* brady-tachy)
BTSH, bTSH
  bovine thyroid-stimulating
    hormone
BTTP
  British Testicular Tumour Panel
BTU
  British thermal unit
BTV 1–24
  bluetongue virus 1–24
BTX
  bactrachotoxin
  benzene, toluene, xylene
  botulinum toxin [Botox]
  brevetoxin (brevotoxin)
  bungarotoxin
BTx
  blood transfusion
BTX-A–BTX-C
  brevetoxin A–C
BU
  base [of prism] up
  below the umbilicus
  Bethesda unit
  biologic unit
  blood urea
  Bodansky unit
  bromouracil
  burn unit

B

Bu
butyl
BUA
blood uric acid
bone ultrasound attenuation
broadband ultrasound (ultrasonic)
attenuation [of bone]
BUB
budding uninhibited by benzimidazole
[gene]
buc, bucc
buccal
BUDS
bilateral upper dorsal sympathectomy
BUE
both upper extremities (*See also* B↑E)
built-up edge
BUEC
balloon uterine elevator cannula
BUEV
Buenaventura virus
BUF
Buffalo [rat]
BUFA
baby up for adoption
BUG
buccal ganglion
BUI
brain uptake index
BULB
bilateral upper lid blepharoplasty
BULIT
bulimia test
BULIT-R
bulimia test revised
BULL
buccal of upper and lingual of lower
bull.
bulletin
let it boil
BUMP
behavioral regression, or upset [in
hospitalized] medical patients [scale]
BUN
blood urea nitrogen
bunion
bun br
bundle branch
BUN:Cr
blood urea nitrogen to creatinine ratio
BUNV
Bunyamwera virus
BUO
bilateral ureteral obstruction
bilirubin of undetermined origin
bleeding of undetermined origin
bruising of undetermined origin
BUQ
both upper quadrants

BUR
backup rate [ventilator]
bilateral ureteral occlusion
bur
bureau
Burd
Burdick [suction]
BURP
backward, upward, rightward pressure
BUS
Bartholin, urethral, and Skene (glands)
(*See also* BSU)
bladder ultrasound
bulbourethral sling
BUSEG
Bartholin, urethral, Skene [glands],
external genitalia
BUSTOP
Burke Stroke Time-Oriented profile
BUT
breakup time
But
butyrate
butyric (acid)
but.
butter [L. *butyrum*]
BUTV
Buttonwillow virus
BUV
backup ventilation
BV
bacilliform virus
bacterial vaginitis (vaginosis)
balloon valvuloplasty
basilic vein
billion volts
biologic value
blood vessel
blood volume (*See also* BLV)
Bracovirus
bronchovesicular
buccoversion
bulboventricular
B&V
binging and vomiting
BVA
best-corrected visual acuity
bioimpedance venous analysis
BVAD
biventricular assist device
BVAS
Birmingham Vasculitis Activity Score
BVAT
Baylor-Video Acuity Tester
Binocular Visual Acuity Test
BVC
British Veterinary Codex
BVD
bovine viral diarrhea

BVD-MD
bovine viral diarrhea mucosal disease
BVDT
Brief Vestibular Disorientation Test
BVDV1–BVDV2
bovine viral diarrhea virus 1–2
BVE
binocular visual efficiency
biventricular enlargement
blood vessel endothelium
blood volume expander (expansion)
BVF
bone volume fraction
bulboventricular foramen
BVFI
bilateral vocal fold [cord] immobility
BVFP
bilateral vocal fold [cord] paralysis
BVH
biventricular hypertrophy
BVI
blood vessel invasion
BVL
bilateral vas [deferens] ligation
BVM
bag-valve-mask [ventilation]
bronchovascular markings
BVMG
Bender Visual-Motor Gestalt [test]
(*See also* BG, BGT, BVMOT)
BVMOT
Bender Visual-Motor [Gestalt Test]
(*See also* BG, BGT, BVMG)
BVO
branch vein occlusion
brominated vegetable oil
BVP
back vertex power [contact lens]
blood vessel prosthesis
blood volume pulse
burst of ventricular pacing
BVR
baboon virus replication
balloon valvuloplasty registry
basal vein of Rosenthal
BVRO
bilateral vertical ramus osteotomy
BVRT
Benton Visual Retention Test
BVRT-R
Benton Visual Retention Test,
Revised
BVS
biventricular support
blanked ventricular sense
BVT
bilateral ventilation tubes

BVTA
biventricular transposed aorta
BV:TV
bone volume to trabecular volume ratio
BVV
bovine vaginitis virus
BW
bacteriologic warfare
bandwidth
bed wetting
below waist
biologic warfare (weapon)
birth weight (*See also* BWt)
bite-wing [radiograph]
bladder washout
blood Wassermann
body water
body weight
B&W
black and white [milk of magnesia and
cascara extract]
BWA
bedwetter admission
BWAS
Barron-Welsh Art Scale
BWAV
Bwamba virus
BWC
bladder wash cytology
BWCS
bagged white cell study
BWD
bacillary white diarrhea
BWF
blackwater fever [color of urine in
malaria]
BWFCM
bladder wash flow cytometry
BWFI
bacteriostatic water for injection
BWGA
birth weight for gestational age
BWM
Bad Wildungen Metz [spinal
instrumentation system]
BWS
battered woman (wife) syndrome
BWST
black widow spider toxin
BWSV
black widow spider venom
BWt
birth weight (*See also* BW)
BWX
bitewing x-ray
bwyv
beet western yellows virus

BX, Bx
biopsy
BXO
balanitis xerotica obliterans
ByCPR
bystander cardiac pulmonary
resuscitation
BYV
bee virus Y
BZ
benzoyl (*See also* Bzl)
NATO code for 3-quinuclidinyl
benzilate [QNB]
BZA
benzylamine

BZD, BZDZ
benzodiazepine
bZIP
basic region-leucine zipper [transcription
factor]
BZK
benzalkonium chloride
Bzl
benzoyl (*See also* BZ)
BZLZ
bian zheng lun zhi [pattern
diagnosis]
Bz-Ty-PABA
benzoyltyrosyl-*p*-aminobenzoic acid
[test]

C

ascorbic acid [vitamin C]
bruised [L. *contusus*] (*See also* cont.)
calculus [dental]
calorie (large) (*See also* Cal)
Campylobacter
Candida
canine [tooth, upper]
capacitance [electrical]
carbon
cardiac
carrier
cast
cathode (*See also* CA, cath, K)
Caucasian (*See also* cauc)
cell
Celsius [temperature scale]
centisimal dilution [homeopathy]
centigrade
central [electrode placement in electroencephalography]
certified (*See also* CRT)
cervical [nerve, vertebra]
cesarean [section]
chest [precordial lead in electrocardiography]
Chlamydia
class
clear
clonus
Clostridium
closure
clubbing
coarse [bacterial colonies]
coefficient (*See also* K)
colored [guinea pig]
color sense
communicating [pacemaker]
complement
complete(d) (completion) (*See also* cpl, compl)
complex
compliance
component
compound(ed) [L. *compositus*] (*See also* comp, CP, cpd)
condition(ed) (conditioning) (*See also* cond)
condyle
constant (*See also* K)
consult(ation) (*See also* cons)
contact
contamination
content

contraction (*See also* contr, contrx, CTX, CTXN, CX)
control
conventionally reared [experimental animal]
convergent (convergence) (*See also* conv)
cornea (*See also* K)
cornu
correct
cortex (*See also* cort)
costa [rib]
coulomb [SI unit of electric charge]
count
criterion [singular] (criteria [plural], criterias [plural])
Cryptococcus
cubic
cubitus
cup
cuspid [canine tooth]
cuticular
cyanosis
cylinder, (cylindrical lens) (*See also* cyl)
cysteine
cytidine
cytochrome
cytosine
[specific] heat capacity
hundred [L. *centum*] (*See also* h)
calorie [large] (*See also* Cal)
rib [L. *costa*]
velocity of light
velocity of sound of blood

C3

Collins solution

3C

craniocerebellocardiac [syndrome] (*See also* CCC)

C6

hexamethonium

C10

decamethonium

[11]C

carbon-11

[12]C

carbon-12

[13]C

carbon-13

[14]C

carbon-14

°C

degree Celsius

C_{Am}
    amylase clearance

C_{in}
    insulin clearance

C_{pah}
    p-aminohippurate clearance

-C
    convexoconcave

c
    about [L. *circa*](*See also* ca)
    calorie [small] (*See also* cal)
    candle (*See also* ca)
    canine [tooth, lower]
    capacity (*See also* cap.)
    capillary blood (subscript)
    carat
    centi- (prefix)
    circumference
    culture [medium]
    cuspid [canine tooth]
    cycle (cyclic)
    meal [L. (*cibus*)]

c̄, c
    with [L. *cum*] (*See also* W, w/, w̄)

CI, CII, CIII, CIV, CV
    DEA controlled substances schedules I
    through V

CA
    anterior commissure [L. *commissure
    anterior*]
    calcium antagonist
    California [rabbit]
    cancer (carcinoma) (*See also* Can)
    cancer antigen
    Candida albicans
    caproic acid
    capsid [protein]
    carbohydrate antigen
    carbonic anhydrase
    cardiac angiography
    cardiac-apnea [monitor]
    cardiac arrest
    cardiac arrhythmia
    carotid artery
    cast
    catecholamine (catecholaminergic)
    (*See also* CAT)
    cathode (*See also* C, cath, K)
    celiac artery
    celiac axis
    cellulose acetate
    central apnea
    cerebral aqueduct
    cerebral atrophy
    chemotactic activity (*See also* CTA)
    child abuse
    cholic acid
    chorioamnionitis
    chromosomal aberration
    chronic anovulation
    chronologic age
    citric acid
    clotting assay
    coagglutination [test]
    coarctation of aorta (*See also* C of A)
    Cocaine Anonymous
    coefficient of absorption [sound]
    cold agglutinin
    collagen antigen
    collagenolytic activity
    colloid antigen
    common antigen
    community acquired
    compressed air
    conception (conceptual) age
    conditioned abstinence
    conditioned air
    condyloma acuminatum
    congenital anomaly
    continuous aerosol
    coracoacromial [muscle, ligament]
    corneal abrasion
    coronary angioplasty
    coronary arrest
    coronary artery
    corpora allata [insect anatomy]
    corpus albicans
    corpus amylaceum
    corrected [echo] area
    cricoarytenoid
    cricoid arch
    croup-associated [virus]
    cytosine arabinoside
    cytotoxic antibody
    NATO code for riot control agent
    bromobenzylcyanide

C of A
    coarctation of aorta (*See also* CA)

CA15.3
    marker for breast carcinoma

C17-1A
    chimeric [mouse antibody] 17-1A

CA242
    marker for pancreatic and colorectal
    carcinoma

CA27.29
    marker for breast carcinoma

CA50
    marker for pancreatic or colorectal
    carcinoma

CA72.4
    marker for gastrointestinal and ovarian
    carcinoma

C&A
    Clinitest and Acetest
    conscious and alert (*See also* C/A)

C/A
    conscious [and] alert (*See also* C&A)

[Ca^{++}]
  intracellular free calcium concentration

Ca
  calcium

Ca$_{2+}$
  calcium ion

C3a
  complement C3a [fragment, component]
  [anaphylatoxin]

C4a
  complement C4a [fragment, component]
  [anaphylatoxin]

C5a
  complement C5a [fragment, component]
  [anaphylatoxin]

ca
  about [L. *circa*] (*See also* c)
  candle (*See also* c)

c-a
  cardioarterial

CA II
  carbonic anhydrase II

CA19-9
  cancer antigen 19-9
  carbohydrate antigen 19-9

^{45}Ca
  calcium-45

^{47}Ca
  calcium-47

CA 125
  cancer antigen 125

CAA
  cardiac allograft atherosclerosis
  carotid audiofrequency analysis
  cerebral amyloid angiopathy
  chloracetaldehyde
  circulating anodic antigen
  coloanal anastomosis
  complementary and alternative
    approach
  computer-assisted assessment
  constitutional aplastic anemia
  coronary artery aneurysm
  crystalline amino acid

CAAS
  cardiovascular angiography analysis
    system
  Children's Attention and Adjustment
    Survey

CAAT
  computer-assisted axial tomography

CAB
  captive air bubble
  catheter-associated bacteriuria
  cellulose acetate butyrate
  combined androgen blockade
  competitive ankle board
    [equipment]

Comprehensive Ability Battery
coronary artery bypass

CABA
  Child and Adolescent Burden
    Assessment

CABBS
  computer-assisted blood background
    subtraction

CABF
  coronary artery blood flow

CaBF
  carotid blood flow

CABG
  coronary artery bypass graft(ing)

CABGS
  coronary artery bypass graft surgery

CaBI
  calcium bone index

CaBP
  calcium-binding protein

CABS
  chronic alcoholic brain syndrome
  continuous ambulatory blood sampler
  coronary artery bypass surgery

CABV
  Cabassou virus

CAC
  cancer cell
  cardiac accelerator center
  cardiac arrest code
  carotid artery canal
  central anterior curve
  chronic active cirrhosis
  circulating anticoagulant
  cold air challenge
  comprehensive ambulatory care
  coronary artery calcification
  cryptogenic autoimmune cirrhosis

CA:C
  convergence to accommodation ratio

CAC/CIC
  chronic active [and] inactive cirrhosis

CACG
  cineangiocardiogram

CACh
  cold air challenge

CACI
  computer-assisted continuous (controlled)
    infusion

CaCl$_2$
  calcium chloride

CaCN
  calcium cyanide

CaCO$_3$
  calcium carbonate

CACS
  cancer, anorexia, cachexia syndrome
  coronary artery calcium score

C

CACT
celite-activated clotting time
computer-assisted corneal topography
CACV
cacao virus
CaCx
cancer of cervix
CAD
cadaver donor
cadaver(ic)
calcium alginate dressing
chronic actinic dermatitis
chronic airways disease
coenzyme A dehydrogenase
cold agglutinin disease
collisionally activated dissociation [mass
spectrometry]
compound absorption device
compressed-air disease
computer-aided detection
computer-aided diagnosis
computer-assisted diagnosis
computer-assisted dialogue
congenital abduction deficiency
coronary artery disease
coronoradiographic documentation
CaD
caldesmon
CADASIL
cerebral autosomal dominant
arteriopathy with subcortical infarcts
and leukoencephalopathy
CAD/CAM
computer-aided design [and]
computer-aided manufacturing
contoured adducted trochanteric [and]
controlled-alignment method
CADD
central axis depth dose
continuous ambulatory drug delivery
CADDS
Columbia Atypical Depression
Diagnostic Scale
CADI
computer-assisted diabetic instruction
[system]
coronary artery disease index
CADL
Communicative Abilities in Daily
Living
CADP
computer-assisted design of prosthesis
CADR
Clean Air Delivery Rate
CADT
Communication Abilities Diagnostic
Test
Ca-DTPA
calcium diethylenetriaminepentaacetate

CAE
caprine arthritis-encephalitis
cellulose acetate electrophoresis
childhood absence epilepsy
chloroacetate esterase
contingent aftereffects
coronary artery embolism (embolization)
CaE
calcium excretion
CAEC
cardiac arrhythmia evaluation center
CAECS
chronic anterior exertional compartment
syndrome
CaEDTA, CaEdTA
calcium disodium edetate
calcium disodium
ethylenediaminetetraacetate
CAEFISS
Canadian Adverse Events Following
Immunization Surveillance System
CAEP
chronotropic exercise assessment
protocol
cortical auditory evoked potential
CAER
caerulein
community awareness and emergency
response
cortical auditory evoked response
CAESAR
Computer-Assisted ENT Surgery [using]
Augmented Reality
computer-assisted evaluation of stenosis
and restenosis [system]
CAEV
caprine arthritis-encephalitis virus
CAF
cell adhesion factor
chronic atrial fibrillation
citric acid fermentation [medium]
combined acetabular and femoral
[navigation in computer-assisted
surgery]
continuous (chronic) atrial fibrillation
contract administration fees
coronary arteriovenous fistula
coronary artery fistula
cortical activation function
CaF
correction of area factor
caf
caffeine
CAFAS
Child and Adolescent Functional
Assessment Scale
CAFET
computer-aided fluency establishment
trainer

CAFF
controlled atrial fibrillation [and] flutter
CAFT
Clinitron air-fluidized therapy
CAG
cholangiograph(y) (cholangiogram)
chronic atrophic gastritis
closed-angle glaucoma
continuous ambulatory gamma globulin
[infusion]
coronary angiograph(y) (angiogram)
coronary arteriography
CaG
calcium gluconate
CagA, cagA
cytotoxin-associated gene product A
CAGE
cut down [on drinking], annoyance,
guilt [about drinking], [need for]
eyeopener [alcoholism screening]
CAGEIN
catheter-guided endoscopic intubation
CAH
camber axis hinge
central alveolar hypoventilation (*See also*
CAHV)
chronic active (aggressive) hepatitis
combined atrial hypertrophy
congenital adrenal (adrenogenital)
hyperplasia
cryptogenic autoimmune hepatitis
cyanacetic acid hydrazide
CaHA
calcium hydroxyapatite
CAHB
chronic active hepatitis B
CAHC
chronic active hepatitis with cirrhosis
CAHD
coronary arteriosclerotic (atherosclerotic)
heart disease
CAHJ
cup arthroplasty of hip joint
CAHM
complex atypical hyperplasia [and]
metaplasia
CAHMR
cataract, hypertrichosis, mental
retardation
CAHS
central alveolar hypoventilation
syndrome
CAHV
central alveolar hypoventilation (*See also*
CAH)
CAI
calcium intake

carbonic anhydrase inhibitor
Career Assessment Inventory
catheter-associated infection
celiac artery infusion
cellular adaptive immunotherapy
chemical accident or incident
Clinical Activity Index
complete androgen insensitivity
computer-assisted instruction
confused artificial insemination
cortical arousal index
Cultural Attitude Inventory
CaI
carotid artery insufficiency
Ca ION
calcium, ionized
CAIS
complete androgen insensitivity
syndrome
CAIV
Caimito virus
cold-attenuated intranasal influenza
vaccine
CaIV
Campoletis aprilis ichnovirus
CAIV-T
cold-adapted influenza virus vaccine,
trivalent
CAL
café au lait [spots]
calcium [test]
calculated average life
caliber
callus
chronic airflow limitation
clinical attachment level
computer-assisted learning
coracoacromial ligament
coronary artery lesion
Cal
calorie [large] (*See also* C)
cal
calorie [small] (*See also* c)
Calb, C$_{alb}$, C/alb/
albumin clearance
calc
calculate(d)
calcif
calcification
CALCR
calcitonin receptor
cal ct
calorie count
CALD
chronic active liver disease
CALH
chronic active lupoid hepatitis

calib
  calibrat(ed)
cal/kg day
  calorie per kilogram per day
cALL
  common leukemia antigen
CALLA, cALLA
  common acute lymphoblastic leukemia
  antigen
CALM
  café au lait macule
cal/oz
  calorie per ounce
CALP
  calponin
  congenital absence of left pericardium
CALS
  café au lait spots
  Checklist of Adaptive Living Skills
CAM
  calf aortic microsome
  cell adhesion (cellular adhesion)
    molecule
  chemical agent monitor
  child-adult mist
  chorioallantoic membrane
  circulating adhesion molecule
  Cognitive Assessment of Minnesota
  complementary and alternative medicine
  computer-assisted (aided) myelography
  Confusion Assessment Method
  content-addressable memory
  contralateral axillary metastasis
  controlled ankle motion
  cystic adenomatoid malformation
C$_{am}$
  amylase clearance
CaM
  calmodulin
CAMAC
  computer-automated measurement and
    control
CAMAK
  cataract, microcephaly, arthrogryposis,
    kyphosis
CAMC
  camera augmented mobile C-arm
  computer applications in medical care
CAMCOG
  Cambridge Cognitive Examination
CAMDEX
  Cambridge Mental Disorders in Elderly
    Examination
CAMFAK
  cataract, microcephaly, failure to thrive,
    kyphoscoliosis
CAMI
  computer-assisted medical
    intervention

CaMKII
  calcium-calmodulin kinase II
CaM-kinase
  calmodulin-dependent protein kinase
CAML
  calcium-signal modulating cyclophilin B
    ligand
  Coarticulation Assessment in Meaningful
    Language
CAMP
  Childhood Asthma Management
    Program
  Christie-Atkins-Munch-Petersen [test]
  computer-assisted menu planning
  concentration of adenosine
    monophosphate
cAMP
  adenosine 3′,5′-cyclic phosphate (cyclic
    AMP)
CAMPI
  computer analysis of mammography
    phantom images
CAMS
  computer-assisted monitoring system
  computerized arrhythmia monitoring
    system
CAMV
  congenital anomaly of mitral valve
CaMV
  cauliflower mosaic virus
CAMVA
  chorioallantoic membrane vascular
    assay
CAN
  cancer (carcinoma) (*See also* CA)
  cardiac autonomic neuropathy
  cardiovascular autonomic neuropathy
  child abuse and neglect
  chronic allograft nephropathy
  continuous albuterol nebulization
  cord [umbilical] around neck
CA/N
  child abuse and neglect
can.
  cannabis
CANA
  circulating antineuronal antibody
  convulsant antidote for nerve agent
CANC, canc
  cancelled
cANCA
  cytoplasmic [type] antineutrophil
    cytoplasmic antibody
CANCERLIT
  Cancer Literature
CANE
  computer-assisted neuroendoscopy
cANP
  c fragment atrial natriuretic peptide

CANP
calcium-activated neutral protease
CANS
central auditory nervous system
computer-assisted neurosurgical
navigational system
CANTAB
Cambridge Neuropsychological Test
Automated Battery
CANT LEAP
cyclosporine, alcohol, nicotinic acid,
thiazides, Lasix, ethambutanol, aspirin,
pyrazinamide [substances causing
hyperuricemia]
CANV
Caninde virus
CAO
carotid artery occlusion
chronic airflow obstruction
chronic airways obstruction
coronary artery obstruction
CAOD
coronary artery occlusive disease
CAOM
chronic adhesive otitis media
CAOS
computer-assisted orthopedic surgery
Ca ox
calcium oxalate
CAP
camptodactyly-arthropathy-pericarditis
[syndrome]
cancer (carcinoma) of prostate
capillary (See also cap.)
capitation
capsule (See also cap., caps.)
carotid Amytal procedure
catabolite activator protein
Cbl-associated protein
cell attachment protein
cellular acetate [and] propionate
cellulose acetate phthalate
central apical part (portion)
Children's Art Project
chloroacetophenone [tear gas, Mace]
cholesteric analysis profile [test]
chronic alcoholic pancreatitis
chronic apical periodontitis
community-acquired pneumonia
complement-activated plasma
compound action potential
computerized automated
psycho-physiologic [device]
continent anal cap
contoured ablation pattern
contraction-associated protein
coronary artery fistula

coupled atrial pacing
cyclic AMP (cAMP) binding protein
cystine aminopeptidase
Ca:P
calcium to phosphorus ratio
cap.
capacity (See also c)
capillary (See also CAP)
capsule (See also CAP, caps.)
CAPA
caffeine, alcohol, pepper, and aspirin
[diet free of]
cancer-associated polypeptide antigen
Child and Adolescent Psychiatric
Assessment
CAPB
cancer of prostate and brain [gene]
central auditory processing battery
CAPD
central auditory processing disorder
chronic (continuous) ambulatory
peritoneal dialysis
continuous abdominoperitoneal
dialysis
CAPE
caffeic acid phenethyl ester
Children's Assessment of Participation
and Enjoyment
Clifton Assessment Procedures for the
Elderly
continuous anatomical passive
exerciser
CAPERS
Computer-Assisted Psychiatric
Evaluation and Review System
CAPM
continuous airway pressure monitoring
CAPP
Clinical Appraisal of Psychosocial
Problems
CAPPS
Current and Past Psychopathology
Scales
CAPR
calcium pyrophosphate
CAPRCA
chronic acquired pure red cell aplasia
CAPS
carbamoyl phosphate synthetase
Children of Aging Parents
[diet free of] caffeine, alcohol, pepper,
spicy foods
caps.
capsule (See also CAP, cap.)
CAPSO
cautery-assisted palatal stiffening
operation

C

CAPTA
Child Abuse Prevention and Treatment Act
CAPV
Capim virus
CAPWA
computerized arterial pulse waveform analysis
CAPYA
child and adolescent psychoanalysis
CAQ
Change Agent Questionnaire
Childhood Asthma Questionnaire
Classroom Atmosphere Questionnaire
Clinical Analysis Questionnaire
CAR
cancer-associated retinopathy
cardiac ambulation routine
carotid artery rupture
cell adhesion regulator
center of mandibular autorotation
chronic articular rheumatism
computer-assisted research
conditioned avoidance response
congenital articular rigidity
CaR
calcium-sensing receptor
car.
carotid
CARA
chronic aspecific respiratory ailment
congenital aregenerative anemia
CAR AMP
carotid pulse amplitude
CARB, carb, carbo
carbohydrate (See also CHO)
carbonate
CARC
chemical agent-resistant coating
CARD
cardiac automatic resuscitative device
cardiology (See also card., cardiol)
catalyzed reporter deposition [test]
card., cardiol
cardiac
cardiology (See also CARD)
card. insuff
cardiac insufficiency
CARE
calcium antagonist in reperfusion
chakra armor release of emotion
Comprehensive AIDS Resources Emergency [Act]
consultation and relational empathy
CARES
Cancer Rehabilitation Evaluation System
CARIFS
Canadian Acute Respiratory Illness and Flu Scale

CARM1
coactivator-associated arginine methyltransferase 1
CAROT
carotene
CA-RP
carbonic anhydrase-related protein
CARS
Childhood Autism Rating Scale
Children's Affective Rating Scale
compensatory antiinflammatory response syndrome
constrained access robotic therapy
CART
Classification and Regression Tree
cocaine and amphetamine regulated transcript [protein]
combined antiretroviral therapy
computer-assisted real-time [transcription]
cart.
cartilage
CARTI
community-acquired respiratory tract infection
CARTOS
computer-assisted reconstruction by tracing of serial sections
CARTT
computer-assisted real-time transcription
CARV
Caraparu virus
CAS
calcarine sulcus
calcific aortic stenosis
Cancer Attitude Survey
carbohydrate-active steroid
cardiac adjustment scale
cardiac surgery
carotid angioplasty and stenting
carotid artery stenosis
carotid artery stenting
carotid artery system
casein
casualty
central anticholinergic syndrome
cerebral arteriosclerosis (atherosclerosis)
Chemical Abstracts Service
Child Assessment Schedule
chronic alcohol syndrome
chronic anovulation syndrome
clinical asthma score
Cognitive Assessment Scale
cold agglutinin syndrome
computer-aided surgery
computer-assisted surgery
Concept-Specific Anxiety Scale
congenital alcohol syndrome
congenital anterior staphyloma

congenital asplenia syndrome
contralateral acoustic stimulation
control adjustment strap
coronary artery scan
coronary artery spasm
Creativity Attitude Survey
Cultural Attitude Scale

cas
castrate(d)
castration

CASA
cancer-associated serum antigen
Child and Adolescent Services
Assessment
computer-aided sperm (semen) analysis
computer-assisted self-assessment

CASE
computer-assisted sensory examination

CASF
coronary arteriosystemic fistula

CASH
classic abdominal Semm hysterectomy
comprehensive assessment of symptoms
and history
cortical androgen-stimulating hormone
corticoadrenal stimulating hormone
cruciform anterior spinal hyperextension
[brace]

CASHD
coronary arteriosclerotic (atherosclerotic)
heart disease

CASI
Cognitive Abilities Screening Instrument

CASL-PI MRI
continuous arterial spin-labeled perfusion
magnetic resonance imaging

CASMD
congenital atonic sclerotic muscular
dystrophy

CASP
calcium urine spot [test]
Child and Adolescent Social Perception
Measure
contoured anterior spinal plate

Ca-SP
calcium urine spot [test]

CASPER
computer-assisted pericardial [puncture,
surgery]

CASPR
contactin-associated protein

CASQ
calsequestrin

CASR
calcium-sensing receptor [protein]

CAS REGN
Chemical Abstracts Service Registry
Number

CASRT
corrected adjusted sinus [node] recovery
time

CASS
California soft spinal system
cataract-alopecia-sclerodactyly syndrome
computer-aided sleep system
computer-assisted stereotactic surgery
continuous aspiration of subglottic
secretions

CASST
child abuse-specific treatment of trauma

CAST
Canterbury Alcoholism Screening Test
cellular antigen stimulation test
childhood accidental spiral tibial
[fracture]
Children of Alcoholics Screening Test
Children's Apperceptive Story-Telling
Test
cognitive assessment screening test
Color Allergy Screening Test
computer automated scan technology

cAST
cytoplasmic aspartate aminotransferase

CASTLE
carcinoma showing thymuslike
differentiation

CASTNO
number of casts [urinalysis]

CAT
California Achievement Test
cancer after transplant(ation)
capillary agglutination test
catalase (*See also* CAT'ase)
cataract (*See also* cat.)
catecholamine (catecholaminergic)
(*See also* CA)
cellular atypia
Children's Apperception Test
Children's Articulation Test
chloramphenicol acetyl transferase
[protein]
chlormerodrin accumulation test
choline acetyltransferase
chronic abdominal tympany
classified anaphylatoxin
Clinical Adaptive Test
Coblation-assisted tonsillectomy
Cognitive Abilities Test
cognitive analytic therapy
coital alignment technique
College Ability Test
computed abdominal tomography
computed (computerized) axial
tomography
computer of average transients
[obsolete]

CAT *(continued)*
computerized transcription
conventional asthma therapy
CAT/5
California Achievement Test, Fifth
Edition
cat.
catalyst
cataract (*See also* CAT)
CAT'ase
catalase (*See also* CAT)
CAT-CAM
contoured adducted trochanter-controlled
alignment method
CATCH-22
cardiac abnormality, abnormal facies,
thymic hypoplasia, cleft palate,
hypocalcemia [chromosome 22q11
microdeletion]
cat c̄ IL, cat. c̄ IOL
cataract with intraocular lens
CAT/CLAMS
Clinical Adaptive Test/Clinical
Linguistic and Auditory Milestone
Scale
CAT-H
Children's Apperception Test, Human
cath
cathartic
catheteri(zation)
catheterize
cathode (*See also* C, CA, K)
CAT-S
Children's Apperception Test,
Supplemental
CATS
cartilaginous autologous septal [graft]
CAT scan
computerized axial tomography scan
CATT
calcium tolerance test
card agglutination trypanosomiasis test
CATUV
Catu virus
CAU
chronic anterior uveitis
cauc
Caucasian (*See also* C)
caud
caudal (*See also* CD)
caut
cauterize (cauterization)
CAUTI
catheter-associated urinary tract infection
CAV
cardiac allograft vasculopathy
Chara australis virus
computer-assisted ventilation
congenital absence of vagina

congenital adrenal virilism
constant angular velocity
croup-associated virus
cav
cavity
CAVB
complete atrioventricular block
CAVC
common atrioventricular canal
CAVD
cardiac allograft vascular disease
complete atrioventricular dissociation
completion, arithmetic problems,
vocabulary, following directions
[battery]
congenital absence (aplasia) of vas
deferens
C(a-VDO$_2$), C(aVDO$_2$)
arteriovenous oxygen difference
CAVE
cerebroacrovisceral early lethality
[phenotype]
CAVG
coronary artery vein graft
CAVH
chronic active viral hepatitis
continuous arteriovenous hemofiltration
CAVH-B
chronic active viral hepatitis, type B
CAVHD
continuous arteriovenous hemodialysis
CAVHDF
continuous arteriovenous
hemodiafiltration
CAVH-NAB
chronic active viral hepatitis non-A
non-B
CA virus
croup-associated virus
CAVLT
Children's Auditory Verbal Learning
Test
CAVLT-2
Children's Auditory Verbal Learning
Test 2
CAVM
cerebral arteriovenous malformation
CAVO
common atrioventricular orifice
CAVR
continuous arteriovenous rewarming
CAVSD
complete atrioventricular septal defect
CAVU
continuous arteriovenous ultrafiltration
CAW
carbonaceous activated water
catalyst altered water
central airways

C_{AW}, C_{aw}
    airways conductance (*See also* GAW)
CAWO
    closing abductory wedge osteotomy
CAX
    central axis [radiotherapy]
CB
    calcium blocker
    cannabinoid receptor, type 1
    carbonated beverage
    carcinoma of breast
    carotid body
    catheterized bladder
    ceased breathing
    centroblastic
    cesarean birth
    chair and bed (*See also* C&B)
    chest-back (*See also* C-B, C/B)
    chocolate blood [agar]
    chondroblast
    chronic blepharitis
    chronic bronchitis
    circumflex branch
    code blue
    color blind
    compensated base
    conjugated bilirubin
    contrast bath
    coracobrachial
    cord blood
    coronary bypass
    custom blocks
    cytochalasin B
C-B, C/B
    chest [and] back (*See also* CB)
C&B
    chair and bed (*See also* CB)
    crown and bridge (*See also* Cr&Br)
Cb
    columbium
cb
    cardboard [or plastic film holder without intensifying screens]
CBA
    carcinoma-bearing animal
    chronic bronchitis with asthma
    Columbia blood agar [test]
    competitive binding assay
    congenital bronchial atresia
    cost-benefit analysis
    cutting balloon angioplasty
    cytochemical bioassay
CBAB
    complement-binding antibody
C-band
    centromeric heterochromatin

CBAS
    carotid bifurcation angioplasty and stenting
CBASP
    Cognitive Behavioral Analysis System of Psychotherapy
CBAVD
    congenital bilateral absence of vas deferens
CBB
    Bethesda-Ballerup group of *Citrobacter*
    complete bed bath
    Coomassie brilliant blue R-250 [stain]
CBBB
    complete bundle branch block
CBBM
    color blindness, blue mono-cone-monochromatic type
CBC
    Camelot Behavioral Checklist
    cerebrobuccal connective
    child behavior characteristics
    complete blood [cell] count (*See also* cbc)
cbc
    complete blood [cell] count (*See also* CBC)
CBCL
    Child Behavior Checklist
    cutaneous B-cell lymphoma
CBCL/2-3
    Child Behavior Checklist for ages 2-3
CBCME
    computer-based continuing medical education
CBCS
    cord blood collection system
CBD
    cannabidiol
    carotid body denervation
    chronic beryllium disease
    closed bladder drainage
    common bile duct
    community-based distribution
CBDC
    chronic bullous disease of childhood
CBDE
    common bile duct exploration
CBDL
    chronic bile duct ligation
CBDM
    common bile duct microlithiasis
CBDS
    Carcinogenesis Bioassay Data System
    common bile duct stone

C

CBE
  clinical breast examination
  congenital biliary ectasia
CBF
  capillary blood flow
  cerebral blood flow
  ciliary beat frequency
  cochlear blood flow
  collagen-binding factor
  core-binding factor
  coronary blood flow
  cortical blood flow
CBFS
  cerebral blood flow studies
CBFV
  cerebral blood flow velocity
  coronary blood flow velocity
  cortical blood flow velocity
CBG
  capillary blood gas
  capillary blood glucose
  cord blood gas
  coronary bypass graft
  corticosteroid-binding globulin
  cortisol-binding globulin
CBG-BC, CB-GBC
  corticosteroid-binding globulin-binding
    capacity
CBGm
  capillary blood glucose monitor
CBGT
  cognitive-behavioral group therapy
CBG$_v$
  corticosteroid-binding globulin variant
CBH
  chronic benign hepatitis
  collimated beam handpiece
  cutaneous basophilic hypersensitivity
CBI
  Career Beliefs Inventory
  Child Behaviors Inventory of
    Playfulness
  continuous bladder irrigation
  convergent beam irradiation
CBIL
  Conjugated bilirubin
CBIP
  Cancer Background Interference
    Procedure
CBIPBG
  Cancer Background Interference
    Procedure for Bender Gestalt
CBIRF
  Chemical Biological Incident Response
    Force [of the U.S. Marine Corps]
CBL
  chronic blood loss
  circulating blood lymphocytes
  [umbilical] cord blood leukocytes

Cbl
  cobalamin
cbl
  chronic blood loss
CBM
  capillary basement membrane
  cryopreserved bone marrow
CBMC
  cord blood mononuclear cell
CBMMP
  chronic benign mucous membrane
    pemphigus
CBMT
  capillary basement membrane thickness
CBMW
  capillary basement membrane width
CBN
  cannabinol
  cellular blue nevus
  central benign neoplasm
  chronic benign neutropenia
CBOC
  completion bed occupancy care
CBP
  calcium-binding protein
  carbohydrate-binding protein
  cardiac bypass
  cardiopulmonary bypass
  casual blood pressure
  chiropractic biophysics
  chlorobiphenyl
  chronic bacterial prostatitis
  chronic benign pain
  cobalamin-binding protein
  color blindness, protan type
  complete breech presentation
  copper-binding protein
  cruciform binding protein
  cyclic adenosine monophosphate
    [cAMP] response element binding
    [CREB] protein
CBPA
  competitive protein-binding assay
CBPM
  certified Bonnie Prudden myotherapy
CBPP
  contagious bovine pleuropneumonia
CBPR
  computer-based patient record
CBPS
  congenital perisylvian syndrome
  coronary bypass surgery
CBPV
  chronic bee paralysis virus
CBR
  carotid bodies resected
  chemical, bacteriologic, radiologic
    [weapon, warfare]
  chemically bound residue

complete bedrest
cord blood registry
crude birth rate

C$_{BR}$
bilirubin clearance

CBRAM
controlled partial rebreathing - anesthesia method

CBRF
child behavior rating form

CBRG
cancer biotherapy study group

CBRN
chemical, biological, radiological, nuclear [weapons, warfare]

CBRNE
chemical, biological, radiological, nuclear, explosive [weapon, warfare]

CBS
capillary blood sugar
cervicobrachial syndrome
child behavioral study
chronic brain syndrome
citrate-buffered saline
coarse breath sounds
colloidal bismuth subcitrate
conjugated bile salts
culture-bound syndrome
cystathionine beta-synthase

CBT
carotid body tumor
certified biofeedback therapy
childhood brain tumor
code blue team
cognitive behavior therapy
computed body tomography
cord blood transplant(ation)
corticobulbar tract

CBTIS
computerized bedside transfusion identification system

CBTP
Cognitive Behavior Therapy Package

CBTR
contralateral breast tumor recurrence

CBU
cumulative breath units

CBV
capillary blood [flow] velocity
catheter balloon valvuloplasty
central blood volume
cerebral blood volume
circulating blood volume
corrected blood volume
cortical blood volume

CBV:CBF
cerebral blood volume to cerebral blood flow ratio

CBVD
cerebrovascular disease

CBVI
computer based video instruction

CBW
chemical and biological warfare
critical bandwidth [range of frequencies]

CBWO
closed base wedge osteotomy

CBX
computer-based examination

Cbx
core biopsy

C-C
convexoconcave

⚠ **CC**
calcaneocuboid
calcium cyclamate
canal catheterization
cardiac catheter(ization)
cardiac contusion
cardiac cycle
cardiovascular clinic
carotid-cavernous
caval catheteriz(ation)
cell culture
cellular compartment
central compartment
cerebral commissure
cerebral concussion
cerebral cortex
cervical cancer
cervical collar
chest circumference
chest compression
chief complaint (*See also* C/C)
cholangiocarcinoma
cholecalciferol
choledochocholedochostomy
chondrocalcinosis
choriocarcinoma (*See also* CCA)
chronic complainer
ciliated cell
circulatory collapse
classical conditioning
clean catch [of urine]
clinical course
closing capacity
coefficient of correlation
collagenous colitis
colony count
colorectal cancer
columnar cells
comfort care
commission-certified [stain]
complicating condition
complications and comorbidities
compound cathartic

CC *(continued)*
    computer calculated
    concave (*See also* Cc)
    congenital cardiopathy
    congenital cataract
    consumptive coagulopathy
    continuing care
    contractile component
    contrast cystogram
    convexo-concave
    coracoclavicular
    cord compression
    coronary care
    coronary collateral
    corpus callosum
    costochondral
    Coulter counter
    cradle cap
    craniocaudal
    craniocervical
    creatinine clearance (*See also* CCR, C_{cr}, C/Cr, CrCl, crcl, CRC)
    critical care
    critical condition
    Crohn colitis
    crus cerebri
    crus communis
    cubic centimeter [Note: Do not use, substitute mL] (*See also* cc, c.c., cm^3, cu cm) ⚠
    cup cell
    current complaint
    current contents
    cytochrome C
    with correction [with glasses] (*See also* cc)

C1–C7
    cervical vertebrae 1–7
C1–C8
    cervical nerves 1–8
C1–C9
    complement 1–9
C/C
    chief complaint (*See also* CC)
    cholecystectomy and [operative] cholangiogram
    complete upper and lower dentures
C&C
    cold and clammy
    confirmed and compatible
Cc
    concave (*See also* CC, cc)
⚠ **cc**
    carbon copy
    condylocephalic
    corrected
    cubic centimeter [NOTE: Do not use, substitute mL] (*See also* cc, c.c., cm^3, cu cm) ⚠

    with correction (with glasses)
    with correction [with glasses] (*See also* CC)
$\overline{cc}$
    with meals [L. *cibum*]
⚠ **c.c.**
    cubic centimeter [note: Do not use Substitute mL] (*See also* cc, CC, cm^3, cu cm) ⚠

CCA
    calcium channel antagonist
    central choroidal apposition
    cephalin cholesterol antigen
    chick-cell agglutination [unit]
    chimpanzee coryza agent
    cholangiocarcinoma
    cholecystic atony
    choriocarcinoma (*See also* CC)
    chromated copper arsenate
    circulating cathodic antigen
    circumflex coronary artery
    colitis colon antigen
    common carotid artery
    concentrated care area
    congenital contractural arachnodactyly
    constitutional chromosome abnormality
CCA-1
    cancer cell-derived blood coagulating activity 1
CC&A
    cardiac catheterization and angiography
CCAB
    complex cognitive assessment battery
CCABA
    cough, cough, allergy, bronchodilator, antiasthmatic
CCAE
    Checklist for Child Abuse Evaluation
CCAI
    Clinical Colitis Activity Index
    Cross-Cultural Adaptability Inventory
CCA-IMT
    common carotid artery intima [and] media thickness
CCAM
    congenital cystic adenomatoid malformation
C-CAM
    cell-cell adhesion molecule
CCAP
    capsule cartilage articular preservation
CCAS
    Comprehensive Career Assessment Scale
CCAT
    Canadian Cognitive Abilities Test
    common carotid artery thrombosis
    conglutinating complement absorption test

CCB
calcium channel blocker
cancellous cellular bone
conventional core biopsy
corn, callus, bunion
CCBD
central cell-binding domain
CCBV
central circulating blood volume
CCC
care-cure coordination
central corneal clouding [grade
0 + −4 +]
central counteradaptive changes
cholangiocellular carcinoma
chronic calculus cholecystitis
chronic catarrhal colitis
clear cell carcinoma
common carotid compression
concurrent care concern
consecutive case conference
continuous curvilinear capsulorrhexis
continuous curvilinear capsulotomy
craniocerebellocardiac [syndrome]
(*See also* 3C)
critical care complex
cylindrical confronting cisterna
CC&C
colony count and culture
CCCC
centrifugal counter-current
chromatography
CC-CKR-5
nonsyncytium-inducing chemokine
CCCP
carbonyl cyanide
m-chlorophenylhydrazone
CCCR
closed-chest cardiac resuscitation
CCCS
condom catheter collecting
system
CCCT
clomiphene citrate challenge test
(*See also* C3T)
closed craniocerebral trauma
CCCU
comprehensive cardiac care unit
CCD
calcified cellular debris
calibration curve data
central collodiaphysial
central core disease
charge-coupled device
childhood celiac disease
chin-chest distance
choriocapillaris degeneration

cleidocranial dysplasia
clinical cardiovascular disease
cortical collecting duct
countercurrent distribution
crossed cerebellar diaschisis
cumulative cardiotoxic dose
CCDA
calcaneocuboid distraction arthrodesis
CCDM
*Control of Communicable Diseases
Manual*
ccDNA
closed circle deoxyribonucleic acid
CCDS
color-coded duplex sonography
CCE
capacitative calcium entry
carboline [and] carboxylic acid ester
chamois contagious ecthyma
cholesterol crystal embolization
chronic cutaneous erythematosus
clear-cell endothelioma
clear-cell ependymoma
clubbing, cyanosis, edema
countercurrent electrophoresis
CCEI
Crown-Crisp Experimental Index
CC-EPT
continuous-combined
estrogen-progestogen therapy
CCF
cancer coagulation factor
cardiolipin complement fixation
carotid cavernous fistula
centrifuged culture fluid
cephalin-cholesterol flocculation
compound comminuted fracture
congestive cardiac failure
critical corresponding frequency
crystal-induced chemotactic factor
CCFA
cycloserine-cefoxitin-fructose agar
CCFAS
compact colony-forming active substance
CCFH
cellular cutaneous fibrous histiocytoma
CCG
cationic colloidal gold
cholecystograph(y) (cholecystogram)
costochondral graft
CCGC
capillary column gas chromatography
CCGG
cytosine-cytosine-guanine-guanine
CCH
C-cell hyperplasia
chromic chloride hemagglutination

CCH *(continued)*
    chronic cholestatic hepatitis
    circumscribed choroidal hemangioma
CCh
    carbamylcholine
CCHB
    congenital complete heart block
CCHD
    cyanotic congenital heart disease
CCHF, C-CHFV
    Crimean-Congo hemorrhagic fever
⚠ **cc/hr**
    cubic centimeter per hour [NOTE: Do
    not use, substitute mL/hr] ⚠
ccHRT
    continuous-combined hormone
    replacement therapy
CCHS
    congenital central hypoventilation
    syndrome
CCI
    cholesterol crystallization inhibitor
    chronic coronary insufficiency
    coherent contrast imaging
    College Characteristics Index
    corrected count increment
    Cronqvist cranial index
CCIC
    contrast chromoscopy using indigo
    carmine
CCJ
    costochondral junction
CCK
    cholecystokinin
CCK-4
    cholecystokinin tetrapeptide
CCK8–CCK8S
    cholecystokinin octapeptide *(See also*
    CCK-OP)
CCK-A–CCK-C
    cholecystokinin A–C
CCK-GB
    cholecystokinin-gallbladder
    [cholecystogram]
⚠ **cc/kg day**
    cubic centimeter per kilogram per day
    [NOTE: Do not use, substitute mL/kg
    per day] ⚠
CCK-LI
    cholecystokinin-like immunoreactivity
CCKNOW
    Crohn and Colitis Knowledge
CCK-OP
    cholecystokinin octapeptide *(See also*
    CCK8, CCK8S)
CCK-PZ
    cholecystokinin-pancreozymin
CCL
    carcinoma cell line

    cardiac catheterization laboratory
    centrocytelike [cell]
    certified cell line
    costoclavicular ligament
    critical carbohydrate level
    critical condition list
CCl4
    carbon tetrachloride
c̄cl
    with contact lenses
CCLE
    chronic cutaneous lupus erythematosus
CCLI
    composite clinical and laboratory
    index
CCLO
    child-centered literary orientation
CCM
    calcium citrate malate
    cerebral cavernous malformation
    cerebrocostomandibular [syndrome]
    chronic cystic mastitis
    congestive cardiomyopathy
    contralateral competing message
    craniocervical malformation
    Crime Classification Manual
    critical care medicine
CC/MCL
    centrocytic mantle cell lymphoma
CCMD-2
    Chinese Classification of Mental
    Disorders, Second Edition
CCMEC
    clear cell myoepithelial carcinoma
CCMM
    conventional cutaneous malignant
    melanoma
CCMS
    cerebrocostomandibular syndrome
    clean-catch midstream [urine] *(See also*
    CCMSU, CCMSUA)
    clinical care management system
CCMSU
    clean-catch midstream [urine] *(See also*
    CCMS, CCMSUA)
CCMSUA
    clean-catch midstream urine (urinalysis)
    (See also CCMS, CCMSU)
CCMT
    catechol methyltransferase
CCN
    caudal central nucleus
    cervical cord neurapraxia
    coronary care nursing
    critical care nursing
CCNS
    cell cycle nonspecific [agent]
CCO
    continuous cardiac output

CcO$_2$
oxygen concentration in pulmonary capillary blood

CCOF
chromosomally competent ovarian failure

C-collar
cervical collar

CCOT
clear cell odontogenic tumor

CCP
chronic calcifying pancreatitis
ciliocytophthoria
colitis cystica profunda
columnar-cell papilloma
complement control protein
continuous cooling pad
continuous coronary perfusion
criminal career profile [psychology]
crippled children's program
crystalloid cardioplegia
cyclic citrullinated peptide
cytidine cyclic phosphate

CCPD
continuous cycling (cyclical) (cycled) peritoneal dialysis
crystalline calcium pyrophosphate dihydrate

CCPDS
centralized cancer patient data system

CCPQ
Children's Comprehensive Pain Questionnaire

CCPR
cerebral cortex perfusion rate (*See also* CPR)
closed chest cardiopulmonary resuscitation
crypt cell production rate

CCPT
chronic calcific pancreatitis of tropics

CCQ
Chronicle Career Quest

CCR
cardiac catheterization recovery
chemokine receptor
complete continuous remission
complex chromosome rearrangement
continuous complete remission
conventional chest radiograph (radiography)
creatinine clearance (*See also* CC, C$_{cr}$, C/cr/, CRC, CrCl, Crcl)
cumulative conception rate

CCR1–CCR11
chemokine receptor 1–11

C$_{cr}$, C/cr/
creatinine clearance (*See also* CC, CCR, CrCl, Crcl, CRC)

CCRN
congenital cartilaginous rest of neck

CCRS
carotid chemoreceptor stimulation

CCRT, CC-RT
computer-controlled conformal radiation therapy
computer-controlled radiotherapy
concurrent chemoradiotherapy

CcRV-W2
Carcinus mediterraneus W2 virus

CCS
cardiac care system
casualty clearing station
celiac artery compression syndrome
cell cycle specific [agent]
central cord syndrome
Cheshire cat syndrome
Children's Coma Score
cholecystosonography
chronic cerebellar stimulation
chronic compartment syndrome
clear-cell sarcoma
Clinical Classification System
cloudy-cornea syndrome
color contrast sensitivity
composite cultured skin
concentration-camp syndrome
costoclavicular syndrome
crippled children's services

CC&S
corneas, conjunctivae, sclerae

CCSA
central centrifugal scarring alopecia
central chemosensitive area

CCSAS
Canadian Cardiovascular Society angina score

CCSC
Canadian Cardiovascular Society classification
Children's Coping Strategies Checklist

CCSCS
central cervical spinal cord syndrome

CCSE
Cognitive Capacity Screening Examination

CCSEQ
Community College Student Experiences Questionnaire

CCSF
carotid-cavernous sinus fistula

CCSK
clear-cell sarcoma of kidney

CCSL
  clear-cell sarcoma of liver
CCSP
  Clara cell secretory protein
CCT
  carotid compression tomography
  central conduction time
  central corneal thickness
  cerebrocranial trauma
  chocolate-coated tablet
  closed cerebral trauma
  closed cranial trauma
  coated compressed tablet
  collision cell technology [imaging]
  combined cortical thickness
  composite cyclic therapy
  computerized cranial tomography
  congenitally corrected transposition [of
    the great vessels]
  controlled clinical trial
  controlled cord traction
  conventional computed tomography
  corrected congenital transposition [of
    the great vessels]
  cortical collecting tubule
  cranial computed tomography
  crude coal tar
  cyclocarbothiamine
  cyclosporine challenge test
cct
  circuit
CCTA
  coronal computed tomographic
    arthrography
CCTD
  craniocarpotarsal dystrophy
CCTDI
  California Critical Thinking Dispositions
    Inventory
CCTET
  contact, control, test, evaluate, treatment
CCTGA
  congenitally corrected transposition of
    the great arteries
CCTP
  coronary care training program
CCT in PET
  crude coal tar in petroleum
CCTST
  California Critical Thinking Skills
    Test
CCTV
  closed-circuit television
CCTV-EEG
  closed-circuit television
    electroencephalogram
CCU
  Cherry-Crandall unit [Serum lipase
    measurement]

CCUA
  clean-catch urinalysis
CCUP
  colpocystourethropexy
CCV
  canine coronavirus
  columnar cell variant
  conductivity cell volume
  critical closing volume
CCVD
  chronic cerebrovascular disease
CCVM
  congenital cardiovascular malformation
CCW
  counterclockwise
  craniocortical width [fetal sonogram
    measure]
Ccw
  chest wall compliance
CCX
  complications
CCY
  cholecystectomy (*See also* chole)
CD
  cluster of differentiation [antigenic
    marker on helper/inducer T-cells]
  cadaver donor
  canine distemper
  carbohydrate dehydratase
  cardiac disease
  cardiac dullness
  cardiac dysrhythmia
  cardiovascular deconditioning
  cardiovascular disease (*See also* CVD)
  Carrel-Dakin [fluid]
  caudad
  caudal (*See also* caud)
  celiac disease
  cell dissociation
  central deposition
  cervical dystonia
  cervicodorsal [spine]
  cesarean delivery
  channel down
  character disorder
  chemical dependency
  chemotactic difference
  childhood disease
  chronic dialysis
  circular dichroism
  civil defense
  closed drainage
  Clostridium difficile
  cluster of differentiation [antigenic cell
    marker] (*See also* CD2–CD72)
  coincidence detection
  collecting duct
  colloid droplet
  color denial

color Doppler
combination drug
common duct
communicable disease
communication deviance
communication disorder
completely denatured
complicated delivery
conduct disorder
conduction defect
conduction disorder
cone down [radiotherapy}
conjugata diagonalis [diagonal conjugate
 of pelvic inlet] [L. *conjugata
 diagonalis*]
consanguineous donor
constant drainage
contact dermatitis
contagious disease
continuous drainage
contrast-detail [imaging]
control diet
convulsive disorder
convulsive dose
copying drawings
corneal dystrophy
cortical dysplasia
Cotrel-Dubousset [rod]
covert dyskinesia
crossed diagonal
cumulative dose
curative dose
current diagnosis
cutdown
cystic duct
cytoplasmic domain
Czapek-Dox [agar]
with the right hand [L. *colla dextra*]
2CD
two-cycle duration
CD2–CD72
cluster of differentiation 2–72 [antigenic
 cell marker] (*See also* CD)
CD4
cluster of differentiation 4 (HIV helper
 cell count)
C4D
complement component 4 deficiency
C7D
complement component 7 deficiency
CD117
c-kit protooncogene
CD$_{50}$
median curative dose
C/D
cigarettes per day
C&D
curettage and desiccation

cystectomy and diversion
cystoscopy and dilation (dilatation)
C:D
cup to disc ratio
Cd
cadmium
cd
candela [SI unit of luminous
 intensity]
condylion [craniometric]
CDA
chenodeoxycholic acid
ciliary dyskinesia activity
cold dry air
complement-dependent antibody
completely denatured alcohol
congenital dyserythropoietic anemia
 [types I–III]
CDAA
chlorodiallylacetamide [herbicide]
CDAC
Clostridium difficile-associated colitis
 (*See also* CDC)
complement-dependent antibody-mediated
 cytotoxicity
CDAD
Clostridium difficile-associated diarrhea
 (disease)
CDAI
Crohn Disease Activity Index
CDAK
Cordis Dow Artificial Kidney
CDAP
continuous distending airway pressure
CDB, C&DB
cough and deep breath
CDBR
computerized diaphragmatic breathing
 retraining
controlled diaphragmatic breathing
CDC
calculated date of confinement
cancer detection center
capillary diffusion capacity
cardiac decompensation
casualty decontamination center
cell-dependent cytotoxicity
cell division cycle
Centers for Disease Control and
 Prevention [U.S. Department of Health
 and Human Services]
Child Dissociative Checklist
choledochocholedochostomy
chronic degenerative disease
chronic disseminated candidiasis
Clostridium difficile-associated colitis
 (*See also* CDAC)
collecting duct carcinoma

CDC *(continued)*
    complement-dependent cytotoxicity
    Crohn disease of colon
CDCA
    choledochocaval anastomosis
CDCC
    complement-dependent cellular
        cytotoxicity
CDCE
    constant denaturant capillary
        electrophoresis
CDCF
    Clostridium difficile culture filtrate
cDCIS
    comedo-type ductal carcinoma in situ
CDCR
    conjunctivodacryocystorhinostomy
CDCV
    Caddo Canyon virus
CDD
    certificate of disability for discharge
    childhood disintegrative disorder
    choledochoduodenostomy
    chronic degenerative disease
    chronic disabling dermatosis
    congenital diaphragmatic defect
    contrast-detail-dose [imaging]
    craniodiaphysial dysplasia
    critical degree of deformation
CDE
    canine distemper encephalitis
    color Doppler energy
    common duct exploration
    cystine dimethyl ester
CDEF
    chemically defined enteral feeding
CDEIS
    Crohn Disease Endoscopic Index of
        Severity
CDER
    Center for Drug Evaluation and
        Research [FDA]
CDEV
    Choristoneura diversuna entomopoxvirus
CDF
    chondrodystrophia fetalis
    chromosomal deoxyribonucleic acid
        (DNA) fingerprint [individual's genetic
        makeup, not testing procedure]
    color flow Doppler
CDFI
    color-coded Doppler flow imaging
    color Doppler flow imaging
CDFR
    cumulative duration of first
        remission
CDG
    carbohydrate-deficient glycoprotein
    central developmental groove

CDGA
    constitutional delay in growth and
        adolescence
CDGD
    constitutional delay in growth and
        development
CDGE
    constant denaturant gel electrophoresis
CDGG
    corneal dystrophy Groenouw type,
        granular
CDGN
    chronic diffuse glomerulonephritis
CDGS
    carbohydrate-deficient glycoprotein
        syndrome
CDH
    ceramide dihexoside
    chondrodysplasia punctata
    chronic daily headache
    chronic disease hospital
    congenital diaphragmatic hernia
    congenital dislocation (dysplasia) of hip
CDI
    cell-directed inhibitor
    central diabetes insipidus
    Children's Depression Inventory
    chronic diabetes insipidus
    clam digger's itch
    color Doppler imaging
    communicative development inventory
    controlled diabetes insipidus
    Cotrel-Dubousset [orthopaedic]
        instrumentation (*See also* CDO)
    cranial diabetes insipidus
CDIC
    Clostridium difficile-induced colitis
cDICA
    Computerized Diagnostic Interview for
        Children and Adolescents
C Diff
    Clostridium difficile
CD4-IgG
    cluster of differentiation 4
        immunoglobulin G
CDILD
    chronic diffuse interstitial lung disease
CDIS
    continuous distention-irrigation system
CDJ
    choledochojejunostomy
CDK
    climatic droplet keratopathy
Cdk1–Cdk6
    cyclin-dependent protein kinase 1–6
CdkI
    cyclin-dependent kinase inhibitor
CdkN2A
    cyclin-dependent kinase inhibitor 2A

CDL
Copying Drawings with Landmarks
CDLC
continuous double-loop closure
CDLE
chronic discoid lupus erythematosus
CDM
Career Decision-Making
change description master
chemically defined medium
childhood dermatomyositis
clinical decision making
clinical development monitor
CDMMS
chorioretinal
dysplasia-microcephaly-mental
retardation syndrome
cDNA
cloned deoxyribonucleic acid [human]
complementary deoxyribonucleic acid
CDNF
ciliary-derived neurotrophic factor
receptor
CDNH
chondrodermatitis nodularis helicis
CDO
controlled depth osteotomy cutter
Cotrel-Dubousset Orthopaedic
[instrumentation] (*See also* CDI)
CDP
certified distinct part
chemical dependence profile
chondrodysplasia punctata
chronic destructive periodontitis
collagenase-digestible protein
complete decongestive physiotherapy
comprehensive discharge planning
computerized dynamic posturography
continuous distending pressure
coronary drug project
crystalline degradation product
cytidine diphosphate (cytidine
5′-diphosphate)
CDPC, CDP-choline
cytidine diphosphate choline
(diphosphocholine)
CDPG, CDP-glyceride
cytidine diphosphoglyceride
CDPP
computerized dynamic platform
posturography
CDPR
chondrodysplasia punctata, rhizomelic
CDPS
common duct pigment stone
CDPS, CDP-sugar
cytidine diphosphosugar

CDPX
X-linked chondrodysplasia punctata
CDQ
corrected development quotient
CDR
calcium-dependent regulator
chronologic drinking record
clinical data repository
Clinical Dementia Rating
complementarity determining region
computed dental radiography
computed digital radiography
continuing disability review
cup to disc ratio
CDR3
third complementarity determining
region
CDR(H)
cup to disc ratio horizontal
CDRS-R
Children's Depression Rating
Scale-Revised
CDR(V)
cup to disc ratio vertical
CDS
caudal dysplasia syndrome
Chemical Data System
Children's Depression Scale
closed-door seclusion
color Doppler sonography
commercial dialysis solution
congenital dermal sinus
cul-de-sac
cumulative duration of survival
CDSACC
code substitution accuracy [subtest]
CDSEFF
code substitution efficiency [subtest]
CDSIACC
code substitution immediate
recall-accuracy [subtest]
CDSPIES
congestive heart failure, drugs, spasm,
pneumothorax, infection, embolism,
drugs [mnemonic for differential
diagnosis]
cd-sr
candela-steradian [unit of lighting]
CDSS
[computer assisted] clinical decision
support system
CDT
carbohydrate-deficient transferrin
carbon dioxide therapy
clock drawing test
Clostridium difficile toxin
combined diphtheria tetanus

CDT *(continued)*
complete decongestive therapy [for lymphedema]
connective discourse tracking
Current Dental Terminology
cystic dysplasia of testis

CDTA
cyclohexenediaminetetraacetic acid

CDTM
collaborative drug therapy management

CDU
cardiac diagnostic unit
chemical dependency unit
color Doppler ultrasonography
cumulative dose unit

CDUS
color Doppler ultrasound

CDUV
Candiru virus

CDV
canine distemper virus

CDY
cystoduodenostomy

CDYN, C_dyn, Cdyn
dynamic compliance [of lung in pulmonary function test]

CE
California encephalitis
capillary zone electrophoresis
capital epiphysis
cardiac emergency
cardiac enlargement
cardiac enzymes
cardioesophageal [junction] (*See also* CEJ)
carotid endarterectomy
catamenial epilepsy
cataract extraction
cell extract
center-edge
central episiotomy
cerebral edema
chemical energy
chemoembolization
chest expansion
chick embryo
cholera exotoxin
cholesterol ester (*See also* chol est, CHE)
cholinesterase (*See also* CHE, CHS)
chorioepithelioma
chromatoelectrophoresis
clinical emphysema
cocaethylene [drug of abuse]
coefficient of error [statistics]
columnar epithelium
community education
conductive education
conical elevation

conjugated estrogens
constant error
constant estrus
consultative examination
continuing education
contractile element
contrast echocardiology
contrast enema
contrast enhancement [imaging]
converting enzyme
cornified epithelium
corrective exercise
crude extract
curettage and electrodesiccation
cystic echinococcosis
cytopathic effect

C&E
consultation and examination
cough and exercise
curettage and electrodesication

Ce
cerium

CEA
carcinoembryonic antigen
carotid endarterectomy
cholesterol-esterifying activity
cost-effectiveness analysis
cranial epidural abscess
crystalline egg albumin
cultured epithelial (epithelium) autograft

CEA-125, CEA 125
carcinoembryonic antigen-125

CEACAM1
carcinoembryonic antigen-related cell adhesion molecule 1

CEA-DT
carcinoembryonic antigen doubling time

CEAL
carcinoembryonic antigenlike [protein]

CEAP
clinical manifestations, etiologic factors, anatomic involvement, pathophysiologic features

CEARP
Continuing Education Approval and Recognition Program

CEAT
chronic ectopic atrial tachycardia

CEB
calcium entry blocker
cotton elastic bandage

CEBD
controlled extrahepatic biliary drainage

C/EBP beta
CCAAT/enhancer binding protein [gene promoter element]

CEBV
chronic Epstein-Barr virus

CEC
  capillary electrochromatography
  ciliated epithelial cell
  contractile electrical complex
  corneal endothelial cell
CECD
  congenital endothelial corneal dystrophy
CECT
  contrast-enhanced computed tomography
CED
  chondroectodermal dysplasia
  chronic energy deficiency
  chronic enthusiasm disorder
  clinically effective dose
  compulsive eating disorder
  congenital ectodermal defect
  convection-enhanced delivery
  cranioectodermal dysplasia
  cultural [and] ethnic diversity
  cystoscopy-endoscopy dilation
CEDIA
  cloned enzyme donor immunoassay
CEE
  central European encephalitis
  chick embryo extract
  conjugated equine estrogens
CEEA
  curved (circular) end-to-end
    anastomosis
CEEC
  calf esophagus epithelial cell
CEEG
  computer-analyzed
    electroencephalography
CEEP
  conjugated equine estrogen plus
    norgestrel
CE-EUS
  contrast-enhanced endoscopic
    ultrasonography
CEEV
  central European encephalitis virus
CEF
  centrifugation extractable fluid
  chick embryo fibroblast
  constant electric field
CEFA
  continuous epidural fentanyl anesthesia
  capillary electrophoresis frontal analysis
    [method]
CE-FAST
  contrast-enhanced Fourier-acquired
    steady state
CEFM
  continuous external fetal monitoring
CEFT
  Children's Embedded Figures Test

CEG
  chronic erosive gastritis
C-EGD
  conventional upper
    esophagogastroduodenoscopy
cEGF
  concentration epidermal growth factor
CEH
  carboxylic ester hydrolase
  cholesterol ester hydrolase
CEHC
  calf embryonic heart cell
CEI
  character education inquiry
  continuous extravascular infusion
  converting enzyme inhibitor
  corneal epithelial involvement
CEID
  crossed electroimmunodiffusion
C1EInh
  complement 1 esterase inhibitor
CE/IOL
  cataract extraction with intraocular lens
CEJ
  cardioesophageal junction (*See also* CE)
  cementoenamel junction
CEK
  chick embryo kidney
CEL
  cardiac exercise laboratory
  chronic eosinophilic leukemia
CelCer1V
  Caenorhabditis elegans Cer1 virus
CELF
  Clinical Evaluation of Language
    Functions
CELI
  Carrow Elicited Language Inventory
CELO
  chicken embryo lethal orphan [virus]
CELP
  chronic erosive lichen planus
  code excited linear prediction
CEM
  central extensor mechanism
  clinical event monitor
  computerized electroencephalographic
    map
  continuous electrocardiographic
    monitoring
  conventional electron microscope
  continuous ultrasonic surgical aspiration
    (CUSA) electrosurgical module
cemf
  counterelectromotive force
C-EMR
  cutting endoscopic mucosal resection

CEMRA, CE-MRA
contrast-enhanced magnetic resonance
angiography
CEMRI, CE-MRI
contrast-enhanced magnetic resonance
imaging
cen
central
centromere
CENMR
capillary electrophoresis nuclear
magnetic resonance
CENOG
computerized
electroneuroophthalmograph(y)
(electroneuroophthalmogram)
CENP
centromere protein
CENT
central (*See also* C)
centimeter (*See also* cm, cent.)
cent.
centimeter (*See also* cm)
CEO
chick embryo origin
chloroethylene oxide
CEOM
chronic exudative otitis media
CEOT
calcifying epithelial odontogenic tumor
CEP
centromere enumeration probe
chronic eosinophilic pneumonia
chronic erythropoietic porphyria
cognitive evoked potential
congenital erythropoietic porphyria
continuing education program
cortical evoked potential
countercurrent electrophoresis
(counterelectrophoresis)
CEPA
chloroethane phosphoric acid
CEPB
Carpentier-Edwards porcine bioprosthesis
CEPH, ceph
cephalic
cephalin
CEPH FLOC, ceph-floc
cephalin flocculation [test]
CER
central episiotomy and repair
ceramide
ceruloplasmin (caeruloplasmin [British])
(*See also* CERULO, CP)
conditioned emotional response
control electrical rhythm
cortical evoked response
CE&R
central episiotomy and repair

CERA
cardiac-evoked response audiometry
continuous erythropoiesis receptor
activator
CERD
chronic end-stage renal disease
CEREC
ceramic reconstruction
chairside economical restorations of
esthetic ceramics
CERP
Continuing Education Recognition
Program
CERS
Crisis Evaluation Referral Service
CERT
composite extrarenal rhabdoid tumor
cert
certificate (*See also* CTF)
certified
CERULO
ceruloplasmin (caeruloplasmin [British])
(*See also* CER, CP)
cerv
cervical (*See also* C)
cervix (*See also* CX)
CES
cardioembolic stroke
cat's-eye syndrome
cauda equina syndrome
central excitatory state
chronic electrophysiologic study
Classroom Environmental Scale
clinical estimation of survival
clitoral enlargement syndrome
cognitive environmental stimulation
Combat Exposure Scale
cranial electrical stimulation
CESD
cholesterol ester storage disease
CES-D
Centers for Epidemiologic Studies
Depression scale
CESI
cervical epidural steroid injection
CESQ
Consumer Experience Of Stigma
Questionnaire
cESS
circumferential end-systolic stress
CET
capital expenditure threshold
cerebral electrotherapy
cholesterol-ester transfer
combination endocrine therapy
computed electroencephalogram (EEG)
tomography
congenital eyelid tetrad
controlled environment treatment

CE-TCCS
contrast-enhanced transcranial
color-coded real-time sonography
CETE
central European tick-borne encephalitis
CETP
cholesteryl ester transfer protein
CEU
congenital ectropion uveae
continuing education unit
contrast-enhanced ultrasound
CEV
California encephalitis virus
CeVD
cerebrovascular disease
CF
calcaneal fibular [ligament]
calf blood flow
calibration factor
cancer free
carbol-fuchsin [stain]
cardiac failure
carotid foramen
carrier-free
cascade filtration
case file
central field
central fossa
characteristic frequency
chemotactic factor
chest and left leg [lead in
electrocardiography]
chick fibroblast
choroid fissure
Christmas factor
chronicity factor
circumflex [coronary artery] (*See also*
CFX, CX, CXA, CxCor)
citrovorum factor
clavicular fracture
climbing fiber
clotting factor
clubfoot
colicin factor
collected fluid
colonization factor
colony-forming
color and form
common femoral [artery]
compare [L. *confer*] (*See also* cf.,
comp)
complementary feeding
complement factor
complement fixing (fixation) (*See also*
C'F, com fix)
completely follicular
complex fixation

computed fluoroscopy
constant frequency
contractile force
coronary flow
correction factor
cough fracture
cough frequency
count fingers [visual acuity test]
(*See also* cf)
coupling factor
cycling fibroblast
cystic fibrosis (*See also* C/F)
CFII
Cohn fraction II
C'F
complement fixing (fixation) (*See also*
CF, com fix)
C&F
cell and flare
chills and fever
curettage and fulguration
Cf
californium
²⁵²Cf
californium-252
cf
centrifugal force
count fingers [visual acuity test]
(*See also* CF)
cf.
compare [L. *confer*] (*See also* CF,
comp)
CFA
cerebrofacioarticular syndrome
clofibric acid [pesticide]
colonization factor antigen
colony-forming assay
common femoral artery
complement-fixing antibody
complete Freund adjuvant
craniofacial abnormality
cryptogenic fibrosing alveolitis
cut-film angiography
cystic fibrosis arthropathy
CFAC
complement-fixing antibody consumption
C-factor
cleverness factor
CFAG
cystic fibrosis antigen
CFA-SFA
common femoral artery [and] superficial
femoral artery
CFB
central fibrous body
CFBRS
Cooper-Farran Behavioral Rating Scale

125

CFC
capillary filtrate collector
capillary filtration coefficient
cardiofaciocutaneous [syndrome]
chlorofluorocarbon
colony-forming capacity
colony-forming cells
continuous-flow centrifugation
CFCL
continuous-flow centrifugation
leukapheresis
CFC-S
colony-forming cells, spleen
CFD
cephalofacial deformity
color-flow Doppler
craniofacial dysostosis
CFDS
craniofacial dysostosis
CFDU
color-flow Doppler ultrasonograph(y)
(ultrasonogram)
CFE
colony-forming efficiency
CFEOM
congenital fibrosis of extraocular
muscles
CFF
critical flicker frequency [test]
critical flicker fusion [test]
critical fusion frequency [test]
cystic fibrosis factor
CFFA
cystic fibrosis factor activity
Cf-Fe
carrier-bound iron [L. *ferrum*]
CFFR
crevicular fluid flow rate
CFFT
critical flicker fusion threshold
CFG
chronic familial granulomatosis
CFH
complement factor H
CFHL
complement factor H-like [protein]
CFI
cardiac function index
chemotactic-factor inactivator
closed-clenched fist injury
color flow imaging
complement fixation inhibition
confrontation fields intact
contour-facilitating instrument
CFIDS
chronic fatigue and immune dysfunction
syndrome
CFIT
Culture-Free Intelligence Test

CFL
cadaveric fascia lata
calcaneofibular ligament
central field loss
CFLB
carbon fiber lamination braid
CFLP
cleavage fragment length polymorphism
CflV
Campoletis flavicincta ichnovirus
CFM
cerebral function monitor
chemotactic factor for macrophage
chlorofluoromethane
close-fitting mask
craniofacial microsomia
cfm
cubic foot per minute
CfMNPV
Choristoneura fumiferana multicapsin
nucleopolyhedrovirus
CFMV
constant flow mechanical ventilation
CFND
craniofrontonasal dysostosis (dysplasia)
CFNG
cross-facial nerve grafting
CFNS
chills, fever, night sweats
craniofrontonasal syndrome
CfoIV
Casinaria forcipata ichnovirus
CFOS
constrained fast orthogonal search
CFOV
circular field of view [radiotherapy]
CFP
chronic false-positive
ciguatera fish poisoning
cystic fibrosis of pancreas
cystic fibrosis protein
CFPD
critical frequency of photic driving
CFQ
Cognitive Failures Questionnaire
CFR
case to fatality ratio
complement-fixation reaction
coronary flow reserve
cyclic flow reduction
CFRD
cystic fibrosis-related diabetes
CFS
call for service
cancer family syndrome
childhood febrile seizure
chronic fatigue syndrome
congenital fibrosarcoma
contoured femoral stem

craniofacial stenosis
craniofacial surgery
crush fracture syndrome
cfs
cubic foot per second
CFSE
crystal field stabilization energy
CFSEI-2
Culture-Free Self-Esteem Inventories,
Second Edition
CFT
capillary filling time
cardiolipin flocculation test
clinical full-time
complement-fixation test
Complex Figure Test
crystal field theory
Culture-Free Test
CFTC
complication-free tumor control
CFTD
congenital fiber-type disproportion
CFTP
Cattell factorial theory of personality
CFTR
cystic fibrosis transmembrane
conductance regulator [gene]
CFU
colony-forming unit
CFUC, CFU-C
colony-forming unit, culture
CFU-E
colony-forming unit, erythrocyte
colony-forming unit, erythroid
CFU-EOS
colony-forming unit, eosinophil
CFU-F
colony-forming unit, fibroblast(oid)
CFU-GEMM
colony-forming unit, granulocyte,
erythrocyte, megakaryocyte,
macrophage
CFU-GM, CFU$_{GM}$
colony-forming unit,
granulocyte-macrophage
CFU-L
colony-forming unit, lymphoid
CFU-Meg
colony-forming unit, megakaryocyte
CFU/mL
colony-forming unit per milliliter
CFU-NM
colony-forming unit,
neutrophil-monocyte
CFU-S
colony-forming unit, spleen
colony-forming unit, stem [cell]

CFUV
Corfou virus
CFV
Chrysanthemum frutescens virus
common femoral vein
CFVR
coronary flow velocity reserve
CFVS
cerebrospinal fluid flow void sign
CFW
calcofluor white stain
cancer-free white [mouse] (*See also*
CFWM)
Carworth farm [mouse], Webster strain
CFWM
cancer-free white mouse (*See also*
CFW)
CFX
circumflex [coronary artery] (*See also*
CF, Cx, CXA, CxCor)
CFX-MARG
circumflex [coronary] artery marginal
[branch]
CFZ
capillary-free zone
CFZC
continuous-flow zonal centrifugation
CG
calcium gluconate
cardiography
Cardio Green [obsolete for IC Green,
indocyanine green injectable dye]
center of gravity (*See also* cg)
central gray [matter]
cholecystograph(y) (cholecystogram)
choriogenic gynecomastia
chorionic gonadotropin (*See also* CGT)
chronic glomerulonephritis (*See also*
CGN)
cingulate gyrus
colloidal gold
contact guarding
control group
cryoglobulin
cystine-guanine [dinucleotide]
NATO code for phosgene [choking
gas]
cg
center of gravity (*See also* CG)
centigram
chemoglobulin
CGA
catabolite gene activator
clonal group A [*Escherichia coli*]
comprehensive geriatric assessment
contact guard assist [physical therapy]
corrected gestational age

C

CgA
chromogranin A
CGAB
congenital abnormality
CGAS
Children's Global Assessment Scale
CGB
chronic gastrointestinal [tract] bleeding
CGC
cumulus-granulosa cell
CGCF
central groove of central fossa
CGCG
central giant cell granuloma
CGCL
central giant cell lesion
CGCOT
central granular cell odontogenic tumor
CGCT
combined germ cell tumor
CGD
chromosomal gonadal dysgenesis
chronic glycogen deficit
chronic granulomatous disease
continuous gastric drip
CGDE
contact glow discharge electrolysis
CGESS
computer-guided endoscopic sinus
surgery
CGF
chronic gavage feeding
CGFH
congenital fibrous histiocytoma
CGG
cytosine-guanine-guanine
[trinucleotide]
CGGE
constant gradient gel electrophoresis
CGH
chorionic gonadotropic hormone
comparative genomic hybridization
CGI
chronic granulomatous inflammation
Clinical Global Impression
(Improvement) (Index) [Scale]
common gateway interface
glycoprotein crystal growth inhibitor
CGI-BP
Clinical Global Impression Bipolar
CGIC
Clinical Global Impression of Change
CGI-S, CGI S
Clinical Global Impression Severity
[Scale]
CGKD
complex glycerol kinase deficiency
CGL
chronic granulocytic leukemia

congenital generalized lipodystrophy
correction with glasses (*See also* c gl)
c gl
correction with glasses (*See also* CGL)
CGLV
Changuinola virus
CGM
central gray matter [spinal cord]
coffee-grounds material
cGMP
cyclic 3′,5′-guanosine monophosphate
CGMS
continuous glucose monitoring system
CGN
chronic glomerulonephritis (*See also*
CG)
compressor-generated nebulizer
convalescent growing nursery
CGNB
composite ganglioneuroblastoma
CG:OQ
cerebral glucose to oxygen quotient
CGP
choline glycerophosphatide
chorionic growth hormone-prolactin
circulating granulocyte pool
Comparative Guidance and Placement
Program
CGPF
cell-growth potentiating factor
CGPP
comparative guidance and placement
program
CGPS
Current Global Psychiatric-Social Status
[rating scale]
CGRH
calcitonin gene-related hormone
CGRP
calcitonin gene-related peptide
CGRS
Clinician's Global Rating Scale
CGS
cardiogenic shock
catgut suture (*See also* CS)
causal genesis syndrome
centimeter-gram-second [system, unit]
(*See also* cgs)
clinical grading scale
computer graphic simulation
corrected gestational age
cgs
centimeter-gram-second [system, unit]
(*See also* CGS)
CGT
chorionic gonadotropin (*See also* CG)
cyclodextrin glucanotransferase
CGTT
cortisone-glucose tolerance test

CGV
Chobar Gorge virus
CGVD
chronic graft vascular disease
c-GVHD
chronic graft-versus-host disease
CGY
cystogastrostomy
cGy
centigray
CH
calcium heparin
calcium hydroxide
case history
casein hydrolysate
cervicogenic headache
chest
chief
child (children) (*See also* Ch, ch)
Chinese hamster
chloral hydrate
cholesterol (*See also* C, Ch, CHOL, chol, chol.)
Christchurch chromosome
chronic
chronic hepatitis
chronic hypertension
cluster headache
common hepatic [duct]
communicating hydrocele
complete healing
concentric hypertrophy
congenital hypothyroidism
continuous heparinization
convalescent hospital
conversion hysteria
coracohumeral
cortical hamartoma
crown-heel [infant or fetus length] (*See also* CHL)
cycloheximide
(wheel)chair (*See also* WC, W/C wh ch)
C-H
carbon-hydrogen
C&H
coarse and harsh [breathing]
cocaine and heroin
CH$_{50}$
(total serum) hemolytic complement
C$_H$
constant domain of [immunoglobulin G] H (heavy) chain
Ch
Chido [antibody]
choline
chromosome (*See also* chr)

cH
hydrogen ion concentration
CHA
chronic hemolytic anemia
common hepatic artery
compound hypermetropic astigmatism
congenital hypoplasia of adrenal glands
congenital hypoplastic anemia
continuous heated aerosols
controlled hypotensive anesthesia
cyclohexyladenosine
cyclohexylamine
ChA
choline acetylase
ChAc, ChAct
choline acetyltransferase
CHAD
cold hemagglutinin disease
CHADD
children and adults with attention deficit disorder
controlled heat-aided drug delivery
CHAF
central hyperalimentation nutrition
CHAG
coralline hydroxyapatite *Goniopora* genus tag
CHAI
continuous hepatic artery infusion
CHAID
chi-square automatic interaction detection
CHAL
chronic haloperidol
CHAMPUS
Civilian Health and Medical Programs of Uniformed Services
CHAMPVA
Civilian Health and Medical Program of Veterans' Administration
CHANDS
curly hair-ankyloblepharon-nail dysplasia syndrome
Chang C
Chang conjunctiva [cells]
Chang L
Chang liver [cells]
CHAOS
congenital high airway obstruction syndrome
coronary artery disease, hypertension, adult-onset diabetes, obesity, stroke
CHAP
Certified Hospital Admission Program
Child Health Assessment Program

CHAQ
Childhood Health Assessment Questionnaire

CHAR
continuous hyperfractionated accelerated radiotherapy

CHARGE
coloboma, heart anomaly, choanal atresia, retardation, genital and ear anomalies [syndrome]

CHARM
chunk acquisition and reconstruction method [computed tomography]

CHART
continuous hyperfractionated accelerated radiotherapy
Craig Handicap Assessment and Reporting Technique

CHARTS
Computerized Healthcare And Record Transfer System

CHAS
continuous hepatic artery syndrome

CHASE
cut holes and sink 'em [chemical weapons disposal operation]

CHAT, ChAT, ChaT
choline acetyltransferase
conversational hypertext access technology

CHATH
chemically hardened air-transportable hospital

CHB
chronic hepatitis B
complete heart block
congenital heart block

ChBFlow
choroidal blood flow

CHBHA
congenital Heinz body hemolytic anemia

CHBMS
Champion health belief model scale

ChBVol
choroidal blood volume

CHC
Canadian Heart Classification
chronic hepatitis C
collapsible holding chamber
community health center
concentric hypertrophic cardiomyopathy

CHCL
congenital healed cleft lip

CHCP
correctional healthcare program

CHCT
caffeine and halothane contracture test

CHD
center hemodialysis
childhood disease
chronic hemodialysis
common hepatic duct
congenital heart defect (disease)
congenital hip dislocation (dysplasia)
congestive heart disease
constitutional hepatic dysfunction
coronary heart disease
cyanotic heart disease

CHE
cholesterol ester (*See also* chol est, CE)
cholinesterase (*See also* CE, CHS)
chronic hepatic encephalopathy
comprehensive health examination

ChE
cholinesterase

CHEC
community hypertension evaluation clinic

CHED
congenital hereditary endothelial dystrophy

CHEDDAR
chief complaint, history [present illness, social, and family], examination, details [of problems and complaints], drugs and dosage, assessment, return [medical history documentation]

CHEF
Chinese hamster embryo fibroblast
contour-clamped homogeneous electric field [electrophoresis]

chem
chemical
chemistry
blood chemistry profile (*See also* chem panel)

CHEMLINE
Chemical Dictionary On-Line

chemo
chemotherapy

chem panel
blood chemistry profile (*See also* chem)

chemrad
chemotherapy and radiotherapy

CHEP
cricohyoidoepiglottopexy

CHERSS
continuous high-amplitude electroencephalogram rhythmical synchronous slowing

CHES
Children's Handwriting Evaluation Scale

CHES-M
Children's Handwriting Evaluation Scale for Manuscript Writing

CHESS
  chemical shift selective suppression
  [technique]
  comprehensive health enhancement
  support system
  Cornell high energy synchrotron source
CHEST
  Chick Embryotoxicity Screening Test
CHF
  chick embryo fibroblast
  chronic heart failure
  congenital hepatic fibrosis
  congestive heart failure
  Crimean hemorrhagic fever
CHFD
  controlled high flux dialysis
CHFDT
  congestive heart failure data tool
CHFV
  combined high-frequency ventilation
CHG, chg
  change(d)
ch gn
  chronic glomerulonephritis
CHGV
  Chagres virus
CHH
  cartilage-hair hypoplasia
χ, Chi
  χ [22nd letter of Greek alphabet
  lowercase]
chi$_2$ (χ_2)
  chi-squared [distribution, test]
chi$_e$ (χ_e)
  electric susceptibility
chi$_m$ (χ_m)
  magnetic susceptibility
CHI
  closed head injury
  creatinine height index
CHIC
  Coping Health Inventory for Children
CHID
  Combined Health Information
  Database
CHIKV
  Chikungunya virus
CHILD
  congenital hemidysplasia with
  ichthyosiform erythroderma and limb
  defects [syndrome]
CHIME
  Collaborative Home Infant Monitoring
  Evaluation
  coloboma, heart anomaly, ichthyosis,
  mental retardation, and ear
  abnormality or epilepsy [syndrome]

CHIMV
  Chim virus
CHINA
  chronic infectious neuropathic agent
CHINS
  child in need of service [petition]
CHIP
  channel-forming integral protein
  comprehensive health insurance plan
  comprehensive hospital infections
  project
  Coping Health Inventory for Parents
  Coping with Health, Injuries, and
  Problems
CHIP-1
  channel-forming integral protein 1
ChIP
  chromatin immunoprecipitation
CHIP-AE
  Child Health and Illness Profile,
  Adolescent Edition
CHIPASAT
  Children's Paced Auditory Serial
  Addition Test
ChIPS
  Children's Interview for Psychiatric
  Disorders
CHIPX
  [X-linked] chronic idiopathic intestinal
  pseudoobstruction
CHIV
  Chilibre virus
chix
  chickenpox (*See also* CHPX, chpx, Cp)
CHK
  Csk homologous kinase
CHL
  Chinese hamster lung
  classic Hodgkin lymphoma
  conductive hearing loss
  crown-heel [infant or fetus] length
  (*See also* CH)
CHLD
  chronic hypoxic lung disease
CHLS
  combined heart and lung surgery
CHM
  complete hydatidiform mole
CHMD
  clinical hyaline membrane disease
CHMIS
  community health management
  information system
CHN
  carbon, hydrogen, nitrogen
  central hemorrhagic necrosis
  child neurology

CHN *(continued)*
Chinese [hamster]
Chinese herb nephropathy
congenital hypomyelinating neuropathy

CHO
carbohydrate (*See also* CARB, carb, carbo)
Chinese hamster ovary
chlorhexidine digluconate
chorea

C$_{H2O}$
clear water
water clearance

choc
chocolate

CHOL, chol, chol.
cholesterol (*See also* CH)

chold
withhold

chole
cholecystectomy (*See also* CCY)

chol est
cholesterol ester (*See also* CE, CHE)

chorio
chorioamnionitis

CHOV
Chaco virus

CHP
capillary hydrostatic pressure
charcoal hemoperfusion
child psychiatry
comprehensive health planning
cricohyoidopexy
cutaneous hepatic porphyria
histiocytic cytophagic panniculitis

CHPB
Canadian Health Prevention Branch

CHPM
chronic hypertrophic pachymeningitis

CHPP
continuous hyperthermic peritoneal perfusion

CHPS
chronic heel pain syndrome

CHPV
Chandipura virus

CHPX, chpx
chickenpox (*See also* chix, Cp)

CHQ
child health questionnaire

CHR
cercaria-Hüllen reaction [lab test for trematode larvae]
cerebrohepatorenal [syndrome]
chromogranin
complete hematologic response

chr
chromosome (*See also* Ch)
chronic (*See also* CH chron)

ChrA
chromogranin A

ChRBC
chicken red blood cell (*See also* CRBC)

CH/RG
Chido/Rodgers [blood group system]

CHRIS
Cancer Hazards Ranking and Information System

CHROMINFO
chromosome information [database]

chron
chronic (*See also* CH, chr)
chronologic(al)

CHRP
coagulation and hemostatic resection of prostate

CHRPE
congenital hypertrophy of retinal pigment epithelium

CHRS
cerebrohepatorenal syndrome
congenital hereditary retinoschisis

CHS
central hypoventilation syndrome
Children's Health Study
cholinesterase (*See also* CE, CHE)
chondroitin sulfate
compression hip screw
congenital hypoventilation syndrome
contact hypersensitivity

CHSD
congenital hyperphosphatasemic skeletal dysplasia

CHS/NP
chronic hyperplastic sinusitis with nasal polyposis

CHSS
cooperative health statistics system

CHT
closed head trauma
combined hormone therapy
congenital hypothyroidism
contralateral head turning

CHTN
Cooperative Human Tissue Network

CHU
closed head unit

CHUK
conserved helix-loop-helix ubiquitous kinase

CHUS
chemotherapy (cancer) [related] hemolytic-uremic syndrome

CHV
canine herpesvirus
Cryphonectria hypovirus

CHVF
chemically viewed functionally

CHVS
chemically viewed structurally
CHVV
Charleville virus
CI
calcium ionophore
cardiac index
cardiac insufficiency
care imprint
cell immunity
cell inhibition
cell interaction [molecule]
cephalic index
cerebral infarct(ion)
cervical incompetence
cesium implant
chain initiating
chemical ionization
chemoimmunotherapy
chemotactic index
chemotherapeutic index
chronically infected
chronic inflammation
clinical investigation
clonus index
closure index
cochlear implant(ation)
coefficient of intelligence
cognitively impaired
colloidal iron
colon inertia
colony inhibition
complete iridectomy
confidence interval
constraint-induced [movement therapy]
contamination index
continuous imaging
continuous infusion
contraindicat(ed) (contraindication)
convergence insufficiency
cord insertion
coronary insufficiency
corrected count increment
crystalline insulin
cumulative incidence
cumulative injury
cytotoxic index
C.I.
Colour Index
Ci
curie
CIA
canine inherited ataxia
chemiluminescent immunoassay
chemotherapy-induced amenorrhea
chemotherapy-induced anemia
chemotherapy-induced diarrhea

chronic idiopathic anhidrosis
chymotrypsin inhibitor activity
collagen-induced arthritis
colony-inhibiting activity
common iliac artery
congenital intestinal aganglionosis
CIAA
competitive insulin autoantibodies
CIAC
chronic idiopathic arthritides of
childhood
CIAED
collagen-induced autoimmune ear
disease
cIAP
cellular inhibitor of apoptosis
CIAS
Chen Internet Addiction Scale
CIB, cib
crying-induced bronchospasm
cytomegalic inclusion body
CIBD
chronic inflammatory bowel disease
CIBHA
congenital inclusion-body hemolytic
anemia
CIBI
continuous intrathecal baclofen infusion
CIBP
chronic intractable benign pain
CIBPS
chronic intractable benign pain
syndrome
CIC
carbachol inhalation challenge
cardioinhibitor center
chronic inactive cirrhosis
circulating immune complex
clean intermittent catheterization
completely in the canal [hearing aid]
complex instability of carpus
constant initial concentration
crisis intervention center (clinic)
CICA
cervical internal carotid artery
CICE
combined intracapsular cataract
extraction
CICI
Hymovich Chronicity Impact and
Coping Instrument
CICLP
chronic ischemic colonic lesion caused
by phlebosclerosis
CICR
calcium-induced calcium release
[process]

C

CID
   carpal instability, dissociative (dissociated)
   cellular immunodeficiency
   central integrative deficit
   cervical immobilization device
   charge injection device
   chemotherapy-induced diarrhea
   chick infective dose
   chronic intestinal dysmotility
   combined immune deficiency (immunodeficiency) [disease]
   cytomegalic inclusion disease (*See also* CMID)

CIDEP
   chemically induced dynamic electron polarization

CIDI
   Composite International Diagnostic Interview [WHO]

CIDNP
   chemically-induced dynamic nuclear depolarization

CIDP
   chronic idiopathic polyradiculopathy
   chronic inflammatory demyelinating polyradiculopathy

CIDPN
   chronic inflammatory demyelinating polyneuropathy
   chronic inflammatory demyelinating polyradiculoneuropathy

CIDS
   cellular immune deficiency (immunodeficiency) syndrome
   combined immunodeficiency syndrome
   continuous insulin delivery system

CIE
   chemotherapy-induced emesis
   congenital ichthyosiform erythroderma
   countercurrent (crossed) immunoelectrophoresis (*See also* CIEP)
   counterimmunoelectrophoresis (*See also* CIEP)

CIEA
   continuous infusion epidural analgesia

CIE-C
   counter immunoelectrophoresis colorimetric

CIE-D
   counter immunoelectrophoresis densitometric

cIEL
   crypt intraepithelial lymphocyte

CIEP
   countercurrent (crossed) immunoelectrophoresis (*See also* CIE)
   counterimmunoelectrophoresis (*See also* CIE)

CIES
   Correctional Institutions Environment Scale

CIF
   cartilage induction factor
   claims inquiry form
   clone-inhibiting factor
   cloning inhibitory factor
   congenital infantile fibrosarcoma

CIFN
   chemotherapy-induced fever and neutropenia

CIG
   cardiointegram
   cigarettes
   cold-insoluble globulin

CIg
   cytoplasmic immunoglobulin

cIgM
   cytoplasmic immunoglobulin M

CIH
   carbohydrate-induced hyperglyceridemia
   children in hospital

CIHD
   chronic ischemic heart disease

Ci-hr
   curie-hour

CIHS
   chronic infantile hypotonic syndrome

CII
   Carnegie Interest Inventory
   continuous insulin infusion

CIIA
   common internal iliac artery

CIIP
   chronic idiopathic intestinal pseudoobstruction

CIIPS
   chronic idiopathic intestinal pseudo-obstruction syndrome

CIIS
   Cattell Infant Intelligence Scale

CIITA
   class II transcriptional activator

CiIV
   Casinaria infesta ichnovirus

CIL
   carbamazepine-induced lupus
   center for independent living

CILP
   cartilage intermediate layer protein

CIM
   cardia-intestinal metaplasia
   changes in menses
   chemotherapy-induced mucositis
   constraint-induced movement [therapy]
   cortically induced movement
   corticosteroid-induced myopathy

Cumulated Index Medicus [obsolete]
cutaneous intolerance to
  mechlorethamine

C-IMC
circumference of chest at inframammary
  crease

CIMF
chronic idiopathic myelofibrosis

Ci/mL
curie per milliliter

CIMS
chemical ionization mass spectrometry
clinical information scale
Conflict in Marriage Scale

CIN
cefsulodin-Irgasan-novobiocin [agar]
cerebriform intradermal nevus
cervical intraepithelial neoplasia
cervical invasive neoplasia
chemotherapy-induced neutropenia
chromosomal instability
chronic interstitial nephritis
conjunctival intraepithelial neoplasia

CIN 1–3
cervical intraepithelial neoplasia, grade
  1–3

C_{IN}, C_{in}
inulin clearance

CINAHL
Cumulative Index to Nursing and Allied
  Health Literature

CINCA
chronic infantile neurological, cutaneous,
  and articular

CIND
carpal instability, nondissociative
cognitive impairment, not dementia

CINE
chemotherapy-induced nausea and
  emesis
cineangiogram

cine-MRI
cine [motion picture] magnetic
  resonance imaging

C1INH
first component of complement

CINV
chemotherapy-induced nausea and
  vomiting

CIO
corticoid-induced osteoporosis

CIOF
chromosomally incompetent ovarian
  failure

CIOH
chronic idiopathic orthostatic
  hypotension

CIP
cellular immunocompetence profile
chronic idiopathic
  polyradiculoneuropathy
chronic inflammatory polyneuropathy
chronic intestinal pseudoobstruction
comprehensive identification process
critical illness polyneuropathy
critical infrastructure protection

CIPA
congenital insensitivity to pain

CIPD
chronic intermittent peritoneal dialysis

CIPF
classic interstitial pneumonitis with
  fibrosis
clinical illness promoting factor

CIPN
chronic idiopathic peripheral
  neuropathy
chronic inflammatory polyneuropathy

CIPO
chronic intestinal pseudoobstruction

CIPS
chronic intestinal pseudoobstructive
  syndrome

CIQ
Community Integration Questionnaire

CIR
continent intestinal reservoir

cir
circuit
circular
circumference (*See also* circ)

circ
circulation
circumcision (*See also* circum)
circumference (*See also* cir)

circ & sen
circulation and sensation

circum
circumcision (*See also* circ)

CIRF
cocaine-induced respiratory failure
contrast-induced renal failure

CIRP
cold-inducible ribonucleic acid-binding
  protein
cooperative institutional research
  program

CIRR
cirrhosis

CIRS-G
Cumulative Illness Rating Scale For
  Geriatrics

CIRT
carbon ion radiotherapy

CIS
carcinoma in situ
catheter-induced spasm
central inhibitory state
clinical information system
clinically isolated syndrome
computer-integrated surgery
continuous interleaved sampling
coronary implant system
cumulative impairment score

CI-S
Simplified Calculus Index

CiS
cingulate sulcus

CISC
clean intermittent self-catheterization

CISD
critical incident stress debriefing

CISE
Children's Inventory of Self-Esteem

CISH
chromagen in situ hybridization

CISI
Cattell Infant Scale Inventory

CIS/ITGCNU
carcinoma in situ [and] intratubular
germ cell neoplasia unclassified

CISM
critical incident stress management

CISMD
California Infant Scale for Motor
Development

CISP
chronic intractable shoulder pain

CISS
Campbell Interest and Skill Survey

CIT
chemotherapy-induced toxicity
citrate (*See also* cit)
cold ischemic (ischemia) time
combined intermittent therapy
conjugated-immunoglobulin technique
constraint-induced therapy
conventional immunosuppressive therapy
conventional insulin therapy
corneal impression test
crisis intervention therapy
critical incident technique

cit
citrate (*See also* CIT)

CITP
capillary isotachophoresis

CITS
Carey Infant Temperature Scale

CIU
chronic idiopathic urticaria

CIV
Carey Island virus
common iliac vein

continuous intravenous [infusion]
(*See also* CIVI)

CIVI
continuous intravenous infusion
(*See also* CIV)

CIVII
continuous intravenous insulin infusion

CIVRA
continuous intravenous regional
anesthesia

CIXU
constant infusion excretory urogram

CJ
conjunctivitis

CJD
Creutzfeldt-Jakob disease

CJR
centric jaw relationship

CJS
costochondral junction syndrome

CK
calf kidney
chicken kidney
cholecystokinin
choline kinase
color kinesis
conductive keratoplasty
contralateral knee (*See also* ck)
creatine kinase
cyanogen chloride
cytokeratin
NATO code for cyanogen chloride
[$CNCl_2$]

CK20
cytokeratin 20

CK$_1$, CK$_2$, CK$_3$
isoenzymes of creatine kinase

ck
check(ed)
contralateral knee (*See also* CK)

CK-BB
creatine kinase brain band [isoenzyme]
(*See also* CPK-BB)

CKC
closed kinetic chain
cold-knife cone (conization)

CKCE
closed kinetic chain exercise

CKD
chronic kidney disease

CKF
co-cancerogenic K factor

CKG
cardiokymograph(y)

c/kg
coulomb per kilogram

CK-ISO
creatine kinase isoenzyme (*See also*
CPKI, CPKISO)

CK-MB
    creatine kinase muscle-band [isoenzyme]
    (*See also* CPK-MB)
    creatine kinase myocardial band
    (*See also* CPK-MB)
CK-MM
    creatine kinase skeletal muscle
    [isoenzyme] (*See also* CPK-MM)
CKPT
    combined kidney and pancreas
    transplant (ahm)
CK-PZ
    cholecystokinin-pancreozymin
CKS
    classic form of Kaposi sarcoma
CKW
    clockwise (*See also* CW)
CL
    capacity of lung
    capillary lumen
    cardinal ligament
    cardiolipin
    cell line
    cellular leiomyoma
    center line
    centralis lateralis
    central line
    central [venous or arterial] line
    cervical line
    chemiluminescence
    chest and left arm [lead in
        electrocardiography]
    childhood leukemia
    cholelithiasis
    cholesterol-lecithin
    chronic leukemia
    cirrhosis of liver
    clamp lamp
    clavicle
    clearance
    clear liquid
    cleft lip
    clinical laboratory
    clonus
    Clostridium
    closure
    clot lysis
    cloudy (*See also* c, cldy)
    complex loading
    compliance of lung
    composite lymphoma
    confidence level
    contact lens (*See also* ctl)
    continence line
    corpus luteum
    cricoid lamina
    criterion level

critical list
current liabilities
cutaneous leishmaniasis
cutis laxa
cycle length
cytotoxic lymphocyte
2C-L
    2-chamber longitudinal
        [echocardiographic view]
C-L
    consultation-liaison [psychiatry]
C_L
    constant domain of immunoglobulin GI
        L (light) chain
Cl
    chloride
cL
    centiliter
CLA
    cerebellar ataxia
    cervicolinguoaxial
    cleft lip and alveolus
    closed loop algorithm
    community living arrangements
    congenital lactic acidosis
    congenital laryngeal atresia
    conjugated linoleic acid
    contralateral local anesthesia
    cutaneous lichen amyloidosis
    cutaneous lymphocyte antigen
    cyclic lysine anhydride
CLAH
    congenital lipoid adrenal
        hyperplasia
C lam
    cervical laminectomy
CLAMS
    Clinical Linguistic and Auditory
        Milestone Scale
CLAP
    contact laser ablation of prostate
CLARE
    contact lens-induced acute red eye
CLAS
    congenital localized absence of skin
CLASH
    cryoglobulinemia, leukemia, arthritis,
        Sjögren syndrome, hepatitis B
        [diseases with vasculitis]
CLASP
    compression locking anchor with
        secondary purchase
class.
    classification
CLASSI
    Cornell Learning and Study Skills
        Inventory

C

CLAV, clav
 clavicle
CLB
 curvilinear body
CLBBB
 complete left bundle branch
 block
CLBC
 contralateral breast cancer
CLBD
 cortical Lewy body disease
CLBP
 chronic low back pain
CLC
 Charcot-Leyden crystal
 cork, leather, celastic (orthotic)
CLCC
 classic large-cell carcinoma
CLCD
 cleidocranial dysostosis
ClCN7
 chloride channel 7 [gene]
CL/CP
 cleft lip and cleft palate
CLCS
 colchicine sensitivity
 Comprehensive Level of Consciousness
 Scale
CLD
 central language disorder
 central low density
 central lung distance
 chloride diarrhea
 chronic liver disease
 chronic lung disease
 congenital limb deficiency
 crystal ligand field
 cytoplasmic lipid droplet
cld
 cleared
 colored
CLDH
 choline dehydrogenase
C-LDP
 complete laparoscopic distal
 pancreatectomy
CLDQ
 Chronic Liver Disease Questionnaire
cldy
 cloudy (See also CL)
CLE
 central hepatic irradiation
 centrilobular emphysema
 clear lens extraction
 columnar-lined esophagus
 congenital lobar emphysema
 constant load exercise
 continuous lumbar epidural
 [anesthesia]

CLED
 cystine-lactose electrolyte-deficient [agar]
CLEF-P
 Clinical Evaluation of Language
 Function Preschool
CLEP
 College-Level Examination Program
 General Examination
CLF
 cardiolipin fluorescence [antibody]
 cholesterol-lecithin flocculation
CLH
 chronic lobular hepatitis
 cleft limb [and] heart [malformation
 syndrome]
 congenital lipoid hyperplasia
 corpus luteum hormone
 cutaneous lymphoid hyperplasia
CLHN
 centrilobular hepatic necrosis
CLI
 Campbell Leadership Index
 corpus luteum insufficiency
 critical limb ischemia
CLi
 lithium clearance
CLIA
 chemiluminescent immunoassay
 Clinical Laboratory Improvement Act
 [1967]
 Clinical Laboratory Improvement
 Amendments [1988]
CLIF
 cloning inhibitory factor
 Crithidia luciliae immunofluorescence
CLIFT
 Crithidia luciliae immunofluorescence
 test
clin
 clinic(al)
CLINHAQ
 Clinical Health Assessment
 Questionnaire
clin path
 clinical pathology (See also CLP, CP)
clin proc
 clinical procedure
ClinSeg
 clinoidal segment [carotid artery]
CLIP
 class II invariant chain-derived peptide
 corticotropinlike intermediate lobe
 peptide
CLKTx
 combined liver and kidney
 transplant(ation)
CLL
 centrocytelike cell
 cholesterol-lowering lipid

chronic lymphocytic (lymphoblastic) (lymphatic) (lymphoid) leukemia
cow lung lavage

CLLE
columnar-lined lower esophagus

cl liq
clear liquid

CLM
capillary-lymphatic malformation

CLMB
cutaneous lineal melanoblastosis

CLML
Current List of Medical Literature

CLMN
complete lower motor neuron [lesion]

clmp
clump(ed)

CLN
centrilobar necrosis
cervical lymph node
neuronal ceroid lipofuscinosis [gene]

CLND
complete lymph node dissection

CLO
Campylobacter-like organism
cod liver oil
congenital lobar overinflation
cyclooxygenase

CLOCK
circadian locomotor output cycles kaput [gene]

C-loop
anatomical shape of duodenum

CLOtest
Campylobacter-like organism test [for *H. pylori*]

CLOT R
clot retraction

CLP
cardiac laboratory panel
cecal ligation and puncture
chymotrypsinlike protein
cleft lip with cleft palate (*See also* CL&P)
clinical pathology (*See also* clin path, CP)
cycle length, paced

CL&P
cleft lip and palate (*See also* CLP)

Clpal
cleft palate (*See also* CP)

CLPD
chronic lymphoproliferative disorder

CLPU
contact lens-induced peripheral ulcer

CLQ
cognitive laterality quotient

CLRB
clinical laboratory read back

CLRO
community leave for reorientation

CLRSS
Composite Laryngeal Recurrence Staging System

CLRT
continuous lateral rotational therapy

CLRV
Cimex lectularius reovirus

CLS
capillary leak syndrome
capillary lymphatic space
community living skills
confused language syndrome

CLSE
calf lung surfactant extract

CLSH
corpus luteum stimulating hormone

CLSL
chronic lymphosarcoma-cell leukemia

CLSM
confocal laser scan(ning) microscopy

cLSO
confocal laser scanning ophthalmoscopy

CLT
chronic lymphocytic thyroiditis
clot lysis time
clotting time
complex lymphedema therapy
cool lace tent

CLTM
continuous long-term monitoring

CLV
Colletotrichum lindemuthianum virus
constant linear velocity

CLVM
complex-combined vascular malformation

CL VOID
clean voided specimen [urine]

CLVP
contact laser vaporization of prostate

clysis
hypodermoclysis

CM
California mastitis [test]
calmodulin
carboxymethylcellulose (*See also* CMC)
cardiac monitor
cardiac murmur
cardiac muscle
cardiac myxoma
cardiomyopathy (*See also* CMP)
carpometacarpal [joint] (*See also* CMC)
castrated male
cavernous malformation

CM *(continued)*
    cell membrane
    center of mass
    central mentum [craniometric]
    centrum medianum
    cerebral malaria
    cerebral mantle
    cervical mucus
    chemotactic migration
    Chick-Martin [test of efficacy of
      bactericidal agent]
    chondromalacia
    chopped meat [medium]
    chronic meningitis
    chylomicron
    circular muscle
    circulating monocyte
    clinical medicine
    coccidioidal meningitis
    cochlear microphonics
    combined mechanical
    combined modality
    common migraine
    community meeting
    competing message
    complete medium
    complications
    conditioned medium
    congenital malformation
    congestive myocardiopathy
    continuous murmur
    contrast material
    contrast medium
    copulatory mechanism
    costal margin
    cow's milk
    culture medium
    cutaneous melanoma
    cystic mesothelioma
    cytometry
    cytoplasmic membrane

C/M
    count per minute (*See also* CPM, cpm)

C&M
    cocaine and morphine

C_m
    maximal clearance

Cm
    curium

cM
    centimorgan

cm
    centimeter (*See also* CENT, cent.)

cm^2
    square centimeter (*See also* sq cm)

cm^3
    cubic centimeter [Note: Do not use,
      substitute mL] (*See also* cc, CC, c.c.,
      cu cm)

CMA
    Candida metabolic antigen
    cerebral microangiopathy
    chronic metabolic acidosis
    complete maturation arrest
    compound myopic astigmatism
    Conflict Management Appraisal
    cow's milk allergy
    cultured macrophages

CMAD
    count median aerodynamic diameter

CMAF
    centrifuged microaggregate filter

CMAI
    Cohen-Mansfield agitation inventory

CMAmg
    corticomedial amygdaloid [nucleus]

CMAP
    compound motor (muscle) action
      potential

CMAS
    Childhood Myositis Assessment Scale
    Children's Manifest Anxiety Scale

C_{max}
    maximal drug concentration

CMB
    carbolic methylene blue
    chloromercuribenzoate

p-CMB
    p-chloromercuribenzoate

CMBBT
    cervical mucous basal body temperature

CMC
    carboxymethylcellulose (*See also* CM)
    care management continuity
    carpometacarpal [joint] (*See also* CM)
    cell-mediated cytotoxicity
    chronic mucocutaneous candidiasis
      (*See also* CMCC)
    closed mitral commissurotomy
    complement-mediated cytotoxicity
    corticomedullary contrast
    critical micelle concentration

CMCA
    care management for chronic addiction

CMCC
    chronic mucocutaneous candidiasis
      (*See also* CMC)

CM-cellulose
    carboxymethylcellulose

CMCJ
    carpometacarpal joint

CMCT
    central motor conduction time

CMCt
    care management continuity [across
      settings]

CMD
    camptomelic dwarfism (dysplasia)

cartilage matrix deficiency
cerebromacular degeneration
childhood muscular dystrophy
common mental disorder
congenital muscular dystrophy
corticomedullary differentiation
count median diameter [particle size of
    microbiologic aerosol]
craniomandibular disorder (dysfunction)
cystoid macular degeneration
cytomegalic disease

CME
cervical mediastinal exploration
cervical mucous extract
continuing medical education
crude marijuana extract
cystoid macular edema

CMEC
central mucoepidermoid carcinoma

CME-MRI
contrast medium-enhanced magnetic
    resonance imaging

CMER
current medical evidence of record

11C-MET-PET
carbon-11 methionine positron emission
    tomography

CM EVA
compression-molded ethylene vinyl
    acetate

CMF
calcium-magnesium free
catabolite modular factor
chondromyxoid fibroma
cortical magnification factor
craniomandibulofacial

CMFE
calcium and magnesium free plus
    ethylenediaminetetraacetic acid
    [medium]

CMFT
cardiolipin microflocculation test

CMFTD
congenital muscle fiber-type
    disproportion

CMG
canine myasthenia gravis
chopped-meat [and] glucose
    [medium]
congenital myasthenia gravis
cyanmethemoglobin
cystometrograph(y) (cystometrogram)

CMGM
chronic megakaryocytic granulocytic
    myelosis

CMGN
chronic membranous glomerulonephritis

CMGS
chopped meat-glucose-starch
    [medium]

CMGT
chromosome-mediated gene transfer

CMH
cardiomyopathy, hypertrophic
congenital malformation of heart

CMHC
community mental health center

cm H₂O
centimeter of water [cuff pressure]

CMHS
Cook-Medley Hostility Score

CMI
carbohydrate metabolism index
Career Maturity Inventory
care management integration
cell-mediated immunity
cell multiplication inhibition
chronically mentally ill
chronic mesenteric ischemia
circulating microemboli index
colonic motility index
combined myocardial infarction
computed maxillofacial imaging
computer-managed instruction
Cornell Medical Index

CMID
cytomegalic inclusion disease (*See also*
    CID)

c/min
cycle per minute

CMIR
cell-mediated immune response

CMIS
common mucosal immune
    system

CMIT
*Current Medical Information and
    Terminology*

CMJ
carpometacarpal joint
cervicomedullary junction
corticomedullary junction

CMK
chloromethyl ketone
congenital multicystic kidney

CML
cell-mediated lymphocytotoxicity
cell-mediated lympholysis
cell-mediated lysis
central motor latency
chronic myeloblastic (myelocytic)
    (myelogenous) (myeloid) leukemia
count median length
cross midline

C

CML AP
　chronic myeloblastic (myelocytic)
　(myelogenous) (myeloid) leukemia
　accelerated phase
CML BC
　chronic myeloblastic (myelocytic)
　(myelogenous) (myeloid) leukemia
　blast crisis
CML CP
　chronic myeloblastic (myelocytic)
　(myelogenous) (myeloid) leukemia
　chronic phase
CMLV
　camelpox virus
CMM
　cell-mediated mutagenesis
　cerebellomedullary malformation
　coordinate measuring machine
　[orthopedic surgery]
　cutaneous malignant melanoma
cmm
　cubic millimeter (*See also* cu mm,
　mm³)
cm/m²
　centimeter per square meter
CMMC
　cervical myelomeningocele
CMME
　chloromethyl methyl ether [carcinogen
　at technical grade]
CMMHN
　cutaneous malignant melanoma of head
　and neck
CMML
　chronic myelomonocytic leukemia
CMMS
　Columbia Mental Maturity Scale
CMN
　caudal mediastinal node
　congenital melanocytic nevus
　congenital mesoblastic nephroma
　cranial motor nuclei
　cystic medial necrosis
CMN-AA
　cystic medial necrosis of ascending
　aorta
CMO
　calculated mean organisms
　capillary membrane oxygenator
　cardiac minute output
　card made out
　chronic mastoid osteomyelitis
　comfort measures only
　conventional mechanical orthosis
　corticosterone methyl oxidase
CMOAT
　canicular multispecific organic anion
　transporter

CMOR
　craniomandibular orthopedic
　repositioning device
CMP
　calorie-protein malnutrition
　captioned media program
　cardiomyopathy (*See also* CM)
　cervical mucus penetration
　chondromalacia patellae
　colorimetric microtiter plate
　competitive medical plans
　complementary medical practice
　complexity of mental processes
　comprehensive (complete) metabolic
　panel (profile)
　comprehensive medical plan
　control measurement point
　cow's milk protein
　crossmodal priming
　cushion mouthpiece
　cytidine monophosphate
CMPD
　chronic myeloproliferative disorder
CMP-FX
　complement fixation
CMPGN
　chronic membranoproliferative
　glomerulonephritis
CMP-NANA
　cytidine
　monophospho-*N*-acetylneuraminic acid
CMPS
　chronic musculoskeletal (myofascial)
　pain syndrome
cmps
　centimeter per second (*See also* cm/s)
CMPT
　cervical mucus penetration test
CMR
　cardiomodulorespirography
　cardiovascular magnetic resonance
　carpometacarpal ratio
　cerebral metabolic rate
　chief medical resident
　chylomicron remnant
　common mode rejection
　congenital mitral regurgitation
　crude mortality ratio
CMRE
　California Marriage Readiness
　Evaluation
CMRG, CMR_glc
　cerebral metabolic rate of glucose
CMRI
　cardiovascular magnetic resonance
　imaging
CMRL
　cerebral metabolic rate of lactate

CMRNG
chromosomally mediated resistant
Neisseria gonorrhoeae

CMRO₂
cerebral metabolic rate of oxygen

CMRP
cervicalmagnetic resonance phlebography

CMRR
common mode rejection ratio [of
amplifiers]

CMRT
chiropractic manipulative reflex
technique

CMS
cardiomediastinal silhouette
Cardiovascular Measurement system
Centers for Medicare and Medicaid
Services
central margin syndrome
central material section
central material supply
cervical mucous solution
cholesterol monitoring system
chromosome modification site
chronic mycelial stomatitis
chronic myelodysplastic syndrome
circulation, motion, sensation
clean, midstream [urinalysis] (*See also*
CMSUA)
click-murmur syndrome
clofibrate-induced muscular syndrome
Clyde Mood Scale
compliance matching stent
Conflict Management Survey
continuous motion syndrome
cortical magnetic stimulation
cytoplasmic male sterility

cm/s
centimeter per second

CMSD
congenital myocardial sympathetic
dysinnervation

CMSE
cow's milk-sensitive enteropathy

CMSS
circulation, motor (ability), sensation,
swelling

CMSUA
clean midstream urinalysis (*See also*
CMS)

CMT
California mastitis test
cancer multistep therapy
carpometatarsal [joint]
catechol methyltransferase
cervical motion tenderness
chemotherapy

chiropractic manipulative therapy
(treatment)
chronic motor tic
circus-movement tachycardia
combined modality therapy
complex motor tic
Concept Mastery Test
Contextual Memory Test
continuous memory test
Current Medical Terminology
cutis marmorata telangiectasis

CMTC
cutis marmorata telangiectatica congenita

CMU
cardiac monitoring unit
chlorophenyldimethylurea
complex motor unit

CMUA
continuous motor unit activity

CMV
Clo Mor virus
continuous mandatory ventilation
continuous mechanical ventilation
controlled mechanical ventilation
conventional mechanical ventilation
cool mist vaporizer
cucumber mosaic virus
cytomegalovirus

CMV-E
cytomegalovirus encephalitis

CMVIg
cytomegalovirus immune globulin
(immunoglobulin)

CMV-IgIV
cytomegalovirus immune globulin
(immunoglobulin) intravenous

CMV-MN
cytomegaloviral mononucleosis

CMVS
culture midvoid specimen

CMV-VE
cytomegalovirus ventriculoencephalitis

CN
calcaneonavicular
calcineurin
caudate nucleus
cellulose nitrate
charge nurse
child nutrition
clinical nursing
cochlear nucleus
congenital nephrosis
congenital nystagmus
cranial nerve (*See also* cr nn)
cyanogen
cyanosis neonatorum
NATO code for 1-chloroacetophenone

C-N
circumference of chest at nipple

C:N
carbon to nitrogen ratio
contrast to noise ratio (*See also* CNR)
carrier to noise ratio

CN −
cyanide radical

CN 1–12, CN I–XII
cranial nerves 1–12 (I–XII)

CN 1, CN I
first cranial nerve [olfactory]

CN 2, CN II
second cranial nerve [optic]

CN 3, CN III
third cranial nerve [oculomotor]

CN 4, CN IV
fourth cranial nerve [trochlear]

CN 5, CN V
fifth cranial nerve [trigeminal]

CN V1
trigeminal [fifth cranial nerve,
ophthalmic division]

CN V2
trigeminal [fifth cranial nerve, maxillary
division]

CN V3
trigeminal [fifth cranial nerve,
mandibular division]

CN 6, CN VI
sixth cranial nerve [abducent]

CN 7, CN VII
seventh cranial nerve [facial]

CN 8, CN VIII
eighth cranial nerve [vestibulocochlear]

CN 9, CN IX
ninth cranial nerve [glossopharyngeal]

CN 10, CN X
tenth cranial nerve [vagus]

CN 11, CN XI
eleventh cranial nerve [accessory]

CN 12, CN XII
twelfth cranial nerve [hypoglossal]

Cn
color naming
cyanide

CNA
calcium nutrient agar
chart not available

CNAF
chronic nonvalvular atrial fibrillation

CNAG
chronic narrow angle glaucoma

CNAP
cochlear nerve action potential
compound nerve action potential
continuous negative airway pressure

CNAV
Canancia virus

CNB
core needle biopsy
cutting needle biopsy

CNBr
cyanogen bromide [poisonous vapor]

CNC
clear no creamy [layer]

CNCbl
cyanocobalamin

CNCH
chondrodermatitis nodularis chronica
helicis

CND
canned
cannot determine
cause not determined
chronic nausea and dyspepsia
congenital neuromuscular disorder

CNDC
chronic nonspecific diarrhea of
childhood
chronic nonsuppurative destructive
cholangitis

CNDI
congenital nephrogenic diabetes
insipidus

CNDO
complete neglect of differential overlap

CNE
chronic nervous exhaustion
concentric needle electrode
could not establish
culture-negative endocarditis

CNEMG
concentric needle electromyography

CNEP
continuous negative extrathoracic
pressure

CNES
chronic nervous exhaustion syndrome

C-NES
conversion nonepileptic seizure

CNF
chronic nodular fibrositis
congenital nephrotic [syndrome],
Finnish

CNFA
clinically nonfunctioning pituitary
adenoma

CNFS
craniofrontonasal syndrome

CNH
central neurogenic hyperventilation

CNHD
congenital nonspherocytic hemolytic
disease

CNI
calcineurin inhibitor
chronic nerve irritation

CNK
cortical necrosis of kidneys
CNL
cardiolipin natural lecithin
chronic neutrophilic leukemia
CNLD
chronic neonatal lung disease
CNLDO
congenital nasolacrimal duct obstruction
CNM
centronuclear myopathy
computerized nuclear morphometry
CNMD
chronic neuromuscular disease
CNMP
chronic nonmalignant pain
CNN
congenital nevocytic nevus
CNNA
culture-negative neutrocytic ascites
cNOS
constitutive nitric oxide synthase
CNP
capillary nonperfusion
chronic nonbacterial prostatitis
constant negative pressure
continuous negative pressure
cranial nerve palsy
C-type natriuretic peptide
cyclic nucleotide phosphodiesterase
CNPAP
continuous nasal positive airway
pressure
CNPAS
congenital nasal pyriform aperture
stenosis
CNPase
cyclic nucleotide phosphohydrolase
CNPB
continuous negative-pressure breathing
CNPS
cardiac nuclear probe scan
CNPV
continuous negative-pressure
ventilation
CNQ
Cancer Needs Questionnaire
Child Neuropsychological Questionnaire
CNR
contrast to noise ratio (*See also* C:N)
coronary nodal rhythm
CNRS
citrated normal rabbit serum
CNRT
corrected sinus nodal recovery time
CNS
central nervous system

coagulase-negative staphylococcus
(*See also* CONS, CoNS)
computerized notation system
congenital nephrotic syndrome
CNSB
coagulase-negative staphylococcus
bacteremia
CNSD
chronic nonspecific diarrhea
CNSHA
congenital nonspherocytic hemolytic
anemia
CNS-L
central nervous system leukemia
CNSLD
chronic nonspecific lung disease
CNT
clean needle technique
Clostridium neurotoxin
continuous nebulization therapy
could not test
current night terrors
cutaneous neural tumor
CNTA
combined neurosurgical and transfacial
approach
CNTF
ciliary neurotrophic factor
CNTHM
conotruncal heart malformation
CNTV
Connecticut virus
CNUV
Chenuda virus
CNV
choroidal neovascularization
conative negative variation
contingent negative variation
cutaneous necrotizing vasculitis
CNVM
choroidal neovascular membrane
CO
calcium oxalate
candidal onychomycosis
carbon monoxide
cardiac output (*See also* Q)
castor oil
casualty officer
central obesity
centric occlusion
cervical orthosis
choline oxidase
coenzyme
community organization
complains (complaining) of
continuous observation
control

CO *(continued)*
corneal opacity
coronary occlusion
crossover
Co
cobalt
Co I, II
coenzyme I, II
co
cutoff
C/O, c/o
check out
complains of
complaints
[in or under] care of
CO_3^{2-}
carbonate
CO_2
carbon dioxide (*See also* CD)
^{57}Co
cobalt-57
^{58}Co
cobalt-58
^{60}Co
cobalt-60
COA
calculated opening area
cervicooculoacusticus [syndrome]
child of alcoholic
coagglutination
coarctation of aorta (*See also* CoA,
coarc)
condition on admission
consent of admission
CoA
coarctation of aorta (*See also* CoA,
coarc)
coenzyme A
COAB
Computer Operator Aptitude
Battery
COACH
cerebellar vermis hypo/aplasia,
oligophrenia, congenital ataxia, ocular
coloboma, hepatic fibrosis
Choosing Outcomes and
Accommodations for Children
COAD
chronic obstructive airway disease
COAG
chronic open angle glaucoma
coagulase
coagulate(d)
coagulation [study, panel] (*See also*
coags)
coag pd
coagulation profile diagnosis
coag pp
coagulation profile presurgery

coags
coagulation panel (*See also* COAG)
coagsc
coagulation screen
coag T
coagulation time
COAL
chronic obstructive airflow limitation
coarc
coarctation of aorta (*See also* CoA,
COA)
COAS
Complete Ophthalmic Analysis System
CoASH
coenzyme A
CoA-SPC
coenzyme A-synthesizing protein
complex
COAT
Children's Orientation and Amnesia
Test
chronic opioid analgesic therapy
COB
chronic obstructive bronchitis
coordination of benefits
COBE
chronic obstructive bullous emphysema
COBRA
Consolidated Omnibus Budget
Reconciliation Act
COBS
cesarean [section]-obtained
barrier-sustained [animals]
chronic organic brain syndrome
COBT
chronic obstruction of biliary tract
COC
calcifying odotogenic cyst
cement-on-crown
chain of custody
coccygeal (*See also* coc)
combined (combination) oral
contraceptive
continuity of care
COCA
Clinician Outreach and Communication
Activity
CO/CI
cardiac output/cardiac index
COCM
congestive cardiomyopathy
CoCN6
cobalticyanide
CO_2 comb
carbon dioxide combining power
CO_2 cont
carbon dioxide content
COCP
combination oral contraceptive pill

Co-Cr-Mo
cobalt-chromium-molybdenum [alloy]
Co-Cr-W-Ni
cobalt-chromium-tungsten-nickel [alloy
metal implant]
COCV
Cocal virus
COD
carotid occlusive disease
cause of death
cementoosseous dysplasia
cerebroocular dysgenesis
chemical oxygen demand
chronic oxygen dependency
coefficient of oxygen delivery
computerized optical densitometry
condition on discharge
CODA
cadaveric organ donor act
Canadian Organ Donors Association
Codependents Anonymous
CODAS
cerebral, ocular, dental, auricular,
skeletal [syndrome]
CoDe
coincidence detection
CODEC
compression and decompression
CODIS
combined deoxyribonucleic acid index
system
CODM
craniooculoorbital dysraphia-
meningocele
COD-MD
cerebroocular dysplasia-muscular
dystrophy
CODO
codocyte
COE
court-ordered examination
coeff
coefficient
COEPS
cortical originating extrapyramidal
system
COF
cementoossifying fibroma
cutoff frequency
CoF
cobra [venom] factor
cofactor
COFHP
chronic oral, facial, head pain
COFS
cerebrooculofacial-skeletal
[syndrome]

COG
center of gravity
clinical obstetrics and gynecology
closed angle glaucoma
cognitive [function tests]
Cognitive Observation Guide
COGN
cognition
COGTT
cortisone-primed oral glucose tolerance
test
COH
control of hemorrhage
controlled ovarian hyperstimulation
COI
Central Obesity Index
combination of isotonics
COIB
Crowley Occupational Interests
Blank
COIF
congenital onychodysplasia of index
finger
COL, col
colicin
colony
color
colored
colostrum
colposcopy
column
cost of living
COL2A1
type II procollagen gene
COLAP
colonoscopic allergen provocation
COLD
chronic obstructive lung disease
COLD A, cold agg
cold agglutinin [titer]
COLDER
character, onset, location, duration,
exacerbation, remission [medical
screening]
COLL, coll
collect(ion) (collective)
colloidal
collat
collateral
collut.
mouthwash [L. *collutorium*]
coll vol
collective volume
COLLYR, collyr.
eyewash [G. *kollyrion*]
col/mL
colony per milliliter

C

color
　　colorimetry [including spectrophotometry and photometry]
　　let it be colored [L. *coloretur*]
colp, colpo
　　colporrhaphy
　　colposcopy
CoLV
　　Cole [vegetable] latent virus
COM
　　calcium oxalate monohydrate
　　chronic otitis media
　　computer output on microfilm
com
　　comminute(d)
　　commit(ment)
COMA
　　congenital ocular motor apraxia [type Cogan]
comb.
　　combine (combination)
COMBI
　　continuous moving bed imaging [magnetic resonance]
COMBIMAN
　　Computerized Biomechanical Man
COME
　　chronic otitis media with effusion
COMF, comf
　　comfortable
com fix
　　complement fixing (fixation) (*See also* CF)
comm
　　commission(er)
　　committee
　　communicable (*See also* commun)
commun
　　communicable (*See also* comm)
commun dis
　　communicable disease
COMP
　　cartilage oligomeric matrix protein
comp
　　comparable
　　comparative
　　compare (*See also* CF, cf.)
　　compensate(d) (compensation)
　　complaint
　　complete
　　complicating
　　complication
　　composition (*See also* compn)
　　compound(ed) (*See also* C)
　　comprehension
　　compress
　　compression
　　computer

compet
　　competition
compl
　　complete(d) (completion) (*See also* C, cpl)
　　complicate(d) (complication) (*See also* complic)
complic
　　complicate(d) (complication) (*See also* compl)
compn
　　composition (*See also* comp)
COMS
　　cerebrooculomuscular syndrome
　　chronic organic mental syndrome
　　clinical outcome management system
COMT
　　catechol-*O*-methyltransferase
COMTRAC
　　computer-based [case] tracing
COMUL
　　complement fixation murine leukosis [test]
CON
　　catheter over needle
　　certificate of need
Con
　　concanavalin
con.
　　against [L. *contra*] (*See also* cont.)
ConA
　　concanavalin A
ConA-HRP
　　concanavalin A horseradish peroxidase
CONAMORE
　　Conflict And Management Of Relationships
conc, concentr
　　concentrate(d) (concentration)
COND
　　cerebroosteonephrodysplasia
cond
　　condense(d) (condensation)
　　condition(ed) (conditioning) (*See also* C)
　　conditional
　　conduction
　　conductivity (*See also* σ)
cond ref
　　conditioned reflex (*See also* CR)
cond resp
　　conditioned response (*See also* CR)
conf
　　conference
congen, cong
　　congenital
congHD
　　congenital heart disease
congr
　　congruent

coniz
conization [of cervix]
conj
conjunctiva [singular] (conjunctivae [plural])
conjunctival
conjug
conjugate(d)
conjugation
CONS, CoNS
coagulase-negative staphylococcus (*See also* CNS)
cons
conservation
conservative
conserve
consultant
consult(ation) (*See also* C)
const
constant
constit
constituent
cont
contain(ing)
contains
contents
continuation
continue
contusions
cont.
against [L. *contra*] (*See also* con.)
bruised [L. *contusus*] (*See also* C)
contag
contagion
contagious
contr
contraction (*See also* C, contrx, CTX, CTXN, CX)
contra
contraindicated
contralat
contralateral
contrib
contributory
contrx
contraction (*See also* C, contr, CTX, CTXN, CX)
conv
convalescent (convalescence) (convalescing)
conventional [rat]
convergent (convergence) (*See also* C)
conv hosp
convalescent hospital
conv strab
convergent strabismus

COOD
chronic obstruction (obstructive) outflow disease
coord
coordinate(d) (coordination)
CO-oximeter
carbon monoxide oximeter
CO-oximetry
carbon monoxide oximetry
COP
capillary osmotic pressure
change of plaster
cicatricial ocular pemphigoid
circumoval precipitin
coatomer protein
coefficient of performance
colloid(al) osmotic pressure
colloid(al) oncotic pressure
cryptogenic organizing pneumonia (pneumonitis)
COP 1
copolymer 1
COPA
cuffed oropharyngeal airway
COPC
community-oriented primary care
COPD
chronic obstructive pulmonary disease
COPE
chronic obstructive pulmonary emphysema
Coping Operations Preference Enquiry
Coping Orientations to Problems Experienced
COPES
Community-Oriented Programs Environment Scale
COPI
California Occupational Preference Inventory
COP$_i$
colloid(al) osmotic pressure in interstitial fluid
COPM
Canadian Occupational Performance Measure
COP$_p$
colloid(al) osmotic pressure in plasma
COPRO
coproporphyria (coproporphyrin) (*See also* CP)
COPS
calcinosis cutis, osteoma cutis, poikiloderma, skeletal abnormalities
California Occupational Preference Survey

COPT
computerized oxygen therapy protocol
COPU
cutaneous oropharyngeal ulceration
CoQ
coenzyme Q [ubiquinone] (*See also* Q)
CoQ$_{10}$
coenzyme Q10
COR
body [L. *corpus*]
cardiac output recorder
cervicoocular reflex
coefficient of reproducibility
conditioned orientation reflex
[audiometry]
coroner
corrosion (corrosive)
cortisone
CoR
corepressor
Cor
Congo red (*See also* CR)
cor
coronary [heart]
CORA
conditioned orientation reflex
audiometry
CORB
counterrotational biopsy [device]
CORD
chronic obstructive respiratory disease
Cor Flow
coronary blood flow
CORLA
clusters of radiolucent areas
CorPP
coronary perfusion pressure
corr
correct(ed) (correction)
correspond(ence)
cort
cortex (*See also* C)
cortical
CORTES
coordinate reduction time encoding
system [digital compression EKG]
CORTIS
cortisol
CORV
Corriparta virus
COS
cheirooral syndrome
childhood-onset schizophrenia
clinically observed seizure
controlled ovarian stimulation
cos
change of shift
COSA
child of substance abuser

Cosm
osmolar clearance
COSTAR
computer-stored ambulatory record
COSTART
Coding Symbols for a Thesaurus of
Adverse Reaction Terms [FDA]
COSY
correlated spectroscopy
COT
colony overlay test
content of thought
continuous oxygen therapy
contralateral optic tectum
court-ordered treatment
critical off-time
CO$_2$T
total carbon dioxide content
COTD
cardiac output by thermodilution
COTE
comprehensive occupational therapy
evaluation
COTX
cast off to x-ray (*See also* COX)
COU
cardiac observation unit
COUP
chicken ovalbumin upstream promoter
COUP-TF
chicken ovalbumin upstream
promoter-transcription factor
COV
coefficient of variation [statistics]
crossover value
CoV
coronavirus
COVESDEM
costovertebral segmentation defect with
mesomelia [syndrome]
CoVF
cobra venom factor
COW
circle of Willis
COWAT
Controlled Oral Word Association Test
COWS
cold-opposite, warm-same [Hallpike
caloric stimulation response]
COX
cast off to x-ray (*See also* COTX)
coxsackievirus
cyclooxygenase
cytochrome c oxidase
COX1–COX5
cyclooxygenase 1–5
COX mRNA
cyclooxygenase messenger
ribonucleoprotein acid

COZ
  cranioorbitozygomatic osteotomy
CP
  canal paresis
  capillary pressure
  carbamide peroxide
  carbamoyl phosphate
  cardiac pacing
  cardiac performance
  cardiac pool
  cardiopulmonary
  Carr-Purcell [sequence, MRI]
  caudate putamen
  cell passaged
  central pit
  centric position
  cephalic presentation
  cerebellopontine
  cerebral palsy
  ceruloplasmin (caeruloplasmin [British])
    (*See also* CER, CERULO)
  cervical probe
  chemically pure (*See also* cp)
  chemical peel
  chemistry profile
  chest pain
  chickenpox
  child psychiatry
  child psychology
  Chlamydia pneumoniae
  chloropurine
  chondrodysplasia punctata
  chondromalacia patellae
  choroid plexus
  chronic pain
  chronic pancreatitis
  chronic polyarthritis
  chronic pyelonephritis
  cicatricial pemphigoid
  circular polarization
  classical pathway
  cleft palate (*See also* Clpal)
  clinical pathology (*See also* clin path,
    CLP)
  closing pressure
  clottable protein
  cochlear potential
  Code of Practice
  cold pack
  cold pressor
  color perception
  combination product
  combining power
  commercially pure
  complete physical
  compound(ed) (*See also* CO, comp, cpd)
  compress(ed)

  congenital porphyria
  constant pressure
  constrictive pericarditis
  coproporphyria (coproporphyrin)
    (*See also* COPRO)
  coracoid process
  cornual pregnancy
  coronal plane
  cor pulmonale
  cortical plate
  costal plaque
  costophrenic [angle]
  coverage probability [radiotherapy]
  C peptide
  creatine phosphate
  creatine phosphokinase
  crosslinked protein
  cross-polarization
  crude protein
  current practice
  cystopanendoscopy
  cystosarcoma phyllodes
  cytosol protein
C + P
  cryotherapy with pressure
C:P
  carbohydrate to protein ratio
  cholesterol to phospholipid ratio
C&P
  compensation and pension
  complete and pain-free [range of
    motion]
  complete and pushing [stage of labor]
  cystoscopy and panendoscopy
    [pyelogram]
C$_p$
  constant pressure
  phosphate clearance (*See also* Cp)
Cp
  chickenpox (*See also* chix, CHPX,
    chpx)
  Corynebacterium parvum
  peak concentration
  phosphate clearance (*See also* C$_p$)
cP
  centipoise
cp
  candlepower [candela] (*See also* CP)
  chemically pure (*See also* CP)
CP II
  c propeptide of type II collagen
CPA
  calcaneal pitch angle
  carboxypeptidase A
  cardiophrenic angle
  cardiopulmonary arrest
  carotid phonoangiography

C

CPA *(continued)*
cerebellopontine angle
chlorophenylalanine
chronic pyrophosphate arthropathy
circulating platelet aggregate
conditioned play audiometry
condylar plateau angle
control, preoccupation, addiction
corneal polarization axis
costophrenic angle
cumulative phase advancement
C3PA
complement 3 proactivator [convertase]
c:pa
crown to pubic arch ratio
CPAB
Computer Programmer Aptitude Battery
CPAC
clusters of pancreatic acinar cells
C-PAC, CPAC
Clinical Probes of Articulation
Consistency
C-PACG
chronic primary angle-closure
glaucoma
CPAD
chronic peripheral arterial disease
CPAF
chlorpropamide-alcohol flushing [trait]
Cpah, C$_{pah}$
p-aminohippurate clearance
p-aminohippuric acid clearance
CPAI
central principal axis of inertia
CPA/OPG
carotid phonoangiography [and]
oculoplethysmography
CPAP
constant (continuous) positive airway
pressure
CPB
carboxypeptidase B
cardiopulmonary bypass
celiac plexus block
competitive protein binding
controlled position brace
CPBA
competitive protein-binding assay
CPBS
cardiopulmonary bypass surgery
CPBV
cardiopulmonary blood volume
CPC
central posterior curve
cerebellar Purkinje cell
cerebral palsy clinic
cetylpyridinium chloride
chest pain center
choroid plexus carcinoma

choroid plexus cyst
chronic passive congestion
circumferential pneumatic compression
clinicopathologic conference
clinicopathologic correlation
committed progenitor cell
conventional papillary carcinoma
corrective pigment camouflage
CP&C
cast, post, and core [dental]
CPCB
continuous psoas compartment block
CPCL
congenital pulmonary cystic
lymphangiectasia
CP-CML
chronic phase chronic myelogenous
leukemia
CPCN
capitated primary care network
CPCP
chronic progressive coccidioidal
pneumonitis
CPCR
cardiopulmonary-cerebral resuscitation
cPCR
competitive polymerase chain reaction
CPCS
circumferential pneumatic compression
suit
clinical pharmacokinetics consulting
service
CPCV
Cacipacore virus
CPD
calcium pyrophosphate deposition
calcium pyrophosphate dihydrate
cephalopelvic disproportion
cerebelloparenchymal disorder
childhood polycystic disease
chorioretinopathy and pituitary
dysfunction
chronic peritoneal dialysis
chronic pulmonary disease
citrate-phosphate-dextrose [solution]
congenital penile deviation
congenital polycystic disease
contact potential difference
contagious pustular dermatitis
continuous peritoneal dialysis
critical point drying
cryopoor plasma
cyclopentadiene
cpd
compound(ed) (*See also* CO,
comp, CP)
cycle per degree
CPD I–IV
cerebelloparenchymal disorder IV

CPDA
citrate-phosphate-dextrose-adenine [type 1, 2]

CPDD
calcium pyrophosphate dihydrate deposition [disease] (*See also* CPPD, CPPDD)

CPDL
cumulative population doubling level

CPDN
cystic partially differentiated nephroblastoma

CPDV
contagious pustular dermatitis

CPE
cardiac (cardiogenic) pulmonary edema
chronic pulmonary emphysema
Clostridium perfringens enterotoxin
clubbing, pitting, edema
compensation, pension, education
complete physical examination (*See also* CPX)
complex partial epilepsy
complicated pleural effusion
corona-penetrating enzyme
cryptogenic partial epilepsy
cystopanendoscopy
cytopathic effect

CPEO
chronic progressive external ophthalmoplegia

CPE-R
Clostridium perfringens enterotoxin receptor

CPET
cardiopulmonary exercise test

CP-EUS
catheter probe-assisted endoluminal ultrasonography

CPEV
Chironomus plumosus entomopoxvirus

CPF
clot-promoting factor
complication probability factor
contraction peak force

C-PF
coronary-pulmonary fistula

CP&FD
cephalopelvic disproportion and fetal distress

CPG
capillary blood gases
cardiopneumographic [recording]
carotid phonoangiogram
clinical practice guidelines
computerized pattern generator
craniopharyngioma

CpG
cytosine phosphate guanine

CPGN
chronic progressive (proliferative) glomerulonephritis

CpGV
Cydia pomonella granulovirus

CPH
carboxypeptidase H
chronic paroxysmal hemicrania
chronic persistent hepatitis
chronic primary headache

CPHD
combined pituitary hormone deficiency

CpHV
caprine herpesvirus

CPI
California Personality Inventory
California Psychological Inventory
Cancer Potential Index
chronic pneumonitis of infancy
Clostridium perfringens enterotoxin iota (ι)
Community Periodontal Index
congenital pain indifference
congenital palatopharyngeal incompetence
constitutional psychopathic inferiority
conventional planar imaging
coronary prognosis (prognostic) index
cysteine proteinase inhibitor

CPIB
chlorophenoxyisobutyrate

CPID
chronic pelvic inflammatory disease

CPIP
chronic pulmonary insufficiency of prematurity
common peak isovolumetric pressure

CPIR
cephalic-phase insulin release

CPIS
clinical pulmonary infection score

CPIT
California Psychological Inventory Test

CPITN
Community Periodontal Index of Treatment Needs [WHO]

CPK
creatine phosphokinase

CPK-BB
creatine phosphokinase brain band [isoenzyme] (*See also* BB, CK-BB)

CPKD
childhood polycystic kidney disease

CPKI, CPKISO
creatine phosphokinase isoenzyme(s)

CPK-MB
  creatine phosphokinase myocardial band
    (*See also* CK-MB)
  creatine phosphokinase muscle band
    [isoenzyme] (*See also* CK-MB, MB,
    MB CK)
CPK-MM
  creatine phosphokinase skeletal muscle
    [isoenzyme] (*See also* CK-MM)
CPL
  caprine placental lactogen
  conditioned pitch level
  congenital pulmonary lymphangiectasia
    (lymphangiectasis)
C:PL
  cholesterol to phospholipid ratio
cpl
  complete(d) (completion) (*See also*
    compl)
cPLA2
  cytosol phospholipase A2
CPLM
  cysteine-peptone-liver infusion medium
CPLS
  cleft palate-lateral synechia syndrome
CPM
  cancer pain management
  central pontine myelinolysis
  chronic progressive myelopathy
  Clinical Practice Model
  cognitive-perceptual-motor
  Colored Progressive Matrices (*See also*
    RCPM)
  confined placental mosaicism
  continue present management
  continuous passive motion [device]
  count per minute (*See also* C/M, cpm)
  cycle per minute (*See also* cpm)
cpm
  count per minute (*See also* C/M, CPM)
  cycle per minute (*See also* CPM)
CPmax
  calculated maximum peak concentration
    [in serum]
  maximum serum concentration [peak]
CP-MCT
  chirp pulse microwave computed
    tomography
CPMDI
  computerized pharmacokinetic-model
    drug infusion
CPMG
  Carr-Purcell-Meiboom-Gill [sequence,
    spin-echo technique]
CPMI
  central principal moment of inertia
CPmin
  minimum serum concentration
    [trough]

CPMM
  constant passive-motion machine
CPMP
  computer-patient management problems
CPMS
  chronic progressive multiple sclerosis
CPN
  carboxypeptidase N
  celiac plexus neurolysis
  chronic polyneuropathy
  chronic pyelonephritis
  cisplatin nephropathy
  common peroneal nerve
CPNC
  chronic progressive nonhereditary
    chorea
cPNET
  central primitive neuroectodermal tumor
CPNM
  corrected perinatal mortality
CPO
  cardiac power output
CPOM
  continuous pulse oximeter monitoring
CPOS
  chest pain order sheet
CPOTHA
  chest pain onset to hospital arrival
CPP
  cancer proneness phenotype
  canine pancreatic polypeptide
  career planning program
  central precocious puberty
  cerebral perfusion pressure
  chest pain policy (protocol)
  choroid plexus papilloma
  chronic pelvic pain
  chronic pigmental purpura
  community psychiatry program
  conditioned place preference
  coronary perfusion pressure
  cranial perfusion pressure
  cryoprecipitate
CPPB
  continuous positive-pressure breathing
CPPD
  calcium pyrophosphate dihydrate
    deposition [disease] (*See also* CPDD,
    CPPDD)
  chest percussion and postural drainage
    (*See also* CP&PD)
CP&PD
  chest percussion and postural drainage
    (*See also* CPPD)
CPPDD
  calcium pyrophosphate deposition
    disease (*See also* CPDD)
CPPS
  chronic pelvic pain syndrome

chronic prostate pain syndrome
chronic prostatitis [and] pelvic pain
  syndrome
cPPT
central polypurine tract
CPPTS
complete pacemaker patient testing
  system
CPPV
continuous positive-pressure ventilation
CPQ
Children's Personality Questionnaire
Conners Parent Questionnaire
CPR
cardiac and pulmonary rehabilitation
cardiopulmonary reserve
cardiopulmonary resuscitation
centripetal rub
cerebral cortex perfusion rate
chlorophenyl red
clinical partial response
cochleopalpebral reflex
computer-based patient record
cortisol production rate
cumulative potency rate
curved multiplanar reformation
customary, prevailing, and reasonable
CPRAM
controlled partial rebreathing anesthesia
  method
CPRCA
constitutional pure red [blood] cell
  aplasia
CPRD
chronic progressive renal disease
CP/ROMI
chest pain, rule out myocardial
  infarction
CPRS
Categorical Pain Relief Scale
Children's Psychiatric Rating Scale
Comprehensive Psychopathological
  Rating Scale
CPS
carbamoyl phosphate synthetase
  [deficiency]
cardioplegic perfusion solution
cardiopulmonary support
cervical pain syndrome
character per second
chest pain syndrome
Child Personality Scale
Child Protective Services (Children's
  Protective Service)
Chinese paralytic syndrome
chronic paranoid schizophrenia
chronic prostatitis syndrome

clinical performance score
clinical pharmacokinetic service
coagulase-positive staphylococcus
complex partial seizure
compliant prestress system
Comrey Personality Scale
constitutional psychopathic state
contagious pustular stomatitis
coronary perfusate (perfusion) solution
count per second (*See also* cps)
C-polysaccharide
cumulative pain score
cumulative probability of success
current population survey
capsular polysaccharide
cps
count per second (*See also* CPS)
cycle per second (*See also* c/s, c/sec)
cPSA
complexed prostate-specific antigen
CPSC
congenital paucity of secondary synaptic
  clefts [syndrome]
CPSCS
California Preschool Social Competency
  Scale
CPSD
carbamoyl phosphate synthetase
  deficiency
corrected pattern standard deviation
  [statistics]
CPSE
complex partial status epilepticus
CPSI
Children's Perception of Support
  Inventory
Chronic Prostatitis Symptom Index
CPSMP
chronic pain self-management program
CPSP
central poststroke pain
CPSR
chronic paranoid schizophrenic reaction
CPT
carnitine palmitoyltransferase
carotid pulse tracing
chest physical therapy (physiotherapy)
child protection team
choline phosphotransferase
chromopertubation
ciliary particle transport
Cognitive Performance Test
cold pressor test
collarless polished tapered [stem, hip
  prosthesis]
combining power test
conjunctival provocation test

C

CPT *(continued)*
  continuous performance task (test)
  corticosteroid pulse treatment
  current perception threshold
  Current Procedural Terminology
CPT1
  carnitine palmitoyltransferase 1
    [deficiency]
CPT2
  carnitine palmitoyltransferase 2
    [deficiency]
CPT-ACC
  continuous performance task accuracy
CPT-EFF
  continuous performance task
    efficiency
CPTH
  chronic posttraumatic headache
  C-terminal parathyroid hormone
CPTN
  culture-positive toxin-negative
CPTP
  culture-positive toxin-positive
CPTX
  chronic parathyroidectomy
CPU
  caudate putamen
  central processing unit
CPUE
  chest pain of unknown etiology
CPV
  canine parvovirus
  Costal Plains virus
  Cotia virus
  cowpox virus
  cytoplasmic polyhedrosis virus
CPVC
  common pulmonary venous channel
CPVD
  congenital polyvalvular disease
cPVL
  cystic periventricular leukomalacia
CPX
  calciphylaxis
  cardiopulmonary exercise
  cleft palate, X-linked
  complete physical examination (*See also*
    CPE)
CPXD
  chondrodysplasia punctata, X-linked
    dominant
CPXR
  chondrodysplasia punctata, X-linked
    recessive
CQ
  circadian quotient
  conceptual quotient
CQA
  concurrent quality assurance

CQDS
  cumulative quality disruption score
CQI
  continuous quality improvement
CQIV
  Calchaqui virus
CR
  calcification rate
  calorie restricted
  capillary refill
  cardiac rehabilitation
  cardiac resuscitation
  cardiac rhythm
  cardiorespiratory
  cardiorrhexis
  caries resistant
  cartilage residue
  case report
  cathode ray
  center of rotation
  central ray
  centric relation
  chemoradiation
  chest and right arm [lead in
    electrocardiography]
  chest roentgenograph(y) (roentgenogram)
  child-resistant [bottle top]
  choice reaction
  chorioretinal
  chronic rejection
  clinical record
  clinical research
  closed reduction
  clot retraction
  coefficient [of fat] retention
  colon resection
  colony-reared [animal]
  colorectal
  complement receptor [1, 2, 3, 3a, 3b,
    4, 5, 5a]
  complete remission
  complete responder
  complete response
  computed radiography
  conditioned reflex (*See also* cond ref)
  conditioned response (*See also* cond
    resp)
  congenital rubella
  Congo red (*See also* Cor)
  contact record
  continuous reinforcement
  controlled release
  controlled respiration
  controlled response
  conversion rate
  conversion reaction
  cooling rate
  corneal reflex
  correct response

correlation [algorithm]
corticoresistant
cranium (cranial) (*See also* cran)
creamed
creatinine (*See also* cre)
cremaster ratio
cresyl red
critical ratio
crown
crown-rump [length] (*See also* CRL)
crutches
Cryptococcus
cycloplegic refraction
NATO code for
   dibenz(b,f)-1:4-oxazepine
CR0–CR10
   category ratio 0–10
C&R
   cardiac and respiratory
   convalescence and rehabilitation
   cystoscopy and retrograde [pyelogram]
C/R
   chorioretinal
   conscious, rational
Cr
   chromium
⁵¹Cr
   chromium-51
CRA
   central retinal artery
   chemotherapy-related amenorrhea
   Chinese restaurant asthma
   chronic rheumatoid arthritis
   cis-retinoic acid
   clinical risk assessment
   colorectal adenocarcinoma
   colorectal anastomosis
   coronary rotational atherectomy
   corticosteroid-resistant asthma
13-CRA
   13-*cis*-retinoic acid
CRAA
   cerebroretinal arteriovenous aneurysm
CRABP
   cellular retinoic acid-binding protein
CRAC
   compliance-related acute complication
   contract relax agonist contract
CRAG
   cerebral radionuclide angiography
CRAg
   Cryptococcus antigen
CRAI
   continuous regional arterial infusion
CRAMS
   circulation, respiration, abdomen, motor,
      speech

cran
   cranium (cranial) (*See also* CR)
CRAO
   central retinal artery occlusion
CRAS
   Clinician Rated Anxiety Scale
CRASH
   corpus callosum hypoplasia, retardation,
      adducted thumbs, spastic paraplegia,
      hydrocephalus [syndrome]
CRB
   chemical, radiological, biological
   congenital retinitis blindness
CRBBB
   complete right bundle branch block
CRBC
   chicken red blood cell (*See also*
      ChRBC)
CRBI
   catheter-related bloodstream infection
CRBP
   cellular retinol-binding protein
Cr&Br
   crown and bridge (*See also* C&B)
CRBSI, CR-BSI
   catheter-related bloodstream infection
CRC
   calcium release channel
   cardiovascular reflex conditioning
   cerebrovascular reserve capacity
   child-resistant container
   clinical research center
   colorectal cancer (carcinoma)
   concentrated red [blood] cell
   creatinine clearance [urine] (*See also*
      CCR, C_{cr}, C/cr/ CrCl, Crcl, CC)
   cross-reacting cannabinoids
CR&C
   closed reduction and cast
CRCC
   chromophobe renal cell carcinoma
   cystic renal cell carcinoma
CrCl, Crcl
   creatinine clearance (*See also* CC, CCR,
      C_{cr}, C/cr/, CRC, CrCl, Crcl)
CR/CO
   centric relation [and] centric occlusion
CRCS
   calciobiotic root canal sealer
   calcium [hydroxide] root canal sealer
   cardiovascular reflex conditioning
      system
CRCT
   creamatocrit
   volume percent of cream in milk
CRCV
   cerebral red blood cell volume

CRD
childhood rheumatic disease
child-restraint device
chorioretinal degeneration
chronic renal disease
chronic respiratory disease
completely randomized design
complete reaction of degeneration
complete remission duration
complex repetitive discharge
cone-rod dystrophy
congenital rubella deafness
contractile ring dysphagia
crown-rump distance [fetal
measurement]

CR-DIP
chronic relapsing demyelinating
inflammatory polyneuropathy

CRDS
curdlan sulfate

CRE
cardiorespiratory endurance
controlled radial expansion
cumulative radiation effect
cyclic adenosine monophosphate
(cAMP) regulatory element

cre
creatinine (See also CR)

CREA-S
creatinine urine spot [test]

CREB
cyclic adenosine monophosphate
(cAMP) response element binding
[protein]

CREB/ATF
cyclic adenosine monophosphate
(cAMP) response element binding
[protein] activation transcription factor

^{51}Cr-EDTA
51-chromium-labeled
ethylenediaminetetraacetate

CREG
cross-reactive (antigen) group

CREM
cyclic adenosine monophosphate
(cAMP)-response element modulator

CRENA
crenated [red blood cells]

crep.
crepitation [L. crepitus]

CREST
calcinosis cutis, Raynaud phenomenon,
esophageal motility disorder,
sclerodactyly, telangiectasia [syndrome]

CRF
cancer-related fatigue
cardiac risk factor
cardiorespiratory function
case report form
chronic renal failure
chronic respiratory failure
coagulase-reacting factor
continuous reinforcement
coronary reserve flow
corticotropin-releasing factor

CRFK
Crandell feline kidney [cells]

CRFR
corticotropin-releasing factor receptor

CRG, CR-gram
cardiorespirogram

CRH
corticotropin-releasing hormone

CRH-BP
corticotropin-releasing hormone-binding
protein

CRH-R1–CRH-R2
corticotropin-releasing hormone receptor
type 1–2

CRHV
cottontail rabbit herpesvirus

CRI
Cardiac Risk Index
Caring Relationship Inventory
catheter-related infection
chronic renal insufficiency
chronic respiratory insufficiency
Composite Risk Index
concentrated rust inhibitor
congenital rubella infection
constant-rate infusion
Coping Resources Inventory
cranial rhythmic impulse
cross-reactive idiotype

CRIB
Clinical Risk Index for Babies

CRIE
crossed radioimmunoelectrophoresis

CRIES
crying [high pitched], requires [oxygen],
increased [vital signs], expression
[grimace], sleepless [last hour]
[neonatal pain assessment]

CRIS
controlled release infusion syndrome

crit
critical
hematocrit (See also h'crit, HCT, Hct)

Crk
cytokinin-regulated kinase

CrkI–CrkII
cytokinin-regulated kinase I–II

CrkL
cytokinin-regulated kinase L

CRL
cell repository line
central right lung
complement receptor location

complement receptor lymphocyte
crown-rump length (*See also* CR)
CRM
canalith repositioning maneuver
certified raw milk
Certified Reference Materials
circumferential resection margins
contralateral remote masking
controlled range of motion
cross-reacting material
crown-rump measurement
CRMI
curved reformatted mandibular image
CRMO
chronic recurrent multifocal
osteomyelitis
CR-MVB
Cramer-Rao minimum variance
bound
CRN
cerebral radiation necrosis
cRNA
chromosomal ribonucleic acid
complementary ribonucleic acid
CRNF
chronic rheumatoid nodular fibrositis
cr nn
cranial nerves [plural] (*See also* CN)
CRO
cathode ray oscilloscope
centric relation occlusion
CROM
cervical range of motion
chronic refractory osteomyelitis
CROP
compliance, rate, oxygenation,
pressure
CROS
contralateral routing of offside signal
CR/OV
colorectal/ovarian
CROW
Charcot restraint orthotic walker
CRP
cyclic adenosine monophosphate
(cAMP) receptor protein
canalith repositioning procedure
chronic recurrent parotitis
chronic relapsing pancreatitis
colorectal polyps
confluent reticulated papillomatosis
corneal reflection pupillometer
corneal-retinal potential
coronary rehabilitation program
C-reactive protein
cross-reacting protein
C&RP
curettage and root planing

CrP
creatine phosphate (phosphocreatine)
CRPA
C-reactive protein antiserum
CRPD
chronic restrictive pulmonary disease
CRPF
chloroquine-resistant *Plasmodium
falciparum*
closed reduction and percutaneous
fixation
contralateral renal plasma flow
CRPP
closed reduction and percutaneous
pinning
CRPS
complex regional pain syndrome
CRPS-2
complex regional pain syndrome type 2
CRQ
Chronic Respiratory Questionnaire
CRR
canal resonance response
CRRT
continuous renal replacement therapy
CrRT
cranial radiotherapy
CRS
Cambridge Research Systems
Carroll self-rating scale
catheter-related sepsis
caudal regression syndrome
Cell Recovery System
central supply room
cherry-red spot
child restraint system
Chinese restaurant syndrome
Clinical Rating Scale
cocaine-related seizure
colorectal surgery
compliance of the respiratory system
congenital rubella syndrome
Conners Rating Scale
continuous running suture
Counter Rotation System (brace)
cryoreductive surgery
cytokine-release syndrome
CRSM
cherry-red spot myoclonus
cranial-sacral respiratory mechanism
CRSP
comprehensive renal scintillation
procedure
CrSp
craniospinal
CRST
calcinosis cutis, Raynaud phenomenon,
sclerodactyly, telangiectasia

CRT
cadaver renal transplant
capillary refill time
cardiac resynchronization therapy
cartilage roof triangle
cathode-ray tube
central reaction time
certified (*See also* C)
chemoradiation therapy
choice reaction time
chromium release test
circuit resistance training
complex reaction time
computed renal tomography
conformal radiation therapy
copper reduction test
coronary radiation therapy
corrected retention time
cortisone resistant thymocyte
cranial radiation therapy
Critical Reasoning Test

cRT-PCR
competitive reverse
   transcription-polymerase chain reaction

CrTr
crutch training (*See also* CT)

CRTX
cast removed take x-ray

CRU
cardiac rehabilitation unit
clinical research unit

CRu
unconfirmed (uncertain) complete
   remission

CRV
central retinal vein
channel catfish reovirus
community-acquired respiratory
   virus
Cowbone Ridge virus

CRVF
congestive right ventricular failure

CRVO
central retinal vein occlusion

CRVS
California Relative Value Studies

CRW
Cosman-Roberts-Wells [stereotactic
   frame]

CRY-AB
cryptococcal antibody

CRY-AG
cryptococcal antigen

cryo
cryoablation
cryoglobulin
cryoprecipitate
cryosurgery
cryotherapy

crys, cryst
crystal
crystalline
crystallinized

CRYST
crystal examination screen

CS
calf serum
camptomelic syndrome
carcinoid syndrome
cardiogenic shock
cardioplegia solution
caries susceptible
carotid sheath
carotid sinus
catgut suture (*See also* CGS)
cat-scratch [disease] (*See also* CSD)
cavernous sinus
celiac sprue
cerebral scintigraphy
cerebrospinal
cervical spine (*See also* C-spine)
cervical stimulation
cesarean section (*See also* C-section,
   C sect)
chemical sympathectomy
chest strap
cholesterol stone
cholesterol sulfate
chondroitin sulfate
chorionic somatomammotropin
chronic schizophrenia
cigarette smoke(r)
citrate synthase
climacteric syndrome
clinical [laboratory] scientist
clinically significant
clinical stage
close supervision
cold storage
completed stroke
completed suicide
compression syndrome
concentrated strength [of solution]
conditioned stimulus
congenital syphilis
conjunctiva [and] sclera [singular]
conjunctivae [and] sclerae [plural]
conjunctival secretion
conscious(ness)
conscious sedation
conservative surgery
Constant Spring [hemoglobin]
contact sensitivity
continue same [treatment]
continuing smoker
continuous stripping
control serum
convalescence

convalescent
coronal suture
coronary sclerosis
coronary sinus
corpus striatum
cortical spoking
corticoid sensitive
corticosteroid
Cost-Stirling [antibody]
cough and sneeze
countershock
crush syndrome
current smoker
current strength
cyclic sedentary
NATO code for o-chlorobenzylidene
  malononitrile

C4S
chondroitin 4 sulfate

C&S
conjunctiva and sclera [singular]
conjunctivae and sclerae [plural]
cough and sneeze
culture and sensitivity
culture and susceptibility

CS$_2$
carbon disulfide

C$_s$
standard clearance (*See also* Cs)
static [lung] compliance (*See also* CST)

Cs
cesium

cS
centistoke [obsolete, use only cSt]

c/s
cycle per second (*See also* cps, c/sec)

^{132}Cs
cesium-132

^{137}Cs
cesium-137

^{139}Cs
cesium-139

CSA
canavaninosuccinic acid
central sleep apnea
chondroitin sulfate A
clinically significant arrhythmia
Cognitive Skills Assessment
colon-specific antigen
colony-stimulating activity
compressed spectral assay
Controlled Substances Act [DEA]
controlled substance analog
corticosteroid sensitive asthma
cross-sectional area

CSAD
cysteine sulfinic acid decarboxylase

CSAP
colon-specific antigen protein
cryosurgical ablation of prostate

CSAR
conservative subtraction-addition
  rhinoplasty

CSAS
central sleep apnea syndrome

CSAVP
cerebral subarachnoid venous pressure

CSB
chemical stimulation of brain
Cheyne-Stokes breathing
contaminated small-bowel
craniosynostosis, Boston type

CSB I&II
chemistry screening batteries I and II

CSBF
coronary sinus blood flow

CSBI
Child Sexual Behavior Inventory

CSBO
complete small-bowel obstruction

CSBS
contaminated small-bowel syndrome

CSC
blow on blow [administration of small
  doses of drugs at short intervals] [Fr.
  coup sur coup]
cardiac sphincter chalasia
central serous chorioretinopathy
central serous choroidopathy
cigarette smoke condensate
collagen sponge contraceptive
cornea, sclera, conjunctiva
crankcase spool catheter
cryogenic storage container
cryopreserved stem cell

C/S & CC
culture and sensitivity and colony count

CSCED
cribriform salivary carcinoma of
  excretory duct

CSCI
continuous subcutaneous infusion

CSCR
central serous chorioretinopathy

CSCS
Children's Self-Concept Scale

C1s
complement 1 protease

CSCT
central somatosensory conduction time
comprehensive support care team

CSD
carotid sinus denervation
cat-scratch disease (*See also* CS)

CSD *(continued)*
celiac sprue disease
cervical spine dislocation
chemical sensitivity disorder
closed suction drainage
combined system disease
conditionally streptomycin dependent
conduction system disease
congenital sodium diarrhea
cortically spreading depression
craniospinal defect
critical stimulus duration
CS&D
cleaned, sutured, and dressed
CSDB
cat-scratch disease bacillus
CSDD
Cornell Scale for Depression, Dementia
CSDH
chronic subdural hematoma
CSDR
Cochrane Database of Systematic
Reviews
CS/DS
chondroitin sulfate [and] dermatan
sulfate
CSE
clinical-symptom/self-evaluation
[questionnaire]
combined spinal [and] epidural
[anesthesia] (*See also* CSEA)
complete surgical exploration
cone-shaped epiphysis
conventional silicone elastomer
conventional spin-echo
coping strategy enhancement
cross-sectional echocardiography
CSEA
combined spinal-epidural anesthesia
c/sec
cycle per second (*See also* cps, c/s)
C-section, C sect
cesarean section (*See also* CS, C/S)
CSEP
cortical somatosensory evoked potential
CSER
cortical somatosensory evoked response
CSF
cancer family syndrome
cerebrospinal fluid
circumferential shortening fraction
colony-stimulating factor
contoured femoral stem
coronary sinus flow
CSF-1
colony-stimulating factor 1
CSF-FTA-ABS
colony-stimulating factor fluorescent
treponemal antibody-absorption

CSFH
cerebrospinal fluid hypotension
CSFI
Cholesterol-Saturated Fat Index
CSF-IFE
cerebrospinal fluid immunofixation
electrophoresis
CSF-MHA-TP
colony-stimulating factor
microhemagglutination *Treponema*
pallidum [test]
CSFP
cerebrospinal fluid pressure
CSFS
coronary slow flow syndrome
CSFs
colony stimulating factor
CSFV
cerebrospinal fluid volume
classical swine fever virus
CSF-VDRL
colony-stimulating factor developed by
Venereal Disease Research Laboratory
CSF-WR
cerebrospinal fluid Wassermann reaction
CSG
chronic simple glaucoma
chronic superficial gastritis
coronary sinus guiding [catheter]
CSGBM
collagenase soluble glomerular basement
membrane
CSGE
conformational sensitive gel
electrophoresis
CSGIT
continuous suture graft inclusion
technique
CSGP
computed strain-gauge plethysmography
CSH
capsular synoviallike hyperplasia
carotid sinus hypersensitivity
chronic subdural hematoma
congenital subluxation of hip
cortical stromal hyperplasia
C-Sh
chair shower
CSHEP
constriction, sclerosis, hemorrhage,
exudate, papilledema
CSHH
congenital self-healing histiocytosis
CSHQ
Children's Sleep Habits Questionnaire
CSI
Calculus Surface Index
cancer serum index
Caregiver Strain Index

cavernous sinus infiltration
cervical spine injury
chemical shift imaging
cholesterol saturation index
continuous subcutaneous infusion
coronary sinus intervention
coronary stenosis index
coronary stent implant(ation)
craniospinal irradiation
CsI
cesium iodide
CSICU
cardiac surgery intensive care unit
CSID
congenital sucrase-isomaltase deficiency
CSII
continuous subcutaneous insulin
infusion
CSIIP
continuous subcutaneous insulin infusion
pump
CSIS
clinical supplies and inventory system
CSL
cardiolipin synthetic lecithin
central sacral line
complex sclerosing lesion
computerized speech laboratory
confocal scanning laser
CSLD
chronic suppurative lung disease
CSLM
confocal scanning microscopy
CSLO
confocal scanning laser ophthalmoscopy
CSLP
cervical spine locking plate
CSLR
crossed straight leg raising
CSLU
chronic stasis leg ulcer
CSM
cardiosynchronous myostimulator
carotid sinus massage
central, steady, maintained [fixation]
cerebrospinal meningitis
cervical spondylotic myelopathy
circulation, sensation, mobility
circulation, sensation, motion
Consolidated Standards Manual
cornmeal, soybean, milk
CSMA
chemical shift misregistration artifact
chronic spinal muscular atrophy
CSMAP
celiac [and] superior mesenteric artery
portography

CSME
clinically significant macular edema
cotton-spot macular edema
CSMEMP
contiguous slice multiecho multiplane
CSMN
chronic sensorimotor neuropathy
CSMP
chloramphenicol-sensitive microsomal
protein
CSMT
capillary refill, sensation, motor
function, temperature
chorionic somatomammotropin
CSN
cardiac sympathetic nerve
carotid sinus nerve
cystic suppurative necrosis
CSNA
congenital sensory neuropathy with
anhidrosis [syndrome]
CSNB
congenital stationary night
blindness
CSNRT, cSNRT
corrected sinus node recovery time
(*See also* CSRT)
CSNS
carotid sinus nerve stimulation
CSO
clinically severe obesity
common source outbreak
copied standing orders
coronary sinus ostium
craniosynostosis (craniostosis)
craniostenosis
crescentic shelf osteotomy
CSOM
chronic serous otitis media
chronic suppurative otitis media
CSOP
coronary sinus occlusion pressure
CSP
Cancer Surveillance Program
carotid sinus pressure
cavum septum pellucidum
cell surface protein
cellulose sodium phosphate
central silent period [nerves]
cervical spine pain
chemistry screening profile
Cooperative Statistical Program
criminal sexual psychopath
cutaneous silent period [nerves]
CSPAMM
complementary spatial modulation of
magnetization [imaging]

CSPG
chondroitin sulfate proteoglycan
CSPI
childhood severity of psychiatric illness
C-spine
cervical spine (*See also* CS)
CSPS
continual skin peeling syndrome
CSQ
College Student Questionnaire
Coping Strategies Questionnaire
CSQI
continuous subcutaneous infusion
CSR
central serous retinopathy
central supply room
Cheyne-Stokes respiration
Communicable Disease Surveillance and
Response
complete subtalar release
continued-stay review
corrected sedimentation rate
corrected survival rate
corrective septorhinoplasty
cortisol secretion rate
cosmetic skin resurfacing
cumulative survival rate
CSRA
cementless surface replacement
arthroplasty
CSRI
Caregiver's School Readiness Inventory
CSRS
cardiac surgery reporting system
CSRT
corrected sinus (node) recovery time
(*See also* CSNRT, cSNRT)
CSS
Canadian Stroke Scale
Cancer Surveillance System
carotid sinus stimulation
carotid sinus syndrome
cause-specific survival
cavernous sinus sampling
cavernous sinus syndrome
chewing, sucking, swallowing
Chronic Sinusitis Survey
chronic subclinical scurvy
coronary sinus stimulation
cranial sector scan
CSSA
carotid stent-supported angioplasty
Cocaine Symptom Severity Assessment
CSSD
central sterile supply department
closed system sterile drainage
corticostriatal spinal degeneration
CSSEP
cortical somatosensory evoked potential

CSSQ
College Student Satisfaction
Questionnaire
CST
cardiac stress test
cardiovascular self-assessment tool
cavernous sinus thrombosis
Christ-Siemens-Touraine (syndrome)
cognitive skill training
Completing Sentence Test
Compton scatter tomography
Conceptual Systems Test
contraction stress test
contrast sensitivity test
convulsive shock therapy
corticospinal tract
cosyntropin stimulation test
craniosacral therapy
craniosacral treatment
static [lung] compliance (*See also* C_s)
cSt
centistokes [metric unit of viscosity]
CSTD
chronic single tic disorder
CSTM
cervical prevertebral soft tissue
measurement
CSTR
complete subtalar release
CSTT
cold-stimulation time test
CSU
catheter specimen of urine
cognition of semantic unit
CSUF
continuous slow ultrafiltration [for renal
failure]
CSV
chick syncytial virus
continuous spontaneous ventilation
CSVD
cerebral small-vessel disease
CSVT
central splanchnic venous thrombosis
CSW
cerebral salt wasting
commercial sex worker
current sleepwalker
CSWSS
continuous spike-waves of slow sleep
[EEG]
CSWT
cardiac shock wave therapy
CT
calcitonin
calf tenderness
calf testis
cardiac tamponade
cardiothoracic

carotid tracing
carpal tunnel
Category Test [psychology]
cationic trypsinogen
cell therapy
cellulose triacetate
census tract
center thickness
cerebral thrombosis
cerebral tumor
cervical traction (*See also* CXTX)
cervicothoracic
chemotaxis (*See also* CTX)
chemotherapy
chest tube
Chlamydia trachomatis
cholera toxin
cholesterol, total
chordae tendineae
chronic thyroiditis
chymotrypsin
circulation time
classic technique
closed thoracotomy
clotting time
coagulation time
coated tablet
cobra toxin
cognitive therapy
coil test
collecting tubule
combined tumor
compressed tablet
computed [axial] tomography
computerized tomography
connective tissue
continue treatment
continuous-flow tub
contraction time
controlled temperature
Coombs test
corneal thickness
corneal transplant(ation)
coronary thrombosis
corrected transposition
correctional transfer
corrective therapy
cortical thickness
cough threshold
cover test
crest time
crutch training (*See also* CrTr)
cystine-tellurite [medium]
cytotechnology
cytotoxic therapy

CT-1
cardiotropin 1

CT1
primary chemotherapy

C3T
clomiphene citrate challenge test
(*See also* CCCT)

4C-T
four-chamber transverse [view]

5C-T
five-chamber transverse [view]

C × T
concentration times time

C&T
color and temperature
counseling and testing

C:T
compression to traction ratio
crossmatch to transfusion ratio

Ct
carboxyl terminal (*See also* C-terminal)
concentration-time product

Ct$_{50}$
concentration-time product for 50% of
exposed group

ct
count

ct0$_2$
concentration of total oxygen

C$_{T-1824}$
T-1824 [Evans blue] clearance

CTA
chemotactic activity (*See also* CA)
chromotropic acid
clear to auscultation
computed tomographic (tomography)
angiography
computed tomography of abdomen
congenital trigeminal anesthesia
cuff tear arthropathy
cystine trypticase agar
cytoplasmic tubular aggregate
cytotoxic assay
menses [L. *catamenia*]

CTAB
cetyltrimethylammonium bromide
(*See also* CTBM)

C-TAB
cyanide tablet

CTAC
Carrow Test for Auditory
Comprehension
cetyltrimethylammonium chloride

CTACK
cutaneous T-cell attracting chemokine

CTAF, CTAFS
conotruncal anomaly face syndrome

CTAL
cortical thick ascending limb

CTAO
cerebral thromboangiitis obliterans

CTAP
clear to auscultation and percussion
computed tomography [during]
angiographic (arterial) portography
connective tissue-activating peptide

CTAS
colonic transabdominal sonography

CTAT
computerized transverse axial
(transaxial) tomography

CTB
calciotraumatic band
ceased to breathe
cholera toxin B
cytotrophoblast

CTBA
cetrimonium bromide

CTBM
cetyltrimethyl-ammonium bromide
(*See also* CTAB)

CTBS
California Test of Basic Skills
Canadian Test of Basic Skills

CTC
Child-Turcotte classification [liver
function]
circular tear capsulotomy
circulating tumor cells
Common Toxicity Criteria
computed tomographic (tomography)
colonography
computer-aided tomographic
cisternography
congenital thrombocytopenia
contaminating tumor cell
Creativity Tests for Children
cultured T cell

CTCL
cutaneous T-cell lymphoma

ctCO$_2$
concentration of total carbon
dioxide

CTD
carpal tunnel decompression
chest tube drainage
chronic tic disorder
clitoral therapy device
close to death
congenital thymic dysplasia
connective tissue disease
corneal thickness depth
cumulative trauma disorder

CT&DB
cough, turn, and deep breath (*See also*
TC&DB)

CTDI
computed tomography dose index

CTDW
continues to do well

CTE
calf thymus extract
chronic traumatic encephalopathy
congenital telangiectatic erythema
cultured thymic epithelium

CTEI
communal traumatic experiences
inventory

CTEM
conventional transmission electron
microscopy

CTEPH
chronic thromboembolic pulmonary
hypertension

C-terminal
carboxyl terminal (*See also* Ct)

CTE: YAG
contrast transesophageal
echocardiography [and]
yttrium-aluminum-garnet [laser
therapy]

CTF
cancer therapy facility
certificate (*See also* cert)
Colorado tick fever
computed tomography fluoroscopy
continuous tube feeding
contrast transfer function
cytotoxic factor

CTFC
corrected thrombosis in myocardial
infarction (TIMI) frame count

CTFS
complete testicular feminization
syndrome

CTFV
Colorado tick fever virus

CTG
cardiotocography
cervicothoracic ganglion
chymotrypsinogen

C:TG
cholesterol to triglyceride ratio

CTGA
complete (corrected) transposition of the
great arteries

CTGF
connective tissue growth factor

CTH
ceramide trihexoside
chronic tension headache
clot to hold
computerized tomographic
holography

CTHA
computed tomographic hepatic
angiography

CTHD
computer-telephony integration [telemedicine]

CTI
certification of terminal illness
coffee table injury
cutaneous tolerance index

CTID
chemotherapy-induced diarrhea

CTL
cervical, thoracic, lumbar
cytolytic T lymphocyte
cytotoxic T lymphocyte

ctl
contact lens (*See also* CL)

CTLA-4
cytotoxic T lymphocyte antigen 4

CTLA4Ig
cytotoxic lymphocyte activation antigen 4 immunoglobulin

CTLC
contact transscleral laser cytophotocoagulation

CTLG
computed tomography lymphography

CTLL
cytotoxic T lymphocyte line

CTLM
computed tomography laser mammography

CTLp
cytotoxic T lymphocyte precursor

CTLSO
cervical-thoracic-lumbar-sacral (cervicothoracolumbosacral) orthosis

CTLV
cross-table lateral view

CTM
cardiac transplant[ation] monitoring
cardiotachometer
cervical tension myositis
Chlamydia transport media
computed tomographic myelography
connective tissue massage
continuous tone masking
cricothyroid muscle

CTMC
connective tissue-type mast cell

CTMM
California Test of Mental Maturity
computed tomographic metrizamide myelography

CTMM-SF
California Test of Mental Maturity-Short Form

CTMP
contrast threshold for motion perception

CT/MPR
computed tomography with multiplanar reconstruction

CT/MR
computerized tomography/magnetic resonance

CT/MRI
computed tomography/magnetic resonance imaging

CTN
calcitonin
chronic transplant nephropathy
computed tomography number

C&TN BLE
color and temperature normal, both lower extremities

cTnC
cardiac troponin C

cTnI
cardiac troponin I

cTNM
clinical staging of tumor, node, metastasis [TNM classification]

cTnT
cardiac troponin T

CTO
cervicothoracic orthosis
chest tube output
chronic total occlusion

CTOPP
Comprehensive Test Of Phonological Processing

CTP
California Test of Personality
carboxyl terminal peptide
Child-Turcotte-Pugh [cirrhosis scoring system]
comprehensive treatment plan
cytidine triphosphate (cytidine 5′-triphosphate)

CTPA
clear to percussion and auscultation

C-TPN
cyclic total parenteral nutrition

CTPP
cerebral tissue perfusion pressure

CTPV
cavernous transformation of portal vein
coal tar pitch volatiles
computerized tomography pulmonary venography

CTPVO
chronic thrombotic pulmonary vascular obstruction

CTQ
childhood trauma questionnaire
Conners Teacher Questionnaire

CTR
    cardiothoracic ratio
    carpal tunnel release (repair)
    cosmetic transdermal reconstruction
    cricotracheal resection
ctr
    center
CTRD
    Cardiac Transplant Research
        Database
CTRS
    carpal tunnel release system
CTRS-28
    Conners Teacher Rating Scale
CT-RT
    chemo- and radiotherapy
CTS
    cardiothoracic surgery
    carpal tunnel syndrome
    Champion Trauma Score
    clitoris tourniquet syndrome
    closed-tube sampling
    composite treatment score
    computed tomographic scan(ner)
    contralateral threshold shift
    corneal topography system
    corticosteroid
CTSI
    computed tomography severity index
CTSIB
    Clinical Test of Sensory Integration and
        Balance
CTSNFR
    corrected time of sinuatrial node
        function recovery
CTSP
    called to see patient
CT/SPECT
    computed tomography/single photon
        emission computed tomography
CTSS
    closed tracheal suction system
CTT
    central tegmental tract
    compressed tablet triturate
    computed transaxial tomography
    cotton thread test
cTT
    cerebral transit time
CTU
    centigrade thermal unit
    computed tomographic urography
    constitutive transcription unit
CTV
    cervical and thoracic vertebrae
    clinical target volume
    clinical tumor volume
    computed tomography
        venography

CTVF
    Comprehensive Test of Visual
        Functioning
CTW
    central terminal of Wilson
    combined testicular weight
CTX
    cerebrotendinous xanthomatosis
    cervical traction
    chemotaxis (*See also* CT)
    chemotoxins
    contraction (*See also* C, contr, contrx,
        CTXN, CX)
    costotendinous xanthomatosis
CTx
    cardiac transplant(ation)
CTXN
    contraction (*See also* C, contr, contrx,
        CTX, CX)
CTZ
    chemoreceptor trigger zone
CU
    casein unit
    cause undetermined
    cause unknown
    chronic undifferentiated
    chymotrypsin unit
    clinical unit
    color unit
    contact urticaria
    control unit
    copper
    Couvelaire uterus [extravasation into
        myometrium]
    cusp
C$_u$
    urea clearance
Cu
    copper [L. *cuprum*]
cu
    cubic (*See also* C)
Cu-7
    Copper-7 [intrauterine contraceptive
        device]
⁶²Cu
    copper-62
⁶⁴Cu
    copper-64
⁶⁷Cu
    copper-67
CUAVD
    congenital unilateral absence of vas
        deferens
CuB
    copper band
CUBS
    compromised urinary bladder syndrome
¹³C-UBT
    carbon-13 urea breath test

^{14}C-UBT
    carbon-14 urea breath test
CUC
    chronic ulcerative colitis
cu cm
    cubic centimeter [Note: Do not use,
        substitute mL] (*See also* cc, CC, c.c.,
        cm^3)
CuCN
    copper cyanide
CUCS
    complex unroofed coronary sinus
CUD
    cause undetermined
    congenital urinary [tract] deformity
    controlled unsterile delivery
CUE
    confidential unit exclusion
    cumulative urinary excretion
CUES
    College and University Environment
        Scales
cu ft
    cubic foot
CUG
    cystidine, uridine, guanidine
    cystourethrograph(y) (cystourethrogram)
CUHB
    chronic unconjugated hyperbilirubinemia
CuHVL
    copper half-value layer
cu in
    cubic inch
CuIUD
    copper intrauterine device
cult.
    culture
CUM
    cumulative report
cu m
    cubic meter (*See also* m^3)
CUMITECH
    Cumulative Techniques and Procedures
        in Clinical Microbiology
cu mm
    cubic millimeter (*See also* cmm, mm^3)
cUMP
    cyclic uridine 3,′5′-monophosphate
CUP
    cancer (carcinoma) of unknown primary
CUPP
    conservative uvulopalatoplasty
CUPS
    cancer (carcinoma) of unknown
        (uncertain) primary site
CUR
    chronic urinary retention

    curettage
    cystourethrorectal
cur.
    curative
    cure
    current
CURL
    compartment of uncoupling receptor and
        ligand
CUS
    carotid ultrasound
    catheterized urine specimen
    chronic undifferentiated schizophrenia
    compression ultrasound
    contact urticaria syndrome
    cranial ultrasound
CUSA
    Cavitron ultrasonic surgical aspirator
    continuous ultrasonic surgical aspiration
cusp.
    cuspid
CUSUM, cusum
    cumulative sum [method]
CUT
    chronic undifferentiated type
        [schizophrenia]
CUTA
    congenital urinary tract anomaly
CUTE
    conventional ultrashort echo time
CuTS
    cubital tunnel syndrome
CUX
    check-up x-ray
cu yd
    cubic yard
Cu/Zn
    copper-zinc
Cu/Zn-SOD
    copper-zinc superoxide dismutase
CV
    cardiac volume
    cardiovascular
    care vigilance
    carotenoid vesicle
    cell volume
    central venous
    cerebrovascular
    cervical vertebra
    closed vitrectomy
    closing volume
    coefficient of variation
    collateralizing vessel
    collecting vein
    color vision
    coma vigil
    common ventricle

C

CV *(continued)*
concentrated volume
conducting vein
conduction velocity
consonant vowel [syllable]
contrast ventriculography
conventional ventilation
conversational voice
corpuscular volume
costovertebral
craniosacral vault
cresyl violet
critical value
crystal violet
curriculum vitae
cutaneous vasculitis
true conjugate [diameter of pelvic inlet]
[L. *conjugata vera*]

C$_v$
heat capacity at constant volume of gas

CV4
craniosacral vault four

C/V
cervical/vaginal
coulomb per volt

Cv, C$_v$
specific heat at constant volume

c/v
cupping and vibrating

c.v.
coefficient of variation [statistics]

cv
conceptional vessel [accupuncture]

CVA
cardiovascular accident
cerebrovascular accident
cervicovaginal antibody
chronic villous arthritis
costovertebral angle
cough variant asthma
cresyl violet acetate

CV A1–A22
human coronavirus A1–22

CVAAS
cold vapor atomic absorption
spectrometry

CVAD
central venous access device

CVAH
congenital virilizing adrenal
hyperplasia

CVAP
cerebrovascular amyloid peptide

CVAS
Colored Visual Analogue Scale

C-Vasc
cerebral vascular [profile study]

CVAT
costovertebral angle tenderness

CVB
chorionic villus biopsy
group B coxsackievirus

CV B1–B6
human coxsackievirus B1–B6

CVBS
congenital vascular-bone syndrome

CVC
calcifying vascular cell
central venous catheter (*See also* CV
cath)
consonant vowel consonant [syllable]

CV cath
central venous catheter (*See also* CVC)

CVCT
cardiovascular computed tomography

CVD
cardiovascular disease (*See also* CD)
cerebrovascular disease
chemical vapor deposition
chronic venous disease
collagen vascular disease
color vision deviant
congenital vascular disorder

cvd
curved

CVE
cerebrovascular episode
cerebrovascular evaluation

CVF
cardiovascular failure
central visual field
cervicovaginal fluid
chronic ventilatory failure
cobra venom factor

CVFn
cardiovascular function

CVG
composite valve graft
contrast ventriculography
coronary vein (venous) graft
cutis verticis gyrata

CVG/MR
cutis verticis gyrata/mental retardation
[syndrome]

CVGV
CSIRO Village virus

CVH
cerebroventricular hemorrhage
cervicovaginal hood
combined ventricular hypertrophy
common variable
hypogammaglobulinemia

CVHD
chronic valvular heart disease

CVI
cardiovascular incident
cardiovascular insufficiency
cerebrovascular incident

cerebrovascular infarct(ion)
cerebrovascular insufficiency
Children's Vaccine Initiative
chronic venous insufficiency
common variable immunodeficiency
  (*See also* CVID)
continuous venous infusion
cortical visual impairment

CVID
common variable immunodeficiency
  (*See also* CVI)

CVIR
Cardiovascular Information Registry

CVIS
cardiovascular imaging system

CVK
computerized videokeratography

CVL
central venous line
cervicovaginal lavage
clinical vascular laboratory

CVLM
caudal ventrolateral medulla

CVLP
chimeric viruslike particles
coronaviruslike particle

CVLT
California Verbal Learning Test

CVLT-II
California Verbal Learning Test II

CVM
cardiovascular malformation
cardiovascular monitor
cerebral venous malformation
childhood visceral myopathy
circular vesicomyotomy
congenital vascular malformation
cryptic vascular malformation

C$_{v,m}$
molar heat capacity at constant volume
  of gas

CVMS
clean voided mid stream

CVMT
cervical-vaginal motion tenderness
Continuous Visual Memory Test

CVN
central venous nutrition
cochleovestibular neurectomy

CVNSR
cardiovascular normal sinus rhythm

CVO
central vein occlusion
central venous oxygen
circumventricular organ
obstetric conjugate [of pelvic inlet]
  [L. *conjugata vera obstetrica*]

CVO$_2$
central venous oxygen content

C$_v$O$_2$
mixed venous oxygen content

CVOD
cerebrovascular obstructive disease

CVP
cardiac valve procedure
cardioventricular pacing
cell volume profile
central venous pressure
cerebrovascular profile

CVR
cardiovascular renal [disease] (*See also*
  CVRD)
cardiovascular resistance
cardiovascular-respiratory
cardiovascular review
cephalic vasomotor response
cerebrovascular reactivity
cerebrovascular resistance
coronary flow velocity reserve
coronary vascular reserve

CVRD
cardiovascular renal disease (*See also*
  CVR)

CVRI
cardiovascular resistance index
coronary vascular resistance index

CVRMED
computer vision, virtual reality, robotics
  in medicine

CVRR
cardiovascular recovery room

CVRS
California Relative Value Studies
cardiovascular and respiratory [elements
  of trauma score]

CVS
cardiovascular surgery
cardiovascular system
cerebral vasospasm
challenge virus strain
chorionic villus sampling
clean-voided specimen
collagen vascular sealing
computer vision syndrome
continuing vegetative state
coronavirus susceptibility
current vital signs
cyclic vomiting syndrome

CVS/CNS
cardiovascular system and central
  nervous system

CVSD
congenital ventricular septal
  defect

CVSF
    conduction velocity of slower
      fibers
CVSMC
    cultured vascular smooth muscle cell
CVST
    cardiovascular stress test
    cerebral venous sinus thrombosis
CVSU
    cardiovascular specialty unit
CVT
    calf vein thrombosis
    central venous temperature
    cerebral venous thrombosis
    congenital vertical talus
CVTMET
    Color Vision Testing Made Easy test
CVTR
    charcoal viral transport medium
CVTS
    cardiovascular-thoracic surgery
CVU
    clean voided urine
CVUG
    cystoscopy and voiding urethrogram
CVV
    Cache Valley virus
CVVH
    continuous venovenous hemofiltration
CVVHD
    continuous venovenous hemodialysis
CVVHDF
    continuous venovenous hemodiafiltration
CW
    cardiac work
    careful watch
    case work
    cell wall
    chemical warfare (weapon)
    chest wall
    circle of Willis
    clockwise (*See also* cw)
    clustered waves
    compare with
    continuous wave (*See also* cw)
    cotton-wool [spots or exudates]
      (*See also* CWS)
    crutch walking
C/W, c/w
    compatible with
    consistent with
CWA
    carcinoma with adenomatous areas
    chemical warfare agent
    cognitive work analysis
CWBTS
    capillary whole blood true sugar
CWD
    cell wall defect(ive)

chronic wasting disease
continuous-wave Doppler
CWDF
    cell wall-deficient form [bacteria]
CWE
    cotton-wool exudates
CWF
    Cornell Word Form
CWH
    cardiomyopathy and wooly-hair coat
      [veterinary syndrome]
CWHB
    citrated whole human blood
CWHTO
    closing wedge high tibial
      osteotomy
CWI
    cardiac work index
CWIF
    cold water immersion foot
CWL
    cutaneous water loss
CWM
    cardiological workspace manager
    comprehensive weight management
CWMS
    color, warmth, movement, sensation
CWOP
    childbirth without pain
CWP
    centimeter of water pressure
    coal workers' pneumoconiosis
    cold wet pack
cWPW
    concealed Wolff-Parkinson-White
      [syndrome]
CWR
    clockwise rotation
CWS
    cell wall skeleton
    chest wall stimulation
    Child Welfare Service
    circumferential wall stress
    cold water soluble
    comfortable walking speed
    cotton-wool spots
CWSN
    Children with Special Health Care
      Needs
CWT
    cold water treatment
cwt
    hundredweight
CWV
    Cape Wrath virus
    closed wound vacuum
CX
    cancel
    cerebral cortex

cervix
chest x-ray (*See also* CXR)
circumflex coronary artery (*See also* CF, CFX, CXA, CxCor)
clearance
complex
complication
contraction (*See also* C, contr, contrx, CTX, CTXN)
controlled expansion
convex
craniohypophysial xanthoma
critical experiment
culture
cylinder axis
NATO code for phosgene oxime

Cx37
connexin 37

Cx43
connexin 43

CXA
circumflex coronary artery (*See also* CF, CFX, CX, CxCor)

CxBx
cervical biopsy

CxCor
circumflex coronary [artery] (*See also* CF, CFX, CX, CXA)

CXCR4
chemokine-related receptor

CXEV
Chorizagrotis auxilliaris entomopoxvirus

CxMT
cervical motion tenderness

CXR
chest x-ray

C × T
concentration multiplied by time

CXTX
cervical traction (*See also* CT)

CY
calendar year
cyanogen (*See also* Cy)

Cy
cyst

cy
copy

CY-BOCS
Children's Yale-Brown Obsessive Compulsive Scale

cyc
cycle
cyclotron

CYE
charcoal yeast extract [medium]

CYFRA 21–1
cytokeratin 19 fragment [tumor marker]

CYL
casein yeast lactate (medium)

cyl
cylinder (cylindrical lens) (*See also* C)

CYN
cyanide

CYNAP
cytotoxicity negative, absorption positive

CYP
cytochrome P450 enzyme
cytochrome pigment
cytochrome protein

CYP19
cytochrome P450 enzyme 19

CYP27
cytochrome P450 enzyme 27

CyP
cyclophilin

CypA
cyclophilin A

CYP1A1
cytochrome P450 enzyme 1A1

CYP11A
cytochrome P450 enzyme 11A

CYP11B1
cytochrome P450 11-beta-hydroxylase

CYP21B
cytochrome P450 enzyme 21B

CYS
cystoscopy

Cys
cysteine

Cys-LT
cysteinyl leukotriene

CYSTO, cysto
cystogram
cystoscopy

CYT
cytochrome

Cyt
cytosine

cyt
cytologic (*See also* cytol)
cytoplasm (cytoplasmic)

cytol
cytologic (*See also* cyt)

cyt ox
cytochrome oxidase

cyt sys
cytochrome system

Cz
central midline placement of electrodes in electroencephalography

CZE
capillary zone electrophoresis

CZI
crystalline zinc insulin

C

D

date
daughter (*See also* da, dau)
day (*See also* d, da)
dead (*See also* d)
dead air space
debye [non-SI and non-CGS unit of electrical dipole moment]
decay
decease(d) (*See also* DEC, decd, dec'd)
deciduous [upper teeth]
decimal reduction time
degree (*See also* d, DEG, deg)
density (*See also* d)
dental
dentin
dependent
depression
dermatologic
dermatology
detail response
deuterium [hydrogen-2]
development(al) (*See also* dev, devel)
deviate (deviation) (*See also* DEV, dev)
dexter [right] (L. *dexter*) (*See also* dex.)
dextro- [right, clockwise] (*See also* d)
dextrorotatory
dextrose
diagnosis (*See also* DG, Dg, diag, DIAGNO, Dx, dx)
diagonal (*See also* diag)
diameter (*See also* dia, diam)
diarrhea (*See also* d)
diastole (*See also* dias)
diathermy
dictated
didymium [mixture of praseodymium and neodymium]
died
difference (*See also* DIFF, diff)
diffusing
diffusion coefficient
dihydrouridine (*See also* hU, hu)
dilate(d)
diminish(ed)
diopter (*See also* diopt, Dptr)
direct treatment
disease (*See also* DIS, DZ)
distal (*See also* dist)
distance
diuresis
diurnal
diverticulum
divorced (*See also* div)
dominant (dominance) (*See also* DOM)
donor
dorsal
dose (dosage) [L. *dosis*] (*See also* d, dos)
drive
drug
dual
duodenum (duodenal)
duration
dwarf
[electric] displacement [field, electric flux density]
give [L. *da*] (*See also* DA)

D1

day one [first day of treatment]
first diagonal branch [coronary artery]
deiodinase type 1

1D

one dimensional

D2

second diagonal branch [coronary artery]
deiodinase type 2

2D

two dimensional

D3

deiodinase type 3

3D

delayed double diffusion [test]
three dimensional

D/3, $^D/_3$
distal third

4D

four dimensional
four prism diopters

D5

dextrose 5% injection

D5/45

dextrose 5% in 0.45% sodium chloride (saline) [injection]

D15

Farnsworth panel D15 color vision test

D50

50% dextrose [injection]

°D

mean dose

D-

note not dictated, save chart for doctor
stereochemical structure

$\overline{D}$

mean dose

2,4-D

2,4-dichlorophenoxyacetic acid

D+

note has been dictated/look for report

D_3
cholecalciferol [vitamin D_3]

D_{beta} (β)
total body bone mineral density

⚠ /d
per day ⚠

⚠ $^1/_d$
daily, one per day ⚠

⚠ $^2/_d$
twice a day ⚠

d
day [L. *dies*] (*See also* D, da)
dead (*See also* D)
deci–
deciduous [lower teeth]
degree (*See also* D, DEG, deg)
density (*See also* D)
deoxyribose
deuteron [nucleus of hydrogen-2]
dextro- [right, clockwise] (*See also* D)
diarrhea (*See also* D)
dose (dosage) [L. *dosis*] (*See also* D, dos)
doubtful
dextro rotatory chemical [relative to rotation of a beam of polarized light]

D-
sterically related to D-glyceraldehyde

d-
dextrorotatary

D5E48
5% dextrose and electrolyte 48% [solution]

D5E75
5% dextrose and electrolyte 75% [solution]

D-A
donor-acceptor

DA
daily activities
dark adaptation [test]
dark agouti [rat]
daytime asthma
decubitus angina
degenerative arthritis
delayed action
delivery awareness
descending aneurysm
descending aorta (*See also* DAo, desc Ao)
developmental age
dextroamphetamine
diabetic acidosis
diagnostic arthroscopy
diastolic augmentation
differentiation antigen
digital angiography
diphenylchlorarsine chloride [Clark 1, chemical weapon agent]

diphenylchlorarsine [riot control agent]
direct admission
direct agglutination
disability assistance
disaggregated
dispense as directed (*See also* DAD)
dissecting aneurysm
diversional activity
dopamine
drug addict(ion)
drug aerosol
ductus arteriosus
give [L. *da*] (*See also* D)

DA1–DA2
distal arthrogryposis type 1–2

D4A
androstenedione

D/A
date of accident
date of admission
digital to analog [converter]
discharge and advise

D&A
dilatation and aspiration

Da
dalton [alternate name for unified atomic mass unit used in biology for mass of large organic molecules]

dA
day of admission
deoxyadenosine (*See also* dAdo)

d(A)
primary donor

da
daughter (*See also* D, dau)
day (*See also* D, d)
deca-

DAA
dead after arrival
decompensated autonomous adenoma
dehydroacetic acid
dementia associated with alcoholism
dialysis-associated amyloidosis
digital auditory aerobics
dissecting aortic aneurysm
double aortic arch

DA/A
drug/alcohol addiction

DAAF
deoxyribonucleic acid amplification fingerprinting

$D_{A-a}O_2$
alveolar-to-arterial oxygen difference

DAB
carcinogenic
days after birth
diaminobenzidine
diaminobutyric acid
dimethylaminoazobenzene

dysrhythmic aggressive behavior
[number of] days after birth

DAB-2
Diagnostic Achievement Battery, Second Edition

DABS
Derogatis Affects Balance Scale

DAC
day activity center
deep abdominal complication
Depressive Adjective Checklist
diazacholesterol
digital-to-analog converter
disabled adult child
disaster assistance center

dac
dacryon [craniometric]

DACA
dissecting aneurysm of coronary artery
Drug Abuse Control Amendments

DACL
Depression Adjective Check List

DACS
density-adjusted cell sorting

DAD
delayed afterdepolarization
diffuse alveolar damage
diode array detector
dispense as directed (See also DA)
drug administration device

DADA
dichloroacetic acid
    diisopropylammonium salt

DADDS
diacetyldiaminodiphenyl sulfone

dAdo
deoxyadenosine (See also dA)

dADP
deoxyadenosine diphosphate

DADPS
diphenylsulfone

DADS
distal acquired demyelinating
    symmetrical [neuropathy]

DAdV
duck adenovirus

DAE
diphenylanthracene endoperoxide
diving air embolism

DAEC
diffusely adherent *Escherichia coli*

DAEM
disseminated acute encephalomyelitis

DAF
decay-accelerating factor
delayed auditory feedback
direct amplification fingerprinting

Draw-A-Family [test]
dural arteriovenous fistula
dynamic axial fixator

DAFM
double aerosol face mask

DAG
diacylglycerol
diffuse antral gastritis
dimeric acidic glycoprotein

DAGT
direct antiglobulin test

DAGV
D'Aguilar virus

DAH
diffuse alveolar hemorrhage
disordered action of heart

DAI
diffuse axonal injury

DAL
diffuse aggressive lymphomas
drug analysis laboratory

daL
decaliter

DALA, d-ALA
delta-aminolevulinic acid

DALE
Developmental Assessment of Life
    Experiences
disability-adjusted life expectancy
Drug Abuse Law Enforcement

DALI
Dartmouth Assessment of Lifestyle
    Instrument

DALM
dysplasia-associated lesion or mass

DALY, DALYs
disability-adjusted life year(s)

DAM
degraded amyloid
diacetylmonoxime
diacetylmorphine [heroin]
discriminant analytic model

dam
decameter

DAMA
discharged against medical advice

DAMIA
direct acute myocardial infarction
    angioplasty

DAMP
deficits in attention, motor control,
    perception

dAMP
deoxyadenosine monophosphate
deoxyadenylic acid

DAN
diabetic autonomic neuropathy

DANA
designed after natural anatomy
drug-induced antinuclear antibodies

DANAOS
Diagnostic and Neuronal Analysis of Skin Cancer

DAN-PSS
Danish Prostate Symptom Score

DANS
1-dimethylamino-naphthalene-5-sulfonic acid

DANTE
delay alternating with nutation for tailored excitation [MRI pulse sequence]

DAO
diamine oxidase
duly authorized officer

DAo
descending aorta (*See also* DA, desc Ao)

DAOM
depressor anguli oris muscle

DAOS
N-ethyl-N-(2-hydroxy-3-sulfopropyl)-3,5-dimethoxyaniline

DAP
data acquisition processor
death-associated protein
delayed afterpolarization
depolarizing afterpotential
diabetes-associated peptide
diastolic arterial (aortic) pressure
diastolic augmentation pressure
dihydroxyacetone phosphate
dipeptidyl aminopeptidase (*See also* DAT)
direct [latex] agglutination pregnancy [test] (*See also* DAPT)
distending airway pressure
Diversity Awareness Profile
dose area product
Draw-A-Person [test] (*See also* DAPT)
dynamic aortic patch

DAPI
4,6-diamidino-2-phenylindole

DAPP-BQ
Dimensional Assessment of Personality Pathology Basic Questionnaire

DAPRE
Daily Adjusted Progressive Resistance Exercise

DAPRU
Drug Abuse Prevention Resource Unit

DAPS
dark-adapted pupil size
Differentiation of Auditory Perception Skill

DAP:SPED
Draw-A-Person Screening Procedure for Emotional Disturbance

DAPST
Denver Auditory Phoneme Sequencing Test

DAPT
diaminophenyl thiazole
direct [latex] agglutination pregnancy test (*See also* DAP)
Draw-A-Person Test (*See also* DAP)

DAQ
Diagnostic Assessment Questionnaire

DAR
daily affective rhythm
data, action, response
death after resuscitation
Diagnostic Assessments of Reading
dual asthmatic reaction

DARC
Duffy antigen receptor for chemokine

DARE
data, action, response, evaluation
Drug Abuse Resistance Education

DARF
direct antiglobulin rosette-forming

DARP
drug abuse rehabilitation program
drug abuse reporting program

D/ART
Depression: Awareness, Recognition, and Treatment

DARTS
Drug and Alcohol Rehabilitation Testing System

DAS
data-acquisition system
day-of-admission surgery
dead air space
dead (died) at scene
death anxiety scale
delayed anovulatory syndrome
developmental apraxia of speech
Differential Ability Scale
distractive auditory stimulus
Dyadic Adjustment Scale

DASA
distal articular set angle

DASE
Denver Articulation Screening Exam
dobutamine-atropine stress echocardiography

DASH
Dietary Approaches to Stop Hypertension [diet]
Disabilities of Arm, Shoulder, and Hand [questionnaire]
Distress Alarm for Severely Handicapped

DASI
Developmental Activities Screening Inventory
Duke Activity Status Index
DASP
double antibody solid phase [immunoassay]
DASS
Depression Anxiety Stress Scale
DAST
Drug Abuse Screening Test
DAT
decision augmentation theory
definitely abnormal tracing (electrocardiogram)
delayed-action tablet
dementia of Alzheimer type
dental aptitude test
Developmental Articulation Test
diet as tolerated
differential agglutination test (titer)
Differential Aptitude Test
digital axial tomography
dipeptidyl aminopeptidase (*See also* DAP)
diphtheria antitoxin
direct agglutination test
direct amplification test
direct antiglobulin [Coombs] test
Disaster Action Team [of Red Cross]
dopamine transporter
DATE
dental auxiliary teacher education
DATI
diastolic amplitude time index
dATP
deoxyadenosine triphosphate
DATT
deep anterior tibiotalar
DATTA
Diagnostic and Therapeutic Technology Assessment
DAU
Dental Auxiliary Utilization
drug abuse urine
dau
daughter (*See also* D, da)
DAV
Drosophila A virus
DAVF
dural arteriovenous fistula
DAVM
dural arteriovenous malformation
DAW
dispense as written
DAWG
demucosalized augmentation with gastric segment

DAWN
Drug Abuse Warning Network
dAXP
total adenine deoxyribonucleotide
DAZ
deleted in azoospermia [gene]
DAZH
deleted in azoospermia homologue [gene]
DAZL
deleted in azoospermia-like [gene]
DB
Baudelocque diameter [external conjugate of pelvis]
database
date of birth (*See also* D/B, DOB)
deep breath
demineralized bone
demonstration bath
dense body
dermabrasion
dextran blue
diabetes (*See also* DIA, diab, db)
diabetic (*See also* dia, diab, db)
diagonal band
diaphragmatic breathing
diet beverage
direct bilirubin (*See also* DBIL, D bili, DBR)
disability (*See also* DIS)
distobuccal
double-blind [study]
dry bulb
duodenal bulb
Dutch belted [rabbit]
D/B
date of birth (*See also* DB, DOB)
dB
decibel
db
diabetes (*See also* DIA, DB, diab)
diabetic (*See also* DB, diab)
DBA
Diamond-Blackfan anemia
dibenzanthracene
Dolichos biflorus agglutinin
duodenal bulb apex
DBAE
dihydroxyborylaminoethyl
DBC
developmental behavior checklist
distal balloon catheter
distance between centers
distobuccal cusp
dye-binding capacity
DB&C
deep breathing and coughing

DBCL
dilute blood clot lysis [method]
DBCP
dibromochloropropane
DBCR
distobuccal cusp ridge
3DBCT
Three-Dimensional Block Construction
Test
DBD
definite brain damage
DNA (deoxyribonucleic acid)-binding
domain
dynamic beam delivery
DBDC
distal bile duct carcinoma
DBDG
distobuccal developmental groove
DBDS
Dementia Behavior Disturbance
Scale
DBE
deep breathing exercise
dibromoethane
diffuse bone endothelioma
DBED
N_1N'-bis-dibenzyl
ethylenediaminediacetic acid
dBEMCL
decibel effective masking contralateral
D5BES
dextrose 5% in balanced electrolyte
solution
DBF
disturbed bowel function
DBFF
distally based fasciocutaneous flap
DBH
dopamine beta hydroxylase
dBHL
decibel hearing level
DBI
development-at-birth index
diffuse brain injury
documented bacterial infection
documented by initials
DBIL, D bili
direct bilirubin (See also DB, DBR)
DBIP
Discrimination by Identification of
Pictures
dBk
decibel above 1 kilowatt
DBKT
Diabetes: Basic Knowledge Test
DBL
distance between lenses
distance between nasal lines
double beta-lactam [drug]

dbl
double
DBM
database management
decarboxylase base Moeller
demineralized bone matrix
diabetic management
dibenzoylmethane
donor breast milk
dBm
decibel above 1 milliwatt
DBMT
displacement bone marrow
transplant(ation)
DBN
downbeat nystagmus
dBnHL
decibel normal hearing level
DBO
distobuccoocclusal
db/ob
diabetic obese [mouse]
DBP
D-binding protein
demineralized bone powder
diastolic blood pressure
di-*tert*-butyl peroxide (See also DTBP)
dibutyl phthalate
distobuccopulpal
Döhle body panmyelopathy
double breech presentation
vitamin D-binding protein
DBPC
dual balloon perfusion catheter
DBPCFC
double-blind placebo-controlled food
challenge
DBR
direct bilirubin (See also DB, DBIL,
D bili)
disordered breathing rate
distobuccal root
DBRI
dysfunctional behavior rating
instrument
DBS
deep bonding system
deep brain stimulation
Denis Browne splint
despeciated bovine serum
dibromosalicil
diffuse brain swelling
diminished breath sounds
direct bonding system
direct brain stimulation
double-burst stimulus
dried blood stain
DBSL
dorsal brain stem lipoma

dBSL
decibel sensation level
dBSPL
decibel sound pressure level
DBSQ
Diabetes Bowel Symptom Questionnaire
DBT
dialectical behavior therapy
disordered breathing time
dry bulb temperature
DBV
Dakar bat virus
DBW
desirable body weight
desired breast width
dry body weight
dBW
decibel above 1 watt
⚠ **DC**
daily census
data communication
daycare
decarboxylase
decrease (*See also* DEC, DECR, decr)
deep compartment
degenerating cell
dendritic cell
dermatochalasis
descending colon
dextran charcoal
dextrocardia
diabetic coma
diagnostic center
diagnostic code
diagonal conjugate
differentiated carcinoma
differentiated cell
diffuse cortical
diffusing capacity
digit copying
dilation catheter
dilation (dilatation) and curettage
(*See also* D&C, D and C)
diphenylarsine cyanide [Clark 2,
chemical weapon agent]
direct and consensual (*See also* D&C,
D and C)
direct Coombs [test]
direct current
discharge(d) (*See also* disch, D/C) ⚠
discomfort
discontinue(d) (*See also* disc., D/C) ⚠
distal colon
distal cusp
distocervical
donor cells
dorsal column

dressing change
dual chamber
duodenal cap
Dupuytren contracture
dynamic compression
dyskeratosis congenita
NATO code for diphenylcyanoarsine
(diphenylarsine chloride)
⚠ **D/C**
diarrhea/constipation
discharge(d) (*See also* DC, disch) ⚠
disconnect
discontinue(d) (*See also* DC, disc) ⚠
D&C, D and C
deep and clear
dilation (dilatation) and curettage
(*See also* DC)
direct and consensual (*See also* DC)
drugs and cosmetics
dC
deoxycytidine
DCA
deoxycholate-citrate agar
deoxycholic acid
dicarboxylic acid
directional color angiography
directional coronary angioplasty
directional coronary atherectomy
disc-condyle adhesion
double cup arthroplasty
DCABG
double coronary artery bypass graft
DCAF
dilated cardiomyopathy and atrial
fibrillation
DCAG
double coronary artery graft
DCAI
desmoplastic cerebral astrocytoma of
infancy
DCAP-BTLS
deformities, contusions, abrasions,
puncture/penetration, burns, tenderness,
lacerations, swelling [EMT assessment
mnemonic]
DC-ART
disease-controlling antirheumatic therapy
DCB
dichlorobenzidine
dilutional cardiopulmonary bypass
distal communicating branch
DC&B
dilation, curettage, and biopsy
DCBE
double-contrast barium enema
DCBF
dynamic cardiac blood flow

DCBGS
direct-current bone growth stimulator

DCC
deleted in colorectal carcinoma
desquamated cornified cell
detected in colon cancer
dextran-coated charcoal
dicyclohexylcarbodiimide (*See also* DCCD)
direct cardiac compression
direct current cardioversion
dorsal calcaneocuboid
dorsal cell column
double concave (*See also* DCc, DDc)
dysgenesis of corpus callosum

DCc
double concave (*See also* DCC, DDc)

DCCD
dicyclohexylcarbodiimide (*See also* DCC)

DCCF
dural carotid-cavernous fistula

DC$_{CO2}$
diffusing capacity for carbon dioxide

DCCV
direct current cardioversion

DCD
Dennis Test of Child Development
developmental coordination disorder

DCE
delayed contrast enhancement
designated compensable event
desmosterol to cholesterol [converting] enzyme

3DCE
three-dimensional contrast-enhanced

DCE-MRI
dynamic contrast-enhanced magnetic resonance imaging

DCF
data collection form
direct centrifugal flotation
dopachrome conversion factor

DCFM
Doppler color flow mapping

DCG
dacryocystography
dynamic (diagnostic) electrocardiograph(y) (electrocardiogram)

DCGI
double-contrast [barium examination of upper] gastrointestinal tract

DCH
delayed cutaneous hypersensitivity

DCHA
dicyclohexylamine

DCHFB
dichlorohexafluorobutane

DCHN
dicyclohexylamine nitrate

DCHS
dysarthria-clumsy hand syndrome

DCI
delayed cerebral ischemia
dichloroisoprenaline
digital cardiac imaging

DCIA
deep circumflex iliac artery [flap]

DCIS
ductal carcinoma in situ

DCIV
deep circumflex iliac vein

dCK
2′-deoxycytidine kinase

DCL
diffuse cutaneous leishmaniasis
digital counter/locator
disseminated cutaneous leishmaniasis

DCLHb
diaspirin-crosslinked hemoglobin

DCLS
deoxycholate citrate lactose saccharose [agar]

DCM
dementia care mapping
dichloromethane
dilated cardiomyopathy
dyssynergia cerebellaris myoclonica

DCML
dorsal column medial lemniscus

dCMP
deoxycytidine monophosphate

dCMP-D
2′-deoxycytidylate deaminase

3D-CMT
three-dimensional computed x-ray microtomography

DCMX
dichloro-*m*-xylenol

DCN
Data Collection Network [medical records]
deep cerebral nucleus
delayed conditioned necrolysis (necrosis)
depressed, cognitively normal
dorsal column nucleus
dorsal cutaneous nerve

DCO
death certificate only
distal clavicle osteolysis

D$_{CO}$
diffusing capacity [of lungs] for carbon monoxide (*See also* DL$_{co}$)

DCOM
dilated cardiomyopathy

DCOP
distal coronary occlusion pressure

DCOR
dopachrome oxidoreductase
DCP
calcium phosphate, dibasic
des-gamma-carboxy prothrombin [serum
marker]
dicalcium phosphate
dichlorophene
discharge planner
dual-chamber pacemaker
dynamic compression plate
DCPC
dichlorodiphenyl methyl carbinol
DCPN
direction-changing positional nystagmus
DCPU
dorsal caudate putamen
DCR
dacryocystorhinostomy
delayed cutaneous reaction
digitally composited radiograph
digitorenocerebral syndrome
direct cortical response
distal cusp ridge
DCRF
data case report forms
3DCRT
three-dimensional conformal radiation
therapy (radiotherapy)
DCS
damage control surgery
decompression sickness
dense canalicular system
diffuse cortical sclerosis
diffuse cutaneous scleroderma
disease control serum
distal coronary sinus
dorsal column (cord) stimulation
(stimulator)
dynamic condylar screw
dyskinetic cilia syndrome
DCSA
double-contrast shoulder arthrography
1D-CSI
one-dimensional chemical-shift imaging
DCSWS
dementia with continuing spike-wave
during slow-wave sleep
DCT
deceleration time
decisional conflict theory
deep chest therapy
direct Coombs test
discrete cosine transform
distal convoluted tubule
diurnal cortisol test
dynamic computed tomography

3D-CTA
three-dimensional computed tomographic
angiography
DCTD
diffuse connective tissue disease
DCTM
delay computer tomographic
myelography
DCTMA
desoxycorticosterone trimethylacetate
3D-CTP
three-dimensional computed tomography
pancreatography
dCTP
deoxycytidine triphosphate
DCTS
dynamic carpal tunnel syndrome
DCU
dichloral urea
DCUS
duplex color ultrasonography
DCV
delayed cerebral vasoconstriction
Drosophila C virus
D2CV
Doppler two-chamber view
[echocardiogram]
D4CV
Doppler four-chamber view
[echocardiogram]
DCW
direct care worker
DCX
double-charge exchange
DCx
double convex
dCYD
2′-deoxycytidine
DD
daily [L. *de die*] (*See also* d.d.)
dangerous drug
day of delivery
D-dimer
death domain
degenerated disc
degenerative disease
delayed diarrhea
delivery date
delusional disorder
dependent drainage
depth dose [x-ray]
Descemet [membrane] detachment
detrusor dyssynergia
developmental disability
development(al) disorder
developmentally delayed (disabled)
dialysis dementia

D

DD *(continued)*
  diaper dermatitis
  diastrophic dysplasia
  died of the disease
  differential diagnosis (*See also* D/D,
    DDX, DDx, diff diag)
  digestive disease
  digestive disorder
  disc diameter
  disc diffusion
  discharged dead
  discharge diagnosis
  Distortion of Dots
  double diffusion
  double dose
  down drain
  drug dependence
  dry dressing
  dual disorder
  Duchenne dystrophy
  due date
  dysthymic disorder
D-D
  duct-to-duct
D1–12
  first through twelfth dorsal vertebrae
    (*See also* T1–T12)
D→D
  discharge to duty
D&D
  debridement and dressing
  diarrhea and dehydration
  drilling and drainage
D/D
  differential diagnosis (*See also* DD,
    DDX, DDx, diff diag)
Dd
  unusual detail response
dD
  confabulated detail response
d.d.
  daily [L. *de die*] (*See also* DD)
DDA
  Dangerous Drugs Act
  digital dermoscopy analyzer
  digital differential analyzer
  digital display alarm
  dorsal digital artery
ddAdo
  2′,3′-dideoxyadenosine
ddATP
  dideoxyadenosine triphosphate
DDB
  donor directed blood
DDC
  dangerous drug cabinet
  dihydrocollidine
  dihydroxyphenylalanine
    decarboxylase

direct display console
diverticular disease of colon
DDc
  double concave (*See also* DCC, DCc)
DDD
  defined daily dose
  degenerative disc disease
  dense-deposit disease
  Denver dialysis disease
  dichlorodiphenyldichloroethane
  digital differential display
  dihydroxydinaphthyl disulfide
  dorsal dural deficiency
  double dose delay
  Dowling Degos disease
  dual [mode], dual [pacing], dual
    [sensing] [atrioventricular universal
    pacemaker]
DDD CT
  double-dose–delay computed tomography
DDDR
  dual [pace], dual [sense], dual
    [response], [programmable] rate [pace
    maker code]
dD/dt
  derived value on apex cardiogram
DDE
  dichlorodiphenyldichloroethylene
  direct data entry
DDF
  difficulty describing feeling
DDFP
  dodecafluoropentane [ultrasound
    contrast]
DDFS
  distant disease-free survival
DDG
  deoxy-D-glucose
ddG
  dideoxyguanosine
DDGB
  double-dose gallbladder [cholecystogram]
DDGE
  denaturing density gradient
    electrophoresis
DDH
  developmental dislocation (dysplasia) of
    hip
  dissociated double hypertropia
DDHT
  dissociated double hypertropia
DDI
  dressing dry and intact
  drug dose intensity
  drug-drug interaction
D-Di
  D-dimer
DDIB
  Disease Detection Information Bureau

DDIS
Dissociative Disorders Interview Schedule
DDLS
disc damage likelihood scale
DDMS
degenerative dense microsphere
diamond dusted membrane scraper
ddN
2′,3′-dideoxynucleoside
dDNA
denatured deoxyribonucleic acid
DDNOS
dissociative disorder not otherwise specified
DDNS
digestive disease and nutrition service
DdNTP
2′,3′-dideoxynucleoside-5′-triphosphate
DDP
density-dependent phosphoprotein
difficult-denture patient
distributed data processing
dual drop pelvis [chiropractic table]
2D DQFC NMR
two-dimensional double quantum filtered correction nuclear magnetic resonance [spectroscopy]
DDR
diastolic descent rate
direct digital radiography
discharged during referral
discoidin domain receptor
DD2R
dopamine D2 receptor
DDRA
dead despite resuscitation attempt
DDREF
dose/dose-rate effective factor
DDS
damaged disc syndrome
dendrodendritic synaptosome
dental distress syndrome
depressed DNA synthesis
dialysis disequilibrium syndrome
directional Doppler sonography
disability determination service
disease disability scale
dodecyl sulfate
double decidual sac
dystrophy-dystocia syndrome
Dds
detail response to small white space
DDSA
duplex Doppler signal analysis

3D-DSA
three-dimensional digital subtraction angiography
DDST
Denver Developmental Screening Test
DDT
dichlorodiphenyltrichloroethane [chlorophenothane, pesticide]
ductus deferens tumor
dye disappearance test
DDTP
drug dependence treatment program
ddTTP
dideoxythymidine triphosphate
DDU
dermodistortive urticaria
DDVP
dimethyldichlorovinyl phosphate [insecticide]
DDW
double distilled water
D5%DW
5% dextrose in distilled water
D/DW
dextrose in distilled water
DdW
detail response elaborating the whole
DDX, DDx
differential diagnosis (*See also* DD, D/D, diff diag)
DE
dendritic expansion
deprived eye
dermal-epidermal [junction]
diagnostic error
dialysis encephalopathy
diatomaceous earth
digestive energy
digitalis effect
dobutamine echocardiograph(y) (echocardiogram)
dose equivalent
dose evaluation
dream elements
drug equivalent
drug evaluation
duodenal exclusion
duration of ejection
2DE
two-dimensional echocardiography
3DE
three-dimensional echocardiography
D&E
diet and elimination
dilation (dilatation) and evacuation
dilation and extraction

de
  edge detail [Rorschach]
DEA
  diethanolamine
  diethylamine
  Drug Enforcement Administration
    [United States Department of Justice]
DEA #
  Drug Enforcement Administration
    number [physicians' federal
    narcotic-prescribing number]
DEA-D, DEAE-D
  diethylaminoethyl dextran
DEAE
  diethylaminoethanol
  diethylaminoethyl [cellulose]
DEAFF
  detection of early antigen fluorescent
    focus
DEB
  diepoxybutane
  diethylbutanediol
  dystrophic epidermolysis bullosa
deb
  debridement
debil
  debility
DEBS
  dominant epidermolysis bullosa simplex
DEC
  decease(d) (*See also* D, decd, dec'd)
  deciduous [upper teeth]
  decimal
  decimeter
  decompose (decomposition)
  decrease (*See also* DC, DECR, decr)
  deoxycholate citrate
  Developmental Evaluation Center
  direction-encoded color mapping
  dynamic environmental conditioning
    [cycle]
  pour off [L. *decanta*]
DEC1
  differentiated embryo-chondrocyte
    expressed gene 1
dec
  decant
  deciduous [lower teeth]
decd, dec'd
  deceased (*See also* D, DEC)
DECEL, decel
  deceleration
  decelerations [labor]
DECG
  differentiated electrocardiogram
DECO
  decreasing consumption of oxygen
decoct
  decoction

DECOMP
  decomposition [EEG, ECG, EKG, EMG
    into separate channels]
  decompose
decon
  decontamination
DECR, decr
  decrease (*See also* DC, DEC)
dec (R)
  decrease, relative
dec-RVKR-cmk
  decanoyl-Arg-Val-Lys-Arg-
    chloromethylketone
    (decanoyl-arginine-valine-lysine-
    arginine-chloromehtylketone) [furin
    inhibitor]
DECU
  decubitus [ulcer]
DECUB, decub.
  decubitus [position]
  lying down [L. *decubitus*]
  decubitus [pressure ulcer]
DED
  date of expected delivery
  defined exposure dose
  delayed erythema dose
  depressive-executive dysfunction
    [syndrome]
  diabetic eye disease
  died in emergency department
DEEDS
  drugs, exercise, education, diet,
    self-monitoring
DEEG
  depth electroencephalograph(y)
    (electroencephalogram)
  deteriorating electroencephalogram
DEEP-IN
  delirium, dementia, depression, drugs;
    eyes and ears; physical performance
    and "phalls" [falls]; incontinence;
    nutrition [screening test for
    geriatrics]
DEET
  diethyltoluamide
  n,n-diethyl-m-toluamide
DEF
  decayed, extracted, filled [permanent
    teeth]
  defecation
  deficiency (deficient) (*See also* defic)
  definite (definition)
  duck embryo fibroblast
2DEF
  two-dimensional [echo-derived] ejection
    fraction
def
  decayed, extracted, filled [deciduous
    teeth]

defib
  defibrillate
defic
  deficiency (deficient)
  deficit
DEFN
  Danubian endemic familial nephropathy
deform.
  deform(ed)
  deformity
DEFS
  detailed evaluation of facial symmetry
DEFT
  driven equilibrium Fourier transform
DEG, deg
  degeneration (*See also* degen)
  degenerative (*See also* degen)
  degree (*See also* D, d)
  diethylene glycol
degen
  degeneration (*See also* DEG)
  degenerative (*See also* DEG)
DEH
  dysplasia epiphysialis hemimelica
DEHFT
  developmental hand function test
DEHP
  diethylhexyl phthalate
dehyd
  dehydrated
  dehydration
DEI
  diffraction-enhanced imaging
  Disease Extent Index
DEIA
  deoxyribonucleic acid-enzyme
    immunoassay
DEJ, dej
  dentinoenamel junction
  dermal-epidermal junction
DEL
  delivered
  deltoid
DEL1
  developmental endothelial locus 1
del
  deletion
  delivery
  delusion
DELFIA
  dissociation enhanced lanthanide
    fluoroimmunoassay
deliq
  deliquescent (deliquescence)
DELIRIUM
  drugs, electrolytes, low [temperature] or
    lunacy, intoxication and intracranial

[processes], retention [of urine or
  feces] or infection, unfamiliar
  [surroundings], myocardial [infarction]
  [mnemonic for evaluation of
  delirium]
δ, delta
  delta [fourth letter of Greek alphabet
    lowercase]
  fourth in a series or group
  heavy chain of immunoglobulin D
Δ, delta
  absence of heat in a reaction
  delta [fourth letter of Greek alphabet
    uppercase]
  delta gap
  difference [mathematics]
  double bond
DELTA
  Descriptive Language for Taxonomy
delta-HCD
  delta (δ) heavy-chain disease
DEM
  Demerol
  Developmental Eye Movement
  diethylmaleate
  drug evaluation matrix
DEMRI
  dynamic enhanced magnetic resonance
    imaging
DEN
  dengue [fever]
  dermatitis exfoliativa neonatorum
  diethylnitrosamine
denat
  denatured
DENM
  direct eighth nerve monitoring
denom
  denominator
DENS
  direct electrical nerve stimulation
DENT
  Dental Exposure Normalization
    Technique
  denti de Chiaie [Chiaie teeth]
dent
  dental
  dentist
  dentistry
  dentition
DENV 1–4
  dengue virus 1–4
DEP
  diatomaceous earth pneumoconiosis
  diesel exhaust particles
  diethyl pyrocarbonate
  dilution end point

D

dep
dependent
deposit
DEPA
depth [of ulcer], extent [of bacterial colonization], phase [of ulcer], associated [etiology]
DEPC
diethylpyrocarbonate
depr
depress(ed)
depression
DEPS
distal effective potassium secretion
DEP ST SEG
depressed ST segment
dept
department
DEQ
Depressive Experiences Questionnaire
digital echo quantification
DER
desmin ensheathment ratio
died in emergency room
disulfiramethanol [and] ethanol reaction
dual-energy radiograph
DeR
degeneration reaction (*See also* DR)
der, deriv
derivative
derive(d)
DERM, Derm, derm
dermatolog(y) (dermatologic)
Dermatology Education by Recall of Mnemonics
DES
dermal-epidermal separation
dialysis encephalopathy syndrome
diethylstilbestrol
diffuse esophageal spasm
disequilibrium syndrome
Dissociative Experiences Scale
doctor's emergency service
drug-eluting stent
dry eye syndrome
dysequilibrium syndrome
dysfunctional elimination syndrome
DESAT, desat
desaturated
DESBRS-II
Devereux Elementary School Behavior Rating Scale II
desc
descendant
descending
descent
desc Ao
descending aorta (*See also* DA, DAo)

DESD
detrusor external sphincter dyssynergia
DESF
dose error sensitivity factor
DESI
drug efficacy study implementation
DESNOS
disorders of extreme stress not otherwise specified
DESS
double-echo steady state
DEST
Denver Eye Screening Test
dichotic environmental sounds test
DET
diethyltryptamine
dipyridamole echocardiography test
dry eye test
Det-6
Detroit-6 [human marrow cell line]
det
determine(d) (*See also* determ)
determ
determination
determine(d) (*See also* det)
detn
detention
detox
detoxification
DEUC
direct electronic urethrocystometry
DEV
deviant
deviate (deviation) (*See also* D, dev)
duck embryo vaccine (virus)
dev
develop
development(al) (*See also* D, devel)
deviate (deviation) (*See also* D, DEV)
devel
development(al) (*See also* D, dev)
DevPd
developmental pediatrics
DEVR
dominant exudative vitreoretinopathy
dex
Dextrostix (*See also* D-stix, DSX)
dex.
right [L. *dexter*] (*See also* D)
DEXA
dual-energy x-ray absorptiometry [scan] (*See also* DXA)
dext
dexterity
DF
day frequency [of voiding]
decapacitation factor [sperm]
decayed and filled [permanent teeth]
decontamination factor

deferred
defibrotide
deficiency factor
defined flora [of an animal]
degree of freedom
dengue [hemorrhagic] fever
dermatofibroma
dermatofibrosis
diabetic father
diabetic fetopathy
diaphragmatic function
diastolic filling
dietary fiber
digital fluoroscopy
discriminant function
disseminated focus [singular] (foci [plural])
distal fossa
distribution factor
dome fragment
dorsiflexion
drug free
dry [gas] fractional [concentration]
dye free

DF-2
dysgonic fermenter 2 [bacillus]

df
decayed and filled [deciduous teeth]
deficient
definite
definition
degrees of freedom

DFA
delayed feedback audiometry
diet for age
difficulty falling asleep
direct fluorescence (fluorescent) antigen (assay) [test]
direct fluorescence (fluorescent) antibody [test]
discriminant function analysis [statistics]
distal forearm
dorsiflexion angle
dorsiflexion assist
hallux dorsiflexion angle

3D FASTER
three-dimensional field echo acquisition [with] short repetition time [and] echo reduction

DFA-TP
direct fluorescent antibody [test] for *Treponema pallidum*
direct fluorescent antibody [test] for *Treponema phagedenis* [Reiter strain]

DFAT-TP
direct fluorescent antibody tissue [test] for *Treponema pallidum*

DFB
dinitrofluorobenzene [Sanger reagent]
dysfunctional [uterine] bleeding

DFC
deletion of final consonants
dry-filled capsule

DFD
defined formula diet
degenerative facet disease

DFDB
demineralized freeze-dried bone

DFDBA
decalcified freeze-dried bone allograft
demineralized freeze-dried bone allograft

DFDCB
decalcified freeze-dried cortical bone

DFDT
difluorodiphenyltrichloroethane [pesticide]

DFE
dietary folate equivalent
diffuse fasciitis with eosinophilia
dilated fundus examination
distal femoral epiphysis

DFECT
dense fibroelastic connective tissue

d$_{FF}$
density of fat mass

d$_{FFM}$
density of fat-free mass

DFG
direct forward gaze

DFI
darkfield illumination
deterioration following improvement
disease-free interval
dye fluorescence index

DFIB
defibrillation

D-FISH
double-fusion fluorescence (fluorescent) in situ hybridization

DFL
dense fibrous lamina

DFLE
disability-free life expectancy

DFM
decreased fetal movement
deep finger massage
deep friction massage

DFMC
daily fetal movement count

DFMR
daily fetal movement record

DFN
distal femoral nail

D

189

DFNA3
deafness, autosomal dominant nonsyndromic sensorineural

DFNB1
deafness, neurosensory, autosomal recessive

DFN3
deafness 3, conductive, with stapes fixation

DFP
diastolic filling pressure (period)
diisopropyl fluorophosphate [insecticide, toxin]

DF³²P
diisopropyl fluorophosphonate radiolabeled with phosphorus-32

DFPP
double filtration plasmapheresis

DFR
designated family respondent
diabetic floor routine
dialysate filtration rate
digital fluororadiography

2DFr
two-dimensional Fourier imaging

3DFr
three-dimensional Fourier imaging

DFRC
deglycerolized frozen red cells

DFS
decayed and filled surfaces [permanent teeth]
Defensive Functioning Scale
disease-free survival
distraction-flexion stage (staging)
Doppler flow study
dynamic flow study

dfs
decayed and filled surfaces [deciduous teeth]

DFSP
dermatofibrosarcoma protuberans

DFT
defibrillation threshold (See also XDT)
dementia of frontal type
discrete Fourier transform
Doppler flow test

2DFT
two-dimensional Fourier transform

3DFT
three-dimensional Fourier transform

DFT₄
dialyzable free thyroxine

DFTT
Digital Finger Tapping Test

DFU
dead fetus in utero

DFV
dengue fever vaccine
diarrhea with fever and vomiting

DFWO
dorsiflexory wedge osteotomy

DG
dark ground
Davis & Geck [manufacturer]
dentate gyrus
diagnosis (See also D, Dg, diag, DIAGNO, Dx, dx)
diastolic gallop
diglyceride
distogingival
documentation guidelines
dorsal glides
downward gaze

Dg
dentate gyrus
diagnosis (See also D, DG, diag, DIAGNO, Dx, dx)

dg
decigram

DGA
dermatoglyphic alteration
DiGeorge anomaly
disseminated granuloma annulare

DGAT
diacylglycerol acyltransferase

DGC
directional gradient concentration
dystrophin-glycoprotein complex

DGCI
delayed gamma camera image

DGCR
DiGeorge chromosome critical region

DGE
delayed gastric emptying
density gradient electrophoresis

dGEMRIC
delayed gadolinium-enhanced magnetic resonance imaging of cartilage

2D-GEMS
two-dimensional gel electrophoresis mass spectrometry

DGER
duodenal gastroesophageal (duodenogastroesophageal) reflux

DGF
delayed graft function
digoxinlike factor

DGGE
denaturing gradient gel electrophoresis

DGHAL
Doppler-guided hemorrhoidal artery ligation
Doppler-guided hemorrhoid artery ligation

DGI
dentinogenesis imperfecta
deoxyglucose imaging
disseminated gonococcal infection
DGJ
deoxygalactonojirimmycin
DGKV
Dera Ghazi Khan virus
DG-L
deep gastric-longitudinal
DGLA
dihomogammalinolenic acid
DGM
ductal glandular mastectomy
dGMP
deoxyguanosine monophosphate
deoxyguanylic acid
DGN
diffuse glomerulonephritis
DGP
deoxyglucose phosphate
DGPG
diffuse proliferative glomerulonephritis
DGR
Dacron graft replacement
duodenogastric reflux
DGS
diabetic glomerulosclerosis
DiGeorge sequence (syndrome)
dysplasia-gigantism syndrome
DGSCR, DGCR
DiGeorge syndrome critical region
[gene 8]
DGSX
X-linked dysplasia-gigantism syndrome
DG-T
deep gastric-transverse
DGT
decaffeinated green tea
dGTP
deoxyguanosine triphosphate
(2-deoxyguanosine 5′-triphosphate)
DGV
dextrose, gelatin, Veronal [solution]
DGVB
dextrose-gelatin-Veronal buffer
DG/VCF
DiGeorge [and] velocardiofacial
[syndromes]
DH
daily habits
day hospital
dehydrocholic acid
dehydrogenase
delayed hypersensitivity
deliberate hypotension
dental habits

dental hygiene
dermatitis herpetiformis
developmental history
diaphragmatic hernia
diffuse histiocytic [lymphoma]
disseminated histoplasmosis
dominant hand
dorsal horn
drug hypersensitivity
ductal hyperplasia
Dunkin-Hartley [guinea pig]
D-H
Dimon-Hughston [intertrochanteric
osteotomy]
D+H
delusions and hallucinations
D:H
deuterium to hydrogen ratio
DHA
dehydroalanine
dehydroascorbic acid
dehydroepiandrosterone (See also
DHEA)
dehydroisoandrosterone
dihydroacetic acid
dihydroacetone
dihydroxyacetone
district health authority
docosahexaenoic acid
DHAP
dihydroxyacetone phosphate
DHA-PUVA
dihydroxyacetone and psoralens plus
ultraviolet [Turbo-PUVA]
DHB
dihydroxybenzoic acid
duck hepatitis B
DHBP
direct His bundle pacing
DHBS
dihydrobiopterin synthetase [enzyme]
DHBV
duck hepatitis B virus
DHC
dehydrocholate
dehydrocholesterol
11-dehydrocorticosterone
DHCA
deep hypothermia (hypothermic)
circulatory arrest
DHCC
dihydroxycholecalciferol
DHCP
dental health care provider
DHCT
dual-phase helical computed
tomography

D

DHD
dissociated horizontal deviation
district health department
donor hepatic duct

DHDA
directed heteroduplex analysis

DHE
dihematoporphyrin ether

DHEA
dehydroepiandrosterone (*See also* DHA)

DHEA-S, DHEAS, DHAS
dehydroepiandrosterone sulfate

DHF
dengue hemorrhagic fever
diastolic heart failure
dorsihyperflexion

DHF-DSS
dengue hemorrhagic fever [and] dengue shock syndrome

DHFK
Dow Hollow Fiber kidney

DHFR
dihydrofolate reductase

DHFS
dengue hemorrhagic fever shock [syndrome]

DHFT
developmental hand-function test

DHGA
dihomogammalinolenic acid

DHI
dihydroisocodeine
dihydroxyindole
Dizziness Handicap Inventory
dynamic hyperinflation

DHIA
dehydroisoandrosterone

DHIC
detrusor hyperactivity with impaired contractility

DHL
diffuse histiocytic lymphoma

DHMA
dihydroxymandelic acid (*See also* DOMA)

DHN
dissociative hysterical neurosis

DHO
deuterium hydrogen oxide

DHODH
dihydroorotate dehydrogenase

DHP
dehydrogenated polymer
dihydroprogesterone
dihydropyridine
dihydroxyacetone phosphate

DHPc
dorsal hippocampus

DHPG
dihydroxyphenylethylene glycol
dihydroxyphenylglycol

DHPLC
denaturing high-performance liquid chromatography

DHPR
dihydropteridine reductase [deficiency]

dhPRL
decidual prolactin

DHPS
dihydropteroate synthase

DHPSA
Dental Health Professional Shortage Area

DHR
delayed hypersensitivity reaction

DHS
delayed hypersensitivity
diabetic hyperosmolar state
duration of hospital stay
dynamic hip screw

D5HS
dextrose 5% in Hartmann solution

DHSI
Digestive Health Status Instrument

DHST
delayed hypersensitivity test

DHT
dehydrotestosterone (dihydrotestosterone)
dihydrothymine
dissociated hypertropia
Dobbhoff tube
domino heart transplant(ation)

DHTF
Dobbhoff tube feeding

DHTR
dihydrotestosterone receptor deficiency

DHZ
degenerating hypertrophied zone

DI
(Beck) Depression Inventory
date of injury
Debris Index [oral hygiene]
defective interfering
degradation index
dental index
dentinogenesis imperfecta
depression inventory
desorption ionization
deterioration index
detrusor instability
diabetes insipidus
diagnostic imaging
diaphragm(atic) (*See also* diaph, DPH)
disability index
disability insurance
dispensing information
distal intestine

distoincisal
DNA (deoxyribonucleic acid) index
donor insemination
dorsal interosseous
dorsoiliacus
dose intensity
double indemnity
double induction
drug information
drug interaction
dyskaryosis index
dyspnea index

3DI
three-dimensional imaging

D&I
debridement and irrigation
dilation and irrigation
dry and intact

D$_I$
insulin dialysance

Di
didymium [rare earth]
Diego [blood group]

di
inside detail [Rorschach]

DIA
depolarization-induced automaticity
desmoplastic infantile astrocytoma
diabetes (*See also* DB, db, diab)
dot immunobinding assay
drug-induced agranulocytosis
drug-induced amenorrhea

Dia
Diego [blood group] antigen

dia
diameter (*See also* D, diam)
diathermy (*See also* diath)

diab
diabetes (*See also* DB, db, DIA)
diabetic (*See also* DB, db)

diag
diagnosis (*See also* D, DG, Dg,
DIAGNO, Dx, dx)
diagnostic
diagonal (*See also* D)
diagram

DIAGNO
diagnosis (*See also* D, DG, Dg, Dx, dx)

DIAL
Developmental Indicators for
Assessment of Learning

DIAL-R
Developmental Indicators for
Assessment of Learning, Revised

DIAM
drug-induced aseptic meningitis

diam
diameter (*See also* D, dia)

diaph
diaphragm(atic) (*See also* DI, DPH)

DIAPPERS
delirium, infection, atrophic urethritis
and vaginitis, pharmaceuticals,
psychological disorders, excessive
output, restricted mobility, stool
impaction

DIAR
dextran-induced anaphylactoid reaction

dias
diastole (*See also* D)
diastolic

DIAS BP
diastolic blood pressure

diath
diathermy (*See also* dia)

DIATH SW
diathermy short wave

DIAZ
diazolidinyl urea

DIB
Diagnostic Interview for Borderlines
difficulty in breathing
disability insurance benefits
dot immunobinding
duodenoileal bypass

DIBC
drug-induced blood cytopenia

DIBS
dead-in-bed syndrome

DIC
diagnostic imaging center
differential interference contrast
[microscopy]
diffuse intravascular coagulation
direct isotope cystography
disposable inner cannula
disseminated intravascular coagulation
(coagulopathy) (*See also* DIVC)
drip infusion cholangiograph(y)
(cholangiogram)
drug information center

dic
dicentric

DICA-C
Diagnostic Interview for Children and
Adolescents Child Version

DICA-P
Diagnostic Interview for Children and
Adolescents Parent Version

DICA-R
Diagnostic Interview for Children and
Adolescents Revised

DICC
drug-induced cicatricial conjunctivitis
dynamic infusion cavernosometry and
cavernosography

DICD
dispersion-induced circular dichroism
DICOM
Digital Imaging and Communications in Medicine [interface]
DICP
demyelinated inflammatory chronic polyneuropathy
DICT
dose-intensive chemotherapy
DID
dead of intercurrent disease
delayed ischemic deficit
dissociative identity disorder
document image decoding
double immunodiffusion [technique]
drug-induced disease
dystonia-improvement-dystonia
DIDA
dimethyl iminodiacetic acid [radiopharmaceutical with ^{99m}Tc]
DIDD
dense intramembranous deposit disease
di-di
dichorionic-diamniotic [twins]
DIDMO, DIDMOA
diabetes insipidus, diabetes mellitus, optic atrophy [syndrome]
DIDMOAD
diabetes insipidus, diabetes mellitus, optic atrophy, deafness [syndrome]
DIDMOHS
drug-induced delayed multiorgan hypersensitivity syndrome
DIDOX
dihydroxybenzohydroxamic acid
DIDS
Dermatology Index of Disease Severity
4,4'-di-isothiocyanatostilbene-2,2'-disulfonic acid
DIE
died in emergency [room]
direct injection enthalpimetry [method]
drug-induced esophagitis
DIEA
deep inferior epigastric artery
DIEAP
deep inferior epigastric artery perforator
DIED
drug-induced esophageal damage
DIEDA
diethyliminodiacetic acid
DIEP
deep inferior epigastric perforator
diabetes in early pregnancy
DIEV
Dicentrarchus labrax encephalitis
DIF
differentiation-inducing factor

difficulty identifying feeling
diffuse interstitial fibrosis
direct immunofluorescence [test]
dose increase factor
DIFF, diff
difference (*See also* D)
different
differential [blood count]
diffusion [coefficient]
diff diag
differential diagnosis (*See also* DD, D/D, DDX, DDx)
DIFP
diffuse interstitial fibrosing pneumonitis
diisopropyl fluorophosphonate
DIF-test
direct immunofluorescence test
DIG
desmoplastic infantile ganglioglioma
digitalis
digitate
digitoxin
digoxigenin
digoxin
drug-induced galactorrhea
DIGGEST
direct imaging of local gradients by group echo selection tomography
DIGS
Diagnostic Interview for Genetic Study
dig. tox
digitalis (digoxin) toxicity
DIH
died in hospital
digoxin-induced hyperkalemia
DIHE
drug-induced hepatic encephalopathy
DIHS
drug-induced hypersensitivity syndrome
DIJOA
dominantly inherited juvenile optic atrophy
DIL
daughter-in-law
dilation (dilatation) (*See also* dilat)
dilute (*See also* dilut)
drug-induced lupus
drug information log
dilat
dilation (dilatation) (*See also* DIL)
DILC
dose-intensity limiting criterion
DILD
diffuse infiltrative lung disease
diffuse interstitial lung disease
drug-induced liver disease
DILE
drug-induced lupus erythematosus

diln
  dilution
DILS
  diffuse infiltrative lymphocytosis
    syndrome
  drug-induced lupus syndrome
dilut
  dilute (*See also* DIL)
DIM
  diminish (*See also* dim.)
  divalent ion metabolism
dim.
  diminish (*See also* DIM)
  one-half [L. *dimidus*]
DIMD
  drug-induced movement disorder
DIMOAD
  diabetes insipidus, diabetes mellitus,
    optic atrophy, deafness
dIMP
  deoxyinosinate monophosphate
DIMS
  disorders of initiating and maintaining
    sleep
DIMSA
  disseminated intravascular multiple
    systems activation
DIN
  ductal intraepithelial neoplasia
DIND
  delayed ischemic neurologic deficit
DIO
  diet-induced obesity
3 alpha-diol G
  3 alpha-diol glucuronide
diopt
  diopter (*See also* D, Dptr)
DIOS
  distal ileal obstruction syndrome
  distal intestinal obstruction
    syndrome
DIP
  desquamative interstitial pneumonia
    (pneumonitis)
  dichlorophenolindophenol
  diffuse interstitial pneumonia
    (pneumonitis)
  digital imaging processing
  diisopropyl phosphate
  diphtheria toxoid vaccine
  diplopia
  distal interphalangeal [joint] (*See also*
    DIPJ)
  drip-infusion pyelogram
  drug-induced parkinsonism
dip.
  diploid

DIPA
  diisopropylamine
DIPant
  diphtheria antitoxin
DIPC
  diffuse interstitial pulmonary
    calcification
  dynamic infusion
    pharmacocavernosometry
DIPD
  daily intermittent peritoneal dialysis
DIPF
  diffuse interstitial pulmonary fibrosis
diph
  diphtheria
diph-tet
  diphtheria-tetanus [toxoid]
diph-tox
  diphtheria toxoid
diph-tox AP
  alum-precipitated diphtheria toxoid
DIPI
  direct intraperitoneal injection
  direct intraperitoneal insemination
DIPJ
  distal interphalangeal joint (*See also*
    DIP)
DIPS
  direct intrahepatic portacaval shunt
DIR
  delivered in room
  direct
  director
  direct treatment
  disturbed interpersonal relationships
  double isomorphous replacement
dir.
  direction [L. *directione*]
DIRD
  drug-induced renal disease
DIS
  Diagnostic Interview Schedule
  digital imaging spectrophotometer
  disability (*See also* DB)
  disabled (*See also* DSBL)
  disease (*See also* D, DZ)
  disease intervention specialist
  dislocate(d) (dislocation) (*See also* disl,
    disloc)
  distance
  distribute(d) (distribution) (*See also* dist)
DI-S
  Debris Index-Simplified [oral hygiene]
DISA-SPECT
  dual-isotope simultaneous acquisition
    single-photon emission computed
    tomography

D

DISASTER
    detect, incident command, scene safety and security, assess hazard, support required, triage and treatment, evacuation, recovery

DISC
    death-inducing signaling complex
    Diagnostic Interview Schedule for Children
    digital interchange standards for cardiology
    disabled infectious single cycle [virus]
    dynamic integrated stabilization chair

DIS-C
    Diagnostic Interview Schedule for Children

DiSC
    differential staining cytotoxicity

disc.
    discontinue(d) (*See also* DC, D/C)

disch
    discharge(d) (*See also* DC, D/C)

DISC-HSV
    disabled infectious single-cycle herpes simplex virus [oncolytic vector]

DISC-R
    Diagnostic Interview Schedule for Children-Revised

DISCUS
    Dyskinesia Identification System: Condensed User Scale

DISE
    driven inversion spin echo

DISH
    diffuse (disseminated) idiopathic skeletal hyperostosis

DISI
    distal intercalated segment instability
    dorsal intercalated segment instability
    dorsiflexed intercalated segment instability

DISIDA
    diisopropyl iminodiacetic acid

disinfect.
    disinfection

disl
    dislocate(d) (dislocation) (*See also* DIS, disloc)

disloc
    dislocate(d) (dislocation) (*See also* DIS, disl)

dism
    dismissed

disod
    disodium

D₅ISOM
    dextrose 5% in Isolyte M

D5ISOP
    5% Dextrose and Isolyte P

DISP, dispo
    disposition

disp
    dispense (dispensary)

DISR
    drug-induced skin reactions

DISS
    Diameter Index Safety System

diss
    dissolve

dissd
    dissolved

dissem
    disseminate(d) (dissemination)

dist
    distal (*See also* D)
    distance
    distillation (*See also* distill.)
    distill(ed)
    distribute(d) (distribution) (*See also* DIS)
    district
    disturbance

dist fr
    distinguished from

distill.
    distillation (*See also* dist)

DIT
    deferoxamine infusion test
    diet-induced thermogenesis
    diiodinated tyrosine
    diiodotyrosine (3,5-diiodotyrosine)
    drug-induced thrombocytopenia

dITP
    deoxyinosine triphosphate

DIU
    death in utero

DiU
    diazolidinyl urea

DIV
    double-inlet ventricle

div
    divergent (divergence)
    divide(d)
    division
    divorce(d) (*See also* D)

DIVA
    digital intravenous angiography

DIVBC
    disseminated intravascular blood coagulation

DIVC
    disseminated intravascular coagulation (*See also* DIC)

div ex
    divergence excess

diz
    dizygotic

DJ
    duodenal juice

DJD
  degenerative joint disease
DJF
  duodenojejunal flexure
DJJ
  duodenojejunal junction
DJOA
  dominant juvenile optic atrophy
DK
  dark
  decay
  degeneration of keratinocyte
  diabetic ketoacidosis (*See also* DKA)
  diet kitchen
  diseased kidney
  dog kidney (cells)
Dk
  diffusion coefficient
  oxygen permeability [ophthalmology]
DKA
  diabetic ketoacidosis (*See also* DK)
  did keep appointment
DKB
  deep knee bend
DKC
  double knee to chest
  dyskeratosis congenita
DKDP
  deuterium with potassium dihydrogen
  phosphate
DKEFS
  Delis-Kaplan Executive Function System
  [psychology]
dkg
  decagram
Dk/L
  oxygen transmissibility [ophthalmology]
dkL
  decaliter
dkm
  decameter
DKP
  dikalium phosphate (dibasic potassium
  phosphate)
  diketopiperazine
DKS
  Damus-Kaye-Stansel [procedure]
DKTC
  dog kidney tissue culture
DKV
  deer kidney virus
DL
  danger list
  dansyl lysine
  deep lobe
  De Lee [catheter]
  developmental level

diagnostic laparoscopy
difference limen [just noticeable
  difference]
diffuse lymphoma
diffusing capacity of lung
directed listening
direct laryngoscopy
disabled list
distolingual
Donath-Landsteiner [antibody] (*See also*
  D-L Ab)
double lumen
drug level
ductal lavage
lethal dose [L. *dosis letalis*]
DL-
  equal quantities of D and L
  enantiomorphs [formerly dl-]
dL
  deciliter
DLa
  distolabial
D-L Ab
  Donath-Landsteiner antibody (*See also*
  DL)
DLaI
  distolabioincisal
DLaP
  distolabiopulpal
DLB
  dementia with Lewy bodies
  diffuse lymphoblastic [non-Hodgkin
  lymphoma]
  direct laryngoscopy and bronchoscopy
  (*See also* DL&B)
DL&B
  direct laryngoscopy and bronchoscopy
  (*See also* DLB)
DLBCL
  diffuse large B-cell lymphoma
DLBD
  diffuse Lewy body disease
DLBL
  diffuse large B-cell lymphoma
DLC
  differential leukocyte count
  distolingual cusp
  double-lumen catheter
  dual-lumen catheter
DLCL
  diffuse large cell lymphoma
DL$_{CO}$
  diffusing capacity of lungs for carbon
  monoxide (*See also* D$_{CO}$)
DL$_{CO_2}$
  diffusing capacity of lungs for carbon
  dioxide

D

DL$_{CO}$^{SB}
single-breath carbon monoxide diffusing capacity of lungs

DL$_{CO}$^{SS}
steady-state carbon monoxide diffusing capacity of lungs

DLCR
distolingual cusp ridge

DLD
date of last drink
developmental language disorder
disease linkage disequilibrium

DLE
decrement-load exercise
delayed light emission
dialyzable leukocyte extract
discoid lupus erythematosus
disseminated lupus erythematosus

D$_1$LE
diagonal 1 lower extremity [exercise]

D$_2$LE
diagonal 2 lower extremity [exercise]

DLEK
deep lamellar endothelial keratoplasty

DLF
digitalislike factor
digoxinlike factor
distolingual fossa
dorsolateral funiculus
ductal lavage fluid

DLG
disseminated lipogranulomatosis
distolingual groove

DLH
dislocated hip

DLI
Digital Libraries Initiative
distolinguoincisal
donor leukocyte (lymphocyte) infusion
double label index

DLIF
digoxinlike immunoreactive factor

DLIS
digoxinlike immunoreactive substance

DLK
deep lamellar keratoplasty
diffuse lamellar keratitis

DLK1
deltalike 1 protein precursor

DLLI
dulcitol lysine lactose iron [agar]

DLMD
Duchenne-like muscular dystrophy

DLMP
date of last menstrual period

DLN
distant lymph nodes

DLNMP
date of last normal menstrual period

DLO
distolinguoocclusal

DL$_{O_2}$
diffusing capacity of lungs for oxygen

D-loop
dextro loop

DLP
delipidized serum protein
developmental learning problems
direct linear plotting
dislocation of patella
distolinguopulpal
dose-length product
double-limb progression
dysharmonic luteal phase
dyslipoproteinemia

DLPD
diffuse lymphocytic poorly differentiated

DLPFC
dorsolateral prefrontal cortex

DLR
distal line of reference

D$_5$LR
dextrose 5% in lactated Ringer [solution]

DLS
daily living skills
digitalislike substance
ductlike structure
dynamic light scattering

DLSC
double lumen subclavian catheter

DLST
drug-induced lymphocyte stimulation test

DLT
decongestive lymphatic therapy
dihydroepiandrosterone loading test
diode laser trabeculoplasty
dorsolateral tract
dose-limiting toxicity
double lung transplant(ation)

DLU
diffused lung uptake

DLV
defective leukemia virus

DLW
doubly labeled water

DLWD
diffuse lymphocytic, well differentiated

DM
adamsite (diphenglomine chlorarsine) [chemical weapon]
dehydrated and malnourished
dermatology
dermatomyositis
Descemet membrane
dextromaltose
diabetes mellitus [type 1, 2]

diabetic mother
diastolic murmur
diffuse mixed
diffusing capacity of alveolar membrane
disease management
distal metastasis
distant metastasis [singular] (metastases [plural])
dopamine
dorsomedial
dose modification
double membrane
double minute [chromosome]
dry matter
duodenal mucosa
dystrophia myotonica
membrane diffusing capacity
myotonic dystrophy
NATO code for diphenylaminearsine (adamsite)

DM-1
diabetes mellitus type 1

DM-2
diabetes mellitus type 2

D$_M$
membrane component of diffusion

dM
decimorgan

dm
decimeter

dm$_2$
square decimeter

dm$_3$
cubic decimeter

DMA
dimethoxyamphetamine
dimethyladenosine
dimethylamine
dimethylaniline
dimethylarginine
dimethylarsinic acid

DMAA
distal metatarsal articular angle

DMAB, DMABA
dimethylaminobenzaldehyde [Ehrlich reagent]

DMAC
dimethylacetamide
disseminated *Mycobacterium avium-intracellulare* complex [dictated/printed *Mycobacterium avium* complex]

DMAIC
disseminated *Mycobacterium avium-intracellulare* complex

DMAP
4-dimethylaminophenol

DMARD
disease-modifying antirheumatic drug

DMAS
deep muscular aponeurotic system
Dementia Mood Assessment Scale
dimethylamine sulfate
Drug Management and Authorization Section

DMAT
Disaster Medical Assistance Team [Department of Homeland Security]

D$_{max}$
maximum density
maximum depth

DMB
data monitoring board
demineralized bone
diffuse microvascular bleeding

DMBA
dimethylbenzanthracene

DMC
diabetes management center
direct microscopic count
double minute chromosome
p,p'-dichlorodiphenyl methyl carbinol (dichlorodiphenylmethylcarbinol)

DMCC
direct microscopic clump count

DMD
Descemet membrane detachment
digital micromirror device
disciform macular degeneration
disease-modifying drug
distal muscular dystrophy
drowsiness monitoring device
Duchenne [de Boulogne] muscular dystrophy
dystonia musculorum deformans

DMD/BMD
Duchenne [de Boulogne] muscular dystrophy/Becker muscular dystrophy

DMDS
dimethyl disulfide

DMDT
dimethoxydiphenyltrichloroethane

DMD w/SRNM
disciform macular degeneration with subretinal neovascular membrane

DME
degenerative myoclonus epilepsy
diabetic macular edema
dimethyl ether
diphasic meningoencephalitis
dropping mercury electrode
drug-metabolizing enzyme
Dulbecco modified Eagle [medium]
durable medical equipment

DMEC
data monitoring and ethics committee
DMEM
Dulbecco modified Eagle medium
DMEPOS
durable medical equipment, prosthetics, orthotics, supplies
DMERC
durable medical equipment regional carrier
DMF
decayed, missing, filled [permanent teeth]
dimethylformamide (*See also* DMFA)
diphasic milk fever
Drug Master File
dmf
decayed, missing, filled [deciduous teeth]
DMFA
dimethylformamide (*See also* DMF)
DMFC
demand minimum functional capacity
DMFFS
distant metastases failure-free survival
DMFS
decayed, missing, filled surfaces [permanent teeth]
dmfs
decayed, missing, filled surfaces [deciduous teeth]
DMFT
decayed, missing, filled teeth [permanent]
dmft
decayed, missing filled teeth [deciduous]
DMG
N,N-dimethylglycine (dimethylglycine)
DMGBL
dimethyl-gamma-butyrolactone
DMH
diffuse mesangial hypercellularity
dimethylhydrazine
DMI
defense mechanism inventory
diabetic muscle infarct(ion)
Diagnostic Mathematics Inventory [psychologic testing]
diaphragmatic myocardial infarct(ion)
direct migration inhibition
DMIPS
dimethylisopropylsilyl
DM Isch
diaphragmatic myocardial ischemia
DMIT
disability management intervention team
DMKA
diabetes mellitus ketoacidosis

DML
diffuse mixed lymphoma
distal motor latency
DMLO
dim light melatonin onset
DMM
diffuse malignant mesothelioma
dimethylmyleran
disproportionate micromelia
DMMA
distal metatarsal articular angle
D0(mm/dd/yy)
day zero [treatment start date]
DMN
dimethylnitrosamine (*See also* DMNA)
dorsal motor nucleus [of vagus never]
dorsomedial nucleus
dysplastic melanocytic nevus
DMNA
dimethylnitrosamine (*See also* DMN)
DMNL
dorsomedial hypothalamic nucleus lesion
DMO
dimethyloxazlidinedione
DMOA
diabetes mellitus-optic atrophy [syndrome]
DMOAD
disease-modifying osteoarthritic drug
DMOOC
diabetes mellitus out of control
DMORT
disaster mortuary operational response team
Disaster Mortuary Team
DMP
dermatopathology
diffuse mesangial proliferation
dimethylphosphate
dimethylphthalate
dura mater prosthesis
DMPA
durable medical power of attorney
DMPC
dimyristoyl phosphatidyl choline
DMPE
3,4-dimethoxyphenyl-ethylamine (dimethoxyphenylethylamine)
DMPG
dimyristoyl phosphatidyl glycerol
DMPH
dysgenetic male pseudohermaphroditism
DMPM
diffuse malignant pleural mesothelioma
DMPP
dimethyl-4-phenylpiperazinium (dimethylphenylpiperazinium)
DMPS
dimercaptopropane-sulfonic acid

dimethylpolysiloxane
dysmyelopoietic syndrome
DMQ
developmental motor quotient
DM-R
decayed plus missing teeth, minus
replaced teeth
DMR
direct myocardial revascularization
distal marginal ridge
DMRF
dorsal medullary reticular formation
D-MRI
dynamic magnetic resonance imaging
3D-MRI
three-dimensional magnetic resonance
imaging
DMS
delayed microembolism syndrome
delayed muscle soreness
demarcation membrane system
dense microsphere
dermatomyositis
diagnostic medical sonography
diffuse mesangial sclerosis
dimethyl sulfate
dimethyl sulfide
dysmyelopoietic syndrome
dms
double minute sphere
DMSA
2,3-dimercaptosuccinic acid
(dimercaptosuccinic acid)
dimethylsuccinic acid
disodium monomethanearsonate
pentavalent dimercaptosuccinate
DMSLT
daytime multiple sleep latency test
DMSO
dimethylsulfoxide
DMT
dermatophytosis
N,N-dimethyltryptamine
(dimethyltryptamine) [psychedelic
drug]
dynamometer muscle testing
DMTU
dimethylthiourea
DMU
dimethanolurea
dual method of use
DMV
diurnal mood variation
dorsal motor nucleus of vagus nerve
DMVA
direct mechanical ventricular
actuation

DMVEC
dermal microvascular endothelial cell
D,M,V,P
disc, macula, vessels, periphery
DMWP
distal mean wave pressure
DMX
diathermy, massage, and exercise
DN
Deiters nucleus
denuded
diabetic nephropathy
diabetic neuropathy
dibucaine number
dicrotic notch
down
duodenum
dysplastic nevus
D&N
distance and near [vision]
D/N
at distance and at near [vision]
D:N
dextrose to nitrogen ratio
Dn
dekanem [10 times nutritional
unit nem]
DNA
deoxyribonucleic acid
did not answer
did not attend
does not apply
do not administer
DNA ds
deoxyribonucleic acid double stranded
DNAP
deoxyribonucleic acid polymerase
dynamic negative airway pressure
DNA-P
deoxyribonucleic acid phosphorus
DNAR
do not attempt resuscitation
DNAse, DNase
deoxyribonuclease
DNA ss
deoxyribonucleic acid single stranded
DNB
dinitrobenzene
dorsal noradrenergic bundle
DNBP
dinitrobutylphenol
DNBT
dinitroblue
DNC
did not come
dinitrocarbanilide
do not close

D

DNCB
dinitrochlorobenzene
DNCP
duct-narrowing chronic pancreatitis
DND
died a natural death
DNE
1,3-dinitrobenzene
Developmental Neurological Evaluation
DNEPTE
did not exist prior to enlistment
DNES
diffuse neuroendocrine system
DNET
dysembryoplastic neuroepithelial tumor
dysplastic neuroepithelial tumor
DNFB
dinitrofluorobenzene [Sanger reagent]
DNFC
does not follow commands
DNH
diffuse nodular hyperplasia
do not hospitalize
DNI
do not intubate
DNIC
diffuse noxious inhibitory control
DNJ
deoxynojirimycin
DNKA
did not keep appointment
DNL
de novo lipogenesis
diffuse nodular lymphoma
disseminated necrotizing
  leukoencephalopathy
DNLL
dorsal nucleus of lateral lemniscus
DNM
descending necrotizing mediastinitis
desmoplastic neurotropic melanoma
DNN
did not nurse
DNOA
diabetic neuropathic osteoarthropathy
DNOC
dinitroorthocresol
DNOCHP
dinitro-*o*-cyclohexyphenol
DNP
Dendroaspis [mamba snake] natriuretic
  peptide
deoxyribonucleoprotein
did not pay
2,4-dinitrophenol (dinitrophenol)
do not publish
dynamic nuclear polarization
DNPH
dinitrophenylhydrazine

DN-PHIP
dominant-negative mutant of pleckstrin
  homology domain-interacting protein
DNPM
dinitrophenol [and] morphine
DNPT
2,4-dinitrophenyl thiocyanate
N,N-dinitrosopentamethylenetetramine
DNR
did not respond
do not report
do not resuscitate
dorsal nerve root
dose nonuniformity ratio
DNS
dansyl (*See also* Dns)
delayed neuropsychological sequela
de novo synthesis
deviated nasal septum
diaphragmatic nerve stimulation
did not show
[doctor] did not see [patient]
do not show
do not substitute
dysplastic nevus syndrome
D5 1/2NS
dextrose 5% in 0.45% sodium chloride
  (saline) injection
D51/2NS
dextrose 5% in 0.45% sodium chloride
  (saline) [injection]
D5NSS
dextrose 5% in normal saline solution
Dns
dansyl (*See also* DNS)
DNT
dermonecrotic toxin
did not test
do not treat
dysembryoplastic neuroepithelial tumor
dnt
do not take
DNTM
disseminated nontuberculous
  mycobacterial [infection]
dNTP
deoxynucleotide triphosphate
diethylnitrophenyl thiophosphate
DNUA
distillable nonurea adductable
DNV
densovirus (densonucleosis virus)
dorsal nucleus of vagus
D-O
directive organic [unity, orientation]
DO
doctor's order
diamine oxidase [histaminase]
diet order

dissolved oxygen
distal occlusal (distoocclusal)
distraction osteogenesis
doctor's orders
drugs only

D/O
disorder

D$_o$
oxygen diffusion

d/o
died of

do.
the same, as before [L. *dicto*]

Do$_2$
oxygen delivery

DOA
date of admission
date of arrival
dead on arrival
depth of anesthesia
diagnostic and operative arthroscopy
differential optical absorption
dominant optic atrophy
driver of automobile
drugs of abuse
duration of action

DOAC
Dubois oleic albumin complex

DOA-DRA
dead on arrival despite resuscitative
attempts

DOB
dangle [legs] out of bed
date of birth (*See also* DB, D/B)
delta over baseline
distal occlusal buccal
Dobrava hantavirus
doctor's order book

DOBI
dynamic optical breast imaging system

DOBV
Dobrava-Belgrade virus
double-outlet both ventricles

DOC
date of conception
death of other cause
deoxycholate
deoxycorticoid
deoxycorticosterone
 (desoxycorticosterone)
11-deoxycorticosterone
diabetes out of control (*See also*
 DOOC)
died of other causes
diet of choice
disorder of cornification
drug of choice
dynamic orthotic cranioplasty

doc
document(ed) (documentation)

DOCA
deoxycorticosterone acetate

DOCLINE
Documents On-Line [National Library
 of Medicine]

DOC-SR
deoxycorticosterone secretion rate

DOD
date of death
date of discharge
day of delivery
dead of disease
dementia [syndrome] of depression
died of disease
dissolved oxygen deficit
drug overdose (overdosage)

DODD
demand oxygen delivery device

DODS
demand oxygen delivery system

DOE
date of examination
desoxyephedrine [drug of abuse]
direct observation evaluation
disease-oriented evidence
dyspnea on exertion

DOES
disorders of excessive somnolence
 (sleepiness)

DOET
dimethoxyethylamphetamine
 [hallucinogen of abuse] (*See also*
 DOM)

DOF
degrees of freedom

DOFOS
disturbance of function occlusion
 syndrome

DOG
distal oblique groove
distraction osteogenesis

DOHb
Döhle bodies

DOI
date of implant [pacemaker]
date of injury
depth of insertion
died of injuries

DO$_2$I
oxygen delivery index

DOL
day of life [followed by number]

dol
dolorimetric unit [of pain intensity]

DOLLS
[Lee] double-loop locking suture

DOLV
double-outlet left ventricle
DOM
deaminated *O*-methyl metabolite
dimethoxymethylamphetamine
(2,5-dimethoxy-4-methylamphetamine)
[hallucinogen of abuse] (*See also*
DOET)
dissolved organic matter
domiciliary
dominant (dominance) (*See also* D)
dom
domestic
DOMA
dihydroxymandelic acid (*See also*
DHMA)
DOMS
delayed-onset muscle soreness
DON
deoxynivalenol [*Fusarium toxin*]
diazo oxonorleucine
DOOC
diabetes out of control (*See also* DOC)
DOOR
deafness, onychoosteodystrophy, mental
retardation [syndrome]
DOP
degenerate oligonucleotide-primed
degenerate oligonucleotide primer
dopamine
DOPA, dopa
dihydroxyphenylalanine
(3,4-dihydroxyphenylalanine)
Dopase
dopamine hydroxylase
DOPC
determined osteogenic precursor cell
DOPE
disease-oriented physician education
DOPP
dihydroxyphenylpyruvate
DOP-PCR
degenerate oligonucleotide primed
polymerase chain reaction
DOPS
diffuse obstructive pulmonary
syndrome
dihydroxyphenylserine
DOR
date of release
diagnostic odd ratio
DORC
Direct Optical Research Company
dors
dorsal
DORV
double-outlet right ventricle
DoRx
date of treatment

DOS
day of surgery
dead on scene
doctor's order sheet
dysosteosclerosis
dos
dose (dosage) [L. *dosis*] (*See also* D, d)
DOSA
day of surgery admission
DOSC
Dubois oleic serum complex
DOSS
Delirium Observation Screening Scale
distal over-shoulder strap
DOST
direct oocyte sperm transfer
DOT
date of transcription
date of transfer
died on (operating) table
directly observed treatment (therapy)
direct oocyte transfer
Doppler ophthalmic test
dose optimized therapy
DOTA
tetraazacyclododecanetetraacetic acid
DOTC
Dameshek oval target cell
DOTP
tetraazacyclododecanetetraacetic
tetramethylene phosphonate
DOTS
directly observed therapy, short
[course]
DOUV
Douglas virus
DOV
date of visit
discharged on visit
distribution of ventilation
Dox
dioxygenase
doz
dozen
DP
data processing
debonding pliers
deep pulse
definitive procedure
degradation product
degree of polymerization
deltopectoral
dementia praecox
dementia pugilistica
dense plate
dental prosthesis
dental prosthodontics
Dermatophagoides pteronyssinus [dust
mite]

desquamative pneumonia
developed pressure
dexamethasone pretreatment
diaphragmatic plaque
diastolic pressure
diffuse precipitation
diffuse pressure
diffusion pressure
digestible protein
diminutive polyp
diphosgene [chemical weapon]
diphosphate
dipropionate
directional preponderance
direct puncture
disability pension
discharge planning
discriminating power
displaced person
distal pancreatectomy
distal phalanx
distal pit
distopulpal
donor's plasma
dorsalis pedis
double pneumonia
driving pressure
dyspnea (*See also* dysp)

D:P
dialysis to plasma [urea ratio]

DP-II
Developmental Profile II

DPA
descending palatine artery
Designed Plan Agencies [medical
    records]
dextroposition of aorta
diphenolic acid
diphenylamine
dipicolinic acid
dual-photon absorptiometry (*See also*
    DPX)
durable power of attorney
dynamic physical activity

DPAHC
durable power of attorney for health
    care

DPAP
diastolic pulmonary artery pressure

D-PAS, dPAS
diastase periodic acid-Schiff

DPB
days postburn
diffuse panbronchiolitis
dynamic pedobarography

DPBS
Dulbecco phosphate-buffered saline

DPC
delayed primary closure
desaturated phosphatidylcholine
direct patient care
discharge planning coordinator
distal palmar crease

dpc
[number of] days post coitus

d-PCI
direct percutaneous coronary
    intervention

DPCRT
double-blind placebo-controlled
    randomized clinical trial

DPD
deoxypyridinoline
depression pure disease
desoxypyridoxine hydrochloride
diffuse pulmonary disease
dihydropyrimidine dehydrogenase
diphenamid [herbicide]
dual-photon densitometry
dysgenetic polycystic disease

D-2PD
dynamic two-point discrimination

Dpd
deoxypyridinoline

DPDA
phosphorodiamidic anhydride

DPDL
diffuse poorly differentiated lymphocytic
    [lymphoma]

DPDT, dpdt
double-pole double-throw [switch]

dP/dt
upstroke pattern on apex cardiogram

DPE
Death Personification Exercise
    [psychology]
dipiperidinoethane

DPEG
dual percutaneous endoscopic
    gastrostomy

DPF
Dental Practitioners' Formulary
    [British]
digital pulsed fluoroscopy
diisopropylphosphorofluoridate

DPFC
distal palmar flexion crease

DPFR
diastolic pressure-flow relationship

DPG
diphosphoglycerate
displacement placentogram

DPGN
diffuse proliferative glomerulonephritis

D

DPGP
diphosphoglycerate phosphatase
DPH
Department of Public Health [state and local governments]
diaphragm(atic) (*See also* DI, diaph)
diphenylhexatriene
ductal papillary hyperplasia
DPI
daily permissible intake
daily protein intake
days postinoculation
dietary protein intake
diphenyleneiodonium
diphtheria-pertussis immunization
Doppler perfusion index
drug-prescribing index
dry powder inhaler
Dynamic Personality Inventory
dynamic pulmonary imaging
DPIF
Drug Product Information File
DPIL
dextrose [percentage], protein [grams per kilogram] Intralipid [grams per kilogram] [parenteral feeding formula]
DPJ
dementia paralytica juvenilis
direct percutaneous jejunostomy
DPL
diagnostic peritoneal lavage
dipalmitoyl lecithin
distopulpolingual
DPLa
distopulpolabial
D5PLM
dextrose 5% and Plasmalyte M injection
DPM
days post mortem
digital phase mapping
disabling pansclerotic morphea
discontinue previous medication
disintegration per minute
dopamine
drop per minute
dual-pedicle dermoparenchymal mastopexy
DPN
deep penetrating nevus
deep peroneal nerve
dermatopolyneuritis
dermatosis papulosa nigra
diabetic peripheral neuropathy
diabetic polyneuropathy
diphosphopyridine nucleotidase [former name for nicotinamide adenine dinucleotide]
dorsal parabrachial nucleus

DPNase
diphosphopyridine nucleotidase
DPNB
dorsal penile nerve block
DPNH
reduced diphosphopyridine nucleotide
DPOA
durable power of attorney
DPOAE
distortion-product otoacoustic emission
DPOAHC
durable power of attorney for health care
DPOC
placebo-controlled oral challenge testing
DPP
dentine phosphoproteins
Diabetes Prevention Program
differential pulse polarography
digital pulse plethysmography
dimethoxyphenylpenicillin
documented poor prognosis
dorsalis pedal pulse (dorsalis pedis pulse)
Dropout Prediction and Prevention
duration of positive pressure
DPPC
dipalmitoyl phosphatidylcholine (dipalmitoylphosphatidylcholine)
DPPIV
dipeptidyl peptidase IV [protein]
DPQ
Dutch Personality Questionnaire
DPR
diagnostic procedure room
doctor to population ratio
dynamic planar reconstructor
DPRHP
duodenum-preserving pancreatic head resection
DPS
delayed primary suture
descending perineum syndrome
disintegration per second
distal perfusion system
dysesthetic pain syndrome
DPSF
diffusion/perfusion snapshot FLASH (fast low-angle shot)
DPST, dpst
double-pole single-throw [switch]
⚠ **DPT**
dehydration, poisoning, trauma
Demerol, Phenergan, and Thorazine ⚠
department
diabetic pseudotabes
dichotic pitch [discrimination] test
diphosphothiamine
diphtheria, pertussis, tetanus [vaccine]

diphtheric pseudotabes
dipropyltryptamine [drug of abuse]
dumping provocation test

DPTA
diethylenetriamine pentaacetic acid
(*See also* DTPA)

DPTI
diastolic pressure-time index

DPTP
diphtheria, pertussis, tetanus,
poliomyelitis [vaccine]

DPTPM
diphtheria, pertussis, tetanus,
poliomyelitis, measles (vaccine)

Dptr
diopter (*See also* D, diopt)

DPTS
delayed pulmonary toxicity syndrome

DPTT
deep posterior tibiotalar

DPU
delayed pressure urticaria

DPUD
duodenal peptic ulcer disease

DPV
disabling positional vertigo
Drosophila P virus

DPVNS
diffuse pigmented villonodular synovitis

DPVS
Denver peritoneovenous shunt
dilated perivascular space

DPVSs
dilated perivascular spaces

DPW
distal phalangeal width

DPX
dual-photon absorptiometry (*See also*
DPA)

DPXA
dual-photon x-ray absorptiometry

DQ
developmental quotient

D&Q
deep and quiet [anterior chamber]

Dq
curvilinear threshold shoulder

3DQCT
three-dimensional quantitative computed
tomography

DQE
detective quantum efficiency

DQF
double quotidian fever

DQFC
double-quantum filtered correlation
spectroscopy

DQFC NMR
double-quantum filtered correlation
nuclear magnetic resonance
spectroscopy

DQFCOSY
double-quantum filtered correlated
spectroscopy

DQOL
diabetes quality of life

DR
degeneration reaction (*See also* DeR)
delivery room
deoxyribose
diabetic retinopathy
diagnostic radiology
diastolic rumble
diffuse redness
digital radiography
dining room
disposable/reusable
distal root
distribution ratio
diurnal rhythm
donor-related
dorsal raphe
dorsal root
dose ratio
drain
dressing (*See also* DRSG, drsg, DSG,
dsg)
drug receptor
drug resistant
dual-chamber rate-responsive
[pacemaker]
reaction of degeneration [muscle fibers]
(*See also* DeR)

Dr
rare detail response [Rorschach]

Dr.
doctor

dr
dram (drachm) [apothecary]
[unusual rare] detail response

DRA
despite resuscitation attempts
dextran-reactive antibody
dialysis-related amyloidosis
digital rotational angiography
disease-resistant antigen
distal rectal adenocarcinoma
distal reference axis
drug-related admission

3DRA
three-dimensional rotational angiography

DRAD
dwarfism with retinal atrophy and
deafness

D

DRAM
de-epithelialized rectus abdominis
muscle [graft]
Distress Risk Assessment Method
dynamic random access memory
DRAMS
Drug Risk Analysis Message System
DRAP
dorsal root action potential
DRAPE
drug-related adverse patient event
DRAT
differential rheumatoid agglutination
test
DRBC
denatured red blood cell
dog red blood cell (*See also* DRC)
donkey red blood cell
DRC
damage risk criteria
dendritic reticulum cell
design rule check
digitorenocerebral [syndrome]
DNA [deoxyribonucleic acid] repair
capacity
dog red [blood] cell (*See also* DRBC)
dorsal radiocarpal ligament
dorsal root, cervical
dose-response curve
dynamic range control
dRCA
distal right coronary artery
DRD
dopa-responsive dystonia
dorsal root dilator
dystrophia retinae pigmentosa-dysostosis
syndrome
DRE
digital rectal examination
DREAM
downstream regulatory element
antagonistic modulator [gene]
DREF
dose reduction effectiveness factor
D reg.
diseased region
DRESS
depth-resolved surface [coil]
spectroscopy
drug rash with eosinophilia and
systemic symptoms
DREZ
dorsal root entry zone
DRF
daily replacement factor [lymphocytes]
digestive-respiratory fistula
dose-reduction factor
DR-FFP
donor-retested fresh frozen plasma

DRFS
distant recurrence-free survival
Dundee rank factor score
DRG
diagnostic related group
dorsal respiratory group [neurons]
dorsal root ganglion
duodenal-gastric reflux gastropathy
DRGE
drainage (*See also* drng)
draining (*See also* drng)
DRI
defibrillation response interval
Dietary Reference Intakes
Discharge Readiness Inventory
dopamine reuptake inhibitor
Doppler Resistive Index
Driver Risk Inventory
dRib
deoxyribose
DRID
double radial immunodiffusion
double radioisotope derivative
DRIFT
drainage, irrigation, fibrinolytic therapy
DRIL
distal revascularization interval ligation
DRIP
delirium and drugs, restricted mobility
and retention, infection and
inflammation and impaction, polyuria
[causes of urinary incontinence]
DRL
differential reinforcement of low
[response rates]
dorsal root, lumbar
dorsoradial ligament
drug-related lupus
D5RL
5% dextrose in Ringer lactate [solution]
DRLST
Del Rio Language Screening Test
DRM
drug-related morbidity
DRMS
drug reaction monitoring system
DRN
dorsal raphe nucleus
drug-related neutropenia
drng
drainage (*See also* DRGE)
draining (*See also* DRGE)
DRnt
diagnostic roentgenology
DRO
differential reinforcement of other
[behavior]
DRP
digoxin reduction product

dorsal root potential
drug-related problem
DRPLA
    dentatorubral-pallidoluysian atrophy
DRQ
    discomfort relief quotient
DRR
    digitally reconstructed radiograph
    dorsal root reflex
    drug regimen review
DRS
    Delirium Rating Scale
    descending rectal septum
    diffuse reflectance spectroscopy
    Disability Rating Scale
    disease-related symptom
    dorsal root, sacral
    drowsiness
    Duane retraction syndrome
    dynamic renal scintigraphy
    Dyskinesia Rating Scale
DRSG, drsg
    dressing (*See also* DR, DSG, dsg)
DRSI
    disease-related symptom improvement
DRSP
    daily record of severity of problems
    drug-resistant *Streptococcus*
      pneumoniae
DRT
    dorsal root, thoracic
    drug-related thrombocytopenia
dRTA
    distal renal tubular acidosis
3DRTP
    three-dimensional radiotherapy
DRUJ
    distal radioulnar joint
DrV
    Diplocarpon rosae virus
DRVV
    dilute Russell viper venom
DRVVT
    dilute Russell viper venom time
DS
    dead [air] space
    deep sedative
    deep sleep
    defined substrate
    delayed sensitivity
    dendritic spine
    density standard
    dental surgery
    deprivation syndrome
    dermatan sulfate
    dermatology and syphilology (*See also*
      D&S)
    desynchronized sleep

dextran sulfate
dextrose [and] saline
dextrose [and] sodium chloride
dextrose stick
diameter stenosis
diaphragm stimulation
diastolic murmur
diencephalic syndrome
difference spectroscopy
diffuse scleroderma
digit span
digit symbol
dilute strength
diopter sphere
dioptric strength
discharge summary
discrimination score
discriminative stimulus
disoriented
disseminated sclerosis
dissolved solids
donor's serum
Doppler sonography
double-stranded
double strength
double subordinance
Down syndrome
driving signal
drug screen
drug store
dry swallow
dumping syndrome
duplex scan
duplex sonography
duration of systole
D5S
    dextrose 5% in saline (sodium chloride)
    [solution]
D51/2S
    5% dextrose in half-normal saline
    (sodium chloride) [injection]
%DS
    percent diameter stenosis
D-S
    Doerfler-Stewart [test]
D&S
    dermatology and syphilology (*See also*
     DS)
    diagnostic and surgical
    dilation and suction
D/S
    dextrose in saline
Ds
    associative detail response to white
    space [Rorschach]
4Ds
    diplopia, dysphagia, dysarthria,
    dysphonia

D

ds
  double-stranded [DNA, RNA]
DSA
  density spectral array
  destructive spondyloarthropathy
  digital subtraction angiography
  digital subtraction arteriography
  disease-susceptible antigen
DSACT, D-SACT
  direct sinuatrial (sinoatrial) conduction
    time
DSAP
  disseminated superficial actinic
    porokeratosis
DSAS
  discrete subaortic stenosis
  discrete subvalvular aortic stenosis
  dynamic subaortic stenosis
DSB
  detachable silicone balloon
  double-strand [DNA, RNA]
    breaks
  drug-seeking behavior
Dsb
  single-breath diffusing [capacity]
DSBB
  double-sheath bronchial brushing
DSBL
  disabled (See also DIS)
DSBT
  donor-specific blood transfusion
DSC
  decussation of superior cerebellar
    [peduncles]
  Developing Skills Checklist
  differential scanning colorimeter
  Down syndrome child
  dynamic susceptibility contrast-enhanced
    [magnetic resonance imaging]
DSCF
  Doppler-shifted constant frequency
DSCG
  disodium cromoglycate
DSC-MRI
  dynamic susceptibility contrast magnetic
    resonance imaging
DSCT
  dorsal spinocerebellar tract
DSD
  degenerative spinal disease
  depressed spectrum disease
  depression sine depression
  depressive spectrum disorder
  detrusor sphincter dyssynergia
  digital selenium drum [radiology]
  discharge summary dictated
  dry sterile dressing
DSDB
  direct self-destructive behavior

DSDDT
  double-sampling dye dilution
    technique
DS-DNA, dsDNA
  double-stranded deoxyribonucleic acid
DSDS
  daughter sites of dimer strands
DSE
  digital subtraction echocardiograph(y)
    (echocardiogram)
  dobutamine stress echocardiography
DSEA
  deep superior epigastric artery
DSF
  dry sterile fluff
DSG, dsg
  dry sterile gauze
  dressing (See also DR, DRSG, drsg)
Dsg
  desmoglein
DSH
  deliberate self-harm
  dexamethasone-suppressible
    hyperaldosteronism
DSHR
  delayed skin hypersensitivity reaction
DSI
  deep shock insulin
  Depression Status Inventory
  digital subtraction imaging
  drug-seeking index
DSIAR
  double-stapled ileoanal reservoir
DS-ICGA
  digital subtraction indocyanine green
    angiography
DSIP
  delta sleep-inducing peptide
DSIS
  dynamic stabilizing innersole system
DSL
  distal sensory latency
3D SLINKY MRA
  three-dimensional time-of flight
    (3DTOF) magnetic resonance
    angiogram
DSL M-U
  distal sensory latency–medianulnar
3D-SLS
  three-dimensional superficial
    liposculpture
dslv
  dissolve
DSM
  degradable starch microsphere
  dextrose solution mixture
  Diagnostic and Statistical Manual of
    Mental Disorders
  digital subtraction mammography

disease state management
dried skim milk
DSMB
Data Safety Monitoring Board
DSM-III
*Diagnostic and Statistical Manual of
Mental Disorders*, 3rd Edition
DSM-III-R
*Diagnostic and Statistical Manual of
Mental Disorders*, Revised Third
Edition
DSM-IV
*Diagnostic and Statistical Manual of
Mental Disorders*, 4th Edition
DSM-IV-TR
*Diagnostic and Statistical Manual of
Mental Disorders*, 4th Edition, Text
Revision
DSNI
deep space neck infection
DSO
diffuse sclerosing osteomyelitis
distal subungual onychomycosis
DSP
decreased sensory perception
delayed sleep phase
diabetic sensorineural polyneuropathy
diarrheic shellfish poisoning
dibasic sodium phosphate
digital signal processing
digital sound processing
digital subtraction phlebography
distal symmetrical polyneuropathy
DSp
digit span
DSPA
Desmodus rotundus [vampire bat]
salivary plasminogen activator
DSPC
desaturated phosphatidylcholine
DSPD
dangerous severe personality disorder
D spine
dorsal spine
DSPN
distal sensory polyneuropathy
distal symmetrical polyneuropathy
DSPS
delayed sleep phase syndrome
DSQ-40
Defense Style Questionnaire 40 [item
version]
DSQL
Dermatology-Specific Quality of Life
DSR
dental stain remover
diffuse syncytial reticulosarcoma

direct suicide risk
distal splenorenal
double simultaneous recording
dynamic spatial reconstructor
DSRCT
desmoplastic small round-cell tumor
DSRF
drainage subretinal fluid
dsRNA
double-stranded ribonucleic acid
DSRS
distal splenorenal shunt
DSS
dengue shock syndrome
dermatitis schistosomiasis
Developmental Sentence Scoring
dextran sodium sulfate
Disability Status Scale
discharge summary sheet
discrete subaortic stenosis
disease-specific survival
distal splenorenal shunt
dosage-sensitive sex [reversal]
double simultaneous stimulation
DSS-AHC
dosage-sensitive sex reversal [and]
adrenal hypoplasia congenita
DSSEP
dermatomal somatosensory-evoked
potential
DSSLR
double seated straight leg raise
DSSN
distal symmetric sensory neuropathy
DSSP
distal symmetric sensory polyneuropathy
DSST
digit symbol substitutional test
DST
daylight saving time
desensitization test
dexamethasone suppression test
digit substitution test
disproportionate septal thickening
donor-specific transfusion
double stapling technique
duodenal secretin test
dural sinus thrombosis
D-stix
Dextrostix (*See also* DSX, dex)
DSTR
distal soft tissue release
DSU
day surgery unit
double setup
DSUH
direct suggestion under hypnosis

DSV

dermal sarcoma virus

digital subtraction ventriculography

DSVNI

Distress Scale for Ventilated Newborn Infants

DSVP

downstream venous pressure

DSWI

deep sternal wound infection

deep surgical wound infection

DSX

Dextrostix (*See also* D-stix, dex)

dysmetabolic syndrome X

DSy

digit symbol

DT

defibrillation threshold

delirium tremens (*See also* DTs)

depression of transmission

dietary thermogenesis

differently tested

diffusion tension (tensor) [imaging]

diphtheria-tetanus [immunization]

diphtheria toxin

diploë thickness

dipole tracing

discharge tomorrow

dispensing tablet

distal tubule

distance test [hearing]

dorsalis tibialis

double tachycardia

doubling time [of tumor size]

dye test

D/T

date/time

date of treatment

due to

D:T

deaths to total ratio

D&T

diagnosis and treatment

dictated and typed

Dt

duration of tetany

dT

deoxythymidine

diphtheria-tetanus [toxoid]

DTA

descending thoracic aorta

differential thermoanalysis

displacement threshold acuity

DTAFA

descending thoracic aorta to femoral artery [bypass]

DTAF-F

descending thoracic aorta femoral-femoral [bypass]

DTaP

diphtheria, tetanus toxoids and acellular pertussis (*See also* DTP, DTPa)

DTB

dedicated time block

DTBN

di-*tert*-butyl nitroxide

DTBP

di-*tert*-butyl peroxide (*See also* DBP)

DTC

day treatment center

differentiated thyroid cancer (carcinoma)

2D-TCCS

two-dimensional transcranial color-coded sonography

DTCD

Dennis Test of Child Development

DT/CEP

Differential Test of Conduct and Emotional Problems

DTD, dtd

delivered total dose

diastrophic dystrophia

dTDP

deoxythymidine diphosphate

thymidine 5′-diphosphate (thymidine diphosphate)

DTE

desiccated thyroid extract

2D TEE

two-dimensional transesophageal echocardiography

DTF

deep temporal fascia

deep temporoparietal fascia

deep transverse friction

desmoid-type fibromatosis

detector transfer function

distal triangular fossa

D-TGA, d-TGA

dextro-transposition of the great arteries

DTH

delayed-type hypersensitivity [reaction]

dTHd, dThd

deoxythymidine

DTI

diffusion tensor imaging [magnetic resonance imaging]

dipyridamole-thallium [cardiac] imaging

direct thrombin inhibitor

Doppler tissue imaging

DTICH

delayed traumatic intracerebral hematoma

delayed traumatic intracerebral hemorrhage

D time

dream time

dTK
2′-deoxy thymidine kinase
DTLA
Detroit Tests of Learning Aptitude
DTLA-3
Detroit Tests of Learning Aptitude, Third Edition
DTLA-A
Detroit Tests of Learning Aptitude, Adult
DTLA-P:2
Detroit Tests of Learning Aptitude Primary, Second Edition
DTM
deep tissue massage
dermatophyte test media
DTMA
deoxycorticosterone trimethylacetate
DTMP, dTMP
de novo thymidylate [synthesis]
deoxythymidylic acid
thymidine 5′-monophosphate
DTMVmax
diastolic transmembrane voltage, maximum
DTN
diphtheria toxin normal
⚠ **DTO**
danger to others
deodorized tincture of opium ⚠
2D TOF
two-dimensional time-of-flight
3DTOF
three-dimensional time-of-flight
DTOGV
dextral-transposition of the great vessels
DTP
differential time to positivity
diphtheria, tetanus toxoid, and acellular pertussis [vaccine] (*See also* DTPa, DTaP)
distal tingling on percussion [Tinel sign]
DTPA
diethylenetriamine pentaacetic acid (*See also* DPTA)
DTPa
diphtheria, tetanus toxoids, acellular pertussis [vaccine] (*See also* DTP, DTaP)
DTPT
dithiopropylthiamine
DTPw, DTwP
diphtheria, tetanus toxoids, whole-cell pertussis [vaccine]
DTR
deep tendon reflex

D-transposition
dextrotransposition
DTRTT
digital temperature recovery time test
DTS
danger to self
dense tubular system
differential temperature sensor
diphtheria toxin sensitivity
discrete time sample
donor transfusion, specific
DTs
delirium tremens (*See also* DT)
3D TSE
three-dimensional turbo-spin echo [images]
DTT
device for transverse traction
diagnostic and therapeutic team
diphtheria-tetanus toxoid
direct transverse reaction
disaccharide tolerance test
dithiothreitol [Cleland reagent]
dTTP
deoxythymidine triphosphate
2′-deoxythymidine 5′-triphosphate
thymidine 5′-triphosphate
DTUS
diathermy, traction, ultrasound
DTV
Dioscorea trifida virus
due to void
DT-VAC
diphtheria-tetanus vaccine
DTVMI
Developmental Test of Visual Motor Integration
DTVP
Developmental Test of Visual Perception
DTVP-2
Developmental Test of Visual Perception, Second Edition
DTwP-HIB
diphtheria, tetanus toxoids, whole-cell pertussis, and *Haemophilus influenzae* type b conjugate [vaccine]
DTX
detoxification
DU
decubitus ulcer
density unknown
depleted uranium
dermal ulcer
developmental unit
diabetic urine
diagnosis undetermined
dialytic ultrafiltration

D

DU *(continued)*
   diazouracil
   diffuse and undifferentiated
   dog unit
   dose unit
   duodenal ulcer
   duplex ultrasound
   duroxide uptake
   Dutch [rabbit]
D&U
   diffuse and undifferentiated
D$_U$
   urea dialysance
dU
   deoxyuridine
du
   dial unit
   du mai channel [acupuncture]
DUA
   dorsal uterine artery
DUB
   Dubowitz [score]
   dysfunctional uterine bleeding
DUBI
   dysfunctional urinary bladder
      instability
DUD
   dihydrouracil dehydrogenase
dUDP
   deoxyuridine diphosphate
DUE
   drug use evaluation
D&UE
   dilation and uterine evacuation
D$_1$UE
   diagonal 1 upper extremity [exercise]
D$_2$UE
   diagonal 2 upper extremity [exercise]
DUF
   Doppler ultrasonic flowmeter
   Drug Use Forecasting
DUG
   drug use guidelines
   dynamic urinary graciloplasty
DUGV
   Dugbe virus
DUI
   driving under influence
DUID
   driving under influence of drugs
DUII
   driving under influence of
      intoxicants
DUIL
   driving under influence of liquor
DUKM
   dialysate urea kinetic modeling
DUL
   diffuse undifferentiated lymphoma

DUM
   dorsal unpaired median [axon, neuron]
   drug use monitoring
dUMP
   deoxyuridine monophosphate
DUN
   dialysate urea nitrogen
DUNHL
   diffuse undifferentiated non-Hodgkin
      lymphoma
duod
   duodenal
   duodenum
DUP
   duodenal ulcer perforation
dup
   duplicate (duplication)
DUQUES
   Duke University quantitative/qualitative
      [cardiac catheterization] evaluation
      system
DUR
   Drug Usage Review
   drug use review
   duration (*See also* D)
   hard [L. *durus*]
dur
   hard [L. *durus*]
DURAC
   duration of anticoagulation
dURD
   2′-deoxyuridine
DUS
   digital ultrasound
   distal urethral stenosis
   Doppler ultrasound
   Doppler ultrasound stethoscope
   duplex ultrasonography
   dynamic ultrasound of shoulder
3DUS
   three-dimensional ultrasound
DUSI-R
   Drug Usage Screening Inventory
      Revised
DUSN
   diffuse unilateral subacute neuroretinitis
      [wipe-out syndrome]
dUTP
   deoxyuridine triphosphate
DUV
   damaging ultraviolet
   degree of voicelessness
DV
   daily value
   dependent variable
   dilute volume [of solution]
   distance vision
   distemper virus
   domestic violence

domiciliary visit
dorsoventral
double vision
3-DV
three-dimensional visualization
D&V
diarrhea and vomiting
discs and vessels [ophthalmology]
ductions and versions
dv/sec
double vibrations per second [unit of
frequency of sound waves]
DVA
developmental venous anomaly
directional vacuum-assisted [biopsy]
distance visual acuity
duration of voluntary apnea [test]
dynamic visual acuity
D/VA
diffusion per unit of alveolar
volume
DVAB
directional vacuum-assisted biopsy
D value
decimal reduction time
DVB
divinylbenzene
DVC
direct visualization of vocal cords
dorsal vagal (vagus) complex
dorsal vein complex [urethra]
DVD
dissociated vertical divergence
double-vessel disease
DVE
duck virus enteritis
DVG
double vein graft
DVH
dose-volume histogram
DVI
atrioventricular sequential pacing
deep venous insufficiency
device-independent
diastolic velocity integral
digital vascular imaging
direct visual inspection
documented viral infection
Doppler [systolic] velocity index
dual-mode, ventricular inhibited
[pacemaker]
DVIS
digital vascular imaging system
DVIU
direct vision internal urethrotomy
DVL
deep vastus lateralis

DVM
digital voltmeter
DVMI
Developmental Test of Visual Motor
Integration
DVMP
disc, vessels, macula, periphery [eye
exam]
DVN
dorsal vagal nucleus
2D-VNQ
two-dimensional variable N-quoit filter
[imaging]
3D-VNQ
three-dimensional variable N-quoit filter
[imaging]
DVP
deep venous pressure
digital volume pulse
DVR
derotational varus osteotomy
digital vascular reactivity
dose-volume relationship
double valve replacement
double ventricular response
DVRT
differential variable reluctance
transducer
DVS
direct vesicoureteral scintigraphy
DVSA
digital venous subtraction angiography
DVSS
dysfunctional voiding scoring system
DVT
deep vein (venous) thrombosis
DVT/PE
deep venous thrombosis [and]
pulmonary embolism
DVTS
deep venous thromboscintigram
DVVC
direct visualization of vocal cords
DVXI
direct vision times one
DW
confabulated whole response
daily weight
deionized water
detention warrant
dextrose in water
diffusion weighted [imaging]
distilled water
doing well
double wrap
dry weight
whole response to detail

215

D-W
    Dandy-Walker [deformity/malformation]
    Danis-Weber [ankle fracture type A, B, C]
D5W
    5% dextrose in water
D10W
    10% dextrose in water
D20W
    20% dextrose in water
D50W
    50% dextrose in water
D70W
    70% dextrose in water
D/W
    dextrose in water
    discussed with
    dry to wet [dressings]
dw
    dwarf [mouse]
DWA
    died from wounds in action [by enemy]
DWCE
    density-weighted contrast enhancement
DWCL
    daily-wear contact lens
DWD
    died with disease
DWDL
    diffuse well-differentiated lymphocytic [lymphoma]
DWI
    diffusion-weighted [magnetic resonance] imaging
    driving while impaired (intoxicated)
DWI/MRI
    diffusion-weighted imaging [and] magnetic resonance imaging
DWI/PI
    diffusion-weighted imaging [and] perfusion imaging
DWM
    Dandy-Walker malformation
DWMHI
    deep white matter hyperintensity
DWMI
    deep white matter infarct(ion)
DWML
    deep white matter lesion
DWRT
    delayed work recall test
DWS
    Dandy-Walker syndrome
    Disaster Warning System
    dorsal wrist syndrome
DWSCL
    daily-wear soft contact lens
DWT
    Dichotic Word Test

dwt
    pennyweight
DWV
    Dandy-Walker variant
DWW
    dynamic wall walk
DX
    Dextran
D&X
    dilation and extraction
Dx, dx
    diagnosis (*See also* D, DG, Dg, diag, DIAGNO)
DXA
    dual-energy x-ray absorptiometry [scan] (*See also* DEXA)
dx cath
    diagnostic catheterization
DXD, Dxd
    diagnosed
    discontinued
DXG
    dioxalane guanine
DxLS
    diagnosis responsible for length of stay
DXR
    deep x-ray
    delayed xenograft rejection
DxRaI
    diagnostic radioiodine [whole body scanning]
DXRT
    deep x-ray therapy (*See also* DXT)
DXT
    deep x-ray therapy (*See also* DXRT)
    dextrose
dXTP
    deoxyxanthine triphosphate
DXV
    Drosophila X virus
D-XYL
    d-xylose
DY
    dense parenchyma
Dy
    dysprosium
dy
    dystrophia muscularis
Dy-DTPA-BMA
    dysprosium diethylenetriaminepentaacetic acid [DTPA]-bis methylamide
DYFS
    Division of Youth and Family Services
dyn
    dynamics
    dynamometer
    dyne
DynA
    dynorphin A

DYNR
  delayed nasal response
dysp
  dyspnea (*See also* DP)
dysph
  dysphagia
DYTRO
  dynamic tone-reducing
    orthosis

DZ
  disease (*See also* D, DIS)
  dizygotic (dizygous)
  dizziness
dz
  dozen
  impedance change
DZT
  dizygotic twins

D

E

air dose
East
edema (*See also* ed)
einstein [unit of light energy concentration]
elastance
electric affinity (*See also* EA, E_O)
electric field vector
electrode potential
electron
eloper
embryo(logy) (*See also* EMB, emb, embryol)
emmetropia
enamel
encephalitis
endangered [animal]
endogenous
endoplasm
enema (*See also* EN, enem)
energy
engorged
Enterococcus
enzyme
eosinophil
epicondyle
epinephrine (*See also* EPI, epineph)
epsilon [fifth letter of Greek alphabet uppercase]
error
erythrocyte (*See also* ERY, eryth)
erythroid
Escherichia (*See also Esch.*)
esophagus (*See also* ES, ESO, eso, esoph)
esophoria [for distance]
ester (*See also* est)
etiology
evaluation
evening
exa-
examiner
expectancy [wave]
expected frequency in a cell of a contingency table
experiment(al) (*See also* EXP, exp, exper, exptl)
expired [air or gas] (*See also* EXP, exp)
expired [died] (*See also* EXP, exp, expir)
extension (*See also* EXT, ext)
extinction [coefficient]
extraction fraction [ratio]
extralymphatic

eye
glutamic acid (glutamate) (*See also* Glu, Glx)
internal energy
mathematical expectation [statistics]
methylenedioxymethamphetamine [MDMA; Ecstasy]
redox potential
vectorcardiography electrode [midsternal]
vitamin E

E_1

estrone

1E–4E

1 plus edema–4 plus edema

E_2

17-beta(β)-estradiol

E_3

estriol

E_4

estetrol

$E°$

standard electrode potential

E'

esophoria [for near]

$E*$

lesion on erythrocyte cell membrane at the site of complement fixation

E'

elbow

E

entgegen [stereo descriptor to indicate configuration at a double bond; opposite] [Ger. *entgegen*]

e

base of natural logarithm
early
egg transfer
elementary charge [electricity]
from [L. *ex*]

e^-

negatron [negative electron]

e^+

positron [positive electron]

EA

early amniocentesis
early antigen
educational age
egg albumin
elbow aspiration
electric affinity (*See also* E, E_o)
electroacoustic analysis
electroacupuncture [analgesia] (*See also* EAC)
electroanesthesia
electrophysiologic abnormality

EA *(continued)*
    embryonic antibody (antigen)
    emergency area
    endocardiographic amplifier
    endotracheal aspirate (aspiration)
    enteral alimentation
    enteroanastomosis
    environmental assessment
    enzymatic active
    epiandrosterone
    epidural anesthesia
    episodic ataxia
    erythrocyte antibody (antiserum)
    esophageal atresia
    esterase activity
    estivoautumnal [malaria]

EA-2
    episodic ataxia type 2

E:A
    early to late diastolic filling ratio

E&A
    evaluate and advise

E→A
    E to A changes [in pulmonary consolidation, vowel E heard as A through stethoscope]

E_a
    energy of activation

ea
    each

EAA
    electroacupuncture analgesia
    electrothermal atomic absorption
    endotoxin activity assay
    essential amino acid
    excitatory amino acid
    excitotoxic amino acid
    extraalveolar air
    extrinsic allergic alveolitis

EAAE
    experimental allergic autoimmune encephalitis

EAAS
    electrothermal atomic absorption spectrophotometry

EAB
    elective abortion
    extraanatomic bypass

EABA
    endogenous avidin-binding activity

EABR
    electrical-evoked auditory brainstem response

EABT
    estrogen add back therapy

EABV
    effective arterial blood volume

EAC
    Ehrlich ascites carcinoma

electroacupuncture [analgesia] *(See also EA)*
    epithelioma adenoides cysticum
    erythema action [spectrum of light]
    erythema annulare centrifugum
    erythrocyte, antibody, complement
    esophageal adenocarcinoma
    expandable access catheter
    external auditory canal

EACA
    epsilon-aminocaproic acid

EACD
    eczematous allergic contact dermatitis

EACS
    exertional anterior compartment syndrome

EAD
    early afterdepolarization
    effective airspace dimension
    extracranial arterial disease

E-ADD
    epileptic attention deficit disorder

eAdHCC
    early advanced hepatocellular carcinoma

EADL
    electronic aid for daily living
    extended activities of daily living

EADS
    early amnion deficit spectrum [syndrome]

EAE
    effective arterial elastance
    experimental allergic (autoimmune) encephalitis
    experimental allergic (autoimmune) encephalomyelitis
    external auditory exostosis

EAEC
    enteroadherent *Escherichia coli*

EAF
    emergency assistance to families
    eosinophilic angiocentric fibrosis

EAG
    electroantennogram
    electroarteriograph(y) (electroatriogram)
    endovascular aortic graft
    experimental autoimmune gastritis
    experimental autoimmune glomerulonephritis

EAggEC, EaggEC
    enteroaggregative *Escherichia coli*

EAHF
    eczema, asthma, hay fever [complex]

EAHLG
    equine antihuman lymphoblast globulin

EAHLS
    equine antihuman lymphoblast serum

EAI
    electronically assisted instruction

Employment and Adaptation Index
erythema ab igne
erythrocyte antibody inhibition

EAL
electronic apex locator
electronic artificial larynx
endoscopic aspiration lumpectomy

EAM
endoscopic aspiration mucosectomy
episodic ataxia with myokymia
external auditory meatus

EAMG
experimental autoimmune myasthenia
gravis

EAN
experimental allergic neuritis

EANG
epidemic acute nonbacterial
gastroenteritis

EAO
experimental allergic orchitis

EAOC
endometriosis-associated ovarian
carcinoma

EAP
Epstein-Barr early region
(EBER)-associated protein
electroacupuncture
Employee Assistance Program
endoscopic access port
erythrocyte acid phosphatase
evoked action potential
extrinsic allergic pneumonia

EAQ
eudismic affinity quotient

e-aq
aqueous electron

EAR
early allergic response
early asthmatic response
electroencephalographic audiometry
endovascular aneurysm repair
estimated average requirement
expired air resuscitation

Ea R
reaction of degeneration [Ger.
Entartungs-Reaktion]

EARD
environmentally associated rheumatic
disorder

EARLY
ergonomic assessment of risk and
liability

ear ox
ear oximetry

EARR
extended aortic root replacement
external apical root resorption

EARS
Early Aberration Reporting System
[Centers for Disease Control]

EART
extended abdominal radiation therapy

EAS
Emotionality Activity Sociability Scale
endoskeletal alignment system
external anal sphincter

EASI
Eczema Area and Severity Index
extraamniotic saline infusion

EASIC
Evaluating Acquired Skills in
Communication

EAST
elevated-arm stress test
enzyme allergosorbent test
external rotation-abduction stress test

EAST1
enteroaggregative *Escherichia coli*
heat-stable enterotoxin 1

eAST
erythrocyte aspartate aminotransferase
activity

EAT
Eating Attitudes Test
ectopic atrial tachycardia
Edinburgh Articulation Test
Education Apperception Test
Ehrlich ascites tumor
electroaerosol therapy
equine assistance therapy
experimental autoimmune thymitis
experimental autoimmune thyroiditis

EATC
Ehrlich ascites tumor cell

EATCL, EATL
enteropathy-associated T-cell lymphoma

EAU
experimental autoimmune uveitis

EAUS
endoanal ultrasound

EAV
electroacupuncture according to Voll
equine abortion virus
extraalveolar vessel

EAVC
enhanced atrioventricular conduction

EAVM
extramedullary arteriovenous
malformation

EAVN
enhanced atrioventricular nodal
[conduction]

EB
elbow bearing
elementary body

E

EB *(continued)*
> endometrial biopsy
> eosinophilic bronchitis
> epidermolysis bullosa
> Epstein-Barr [virus]
> escape beat
> esophageal body
> ethidium bromide [dye]
> Evans blue [dye]

EBA
> early bacterial activity
> electron beam angiography
> epidermolysis bullosa acquisita
> epidermolysis bullosa atrophicans
> ethoxybenzoic acid
> extrahepatic biliary atresia

EBB
> electron beam boosts
> endobronchial brachytherapy
> equal breaths bilaterally

EBBS
> equal bilateral breath sounds

EBC
> early [stage] breast cancer
> endoscopic brush cytology
> esophageal balloon catheter

EBCT
> electron beam computed tomography

EBD
> emotional and behavioral difficulties
> endocardial border delineation
> endoscopic balloon dilation
>   (dilatation)
> epidermolysis bullosa dystrophica
> evidence-based decision [making]
> extragenital Bowen disease

EBDA
> effective balloon-dilated area

EBDD
> epidermolysis bullosa dystrophica,
>   dominant

EBDR
> epidermolysis bullosa dystrophica,
>   recessive

EBE
> equal bilateral expansion
> Excluder bifurcated endoprosthesis

EBEA
> Epstein-Barr [virus] early antigen

EBER
> electron beam electroreflectance
> Epstein-Barr early region [protein]
> Epstein-Barr early RNA [gene, probe
>   for test]
> Epstein-Barr [virus]-encoded ribonucleic
>   acid

EBER ISH
> Epstein-Barr virus-encoded RNA in situ
>   hybridization

EBF
> elastic band fixation
> erythroblastosis fetalis *(See also* EF)

E-BFU
> erythroid blood-forming unit

EBG
> electroblepharograph(y)
>   (electroblepharogram)

EBGS
> electrical bone-growth stimulation
>   (stimulator)

EBH
> epidermolysis bullosa hereditaria

EBI
> electronic bone stimulation
> erythroblastic island
> estradiol-binding index
> external beam irradiation

EBIORT, EB-IORT
> electron-beam intraoperative radiation
>   therapy (radiotherapy)

EBK
> embryonic bovine kidney

EBL
> endoscopic band ligation
> erythroblastic leukemia
> estimated blood loss

EBL-1
> European bat lyssavirus 1

eBL
> endemic Burkitt lymphoma

EBLL
> elevation of blood lead level

EBL/S
> estimated blood loss/surgery

EBLV
> European bat lyssavirus

EBM
> electrophysiologic behavior modification
> epidermolysis bullosa, macular type
> evidence-based medicine *(See also*
>   E-BM)
> expressed breast milk

E-BM
> evidence-based medicine *(See also*
>   EBM)

EBNA
> Epstein-Barr [virus] nuclear antigen

EBNe
> Epstein-Barr nasopharyngeal carcinoma

EBNS
> endoscopic bladder neck suspension

EBO
> Ebola [disease or virus]
> evidence-based outcome

E/BOD
> electrolyte biochemical oxygen demand

EBO-R
> Ebola Reston [virus]

EBOV
Ebola virus
EBO-Z
Ebola Zaire virus
EBP
epidural blood patch
erythroblastopenia
esophageal balloon procedure
estradiol-binding protein
EBPS
Emotional and Behavior Problem
Scale
EBR
embolus to blood ratio
external beam radiotherapy
eye-blink rate
EBRs
evidence-based recommendation
EBRT
electron-beam radiotherapy
external beam radiation therapy
EBS
elastic back strap
electrical brain stimulation
empiric bayesian screening [mathematic
modeling]
epidermolysis bullosa simplex
estrogen binding site
EBSB
equal breath sounds bilaterally
EBSD
endoscopic balloon sphincter dilation
EBSL
external branch of superior laryngeal
[nerve]
EBSS
Earle balanced salt solution
EBT
early bedtime
electron beam tomography
erythromycin breath test
external beam [photon] therapy
EBUS
endobronchial ultrasound
(ultrasonography)
EBV
effective blood volume
electron boost volume
Epstein-Barr virus
estimated (effective) blood
volume
EB-VCA
Epstein-Barr viral capsid antigen
EBVS
Epstein Barr virus susceptibility
EBZ
epidermal basement zone

EC
effect of closing [of eyes in
electroencephalography]
effective concentration
ejection click
electrical cardioversion
electrocautery
electrochemical
electron capture
embryonal carcinoma
emergency contraception
emetic center
endocervical
endometrial carcinoma
endothelial cell
enteric-coated [tablet] (*See also* ECT)
entering complaint
enterochromaffin cell
entorhinal cortex
entrance complaint
environmental complexity
Enzyme Commission
enzyme-treated cell
epidermal cell
epithelial cell
equalization-cancellation [model,
hearing]
Escherichia coli
esophageal candidiasis
esophageal carcinoma
ether-chloroform [mixture, obsolete]
Euro-Collins [solution]
excitation-contraction
excitatory center
experimental control
external carotid
external conjugate [pelvis]
extracapsular
extracellular
extracellular compartment
extracellular concentration
extracorporeal
extracranial
extruded cell
eye care
eyes closed
EC50, EC$_{50}$
median effective concentration
[concentration of substance in medium
to produce effect in 50% of test
organisms]
E:C
estriol to creatinine ratio
estrogen to creatinine ratio
ECA
electric control activity
electrocardioanalyzer

E

ECA *(continued)*
    endothelial-cell antibody
    enteric-coated aspirin [tablet]
    enterobacterial common antigen
    epidemiologic catchment area
    ethylcarboxylate adenosine
    external carotid artery
E-CABG
    endarterectomy and coronary artery
      bypass graft(ing)
    endoscopic coronary artery bypass
      graft(ing)
ECAD
    extracorporeal albumin dialysis
    extracranial carotid arterial disease
E-cad
    E-cadherin
ECAF
    extension corner avulsion fracture
ECAM
    energy conservation and activity
      management
ECAO
    enterocytopathogenic avian orphan
      [virus]
ECaP
    exceptional cancer patient
ECASA
    enteric-coated acetylsalicylic acid
      [aspirin]
ECAT
    emission computer-assisted tomography
    emission computerized axial
      tomography
ECB
    electric cabinet bath
ECBD
    exploration of common bile duct
ECBI
    Eyberg Child Behavior Inventory
ECBO
    enterocytopathogenic bovine orphan
      [virus]
ECBP
    extracorporeal bypass pump
ECBV
    effective circulating blood volume
ECC
    early childhood caries
    edema, clubbing, cyanosis
    electrocorticograph(y)
      (electrocorticogram)
    embryonal cell carcinoma
    emergency cardiac care
    Emergency Communications Center
    endocervical cone
    endocervical curettage
    enterochromaffin cell
    estimated creatinine clearance

    external cardiac compression
    extracapsular cataract
    extracorporeal circulation
    extrusion of cell cytoplasm
ECCE
    extracapsular cataract extraction
    (*See also* XCCE)
ECCL
    encephalocraniocutaneous lipomatosis
ECCO
    enterocytopathogenic cat orphan
      [virus]
ECCO$_2$R
    extracorporeal carbon dioxide removal
ECD
    E-cadherin
    ectrodactyly
    electrochemical detection (detector)
    electron capture detector
    endocardial cushion defect
    endothelial cell density
    endothelial corneal dystrophy
    enzymatic cell dispersion
    equivalent current dipole
    ethyl cysteinate dimer
    excision, curettage, drilling
      [osteochondral lesion]
    extended criteria donor
    external cardioverter-defibrillator
    extracellular domain
    extracranial carotid disease
    extracranial Doppler sonography
ECDB
    encourage to cough and deep breathe
ECDO
    enterocytopathogenic dog orphan
      [virus]
ECE
    early childhood education
    endocervical ecchymosis
    endothelin-converting enzyme
    equine conjugated estrogen
    extracapsular extension
ECE1
    endothelin-converting enzyme
ECEMG
    evoked compound electromyography
ECEO
    enterocytopathogenic equine orphan
      [virus]
ECES
    Education and Career Exploration
      System
ECF
    East Coast fever
    effective capillary flow
    eosinophil (eosinophilic) chemotactic
      factor
    epicanthic fold

erythroid colony formation
Escherichia coli filtrate
executive cognitive function(ing)
extended care facility
extracardial Fontan [procedure]
extracellular fluid
extracytoplasmic function
ECFA, ECF-A
eosinophil chemotactic factor of
anaphylaxis
ECF-C
eosinophilic chemotactic factor
complement
ECFV
extracellular fluid volume (*See also*
EFV)
ECG
electrocardiograph(y) (electrocardiogram)
(*See also* EKG)
ECGE
extracorporeal gas exchange
ECGF
endothelial cell growth factor
ECGS
endothelial cell growth supplement
ECGT
epiphysial chondromatous giant cell
tumor
ECH
epichlorohydrin
echino
echinocyte
ECHO
enteric cytopathogenic human orphan
[virus]
echo
echocardiogram echocardiograph(y)
echoencephalograph(y)
(echoencephalogram)
echoventriculometry
echoCG
echocardiograph(y) (echocardiogram)
echo EG
echoencephalograph(y)
(echoencephalogram) (*See also* echo)
ECHOG, ECochG
electrocochleography (*See also* ECoG)
ECHO-RV
echocardiography-radionuclide
ventriculography
echo-VM
echoventriculometry
ECI
electrocerebral inactivity
ensemble contrast imaging
eosinophilic cytoplasmic inclusion
extracorporeal irradiation [of blood]
(*See also* ECIB)

ECIB
extracorporeal irradiation of blood
(*See also* ECI)
ECIC
external carotid and internal carotid
extracranial-intracranial
ECIL
extracorporeal irradiation of lymph
ECIS
endometrial carcinoma in situ
ECK
extracellular kalium (potassium)
ECKI
Escherichia coli K1
ECL
electrochemiluminescence
electrogenerated chemiluminescence
emitter-coupled logic
enhanced chemiluminescence
enterochromaffin-like [cell]
euglobin (euglobulin) clot lysis [test]
extent of cerebral lesion
extracapillary lesion
ECLA
excimer laser coronary angioplasty
extracorporeal lung assist
ECLAM
European Consensus Lupus Activity
Measure
eclec
eclectic
ECLIA
electrochemiluminescence immunoassay
ECLiPS
encoded combinatorial libraries in
polymeric support [chemistry]
ECLoma
enterochromaffin-like gastric carcinoid
tumor
ECLP
extracorporeal liver perfusion
ECLRS
electronic clinical laboratory reporting
system
ECLS
extracorporeal life support
ECLT
euglobulin clot lysis time
ECM
embryonic chick muscle
endoscope-controlled microsurgery
erythema chronicum migrans
esophagocardiomyotomy
external cardiac massage
external chemical messenger
extracellular material
extracellular matrix
extracolonic malignancy

E

ECM:BCM
extracellular mass to body cell mass ratio

ECMO
enterocytopathogenic monkey orphan [virus]
extracorporeal membrane oxygenation (oxygenator)

ECMP
enterocoated microspheres of pancrelipase

ECN
epithelioid combined nevi

ECN-CC
epithelioid combined nevi Carney complex

ECN-DPN
epithelioid combined nevi deep penetrating nevus

EC No.
Enzyme Commission Number

ecNOS
endothelial constitutive nitric oxide synthase (synthetase)

ECoG
electrocochleography (*See also* ECHOG, ECochG)
electrocorticograph(y) (electrocorticogram)

E. coli
Escherichia coli

ECOM
endotracheal cardiac output monitor(ing)

ECOR
extracorporeal carbon dioxide removal

ECOtox
Escherichia coli [heat-labile toxin] vaccine

ECP
ectrodactyly-cleft palate [syndrome]
effective conduction period
effector cell precursor
electronic claims processing
emergency care provider
emergency contraceptive pill
endocardial potential
endoscopic cyclophotocoagulation
eosinophil (eosinophilic) cationic protein
erythrocyte coproporphyrin
erythroid committed precursor
erythropoietic coproporphyria
Escherichia coli polypeptide
exercise cardiac power
external cardiac pressure
external counterpulsation
extracorporeal photochemotherapy
extracorporeal photopheresis
free cytoporphyrin in erythrocyte

ECPD
external counterpressure device

ECPL
endocavitary pelvic lymphadenectomy

ECPO
enterocytopathogenic porcine orphan [virus]

ECPOG
electrochemical potential gradient

ECPP
extracorporeal photophoresis

ECPR
external cardiopulmonary resuscitation

ECR
electrocardiographic response
emergency chemical restraint
endocervical resection
evoked cortical response
extensor carpi radialis [muscle]

ECRB
extensor carpi radialis brevis [muscle]

ECRL
extensor carpi radialis longus [muscle]

ECRO
enterocytopathogenic rodent orphan [virus]

ECS
elective cosmetic surgery
electrocerebral silence
electroconvulsive shock
electronic claims submission
epileptic confusional state
extracapsular spread
extracellular-like, calcium-free solution
extracellular space

E2CS
Edinburgh 2 Coma Scale

ECSO
enterocytopathogenic swine orphan [virus]

EC-SOD
extracellular superoxide dismutase

ECSP
epidermal cell surface protein

ECST
electroconvulsive shock therapy (treatment)

ECT
ecarin clotting time [test]
ectomesenchymal chondromyxoid tumor
electrochemotherapy
electroconvulsive therapy
emission computed tomography
enhanced computed tomography
enteric-coated tablet (*See also* EC)
euglobulin clot test
European compression technique [bone screw and internal fixation]

extended code therapy
extracellular tissue

ect

ectopic

ECT$_{50}$

effective concentration and time [that causes an effect in 50% of subjects, chemical weapons]

ECTA

esophageal gastric tube airway
Everyman Contingency Table Analysis

ECTEOLA

epichlorohydrin and triethanolamine [medium]

ECTR

endoscopic carpal tunnel release

EC-TRICKS

elliptical centric-time resolved imaging of contrast kinetics

ECU

electrocautery unit
extensor carpi ulnaris
extracorporeal ultrafiltration

ECV

effective circulating volume
emergency center visit
endocardial ventriculotomy
esophageal collateral vein
external cardioversion
external cephalic version
extracellular [fluid] volume
extracorporeal volume

ECVA

extracranial vertebral artery

ECVD

extracellular volume depletion
extracellular volume of distribution

ECVE

extracellular volume expansion

ECW

extracellular water

ED

early differentiation
eating disorder
ectodermal dysplasia
ectopic depolarization
edge detection
education
effective diameter
effective dose
elbow disarticulation
electrodiagnosis (*See also* EDX, EDx, El Dx)
electrodialysis
electron diffraction
elemental diet
embryonic death

emergency department
emotional defensiveness
emotional disorder
emotional disturbance
emotionally disturbed
end diastole
entering diagnosis
Entner-Doudoroff [metabolic pathway]
enzyme deficiency
epidural
epileptiform discharge
epithelial defect
equilibrium dialysis
equine dermis [cells]
equivalent dose
erectile dysfunction
erythema dose
ethyldichloroarsine [chemical weapon]
ethylenediamine
evidence of disease
exertional dyspnea
exit dose
extensive disease
extensor digitorum [muscle]
external diameter
exertional dyspnea
extra-low dispersion

E-D

ego-defense

ED$_{50}$

median effective dose

E$_d$

depth dose

ed

edema (*See also* E)

EDA

elbow disarticulation
electrodermal activity
electrodermal audiometry
electrolyte-deficient agar
electron donor-acceptor [interaction]
end-diastolic area

EDA+

extradomain A positive

EDAM

electron-dense amorphous material

EDAMS

encephaloduroarteriomyosynangiosis

EDAP

emergency department approval for pediatrics

EDAS

encephaloduroarteriosynangiosis

EDAX

energy-dispersive x-ray analysis

E

EDB
early dry breakfast
ethylene dibromide
extensor digitorum brevis
[muscle]
EDBP
erect diastolic blood pressure
EDC
effective dynamic compliance
electrodesiccation and curettage
(*See also* ED&C)
emergency decontamination center
end-diastolic count
endocrine disrupting chemical
estimated date of conception
estimated date of confinement
expected date of confinement
expected delivery, cesarean
extensor digitorum communis
[muscle]
ethyl cysteinate dimer
ED&C
electrodesiccation and curettage
(*See also* EDC)
EDCF
endothelium-derived constricting factor
EDCI
energetic dynamic cardiac
insufficiency
E-DCIS
endocrine ductal carcinoma in situ
EDCP
eccentric dynamic compression plate
(plating)
EDCS
end-diastolic chamber stiffness
end-diastolic circumferential stress
EDCT
early distal proximal tubule
EDD
effective drug duration
end-diastolic diameter
end-diastolic dimension
endothelium-dependent dilation
enzyme-digested delta [endotoxin]
esophageal detection device
estimated discharge date
estimated due date
expected date of delivery
extended daily dialysis
EDDA
expanded duty dental auxiliary
EDE
eating disorders examination
EDe
erosion depth
EDEN
Evaluative Disposition [toward the]
Environment

edent
edentulous
ED-ES
endolymphatic duct [and] endolymphatic
sac
EDF
elongation, derotation, [lateral] flexion
end-diastolic flow
erythroid differentiation factor
extradural fluid
EDG
electrodermography
electrodynogram
EdGr
Edmondson grade (grading)
EDH
epidural hematoma
extradural hematoma
EDHF
endothelium-derived hyperpolarizing
factor
EDI
Eating Disorder Inventory
electrodeionization
estimated daily intake
EDI-2
Eating Disorder Inventory, 2nd edition
EDICP
electron-dense iron-containing particle
EDIE
extended deep inferior epigastric [artery
flap]
EDIM
epidemic disease of infant mice
epizootic diarrhea of infant mice
EDit
electric differential therapy
EDITAR
extended-duration topical arthropod
repellent
EDL
end-diastolic load
end-diastolic [segment] length
estimated date of labor
extensor digitorum longus [muscle]
ED/LD
emotionally disturbed and learning
disabled
EDLF
endogenous digitalislike factors
EDLS
endogenous digitalislike substance
EDM
early diastolic murmur
electronic daily monitor
esophageal Doppler monitor
extensor digiti minimi [muscle]
extramucosal duodenal myotomy
multiple epiphysial dysplasia

EDMA
ethylene glycol dimethacrylate
euclidean distance matrix analysis
EDMD
Emery-Dreifuss muscular dystrophy
EDN
electrodesiccation
eosinophil-derived neurotoxin
EDNF
endogenous digitalislike natriuretic
factor
EDNO
endothelium-derived nitric oxide
EDNOS
eating disorders not otherwise specified
EDOC
estimated date of confinement
EDP
electron-dense particle
electronic data processing
end-diastolic pressure
endoscopic digital pancreatography
EDPA
Erhardt Developmental Prehension
Assessment
ethyl diphenylpropenylamine
EDPCS
exertional deep posterior compartment
syndrome
EDPS
esophageal-directed pressure support
EDQ
extensor digiti quinti
EDR
early diastolic relaxation
effective direct radiation
electrodermal response [biofeedback]
electrodialysis with reversed [polarity]
escalating dose regimen
exposure data recognizer
extreme drug resistance
EDRA
electrodermal response audiometry
EDRF
endothelial derived relaxant factor
endothelium-derived relaxing factor
EDS
edema disease of swine
egg drop syndrome
Ego Development Scale
electrodermal screening
energy-dispersive spectrometer
energy dispersive x-ray spectroscopy
epigastric distress syndrome
excessive daytime sleepiness
extended data stream
extradimensional shift

EDSS
Expanded Disability Status Scale
(Score)
EDT
emergency department thoracotomy
end-diastolic [cardiac wall] thickness
erythrocyte density test
exposure duration threshold
EDTA
ethylenediaminetetraacetic acid (*See also*
EDTAC)
EDTAC
ethylenediaminetetraacetic acid (*See also*
EDTA)
EDTMP
ethylenediamine tetramethylene
phosphoric acid
EDV
end-diastolic velocity
end-diastolic volume
epidermal dysplastic verruciformis
EDVA
Erhardt Developmental Vision
Assessment
EDVI
end-diastolic volume index
EDW
estimated dry weight
EDWGT
emergency drinking water germicidal
tablet
EDWTH
end-diastolic wall thickness
EDX, EDx
electrodiagnosis (*See also* ED, El Dx)
EDXA
energy-dispersed x-ray analysis
energy-dispersive x-ray analysis
EDXRF
energy-dispersive x-ray fluorescence
EDxTM
energy diagnostic treatment method
E$_{dyn}$
respiratory system elastance
E-E
end-to-end [anastomosis] (*See also* EE)
erythema-edema [reaction]
EE
electrosurgical excision
embryo extract
emetic episode
end-expiration
end-to-end [anastomosis] (*See also* E-E)
end-to-end [bite, occlusion]
energy expenditure
Enterobacteriaceae enrichment [broth]
equine encephalitis

E

EE *(continued)*
  erosive esophagitis
  esophageal endoscopy
  exchange efficiency
  exercise echocardiogram
  expressed emotion
  external ear
  eyes and ears (*See also* E&E)
E&E
  eyes and ears (*See also* EE)
EEA
  electroencephalic audiometry
  elemental enteral alimentation
  end-to-end anastomosis
  energy expended with activity
EEC
  ectrodactyly, ectodermal [dysplasia],
    clefting [syndrome]
  endogenous erythroid colony
  endometrioid endometrial carcinoma
  enteropathogenic *Escherichia coli*
  enterovirulent *Escherichia coli*
EECD
  endothelial-epithelial corneal dystrophy
EECG
  electroencephalograph(y)
    (electroencephalogram) (*See also*
    EEG)
EECP
  enhanced external counterpulsation
EECS
  extraembryonic celomic space
EED
  erythema elevatum diutinum
EEDQ
  ethoxycarbonylethoxydihydroquinoline
    [chromatic resin]
EEE
  Eastern equine encephalitis
    (encephalomyelitis)
  edema, erythema, exudate
  estimated energy expenditure
  experimental enterococcal endocarditis
  external eye examination
EEEP
  end-expiratory esophageal pressure
EEEV
  eastern equine encephalitis
    (encephalomyelitis) virus
EEG
  electroencephalograph(y)
    (electroencephalogram)
EEGA
  electroencephalographic audiometry
EEG-CSA
  electroencephalography with
    computerized spectral analysis
EEGF
  esophageal epidermal growth factor

EEHS
  emergency evacuation hyperbaric
    stretcher
EEJ
  electroejaculation
EEL
  external elastic lamina
EELS
  electron energy loss spectroscopy
EELV
  end-expiratory lung volume
EEM
  ectodermal dysplasia, ectrodactyly,
    macular dystrophy [syndrome]
  erythema exudativum multiforme
  external elastic membrane
  [Test for] Examining Expressive
    Morphology
EEMG
  evoked electromyograph(y)
    (electromyogram)
EEN
  estimated energy needs
EENT
  eyes, ears, nose, throat
EEO
  electroendoosmosis
  electroendosmosis
EEP
  end-expiratory phase
  end-expiratory pressure
  equivalent effective photon
E-EPE
  established extraprostatic extension
EEPI
  extraretinal eye position information
EEPLND
  extraperitoneal endoscopic pelvic lymph
    node dissection
EER
  electroencephalographic response
  extended endocardial resection
EERP
  extended endocardial resection
    procedure
EERS
  ears education and retraining system
EES
  endometrial stromal sarcoma
  ethyl ethanesulfate
  expandable esophageal stent
EESG
  evoked electrospinogram
EET
  early exercise testing
  epoxyeicosatrienoic [acid]
EEV
  elastic equilibrium volume
  encircling endocardial ventriculotomy

EF

eccentric fixation
ectopic focus
edema factor
ejection fraction
elastic fiber
elastic fibril
electric field
elongation factor
embryofetal [alcohol syndrome]
embryo fibroblast
emergency facility
emotional factor
encephalitogenic factor
endothoracic fascia
endurance factor
eosinophilic fasciitis
epithelial focus
equivalent focus
erythroblastosis fetalis (*See also* EBF)
erythrocytic fragmentation
escape focus
essential findings
exophthalmic factor
exposure factor
extended field [radiation therapy]
extrafine
extra food
extrinsic factor

EF-4

eugonic fermenter 4 [bacteria]

EFA

essential fatty acid
extrafamily adoptee

EFAD

essential fatty acid deficiency

EFAS

embryofetal alcohol syndrome

EFBW

estimated fetal body weight

EFC

elastin fragment concentration
endogenous fecal calcium

EFD

episode-free day

EFE

endocardial fibroelastosis
epidemic fatal encephalopathy

EFF

electromagnetic focusing field [probe]

eff

efface
effect(ive) (*See also* effect.)
efferent (*See also* effer)

efficient
effusion

effect.

effective (*See also* eff)

effer

efferent (*See also* eff)

EFFU

epithelial focus-forming unit

EF-G

elongation factor G [protein]

EFG

electric field gradient

EFGR

epidermal growth factor receptor

efgre

enhanced fast gradient echo

EFH

explosive follicular hyperplasia

EFHBM

eosinophilic fibrohistiocytic [lesion of] bone marrow

EFHL

essential familial hyperlipemia

EFI

elderly functionally impaired
extended-field radiation

EFL

effective focal length
external fluid loss

EFM

elderly fibromyalgia
electronic fetal monitoring
external fetal monitoring

EF/M

electrostatic force microscopy

EFMM

external fetal-maternal monitor

EFMT

electric field mediated transfer

EFOV

extended field-of-view [technique]

EFP

effective filtration pressure
endoneural fluid pressure
equine-facilitated psychotherapy

EFPS

epicardial fat pad sign

EFR

effective filtration rate
extended field radiation

E FRAG

erythrocyte fragility [test]

EFRT

extended field radiotherapy

EFS

electric field stimulation
event-free survival

E

EFT
Embedded Figures Test
emotional freedom technique
Ewing family of tumors
extended family therapy

EFV
extracellular fluid volume (*See also* ECFV)

EFVC
expiratory flow-volume curve

EFW
estimated fetal weight

EF/WM
ejection fraction [and] wall motion

EG
enteroglucagon
eosinophilic gastroenteritis (*See also* EGE)
eosinophilic granuloma
esophagogastrectomy
esophagogastric
external genitalia

e.g.
for example [L. *exempli gratia*]

EGA
esophageal gastric [tube] airway
estimated gestational age

EGAT
Educational Goal Attainment Test

EGBPS
equilibrium-gated blood pool study

EGBT
esophagogastric balloon tamponade

EGBUS, EG/BUS
external genitalia, Bartholin, urethral, Skene [glands] (*See also* EXGBUS)

EGC
early gastric cancer (carcinoma)
endocrine granule constituent
epithelioid-globoid cell

EGCG
epigallocatechin gallate

EGCT
extragonadal germ cell tumor

EGCUS
early gastric cancer of upper stomach

EGD
endocervical glandular dysplasia
esophagogastroduodenoscopy

EGDF
embryonic growth and development factor

EGDT
early goal-directed therapy
esophagogastric devascularization and transection

EGE
eosinophilic gastroenteritis (*See also* EG)

EGF
early graft failure
endothelial growth factor
epidermal growth factor

eGFP
enhanced green fluorescent protein

EGFR
epidermal growth factor receptor

EGFR-TKI
epidermal growth factor tyrosine kinase inhibitor

EGG
electrogastrograph(y) (electrogastrogram)
electroglottograph(y) (electroglottogram)

EGGCT
extragonadal germ cell tumor

EGH
equine growth hormone

EGI
endogenous glutamic acid decarboxylase (GAD) inhibitor

EGJ
esophagogastric junction

EGL
eosinophilic granuloma of lung

EGLT
euglobulin lysis time

EGM
electrogram
electrogustometry
extracellular granular material
extraglandular manifestation
extraglomerular mesangium

EGN
experimental glomerulonephritis

EGNB
enteric gram-negative bacillary [meningitis, parotitis]
enteric gram-negative bacillus

EGOT
erythrocyte (erythrocytic) glutamic oxaloacetic transaminase

EGP
endogenous glucose production

EGP-2
epithelial glycoprotein 2

EGR
early growth response
erythema gyratum repens
erythrocyte glutathione reductase

EGRA
equilibrium-gated radionuclide angiography

EGS
electric galvanic (electrogalvanic) stimulation
ethylene glycol succinate
extragonadal seminoma

EGT
  ethanol gelation test
  exuberant granulation tissue
EGTA
  esophageal gastric (esophagogastric)
    tube airway
  ethyleneglycoltetraacetic (ethylene glycol
    tetraacetic) acid
EH
  early healed
  eccentric hypertrophy
  educationally handicapped
  emotional handicap
  emotionally handicapped
  endometrial hyperplasia
  enlarged heart
  enteral hyperalimentation
  environment and heredity (*See also*
    E&H)
  Entamoeba histolytica
  epidermolytic hyperkeratosis
  epidural hematoma
  epithelioid hemangioendothelioma
  epoxide hydratase
  esophageal hiatus
  essential hypertension
  external hyperalimentation
  extramedullary hematopoiesis
E&H
  environment and heredity (*See also* EH)
Eh
  oxidation-reduction potential (*See also*
    E_o+, E^o, ORP)
EHAA
  epidemic hepatitis-associated antigen
EHB
  elevate head of bed
  entrance heart beat
  extensor hallucis brevis
EHBA
  extrahepatic biliary atresia
EHBD
  extrahepatic bile duct
EHBDA
  extrahepatic bile duct atresia
EHBF
  estimated hepatic blood flow
  exercise hyperemia blood flow
  extrahepatic blood flow
EHBT
  extrahepatic biliary tree
EHC
  enterohepatic circulation
  enterohepatic clearance
  essential hypercholesterolemia
  extended health care
  extrahepatic cholestasis

eHCC
  early hepatocellular carcinoma
EH-CF
  Entamoeba histolytica-complement
    fixation
EHCR
  electronic health care record
EHD
  electrohemodynamic
  epizootic hemorrhagic disease
EHDV
  epizootic hemorrhagic disease virus 1–8
EHE
  epithelioid hemangioendothelioma
EHEC
  enterohemorrhagic *Escherichia coli*
EHF
  electrohydraulic fragmentation
  epidemic hemorrhagic fever
  exophthalmos-hyperthyroid factor
  extremely high factor
  extremely high frequency
EHG
  electrohysterograph(y)
    (electrohysterogram)
EHH
  episodic hypothermia with
    hyperhidrosis
  esophageal hiatal hernia
EHI
  Edinburgh Handedness Inventory
  exertional heat illness
EHK
  epidermolytic hyperkeratosis
EHL
  effective half-life [of radioactive
    substance]
  electrohydraulic lithotripsy
  endogenous hyperlipidemia
  endoscopic hemorrhoid ligation
  Environmental Health Laboratory
  essential hyperlipidemia
  extensor hallucis longus
EHLL
  epithelial hyperplastic laryngeal
    lesion
EHM
  embryonic heart motion
  extrahepatic metastasis
EHME
  Employee Health Maintenance
    Examination
EHMS
  electrohydrodynamic ionization mass
    spectrometry
EHO
  extrahepatic obstruction

E

EHP
Environmental Health Perspectives
excessive heat production
extra high potency

EHPH
extrahepatic portal hypertension

EHPO
extrahepatic portal vein obstruction

EHPT
Eddy hot plate test

EHPVO
extrahepatic portal vein obstruction

EHR
electronic healthcare record

EHS
employee health service
exertional heat stroke

EHSDS
Experimental Health Services Delivery
System

EHT
electrohydrothermal
essential hypertension

EHV
Edge Hill virus
electric heart vector
equine herpesvirus

EI
Edmonton injector
electrical injury
electrolyte imbalance
electron impact
electron ionization
emotionally impaired
endovascular irradiation
environmental illness
enzyme immunoassay
enzyme inhibitor
eosinophilic index
erythema infectiosum
excretory index
exercise-induced
extensor indicis
external ilium
external intervention

E of I
evidence of insurability

E:I
expiration to inspiration ratio
expiratory to inspiratory ratio

E&I
endocrine and infertility

EIA
electroimmunoassay
enteroinsular axis
enzymatic immunoassay
enzyme immunosorbent assay
enzyme-linked immunosorbent assay
enzyme-multiplied immunoassay

equine infectious anemia
exercise-induced anaphylaxis
(asthma)
external iliac artery

EIA-2
second-generation enzyme immunoassay

EIAB
extracranial-intracranial arterial bypass

EIAC
enzyme-inducing anticonvulsant

EIB
electrophoretic immunoblotting
erythema induration of Bazin
exercise-induced bronchoconstriction
exercise-induced bronchospasm

EIC
early ischemic change
elastase inhibition capacity
electrical impedance cardiography
endometrial intraepithelial carcinoma
enzyme immunochromatography
enzyme inhibition complex
epidermal inclusion cyst
extensive intraductal carcinoma
extensive intraductal component

EICA
extracranial to intracranial artery
[bypass]

EICDT
Ego-Ideal and Conscience Development
Test

EICL
Eldercare Initiative in Consumer Law

EICT
external isovolumic contraction time

EID
egg-infectious dose
electroimmunodiffusion
electronic induction desorption
electronic infusion device
emergency infusion device

EIDC
extreme intervertebral disc collapse

EIDCR
endoscopic intranasal
dacryocystorhinostomy

EIEC
enteroinvasive *Escherichia coli*

EIEE
early infantile epileptic encephalopathy

EIF, eIF
erythrocyte initiation factor
eukaryotic initiation factor

EIFT
embryo intrafallopian transfer

EII
electrical impedance imaging

EIL
elective induction of labor

EILV
  end-inspiratory lung volume
EIM
  excitability-inducing material
  extraintestinal manifestation
EIMS
  electron ionization mass spectrometry
EI/MV
  endotracheal intubation and mechanical
    ventilation
EIN
  endometrial intraepithelial neoplasia
  epiphysial ischemic necrosis
EIO
  exploratory insight-oriented
    psychotherapy
EIOA
  excessive intake of alcohol
EIP
  early intervention program
  elective interruption of pregnancy
  end-inspiratory pause
  end-inspiratory pressure
  extensor indicis proprius [muscle]
EIPS
  endogenous inhibitor of prostaglandin
    synthase
EIPV, eIPV
  enhanced inactivated polio vaccine
EIR
  early ischemic recurrence
  entomological inoculation rate
EIRDS
  exercise-induced respiratory distress
    syndrome
EIRnv
  extraincidence rate in nonvaccinated
    [groups]
EIRP
  effective isotropic radiated power
EIRv
  extraincidence rate in vaccinated
    (groups)
EIS
  electrical impedance scanning
  endoscopic injection sclerotherapy
  Environmental Impact Statement
  Epidemic Intelligence Service
    [CDC]
EISA
  electroencephalogram interval spectrum
    analysis
EIT
  electrical impedance tomography
  erythroid iron turnover
EITB
  enzyme-linked immunotransfer blot

EIU
  enzyme-linked immunosorbent assay
    (ELISA) unit
EIV
  external iliac vein
EJ
  ejection [fraction]
  elbow jerk
  external jugular
EJB
  ectopic junctional beat
EJN
  extended jaundice of newborn
EJP
  excitatory junction potential
EJV
  external jugular vein
EK
  electrophoretic karyotyping
  enterokinase
  erythrokinase
Ek
  kinetic energy [of particle]
EKC
  epidemic keratoconjunctivitis
EKG
  electrocardiograph(y) (electrocardiogram)
    (*See also* ECG)
EKO
  echoencephalograph(y)
    (echoencephalogram)
eKru
  equivalent residual renal urea
    clearance
EKS
  epidemic Kaposi sarcoma
EKV
  erythrokeratodermia variabilis
EKY
  electrokymograph(y) (electrokymogram)
EL
  early latent
  effective level
  egg lecithin
  elastic limit
  electrolarynx
  electroluminescence
  elixir (*See also* elix)
  elopement
  erythroleukemia
  exercise limit
  exploratory laparotomy
  external lamina
E-L
  external lid
El
  elastase

E

ELA
  endotoxinlike activity
  excimer laser-assisted angioplasty
ELAD
  extracorporeal liver assist device
ELAFF
  extended lateral arm free flap
E-LAM, ELAM
  endothelium (endothelial)-leukocyte
    adhesion molecule
ELAM-1
  endothelial-leukocyte adhesion molecule
    1
ELAS
  extended lymphadenopathy syndrome
E-LASIK
  epithelial laser-assisted intrastromal
    keratomileusis
ELAT
  enzyme-linked antiglobulin test
ELB
  early light breakfast
elb
  elbow
ELBF
  estimated liver blood flow
ELBNS
  extraperitoneal laparoscopic bladder
    neck suspension
ELBW
  extremely low birth weight
ELBWI
  extremely low birth weight infant
ELC
  earlobe crease
ELCA
  excimer laser coronary angioplasty
ELD
  egg lethal dose
  end-of-life decision
  energy level diagram
ELDH
  extraforaminal lumbar disc herniation
El Dx
  electrodiagnosis (*See also* ED, EDX,
    EDx)
ELEC
  elective
elec, elect.
  electric(ity)
  electuary [confection]
elem
  elementary
elev
  elevate(d)
  elevation
  elevator
ELF
  elective low forceps [delivery]

  endoscopic laser foraminotomy
  epithelial lining fluid
  extra low frequency
  extremely low frequency
ELFA
  enzyme-linked fluorescent immunoassay
ELFD
  epithelial lining fluid desensitization
ELG
  eligible
  endoluminal gastroplication
  endoluminal graft
elgon
  electrogoniometer
ELH
  egg-laying hormone
  endolymphatic hydrops
ELI
  endomyocardial lymphocytic infiltrates
  Environmental Language Inventory
  exercise lability index
  extra-low interstitial [alloy for
    implant]
ELIA
  enzyme-labeled immunoassay
ELICT
  enzyme-linked immunocytochemical
    technique
ELIEDA
  enzyme-linked immunoelectrodiffusion
    assay
ELIFA
  enzyme-linked immunofiltration assay
ELIG
  eligible
elim
  elimination
ELISA
  enzyme-linked immunosorbent
    (immunoabsorbent) assay
ELISA-I–ELISA-II
  enzyme-linked immunosorbent assay I,
    II
ELISPOT
  enzyme-linked immunospot [assay]
ELITT
  endometrial laser intrauterine thermal
    therapy
elix
  elixir (*See also* EL)
ELK
  endothelial lamellar keratoplasty
ELLIP
  elliptocyte
ELM
  Early Language Milestone [Scale]
  epiluminescence (epiluminescent)
    microscopy
  external laryngeal manipulation

external limiting membrane
extravascular lung mass
ELMS
    epithelioid leiomyosarcoma
ELMT
    elements [on urinalysis]
ELN
    elastin
ELND
    elective lymph node dissection
ELOP
    estimated length of program
ELOS
    estimated length of stay
    extralymphatic organ site
ELP
    early labeled peak
    elastaselike protein
    electrophoresis
    endogenous limbic potential
    endogenous lipid pneumonia
    enterocolic lymphocytic phlebitis
    eruptive lingual papillitis
    Estimated Learning Potential
    exogenous lipoid pneumonia
    extracorporeal liver perfusion
ELPS
    excessive lateral pressure syndrome
ELR
    elevating leg rest
    Equal Listener Response [scale]
ELS
    electron loss spectroscopy
    endolymphatic sac
    extracorporeal life support
    extralobar sequestration
ELSD
    evaporative light scattering detection
ELSI
    ethical, legal, social implications
ELSS
    emergency life support system
ELT
    endless loop tachycardia
    endoscopic laser therapy
    euglobulin lysis test (time)
El Tor vibrio
    Vibrio cholerae biotype El Tor
ELU
    extended length of utterance
ELUS
    endoluminal rectal ultrasonography
ELV
    erythroid leukemia virus
ELVIS
    Enzyme Linked Virus Inducible
    System

ELVT
    endolaser venous therapy
EM
    early memory
    effective masking
    ejection murmur
    electromagnetic (*See also* em)
    electromechanical
    electron micrograph
    electron microscopy (microscope)
      (*See also* EMC, E-MICR)
    electrophoretic mobility
    emergency medicine
    emmetropia [normal vision]
    emotional [disorder]
    emotionally [disturbed]
    emphysema (*See also* emph)
    eosinophilia-myalgia [syndrome]
    erythema migrans
    erythema multiforme
    erythrocyte mass
    esophageal manometry
    esophageal motility
    excreted mass
    extensive metabolizers
    external monitor
    extraordinary meridian
E-M
    Embden-Meyerhof [glycolytic
    pathway]
    eosinophilia-myalgia [syndrome]
E&M
    endocrine and metabolic
    Evaluation and Management [codes]
e:m
    electron charge to mass ratio
em
    electromagnetic (*See also* EM)
EMA
    early morning awakening
    efferent motor aphasia
    elastic mandibular advancement
    electromagnetic articulography
    electronic microanalyzer
    emergency assistance
    endomysial antibody
    epithelial membrane antigen
EMAD
    equivalent mean age at death
EMAG
    environmental metaplastic atrophic
    gastritis
EMAP
    evoked muscle action potential
EMAP II
    endothelial-monocyte activating
    polypeptide II

E

EPMH
extrapyramidal muscular hypertrophy

EPMR
electronic patient medical record

EPN
emphysematous pyelonephritis
estimated protein needs

EPO
Epidemiology Program Office [Centers for Disease Control]
epoetin alfa
erythropoietin
evening primrose oil
exclusive provider organization

EPOC
excess postexercise oxygen consumption

EPP
endplate potential
equal-pressure point
erythropoietic porphyria
erythropoietic protoporphyria
extrapleural pneumonectomy
extrapulmonary pneumocystosis

EPPB
end positive-pressure breathing

EPPER
eosinophilic, polymorphic, pruritic eruption associated with radiotherapy

EPPK
epidermolytic palmoplantar keratoderma

EPPROM
extremely preterm premature rupture of membranes

EPPS
Edwards Personal Preference Schedule

EPQ
Eysenck Personality Questionnaire

EPR
early-phase reaction
early progressive resistance
Einstein-Podolsky-Rosen [paradox]
electronic prescription record
electron paramagnetic resonance
electrophrenic respiration
emergency physical restraint
enhanced permeability and retention
estimated protein requirement
estradiol production rate
evoked potential response
extraparenchymal resistance
extrapyramidal reaction

EPROM
erasable programmable read-only memory

EPS
early and periodic screening
early progressing stroke
ear, patella, short stature [syndrome]
elastosis perforans serpiginosa
electrolyte-polyethylene glycol solution
electrophysiologic study
endoscopic pancreatic sphincterotomy
endoscopic pancreatic stent(ing)
enzymatic pancreatic secretion
exophthalmos-producing substance
expressed prostatic secretions
extrapulmonary shunt
extrapyramidal symptom
extrapyramidal syndrome
extrapyramidal system

EPSA
early postoperative suture adjustment
evoked potential signal averaging

EPSCCA
extrapulmonary small-cell carcinoma

EPSD
E-point to septal distance [vectorcardiogram]

EPSDT
Early and Periodic Screening, Diagnosis, and Treatment [program]

EPSE
extrapyramidal side effect (*See also* EPS)

EPSEM
equal probability of selection method

ε, epsilon
dielectric constant
epsilon [fifth letter of Greek alphabet lowercase]
extinction coefficient
fifth in a series or group
heavy chain of immunoglobulin E
[molar] absorption coefficient
molar absorptivity [avoid use in place of molar absorption coefficient]
[molar] extinction coefficient
permittivity
specific absorptivity [Beer law]

EPSI
echo planar spectroscopic imaging

EPSP
excitatory postsynaptic potential

EPSS
E-point to septal separation [vectorcardiogram]

EPT
early pregnancy test
Eidetic Parents Test
electroporation therapy [oncology]
endocrine pancreatic tumor
endoscopic papillotomy
endpoint temperature
estrogen-progesterone therapy

EPTE
existed prior to enlistment

EPTFE, E-PTFE ePTFE, e-PTFE
expanded polytetrafluoroethylene

EPTS
existed prior to service
EPV
epidemic paralytic vertigo
EPWF
epidural pressure waveform
EPX
eosinophil protein X
EPXMA
electron probe x-ray microanalyzer
EQ
Education Quotient [annual report]
encephalization quotient
energy quotient
equal
equal to
equation (*See also* eqn)
equivalent (equivalency) (*See also* equiv)
equilibrium
external qigong
EQA
external quality assessment
eqn
equation (*See also* EQ)
EQP
extensor quinti proprius
equip.
equipment
equiv
equivalent (equivalency) (*See also* EQ)
equivocal
ER
early repolarization
early reticulocyte
efficacy ratio
ejection rate
electroresection
emergency room
endoplasmic reticulum
end range
enhanced reactivation
enhancement ratio
environmental resistance
epigastric region
equine rhinopneumonia
equivalent roentgen [unit]
erythrocyte receptor
esophageal rupture
estradiol receptor
estrogen receptor
evoked response
expiratory reserve
extended external rotation
extended release [tablet]
extended resistance
external reduction
external resistance
external rotation

extraction ratio
eye research
ER alpha (α)
estrogen receptor alpha (α)
ER beta (β)
estrogen receptor beta (β)
ER−
decreased estrogen receptor
estrogen receptor-negative
ER+
estrogen receptor-positive
increased estrogen receptor
E&R
equal and reactive
equal and regular
examination and report
Er
erbium
ERA
echo record access
electrical response activity
electric response audiometry
electroencephalic response
audiometry
endometrial resection and ablation
estradiol receptor assay
estrogen receptor assay
evoked-response audiometry
%ERAD
eradication rate
ERAF
early recurrence of atrial fibrillation
ERAS
Electronic Residency Application
Service
ERB
ethnic relational behavior
ERBAC
excimer laser, rotational atherectomy,
balloon angioplasty
ERBD
endoscopic retrograde biliary drainage
ERBF
effective renal blood flow
ERC
endoscopic retrograde cholangiograph(y)
(cholangiogram)
enterocytopathogenic human
orphan-rhinocoryza [virus]
erythropoietin-responsive cell
(pupils) equal, reactive, contracting
ERCCE
endoscopic retrograde
cholecystoendoprosthesis
ERCP
endoscopic retrograde
cholangiopancreatograph(y)
(cholangiopancreatogram)

E

ErCr: YAG
    erbium chromium:
      yttrium-aluminum-garnet [laser]
ERCT
    emergency room computerized
      tomography
ERD
    early retirement with disability
    event-related desynchronization
    evoked-response detector
    external reactive depression
    exudative retinal detachment
ERE
    estrogen-receptor element
    estrogen-response element
    external rotation in extension
ERF
    edge response function
    esophagorespiratory fistula
    external rotation in flexion
erf
    error function
ERFC, E-RFC
    erythrocyte rosette-forming cell
ERG
    electrolyte replacement with glucose
    electron radiography
    electroretinograph(y) (electroretinogram)
    existence, relatedness, growth theory
erg
    energy unit [CGS system]
ERGIC
    endoplasmic reticulum Golgi
      intermediate compartment
ERH
    egg-laying release hormone
    experimental renal hypertension
ERHD
    exposure-related hypothermia death
ERI
    electric (elective) replacement indicator
    Employee Reliability Inventory
    Environmental Response Inventory
    erythrocyte rosette inhibitor
ERIA
    electroradioimmunoassay
ER by ICA
    estrogen receptor by
      immunocytochemistry assay
ERIG
    equine rabies immune globulin
      (immunoglobulin)
ER/IR
    external rotation [and] internal rotation
ERISA
    Employee Retirement Income Security
      Act
ERK
    extracellular signal-regulated kinase 1,2

ERL
    effective refractory length
ERLND
    elective regional lymph node dissection
ERM
    electrochemical relaxation method
    epiretinal membrane
    extended radical mastectomy
ERMBT
    erythromycin breath test
ERMS
    embryonal rhabdomyosarcoma
    exacerbating-remitting multiple sclerosis
ERNA
    early return to normal activities
    equilibrium radionuclide angiography
      (angiocardiography)
ERO
    effective regurgitant orifice
ERP
    early receptor potential
    effective refractory period
    endocardial resection procedure
    endoscopic retrograde pancreatograph(y)
      (pancreatogram)
    endoscopic retrograde
      parenchymography
    equine rhinopneumonitis
    estrogen-receptor protein
    event-related [brain] potential
    exposure and response prevention
ERPC
    evacuation of retained products of
      conception
ERP-CT
    computed tomography under endoscopic
      retrograde pancreatography
ERPD
    endoscopic retrograde
      pancreaticoduodenography
ERPF
    effective renal plasma flow
ERPG
    emergency response planning guideline
ERPLV
    effective refractory period of left
      ventricle
ERPM
    early receptor potential mottling
ERPP
    endoscopic retrograde parenchymography
      of pancreas
ER/PR
    estrogen receptor [and] progesterone
      receptor
ERR, err.
    error
ERRT
    extrarenal rhabdoid tumor

ERS
endoscopic retrograde sphincterotomy
evacuation of retained secundines
[afterbirth]
extended, rotated, sidebent
ERSL
extended, rotated, sidebent left
ERSNA
efferent renal sympathetic nerve activity
ERSP
event-related slow-brain potential
ERSR
Electronic Regulatory Submission and
Review
extended, rotated, sidebent right
ERSS
Edinburgh Rehabilitation Status Scale
ERT
electronic textbook of radiology
emergency response to terrorism
emergency room thoracotomy
emergent resuscitative thoracotomy
esophageal radionuclide transit
estrogen replacement therapy
external radiation therapy
[pancreatic] enzyme replacement
therapy
ERTD
emergency room triage documentation
ERU, ERUS
endorectal ultrasound
ERV
early revascularization
endogenous retrovirus
equine rhinopneumonitis virus
Estero Real virus
expiratory reserve volume
e-RX
electronic prescription
ERY
erysipelas
erythrocyte (*See also* E, eryth)
Er: YAG
erbium: yttrium-aluminum-garnet
[laser]
eryth
erythema
erythrocyte (*See also* E, ERY)
ES
Ego Strength [test]
ejection sound
elastic stockings
elastic suspensor
electrical stimulation
electrical stimulus
electrophilic stress
electroshock

electrospray
electrotherapy system
elopement status [psychology]
embryonic stem [cells]
emergency service
emission spectrometry
endometritis-salpingitis
endoscopic sclerosis
endoscopic sclerotherapy
endoscopic sphincterotomy
end stage
end systole
end-to-side [anastomosis] (*See also* E-S,
ETS)
environmental stimulation
enzyme substrate
epileptic syndrome
epithelial (epithelioid) sarcoma
esophageal scintigraphy
esophagus (*See also* E, ESO, eso,
esoph)
esophoria
esterase (*See also* EST)
Ewing sarcoma
excretory-secretory
exfoliation syndrome
Expectation Score
experimental study
ex-smoker
exterior surface
extracapsular spread
extra strength
extrasystole
E-S
end-to-side [anastomosis] (*See also* ES,
ETS)
Es
einsteinium
^{255}Es
einsteinium-255
ESA
Early School Assessment
early systolic acceleration
endocardial surface area
end-systolic area
end-to-side anastomosis
epididymal sperm aspiration
ethmoid sinus adenocarcinoma
evidence of sexual abuse
ESAC
extrastructurally abnormal chromosome
ESADDI
estimated safe and adequate daily
dietary intake
ESAF
endothelial cell-stimulating angiogenesis
factor

E

ESAP
evoked sensory [nerve] action potential
ESAS
Edmonton Symptom Assessment Scale
ESAT
extrasystolic atrial tachycardia
ESB
Effective School Battery
electric stimulation of the brain
ESBL
extended-spectrum beta-lactamase
[inhibitor, protein]
ESBLPE
extended-spectrum
beta-lactamase-producing
Enterobacteriaceae
ES/BS
erosion surface per bone surface
ESC
electromechanical slope computer
embryonic stem cell
end-systolic count
enhanced serum cortisol
epidural spinal cord [stimulation]
erythropoietin-sensitive stem cell
ESCA
electron spectroscopy for chemical
analysis
ESCC
electrolyte steroid cardiopathy by
calcification
epidural spinal cord compression
esophageal squamous cell carcinoma
ESCH
electrolyte steroid-produced cardiopathy
[characterized by] hyalinization
Esch.
Escherichia (See also E)
ESCN
electrolyte and steroid cardiopathy with
necrosis
ESCS
Early Social Communication Scale
electrical spinal cord stimulation
ESD
electronic summation device
electron-stimulated desorption
emission spectrometric detector
end-systolic diameter (dimension)
environmental sex determination
esophagus, stomach, duodenum
exoskeletal device
ESE
electrostatic unit [Ger. *electrostatische
Einheit*]
endoscopic excision
exon splice enhancer
ESEG
echosonoencephalogram

ESEP
elbow sensory potential
extreme somatosensory evoked potential
ESF
electrosurgical filter
erythropoiesis (erythropoietic)
stimulating factor
external skeletal fixation
ES-FISH
extra signal fluorescent in situ
hybridization
ESFL
end-systolic force-length [relationship]
ESFT
Ewing sarcoma family of tumors
ESG
electrospinogram
endovascular stent graft
estrogen
exfoliation syndrome glaucoma
ESGD
end-to-side gastroduodenostomy
ESHD
end-stage heart disease
ESI
Ego State Inventory
electrospray ionization
enamel surface index
enzyme substrate inhibitor
epidural steroid injection
extent of skin involvement
ESIC
electrical stimulation-induced
contractions [DVT prevention]
ESIMS, ESI-MS
electrospray ionization mass
spectrometry
ES-IMV
expiration-synchronized intermittent
mandatory ventilation
ESIN
elastic stable intramedullary nailing
ESKD
end-stage kidney disease
ESL
end-systolic [segment] length
English as a second language
extracorporeal shockwave lithotripsy
ESLD
end-stage liver disease
end-stage lung disease
ESLF
end-stage liver failure
ESM
ejection systolic murmur
endolymphatic stromal myosis
endothelial specular microscope
ESMS
electrospray mass spectrometry

ESN
educationally subnormal
endometrial stromal nodule
estrogen-stimulated neurophysin

ESN(M)
educationally subnormal moderate

ESN(S)
educationally subnormal severe

ESO, eso
electrically stimulated osteogenesis
electrospinal orthosis
embolic signal onset
esophagoscopy (*See also* esoph)
esophagus (*See also* E, ES, esoph)
esotropia (*See also* ET, ST)

ESO/D
esotropia at distance

ESO/N
estropia at near

esoph
esophagoscopy (*See also* ESO, eso)
esophagus (*See also* E, ES, ESO, eso)

esoph steth
esophageal stethoscope

ESP
Early Speech Perception Test
Early Surveillance Project
early systolic paradox
early systolic peak
effective sensory projection
effective systolic pressure
electrosensitive point
electrosurgical pencil
endometritis-salpingitis-peritonitis
end-systolic pressure
eosinophil stimulation promoter
epidermal soluble protein
especially (*See also* esp)
evoked synaptic potential
extended supraplatysmal plane
extramedullary solitary plasmacytoma
extrasensory perception

esp
especially (*See also* ESP)

ESPA
electrical stimulation-produced analgesia

ESP:ESV
end-systolic pressure to end-systolic
volume ratio

ESPI
electronic speckle pattern interferometry

ESPLR
end-systolic pressure-length
relationship

ES/PNET
Ewing sarcoma [and] peripheral
neuroectodermal tumor

ESPQ
Early School Personality Questionnaire

ESPVR
end-systolic pressure-volume relationship

ESQ
early signs questionnaire

ESR
electric skin resistance (response)
electron spin resonance
erythrocyte sedimentation rate

ESRD
end-stage renal disease

ESRF
end-stage renal failure

ESRRL
extension, sidebent right, rotated left

ESRS
extrapyramidal symptom rating scale

ESS
emotional, spiritual, social
empty sella [turcica] syndrome
endometrial stromal sarcoma
endoscopic sinus surgery
endostreptosin
end-systolic [left ventricular] stress
end-systolic stress
Epworth Sleepiness Scale (Score)
erythrocyte-sensitizing substance
European Stroke Scale
euthyroid sick syndrome
excited skin syndrome
expiratory standstill

ess
essence
essential

ESSENCE
Electronic Surveillance System for the
Early Notification of
Community-Based Epidemics

ESSF
external spinal skeletal fixation
(fixator)

ess neg
essentially negative

EST
Eastern Standard Time
electric shock (electroshock) therapy
electric shock (electroshock) threshold
electric shock (electroshock) treatment
electrostimulation therapy
endodermal sinus tumor
endoscopic sphincterotomy
Erhard Seminar Training
established patient
esterase (*See also* ES)
exercise stress test
expression sequence tagged

E

E$_{st}$
 static elastance
est
 ester (*See also* E)
 estimate(d) (estimation)
esth
 esthetic
E-stim
 electrical stimulation
ESTN, estn
 epithelioid soft-tissue neoplasm
ESU
 electrosurgery (electrosurgical) unit
  [Bovie]
E-sub
 excitor substance
ESUE
 emergency screening ultrasound
  examination
ESV
 end-systolic [ventricular] volume
 esophageal valve
ESVH
 endoscopic saphenous vein harvesting
ESVI
 end-systolic volume index
ESVS
 endoscopic vascular surgery
 epiurethral suprapubic vaginal
  suspension
ESWI
 end-systolic wall index
ESWL
 electrohydraulic shock wave lithotripsy
 extracorporeal shock wave lithotripsy
ESWS
 end-systolic wall stress
ESWT
 end-systolic wall thickness
 extracorporeal shock wave therapy
ESY
 expressed sequence tag
ET
 Ebbinghaus test [sensory or congnitive
  illusion]
 edema toxin
 edge thickness
 educational therapy
 effective temperature
 ejection time
 embryo transfer
 endometrial thickness
 endothelin
 endotoxin
 endotracheal [tube] (*See also* ETT,
  ENDO, Endo)
 end-tidal
 endurance time
 enterostomal therapy

enterotoxin
epidermolytic toxin
epithelial tumor
esotropia (esotropic) (*See also* ESO, eso,
 ST)
essential thrombocythemia
essential tremor
estrogen therapy
ethanol (*See also* ETH, EtOH)
etiocholanolone test
etiology (*See also* etio, etiol)
eustachian tube
Ewing tumor
exchange transfusion
exercise test
exercise treadmill
expiration time
exploratory thoracoscopy
extracellular tachyzoite
ET1–ET4
 endothelin 1–4
ET′, ET−, ET$_1$
 esotropia at near
 esotropia for near
 near esotropia
E(T)
 intermittent esotropia
ET@20′
 esotropia at 20 feet (6 meters) [infinity]
E:T
 effector to target ratio
E(T′)
 intermittent esotropia at near
 intermittent near esotropia
ET$_3$
 erythrocyte triiodothyronine [thyroid
  function test]
ET$_4$
 effective thyroxine [test]
Et
 ethyl
η, eta
 absolute viscosity
 eta [seventh letter of Greek alphabet
  lowercase]
ETA
 eicosatetraenoic acid
 electron-transfer agent
 endotracheal airway
 endotracheal aspirate
 estimated time of arrival
 exfoliative toxin A
EtA
 endothelin A
ETAB
 extrathoracic-assisted breathing
ETAC
 electrothermally assisted
  capsulorrhaphy

et al.
　and others [L. *et alii*]
ETAP
　epidemic tropical acute polyarthritis
EtB
　endothelin B
ETBA
　endoscopic transaxillary breast
　　augmentation
ETBD
　etiology to be determined
E₂TBG
　estradiol-testosterone-binding globulin
ETC
　electrothermal capsulorrhaphy
　endoscopic tissue culture
　esophageal (esophagotracheal)
　　combination tube
　esophagotracheal Combitube
　estimated time of conception
ETc
　corrected ejection time
etc.
　and so forth [L. *et cetera*]
ETCD
　endoscopic transpapillary cyst drainage
　external tachyarrhythmia control device
ETCG
　endoscopic transpapillary catheterization
　　of gallbladder
ETCL
　enteropathy-associated T-cell lymphoma
ETCO₂
　end-tidal carbon dioxide [concentration]
ETD
　endoscopic transformational discectomy
　estimated time of death
　eustachian tube dysfunction
　eye-tracking dysfunction
ETDLA
　esophageal-tracheal double lumen airway
ETD(V)
　extrapolated tolerance dose volume
　　[radiotherapy]
ETE
　end-to-end [anastomosis]
　external tissue expander
ETEC
　enterotoxic (enterotoxigenic) *Escherichia
　　coli*
E-test
　epsilometer test
ET-1–ET-3
　endothelin 1–3
ETF
　electron transfer flavoprotein
　eustachian tube function
　extension teardrop fracture

ETF-DH
　electron transfer flavoprotein
　　dehydrogenase
ETFE
　ethylene tetrafluor ethylene
　　(tetrafluoroethylene)
ETFVL
　exercise tidal flow-volume loop
ETG
　episodic treatment group
ETH
　ethanol (*See also* ET, EtOH)
　ethmoid
eth
　ether (*See also* Et₂O)
ETI
　ejective time index
　endotracheal intubation
ETIO
　etiocholanolone
etio, etiol
　etiology (*See also* ET)
ETK
　erythrocyte transketolase
　every test known
ETKTM
　every test known to mankind
ETL
　echo train length
　expiratory threshold load
ETLE
　extratemporal lobe epilepsy
ETLT
　equal to or less than
ETN
　ethanol-induced tumor necrosis
Et₃N
　triethylamine
ET-NANBH
　enterically transmitted non-A, non-B
　　hepatitis
ETO
　estimated time of ovulation
　eustachian tube obstruction
EtO
　ethylene oxide
Et₂O
　ether (*See also* eth)
E-TOF
　electron time-of-flight
EtOH
　ethyl alcohol (ethanol) [consumption,
　　dependency] (*See also* ET, ETH)
ETOP
　elective termination of pregnancy
　　(*See also* ETP)
EtOx
　ethylene oxide (*See also* EO)

E

ETP
elective termination of pregnancy
(*See also* ETOP)
electron transport particle
entire treatment period
eustachian tube pressure

ETPS
electrotherapeutic point stimulation

ETR
effective thyroxine ratio
epitympanic recess
estimated thyroid ratio

ETS
educational testing service
electrical transcranial stimulation
electronic transimpedance scanning
electrosleep therapy
elevated toilet seat
endoscopic transthoracic
symphathectomy
endotracheal suction
end-to-side [anastomosis] (*See also* ES,
E-S)
environmental tobacco smoke

ETT
endotracheal tube (*See also* ET, ENDO,
Endo)
endurance treadmill test
epinephrine tolerance test
esophageal transit time
exercise tolerance test
exercise treadmill test
extrathyroidal thyroxine
eye tracking test

ETTH
episodic tension-type headache

ET-TL
endotracheal tube-Trachlight unit

ETT-Tl
exercise treadmill test with
thallium

ETV
educational television
extravascular thermal volume

ETYA
eicosatetroenoic acid

EU
Ehrlich unit
endotoxin unit
entropy unit
enzyme unit
equivalent unit
esophageal ulcer
esterase unit
etiology unknown
European Union
excretory urograph(y) (urogram)
(*See also* EXU, ExU)
expected utility

Eu
europium
euryon [craniometric]

EUA
examination under anesthesia

EUAL
external ultrasound-assisted lipoplasty

EUBV
Eubenangee virus

EUCD
emotionally unstable character disorder

EUD
external urinary device

EUG
extrauterine gestation

EUL
expected upper limit
extrauterine life [outside of uterus]
extra uterine life [length of time]

EUM
external urethral meatus

EUP
extrauterine pregnancy

EUPF
extended uvulopalatal flap

EUS
echoendoscopy
endorectal ultrasound (ultrasonography)
endoscopic ultrasound (ultrasonography)
esophageal ultrasound
external urethral sphincter

EUS-CPN
endosonography-guided celiac plexus
neurolysis

EUS-FNA
endoscopic ultrasound-guided fine-needle
aspiration

eust
eustachian

EUV
extreme ultraviolet [wavelength]

EV
ejected volume
emergency vehicle
enterovirus
epidermodysplasia verruciformis
esophageal varix [singular] (varices
[plural])
evert(ed) (eversion) (*See also* ever.)
evoked [response]
excessive ventilation
expected value
extravascular

EV71
enterovirus 71

eV
electron volt

EVA
American eel virus

enlarged vestibular aqueduct
[syndrome]
Entry and Validation Application
ethylene vinyl acetate
ethyl violet azide [broth]
EVAC, evac
evacuate(d) (evacuation)
EVAc
ethylene-vinyl acetate copolymer
eval
evaluate(d) (evaluation)
EVAN
ergonomic vascular access needle
evap
evaporate(d) (evaporation)
EVAR
endovascular aneurysm repair
EVAS
enlarged vestibular aqueduct syndrome
EVB
esophageal variceal bleeding
EVCI
expected value of clinical information
EVD
external ventricular drainage
extravascular (lung) density
EVE
endoscopic vascular examination
eve
evening
ever.
evert(ed) (eversion) (*See also* EV)
EVEV
Everglades virus
EVF
ethanol volume fraction
EVG
elastica van Gieson [stain]
electroventriculograph(y)
(electroventriculogram)
electrovomerogram
endovascular grafting
EVH
endoscopic vein harvesting
esophageal variceal hemorrhage
EVI
endocardium, vascular (structures)
interstitium [of striated muscle]
EVL
endoscopic variceal ligation
EVLT
endovenous laser treatment
EVLW
extravascular lung water
EVM
electronic voltmeter
extravascular mass

eye, verbal, motor [Glasgow Coma
Scale]
evol
evolution
EVP
episcleral venous pressure
evoked visual potential
EVR
endocardial viability ratio
endovascular repair
evoked visual response
EVRS
early ventricular repolarization syndrome
EVS
endoscopic variceal sclerosis
(sclerotherapy)
esophageal variceal sclerotherapy
EVSD
Eisenmenger ventricular septal defect
EVTV
extravascular thermal volume
EVUS
endovaginal ultrasound
EVV
Everglades virus
EVXX
exudative vitreoretinopathy X-linked
EW
Edinger-Westphal [nucleus]
emergency ward
estrogen withdrawal
expiratory wheeze
ew
elsewhere
EWB
emotional well-being
estrogen withdrawal bleeding
EWBH
extracorporeal whole body
hyperthermia
EWCL
extended-wear contact lens
EWE
Eastern and Western encephalomyelitis
[vaccine]
EWHO
elbow-wrist-hand orthosis
EWI
Experiential World Inventory
EWL
egg-white lysozyme
estimated weight loss
evaporation (evaporative) water loss
EWS
Ewing sarcoma
EWSCL
extended-wear soft contact lens

E

EWS-PNET
Ewing sarcoma primitive
neuroectodermal tumor
EWS-WT1
Ewing sarcoma Wilms tumor 1
EWT
erupted wisdom teeth
esophageal wall thickness
EX
exacerbation
exaggerate(d) (*See also* exag)
examine(d) (examination) (*See also* exam)
excision (*See also* exc)
exercise (*See also* E, exer)
exophthalmos (*See also* EXOPH)
exposure (*See also* EXP)
external movement
extract(ion) (*See also* EXT)
extra point [acupuncture]
E(X)
expected value of random
variable X
ex
example [singular]
EXAFS
extended x-ray absorption fine structure
[spectroscopy]
exag
exaggerate(d) (*See also* EX)
exam
examine(d) (examination) (*See also* EX)
Ex-B
extra point back trunk [acupuncture]
EXBF
exercise hyperemia blood flow
exc
except (*See also* X)
excision (*See also* EX)
Ex-CA
extra point chest and abdomen
[acupuncture]
exch
exchange
EXD
ethylxanthic disulfide
ExD
exertional dyspnea
EXEC 22
executive 22 chemistry profile
exec
executive
Ex-ECG
exercise stress electrocardiography
Ex-Echo
exercise stress echocardiography
ExEF
ejection fraction during exercise

EXELFS
extended energy loss fine structure
[spectroscopy]
exer
exercise (*See also* EX)
ExFHR
external fetal heart rate
EX-FI-RE
external fixation reduction
EXGBUS
external genitalia, Bartholin, urethral,
Skene [glands] (*See also* EGBUS,
EG/BUS)
Ex-HN
extra point on the head and neck
[acupuncture]
EXH VT
exhaled tidal volume
exist.
existing
EXIT
ex utero intrapartum tracheloplasty
ex utero intrapartum treatment
ex lap
exploratory laparotomy (*See also* exp
lap)
Ex-LE
extra point lower extremity
[acupuncture]
EXO
exonuclease
exophoria
EXOPH
exophthalmos (*See also* EX)
EXP
expect(ed)
expectorant (*See also* expecm expect.,
expt)
experience(d)
experiment(al) (*See also* E, exper, exptl)
expiration (*See also* E, expir)
expiratory (*See also* E, expir)
expire(d) (*See also* E, expir)
exploration
exploratory
exponent
exponential [function]
expose(d)
exposure (*See also* EX, X)
ExPEC
extraintestinal pathogenic *Escherichia
coli*
expec, expect.
expectorant (*See also* EXP)
exper
experiment(al) (*See also* E, EXP, exptl)
ExPGN
extracapillary proliferative
glomerulonephritis

expir
    expiration (*See also* E, EXP)
    expiratory (*See also* E, EXP)
    expire(d) (*See also* E, EXP)
exp lap
    exploratory laparotomy (*See also* ex lap)
expn
    expression
expt
    expectorant (*See also* expec, expect., EXP)
exptl
    experimental (*See also* E, EXP, exper)
ExREM
    external radiation equivalent man [dose]
EXS
    externally supported
    extrinsically supported
EXT
    exchange transfusion
    exercise test (*See also* XT, xt)
    extension (*See also* E)
    external
    extract(ed) (*See also* EX, extd, XT, xt)
    extract(ion) (*See also* EX)
    extremity (*See also* extr)
ext aud
    external auditory
extd
    extended
    extracted (*See also* EXT, XT, xt)
EXT-DCR
    external dacryocystorhinostomy
ext fd
    fluid extract (*See also* FE, fld ext, fldxt)
ext FHR
    external fetal heart rate [monitoring]
ext mon
    external monitor

extr
    extremity (*See also* EXT)
extrap
    extrapolate
    extrapolation
extrav
    extravasation
ext rot
    external rotation
EXTUB
    extubation
EXU, ExU
    excretory urograph(y) (urogram) (*See also* EU)
Ex-UE
    extra point upper extremity [acupuncture]
exx
    examples [plural]
EY
    egg yolk
    epidemiology year
EYA
    egg yolk agar
EYAV
    Eyach virus
EYCAT
    egg yolk-cobalamin absorption test
EYES
    Early Years Easy Screen
EZ
    Edmonston-Zagreb [measles vaccine]
    epileptogenic zone
Ez
    eczema
EZ-HT
    Edmonston-Zagreb high-titer [measles vaccine]
EZW
    embedded zero tree wavelet [picture archiving and communication]

E

F

bioavailability
brother [L. *frater*]
facial
facies
factor (*See also* Fac)
Fahrenheit
failure
fair
false
family (*See also* Fam, fam)
farad
faraday [constant]
farad [electrical capacity]
fascia
fasting (test)
fat (dietary)
father (*See also* FR, FTR)
fecal
feces
Fellow
female (*See also* FEM)
fermentative
fertility [factor, F plasmid]
fetal
fibroblast
fibrous [protein]
filament (*See also* fil)
filial generation
fine
finger
firm
first degree of fineness of abrasive
  particles
fissure
flex(ed) (flexion) (*See also* f)
flow
fluid (*See also* FL, FLD, fld)
fluorine
flutter wave
focal length
focus
foil
fontanelle
foramen
force
forma
form response
formula
formulary
fossa
fraction(al) (*See also* fract, FX)
fractional [composition of gas in gas
  phase]

fragment of antibody
free
French [catheter size]
frequency (*See also* f, freq)
from
frontal electrode placement in
  electroencephalography
full (diet)
function (*See also* fn, FXN)
fundus [singular] (fundi [plural])
fusion beat
Helmholtz free energy
hydrocortisone (compound F)
inbreeding coefficient
make (*See also* f.)
phenylalanine (*See also* Phe)
son [L. *filius*]
variance ratio [statistics]
vectorcardiography electrode
  [left foot]
visual field (*See also* VF, Vf, VFD)

F0, F$_0$

fundamental frequency

F$_1$

first filial generation

FI–FXIII

factor I–XIII [blood]

F1.2

prothrombin fragment 1.2

F$_2$

second filial generation

F3-dT

trifluorothymidine

14F

14-hour fast required

F344

Fischer 344 [rat]

/F

full lower denture (*See also*
  FLD)

F/

full upper denture (*See also*
  FUD, Fu Dtr)

F$^+$

bacterial cell with an F plasmid

F′

hybrid F plasmid
secondary focal point [of lens]

°F

degree Fahrenheit

F+

good form response

(F)

final

F⁻
  bacterial cell lacking an F plasmid
  fluoride
  poor form response

f
  fundamental [atomic orbital with
    angular momentum quantum number
    3]
  femto-
  fingerbreadth (*See also* FB, fb)
  fission
  flex(ed) (flexion) (*See also* F)
  formyl
  fostered [experimental animal]
  frequency (*See also* F, freq)
  frequently
  fugacity
  respiratory frequency

f.
  let it be made [L. *fiat*]

F=
  firm and equal

FA
  failure analysis
  false aneurysm
  Families Anonymous
  Fanconi anemia
  far advanced
  fatty acid
  febrile antigen
  femoral anteversion
  femoral artery
  fertilization antigen
  fetal age
  fetus active
  fibrinolytic activity
  fibroadenoma
  fibrosing alveolitis
  field ambulance
  filterable agent
  filtered (filterable) air
  first aid
  fluorescein angiography
  fluorescent antibody [stain]
  fluorescent assay
  fluoroalanine
  folic acid
  folinic acid
  follicular area
  foramen
  forearm
  fortified aqueous [solution]
  fractional anisotropy
  free acid
  frequent [episodic] asthma
  Freund adjuvant
  Friedreich ataxia
  functional activities
  fusaric acid

FA-1
  fertilization antigen 1

F/A
  fetus active

fa
  fatty [rat]

FAA
  febrile antigen agglutination
  flavone acetic acid
  folic acid antagonist
  formaldehyde, acetic acid, alcohol
    [solution]

FAAD
  fetal activity acceleration determination

FAAH
  fatty acid amide hydrolase

FAAP
  family assessment adjustment pass

FAASOL
  formalin, acetic, alcohol solution

FAB
  Fanconi anemia B [gene]

FAB
  fast atom bombardment
  formalin ammonium bromide
  French-American-British [leukemia
    classification system]
  functional arm brace

Fab
  fragment antigen binding

faber
  flexion, abduction, external rotation

fabere
  flexion, abduction, external rotation,
    extension

FABF
  femoral artery blood flow

FAB L1
  acute lymphoblastic (lymphocytic)
    (lymphoid) (lymphatic) (lymphoblastic)
    leukemia (ALL) (*See also* L1)

FAB L2
  acute lymphoblastic (lymphocytic)
    (lymphoid) (lymphatic) (lymphoblastic)
    leukemia (ALL) (*See also* L2)

FAB L3
  acute lymphoblastic (lymphocytic)
    (lymphoid) (lymphatic) (lymphoblastic)
    leukemia (ALL) [Burkitt type]
    (*See also* L3)

FAB M0
  acute myeloid (myeloblastic)
    (granulocytic) (myelogenous)
    (myelocytic) leukemia (AML), without
    maturation [undifferentiated] (*See also*
    M0)

FAB M1
  acute myeloid (myeloblastic)
    (granulocytic) (myelogenous)

(myelocytic) leukemia (AML) with
minimal maturation (*See also* M1)

FAB M2
acute myeloid (myeloblastic)
(granulocytic) (myelogenous)
(myelocytic) leukemia (AML) with
maturation (*See also* M2, AML)

FAB M3
acute promyelocytic leukemia (APL)
(*See also* M3, APL, AProl)

FAB M4
myelomonocytic leukemia (*See also*
M4)

FAB M4 eos
myelomonocytic leukemia with
eosinophilia (*See also* M4 eos)

FAB M5
monocytic leukemia (*See also* M5)

FAB M6
erythroid leukemia (*See also* M6)

FAB M7
megakaryoblastic leukemia (*See also*
M7)

FAB/MS
fast atom bombardment mass
spectrometry

FABP
fatty acid-binding protein
finger arterial blood pressure
folic acid-binding protein

FABP2
fatty acid-binding protein 2

FABP$_{pm}$
plasma membrane fatty acid binding
protein

FABQ
Fear Avoidance Beliefs Quest

FAC
familial adenomatosis coli
femoral arterial cannulation
ferric ammonium citrate
fetal abdominal circumference
fractional area change
fractional area concentration
free available chlorine
functional aerobic capacity
Functional Ambulation Categories

FAC
Fanconi anemia C [gene]

Fac
factor (*See also* F)

FACA
Fanconi anemia complementation group
A [gene product]

FACB
Fanconi anemia complementation group
B [gene product]

Facb
fragment antigen and complement
binding

FACC
Fanconi anemia complementation group
C [gene product]

FACD
Fanconi anemia complementation group
D [gene product]

FACE
fluorophore-assisted carbohydrate
electrophoresis

FACES
Family Adaptability and Cohesion
Evaluation Scale
[unique] facies, anorexia, cachexia, eye,
and skin [syndrome]

FACES-III, FACES III
Family Adaptability and Cohesion Scale
III

FACH
forceps to aftercoming head

FACO$_2$
fraction of alveolar carbon dioxide

FACS
Facial Action Coding System
fluorescence-activated cell sorter
(sorting)
fluorescent-activated cell sorting

FACScan
fluorescence-activated cell sorter scan

FACT
Flanagan Aptitude Classification
Test
focus angioplasty catheter technology
focused appendix computed
tomography
Functional Acuity Contrast Test
Functional Assessment of Cancer
Therapy

FACT-B
Functional Assessment of Cancer
Therapy Breast

FACT-F
Functional Assessment of Cancer
Therapy Fatigue

FACT-G
Functional Assessment of Cancer
Therapy General

FACT-HN
Functional Assessment of Cancer
Therapy Head and Neck

F-actin
filamentous actin

FACT-L
Functional Assessment of Cancer
Therapy Lung

F

FACT-O
  Functional Assessment of Cancer
    Therapy Ovarian
FACT-P
  Functional Assessment of Cancer
    Therapy Prostate
FACWA
  familial amyotrophic chorea with
    acanthocytosis
FAD
  familial Alzheimer dementia (disease)
  familial autonomic dysfunction
  Family Assessment Device
  Fanconi anemia D [gene]
  fetal abdominal diameter
  fetal activity-acceleration determination
  flavin adenine dinucleotide (*See also*
    FADN)
  floating alveolar device
FADD
  fas-associated death domain [protein]
FADF
  fluorescent antibody dark-field
FADH$_2$
  flavin adenine dinucleotide [reduced
    form]
fadir
  flexion, adduction, internal rotation
fadire
  flexion, adduction, internal rotation,
    extension
FADN
  flavin adenine dinucleotide (*See also*
    FAD)
FADS
  factor analysis of dynamic series
  fetal akinesia deformation sequence
FADU
  fluorometric analysis of DNA
    unwinding
FAE
  Fanconi anemia E [gene]
  fetal alcohol effect
  Fogarty arterial embolectomy
FAF
  fatty acid free
  fibroblast-activating factor
FAG
  fundic atrophic gastritis
FAGA
  full-term appropriate for gestational age
FAH
  fumarylacetoacetase hydrolase [gene]
  fumarylacetoacetate hydrolase [gene]
FAHI
  functional assessment of human
    immunodeficiency
FAI
  Fatigue Assessment Instrument

first aid instruction
  functional aerobic impairment
  functional assessment inventory
FA/ICGA
  fluorescein angiography [and]
    indocyanine green angiography
FAIDS
  feline acquired immunodeficiency
    syndrome
FAIR
  flow-sensitive alternating inversion
    recovery
FAJ
  fused apophysial joints
FAK
  focal adhesion kinase
FAL
  femoral arterial line
  functional and anatomic loading
FALG
  fowl antimouse lymphocyte globulin
FALL
  fallopian
FALP
  fluoroscopic-assisted lumbar puncture
FALS
  familial amyotrophic lateral sclerosis
FAM
  full allosteric modulators
  functional assessment measure
Fam, fam
  familial
  family (*See also* F)
FAMA
  fluorescent antibody to membrane
    antigen [test]
fam doc
  family doctor (*See also* FD)
FAME
  fast acquisition multiple excitation
  fast acquisition with multiphase
    (enhanced fast gradient echo) efgre
  fatty acid methyl ester
  finger-assisted malar elevation
fam hist
  family history (*See also* FH, FHx)
FAMM
  facial artery musculomucosal
    (myomucosal) [flap]
  familial atypical multiple melanoma
FAM-M
  familial atypical mole and melanoma
FAMMM
  familial atypical multiple-mole
    melanoma [syndrome]
fam per par
  familial periodic paralysis
fam phys
  family physician (*See also* FP)

FAN
finger tension
fuchsin, amido black, naphthol yellow
[stain]
FANA
fluorescent antinuclear antibody [assay]
FANCAP
fluids, aeration, nutrition,
communication, activity, pain
[nursing]
FANCAS
fluids, aeration, nutrition,
communication, activity, stimulation
[nursing]
FANG
fluorescent angiography
FANPT
Freeman Anxiety Neurosis and
Psychosomatic Test
FANSS&M
fundus anterior, normal size and shape,
and mobile
FAO
fatty acid oxidation
FAP
familial adenomatous polyposis
familial amyloid (amyloidotic)
polyneuropathy
flatter add plus [rule in optometry]
fatty acid poor
fatty acids polyunsaturated
femoral artery pressure
fibrillating action potential
fixed action pattern
functional ambulation profile
fap-1
fas-associated phosphatase 1
FAPA
fever, adenitis, pharyngitis, aphthous
ulcers
FAPD
fibrosing alopecia in a pattern
distribution
FAQ
Family Attitudes Questionnaire
frequently asked question(s)
FAR
flight aptitude rating
fractional albuminuria rate
frontal arousal rhythm
F^{AR}
immediate good function followed by
accelerated rejection
far.
faradic
FARI
filtered atrial rate interval

FARS
Fatal Accident Reporting System
FARV
Farallon virus
FAS
fatty acid synthase (synthetase)
femoral access stabilization
fetal akinesia sequence
fetal alcohol syndrome
fluorescent actin staining
FASAY
functional analysis of separated alleles
in yeast
FASC
fluorescent-activated substrate conversion
free-standing ambulatory surgical center
fasc
fascicle
fasciculation
fasciculus [singular] (fasciculi [plural])
FASD
fetal alcohol spectrum disorders
FASE
fast asymmetric spin echo
FASF
Factor Analyzed Short Form
FASIAR
follicle aspiration, sperm injection,
assisted rupture
FasL, Fas-L
Fas ligand
FASPS
familial advanced sleep-phase syndrome
FASS
foot and ankle severity scale
FAST
Fein Articulation Screening Test
fetal acoustic stimulation testing
Filtered Audiometer Speech Test
flow-assisted short-term [catheter]
Flowers Auditory Screening Test
fluorescent allergosorbent test
fluorescent antibody staining technique
fluoroallergosorbent test
focused abdominal sonography for
trauma
focused assessment by sonography for
trauma
Fourier-acquired steady-state technique
Frenchay Aphasia Screening Test
Functional Assessment Staging
FASTER
field echo acquisition with short
repetition time and echo reduction
FAT
Family Apperception Test
family attitudes test

F

FAT *(continued)*
  fast axoplasmic transport
  fatty acid translocase
  female athlete triad
  feminizing adrenal tumor
  Fetal Activity Test
  fluorescent antibody technique (test)
  food awareness training
  function, appearance, time
FATG
  fat globule
FATP
  fatty acid transport protein
F1F.-ATP
  adenosine triphosphate synthase
FATS
  face and thigh squeeze [position for
    bag mask ventilation]
  fast adiabatic trajectory in steady
    state
FATSA
  Flowers Auditory Test of Selective
    Attention
FATWO
  female adnexal tumor of probable
    wolffian origin
FAV
  facioauriculovertebral [syndrome]
  feline ataxia virus
  floppy aortic valve
  fowl adenovirus
FAVA
  facioauriculovertebral anomaly
FAVD
  forceps-assisted vaginal delivery
FAVS
  facioauriculovertebral spectrum
FAXT
  fast axoplasmic transport
FAZ
  foveal avascular zone
FB
  factor B [complement]
  fascicular block
  fasting blood
  feedback
  fiberoptic bronchoscope (bronchoscopy)
    (*See also* fib. bronc, FOB)
  fingerbreadth (*See also* f, fb)
  flexible bronchoscope
  foreign body
F/B
  followed by
  forward/backward
  forward bending
fb
  fingerbreadth (*See also* f, FB)
f-b
  face-bow

FBA
  fecal bile acid
  fluorescent bacteriophage assay
FBAO
  foreign body airway obstruction
FBC
  full blood count
  functional bactericidal concentration
⚠ **FBCOD**
  foreign body of cornea, oculus dexter
    [right eye] ⚠
⚠ **FBCOS**
  foreign body of cornea, oculus sinister
    [left eye] ⚠
FBCP
  familial benign chronic pemphigus
FBD
  failed biopsy detection
  familial British dementia
  fibrocystic breast disease
  functional bowel disease (disorder)
    (distress)
FbDP
  fibrin/fibrinogen degradation product
    [test] (*See also* FDP)
FBDSI
  Functional Bowel Disorder Severity
    Index
FBE
  full blood examination
FBEC
  fetal bovine endothelial cell
FBEP
  Fort Bragg evaluation project
FBF
  fair breastfeed
  forearm blood flow
FBG
  fasting blood glucose
  fibrinogen (*See also* FG, FGN, FI,
    FIB)
  foreign body-type granuloma
FBH
  familial benign hypercalcemia
FBHH
  familial benign hypocalciuric
    hypercalcemia
FBI
  fat-blood interface
  flossing, brushing, irrigation
  foodborne illness
  full bony impaction
FBL
  fecal blood loss
  focal brain lesion
  follicular basal lamina
FBM
  fetal bone marrow
  fetal breathing movement

foreign body, metallic
fresh bone marrow

FBP
familial benign pemphigus
femoral blood pressure
fibrin (fibrinogen) breakdown product
filtered back projection
folate-binding protein
fructose-bisphosphatase

FBPM
forward-backward Prony method
[spectral analysis]

FBR
fresh-blood reaction [Ger. *Frischblut*]

FBRCM
fingerbreadth below right costal
margin

FBS
failed back syndrome
fasting blood glucose
fasting blood sugar
feedback signal
feedback system
fetal bovine serum
foreign body sensation [eye]

FBSE
full-body skin examination

FBSS
failed back surgery syndrome

FBT
family-based treatment

FBU
fingers below umbilicus [measurement]
(*See also* F↓U)

FBV
fiber bundle volume

FBW
fasting blood work

FC
family conference
fasciculus cuneatus
fast component [of neuron]
febrile convulsion
fecal coli [broth]
feline conjunctivitis
female child
ferric citrate
fever, chills
fibrocystic
fibrocyte
film-coated
finger clubbing
finger counting
flexion contracture
flow compensation
flow cytometry
foam cuffed [tracheal or endotrachael
tube]

Foley catheter (*See also* F cath)
follows commands
form [response determined by] color
foster care
free cholesterol
frontal cortex
functional capacity
functional castration
functional class

F/C
facilitated communication
fever and chills

F&C
flare and cells (*See also* F+C)
foam and condom

F+C
flare and cells (*See also* F&C)

Fc
centroid frequency
fragment, crystallizable [of
immunoglobulin]
shading response to black areas
[Rorschach test]
shading response to gray areas
[Rorschach test]

Fc′
fragment crystallized in minute
quantities [immunoglobulin]
shade response to light gray area
[Rorschach test]

fc, ftc
footcandle [unit of illuminance]

FCA
Federal False Claims Act
ferritin-conjugated antibody
fracture, complete, angulated
Freund complete adjuvant
functional capacity assessment

FCAH
familial cytomegaly adrenocortical
hypoplasia [syndrome]

F cath
Foley catheter (*See also* FC)

FCBD, FCDB
fibrocystic breast disease
fibrocystic disease of breast

FCC
familial cerebral cavernoma
familial colon (colonic) cancer
family centered care
femoral cerebral catheter
follicular center cell
fracture complete and compound
fracture compound and comminuted

fcc
face-centered-cubic

f/cc
fiber per cubic centimeter [of air]

F

FCCA
familial congenital cardiac abnormality
Final Comprehensive Consensus
Assessment
FCCC
fracture complete, compound,
comminuted
FCCL
follicular center cell lymphoma
FCCP
carbonyl cyanide
p-(trifluoromethoxy)phenylhydrazone
FCD
familial corneal dystrophy
fecal containment device
feces collection device
fibrocystic disease (dysplasia)
final consonant deletion
focal cytoplasmic degradation
fracture complete and deviated
FCE
fibrocartilaginous embolism
functional capacity evaluation
FCF
fetal cardiac frequency
fibroblast chemotactic factor
FCFC
fibroblast colony-forming cells
FCFD
fluorescence capillary-fill device
FCG
fifth cusp groove
French catheter gauge
FCH
familial clitoral hypertrophy
fetal cystic hygroma
fibrosing cholestatic hepatitis
folliculosebaceous cystic
hamartoma
FCHL
familial combined hyperlipidemia
FCI
fixed cell immunofluorescence
flow cytometric immunophenotyping
food-chemical intolerance
FCIS
Flint Colon Injury Scale
FCL
fibular collateral ligament
follicle center lymphoma [cell]
fcly
face lying [position]
FCM
facial choreic movement
fetal cardiac motion
fibroblast-conditioned medium
flow cytometry (cytometric)
FCMC
family-centered maternity care

FCMD
Fukuyama congenital muscular
dystrophy
FCMN
family-centered maternity nursing
F/C/N/V
fever, cough, nausea, vomiting
FCOD
focal cementoosseous dysplasia
⚠ **FCOU**
finger count, both eyes ⚠
FCP
fasting chemistry profile
femoral hole coronal positioning
final common pathway
florid cutaneous papillomatosis
flow cytometric platelet
formocresol pulpotomy
Functional Communication Profile [of
aphasic adults]
functional conduction period
FCPD
fibrocalculous pancreatic diabetes
FCR
flexor carpi radialis [muscle]
fractional catabolic rate
Fuji computed radiography
FcR
fragment, crystallizable [of
immunoglobulin] receptor
FCRA
fecal collection receptacle assembly
FCRB
flexor carpi radialis brevis [muscle]
FCRT
fetal cardiac reactivity test
focal cranial radiation therapy
FCS
facial cosmetic surgery
faciocutaneoskeletal
familial centrolobar sclerosis
fecal containment system
feedback control system
fetal calf serum
fever, chills, sweating
fluorescence correlation spectroscopy
foot compartment syndrome
full cervical spine
FCS-ML
fluorescence correlation spectroscopy
magnifying light
FCSNVD
fever, chills, sweating, nausea, vomiting,
diarrhea
FCSW
female commercial sex worker
FCT
fever clearance time
fluorescein clearance test

food composition table
food control training

FCU
flexor carpi ulnaris [muscle]

FCV
feline calicivirus

FCVD
fracture complete, varus deformity

FCx
frontal cortex

FCXM
flow cytometric cross-matching
flow cytometry crossmatch

FD
failure to descend
familial dysautonomia
family doctor (*See also* fam doc)
fan douche
fatal dose
feeding disorder
fetal danger
fetal demise
fetal distress
fibrinogen derivative
fibrous dysplasia
field desorption
fixed and dilated (*See also* F&D)
flexor digitorum [muscle]
fluorescence depolarization
focal disease
focal distance
Folin-Denis [assay]
follicular diameter
food diary
foot drape
forceps delivery
fractal dimension
fracture-dislocation
freedom from distractibility
free drain
freeze-dried
frequency deviation
full denture
fully dilated
functional deficits

F/D
fracture/dislocation (*See also* Fx-dis)

F&D
fixed and dilated (*See also* FD)

FD$_{50}$
median fatal dose

Fd
animo-terminal portion of heavy chain of immunoglobulin
ferredoxin
fundus

FDA
Food and Drug Administration
Frenchay Dysarthria Assessment
frontodextra (right front) anterior [fetal position] (*See also* RFA)

FDACL
first definite apical clearance lens [contact lens fitting]

FDB
familial defective apolipoprotein B
first-degree burn
flexor digitorum brevis [muscle]

FDBL
fecal daily blood loss

FDC
fixed-dose combination
flexor digitorum communis [muscle]
follicular dendritic cell
frequency dependence of compliance

FDCT
Franck Drawing Completion Test

FddA
2′β-fluoro-2′,3′-dideoxyadenosine

FddaraA
2′,3′-dideoxy-2′-fluoro-9-beta-D-arabinofuranosyladenine

FDDB
freeze-dried demineralized bone

FDDC
ferric dimethyldithiocarbonate

FDDNP
fluorine-18 2-dialkylamino-6-acylmalononitrile substituted naphthalenes

FDDQ
Freedom from Distractibility Deviation Quotient

FDDS
Family Drawing Depression Scale

FDE
female day equivalent
final drug evaluation
first episode of depression
fixed drug eruption

FDF
fast death factor
flexor digitorum profundus [tendon]
further differentiated fibroblast

FDFG
free dermal-fat graft

FDFQ
Food/Drink Frequency Questionnaire

FDG
feeding (*See also* fdg)
fluorodeoxyglucose
freeze-dried gel

F

fdg
feeding (*See also* FDG)
FDGF
fibroblast-derived growth factor
FDG-PET
fluorodeoxyglucose [dual-head] positron emission tomography
FDGS
feedings
FDH
familial dysalbuminemic hyperthyroxinemia
focal dermal hypoplasia
FDI
Facial Disability Index
fibrillation detection interval
first dorsal interosseus [muscle]
food-drug interaction
frequency domain imaging [ultrasound]
frequency-duration index
Functional Disability Index
FDICT
frequency-difference interferential current therapy
FDIP
Facial Disability Index Physical
FDIS
Facial Disability Index Social
FDIU
fetal death in utero
FDL
flexor digitorum longus [muscle]
fluorescein dilaurate
FDLMP
first day of last menstrual period
FDLV
fer-de-lance virus
FDM
fetus of diabetic mother
fibrous dysplasia of mandible
flexor digiti minimi [muscle]
FDMA
first dorsal metatarsal artery
FDNB
fluorodinitrobenzene [Sanger reagent]
FDNS
familial dysplastic nevus syndrome
FDP
factitious disorder by proxy
fibrin/fibrinogen degradation product [test]
fixed-dose procedure
flexor digitorum profundus [muscle]
fructose diphosphate
frontodextra (right frontal) posterior [fetal position] (*See also* RFP)
FDPALD
fructose diphosphate aldolase

FDPase
fructose diphosphatase
FDPCA
fixed-dose patient-controlled analgesia
FD-PET
fluorodopa-positron emission tomography
FDQB
flexor digiti quinti brevis [muscle]
FDR
first-dose reaction
fractional disappearance rate
frequency dependence of resistance
FDS
for duration of stay
fetal distress syndrome
fiberduodenoscope
fiber duodenoscope
flexor digitorum sublimis [muscle]
flexor digitorum superficialis [muscle]
FDT
forced duction test
frequency doubling technology
right frontal transverse [fetal position] [L. *frontodextra transversa*] (*See also* RFT)
FDT-MD
frequency doubling technology mean deviation
FDT-PSD
frequency doubling technology pattern standard deviation
FDTVMP
Frostig Developmental Test of Visual Motor Perception
FDTVP
Frostig Developmental Test of Visual Perception
FdUMP
fluorodeoxyuridylate
5-FDUMP
5-fluorodeoxyuridylate
FDV
Fiji disease virus
Friend disease virus
FDZ
fetal danger zone
FE
fat embolism
fatty ester
fecal emesis
female escutcheon
fetal erythroblastosis
fibroepithelioma
field echo
fluid extract (*See also* ext fd, fld ext, fldxt)
fluorescing erythrocyte
forced expiration

forced expiratory [volume, flow, capacity]
formalin and ethanol
freely eating
frequency encode
frozen embryo

Fe
iron [L. *ferrum*]

^{52}Fe
iron-52

^{55}Fe
iron-55

^{59}Fe
iron-59

FEA
familial erythroblastic anemia
finite element analysis

FEAR
feeling [frightened], expecting [bad things to happen], attitudes [and actions that help], results [and reward]

FEAST
feeding education and support team

feb
febrile

feb agg
febrile agglutinin

FEBP
fetal estrogen-binding protein

FEC
familial erythrocytosis
Feasibility Evaluation Checklist
forced expiratory capacity
free erythrocyte coproporphyrin (*See also* FECP)
free-standing emergency center
Friend erythroleukemia cell

FECG
fetal electrocardiogram

FeCh
ferrochelatase

FECO$_2$, F$_{ECO2}$
fraction of expired carbon dioxide

FECP
free erythrocyte coproporphyrin (*See also* FEC)

FECSR
flexion-extension cervical spine radiography

FECT
fibroelastic connective tissue

FECV
functional extracellular [fluid] volume

FED
fish-eye disease

FeD, Fe def
iron [ferrum] deficiency

FEE
Far-Eastern equine encephalitis
forced equilibrating expiration

FEEG
fetal electroencephalograph(y) (electroencephalogram)

Fe-EHPG
iron ethylene bis 2-hydroxy phenyl glycine

FEER
field even echo rephasing [sequence]

FEES
fiberoptic (flexible) endoscopic evaluation (examination) of swallowing

FEESST, FEEST
fiberoptic (flexible) endoscopic evaluation of swallowing with sensory testing

FEF
Family Evaluation Form
forced expiratory flow
frontal eye field

FEF$_{25-75\%}$
mean midexpiratory flow rate

FEF$_{50}$
forced expiratory flow after 50% of vital capacity has been expelled

FEF$_{50}$:FIF$_{50}$
expiratory flow to inspiratory flow ratio at 50% of forced vital capacity

FEFmax
maximal forced expiratory flow

FEFV
forced expiratory flow volume

FEH
focal epithelial hyperplasia

FEIA
fluorescent enzyme immunoassay

FEIBA
factor VIII inhibitor bypassing activity

FEK
fractional excretion of potassium

FEKG
fetal electrocardiograph(y) (electrocardiogram)

FEL
familial erythrophagocytic lymphohistiocytosis

FELC
Friend erythroleukemia cell

FELI
fractional excretion of lithium

FeLV
feline leukemia virus

FEM
female (*See also* F)
feminine

F

FEM *(continued)*
  femoral (*See also* fem)
  femur (*See also* fem)
  finite element method (modeling)
  fluid-electrolyte malnutrition
femA
  factor essential for methicillin resistance
FEM-FEM
  femoral-femoral [bypass]
FEM-POP
  femoral-popliteal [bypass] (*See also* F-P)
FEM-TIB
  femoral-tibial [bypass]
FEN
  fluids, electrolytes, nutrition
FENa, FE$_{Na}$
  fractional excretion of sodium
FENIB
  familial encephalopathy with neuroserpin
  inclusion bodies
FENO
  fractional exhaled nitric oxide
FEN-PHEN
  fenfluramine and phentermine
FENS
  field-electrical neural stimulation
FEO
  familial expansile osteolysis
Fe$_3$O$_4$
  magnetite
F$_{EO2}$
  fractional concentration of oxygen in
  expired gas
FEOM
  full extraocular motion (movement)
FEP
  fluorinated ethylene-propylene
  [polymer]
  free erythrocyte porphyrin
  (protoporphyrin)
  functional exercise program
FEPB
  functional electronic peroneal brace
F-EPE
  focal extraprostatic extension
FEPP
  free erythrocyte protoporphyrin (*See also*
  FEP)
FER
  familial exudative retinopathy
  flexion, extension, rotation
  fractional esterification rate
  frozen embryo replacement
FERG
  focal electroretinogram
fERG
  flash electroretinogram
FERR
  ferritin

fert
  fertility
  fertilize(d)
FES
  Falls Efficacy Scale
  Family Environment Scale
  fat embolism syndrome
  flame emission spectroscopy
  floppy eyelid syndrome
  fluoroestradiol
  forced expiratory spirogram
  functional electrical stimulation
  functional endoscopic sinus (*See also*
  FESS)
FESA
  finite element stress analysis
FESE
  flexible endoscopic swallowing
  examination
FESEM
  field emission scanning electron
  microscopy
FeSO$_4$
  ferrous sulfate
FESS
  functional endoscopic sinus surgery
  (*See also* FES)
FET
  familial essential tremor
  field-effect transistor
  finger extension test
  Fisher exact test [statistics]
  fixed erythrocyte turnover
  forced expiratory time
fet
  fetus
FETE
  Far Eastern tick-borne encephalitis
FETENDO
  fetal endoscopic [surgery]
FETI
  fluorescence energy transfer
  immunoassay
  fluorescence excitation transfer
  immunoassay
Fe:TIBC
  iron to total iron-binding capacity ratio
FETs
  forced expiratory time in seconds
FEU
  fibrinogen equivalent unit
FEUO
  for external use only
Fe-UR
  iron in urine
FEV
  forced expiratory volume
FEV-1, FEV$_1$
  forced expiratory volume at one second

fev
 fever
FEVB
 frequency ectopic ventricular beat
FEV:FVC
 forced expiratory volume timed to
  forced vital capacity ratio
FEV$_1$:FVC
 forced expiratory volume in one second
  to forced vital capacity ratio
FEVR
 familial exudative vitreoretinopathy
FEV$_t$
 forced expiratory volume timed
FEV$_1$:VC
 one-second forced expiratory volume to
  vital capacity ratio
FEXE
 formalin, ethanol, xylol, ethanol [lab
  method]
FeZ
 iron zone
FF
 factitious fever
 fat free
 father factor
 fear of failure
 fecal frequency
 femorofemoral
 fertility factor
 fibrillation-flutter
 fibrofolliculoma
 fibrotic focus
 fields of Forel [H fields of
  subthalamus]
 filtration factor
 filtration fraction
 fine fiber
 fine fraction
 finger flexion
 finger-to-finger (*See also* FTF, f-f, f→f)
 five-minute format
 fixation fluid
 fixing fluid
 flatfoot
 flip-flop [electronic logic circuitry]
 fluorescent focus
 follicular fluid
 force fluids
 forearm flow
 formula fed
 forward flexion
 foster father
 free fraction
 fresh frozen
 fundus firm
 further flexion

 second finest degree of abrasive
  particles
F:F
 Functional Intact Fibrinogen [test]
F&F
 filiform [bougie] and follower
 fixes and follows [eyes]
F/F
 face to face
^{18}F
 fluorine 18
^{19}F
 fluorine 19
fF
 ultrafine fiber
 ultrafine fraction
ff
 following
f-f, f→f
 finger-to-finger (*See also* FF, FTF)
FFA
 female-female adaptor
 frontal fibrosing alopecia
 fundus fluorescein angiogram
 fusiform face area [brain area specific
  for face recognition]
 [unesterified] free fatty acid (*See also*
  UFA)
FFAP
 free fatty-acid phase
FFAT
 Free-Floating Anxiety Test
FFB
 fast feedback
 flexible fiberoptic bronchoscopy
FFC
 fixed flexion contracture
 free from chlorine
FFCS
 forearm flexion control strap
FFD
 fat-free diet
 focal film distance
 focus film (film-focus) distance
 forward fluorescence detector
FFDCA, FDCA, FDEC
 Federal Food, Drug, and Cosmetic Act
  [FDA]
FFDD
 focal facial dermal dysplasia
FFDD II
 focal facial dermal dysplasia II
^{18}F-FDG
 2-(fluorine-18) fluoro-2-deoxy-D-glucose
^{18}F-FDG-PET
 2-(fluorine-18) fluoro-2-deoxy-D-glucose
  positron emission tomography

F

FFDM
freedom from distant metastases
free of distant metastases
full field digital mammography

FFDR
full florid diabetic retinopathy

FFDW
fat-free dry weight

FFE
fast-field echo
fecal fat excretion
flexible fiberoptic endoscope
free flow electrophoresis

FFEM
freeze fracture electron microscopy

FFF
fast Fourier flow
field-flow fractionation
finest degree of abrasive particles
flicker fusion frequency [test]
fuzzy functional form [protein]

FFG
free fat graft

FFI
family function index
fast food intake
fatal familial insomnia
Foot Function Index
free from infection
fundamental frequency indicator

FFIT
fluorescent focus inhibition test

FFL
fetal foot length
flexible fiberoptic laryngoscopy
floral variant of follicular lymphoma

FFM
fat and fat-free mass
fat-free [body] mass
five-finger movement
freedom from metastases
friction force microscopy
full frequency music

FFN
fetal fibronectin

FFP
fast Fourier projection
flexible fluoropolymer
freedom from progression
free of progression
fresh frozen plasma

FFPB
flexible fiberoptic bronchoscopy with
protected brush

FFPE
formalin-fixed paraffin-embedded

FFQ
fecal fat quantitation
food frequency questionnaire

FFR
familial foveal retinoschisis
fixed frequency response
fractional flow reserve
freedom from relapse
free of recurrence
frequency-following response

FFR$_{myo}$
myocardial fractional flow reserve

FFROM
full, free range of motion

FFr-TMS
fast-frequency repetitive transcranial
magnetic stimulation

FFS
failure of fixation suppression
failure-free survival
fat-free solid
fat-free supper
fee for service
five-factor score
flexible fiberoptic sigmoidoscopy

FFT
fast Fourier transform
flicker fusion test
flicker fusion threshold
free-floating thrombus

FFTDWB
flatfoot touchdown weightbearing

FFTP
first full-term pregnancy

FFU
femur-fibula-ulna [syndrome]
focus-forming unit

FF1/U
fundus firm 1 cm above umbilicus

FF2/U
fundus firm 2 cm above umbilicus

FFU/1
fundus firm 1 cm below umbilicus

FFU/2
fundus firm 2 cm below umbilicus

FF@u
fundus firm at umbilicus

FFW
fat-free weight

FFWC
fractional free-water clearance

FFWW
fat-free wet weight

FG
fasciculus gracilis
fast-glycolytic [muscle fiber]
fast green [stain]
Feeley-Gorman [agar]
fibrin glue
fibrinogen (*See also* FBG, FGN, FI,
FIB)
field gain

Flemish giant [rabbit]
French gauge
fusiform gyrus

fg
femtogram

FGA
first-generation antibiotic
first-generation antipsychotic

FGAR
formylglycinamide ribonucleotide
N-formylglycinamide ribotide

FGB
fully granulated basophil

FGC
familial gigantiform cementoma
fibrinogen gel chromatography
full gold crown

FGD
familial glucocorticoid deficiency
fatal granulomatous disease

FGDS
fibrogastroduodenoscopy

FGDY
faciogenital dysplasia

FGF
father's grandfather
fibroblast (fibroblastic) growth factor
fresh gas flow

FGFa
fibroblast growth factor, acidic (*See also*
aFGF, a-FGF)

FGFR 1–5
fibroblast growth factor receptor 1–5

FGG
focal global glomerulosclerosis
fowl gamma globulin
free gingival groove

FGID
functional gastrointestinal disorder

FGL
fasting gastrin level
fasting glucose level

FGLU
fasting glucose

FGM
father's grandmother
female genital mutilation (*See also*
FGTM)

FGN
fibrinogen (*See also* FBG, FG, FI,
FIB)
focal glomerulonephritis

FGP
fundic gland polyp

FGR
familial glucocorticoid resistance
fetal growth restriction

FGRN
finely granular

FGS
Facial Grading System
fibrogastroscopy
focal glomerular sclerosis

FGT
female genital tract
fluorescent gonorrhea test

FGTCS
female genital tract carcinosarcoma

FGTM
female genital tract mutilation (*See also*
FGM)

FH
facial hemihyperplasia
familial hypercholesterolemia (*See also*
FHC)
familial hypertension
family history (*See also* fam hist, FHx)
fasting hyperbilirubinemia
favorable histology
femoral hernia
femoral hypoplasia
fetal head
fetal heart
fibromuscular hyperplasia (*See also*
FMH)
Ficoll-Hypaque [technique]
flat hyperplasia
[Boston] Floating Hospital
follicular hyperplasia
Frankfort horizontal [plane of skull]
fundal height

FH⁻
family history negative (*See also* FHN)

FH⁺
family history positive (*See also* FHP)

FH₄
tetrahydrofolic acid

fh
fostered by hand [experimental animal]

FHA
familial hemolytic anemia
familial hypoplastic anemia
filamentous hemagglutinin
filterable hemolytic anemia
fimbrial hemagglutinin
functional hypothalamic amenorrhea

FHB
flexor hallucis brevis [muscle]

FHBL
familial hypobetalipoproteinemia

FHC
familial hypercholesterolemia (*See also*
FH)
familial hypertrophic cardiomyopathy

F

FINCC
familial idiopathic nonarteriosclerotic cerebral calcification

FIND
follow up intervention for normal development

F-insulin
fibrous insulin

FIO₂, FiO2, FiO₂, FI$_{O_2}$
fraction of inspired oxygen [in gas]

FIP
feline infectious peritonitis
fibrosing interstitial pneumonitis
flatus in progress

FIPA
familial intestinal polyatresia [syndrome]

FIPC
favorable or intermediate prognosis cytogenetics

FIPT
focal intraretinal periarteriolar transudate

FIPV
feline infectious peritonitis virus

FIQ
Fibromyalgia Impact Questionnaire
full-scale intelligence quotient

FIR
far infrared
fold increase in resistance

FIRDA
frontal intermittent rhythmic delta activity [EEG]

FIRFT
fast inversion-recovery Fourier transform

FIRI
fasting insulin resistance index

FIRM
Family Inventory of Resources for Management

FIRO-B
Fundamental Interpersonal Relations Orientation Behavior

FIRO-F
Fundamental Interpersonal Relations Orientation Feelings

FIS
fiberoptic injection sclerotherapy
forced inspiratory spirogram

FISC
Facial Impairment Scales for Children

FISCA
Functional Impairment Scale for Children and Adolescents

FISH
fluorescent in situ hybridization

FISP
fast imaging with steady-state precession

FISP-3D MRI
fast-imaging steady state precession three-dimensional magnetic resonance imaging

FISS
Flint Infant Security Scale

fiss.
fissure

fist.
fistula

FISTS
fighting, injuries, sex, threats, self-defense

FIT
fibrous intimal thickening
Flanagan Industrial Test
food intolerance testing
Footwear Integration Technology
Fracture Intervention Trial
fusion-inferred threshold [test]

FITC
fluorescein isothiocyanate

FITT
frequency, intensity, time, type [exercise]

FIUO
for internal use only

FIV
feline immunodeficiency virus
forced inspiratory volume

FIV₁
forced inspiratory volume in one second

FIVC
forced inspiratory vital capacity

FIVE
familial isolated vitamin E [deficiency]

F-J
Fisher-John [melting point method]

F-JAS
Fleishman Job Analysis Survey

FJB
facet joint block

FJD
facet joint disease

FJN
familial juvenile nephrophthisis

FJN-MCD
familial juvenile nephrophthisis-medullary cystic disease

FJP
familial juvenile polyposis

FJRM, FJROM
full joint range of motion (movement)

FJS
finger joint size

FJV
first jejunal vein

FK
feline kidney

filamentary keratitis
functioning kasai [Belgian Congo anemia]
FKA
failed to keep appointment
formally known as
FKBP
FK-binding protein
FKBP12
FK-binding protein 12
FKE
full knee extension
FKGL
' Flesh-Kincaid Grade Level [score]
FKHR
forkhead transcription factor (forkhead box protein O1A) [FOXO1a gene]
FL
factor level
false lumen
fatty liver
feline leukemia
femoral length
femur length
fetal length
fibers of Luschka
fibroblastlike
fibrolamellar
filtered load
filtration leukapheresis
flank
flexible
flexion
flow limitation
fluid (*See also* F, FLD, fld)
fluorescein
fluorescent (fluorescence) (*See also* fluor, fluores)
flutter
focal laser
focal length
follicle lysis
follicular lymphoma
frontal lobe
full liquids [diet]
functional length
FL-2
feline lung [cell]
F/L
father-in-law (*See also* FIL)
fL
femtoliter
FLA
fluorescent-labeled antibody
free-living ameba
frontolaeva (left front) anterior [fetal position] (*See also* LFA)

18F-labeled
fluorine-18 labeled
FL:AC
femur length to abdominal circumference ratio
flac
flaccid
flaccidity
FLACC
face, legs, activity, cry, consolability
FLAIR
fluid attenuated (attenuation) inversion recovery
FLAK
flow artifact killer
Fl Ang
fluorescein angiography
FLAP
5-lipoxygenase-activating protein
FLASH
fast low-angle shot
FLAV
Flanders virus
FLB
four-layer bandage
funny-looking beat [heart]
FLBS
funny-looking baby syndrome
FLC
fatty liver cell
fetal liver cell
follicular large cell lymphoma
Friend leukemia cell
FLCOD
florid local cementoosseous dysplasia
FLD
fatty liver disease
fibrotic lung disease
fluid (*See also* F, FL, fld)
full lower denture (*See also* /F)
fld
field
fluid (*See also* F, FL, FLD)
fld ext
fluid extract (*See also* ext fd, FE, fidxt)
fl dr
fluid dram
fld rest.
fluid restriction
fl drs
fluff dressing
fldxt
fluid extract (*See also* ext fd, FE, fld ext)
FLE
frontal lobe epilepsy

F

FLES
Fairview Language Evaluation Scale
FLET
Fairview Language Evaluation Test
FLEV
Flexal virus
FLEX
Federation Licensing Examination [United States Medical Licensing]
flex.
flexion
flexor
flex sig
flexible sigmoidoscopy
FLF
funny-looking facies
FLGA
full-term, large for gestational age
FLH
focal lymphoid hyperplasia
FL-HCC
fibrolamellar hepatocellular carcinoma
FLI
fluorescent light intensity
FLIC
Functional Living Index Cancer
FLICE
FADD-like interleukin-1 beta converting enzyme
FLIE
Functional Living Index-Emesis
FLIP
FLICE-like inhibitory protein
FLIT
Figurative Language Interpretation Test
FLK
funny-looking kid
FLKS
fatty liver and kidney syndrome
FLM
fasciculus longitudinalis medialis
fetal lung maturity
fluorescence lifetime imaging
FLN
fluorescence-lactose-denitrification medium
floc, flocc
flocculation
flor.
flowers [mineral substance in powdery state after sublimation] [L. *flores*]
fl oz
fluid ounce
FLP
fasting lipid profile
Functional Limitation Profile
frontolaeva (left front) posterior [fetal position] [L. *frontolaeva posterior*] (*See also* LFP)

FLPD
flashlamp pulsed dye laser
FLR
funny-looking rash
FL REST
fluid restriction
FLS
fatty liver syndrome
fibroblastlike synoviocyte
fibrous long-spacing [collagen]
flashing lights and/or scotoma
flow-limiting segment
flulike syndrome
Functional Life Scale
FLSA
follicular lymphosarcoma
FLSP
fluorescein-labeled serum protein
FLT
3′fluoro-2′,3′-dideoxythymidine
fluorothymidine
frontolaeva (left frontal) transverse [fetal position] [L. *frontoloaeva transversa*] (*See also* LFT)
FLTA
Fullerton Language Test for Adolescents
FLTAC
Fisher-Logemann Test of Articulation Competence
Fl tx
fluoride treatment
flu
influenza
flu A
influenza A
fluor
fluorescent (fluorescence) (*See also* FL, fluores)
fluoroscopy (*See also* fluoro, FX)
fluores
fluorescent (fluorescence) (*See also* FL, fluor)
fluoro
fluoroscopy (*See also* fluor, FX)
FLUP
front-loading ultrasound probe
fl up
flareup
follow up (followup) (*See also* FU, F/U FUP)
FLUTE
fat and long T2 suppressed ultrashort echo time
FLV
feline leukemia virus
Friend leukemia virus
FLW
fasting laboratory work

FM
    face mask
    facilities management
    fathom
    fat mass
    feedback mechanism
    fetal monitor
    fetal movement
    fibrin monomer
    fibromuscular
    fibromyalgia
    Fielding-Magliato [classification of femoral shaft fractures]
    filtered mass
    fine motor
    flavin mononucleotide
    floor manager
    flowmeter
    fluid movement
    fluorescent microscopy
    foramen magnum
    foreign matter
    forensic medicine
    formerly married
    foster mother
    fragrance mix
    frequency modulation
    Friend-Moloney [antigen]
    functional movement
    fusobacteria microorganisms
F&M
    firm and midline [uterus]
Fm
    fermium
²⁵⁵Fm
    fermium-255
fm
    femtometer
    from (*See also* fr)
FMA
    familial microcytic anemia
    Frankfort mandibular [plane] angle
    functional motor activity
FMAC
    fetal movement acceleration test
FMAIT
    fetomaternal alloimmune thrombocytopenia
FMAP
    feeding mean arterial pressure
FMB
    full maternal behavior
FMC
    fetal movement count
    fine-motor coordination
    focal macular choroidopathy

FMCG
    fetal magnetocardiography
FMD
    familial metaphysial dysplasia
    family medical doctor
    fibromuscular dysplasia
    flow-mediated dilation
    foot-and-mouth disease
    foramen magnum decompression
    frontometaphyseal dysplasia
FMDV
    foot-and-mouth disease virus
FME
    full-mouth extraction
FMEL
    Friend murine erythroleukemia
FMEN
    familial multiple endocrine neoplasia
fMet
    N-formylmethionine
FMF
    familial Mediterranean fever
    fetal movement felt
    flow microfluorometry
    forced midexpiratory flow
FMFD
    familial multiple coagulation factor deficiency [factors II, VII, IX, X, protein C, and protein S]
FMFD1
    familial multiple factor deficiency 1
FMG
    fibrin matrix gel
    fine mesh gauze
    foreign medical graduate
FMH
    familial hemiplegic migraine
    family medical history
    fat-mobilizing hormone
    fetal-maternal (fetomaternal) hemorrhage
    fibromuscular hyperplasia (*See also* FH)
    first metatarsal head
FMI
    fat mass index
    fixed mandibular implant
    Foods and Moods Inventory
FMIA
    Frankfort mandibular incisor angle
FMISO
    F-misonidazole [scan]
FMIV
    forced mandatory intermittent ventilation
FML
    flail mitral leaflet
FMLA
    Family and Medical Leave Act of 1993 [U.S. Department of Labor]

F

FMLH
familial hemophagocytic lymphophistiocytosis

fMLP
fMet-Leu-Phe (formyl methionyl leucyl phenylalanine)

FMN
first malignant neoplasm
flavin mononucleotide
frontomaxillonasal [suture]

FMNH$_2$
reduced flavin mononucleotide

FMO
flavin-containing monooxygenase metabolic system

FMOA
full mouth odontectomy and alveoloplasty

FMOC-Leu
N-(9-fluorenylmethoxycarbonyl)-L-leucine

fmol
femtomole

fmol/mg
femtomole per milligram

FMP
family member presence
fasting metabolic panel
final menstrual period
first menstrual period
functional maintenance program

FMPA
full-mouth periapicals [dental x-ray]

FMPIR
fast multiplanar inversion recovery [imaging]

FMPP
familial male precocious puberty

FMPSPGR
fast multiplanar spoiled gradient-recalled [imaging]

FMR
familial mental retardation
fetal movement record
focused medical review
Friend-Moloney-Rauscher [antigen]
functional magnetic resonance [imaging]
functional mitral regurgitation

FMR1
fragile mental retardation 1 protein [gene]

FMR2
fragile site mental retardation 2 [gene]

fMRA
functional magnetic resonance angiography

FMRD
full-mouth restorative dentistry

fMRI
functional magnetic resonance imaging

FMRP
fragile X mental retardation protein

FMS
false memory syndrome
fat-mobilizing substance
fatty meal sonogram
fibromyalgia syndrome (*See also* FS)
full-mouth series [dental x-ray]

F&MS
frontal and maxillary sinuses

FMSTB
Frostig Movement Skills Test Battery

FMT
fetal mesencephalic tissue
floating mass transducer
fluorescein meniscus time
functional maintenance therapy
functional muscle test

FMTC
familial medullary thyroid cancer (carcinoma)

FMU
first morning urine

FMULC
free monoclonal urinary light chain

FMV
floppy mitral valve
flow-mediated vasodilation
Fort Morgan virus

FMX
full-mouth x-ray

FN
facial nerve
false negative (*See also* Fneg)
fastigial nucleus
febrile neutropenia
fecal nitrogen
femoral neck
fibronectin
final nitrogen
finger-to-nose [neurologic coordination test] (*See also* F-N, F→N, FNT, FTN, F to N)
fluoride number

F-N, F to N, F→N
finger-to-nose [neurologic coordination test] (*See also* FN, FNT, FTN)

F/N
fluids and nutrition

fn
function (*See also* F, FXN)

FNA
femoral neck anteversion
fine-needle aspiration
Functional Needs Assessment

FNa
filtered sodium

FNAB
fine-needle aspiration biopsy

FNAC
fine-needle aspiration cytology
FNB
femoral nerve block
fine-needle biopsy
flat nasal bridge
FNBMD
femoral neck bone mineral density
FNC
fatty nutritional cirrhosis
FNCJ
fine-needle catheter jejunostomy
FND
febrile neutrophilic dermatosis
focal neurological deficit
frontonasal dysplasia
functional neck dissection
f-NE
free norepinephrine
Fneg
false negative (*See also* FN)
FNF
false-negative fraction
femoral neck fracture
finger-nose-finger [coordination test]
FNH
focal nodular hyperplasia
follicular nodular hyperplasia
FNHJ
familial nonhemolytic jaundice
FNHL
follicular non-Hodgkin lymphoma
FNHTR
febrile nonhemolytic transfusion react
FNI
facial nerve injury
FNIC
Food and Nutrition Information Center
FNL
familial neurovisceral lipidosis
f-NM
free normetanephrine
FN-MCD
familial nephronophthisis-medullary
cystic disease
FNMTC
familial nonmedullary thyroid
carcinoma
fn p
fusion point
FNR
false-negative rate
FNS
food and nutrition services
functional neuromuscular stimulation
F/NS
fever and night sweats

FNSD
face near straight down [infant sleep
position]
FNT
false neurochemical transmitter
finger-to-nose test [neurologic
coordination] (*See also* FN, F-N,
F→N, FTN, F to N)
FNTC, FNTHC
fine-needle transhepatic cholangiography
(cholangiogram)
FO
familial occurrence
fast oxidative
fiberoptic
focus out
foot orthosis
foramen ovale
forced oscillation
foreign object
frontooccipital [fetal position]
Fo
foment(ation) (fomenting)
phonation
FOAM
fluorescence overlay antigen mapping
FOAR
faciooculoacousticorenal [syndrome]
FOAVF
failure of all vital forces
FOB
father of baby
fecal occult blood
feet out of bed
fiberoptic bronchoscope (bronchoscopy)
(*See also* FB, fib. bronc)
foot of bed
foreign object [and/or] body
FOBT
fecal occult blood test
FOC
father of child
fluid of choice
frequency of contact [scale]
frontooccipital circumference
FOCALCROS
focal contralateral routing of signals
FOCF
first observation carried forward
FOCMA
feline oncornavirus-associated cell
membrane antigen
FOCS
familial ovarian cancer syndrome
△ **FOD**
familial osseous dystrophy
fatty acid oxidation disorder

F

FOD *(continued)*
fixing right eye ⚠
focus object distance
free of disease
FOE
Fecal Odor Eliminator
fiberoptic examination
FOEB
feet over edge of bed
FOG
fast-oxidative-glycolytic [fiber]
full-on gain
FOH
family ocular history
FOI
flight of ideas
FOIA
Freedom of Information Act [U.S.
Department of Justice]
FOID
fear of impending doom
FOL
fiberoptic laryngoscopy
fiberoptic light
fol
following
Fol cath
Foley catheter
FOM
figure of merit [measure of diagnostic
value per radionuclide radiation dose]
floor of mouth
FOMV
Fomede virus
FONAR
field focused nuclear magnetic
resonance
FONSI
finding of no significant impact
FOO
family of origin
foreign object obstruction
FOOB
fell out of bed
FOOSH
fall on outstretched hand
FOP
fasting office profile
fiberoptic probe
fibrodysplasia ossificans progressiva
forensic pathology
FOPR
full outpatient rate
FOPS
fiberoptic proctosigmoidoscopy
FOPT
fibroosseous pseudotumor
FO-PT
fiberoptic phototherapy

FOR
forensic
for.
foreign
formula (*See also* form.)
form.
formula (*See also* for.)
FORMIL
foreign military
FORV
Forecariah virus
⚠ **FOS**
fiberoptic sigmoidoscopy
(sigmoidoscope)
fissura orbitalis superior
fixing left eye ⚠
force of stream [urine]
fractional osteoid surface
fructooligosaccharide
full of stool
future order screen
FOSQ
Functional Outcomes of Sleep
Questionnaire
FOT
Finger Oscillation Test
forced oscillation technique
form of thought
frontal outflow tract
found.
foundation
FOUR
full outline of unresponsiveness [eye,
motor, brainstem, respiratory functions
in trauma]
four Rs
remove, replace, reinoculate, repair
FOV
field of view
FOVI
field of vision intact
FOW
fenestration open window
[thoracostomy]
FOZR
front optic zone radius
F-P
femoral-popliteal (*See also* FEM-POP)
FP
facial palsy
fall precautions
false-positive
familial porencephaly
family physician (*See also* fam phys)
family planning
family practice
family presence
Fanconi pancytopenia
femoropopliteal [bypass]

fibrinolytic potential
fibrinopeptide
fibrous proliferation
filling pressure
filter paper
final pressure
first pass
fixation protein
flat plate
flavin phosphate
flavoprotein
flexor profundus
fluid pressure
fluorescence polarization
food poisoning
foot process
forearm pronated (*See also* fp)
freezing point (*See also* fp)
frontoparietal
frontopolar
frozen plasma
full period
fundal pressure
fundus photo
fusion point

F-6-P
fructose-6-phosphate

F:P
fluid to plasma ratio
fluorescein to protein ratio

Fp
filtered phosphate
frontal polar electrode placement
[electroencephalography]

fp
flexor pollicis
forearm pronated (*See also* FP)
freezing point (*See also* FP)

FPA
fibrinopeptide A
filter paper activity
fluorophenylalanine
foot progression angle
frontopolar artery

fpa
far point of accommodation

FPAA
female pattern androgenetic alopecia

FPAL
fluorescein-potentiated argon laser
therapy
full-term (deliveries), premature
(deliveries), abortion(s), living
(children)

FPB
femoral-popliteal (femoropopliteal)
bypass

fibrinopeptide B
flexor pollicis brevis [muscle]

FPC
familial paroxysmal choreoathetosis
familial polyposis coli
fibered platinum coil
fish protein concentrate
forced pair copulation
frozen packed cells

FPCL
fibroblast-populated collagen lattice

FPD
fetopelvic disproportion
fine-particle dose
fixed partial denture
flame photometric detector

FPDD
familial pure depressive disease

FPDL
flashlamp-pumped pulsed-dye laser
(*See also* FPPDL)

FPDM
fibrocalculous pancreatic diabetes
mellitus

FPDVP
Frostig Program for the Development of
Visual Perception

FPE
fatal pulmonary embolism
first-pass effect

^{18}F-PET
fluoride-18 positron emission
tomography

FPF
false-positive fraction
fibroblast pneumocyte factor

FPG
fasting plasma glucose
fluorescence plus Giemsa [stain]
focal proliferative glomerulonephritis
(*See also* FPGN)

FPGN
focal proliferative glomerulonephritis
(*See also* FPG)

FPH
familial progressive hyperpigmentation
female pseudohermaphroditism

FPH$_2$
flavin phosphate, reduced

FPHA
family planning health assistant

FPHE
formaldehyde-treated
pyruvaldehyde-stabilized human
erythrocytes
formalin-treated pyruvaldehyde-stabilized
human erythrocytes

F

FPHx
family psychiatric history
FPI
femoral pulsatility index
fluid percussion injury
formula protein intolerance
Freiburger Personality Inventory
FPIA
fluorescent (fluorescence) polarization
immunoassay
FPIES
food protein-induced enterocolitis
syndrome
FPIR
first-phase insulin response
FPK
fructose-6-phosphokinase
FPL
fasting plasma lipid
final printed labeling
flexor pollicis longus [muscle]
fluorescent pulsed light
FPLA
fibrin plate lysis area
FPLC
fast protein liquid chromatography
FPLD
familial partial dystrophy
FPLV
feline panleukopenia virus
FPM
filter paper microscopic (test)
first-pass metabolism
full passive movements
fpm
foot per minute
FPMA
first plantar metatarsal artery
FPN
ferric chloride, perchloric acid, nitric
acid [solution]
FPNA
first-pass nuclear angiocardiography
FPO
faciopalatoosseous
fetal pulse oximetry
freezing point osmometer
FPOR
follicle puncture for oocyte retrieval
FPP
familial paroxysmal polyserositis
familial periodic paralysis
ferriprotoporphyrin
free portal pressure
FPPDL
flashlamp-pumped pulsed-dye laser
(*See also* FPDL)
FPPH
familial primary pulmonary hypertension

FPR
facilitated positional release
false-positive rate
fastigial pressor response
fluorescence photobleaching recovery
fractional proximal resorption
Functional Performance Record
FPRNA, FPRA
first-pass radionuclide angiograph(y)
(angiogram)
FPS
facial plastic surgery
fetal PCB (polychlorinated biphenyl)
syndrome
footpad swelling
fps
foot per second
foot-pound-second [system, unit]
frame per second
fPSA
free prostate specific antigen
FPSLT
Fluharty Preschool Speech and
Language Screening Test
FPT
fixed parenchymal turnover
FPU
fetoplacental unit
FPV
Facey's Paddock virus
feline panleukopenia virus
fowl plague virus
FPVB
femoral-popliteal vein bypass
FQ
fear questionnaire
fluoroquinolones
FQHC
Federally Qualified Health Center
FR
failure rate (contraception)
fair
father (*See also* F, FTR)
Federal Register
feedback regulation
fibrinogen related
first responder
Fisher-Race [notation, statistics]
fixed ratio
flattening ratio
flocculation reaction
flow rate
fluid restriction
fluid resuscitation
fluid retention
folate receptor
fractional reabsorption
free radical
frequency encode

frequency of respiration
frequent relapses
frothy
full range
functional reach
functional residual [capacity]
reticular formation [L. *formatio reticularis*]

F2R
factor II receptor

FR3
third framework region

F/R
fire/rescue

F&R, F and R
force and rhythm [of pulse]

Fr
francium
franklin [CGS unit of electrical charge]
French scale

fr
fried
from (*See also* fm)

FRA
fall risk assessment
fibrinogen-related antigen
fibrin-related antigen
fluorescent rabies antibody
fragile
fragile chromosome site
fragile gene

frac
fracture (*See also* fract, frx, Fx, FXR)

FRACAS
fracture computer-aided surgery

fract
fraction(al) (*See also* F, FX)
fracture (*See also* frac, frx, Fx, FXR)

FRACTS
fractional urines (*See also* fxur)

frag
fragile
fragility
fragment

FRALE
frangible anchor-linker effector

FRAP
family risk assessment program
FK-binding protein rapamycin-associated protein
fluorescence recovery after photobleaching

FRAST
Free Running Asthma Test

FRAT
free radical assay technique

FRAX, fra(X)
fragile X [chromosome, gene, syndrome]

FRAXA
X-linked first site of fragility [gene locus]

FRAXE
X-linked second site of fragility [gene locus]
fragile site, folic acid type, rare, FRA(X) (q 28)
mental retardation, X-linked, associated with fragile site FRAXE

FRAXE1
X-linked mental retardation-fragile site 1

FRAX-MR
fragile X [chromosome] mental retardation

FRBB, Fr BB
fracture of both bones (*See also* Fx BB)

FRBS
fast red B salt

FRC
feedback reduction circuit
frozen red cell
functional reserve (residual) capacity [of lungs]

FRCD
fixed ratio combination drugs

FRD
flexion, rotation, drawer [test]

FRE
Fischer rat embryo
flow-related enhancement

FRED
fog reduction elimination device

frem.
vocal fremitus [L. *fremitus vocalis*]

freq
frequency (*See also* F, f)
frequent

FRET
fluorescence (fluorescent) resonance energy transfer

FRF
fasciculus retroflexus
filtration replacement fluid

FRFC
functional renal failure of cirrhosis

FRG
Functional Related Groups

FRH
follitropin-releasing hormone

FRHS
fast-repeating high sequence

F

frict
friction [rub]
Fried
Friedman [test for pregnancy]
FRIV
Frijoles virus
FRJM
full range joint motion (movement)
FRM
full range of motion (*See also* FROM)
FRN
fetal rhabdomyomatous nephroblastoma
fully resonant nucleus
FRNS
frequently relapsing nephrotic syndrome
FRNT
focus-reduction neutralization test
FROA
full range of affect
FROD
fat removal orbital decompression
FRODO
flow respiratory artifact obliteration with
directed orthogonal pulses
FROM
full range of motion (*See also* FRM)
FROMAJE
functioning, reasoning, orientation,
memory, arithmetic, judgment, emotion
[mental status evaluation]
FROS
front routing of signals
FRP
familial recurring polyserositis
follicle regulatory protein
formaldehyde-releasing preservative
frizzled related protein
functional refractory period
FRPS
functional resting position splint
FR r, fr r
friction rub
FRS
facial reconstructive surgery
ferredoxin-reducing substance
first rank symptoms [of
schizophrenia]
flexed, rotated, sidebent
fluid retention syndrome
fusion and reconstruction system
FRSL
flexed, rotated, sidebent left
FRSR
flexed, rotated, sidebent right
FRT
Family Relations Test
full recovery time
FRTL-5
Fischer rat thyroid line 5

Fru
fructose
FRV
functional residual volume
frx
fracture (*See also* frac, fract Fx, FXR)
FS
[drug] for skin
factor of safety
feminization syndrome
fetoscope
fibromyalgia syndrome (*See also* FMS)
fibrosarcoma
fibrous synovium
field stimulation
fine structure
fingerstick
fire setter [psychology]
flexible sigmoidoscopy
focal spot
fogo selvagem
food service
forearm supination
foreskin
Fourier series
fractional shortening
fracture, simple
fracture site
fragile site
Friesinger score [coronary]
frozen section (*See also* FZ)
full-scale [IQ test]
full and soft [diet] (*See also* F&S)
full strength
functional shortening
functional status
function study
[human] foreskin (cells)
F/S
female, spayed [animal]
frozen section
F&S
full and soft [diet] (*See also* FS)
FSA
familial splenic anemia
fetal sulfoglycoprotein antigen
frozen section assay
FSAD
female sexual arousal disorder
FSALO
Fletcher-Suit afterloading ovoids
[gynecologic cancer treatment]
FSALT
Fletcher-Suit afterloading tandem
[gynecologic cancer treatment]
FSB
fetal scalp blood
Fokes sentence builder
full spine board

FSBG
    fingerstick blood gas
    fingerstick blood glucose
FSBM
    full-strength breast milk
FSBP
    finger systolic blood pressure
FSBS
    fingerstick blood sugar
FSBT
    Fowler single breath test
FSC
    Fatigue Symptom Checklist
    flexible sigmoidoscopy
    Forer Sentence Completion (Test)
    forward scatter
    fracture simple, comminuted
    fracture, simple, complete
    free secretory component
FSCC
    fracture simple, complete, comminuted
FSCR
    flexible surface-coil-type resonator
FSD
    face-straight-down [infant sleep position]
    female sexual dysfunction
    Fletcher-Suit-Delclos [applicator]
    focus-skin distance
    fracture simple and depressed
    full-scale deflection
FS-DFSP
    fibrosarcomatous variant of
      dermatofibrosarcoma protuberans
FSDQ
    Frost Self-Description Questionnaire
FSE
    fast spin echo
    fetal scalp electrode
    filtered smoke exposure
FSF
    fibrin stabilizing (stabilization) factor
FSFD
    female sexual function diagnostic
FSFI
    Female Sexual Function Index
FSG
    fasting serum glucose
    focal sclerosing (segmental)
      glomerulonephritis (*See also* FSGN)
FSGA
    full-term, small for gestational age
FSGHS
    focal segmental glomerular hyalinosis
      and sclerosis
FSGN
    focal sclerosing (segmental)
      glomerulonephritis (*See also* FSG)

FSGO
    floating spherical gaussian orbital
FSGS
    focal segmental glomerular sclerosis
      (glomerulosclerosis)
FSGSH
    focal segmental glomerular sclerosis and
      hyalinosis
FSH
    facioscapulohumeral [muscular
      dystrophy]
    focal and segmental hyalinosis
    follicle-stimulating hormone (follitropin)
FSHD
    facioscapulohumeral [muscular]
      dystrophy
FSH/LR-RH
    follicle-stimulating hormone and
      luteinizing hormone-releasing hormone
FSHMD
    facioscapulohumeral muscular dystrophy
FSH-RF
    follicle-stimulating hormone-releasing
      factor
FSH-RH
    follicle-stimulating hormone-releasing
      hormone
FSHSMA
    facioscapulohumeral spinal muscular
      atrophy
FSI
    fasting serum insulin
    Fatigue Symptom Inventory
    foam stability index
    Functional Status Index
FSIA
    foot shock-induced analgesia
FSIQ
    Full-Scale Intelligence Quotient
FSIVGTT
    frequently sampled intravenous glucose
      tolerance test
FSL
    fasting serum level
    fixed slit lamp
FSM
    functional status measure
F-SM/C
    fungus, smear, culture
FSMD
    facioscapulohumeral muscular dystrophy
FSME
    Fruhsommer meningoencephalitis
FSN
    functional stimulation, neuromuscular
FSO
    for screws only [prosthetic cups]

F

FSpO₂
fetal arterial oxygen saturation
F-SP
special form [taxonomy] [L. *forma specialis*]
FSP
familial spastic paraplegia
femoral hole sagittal positioning
fibrinogen split product
fibrinolytic split product
fibrin split product
fine suspended particulate
free secretory piece
FSPB
finite-size pencil beam [radiation]
FSPG
focal segmental proliferative glomerulonephritis
FSPGR
fast spoiled gradient-recalled
FSQ
Functional Status Questionnaire
FSR
film screen radiography
force-sensing retractor
fractionated stereotactic radiosurgery
fragmented sarcoplasmic reticulum
fusiform skin revision
FSRRL
flexion, sidebent right, rotated left
FSRT
fractionated stereotactic radiotherapy
FSS
Familiar Sensory Stimulation
Fear Survey Schedule
fetal scalp sampling
Flinders Symptom Score
focal segmental sclerosis
French steel sound
frequency-selective saturation
front support strap
full-scale score
functional systems scale
FSSE
fat-suppressed spin-echo
FSST
Full-Scale Score Total
FST
fludrocortisone suppression testing
foam stability test
FSU
functional spinal unit
functional subunit
FSUM
focused segmented ultrasound machine
FSV
feline fibrosarcoma virus
Fort Sherman virus
forward stroke volume

FSW
female sex worker
field service worker
flexible spiral wire
fsw
feet of sea water [conventional unit of pressure]
FT
Fallot tetralogy
false transmitter
family therapy
farnesyl transferase
fast twitch
feeding tube
ferritin
ferromagnetic tamponade
fetal tonsil
fibrous tissue
filling time
finger tapping
fingertip
flexor tendon
fluidotherapy
followthrough [after barium meal]
formol toxoid
Fourier transform
free testosterone
free thyroxine
frontotemporal
full term
function test
FT₃
free triiodothyronine
FT₄
free [unbound] thyroxine
ft
foot [singular] (feet [plural])
FTA
femorotibial angle
fluorescent titer antibody
fluorescent treponemal antibody [test] (*See also* FTAT)
FTA-ABS, FTA-Abs
fluorescent (fluorescence) treponemal antibody absorption [test]
FTA-ABS-DS
fluorescent (fluorescence) treponemal antibody absorption doublestaining
F-TAG
fast-binding target-attaching globulin
FTAS
familial testicular agenesis syndrome
FTase
farnesyl-transferase
FTAT
fluorescent treponemal antibody test (*See also* FTA)

FTB
 fingertip blood
 front-to-back [visualization in 3D
  reconstruction and virtual reality]

FTBD
 fit to be detained
 full term, born dead

FTBE
 focal tick-borne encephalitis

FTBI
 fractionated total body irradiation

FTBS
 Family Therapist Behavioral Scale

FTC
 fallopian tube carcinoma
 fibulotalocalcaneal
 follicular thyroid carcinoma
 frames to come [optometry]
 frequency threshold curve
 full to confrontation [visual fields]

fTCD
 functional transcranial Doppler
  sonography

FTD
 failure to descend
 femoral total density
 frontotemporal degeneration (dementia)
 full-term delivery

FTDP-17
 frontotemporal dementias with
  parkinsonism linked to chromosome
  17

FTDS
 familial testicular dysgenesis
  syndrome

FTE
 failure to engraft
 functional tissue engineering

FTEQ
 Functional Time Estimation
  Questionnaire

FTF
 finger-to-finger [test] (*See also* FF, f-f,
  f→f)
 free thyroxine fraction

FTFTN
 finger-to-finger-to-nose [test]

FTG
 full-thickness graft

FTHA
 14-18F-fluoro-6-thia-heptadecanoic acid
  [fatty acid tracer]

FTI
 farnesyltransferase inhibitor
 force-time integral

FT$_3$I
 free triiodothyronine index

FT$_4$I
 free thyroxine index

FTIR
 Fourier transform infrared
  [spectroscopy]
 functional terminal innervation ratio

FTIUP
 full-term intrauterine pregnancy

FTJ
 femorotibial joint

FTKA
 failed to keep appointment

FTLB
 full-term live birth

ft · lb
 foot pound [traditional unit of work]

ft · lb/s
 foot pound per second [traditional unit
  of force]

FTLD
 frontotemporal lobar degeneration

FTLE
 full-thickness local excision

FTLFC
 full-term living female child

FTLMC
 full-term living male child

FTM
 fluid thioglycolate medium
 fractional test meal

FTMH
 full thickness macular hole

FTMS
 Fourier transform mass spectrometer

FTN
 finger to nose [neurologic coordination
  test] (*See also* FN, F-N, F→N, FNT,
  F to N)

FTNB
 full-term newborn

FTND
 Fagerstrom Test for Nicotine
  Dependence
 full-term normal delivery

FTNS
 functional transcutaneous nerve
  stimulation

FTNSD
 full-term normal spontaneous
  delivery

FTO
 fructose-terminated oligosaccharide
 fulltime occlusion [eye patch]

FTOC
 fetal thymus organ culture

FTOZ
 frontotemporal orbitozygomatic

F

FTP
    failure to progress [in labor]
    full-term pregnancy

ft · pdl
    foot poundal [unit of work]

F:T PSA, fTPSA
    free to total prostate-specific antigen
    ratio

FTQ
    Fagerstrom tolerance questionnaire

FTR
    failed to report
    failed to respond
    father (*See also* F, FR)
    force translation [neurostimulation]
    fractional turnover rate
    for the record

FTRAM
    free transverse rectus abdominis
    myocutaneous [flap]

FTS
    face-to-side
    Family Tracking System
    feminizing testis syndrome
    fetal tobacco syndrome
    fingertips
    fissured tongue syndrome
    flexor tenosynovitis
    serum thymic factor [Fr. *facteur*
    thymique serique]

FTSD
    full-term spontaneous delivery

FTSG
    full-thickness skin graft

FTSP
    fallopian tube sperm perfusion

FTT
    failure to thrive
    fat tolerance test
    fetal tissue transplant
    Finger-Tapping Test
    fraternal twins raised
    together
    fructose tolerance test

FTU
    fingertip unit
    fluorescence thiourea

Ftube
    feeding tube

FTUPLD
    full-term uncomplicated pregnancy,
    labor, delivery

FTV
    fetal thrombotic vasculopathy
    functional trial visit

FTVD
    full term vaginal delivery

FTW
    failure to wean

FTX
    field training exercise

FU
    fat unit
    fecal urobilinogen
    femoral vein cannulation
    finsen unit [ultraviolet light intensity]
    followup (*See also* F/U, FUP, fl up)
    fractional urinalysis
    fraction unbound
    fundus [at umbilicus] (*See also* F/U)

F↓U
    fingers below umbilicus [measurement]
    (*See also* FBU)

F/U
    followup (*See also* FU, FUP, fl up)
    fundus at umbilicus (*See also* FU)

F↑U
    fingers above umbilicus [measurement]

F&U
    flanks and upper quadrants

FU-I
    first set of followup data

FU-II
    second set of followup data

FUA
    flat and upright [x-ray of] abdomen

FUB
    found under bridge
    functional uterine bleeding

FUC
    fucosidase

Fuc
    fucose

FUCA
    alpha-L-fucosidase

FU$_{CO}$
    functional uptake of carbon monoxide

FUD
    fear, uncertainty, doubt
    fever, vomiting, diarrhea
    frequency, urgency, dysuria
    full upper denture (*See also* F/, FU Dtr)

FUDS
    fluorourodynamic study

FUDT
    forensic urine drug testing

FU Dtr
    full upper denture (*See also* F/, FUD)

FUE
    fever of unknown etiology

FUFA
    free volatile fatty acid

FU/FL
    full upper, full lower [denture]

FUL
    federal upper limit [Medicaid drug
    reimbursement]
    functional urethral length

fulg
    fulguration
FU/LP
    full upper denture, lower partial denture
FUM
    fumarase
    fumarate
    fumigation
FUMP
    fluorouridine monophosphate
FUN
    followup note
func, funct
    function(al)
FUNG-C
    fungus culture
FUNG-S
    fungus smear
FUO
    fever of unknown (undetermined) origin
FUOV
    followup office visit
FUP
    followup (*See also* fl up, F/U, FU)
    follow up (*See also* fl up, F/U, FU)
    follow-up (*See also* fl up, F/U, FU)
fu p
    fusion point
FUR
    fluorouridine
FUS
    feline urologic syndrome
    first-use syndrome
    fusion
FUT
    fibrinogen uptake test
FUTE
    fat-suppressed ultrashort echo time
FUV
    follow-up visit
FV
    femoral vein
    flow velocity
    flow volume
    fluid volume
    formaldehyde vapors
F(v)
    velocity distribution function
f:V$_t$
    frequency to tidal volume ratio
FVA
    four-vessel arteriography
    Friend virus anemia
FVC
    false vocal cord
    filled voiding flow rate (*See also* FVFR)
    forced vital capacity

FVCA
    forced vital capacity analysis
FVD
    fibrovascular tissue on disc
FVE
    fibrovascular tissue elsewhere
    forced volume, expiratory
fVEP
    flash visual evoked potential
FVFR
    filled voiding flow rate (*See also* FVC)
FVH
    focal vascular headache
    fulminant viral hepatitis
FVL
    factor V (5) Leiden [mutation]
    femoral vein ligation
    flexible video laparoscope
    flow-volume loop
    force, velocity, length
    functional visual loss
FVM
    familial visceral myopathy
FVN
    familial visceral neuropathy
FVOP
    finger venous opening pressure
FVP
    fast venous pressure
    Friend virus polycythemia
FVPTC
    follicular variant of papillary thyroid carcinoma
FVR
    feline viral rhinotracheitis
    forearm vascular resistance
    fractional velocity reserve
FVS
    fetal valproate syndrome
    fetal varicella syndrome
FVU
    first-void urine
FVWs
    flow-velocity waveforms [umbilical artery Doppler]
FW
    Felix-Weil [reaction]
    fetal weight
    Folin and Wu [method]
    forced whisper
    fracturing wall
    fragment wound
F/W
    followed with
Fw
    fibrillatory (flutter) wave

F

fw
　fresh water
FWB
　full weightbearing
　functional well-being
FWCA
　functional work capacity assessment
FWD
　fairly well developed
FWHM
　full width [of line-spread function] half
　　maximal [height]
　full width [of photopeak measured at]
　　half maximal [count] [tomography]
FWM
　Folin-Wu method (*See also* FW)
FWOC
　fine without changing
FWR
　Felix-Weil reaction
FWS
　fetal warfarin syndrome
FWW
　front wheel walker
FX
　factor X
　fluoroscopy
　fornix
　fraction(al) (*See also* F, fract)
　friction
　frozen section
Fx
　fracture (*See also* frac, fract, frx, FXR)
Fx BB
　fracture of both bones (*See also* FRBB,
　　Fr BB)

Fx-dis
　fracture-dislocation (*See also* F/D)
FXN
　function (*See also* F, fn)
FXR
　fracture (*See also* frac, fract, frx,
　　Fx)
FXS
　fragile X syndrome
fxur
　fractional urines (*See also*
　　FRACTS)
FY
　fiscal year
　full year
FYA
　Duffy antigen A positive phenotype
FYAN
　Duffy antigen A negative phenotype
FYB
　Duffy antigen B positive phenotype
FYBN
　Duffy antigen B negative phenotype
FYC
　facultative yeast carrier
FYI
　for your information
FZ
　focal zone
　frontozygomatic
　frozen section (*See also* FS)
Fz
　frontal midline placement of electrodes
　　[electroencephalography]
FZRC
　frozen section red [blood] cell

G

gallop [heart sound]
ganglion (See also gang, gangl)
gap [cell cycle]
gas (See also g)
gastrin
gastrostomy
gauge [of needle] (See also g, ga)
gauss
gender (See also GEN)
general factor [single variance common to different intelligence tests]
geometric efficiency
Gibbs free energy
Giemsa [banding stain]
giga-
gingiva(l) (See also GING, ging)
glabella (See also Gl)
globular [protein] (See also glob.)
globulin (See also glob.)
glucose (See also Glc, GLU, gluc)
glycogen
gold [inlay]
gonidial [colony]
good (See also gd)
goose
grade (See also gr)
Grafenberg [spot]
Gram [stain] (See also GS)
gravid (See also GR)
gravida [pregnant]
Greek (See also Gr)
green (See also GRN, Grn)
Gross [leukemia antigen]
guanine (See also Gua)
gynecology

G0, G₀

gap zero [quiescent phase of cells leaving mitotic cycle]
gravida 0, never pregnant

G1, G₁

first pregnancy
gap₁ [presynthetic gap phase of cells prior to DNA synthesis]
grid 1 [in electroencephalography]
first pregnancy (primigravida)
well-differentiated [TNM histologic classification]

G1–G6

grade 1–6 [heart murmur]

G2, G₂

gap₂ [postsynthetic gap phase of cells following DNA synthesis]
grid 2 [in electroencephalography]

moderately differentiated [TNM histologic classification]
second pregnancy (secundigravida)

G3, G₃

poorly differentiated [TNM histologic classification]
third pregnancy (tertigravida)

G4, G₄

undifferentiated [TNM histologic classification]

G+

guaiac positive
gram-positive (See also GM+, GP, gr+, GrP)

G−

guaiac negative
gram-negative (See also GM−, GN, gr−, GrN)

g

acceleration due to gravity, 9.80665 m/s^2
gas (See also G)
gauge [of needle] (See also G, ga)
gram [unit of weight]
gravity [unit force of acceleration]
group (See also GP, grp)

g%

gram percent

_g_

relative centrifugal force

GII

Generation II [orthotic]

GA

Gamblers Anonymous
gastric analysis
gastric antrum
general anesthesia (See also GEA, gen-an)
general angiography
general appearance
genetic algorithm
gentisic acid
gestational age
Getting Along [psychologic test]
ginger ale (See also G'ale)
gingivoaxial
glucoamylase
glucose/acetone
glucuronic acid
glycyrrhetinic acid
Golgi apparatus
granulocyte adherence
granulocyte agglutination
granuloma annulare
guessed average

G

GA *(continued)*
gut-associated
gyrate atrophy
NATO code for tabun
G:A
globulin to albumin ratio
Ga
gallium
⁶⁷Ga
gallium-67
⁶⁸Ga
gallium-68
ga
gauge [of needle] *(See also* G, g)
GAA
alpha (α)-glucosidase
glacial acetic acid
glutamic acid codon
gossypol acetic acid
GAAS
Goldberg Anorectic Attitude Scale
Gab-1
growth factor receptor-bound protein 2
(Grb2)-associated binder 1
GABA
gamma-aminobutyric acid
gamma-aminobutyric acidemia
GABA/BZD
gamma-aminobutyric acid/benzodiazepine
[receptor]
GABA-T
gamma-aminobutyric acid
transaminase
GABEB
generalized atrophic benign
epidermolysis bullosa
GABHS
group A beta (β) hemolytic
streptococcus *(See also* GABS)
GABOA, GABOB
gamma-amino-beta-hydroxybutyric
acid
hydroxyl derivative of GABA
GABS
group A beta (β) hemolytic
streptococcus *(See also* GABHS)
GAD
generalized anxiety disorder
glutamate decarboxylase
glutamic acid decarboxylase
GAD65
glutamic acid decarboxylase 65
GADH
gastric alcohol dehydrogenase
GADS
gas atomized dispersion strengthened
gonococcal arthritis/dermatitis syndrome
GAE
granulomatous amebic encephalitis

GAEB
good air entry bilaterally
GAEL
Grammatical Analysis of Elicited
Language
GAF
geographic adjustment factors
giant axon formation
glia-activating factor
global assessment of functioning
GAFT
glutamine-fructose-6-phosphate-
amidotransferase
GAG
glycosaminoglycan
GAGPS
glycosaminoglycan polysulfate
GAGS
global acne grading system
GAGUA
glycosaminoglycan uronate
GAHM
genioglossus [muscle] advancement and
hyoid myotomy
GAHS
galactorrhea amenorrhea
hyperprolactinemia syndrome
GAI
guided affective imagery
GAIPAS
General Audit Inpatient Psychiatric
Assessment Scale
GAIT
great toe arthroplasty implant technique
GAL
galactose
galactosemia
galactosyl
glucuronic acid lactone
Gal
galactose
gal.
gallon [L. *congius*]
GA LAW
glucose, age, LDH (lactate
dehydrogenase), AST (aspartate
aminotransferase), WBC (white blood
cells) [laboratory tests]
G-ALB
globulin-albumin
GALC
galactocerebrosidase deficiency
GALE
uridine diphosphate-galactose-4-
epimerase deficiency
G'ale
ginger ale *(See also* GA)
GALF
glycyrrhetinic acid like factor

GALK
    galactokinase
gal/min
    gallon per minute
GalN
    galactosamine
GalNAc
    N-acetyl-D-galactosamine
GALOP
    gait disorder, autoantibody, late-age
    onset, polyneuropathy
gal-1-P
    galactose-1-phosphate
GALS
    gait, arms, legs, spine
GALT
    galactose-1-phosphate uridyltransferase
    [enzyme]
    gastrointestinal-associated
    (gut-associated) lymphoid tissue
    gut-associated lymphoepithelial tissue
GalTase
    4-galactosyltransferase
GAL TT
    galactose tolerance test
GALV
    gibbon ape leukemia virus
GaLV
    gibbon ape lymphosarcoma virus
Galv, galv
    galvanic
    galvanism
    galvanized
GAM
    gene-activated matrix [singular]
    (matrices [plural])
GAMA
    General Ability Measure for Adults
GAMG
    goat antimouse immunoglobulin G
γ
    activity coefficient
    carbon separated from the carboxyl
    group by two other carbon atoms
    chain of fetal hemoglobin
    constituent of gamma protein plasma
    fraction
    gamma [third letter of Greek alphabet
    lowercase]
    gamma photon [gamma ray]
    10^{-4} gauss
    heavy chain of immunoglobulin G
    monomer in fetal hemoglobin
    plasma gamma (γ) [protein, globulin]
Γ
    gamma [third letter of Greek alphabet
    uppercase]

gamma(γ)-BHC
    gamma-benzene hexachloride (*See also*
    GBH)
gamma(γ)-GTP
    gamma-glutamyl transpeptidase
gamma(γ)-HCD
    gamma-heavy-chain disease
gamma(γ)-HCH
    hexachlorocyclohexane (*See also* HCC,
    HCH)
gamma(γ)-MSH
    gamma-melanocyte-stimulating hormone
gamma-T, γ-T
    gamma(γ)-tocopherol
GAMT
    guanidinoacetate methyltransferase
GAMV
    Gamboa virus
GAN
    giant axonal neuropathy
gang, gangl
    ganglion (*See also* G)
    ganglionic
GANS
    granulomatous angiitis of central
    nervous system
GANT
    gastrointestinal autonomic nerve tumor
GAP
    Gardner Analysis of Personality
    [Survey]
    general all purpose
    glans approximation procedure
    glyceraldehyde phosphate
    gonadotropin-releasing
    hormone-associated peptide
    growth-associated protein
    GTPase-activating protein
    guanosine triphosphate-activating protein
GAP-43
    growth-associated protein 43
GAPD, GAPDH
    glyceraldehyde phosphate dehydrogenase
    glyceraldehyde-3-phosphate
    dehydrogenase
GAPO
    growth retardation, alopecia,
    pseudoanodontia, optic atrophy
    [syndrome]
GAPS
    Guidelines for Adolescent Preventive
    Services
GAR
    genitoanorectal [syndrome]
    goat antirabbit gamma globulin
    (*See also* GARGG)
    gonococcal antibody reaction

G

GARD
gastroesophageal antireflux device
glenoid articular rim disruption
GARF
Global Assessment of Relational
Functioning
GARFT
glycinamide ribonucleotide formyl
transferase
garg
gargle
GARGG
goat antirabbit gamma globulin
(*See also* GAR)
GARP
globally optimized alternating-phase
rectangular pulse
GARS
Gait Abnormality Rating Scale
GARS-M
Gait Abnormality Rating Scale Modified
GART
genotypic antiretroviral resistance testing
GAS
galactorrhea-amenorrhea syndrome
gastric acid secretion
gastroenterology
gene-activating sequence
general adaptation syndrome
generalized arteriosclerosis
ginseng abuse syndrome
Glasgow Assessment Schedule
Goal Attainment Scale
group A *Streptococcus*
GaS
gallium scan
GASA
glove and stocking anesthesia
growth-adjusted sonographic age
Gas Anal F&T
gastric analysis, free and total
GASP
gastric augment and single pedicle tube
GAST
gonadotropin agonist stimulation test
gastro
gastroenterology
gastrointestinal
gastroc
gastrocnemius [muscle]
GASTS
group A streptococcal toxic shock
GAT
gas antitoxin
gelatin agglutination test
geriatric assessment team
Gerontological Apperception Test
Goldmann applanation tonometer
(tonometry)

group adjustment therapy
GATase
6-alkyl guanine alkyl transferase
GATB
General Aptitude Test Battery
GAV
Grand Arbaud virus
gav
gavage
GAVE
gastric antral vascular ectasia
GAX
glutaraldehyde cross-linked collagen
GAZT
glucuronide derivative of
azidothymidine
GB
gallbladder
gallbladder channel [acupuncture]
(*See also* gb)
gingival bleeding
glass bead
glial bundle
goofball [barbiturate pill]
NATO code for sarin
G&B
good and bad [days]
gb
gallbladder channel [acupuncture]
(*See also* GB)
GBA
ganglionic blocking agent
gingivobuccoaxial
GBBS
group B beta (β)-hemolytic
streptococcus
GBCA
gallbladder carcinoma
GBCE
Grassi Basic Cognitive
Evaluation
GBD
gallbladder disease
gender behavior disorder
glassblower's disease
global burden of disease
granulomatous bowel disease
GBEF
gallbladder ejection fraction
GBER
gallbladder ejection rate
GBF
gingival blood flow
good breastfeed
GBG
glycine-rich beta(β)-glycoprotein
gonadal steroid-binding globulin
GB-GI
gallbladder-gastrointestinal

GBH
gamma(γ)-benzene hexachloride
(*See also* gamma-BHC)
gamma(γ) hydroxybutyrate (*See also* GHB)
graphite, benzalkonium, heparin
grievous bodily harm

GBI
gingival bleeding index
globulin-bound insulin

GBIA
Guthrie bacterial inhibition assay

GBL
gamma(γ)-butyrolactone
glomerular basal lamina

GBLC
geometric broken line closure [scar revision]

GBM
glioblastoma multiforme
glomerular basement membrane

GBMI
guilty but mentally ill

GBO
gastric bacterial overgrowth

GBP
galactose-binding protein
gastric bypass procedure
gated blood pool

GBPS
gallbladder pigment stones
gated blood-pool study

GBq
gigabecquerel

GBR
gamma band response [audiology]
good blood return
guided bone regeneration

GBS
gallbladder series
gastric bypass surgery
glycerine-buffered saline
group B streptococcal sepsis
group B streptococcus

GBSS
Grey balanced saline solution

GBT
gastric bleeding time

GBV
GB virus

GBV-C
GB virus C [hepatitis G virus]

GBV-C/HGV
GB virus C/hepatitis G virus

GBV-C/HGV-RNA
GB virus C/hepatitis G virus ribonucleic acid

GBW
generalized body weakness

GBX
gall bladder extraction

GC
ganglion cell
gas chromatography
gastric cancer (carcinoma)
gel chromatography
general circulation
general closure
general condition
geriatric care
geriatric chair
germinal center
giant cell
gingival crevice
gingival curettage
gliomatosis cerebri
glucocorticoid
glycocholate
goblet cell
Golgi complex
goniocurettage
gonococcus (*See also* GN)
gonorrhea
gonorrhea culture
good condition
graham cracker
granular cast
granular cyst
granule cell
granulocyte cytotoxic [function]
granulomatous colitis
granulosa cell
group-specific component
guanine cytosine
guanylcyclase

G−C
gram-negative coccus (*See also* GNC)

G+C
gram-positive coccus (*See also* GPC)

Gc
gigacycle
group-specific component

GCA
gastric cancerous area
germinal cell aplasia
ghost cell ameloblastoma
giant cell arteritis

g-cal
gram calorie [small calorie]

GCB
gonococcal base

GCBM
glomerular capillary basement

GCBP
gated cardiac blood pool

G

GCC
giant cell collagenoma
glassy-cell carcinoma
goblet cell carcinoid
granular-cell carcinoma
guanylyl cyclase C

GCD
geometric center distance
giant colonic diverticulum
graft coronary disease
granular corneal dystrophy

GCDAS
Gesell Child Development Age Scale

GCDFP
gross cystic disease fluid protein

GCDP
gross cystic disease protein

GCE
general conditioning exercise

GCF
giant cell fibroblastoma
gingival crevicular fluid
greatest common factor

GCFT
gonococcal complement-fixation
test
gonorrhea complement-fixation test

G-CFU
granulocyte colony-forming unit

GCH
giant cavernous hemangioma
giant cell hepatitis

GCI
General Cognitive Index
gestational carbohydrate intolerance
global cerebral ischemia

GCII
glucose-controlled insulin infusion

GCIIS
glucose controlled insulin infusion
system

GCIS
[isolated] gland carcinoma in situ

GCKD
glomerulocystic kidney disease

GCL
generalized congenital lipodystrophy
giant-cell leukemia

GCLO
gastric campylobacterlike organism

GCM
geriatric care manager
giant-cell myocarditis
good, central, maintained
good control maintained

g-cm
gram-centimeter

GCMB
granular-cell myoblastoma

GCMD
generalized cardiovascular metabolic
disease

GCMN
giant congenital melanocytic nevus

GCMS
granular-cell myosarcoma

GC-MS, GC/MS
gas chromatography-mass spectrometry

GCN
giant cerebral neuron

GCNF
granular-cell neurofibroma

GCNM
good, central, not maintained

GCOP
glucocorticoid-induced osteoporosis

GCP
good clinical practices

GCPS
Greig cephalopolysyndactyly syndrome

GCR
gastrocolonic response
glucocerebrosidase
glucocorticoid receptor
Group Conformity Rating

GCRH
glucose counterregulatory hormone

GCRS
gynecological chylous reflux syndrome

GCS
general clinical service
Generalized Contentment Scale
giant-cell sarcoma
Glasgow Coma Scale (Score)
glucocorticosteroid
glutamylcysteine synthetase
graduated compression stockings
gram-centimeter-second [system of
measurement]

Gc/s
gigacycle per second

GCSA
Gross cell surface antigen

GCSE
generalized convulsive status epilepticus

GCSF, G-CSF
granulocyte colony-stimulating factor

G-CSF-R
granulocyte colony-stimulating factor
receptor

GCS-HS
glutamylcysteine synthetase heavy
subunit

GCST
Gibson-Cooke sweat test

GCT
general care and treatment
General Clerical Test

germ-cell tumor
giant-cell thyroiditis
giant-cell transformation
giant-cell tumor
granular cell tumor
granulosa cell tumor

GC(T)A
giant-cell [temporal] arteritis

GCTB
giant-cell tumor of bone

GCT-LMP
giant-cell tumor of low malignant potential

GCTSPS
germ-cell tumor with synchronous lesions in pineal and suprasellar regions

GCTTS
giant-cell tumor of tendon sheath

GCU
gonococcal urethritis

GCV
great cardiac vein

GCVF
great cardiac vein flow

GCW
glomerular capillary wall

GCX
giant-cell xanthoma

GCY
gastroscopy

GD
gastric distension
gastroduodenal
general diagnostics
general duties
generalized delays
gestational day
gestational diabetes [mellitus] (*See also* GDM)
given dose
glare disability
global deviation
gonadal dysgenesis
gravely disabled
Graves disease
growth and development (*See also* G&D, G and D)
NATO code for soman

G&D, G and D
growth and development (*See also* GD)

Gd
gadolinium

¹⁵³Gd
gadolinium 153

gd
good (*See also* G)

GDA
gastroduodenal artery
germine diacetate
Graves disease autoantigen

GDB
gas-density balance
Guide Dogs for the Blind

Gd-BOPTA
gadobenate dimeglumine
gadolinium benzylopropionic tetracetate

GDC
giant dopamine-containing cell
Guglielmi detachable coil

Gd-CDTA
gadolinium cyclohexanediaminetetraacetic acid

GDD
glaucoma drainage device

Gd-DOTA
gadolinium tetraazacyclododecanetetraacetic acid

Gd-DTPA
gadolinium-diethylenetriamine pentaacetic acid
gadopentetate dimeglumine

Gd-DTPA-BMA
gadodiamide
gadolinium diethylenetriamine pentaacetic acid bis methylamide

Gd-EDTA
gadolinium ethylenediaminetetraacetic acid
gadolinium ethylenediamine tetraacetic acid

Gd-EOB-DTPA
gadolinium ethoxybenzyl diethylenetriamine pentaacetic acid

GDF
growth differentiation factor

GDF-9
growth differentiation factor 9

GD FA
grandfather (*See also* GF, GR-FR)

Gd-FMPSPGR
gadolinium fast multiplanar spoiled gradient

GDH
glucose dehydrogenase
glutamate dehydrogenase (*See also* GLD, GLDH)
glutamic acid dehydrogenase
glycerophosphate dehydrogenase
gonadotropic hormone (*See also* GTH)
growth and differentiation hormone [insects]

Gd-HP-DO3A
gadoteridol [contrast agent]

G

GDID
genetically determined immunodeficiency disease

GDJ
gastroduodenal junction

g/dL
gram per deciliter

GDM
gestational diabetes mellitus (*See also* GD)

Gd-MRI
gadolinium-enhanced magnetic resonance imaging

GDMS
glow discharge mass spectrometry

GDN
glyceryl dinitrate

gdn
guardian

gDNA
genomic deoxyribonucleic acid

GDNF
glial cell derived neurotrophic factor

GDP
gamma (γ)-detecting probe
gastroduodenal pylorus
gel diffusion precipitin
guanosine diphosphate (guanosine 5′-diphosphate)

GDR
glucose disposal rate

GDS
Geriatric Depression Scale
Gesell Developmental Scale (Schedules)
Global Deterioration Scale
Gordon diagnostic system
gradual dosage schedule

GDSS
Glasgow Dyspepsia Severity Score

GDT
gel development time
goal-directed therapy

GDU
gastroduodenal ulcer

GDV
gastric dilatation and volvulus [of dogs]

GDW
glass-distilled water

GE
gainfully employed
gastric emptying
gastroemotional
gastroenteritis
gastroenterology
gastroenterostomy
gastroesophageal
gastrointestinal endoscopy
gel electrophoresis
General Electric

generalized epilepsy
generator of excitation
genome equivalent
glandular epithelium
group exercise
NATO code for nerve agent isopropyl ethylphosphonofluoridate

G:E
granulocyte to erythroid ratio

Ge
Gerbich [blood group system]
germanium

GEA
gastroepiploic artery
general anesthesia (*See also* GA, gen-an)

GEB
gum elastic bougie

GEBT
gastric emptying breath test

GEC
galactose elimination capacity
glomerular epithelial cell

GED
General Education Development [high school equivalency]
graduated electronic decelerator

GEE
gait energy expenditure
Global Evaluation of Efficacy
glycine ethyl ester
graft enteric erosion

GEF
gastroesophageal fundoplication
glossoepiglottic fold
gonadotropin-enhancing factor
graft enteric fistula

GEFT
Group Embedded Figures Test

GEGB
Garren-Edwards gastric bubble

GEH
glycerol ester hydrolase

GEI
Grief Experience Inventory

GEIN
gradual elongation intramedullary nailing

GEJ
gastroesophageal junction

gel.
gelatin

GELS
gravity extension locking system

GEM
generalized erythema multiforme

GEMM
granulocyte, erythrocyte, monocyte, megakaryocyte

GEMM-CFC
granulocyte, erythrocyte, monocyte, megakaryocyte colony-forming cell

GE-MRI
gradient echo magnetic resonance imaging

GEMS
gel electrophoresis mass spectrometry
good emergency mother substitute

GEMSS
glaucomalike ectopia, microspherophakia, stiffness, shortness [syndrome]

GEMU
geriatric evaluation and management unit

GEN
gender (*See also* G)
generation
general (*See also* gen'l)
genetics (*See also* genet)
genital (*See also* genit)
gradual elongation nailing

gen.
genus [singular]

gen-an
general anesthesia (*See also* GA, GEA)

gen-endo
general anesthesia with endotracheal intubation

genet
genetic
genetics (*See also* GEN)

gen. et sp. nov.
new genus and species [L. *genus et species nova*]

genit
genital (*See also* GEN)
genitalia

gen'l
general (*See also* GEN)

gen. nov.
new genus [L. *genus novum*]

gen proc
general procedure

GENPS
genital neoplasm-papilloma syndrome

GEO
genetically engineered (enhanced) organism

GEP
gastric emptying procedure
gastroenteropancreatic
gel electrophoresis
granulin-epithelin precursor
gustatory evoked potential

GEPA
gastroepiploic artery

GEPG
gastroesophageal pressure gradient

GEQ
generic equivalent

GER
gastroesophageal reflux
geriatrics (*See also* geriat)
granular endoplasmic reticulum

Ger
German

GERD
gastroesophageal reflux disease

geriat
geriatric
geriatrics (*See also* GER)

GERL
Golgi endoplasmic reticulum lysosome

geront
gerontologic
gerontology

GERV
Germiston virus

GES
gastric emptying scintigraphy
Gifted Evaluation Scale
glucose-electrolyte solution
Group Encounter Scale (Survey)
Group Environment Scale

GE SPECT
gradient-echo single-photon emission computed tomography

GEST, gest
gestation(al)

GET
gastric emptying time
general endotracheal [anesthesia]
generalized essential telangiectasia
graded [treadmill] exercise test

GET1/2, GET$^1/_2$
gastric emptying half-time

GETA
general endotracheal anesthesia

GETV
gadolinium-enhancing tumor volume
Getah virus

GEU
geriatric evaluation unit
gestation, extrauterine

GeV
gigaelectron volt

GEWS
Gianturco expandable wire stent

GEX
gas exchange

G

GF
  gastric fistula
  gastric fluid
  germ-free
  girlfriend
  glass factor [tissue culture]
  globule fibril
  glomerular filtrate (filtration)
  gluten-free
  grandfather (*See also* GR-FR, GD FA)
  growth factor
  growth failure
  growth fraction
  NATO code for (nerve agent) cyclosarin
    (cyclohexyl methylphosphonofluoridate)
G-F
  globular-fibrous (protein)
gf
  gram-force
GFA
  glial fibrillary acidic [protein]
  global force applicator
GFAAS
  graphite furnace atomic absorption
    spectrometry
GFAP
  glial fibrillary acidic protein
GF-BAO
  gastric fluid, basal acid output
GFCL
  Goldmann fundus contact lens
GFD
  gluten-free diet
  Goodenough Figure Drawing
GFE
  gas-fluid exchange
GFFF
  gravitational field-flow fractionation
GFFS
  glycogen- and fat-free solid
GFH
  glucose-free Hanks [solution]
GFI
  glucagon-free insulin
  ground-fault interrupter
GFJ
  grapefruit juice (*See also* GJ)
GFL
  giant follicular lymphoma
GFLB
  giant follicular lymphoblastoma
GFM
  gingival fibromatosis
  good fetal movement
GFP
  gamma-fetoprotein
  gel-filtered platelet
  glomerular-filtered phosphate
  green fluorescence (fluorescent) protein

GFPM
  gastric first-pass metabolism [of ethanol]
GFR
  glomerular filtration rate
  growth factor receptor
  grunting, flaring, retracting [breathing]
GFS
  glaucoma filtering surgery
  global focal sclerosis
GFT
  gradient field transform
GFTA
  Goldman-Fristoe Test of Articulation
GFV
  Gabek Forest virus
G-F-W
  Goldman-Fristoe-Woodcock [Auditory
    Skills Test Battery]
GG
  galloping gangrene
  gamma globulin
  genioglossus
  glyceryl guaiacolate
  glycylglycine
  guar gum
G=G
  grips equal and good
GGA
  general gonadotropic activity
  ground-glass attenuation
GGCT
  ground-glass clotting time
GGE
  Gastrografin enema
  generalized glandular enlargement
  gradient gel electrophoresis
ggELISA
  glycoprotein-based enzyme-linked
    immunosorbent assay
GGFC
  gamma globulin-free calf [serum]
GGG
  glycine-rich gamma-glycoprotein
GGM
  glucose-galactose malabsorption
GGO
  ground-glass opacification (opacity)
GGPNA
  gamma-glutamyl-*p*-nitroanilide
GGPP
  geranylgeranylpyrophosphate
GGS
  glands, goiter, stiffness [of neck]
  group G streptococcus
GGT
  gamma (γ)-glutamyltransferase (gamma
    glutamyl transferase)
GGTase
  geranylgeranyltransferase

GGTP
gamma (γ)-glutamyl transpeptidase
GGU
giant gastric ulcer
GGV
Gan Gan virus
GgV-019/6A
Gaeumannomyces graminis virus 019/6A
GGVB
glucose-gelatin Veronal buffer [medium]
GgV-87-1-H
Gaeumannomyces graminis virus 87-1-H
GgV-T1-A
Gaeumannomyces graminis virus T1-A
GGYV
Gadget's Gully virus
GH
general health
general hospital
genetically hypertensive [rat]
genetic hemochromatosis
genetic hypertension
geniohyoid
gingival hyperplasia
glenohumeral
good health
growth hormone
GH3
Gerovital
GHA
glucoheptanoic acid
glucoheptonate acid
GHAQ
General High Altitude Questionnaire
GHB
gamma hydroxybutyrate (*See also* GBH)
gamma (γ)-hydroxybutyrate
GHb
glycosylated hemoglobin
GHBA
gamma (γ)-hydroxybutyric acid
GHBP
growth hormone-binding protein
GHBSS
gelatin Hanks buffered salt solution
GHCH
giant hepatic cavernous hemangioma
GHD
growth hormone deficiency
GHDA
growth hormone deficiency [syndrome]
in adults
GHDD
Ghoshal hematodiaphysial dysplasia
GHDT
Goodenough-Harris Drawing Test
GHF
growth hormone failure

GHHOS
Glasgow Homeopathic Hospital
Outcome Scale
GHI
growth hormone insensitivity
(insufficiency)
GHIH, GH-IH
growth hormone-inhibiting (inhibitory)
hormone
GHJ, G-H jt
glenohumeral joint
GHK
Goldman-Hodgkin-Katz [equation]
GHL
glenohumeral ligament
GHLC
glenohumeral ligament complex
GH-N
growth hormone normal
GHP
gated heart [blood] pool [scan]
GHPP
Genetically Handicapped Persons
Program
GHPQ
General Health Perception
Questionnaire
GHQ
General Health Questionnaire
GHR
granulomatous hypersensitivity
reaction
growth hormone receptor
GHRD
growth hormone receptor deficiency
GHRF, GH-RF
growth hormone-releasing factor
(*See also* GRF)
GHRH, GH-RH
growth hormone-releasing hormone
(*See also* GRH)
GHRH-GH-IGF
growth hormone-releasing
hormone–growth hormone-insulinlike
growth factor
GHRH-R
growth hormone-releasing hormone
receptor
GHRIF, GH-RIF
growth hormone release-inhibiting factor
(*See also* GRIF)
GHRIH, GH-RIH
growth hormone release-inhibiting
hormone
GHRP
growth hormone-releasing peptide
GHRP-5
growth hormone-releasing peptide 5

G

GHS
  growth hormone secretagogue
GHSR
  growth hormone secretagogue receptor
GHST
  growth hormone stimulation test
GHT
  geniculohypothalamic tract
  Glaucoma Hemifield Test
GHTN
  gestational hypertension
GHV
  goose hepatitis virus
  growth hormone variant
GHz
  gigahertz
GI
  gastrointestinal
  gelatin infusion [medium]
  gender identity
  General Inquiry
  Gingival Index
  glomerular index
  glucose intolerance
  glycemic index
  granuloma inguinale
  growth inhibiting (inhibition)
  guided imagery
Gi
  good impression [California
    Psychological Inventory]
G$_i$
  G inhibiting [protein]
gi
  gill [$^1/_4$ pint]
GIA
  gastrointestinal anastomosis
  gastrointestinal anisakiasis
  gastrointestinal assistant
  Global Institute for Asthma
GIB
  gastric ileal bypass
  gastrointestinal bleeding
GIBF
  gastrointestinal bacterial flora
GIC
  gastric interdigestive contraction
  general immunocompetence
GICA
  gastrointestinal cancer antigen
  gastrointestinal cancer-associated antigen
GID
  gastrointestinal distress
  gender identity disorder
GIDA
  gastrointestinal diagnostic area
GIF
  glycosylation-inhibiting factor

  gonadotropin-inhibitory factor
    [somatostatin]
  growth hormone-inhibiting factor
GIFAM
  giant intracanalicular fibroadenomyxoma
GIFT
  gamete intrafallopian transfer
  gastrointestinal fibrous tumor
  granulocyte immunofluorescence test
GIGT
  gastrointestinal glial/schwannoma tumor
GIH
  gastric-inhibitory hormone
  gastrointestinal hemorrhage
  gastrointestinal hormone
  glucose-dependent insulinotropic
    hormone
  growth-inhibiting hormone
GIK
  glucose-insulin-potassium [solution]
GIL
  gastrointestinal [tract] lymphoma
GILCU
  gradual increase in length and
    complexity of utterance
GILT
  gastrointestinal leiomyogenic tumor
GIM
  gonadotropin-inhibiting material
  gonadotropin-inhibitory material
  guided imagery and music
GING, ging
  gingiva(l) (*See also* G)
  gingivectomy (*See also* GV, GVTY)
GINSEST
  generalized interferography using spin
    echoes and stimulated echoes
g-ion
  gram-ion
GIOP
  glucocorticoid (steroid)-induced
    osteoporosis
GIP
  gastric inhibitory peptide (polypeptide)
  gastrointestinal polyposis
  giant-cell interstitial pneumonia
    (pneumonitis)
  glucose-dependent insulinotropic peptide
  glucose-dependent insulin-releasing
    peptide
  glucose insulin, potassium [solution]
  gonorrheal invasive peritonitis
GIPACT
  gastrointestinal pacemaker cell tumor
GIPU
  gastrointestinal postburn ulcer
  gastrointestinal procedure unit
GIQLI
  Gastrointestinal Quality of Life Index

GIR
    Global Improvement Rating
    glucose infusion rate
GIRMS
    gas isotope ratio mass spectrometry
GIS
    gas in stomach
    gastrointestinal series
    gastrointestinal symptom
    gastrointestinal system
    Gender Identity Service
GISA
    glycopeptide-insensitive *Staphylococcus*
        aureus
GIST
    gastrointestinal smooth [muscle] tumor
    gastrointestinal stromal tumor
GIT
    gastrointestinal tract
    glucose infusion test
    glutathione-insulin transhydrogenase
GITS
    gastrointestinal therapeutic system
    gut-derived infectious toxic shock
GITT
    gastrointestinal transit time
    glucose insulin tolerance test
GITUP
    glansplasty (glanuloplasty) and in situ
        tubularization of urethral plate
GIT-V
    Groningen Intelligence Test, short form
GIV
    gastrointestinal virus
    Great Island virus
giv
    give(n)
GIWU
    gastrointestinal workup
GJ
    gap junction
    gastric juice
    gastrojejunostomy
    grapefruit juice (*See also* GFJ)
GJAV
    Guajara virus
GJIC
    gap junction intercellular communication
GJLO
    gastrojejunal loop obstruction
GJT
    gastrojejunostomy tube
    glomus jugulare tumor
GK
    galactokinase
    Gamma Knife
    glomerulocystic kidney

glucokinase
    glycerol kinase
GKA
    glucokinase activator
    guinea pig keratocyte
GKD
    glycerol kinase deficiency
GKI
    glucose-potassium-insulin
GKMDT
    Graham-Kendall Memory for Designs
        Test
GKNa, GKN
    glucose-potassium-sodium [solution]
GKRS
    Gamma Knife radiosurgery
GKS
    Gamma Knife surgery
GL
    gastric lavage
    germline
    gland (*See also* gl)
    glaucoma (*See also* glau, glc)
    glomerular layer
    glucagon (*See also* Gln, GN)
    glycolipid
    glycosphingolipoid
    granular layer
    greatest length [fetus]
    gustatory lacrimation
Gl
    glabella (*See also* G)
g/L
    gram per liter
gl
    gland (*See also* GL)
    glandular (*See also* gland.)
GLA
    alpha (α)-galactosidase [gene]
    gamma (γ) linolenic acid
    gene-linkage analysis
    giant left atrium
    gingivolinguoaxial
    D-glucaric acid
    glucose-lowering agents
Gla
    4-carboxyglutamate
    4-carboxyglutamic acid
    gamma-carboxyglutamic acid
glac
    glacial
GLAD
    glenolabral articular disruption [lesion]
    gold-labeled antigen detection
        (technique)
gland.
    glandular (*See also* gl)

G

GLAT
galactose [enzyme] activator
glau
glaucoma (*See also* GL, glc)
GLB
gay, lesbian, bisexual
GLB-1
beta-galactosidase 1
GLBT
gay, lesbian, bisexual, transgender
(*See also* LGBT)
GLC
gas-liquid chromatography
Glc
glucose (*See also* G, GLU, gluc)
glc
glaucoma (*See also* GL, glau)
GlcA
gluconic acid
GLC/MS
gas-liquid chromatography/mass
spectrometry
GlcN
glucosamine
GlcNAc
N-acetylglucosamine
GlcUA
glucuronic acid
GLD
glanders (*Actinobacillus mallei*) vaccine
globoid leukodystrophy
glutamate dehydrogenase (*See also*
GLDH, GDH)
GLDH
glutamate dehydrogenase (*See also* GLD,
GDH)
GLF
ground-level fall
GLH
germinal layer hemorrhage
giant lymph node hyperplasia
glossolabial hemispasm
GLI
glicentin
glucagonlike immunoreactivity
GLIIRA
green light induced infrared absorption
GLIM
generalized linear interactive model(ing)
GLIO, glio
glioblastoma
glioma
GLIP
glucagonlike insulinotropic peptide
GLL
glabellolambda line [craniometric]
glycolipid lipidosis
GLM
general linear model

GLMA
gastric laryngeal mask airway
GLMM
generalized linear mixed model
GLN
glomerulonephritis
Gln
glucagon (*See also* GL, GN)
glutamine (*See also* Q)
GLNH
giant lymph node hyperplasia
GLNS
gay lymph node syndrome [obsolete]
GLO, glo
glyoxalase
glob.
globular [protein] (*See also* G)
globulin (*See also* G)
GLOC
gravity induced loss of consciousness
GLOF
global level of functioning
GLOM
glenolabral ovoid mass
GLORIA
gold-labeled optical rapid immunoassay
GLOV
Gray Lodge virus
GLP
glucagonlike peptide
glucose-L-phosphate
glycolipoprotein
good laboratory practice
grid laser photocoagulation
group-living program
GLP 1, 2
glucagonlike peptide 1, 2
Glp
5-oxoproline
GLPC
gas-liquid phase chromatography
GLPD
granular lymphocyte-proliferative
disorder
GLPP
glossolabiopharyngeal paralysis
GL-PP
glucose, postprandial
GLPT
glutamate pyruvate transaminase
GLR
graphic level recorder
gravity lumbar reduction
GLS
gait lock splint
generalized lymphadenopathy syndrome
guinea [pig] lung strip
GLSH
glucose, lactalbumin, serum, hemoglobin

GLTN
glomerulotubulonephritis
GLTT
glucose-lactate tolerance test
GLU
glucose (*See also* G, Glc, gluc)
glucuronidase
GLU-5
five-hour glucose tolerance test
Glu
glutamic acid (glutamate) (*See also* E, Glx)
GluA
glucuronic acid
GLUC
glucosidase
gluc
glucose (*See also* G, Glc, GLU)
GLUC-S
[urine] glucose spot [test]
glucur
glucuronide
glu ox.
glucose oxidase
GluR1
glutamide receptor subunit
GLUS
granulomatous lesions of unknown significance
GLUT
glucose transporter
GLUT1–GLUT15
glucose transporter 1-15
glut
gluteus
GLV
Gross leukemia virus
Gumbo Limbo virus
Glx
glutamic acid (*See also* E, Glu)
glutaminyl and/or glutamyl [indicates uncertainty between Glu and Gln] (*See also* Z)
GLY
glycerite (*See also* glyc)
glycerol (*See also* glyc)
glycyl
Gly
glycine (*See also* G)
glyc
glyceride
glycerin
glycerite (*See also* GLY)
glycerol (*See also* GLY)
GM
gastric mucosa
Geiger-Müller [counter]
general medical

general medicine
genetically modified
genetic manipulation
geometric mean
giant melanosome
gingival margin
grand mal
grandmother (*See also* GR-MO)
grand multiparity
granulocyte-macrophage
granulocyte-monocyte
gray matter
growth medium
monosialoganglioside [genetic marker]
GM+
gram-positive (*See also* G+, GP, gr+, GrP)
GM−
gram-negative (*See also* G−, GN, gr−, GrN)
Gm
allotype marker on heavy chains of immunoglobins
g/m
gallon per minute
g-m
gram-meter
GMA
glyceral methacrylate
glycol methacrylate
goat's milk anemia
gross motor activity
GMAV
Guama virus
GMB
gastric mucosal barrier
granulomembranous body
GMBF
gastric mucosal blood flow
GMC
general medical clinic
general medical condition
geometric mean concentration
giant migrating contraction
globulomaxillary cyst
grivet monkey cell
GMCD
grand mal convulsive disorder
GM-CFU
granulocyte-macrophage colony-forming unit
GM-CSA
granulocyte-macrophage colony-stimulating activity
GM-CSF
granulocyte-macrophage colony-stimulating factor

G

GMCU
gracilis myocutaneous unit
GMD
geometric mean diameter
glycopeptide moiety [modified]
derivative
GMDS
Griffiths Mental Developmental
Scale
GME
gaseous microembolus
graduate medical education
GMEPP
giant miniature endplate potential
GMER
gastric mucosal ectopia in rectum
GMF
glia maturation factor
GMFCS
Gross Motor Function Classification
System [cerebral palsy level I–V]
GMFM
Gross Motor Function Measure
GMH
germinal matrix hemorrhage
GMK
green monkey kidney [cells]
GML
glabellomeatal line
gut mucosal lymphocyte
g/mL
gram per milliliter
GMLOS
geometric mean length of stay
GMM
giant mammary myxoma
GMN
gradient moment nulling
GMO
genetically modified organism
g-mol
gram-molecule
GMP
gated stress myocardial perfusion
general medical panel
Good Manufacturing Practices
guanosine monophosphate (guanosine
5′-monophosphate)
guanylic acid [reductase, synthetase]
G-MP
G-myeloma protein
3′,5′-GMP
guanosine 3′,5′-cyclic phosphate
GMP-K
guanylate kinase
GMR
gallop, murmur, rub
gradient moment reduction (rephasing)
[magnetic resonance]

GMRH
germinal matrix related hemorrhage
GMS
galvanic muscle stimulation
general medicine and surgery (See also
GM&S)
geriatric mental state
glyceryl monostearate
goniodysgenesis, mental retardation,
short stature
grand mal seizure
Grocott-Gomori methenamine silver
[stain]
GM&S
general medicine and surgery (See also
GMS)
GMSPS
Glasgow Meningococcal Septicemia
Prognostic Score
GMT
geometric mean titer
gingival margin trimmer
Greenwich Mean Time
GMV
gram-molecular volume
GMW
gram-molecular weight
GN
ganglioneuroma
gaze nystagmus
glomerulonephritis
glucagon (See also GL, Gln)
gnotobiote
gonococcus (See also GC)
gram-negative (See also G−, GM−,
gr−, GrN)
G:N
glucose to nitrogen [ratio in urine or
water]
Gn
gnathion [craniometric]
gonadotropin
GNA
Galanthus nivalis agglutinin
general nursing assistance
GNB
ganglioneuroblastoma
gram-negative bacillus
gram-negative bacteremia
GNBL
ganglioneuroblastoma
GNBM
gram-negative bacillary meningitis
GNC
general nursing care
glandular neck cell
gram-negative coccus (See also G−C)
GNCA
gastric noncancerous area

GND
  gram-negative diplococcus
gnd
  ground
GNG
  generalized nephrographic
GNID
  gram-negative intracellular diplococcus
GNIP
  glycogenin-interacting protein
GNR
  gram-negative rod (*See also* G–R)
GNRF
  guanine nucleotide-releasing factor
GnRF
  gonadotropin-releasing factor (*See also* GRF)
GnRH, Gn-RH
  gonadotropin-releasing hormone (*See also* GRH)
GnRHa
  gonadotropin-releasing hormone agonist
GnRH-R
  gonadotropin-releasing hormone receptor
GNRP
  guanine nucleotide regulatory protein
GNS
  gram-negative sepsis
G/NS
  glucose in normal saline
GnSAF
  gonadotropin surge attenuating factor
GΩ
  gigaohm [one billion ohms]
GO
  generalized obesity
  geroderma osteodysplastica
  glucose oxidase (*See also* GOD)
  gonorrhea
  Graves ophthalmopathy
  gynecooncology
G&O
  gas and oxygen
Go
  Golgi
  gonion [craniometric]
GOA
  generalized osteoarthritis
GOAT
  Galveston Orientation and Amnesia Test
GOBAB
  gamma-hydroxy-beta-aminobutyric acid
GOBI
  growth monitoring, oral rehydration, breast feeding, immunization
GOCL-II
  Gordon Occupational Checklist-II

GOCS
  Global Obsessive-Compulsive Scale
GOD
  generation of diversity
  glucose oxidase (*See also* GO)
GOD/POD
  glucose oxidase-peroxidase [method]
GOE
  gas, oxygen, ether [anesthesia]
GOH
  geroderma osteodysplastica hereditaria
GOI
  glycerol-3-phosphate oxidase
GOLD
  Global Initiative Chronic Obstructive Lung Disease [COPD severity staging]
GOLPH
  Giannetti Online Psychosocial History
GOM
  granular osmiophilic material
GOMBO
  growth retardation, ocular abnormalities, microcephaly, brachydactyly, oligophrenia
GOMV
  Gomoka virus
GON
  gonococcal ophthalmia neonatorum
  greater occipital neuritis
GONA
  glaucomatous optic nerve atrophy
GOND
  glaucomatous optic nerve damage
gonio
  gonioscopy
GOO
  gastric outlet obstruction
GO-POG
  gonion to pogonion [craniometric]
GOQ
  glucose oxidation quotient
GOR
  gastroesophageal reflux
  general operating room
GORD
  gastro-oesophageal reflux disease [British]
GORT
  Gilmore Oral Reading Test
  Gray Oral Reading Test
GORT-3
  Gray Oral Reading Test, Third Edition
GORT-R
  Gray Oral Reading Test-Revised
GORV
  Gordil virus

G

GOS
    galactose oxidase-Schiff [reaction]
    galactose oxidase and Schiff
      reagent
    Glasgow Outcome Scale (Score)

GOSV
    Gossas virus

GOT
    glucose oxidase test
    glutamic-oxaloacetic transaminase
    goals of treatment

GOTM, GOT-M
    glutamic-oxaloacetic transaminase,
      mitochondrial

GOT-S
    glutamic-oxaloacetic transaminase,
      soluble

govt
    government

GOX
    glucose oxidation

GP
    gastroplasty
    general paralysis
    general paresis
    general practice
    general practitioner
    general proprioception
    general purpose
    genetic prediabetes
    geometric progression
    globus pallidus
    glucose phosphate
    glucose polymer
    glucose production
    glutathione peroxidase (*See also*
      GPx)
    glycerophosphate
    glycopeptide
    glycoprotein
    gram-positive (*See also* GM+, gr+,
      GrP)
    grandparent
    group (*See also* g, grp)
    guinea pig
    gutta-percha

G/P
    gait practice
    gravida/para

G-1,6-P
    glucose-1,6-phosphate

G3P, G-3-P
    glyceraldehyde 3-phosphate

G6P
    glucose-6-phosphate

gp
    gene product
    glycoprotein
    glycosylated protein

gp 41
    glycosylated protein spanning viral
      envelope

GPA
    gelatin particle agglutination
    global program on AIDS
    glutaraldehyde, picric acid, acetic acid
    grade point average
    gravida, para, abortus
    guinea pig albumin

GPAC
    gram-positive anaerobic coccus

GPAIS
    guinea pig antiinsulin serum

G6PASE, G-6-Pase
    glucose-6-phosphatase

G3PAT
    glycerol-3-phosphate acyltransferase

GPB
    glossopharyngeal breathing
    gram-positive bacillus
    gram-positive bacteremia

GPBB
    glycogen phosphorylase isoenzyme
      BB

GPBP
    guinea pig myelin-basic protein

GPC
    gastric parietal cell
    gel permeation chromatography
    giant papillary conjunctivitis
    glycerophosphorylcholine
      (glycerolphosphorylcholine)
    G-protein coupled
    gram-positive coccus (*See also* G+C)
    granular progenitor cell
    guinea pig complement

GPCL
    gas permeable contact lens

GPCR
    G protein-coupled receptor

GPC:TP
    glycerophosphorylcholine to total
      phosphate ratio

GPD
    glycerophosphate dehydrogenase
    guinea pig dander

G6PD, G-6-PD
    glucose-6-phosphate dehydrogenase
      [deficiency]

G6PDA
    glucose-6-phosphate dehydrogenase,
      variant A

G3PDH
    glyceraldehyde-3-phosphate
      dehydrogenase

GPE
    glycerylphosphorylethanolamine
    guinea pig embryo

gpELISA
glycoprotein-based enzyme-linked immunosorbent assay

GPF
glomerular plasma flow
granulocytosis-promoting factor
greater palatine foramen

GPGG
guinea pig gamma globulin

GPGL
gamma probe guided lymphoscintigraphy

GPH
giant papillary hypertrophy
gonococcal perihepatitis

GPHN
giant pigmented hairy nevus

GPI
general paralysis (paresis) of insane
Gingival-Periodontal Index
glucose phosphate isomerase
glucose-6-phosphate isomerase
glycosylphosphatidylinositol
Gordon Personal Inventory
gram-positive identification
guinea pig ileum

GPIIa
glycoprotein IIa

GPIIb
glycoprotein IIb

GPIIb/IIIa
glycoprotein IIb-IIIa [inhibitor]

GPIPID
guinea pig intraperitoneal infectious dose

GPI-PLD
glycosylphosphatidylinositol specific phospholipase D

GPJ
glossopalatal junction

GPK
guinea pig kidney [antigen]

GPKA
guinea pig kidney absorption [test]

GPLP
glossopalatolabial paralysis

G-PLT
giant platelets

Gply
gingivoplasty

GPM
general preventive medicine
giant pigment melanosome

GPMAL
gravida, para, multiple births, abortions, live births

GPMT
guinea pig maximization test

GPN
glossopharyngeal nerve
glossopharyngeal neuralgia

GPO
group purchasing organization

GPOA
primary open angle glaucoma

GPP
glossopharyngeal paralysis
Gordon Personal Profile

GPPI
Gordon Personal Profile Inventory

GPPQ
General Purpose Psychiatric Questionnaire

GPR
glucose production rate
good partial response
gram-positive rod (*See also* G+R)
Grenoble-Paris-Rennes [epilepsy]

GPRBC
guinea pig red blood cell

GPRL
gamma probe radiolocalization

GPRVS
giant prosthetic reinforcement of visceral sac

GPS
gravitational platelet separation
gray platelet syndrome
guinea pig serum (spleen)

GP-ST
group A streptococcus direct test

GPT
glutamic-pyruvic transaminase
guinea pig trachea

GpTh
group therapy (*See also* GT)

GPTSM
guinea pig tracheal smooth muscle

GPU
guinea pig unit

GPUT
galactose phosphate uridyl transferase

GPx
glutathione peroxidase (*See also* GP)

GQAP
general question-asking program

GR
gamma (γ) ray (roentgen)
gastric resection
gastric retention
generalized rash
general relief
general research

GR *(continued)*
glucocorticoid receptor
glucose response
gluthathione reductase (*See also* GSR)
good recovery
granulocyte
gravid (*See also* G)
growth rate
[pulse] generated runoff

G−R
gram-negative rod (*See also* GNR)

G+R
gram-positive rod (*See also* GPR)

Gr
Greek (*See also* G)

gr
grade (*See also* G)
graft
grain
gray
great
gross (*See also* GRS)

gr+
gram-positive (*See also* G+, GM+, GP, GrP)

gr−
gram-negative (*See also* G−, GM−, GN, GrN)

GRA
gated radionuclide angiography
glucocorticoid-remediable aldosteronism
gonadotropin-releasing agent

grad.
gradient
gradual(ly)
graduate

GRAE
generally regarded as effective

gran
granular
granulate(d)
granule

GRAPPA
generalized autocalibrating partially parallel acquisition

GRAS
Generally Recognized As Safe

GRASE
Generally Recognized as Safe and Effective

GRASS
gradient-recalled acquisition in steady state
gradient-refocused acquisition in steady state

grav
gravida [pregnant] (*See also* G)

grav ō
no pregnancies

GRB
general reading backwardness

GRB2
growth factor receptor-bound protein 2

GRBAS
grade, rough, breathy, asthenic, strained [voice quality]

GRC
gastric remnant cancer

GRD
beta-glucuronidase (*See also* GRS, GUSB)
gastroesophageal reflux disease
gender role definition

grd
ground

GRE
glucocorticoid response element
glycopeptide-resistant enterococcus
graded resistive exercise
gradient recall(ed) (refocused) echo [imaging technique]
graduated resistance exercise
Graduate Record Examination

GREAT
ghost reduction by equalized acquisition triplets [imaging]
Graduate Record Examination Aptitude Test

GRF
gelatin, resorcinol, formaldehyde
gonadotropin-releasing factor (*See also* GnRF)
growth hormone-releasing factor (*See also* GHRF, GH-RF)

GRFoma
growth hormone-releasing factor tumor

GR-FR
grandfather (*See also* GF, GD FA)

GRG
glycine-rich glycoprotein

GRH
glucocorticoid-remediable hyperaldosteronism
gonadotropin-releasing hormone (*See also* GnRH)
growth hormone-releasing hormone (*See also* GHRH, GH-RH)

GRID
gay-related immunodeficiency disease [obsolete]

GRIF
growth hormone release-inhibiting factor (*See also* GHRIF, GH-RIF)

GRIMS
Golombok-Rust Inventory of Marital State

GRIP 1
glucocorticoid receptor-interacting protein 1

GRKP
gentamicin-resistant *Klebsiella pneumoniae*

GRL
granular layer

GR-MO
grandmother (*See also* GM)

GRN
granule
green (*See also* G, Grn)

GrN
gram-negative (*See also* G−, GM−, GN, gr−)

Grn
glycerone
green (*See also* G, GRN)

GRO
growth-related oncogene

GROPE
generalized compensation for resonance offset and pulse length errors [imaging]

gros
coarse [L. *grossus*]

GROV
Guaroa virus

GRP
gastrin-releasing peptide
glycine-rich RNA-binding protein

GrP
gram-positive (*See also* G+, GM+, GP, gr+)

grp
group (*See also* g, GP)

GRPP
glicentin-related pancreatic polypeptide

GRPR
gastrin-releasing peptide receptor

GRPS
glucose-Ringer-phosphate solution

GRS
beta-glucuronidase (*See also* GRD, GUSB)
Graphic Rating Scale
gross (*See also* gr)

GRSA
glycopeptide-resistant *Staphylococcus aureus*

GRS&MIC
gross and microscopic

GRT
gastric residence time
giant retinal tear
glandular replacement therapy

good response to treatment
grasp and release test
group randomized trial
Group Reading Test

GRTH
generalized resistance to thyroid hormone

GrTr
graphite treatment

GRV
gastric residual volume

GRW
giant ragweed [test]

GRWR
graft-to-recipient weight ratio

gr wt
gross weight

GS
gallstone
gastric shield
gastrocnemius [and] soleus [muscles]
generalized seizure
general surgery
gestational sac
gestational score
Gleason score
gliosarcoma
glomerular sclerosis
glucagon secretion
glutamine synthetase
gluteal sets
goat serum
graft survival
Gram stain (*See also* G)
granulocyte substance
granulocytic sarcoma
grip strength
group section
group specific (*See also* gs)
gut sutures

G/S
glucose and saline

G&S
gait and stance

G$_s$
G-stimulating protein

gs
group specific (*See also* GS)

g/s
gallon per second

GSA
galactosyl [human] serum albumin
general somatic afferent [nerve]
Gross [sarcoma] virus antigen
group-specific amplification
group-specific antigen
guanidinosuccinic acid

G

GSA65
Giardia-specific antigen 65
GSAP
greatest single allergen present
GSB
graduated spinal block
Gschwend, Scheier, Bahler [elbow
arthroplasty]
GSBG
gonadal steroid-binding globulin
GSC
gas-solid chromatography
gravity settling culture [plate]
greater saphenous vein
G-SC
guanosine-coupled spleen cell
GSCN
giant serotonin-containing neuron
GSD
gallstone disease
genetically significant dose [mutagenic
radiation]
glutathione synthetase deficiency
glycogen storage disease [type Ia, Ib,
II–VII] (*See also* GT1-GT10)
GSE
general somatic efferent [nerve]
genital self-examination
gluten-sensitive enteropathy
grips strong and equal
GSENSE
generalized sensitivity encoding
(SENSE)
GSF
galactosemic fibroblast
genital skin fibroblast
GSH
glomerulus-stimulating hormone
glutathione
golden Syrian hamster
Green-Seligson-Henry [orthopedic nail]
growth-stimulating hormone
GSHP
reduced glutathione peroxidase
GSI
genuine stress incontinence
Global Severity Index
Group Styles Inventory
GSI-BSI
Global Severity Index of Brief
Symptom Inventory
GSIS
glucose-stimulated insulin secretion
GSK
glycogen synthetase kinase
GSK3
glycogen synthase kinase 3
GSL
goniosynechialysis

GSM
gray-scale median
GSMD
gestational sac and maternal date
GSMS
Great Smoky Mountains Study of Youth
GS-MS
gas spectrography-mass
spectrophotometry
GSN
giant serotonin-containing neuron
GSNO
S-nitrosoglutathione
GSP
galvanic skin potential
generalized social phobia
general survey panel
glycogen synthetase phosphatase
glycosylated serum protein
GSPECT
gated single-photon emission computed
tomography
GSPN
greater superficial petrosal neurectomy
GSR
galvanic skin resistance (response)
gastrosalivary reflex
generalized Shwartzman reaction
glutathione reductase (*See also* GR)
gunshot residue
GSRA
galvanic skin response audiometry
GSRS
Gastrointestinal Symptom Rating Scale
GSS
gamete-shedding substance
gestational sac size
gloves and socks syndrome
GSSG
glutathione disulfide
oxidized glutathione
GSSI
Global Sexual Satisfaction Index
GSSR
generalized Sanarelli-Shwartzman
reaction
GST
glutathione-S-transferase
gold salt therapy
graphic stress telethermometry
graphic stress thermography
group striction
GSTF
glucose-sensitive transcription factor
GSUI
genuine stress urinary incontinence
GSV
golden shiner virus
great saphenous vein

GSVT
greater saphenous vein thrombophlebitis
GSW
gunshot wound
GSWA
gunshot wound to abdomen
GSWH
gunshot wound to head
GT
gait
gait training
galactosyl transferase
gamma-glutamyl transferase
Gamow-Teller [strength]
gastrostomy tube (*See also* G-tube)
generation time (*See also* Tg)
gene therapy
genetic therapy
gingiva treatment
Glanzmann thrombasthenia (*See also* GTA)
glucagon test
glucose tolerance
glucose transport
glucuronyl transferase
glutamyl transpeptidase
glycityrosine
grand total
granulation tissue (*See also* g/t)
greater trochanter
great toe
green tea
group tension
group therapy (*See also* GpTh)
GT1-GT10
glycogen storage disease, types 1 to 10
G&T
gowns and towels
⚠ **gt.**
drop [L. *gutta*] [apothecary] ⚠
g/t
granulation time
granulation tissue (*See also* GT)
GTA
Glanzmann thrombasthenia (*See also* GT)
global transient amnesia
glutaraldehyde
GTAM
Gore-Tex augmentation material (membrane)
GTB
gastrointestinal tract bleeding
GTC
generalized tonic-clonic
GTCS
generalized tonic-clonic seizure

GTD
gestational trophoblastic disease
GTE
general therapeutic exercise
green tea extract
GTF
gastrostomy tube feeding
glucose tolerance factor
glucosyltransferase
GTH
gonadotropic hormone (*See also* GDH)
GTHR
generalized thyroid hormone resistance
GTI
genital tract infection
GTL
glomerular tip lesion
GTM
generalized tendomyopathy
GTN
gestational trophoblastic neoplasia (neoplasm)
glomerulotubulonephritis
glyceryl trinitrate (nitroglycerin)
GTO
Golgi tendon organ
GTP
deoxyguanosine triphosphate
glutamyl transpeptidase
green tea polyphenol
guanosine triphosphate (guanosine 5′-triphosphate)
guanyltriphosphate
GTPase
guanosine triphosphatase
GTR
galvanic tetanus ratio
generalized time reflex
granulocyte turnover rate
gross total resection
guided tissue regeneration
GTS
glucose transport system
guided trephine system
GTSTD
Grid Test of Schizophrenic Thought Disorder
GTT
gelatin-tellurite-taurocholate [agar]
gestational transient thyrotoxicosis
gestational trophoblastic tumor
glucose tolerance test
⚠ **gtt.**
drops [L. guttae] [apothecary] ⚠
GTT3H
glucose tolerance test 3 hours

G

G-tube
 gastrostomy tube (*See also* GT)
GTV
 gross tumor volume
GU
 gastric ulcer
 gastric upset
 genitourinary
 glucose uptake
 glycogenic unit
 gonococcal urethritis
 gravitational ulcer
GUA
 group of units of analysis [statistics]
Gua
 guanine (*See also* G)
GUAR
 guarantor
GUD
 genital ulcer disease
GUI
 genitourinary infection
guid
 guidance
GUK
 guanylate kinase
GULHEMP
 general [physique], upper [extremity],
  lower [extremity], hearing, eyesight,
  mentality, personality
Guo
 guanosine
GURV
 Gurupi virus
GUS
 genitourinary sphincter
 genitourinary system
GUSB
 beta-glucuronidase (*See also* GRD,
  GRS)
guttat.
 guttatim [drop by drop]
GV
 gastric volume
 gentian violet
 germinal vesicle
 gingivectomy (*See also* GING, ging,
  GVTY)
 granulosis virus
 Gross virus
 growth velocity
gv
 governing vessel [acupuncture]
GVA
 general visceral afferent [nerve]
GVB
 gelatin-Veronal buffer
GVBD
 germinal vesicle breakdown

GVD
 graft vessel disease
GVE
 gastric vascular ectasia
 general visceral efferent [nerve]
GVF
 Goldman visual fields
 good visual fields
GVH
 generalized visceral hypersensitivity
 graft versus host
GVHD, GvHD
 graft-versus-host disease [grade 1–4]
GVHR
 graft-versus-host reaction (response)
GVL
 graft-versus-leukemia [effect]
GVM
 graft-versus-malignancy
GVS
 gastric vertical stapling
GVSDS
 growth velocity standard deviation
  score
GVT
 graft-versus-tumor
GVTY
 gingivectomy (*See also* GING, ging,
  GV)
GW
 gastric wrap
 general ward
 germ warfare
 gigawatt
 glycerin in water
 gradual withdrawal
 group work
 guidewire
 gunshot wound
G&W
 glycerin and water
G/W
 glucose in water
GWA
 gunshot wound of abdomen
GWAFD
 Genée-Wiedemann acrofacial dysostosis
GWBI
 General Well-Being Index
GWBS
 global ward behavior scale
GWD
 Guinea worm disease
GWE
 glycerin and water enema
GWG
 generalized Wegener granulomatosis
GWMFT
 Graded Wolf Motor Function Test

GWS
Gulf War syndrome
GWT
gunshot wound of throat
GWX
guide wire exchange
GX
cannot be assessed [TNM histologic classification]
GXM
glucuronoxylomannan
GXP
graded exercise program
GXT
graded exercise test
GXT EKG
graded exercise test electrocardiogram

Gy
gray [unit of absorbed dose of ionizing radiation]
GYN, gyn
gynecologic
gynecology
GYS
guaranteed yield strength
GZAS
Guilford-Zimmerman Aptitude Survey
GZII
Guilford-Zimmerman Interest Inventory
GZPT
Guilford-Zimmerman Personality Test
GZTS
Guilford-Zimmerman Temperament Survey

G

H

deflection in His bundle in electrogram [spike]

draft, drink [L. *haustus*] (*See also* haust., ht.)

electrically induced spinal reflex

eta [seventh letter of Greek alphabet uppercase]

Haemophilus

Hauch [motile bacteria with flagellum]

head

heart (*See also* HT)

heavy

heelstick (*See also* HS)

height (*See also* ht, Hgt)

Helicobacter

hemagglutination (*See also* HA)

hemisphere (*See also* hemi)

hemolysis (*See also* HEM, hem, HL)

hemolytic (*See also* HEM, hem)

henry [electric inductance]

hernia (*See also* her., hern)

herniate(d) (herniation) (*See also* her., hern)

heroin

high (*See also* h)

hippocampus (*See also* HC)

histidine (*See also* His)

history (*See also* hist, Hx, Hy)

Hoffmann [reflex] (*See also* Hoff)

Holzknecht [unit]

homosexual

horizontal (*See also* h, hor, horiz)

hormone (*See also* horm)

horse [slang for heroin] (*See also* Ho)

hot

Hounsfield [unit] (*See also* HU)

hour (*See also* h, HR, hr)

human (*See also* h, hu)

husband (*See also* husb, HSB)

hydrogen

hydrolysis

hygiene (*See also* hyg)

hygienic (*See also* hyg)

hyperopia (hypermetropia) (*See also* h, Hy)

hyperopic (*See also* Hy)

hyperphoria (*See also* HP)

hyperplasia

hypothalamus (*See also* HT, HTH, hyp)

magnetic field strength

NATO code for impure sulfur mustard (mustard gas dichlorodiethyl sulfide)

objective angle

hypodermic [injection] (*See also* hypo, (H))

region of sarcomere containing only myosin filaments [Ger. *heller* lighter]

vectorcardiography electrode [neck]

(H)

hip

hypodermic [injection] (*See also* H, hypo)

H^+

hydrogen ion

H_0

null hypothesis

^1H

hydrogen 1 isotope [protium] [light hydrogen]

H_1

alternative hypothesis

histamine [receptor type] 1

^2H

hydrogen 2 isotope [deuterium] [heavy hydrogen]

H_2

histamine 2

histamine [receptor type] 2

^3H

hydrogen 3 isotope [tritium]

H

specific enthalpy [heat content, thermodynamics]

h

hand-rearing [of experimental animals]

hecto-

heteromorphic [region]

high (*See also* H)

horizontal (*See also* H, hor, horiz)

hour (*See also* H, HR, hr)

human (*See also* H, hu)

human response

hundred

negatively staining region of chromosome

specific enthalpy

h2

heritability

h

Planck constant [physics]

HA

hallux abductus

halothane anesthesia

H antigen

harm avoidance

Hartley [guinea pig]

headache (*See also* H/A)

hearing aid

HA *(continued)*
  heart attack
  heated
  heated aerosol *(See also* ht aer)
  height age
  hemadsorbent
  hemadsorption [test]
  hemagglutinating activity
  hemagglutinating antibody
  hemagglutinating antigen
  hemagglutination *(See also* H)
  hemolytic anemia
  hemophiliac with adenopathy
  hepatic adenoma
  hepatic artery
  hepatitis A *(See also* hep)
  hepatitis-associated [virus]
  herpangina
  heterophil (heterophile) antibody
    (See also het)
  high anxiety
  hippocampal asymmetry
  hippuric acid
  histamine *(See also* Hi)
  histidine ammonialyase
  histocompatibility antigen
  Horton arteritis
  hospital acquired
  hospital administration *(See also* HAD)
  hospital admission
  household activity
  hyaluronan
  hyaluronic acid
  hydroxyanisole
  hydroxyapatite (hydroxylapatite)
  hyperalimentation *(See also* HAL,
    hyperal, hyper-al)
  hyperandrogenic anovulation
  hyperandrogenism
  hypermetropic astigmatism
  hyperopia, absolute
  hypersensitivity alveolitis
  hypoplastic aorta
  hypothalmic amenorrhea
HA1–HA2
  hemadsorption type 1, 2
H/A
  headache *(See also* HA)
  holding area
H:A
  head to abdomen ratio [fetal]
  height to age ratio
Ha
  hahnium
H/a
  home with advice
HAA
  hearing aid amplifier
  hemolytic anemia antigen

  hepatitis A antibody *(See also* HAAb)
  hepatitis A antigen *(See also* HAAg)
  hepatitis-associated antigen
  hepatitis-associated aplastic anemia
  heterocyclic aromatic amine
  hospital activity analysis
HAAb
  hepatitis A antibody *(See also* HAA)
HAAg
  hepatitis A antigen *(See also* HAA)
HAAP
  HTLV-1-associated arthropathy
HAART
  highly active antiretroviral therapy
    (treatment)
HAAS
  Havighurst Activities and Attitudes
    Scale
HAb
  heart antibody
HABA
  hydroxyazobenzoic acid
  hydroxybenzeneazobenzoic acid
HABF
  hepatic artery blood flow
HAb/HAd
  horizontal abduction/adduction
HAC
  human artificial chromosome
HAc
  acetic acid
HACA
  human antichimeric antibodies
HACCP
  Hazard Analysis Critical Control
    Point(s)
HACE
  hepatic artery chemoembolization
  high-altitude cerebral edema
HACEK
  Haemophilus aphrophilus, Actinobacillus
    actinomycetemcomitans,
    Cardiobacterium hominis, Eikenella
    corrodens, and Kingella kingae
HAChT
  high-affinity choline transport
HACR
  hereditary adenomatosis of colon and
    rectum
HACS
  hyperactive child syndrome
HAD
  hearing aid dispenser
  hemadsorption [test] *(See also* HA)
  HIV (human immunodeficiency
    virus)-associated dementia
  hospital administration *(See also* HA)
  Hospital Anxiety and Depression [scale]
    (See also HADS)

human adjuvant disease
hypertonic acetate dextran
hypophysectomized alloxan diabetic

HADD
hydroxyapatite deposition disease

HAd-I
hemadsorption inhibition

HADS
Hospital Anxiety and Depression Scale
(*See also* HAD)

HadV 1-51
human adenovirus 1–51

HadV A, B, C, D, E, F
human adenovirus A, B, C, D, E, F

HAE
health appraisal examination
hearing aid evaluation
hepatic artery embolization
herb-related adverse event
hereditary angioedema (angioneurotic)
edema (*See also* HANE)

HAEC
Hirschsprung-associated enterocolitis
human aortic endothelial cell

HAEM
herpes (simplex)-associated erythema
multiforme

HAF
hepatic arterial flow
hyperalimentation fluid

HaF
Hageman factor [factor XII] (*See also*
HF)

HAFM
hospital-acquired *Plasmodium falciparum*
malaria

HAFOE
high air flow with oxygen entrainment

hAFP
human alpha (α)-fetoprotein

HAG
heat-aggregated globulin
Histoplasma capsulatum antigen

HAGG
hyperimmune antivariola gamma (γ)
globulin

HAGL
humeral avulsion of glenohumeral
ligament

HAH
high-altitude headache

HAHTG
horse antihuman thymus globulin

HAI
hemagglutination inhibition [titer]
(*See also* HI)
hepatic arterial infusion

hepatitis activity index
histologic activity index
history activity index
hospital-acquired infection

HAIC
hepatic arterial infusional chemotherapy

H&A Ins
health and accident insurance

HAIR-AN, HAIRAN
hirsutism, androgen excess, insulin
resistance, acanthosis nigricans
[syndrome]
hyperandrogenism, insulin resistance,
acanthosis nigricans [syndrome]

HaK
hamster kidney

HAL
hand-assisted laparoscopy
hemorrhoidal artery ligation
hepatic artery ligation
hip axis length
hyperalimentation (*See also* HA, hyperal,
hyper-al)
hypoplastic acute leukemia

HALE
health-adjusted life expectancy

HALF
hyperacute liver failure

HALK
hyperopic automated lamellar
keratoplasty

halluc
hallucination

HALN
hand-assisted laparoscopic [radical]
nephrectomy (*See also* HALRN)

HALNU
hand-assisted laparoscopic
nephroureterectomy

HALO
hemorrhage, abruption, labor, placenta
previa with mild bleeding
hours after light onset

HALP
hyperalphalipoproteinemia

HALRI
hospital-acquired lower respiratory
infections

HALRN
hand-assisted laparoscopic radical
nephrectomy (*See also* HALN)

HALS
hand-assisted laparoscopic surgery
Health and Activity Limitation Survey

HALT
Heroin Antagonist And Learning
Therapy [program]

H

319

HALV
    human AIDS lymphotropic virus
HaLV
    hamster leukemia virus
HAM
    hearing aid microphone
    helical axis of motion
    human albumin microsphere
    human alveolar macrophage
    human T-cell lymphotropic virus 1
        (HTLV-1) associated myelopathy
    hypoparathyroidism, adrenal insufficiency
        (Addison disease) mucocutaneous
        candidiasis [syndrome]
HAM-56
    human alveolar macrophage 56
HAMA
    Hamilton Anxiety [Scale]
    human antimouse (antimurine) antibody
HAMD
    Hamilton Depression [Scale]
HAMM
    human albumin minimicrosphere
hams.
    hamstrings (See also HS)
HaMSV
    Harvey murine sarcoma virus
HAM/TSP
    HTLV-1-associated myelopathy or
        tropical spastic paraparesis
HAN
    Health Alert Network
    heroin-associated nephropathy
    hyperplastic alveolar nodule
HANA
    hemagglutinin neuraminidase
handicp
    handicapped (See also HC, HCAP, HP)
HANE
    hereditary angioneurotic edema (See also
        HAE)
HANES
    health and nutrition examination survey
hANF
    human atrial natriuretic factor
hANP
    human atrial natriuretic peptide
HAO
    hearing aid orientation
HAODM
    hypoplasia of anguli oris depressor
        muscle
HAP
    hazardous air pollution
    hearing aid problem
    held after positioning
    hepatic arterial-dominant phase
    hepatic arterial phase
    heredopathia atactica polyneuritiformis

high-amplitude peristalsis
    histamine acid phosphate
    home antibiotic program
    hospital-acquired pneumonia
    humoral antibody production
    hydrolyzed animal protein
    hydroxyapatite fractionation procedure
    hyperthermic antiblastic perfusion
HA-P
    hemagglutinin-protease
HAP1
    huntingtin-associated protein 1
HAPA
    hemagglutinating antipenicillin antibody
HAPC
    high-amplitude peristaltic contraction
        [esophagus]
    hospital-acquired penetration contact
HAPD
    home automated peritoneal dialysis
HAPE
    high-altitude pulmonary edema
HAPE-r
    high-altitude pulmonary edema, resistant
HAPE-s
    high-altitude pulmonary edema,
        susceptible
HA-PI
    hepatic arterial pulsatility index
HAPO
    high-altitude pulmonary oedema
        [British]
HAPS
    hepatic arterial perfusion scintigraphy
HAPTO
    haptoglobin (See also HP, Hp, Hpt)
HAPVC
    hemianomalous pulmonary venous
        connection
HAPVD
    hemianomalous pulmonary venous
        drainage
HAPVR
    hemianomalous pulmonary venous return
HAQ
    Headache Assessment Questionnaire
    [Stanford] Health Assessment
        Questionnaire
HAQ DI
    Health Assessment Questionnaire
        Disability Index
HAR
    high-altitude retinopathy
    hyperacute rejection
Har
    homoarginine
HARD
    hydrocephalus, agyria, retinal dysplasia
        [syndrome]

HARD+/-E
 hydrocephalus, agyria, retinal dysplasia
 with or without encephalocele
 [syndrome]
HARDI
 high-angular resolution
 diffusion-weighted imaging
HAREM
 heparin assay rapid easy method
HARH
 high-altitude retinal hemorrhage
HARM
 heparin assay rapid method
harm.
 harmonic
HARP
 harmonic phase
 homeless and at-risk population
 Hospital Admission Risk Profile
 hypobetalipoproteinemia, acanthocytosis,
 retinitis pigmentosa, pallidal
 degeneration [syndrome]
HARPPS
 heat, absence of use, redness, pain, pus,
 swelling [symptoms of infection]
HARS
 Hamilton Anxiety Rating Scale
 HIV (human immunodeficiency virus)
 associated adipose redistribution
 syndrome
HART
 hyperfractionated accelerated radiation
 therapy
HAS
 Hamilton Anxiety Scale
 headache associated with sexual
 activity
 health advisory service
 high-amplitude sucking [technique]
 highest asymptomatic [dose]
 hospitalized attempted suicide
 hydrocephalus due to stenosis of
 aqueduct of Sylvius
 hyperalimentation solution
 hypertensive arteriosclerosis
 (atherosclerosis)
HASCHD
 hypertensive atherosclerotic
 (arteriosclerotic) coronary heart
 disease
HASCI
 head and spinal cord injury
HASCVD
 hypertensive atherosclerotic
 (arteriosclerotic) cardiovascular disease
HASH
 human achaete-scute homolog

HASHD
 hypertensive atherosclerotic
 (arteriosclerotic) heart disease
HASMC
 human aortic smooth muscle cell
HAsP
 health aspects of pesticides [bulletin]
HASS
 highest anxiety subscale score
HAST
 high-altitude simulation test
HASTE
 half-Fourier acquisition single-shot turbo
 spin-echo
HAstV1–HAstV7
 human astrovirus serotype 1–7
HAT
 Halstead Aphasia Test
 handgrip apexcardiographic test
 harmonic attenuation table (test)
 head, arms, trunk
 heparin-associated thrombocytopenia
 hepatic artery thrombosis
 heterophil (heterophile) antibody titer
 histone acetyltransferase
 home asthma telemonitoring
 hormone ablative therapy
 hospital arrival time
 human African trypanosomiasis
 [sleeping sickness]
 hyperazotemia
 hypoxanthine aminopterin thymidine
 [medium]
 hypoxanthine, azaserine, thymidine
 [medium]
HATG
 horse antihuman thymocyte globulin
HATH
 Heterosexual Attitudes Toward
 Homosexuality [scale]
H⁺-ATPase
 hydrogen adenosine triphosphatase
HATT
 heparin-associated thrombocytopenia and
 thrombosis
HATTS
 hemagglutination treponemal test for
 syphilis
HAU
 hemagglutinating unit
haust.
 draft, drink [L. *haustus*] (*See also* H,
 ht.)
HAV
 hallux abductovalgus
 hemadsorption virus
 hepatitis A vaccine (virus)

H

HAVAB
   hepatitis A virus antibody
HAV-HBV
   hepatitis A virus and hepatitis B virus
   vaccine
HAVS
   hand-arm vibration syndrome
HAWIC
   Hamburg-Wechsler Intelligence Test for
   Children
HAZ
   height for age Z-score
HAZMAT
   hazardous material
HAZV
   Hazara virus
HAZWOPER
   Hazardous Waste Operations and
   Emergency Response
HB
   head backward
   health board
   heart-beating [donor] (*See also*
   HBD)
   heart block
   heel to buttock
   held backward
   hemolysis blocking
   hepatitis B (*See also* hep)
   His bundle
   histamine blocker
   hold breakfast
   hospital-based
   hospital bed
   housebound
   hybridoma bank
   hyoid body
HB1°
   first-degree heart block
HB2°
   second-degree heart block
HB3°
   third-degree heart block
Hb
   hemoglobin (*See also* Hgb)
HbA, Hb A
   hemoglobin A [adult, α-chain]
   normal adult hemoglobin
HbA°
   hemoglobin determination
HbA$_1$
   major component of adult hemoglobin
HbA$_{1c}$
   glycosylated hemoglobin [major
   fraction]
HbA$_2$
   minor fraction of adult hemoglobin
HBAb
   hepatitis B antibody

HBAC
   hyperdynamic beta-adrenergic
   circulatory
HBAg
   hepatitis B antigen
HbAS
   heterozygosity for hemoglobin A and
   hemoglobin S [sickle-cell trait]
HBB
   hospital blood bank
   hydroxybenzylbenzimidazole
HbB
   hemoglobin B [B chain]
HbBart
   hemoglobin Bart
HbBC
   hemoglobin-binding capacity
HBBW, HB/BW
   hold breakfast for blood work
HBC
   hereditary breast cancer
   hit by car
   hyperimmune bovine concentrate
HB$_c$
   antibody to hepatitis B core antigen
HbC, Hb C
   hemoglobin C
HB$_c$Ab, HB$_{cAb}$, HBcAb
   antibody to hepatitis B core antigen
HB$_c$Ag, HB$_{cAg}$, HBcAg
   hepatitis B core antigen
HBCG
   heat-aggregated bacille Calmette-Guérin
Hb$_{Chesapeake}$
   hemoglobin Chesapeake
HbCO
   carboxyhemoglobin (carbon monoxide
   hemoglobin)
HbCO$_2$
   carbaminohemoglobin (carbon dioxide
   hemoglobin)
HbCS
   hemoglobin Constant Spring
HBCT
   helical biphasic contrast-enhanced CT
HbCV
   Haemophilus b conjugate vaccine
HBD
   has been drinking
   heart-beating donor (*See also* HB)
   hormone-binding domain
   hydroxybutyric dehydrogenase
   hypophosphatemic bone disease
HbD
   hemoglobin D (δ chain)
HBDH
   hydroxybutyrate dehydrogenase
HBDT
   human basophil degranulation test

HBE
His bundle electrogram
human bronchial epithelial [cells]
hypopharyngoscopy, bronchoscopy,
  esophagoscopy
HbE, Hb E
hemoglobin E (ε chain)
HBE₁
His bundle electrogram, distal
HBE₂
His bundle electrogram, proximal
HBₑ
hepatitis B e [type]
HBₑAb, HBₑAb
antibody to hepatitis B e antigen
HBₑAg, HBeAg
hepatitis B e antigen
HBEC
human brain endothelial cell
HBED
hydroxybenzylethylene-diamine diacetic
  acid
HB-EGF
heparin-binding EGF-like growth factor
HBF
hand blood flow
hemispheric blood flow
hemoglobinuric bilious fever
hepatic blood flow
hypothalamic blood flow
HbF, Hb F
fetal hemoglobin (hemoglobin F)
HbG1
hemoglobin Gower 1 [embryonic]
HbG2
hemoglobin Gower 2 [embryonic]
HBGA
had it before, got it again
HBGF
heparin-binding growth factor
HBGF-1
heparin-binding growth factor 1
HBGF-2
heparin-binding growth factor 2
HBGM
home blood glucose monitoring
HBGS
House-Brackmann Grading Scale [facial
  nerve]
HbH, Hb H
hemoglobin H
HBHC
home-based hospital care
Hb-Hp
hemoglobin-haptoglobin [complex]
HBI
Harvey-Bradshaw Index [Crohn disease]

hemibody irradiation
hepatobiliary imaging
high serum-bound iron
human blood index
Hutchins Behavior Inventory
HBID
hereditary benign intraepithelial
  dyskeratosis
HBIg
hepatitis B immune globulin
  (immunoglobulin)
hyperimmune serum globulin
HBIR
Hering-Breuer inflation reflex
Hb$_{Kansas}$
mutant hemoglobin with low affinity for
  oxygen
HBL
hepatoblastoma
HBLA
human B-lymphocyte antigen
Hb$_{Lepore}$
hemoglobin Lepore
HBLLSB
heard best at left lower sternal border
HBLP
hyperbetalipoproteinemia
HBLUSB
heard best at left upper sternal border
HBLV
human B lymphotropic virus
HBM
Health Belief Model
human bone marrow
hypertonic buffered medium
HbM, Hb M
hemoglobin M
HBME-1
human mesothelial cell membrane
HBMEC
human brain microvascular endothelial
  cell
HbMet
methemoglobin (*See also* Met-Hb)
HBNF
heparin-binding neurotrophic factor
hBNP
human B-type natriuretic peptide
HBO, HBO₂
hyperbaric oxygen (oxygenation)
  (therapy) (*See also* HBOT)
HbO₂
oxygenated hemoglobin
  (oxyhemoglobin)
HBOC
hereditary breast and ovarian
  cancer

H

HbOC
hepatitis B oligosaccharide-CRM197 vaccine

HBOT
hyperbaric oxygen therapy (*See also* HBO, HBO$_2$)

HBP
heartbeat period
helix-bundle peptide
hepatic binding protein
high blood pressure
hysterical back pain

Hbp
hemoglobin protease

HbP, Hb P
primitive (fetal) hemoglobin

Hb Portland
embryonic form of hemoglobin

HBPM
home blood pressure monitoring

HBQ
human health and behavior questionnaire

HBr
hydrobromic acid

HbR
methemoglobin reductase

HBS
headless bone screw
Health Behavior Scale
hyperkinetic behavior syndrome

HB$_S$
hepatitis B surface [antibody, antigen]

HbS, Hb S
hemoglobin S
sickle cell hemoglobin
sulfhemoglobin (*See also* SHb, S-Hb, SULFHb)

HB$_S$A
hepatitis B surface associated

HB$_s$Ab, HB$_{sAb}$, HBsAb
antibody to hepatitis B surface antigen

HB$_s$Ag, HB$_{sAg}$, HBsAg
hepatitis B surface antigen

HBsAg/adr
hepatitis B surface antigen manifesting group-specific determinant *a* and subtype-specific determinants *d* and *r*

HBSC
hemopoietic blood stem cell

HbSC, HbsC
sickle cell hemoglobin C

HBSS
Hanks balanced salt solution

HbSS
homozygosity for hemoglobin S
homozygous hemoglobin S

HBSSG
Hanks balanced salt solution plus glucose

HbS-Thal
hemoglobin S-thalassemia (sickle thalassemia)

HBT
hereditary benign tumor
home-based telemetry
human [blood] bilayer Tween [agar]
human brain thromboplastin
human breast tumor
hydrogen breath test

HBV
hepatitis B vaccine
hepatitis B virus
honeybee venom

HBVig
hepatitis B virus immune globulin

HBVP
high biological value protein

HBVV
hepatitis B virus vaccine

HBW
high birth weight

H:BW
heart to body weight ratio

HbZ
hemoglobin Z (zeta, Zurich, ξ chain)

HC
hair cell
hair count
hairy cell
handicapped (*See also* HCAP, HCP, handicp)
head check
head circumference
head compression
health care
healthy control
heart catheter(ization)
heart cycle
heat conservation
heavy chain
heel cord
hemochromatosis
hemoglobin concentration
hemorrhage, cerebral
hemorrhagic colitis
heparin cofactor
hepatic catalase
hepatic coma
hepatitis C (*See also* hep)
hepatocellular cancer (carcinoma) (*See also* HCC)
hereditary coproporphyria (*See also* HCP)
Hickman catheter
high calorie [diet] (*See also* hi-cal)

hippocampus (*See also* H)
histamine challenge
histochemistry
home call
home care
home collection
homocystinuria (*See also* HCU)
hospital course
hospitalized controls
hot compress
house call
Huntington chorea
hyaline cast
hybrid capture [assay] (*See also* HCA)
hydranencephaly
hydraulic concussion
hydrocarbon
hydrocephalus
hydroxycorticoid (*See also* HOC)
hyoid cornu
hypercholesterolemia
hypertrophic cardiomyopathy
NATO code for military obscurant
   smoke [zinc oxide, hexachloroethane,
   grained aluminum]

HCII
heparin cofactor II

4-HC, 4HC
4-hydroperoxycyclophosphamide

H&C
hot and cold

Hc
hydrocolloid

HCA
heart cell aggregate
heel cord advancement
hepatocellular adenoma
heterocyclic antidepressant
hybrid capture assay (*See also* HC)
hypercalcemia
hypochromic anemia (*See also*
   HchA)
hypoplastic congenital anemia
hypothalamic chronic anovulation
hypothermic circulatory arrest

HC:AC
head circumference to abdominal
   circumference ratio

HCAEC
human coronary artery endothelial cell

HCAO
hepatitis C-associated osteosclerosis

HCAP
handicapped (*See also* HC, HCP,
   handicp)

HCB
hexachlorobenzene

HCBR
human carbonyl reduction

HCC
heat conservation center
hepatitis contagiosa canis [virus]
hepatocellular cancer (carcinoma)
   (*See also* HC)
hepatocellular carcinoma cell [line]
hexachlorocyclohexane (*See also* HCH,
   gamma (γ) HCH)
history of chief complaint
hydroxycholecalciferol

25-HCC
25-hydroxycholecalciferol

HCCA
hilar cholangiocarcinoma

HCCAA
hereditary cysteine C amyloid
   angiopathy

HCCC
hyalinizing clear cell carcinoma

HCC-CC
clear cell hepatocellular carcinoma

HCD
h-caldesmon [antibody]
health care delivery
heavy-chain disease [protein]
herniated cervical disc
high caloric density
high carbohydrate diet (*See also*
   HICHO)
higher cerebral dysfunction
homologous canine distemper
   [antiserum]
hydrocolloid dressing
hysterical conversion disorder

HCDVA
high-contrast distance visual acuity

HCE
human chorionic ehrlichiosis
hypoglossal carotid entrapment

H(c)ELISA
competitive hemagglutinin
   enzyme-linked immunosorbent
   assay

HCF
hereditary capillary fragility
high carbohydrate food
high-carbohydrate, high-fiber [diet]
   (*See also* HCHF)
highest common factor
Horsley-Clarke stereotactic frame
hypocaloric feeding

HCFA
Health Care Financing Administration
   [obsolete, now Centers for Medicare
   and Medicaid Services]

H

HD$_{50}$
hemolyzing dose of complement that lyses 50% of sensitized erythrocytes

Hd
human figure parts response [Rorschach]

HDA
heteroduplex analysis
high-dose arm
histiocytic dermoarthritis
hydroxydopamine (See also HD)

HDAC
histone deacetylase

HDAg
hepatitis D antigen

HDBQ
Hilton Drinking Behavior Questionnaire

HDC
habilitative day care
hand drive control
high-dose chemotherapy (See also HDCh, HDCT)
histidine decarboxylase (See also HD)
human diploid cell
hyperdiploid cell
hypodermoclysis

HDC-ABMT
high-dose chemotherapy with autologous bone marrow transplant(ation)

HDC-ASCR
high-dose chemotherapy with autologous [bone marrow or] stem cell rescue

HDC-ASCS
high-dose chemotherapy with autologous stem cell support

HDCC
high-dose combination chemotherapy

HDCh
high-dose chemotherapy (See also HDC, HDCT)

HDCS
human diploid cell strain (system)

HDC-SCR
high-dose chemotherapy and stem cell rescue

HDCT
high-dose chemotherapy (See also HDC, HDCh)

HDCV
human diploid cell (rabies) vaccine

HDD
half-dose depth
high-dose depth

HDDS
high-dose dexamethasone suppression [test]

HDE
higher-dose therapy with epinephrine
Humanitarian Device Exemption [FDA]

HDF
hemodiafiltration
hereditary dysfibrinoginemia
high dry field
host defensive factor
human diploid fibroblast

HDFL
human development and family life

HDG
high-dose group
hydrogel [dressing]

HDGC
hereditary diffuse gastric cancer

HDGF
hepatoma-derived growth factor

HDH
heart disease history
high density humidity
Hostility and Direction of Hostility [questionnaire] (See also HDHQ)

HDHQ
Hostility and Direction of Hostility Questionnaire (See also HDH)

HDI
hemorrhagic disease of infants
high-definition image (imaging)
histologically detectable iron
histone deacetylase inhibitor

HDIC
hepatodiaphragmatic interposition of colon

HDIR
high isodose range [radiosurgery]

HDIT
high-dose immunosuppressive therapy

HDIVIg
high-dose intravenous immunoglobulin

HDL
high-density lipoprotein

HDLBP
high-density lipoprotein binding protein

HDL-C, HDLC
high-density lipoprotein-cholesterol [complex]

HDL-c
high-density lipoprotein-cell surface [receptor]

HDLP
high-density lipoprotein

HDLS
hereditary diffuse leukoencephalopathy with spheroids

HDLW
hearing distance, left, watch [distance from watch, heard by left ear]

HDM
hexadimethrine
high-dose morphine

home-delivered meals
house dust mite

HDMEC
human dermal microvascular endothelial cell

HDMFP
house dust mite fecal pellet

HDN
[ABO] hemolytic disease of the newborn
hemorrhagic disease of newborn
heparin dosing nomogram
high-density nebulizer

hDNA
deoxyribonucleic acid, histone

HDNS
hereditary dysplastic nevus syndrome
Hodgkin disease nodular sclerosis

HDoov
Humpty Doo virus

HDP
hexose diphosphate
high-definition power
high-density polyethylene
hydroxydimethylpyrimidine [imaging agent]
hydroxymethylene diphosphonate [imaging agent]

HDPA
high-dose pulse administration

HDPAA
heparin-dependent platelet-associated antibody

HDPC
handpiece

HDPE
high-density polyethylene

HDR
heparin dose response
high dose radiation
high dose rate
husband to delivery room
hysteric dissociative reaction

HDRA
histoculture drug response assay

HDRB
high dose rate brachytherapy

HDRF
Heart Disease Research Foundation

HDRS
Hamilton Depression Rating Scale (*See also* HDS)

HDRV
human diploid [cell strain] rabies vaccine

HDRW
hearing distance, right, watch [distance from watch, heard by right ear]

HDS
Hamilton Depression [Rating] Scale (*See also* HDRS)
healthcare data systems
health data services
health delivery system
hematuria-dysuria syndrome
herniated disc syndrome
HIV Dementia Scale
hospital discharge survey

HDSCR
health deviation self-care requisite

HDT
habilitative day treatment
hand dynamometer test
hearing distraction test
high-dose therapy

HDU
head-drop unit [curare standard]

HDV
hemorrhagic disease virus
hepatitis D (delta) (δ) virus

HDVD
high-definition video display

HDW
hearing distance [with] watch
reticulocyte hemoglobin distribution width

HDYF
how do you feel

HE
half-scan with extrapolation
hard exudate
health educator
Hektoen enteric [agar]
hemagglutinating encephalomyelitis
hematoxylin and eosin (*See also* H&E)
hemoglobin electrophoresis
hepatic encephalopathy
hepatitis E (*See also* hep)
hereditary elliptocytosis
hollow enzyme
human ehrlichiosis
human enteric [virus]
hyperextension
hypertensive encephalopathy
hypogonadotropic eunuchoidism
hypophysectomy
hypoxemic episode

H-E
heat exchanger

H&E, H and E
hematoxylin and eosin [stain] (*See also* HE)
hemorrhage and exudate
heredity and environment

H

He
   Hedstrom number [turbulence]
   helium
³He
   helium-3
⁴He
   helium-4
he
   heart channel (acupuncture)
HEA
   health
   hereditary elliptocytic anemia
   hexone-extracted acetone
   human erythrocyte antigen
HEAD
   high-throughput extraction amplification
      and detection
HEADS FIRST
   home, education, abuse, drugs, safety,
      friends, image, recreation, sexuality,
      threats
HEADSS
   home [life], education [level], activities,
      drug [use], sexual [activity], suicide
      [ideation/attempts] [adolescent medical
      history]
HEAL
   Health Education Assistance Loan
HEAR
   hospital emergency ambulance radio
HEART
   human energetic assessment and
      restorative technic
HEAT, hEAT
   human erythrocyte agglutination test
HEB
   hematoencephalic barrier [blood-brain
      barrier]
   hydrophilic emollient base
HEC
   hamster embryo cell
   health education center
   health evaluation center
   highly emetogenic chemotherapy
   human endothelial cell
   hydroxyergocalciferol
HED
   Haut-Einheits-Dosis [unit skin dose of
      radiation]
   hereditary ectodermal dysplasia
   hidrotic ectodermal dysplasia
   human embryoid-body derived
      [cell]
   hydrotropic electron donor
   hydroxyephedrine
   hypohidrotic ectodermal dysplasia
HEDH
   hypohidrotic ectodermal dysplasia with
      hypothyroidism

HEDIS
   Health (Plan) Employer Data and
      Information Set
HEDP
   hydroxyethylidene-1,1-diphosphonic acid
HEDSPA
   ⁹⁹ᵐTc-etidronate [bone-imaging agent]
HEENT
   head, ears, eyes, nose, throat
HEEP
   health effects of environmental
      pollutants
HEF
   hamster embryo fibroblast
   human embryo fibroblast
HeFH
   heterozygous familial
      hypercholesterolemia (*See also* hFH)
HEG
   hemorrhagic erosive gastritis
hEGF, h-EGF
   human epidermal growth factor
HEHR
   highest equivalent heart rate
HEI
   high-energy intermediate
   highly exposed individual
   homogeneous enzyme immunoassay
   human embryonic intestine [cell]
HEIR
   health effects of ionizing radiation
   high-energy ionizing radiation
HEIS
   high-energy ion scattering
HEK
   human embryo (embryonic) kidney
      [cell]
HEL
   Helicobacter pylori vaccine
   hen egg-white lysozyme
   human embryo lung [cell culture]
   human erythroleukemia line
HeLa
   continuously cultured carcinoma cell
      line used for tissue cultures [named
      for patient, Henrietta Lacks]
HELF
   human embryonic lung fibroblast
heliox
   helium and oxygen
   helium-oxygen mixture
HELLP
   hemolysis, elevated liver enzymes, low
      platelets
HELM
   helmet cell
HELP
   Hawaii Early Learning Profile
   Health Education Library Program

Health Emergency Loan Program
Health Evaluation and Learning
  Program
heat escape lessening posture
heparin-induced extracorporeal
  low-density lipoprotein precipitation
Heroin Emergency Life Project
Hospital Equipment Loan Project
HEM, hem
  hematology (*See also* hemat)
  hematuria
  hematuric
  hemolysis (*See also* H, HL)
  hemolytic (*See also* H)
  hemophilia
  hemorrhage (*See also* hemorr)
  hemorrhoid
  high-electrolyte meal
  hypertensive emergency
HEMA
  hydroxyethylmethacrylate
  2-hydroxyethyl methacrylate
hemat
  hematology (*See also* HEM, hem)
hematem
  hematemesis
HEMB
  hemophilia B
hemi
  hemiparalysis
  hemiparesis (*See also* HP)
  hemiplegia (*See also* HP)
  hemisphere (*See also* H)
HEMO
  hemodialysis (*See also* HD)
hemocyt, hemocyt.
  hemocytometer
hemorr
  hemorrhage (*See also* HEM, hem)
HEMOSID
  hemosiderin
HEMPAS
  hereditary erythroblastic multinuclearity
    with positive acidified serum
HEMRI
  hereditary multifocal relapsing
    inflammation
He-MRI
  helium magnetic resonance imaging
HEMS
  helicopter emergency medical services
HEN
  hemorrhages, exudates, and/or
    nicking
  home enteral nutrition
He-Ne, HeNe
  helium-neon

HEP
  hemoglobin electrophoresis
  hemolysis end point
  hemorrhage, exudates, papilledema
  heparin (*See also* H, HP)
  hepatic
  hepatitis (*See also* hep)
  hepatoerythrocytic porphyria
  hepatoerythropoietic porphyria
  hepatoma
  high egg passage [virus]
  high-energy phosphate
  histamine equivalent prick
  home exercise program
HEp
  human epithelial [cell]
HEp-1
  human cervical carcinoma cells
HEp-2
  human laryngeal tumor cells
hEP
  human endorphin
hep
  hepatitis A–G (*See also* HA, HB, HC,
    HD, HE)
HEPA
  hamster egg penetration assay
  high-efficiency particulate air [filter]
  high-efficiency particulate arresting
    [filter]
HEP-AC
  hepatitis battery-acute
hep cap
  heparin cap
Hep/Clav
  hepatoclavicular
HEPES
  N-[2-hydroxyethyl]piperazine
  N′-[2-ethanesulfonic acid]
hep lock
  heparin lock (*See also* HL, H/L)
HEPM
  human embryonic palatal mesenchymal
    [cell]
HEPOD
  hereditary expansile polyostotic
    dysplasia
HER
  healing energy research
  hemorrhagic encephalopathy of
    rats
HER2
  human epidermal growth receptor 2
her.
  hernia (*See also* H, hern)
  herniat(ed) (herniation) (*See also* H,
    hern)

H

hered
    hereditary
    heredity
HERF
    high-energy radiofrequency
HERG
    human ether-a-go-go-related gene
hern
    hernia (*See also* H, her.)
    herniat(ed) (herniation) (*See also* H, her.)
HER2/neu
    breast cancer gene
HERP
    human exposure [dose]/rodent potency
HERS
    Health Evaluation and Referral Service
hERV
    human endogenous retrovirus
hERV-E
    human endogenous retrovirus E
hERV-K
    human endogenous retrovirus K
HES
    [acute] hypereosinophilic syndrome
    health examination survey
    hematoxylin-eosin stain
    hetastarch [hydroxyethyl starch; Hespan]
    human embryonic skin
    human embryonic spleen
    hydroxyethyl starch [solution]
    hypereosinophilic syndrome
hES
    human embryonic stem [cell]
HESX1
    homeobox gene expressed in embryonic stem ES cells
HET
    Health Education Telecommunications
    helium equilibration time
het
    heterophil (heterophile) [antibody] (*See also* HA)
    heterozygous
HETE
    hydroxyeicosatetraenoic (acid)
12-HETE
    12-hydroxyeicosatetraenoic acid
15-HETE
    15-hydroxyeicosatetraenoic acid
20-HETE
    20-hydroxyeicosatetraenoic acid
HETF
    home enteral tube feeding
HETP
    height equivalent to theoretical plate [gas chromatography]

HE-TUMT
    high-energy transurethral microwave thermotherapy
HEV
    health and environment
    hemagglutination encephalomyelitis virus
    hemorrhagic endovasculitis
    hemorrhagic endovasculopathy
    hemorrhagic enteritis virus
    hepatitis E vaccine
    hepatitis E virus
    hepatoencephalomyelitis virus
    high-endothelial venule
    human enteric virus
HEVI
    hibernal epidemic viral infection
HeV
    hepatitis virus
HEV A–D
    human enterovirus A–D
HEV b1
    rubber elongation factor B1 [allergen protein of natural latex]
HEV b6.02
    hevein [allergen protein of natural latex]
HEW
    Health, Education, and Welfare [United States Department of]
HEX
    hexosaminidase [gene]
HEx
    hard exudate
HEX A
    hexosaminidase A [alpha (α) subunit]
HEX B
    hexosaminidase B [beta (β) subunit]
HF
    Hageman factor [factor XII] (*See also* HgF)
    half (*See also* hf, S, sem., semi, ss)
    haplotype frequency
    hard feces
    hard fibroma
    hard filled [capsule]
    harlequin fetus
    harvest fluid
    hay fever
    head of fetus
    head forward
    heart failure
    helper factor
    hemofiltration
    hemorrhagic factor
    hemorrhagic fever
    hepatocyte function
    high-fat [diet]
    high flow
    high frequency (*See also* HFR)
    hippocampal formation

hollow fiber
hollow filter [dialyzer]
hot flash
hot fomentation
house formula
human fibroblast
humidifier fever
hydrogen fluoride [catalyst]
hyperflexion

H/F
HeLa/fibroblast [hybrid cell line]

Hf
hafnium

hf
half (*See also* HF, S, sem., semi, ss)

HFA
high-functioning autism
hydrofluoroalkane
hyperfolicacidemia

H-FABP
heart fatty acid binding protein

HFAK
hollow-fiber artificial kidney

HFAS
hereditary flat adenoma syndrome

HFB
high-frequency band
human fetal brain

HFBA
heptafluorobutyric anhydride

HFC
hand-filled capsule
high-frequency current
histamine-forming capacity
hydrofluorocarbon

HFCB
horizontal flow clean bench

HFCC
high-frequency chest compression

HFCS
high-fructose corn syrup

HFCWC
high-frequency chest wall
compression

HFCWO
high-frequency chest wall oscillation

HFD
hemorrhagic fever of deer
high-fiber diet
high forceps delivery
high-frequency discharge
high-frequency Doppler
Human Figure Drawing

HFDD
human fibroblast-derived dermis

HFDK
human fetal diploid kidney [cell]

HFDL
human fetal diploid lung [cell]

HFEA
Human Fertilization and Embryology
Authority

HFEC
human foreskin epithelial cell

HFEE
high-frequency epicardial
echocardiography

HFF
high-filter frequency
human foreskin fibroblast

HFFI
high-frequency flow interruption

HFG
hand-foot-genital [syndrome]

HFGC
human fetal glial cell

hFGF
human fibroblast growth factor

HFH
hemifacial hyperplasia
homozygous familial
hypercholesterolemia

hFH
heterozygous familial
hypercholesterolemia (*See also* HeFH)

HFHL
high-frequency hearing loss

HFI
half-Fourier imaging
Hand Functional Index
hereditary fructose intolerance
high fat intake
human fibroblast interferon (*See also*
HFIF)

HFIF
human fibroblast interferon (*See also*
HFI)

HFJ
high-frequency jet

HFJV
high-frequency jet ventilation

HFK
human foreskin keratinocyte

HFL
human fetal lung [fibroblast]

HFLL
hemosiderotic fibrohistiocytic lipomatous
lesion

HFL-TMS
high-frequency left-sided repetitive
transcranial magnetic stimulation

H flu
Haemophilus influenzae (*See also* HI,
HIF)

H

HFM
    hand-foot-and-mouth [disease] (*See also* HFMD)
    hemifacial microsomia (*See also* HM)
HFMD
    hand-foot-and-mouth disease (*See also* HFM)
HFO
    hard food orientation
    high-frequency oscillation (oscillatory)
HFOC
    high-flow oxygen conserver
HFOV
    high-frequency oscillatory ventilation
HFP
    hepatic functional panel
    Hoffa fat pad
    hypofibrinogenic plasma
HFPP
    high-frequency positive pressure
HFPPV
    high-frequency positive-pressure ventilation
HFPV
    high-frequency percussive ventilation
HFR
    high frequency (*See also* HF)
Hfr
    high-frequency recombination
HFRS
    hemorrhagic fever with renal symptoms
    hemorrhagic fever with renal syndrome
HFRT
    hyperfractionated radiotherapy
HFS
    hand-foot-skin [reaction]
    hand-foot syndrome
    hemifacial spasm
hfs
    hyperfine structure
hFSH
    human-derived follicle-stimulating hormone
    human follicle-stimulating hormone
HFST
    hearing-for-speech test
HFT
    hemofiltration therapy
    high-frequency transduction
    high-frequency transfer
HFU
    hand-foot-uterus [syndrome]
    high-intensity focused ultrasound
HFUPR
    hourly fetal urine production rate
HFUPS
    high-frequency ultrasound probe sonography

HFV
    hepatitis F virus
    high-frequency ventilation
    high-fruit/vegetable [diet]
    human foamy virus
HFX RT
    hyperfractionated radiation therapy
HG
    handgrasp
    handgrip [exercise]
    Harris-Galante [porous acetabular component] (*See also* HGP)
    herpes genitalis
    herpes gestationis
    Heschl gyrus
    high glucose
    high grade
    human gonadotropin
    human growth [factor] (*See also* HGF, hGF)
    hyperemesis gravidarum
    hypoglycemia
H/G
    human granulocyte colony-stimulating factor recombinant [protein]
Hg
    mercury [L. *hydrargyrum* silver water] (*See also* hydrarg.)
Hg2+
    inorganic mercury
^{195m}Hg
    mercury-195m
hg
    hectogram
HGA
    high-grade astrocytomas
    homogentisate
    homogentisic acid
Hgb
    hemoglobin (*See also* Hb)
Hgb ELECT
    hemoglobin electrophoresis
HGBV
    hepatitis GB virus
HGC
    hard gel capsule
HgCl2
    mercury chloride
HgCN
    mercury cyanide
HGD
    high-grade dysplasia
HGE
    human granulocytic ehrlichiosis
    human granulocytotropic ehrlichiosis
HGES
    handgrasp equal and strong
HGF
    hematopoietic growth factor

hepatocyte growth factor (*See also* HPG)

human growth factor (*See also* HG, hGF)

hyperglycemic-glycogenolytic factor

hGF
human growth factor (*See also* HG, HGF)

HGF/SF
hepatocyte growth factor/scatter factor

HGG
herpetic geniculate ganglionitis
hypogammaglobulinemia

hGG
human gamma globulin

hGH
human [pituitary] growth hormone (somatotropin)

HGI
Human Genome Initiative

HGM
hog gastric mucin
home glucose monitoring
human glucose monitoring

HGMCR
human genetic mutant cell repository

HGN
hypogastric nerve

HGNT
high-grade neuroendocrine tumor

HGO
hepatic glucose output
hip guidance orthosis
human glucose output

HGP
Harris-Galante porous [acetabular component] (*See also* HG)
hepatic glucose production
Human Genome Project
hyperglobulinemia purpura

HGPIN
high-grade prostatic intraepithelial neoplasia

HGPRT, HG-PRTase
hypoxanthine-guanine phosphoribosyltransferase [deficiency]

HGPS
hereditary giant platelet syndrome

HGS
handgrip strength
human genome sequence

HGSHS
Harvard Group Scale of Hypnotic Susceptibility

HGSHS:A
Harvard Group Scale of Hypnotic Susceptibility, Form A

HGSIL
high-grade squamous intraepithelial lesion

Hgt
height (*See also* H, ht)

HGV
hepatitis G vaccine
hepatitis G virus

HH
halothane hepatitis
hand held
hard of hearing (*See also* HOH)
head hood
healthy hemophiliac
hereditary hemochromatosis
hiatal hernia
holistic health
home health
home help
home hyperalimentation
homonymous hemianopia (hemianopsia)
household
hydroxyhexamide
hypergastrinemic hyperchlorhydria
hyperhidrosis
hyperhomocysteinemia
hypogonadotropic hypogonadism
hyporeninemic hypoaldosteronism

H-H
head-to-head sperm agglutination

H/H, H&H
hemoglobin and hematocrit

Hh
hemopoietic histocompatibility

HHA
health hazard appraisal
hereditary hemolytic anemia
home health agency
hypogonadotropic hypogonadism-anosmia syndrome
hypothalamic-hypophysial-adrenal [system]

HHAA
hypothalamohypophyseoadrenal axis

HH Assist
hand-held assistance

HHAV
human hepatitis A virus

HHb
hypohemoglobin
reduced hemoglobin
un-ionized (nonionized) hemoglobin

HHC
home health care
hypocalciuric hypercalcemia

H

HHCA
hypothermic hypokalemic cardioplegic arrest

HHCS
high-altitude hypertrophic cardiomyopathy syndrome

HHD
handheld dynamometer
high heparin dose
home hemodialysis
hypertensive heart disease (*See also* HTHD)

HHE
health hazard evaluation
hemiconvulsion-hemiplegia-epilepsy [syndrome]

HHF-35
muscle-specific actin (*See also* MSA)

HHFM
high-humidity face mask

HHG
hypertrophic hypersecretory gastropathy
hypogonadotropic hypogonadism

HHH
hyperammonemia, hyperornithinemia, homocitrullinuria [syndrome]
hypermethionemia, hyperammonemia, homocitrullinemia [syndrome]

HHHH
hereditary hemihypotrophy-hemiparesis-hemiathetosis [syndrome]

HHHO
hypotonia, hyperphagia, hypogonadism, obesity [syndrome]
hypotonia, hypomentia, hypogonadism, obesity [syndrome]

HHI
hereditary hearing impairment

HHIE, HHIE-S
Hearing Handicap Inventory for the Elderly

HHLL
histocytoid hemangioma-like lesion

HHM
hemohydrometry
high-humidity mask
humoral hypercalcemia of malignancy

H-Hm
compound hypermetropic astigmatism

HHN
handheld nebulizer
hyperosmolar hyperglycemic nonketotic [syndrome] (*See also* HHNS)

HHNC, HHNK
hyperosmolar hyperglycemic nonketotic [coma] (*See also* HHNKC)

HHNKC
hyperosmolar hyperglycemic nonketotic coma (*See also* HHNC, HHNK)

HHNKS
hyperglycemic hyperosmolar nonketotic syndrome (*See also* HHN)

HHP
holistic health practitioner

HHPA
hexahydrophthalic anhydride

HHPC
hyperoxic-hypercapnic

HHPS
hypothalamohypophysial portal system

HHRH
hypothalamic hypophysiotropic-releasing hormone
[syndrome of] hereditary hypophosphatemic rickets with hypercalciuria

HHS
Harris hip score
Health and Human Services [United States Department of]
Hearing Handicap Scale
hereditary hemolytic syndrome
history of heavy smoking
human hypopituitary serum
hyperglycemic hyperosmolar syndrome
hyperkinetic heart syndrome

HHT
head halter traction (*See also* HHTx)
hereditary hemolytic telangiectasia
hereditary hemorrhagic telangiectasia
heterotopic heart transplant(ation)
hydroxyheptadecatrienoic (acid)
hypertensive hypervolemic therapy

HHTA
hypothalamohypophyseothyroidal axis

HHTC
high-humidity tracheostomy collar

HHTM
high-humidity tracheostomy mask

HHTS
high-humidity tracheostomy shield

HHTx
head halter traction (*See also* HHT)

HHV
human herpesvirus [1–9, 6A, 6B]

HHW
handheld weight

HI
Haemophilus influenzae (*See also* H flu, HIF)
harmonic imaging
hazard index
head injury
health insurance
hearing impaired
heart infusion
heat inactivated
heat input

hemagglutination inhibition [titer]
  (*See also* HAI)
hemorrhagic infarction
hepatic insufficiency
hepatobiliary imaging
high impulsiveness
homicidal ideation
hormone independent
hormone insensitive
hospital induced
hospital insurance
human insulin
humoral immunity
hydrogen iodide
hydroxyindole
hyperglycemic index
hypoglycemic index
hypomelanosis of Ito
hypothermic ischemia

HI 30
human [urinary trypsin] inhibitor
  [bikunin]

Hi
histamine (*See also* HA)

HIA
hallux interphalangeus angle
heat infusion agar
hemagglutination (hemagglutinating)
  inhibition antibody
hemagglutination inhibition assay
hyperventilation-induced asthma

HIAA
hydroxyindoleacetic acid (*See also*
  OH-IAA)

5-HIAA
5-hydroxyindoleacetic acid

21-HIAA
21-hydroxyindoleacetic acid

HIAD
high-impact aerobic dance

HIAP
human intracisternal A-type particle

HIB
Haemophilus influenzae type b [vaccine]
  (*See also* HITB, Hib)
heart infusion broth
hemolytic immune body
hyperpnea-induced bronchoconstriction
hypoxia, intussusception, brain [mass]

Hib
Haemophilus influenzae type b

HIB$_{cn}$
Haemophilus influenzae type b
  conjugate vaccine

HIB$_{HbOC}$
Haemophilus influenzae type vaccine
  oligosaccharide-CRM197 vaccine
  conjugate

HIB$_{PRP-D}$
Haemophilus influenzae type b vaccine,
  PRP-D conjugate vaccine

HIB$_{PRP-OMP}$
Haemophilus influenzae type b vaccine,
  PRP-OMP conjugate vaccine

HIB$_{PRP-T}$
Haemophilus influenzae type b vaccine,
  PRP-T conjugate vaccine

HIBps
Haemophilus influenzae type b
  polysaccharide vaccine

HIC
handling-induced convulsion
hepatic iron concentration
Human Investigation Committee
Humphriss immediate contrast
  [refraction]

hi-cal
high caloric
high calorie [diet] (*See also* HC)

HIC-CPR
high-impulse compression
  cardiopulmonary resuscitation

H-ICD-A
International Classification of Diseases,
  Adopted Code for Hospitals

HICH
hypertensive intracranial hemorrhage

HICHO
high carbohydrate [diet] (*See also*
  HCD)

HiCN
hemoglobincyanide

HiCn
cyanmethemoglobin

HI-CPR
high-impulse cardiopulmonary
  resuscitation

HID
headache, insomnia, depression
  [syndrome]
herniated intervertebral disc
high iron diamine
human infectious dose
hyperimmunoglobulinemia syndrome
hyperkinetic impulse disorder

HIDA
hepatic 2,6-dimethyliminodiacetic acid
hepatoiminodiacetic acid

HID/AB
high-iron diamine/Alcian blue

HIDS
hyperimmunoglobulinemia D syndrome

HIE
human intestinal epithelium
hyperimmunoglobulin E
hypoxic-ischemic encephalopathy

H

HIER
heat-induced epitope retrieval
HIES
hyperimmunoglobulin E syndrome
HIF
Haemophilus influenzae (*See also* HI, H flu)
higher integrative function
higher intellectual function
Histoplasma inhibitory factor
Historical Information Form
HIV-inducing factor
hypoxia inducible factor
HIF1
hypoxia inducible factor 1
HIF1 alpha (α)
hypoxia inducible factor 1 alpha (α)
HIFBS
heat-inactivated fetal bovine serum
HIFC
hog intrinsic factor concentrate
HIFCS
heat-inactivated fetal calf serum
HIFT
high-frequency ventilation trial
HIFU
high-intensity focused ultrasonography
high-intensity focused ultrasound
HIg
hyperimmunoglobulin
HIH
Halsted inguinal herniorrhaphy
hypertensive intracerebral hemorrhage
HIHA
high impulsiveness high anxiety
HIHARS
hyperventilation-induced high-amplitude
rhythmic slowing
HII
hemagglutination inhibition immunoassay
hepatic iron index
HIIC
heated intraoperative intraperitoneal
chemotherapy
hyperthermic intraperitoneal antiblastic
perfusion
hyperthermic intraperitoneal
intraoperative chemotherapy
HIIN
hypertrophic interstitial infantile neuritis
HIL
hypoxic-ischemic lesion
HILA
high impulsiveness low anxiety
HILP
hyperthermic isolated limb perfusion
HIM
health information management
hemopoietic inductive microenvironment

hepatitis-infectious mononucleosis
hexyl-insulin monoconjugate
Hill Interaction Matrix [psychologic test]
hyper-immunoglobulin M (IgM) syndrome
HIMC
hepatic intramitochondrial crystalloid
HIMT
hemagglutination inhibition morphine test
Hind II, Hind III
restriction endonucleases from *Haemophilus influenzae*
H inf
hypodermoclysis infusion
HINI
hypoxic-ischemic neuronal injury
HINT
Harris Infant Neuromotor Test
Hint.
Hinton [flocculation test for syphilis]
HIO
health insuring organization
hepatic iron overload
hole-in-one [technique]
hypoiodism
hypoiodite [salt of hypoiodous acid]
HIOMT
hydroxyindole-*O*-methyltransferase
HIOS
high index of suspicion (*See also* HIS)
HIP
health illness profile
health insurance plan
homograft incus prosthesis
hospital insurance program
humoral immunocompetence profile
hydrostatic indifference point
Hypnotic Induction Profile
HIP1
huntingtin-interacting protein 1
HIPA
heparin-induced platelet activation [assay]
heparin-induced platelet aggregation
HIPAA
Health Insurance Portability and Accountability Act [of 1996]
Hip B
Hippocratic baldness
HIPC
hormone independent prostate cancer
HiPIP
high-potential iron protein
HIPO
hemihypertrophy, intestinal web, preauricular skin tag, and congenital corneal opacity [syndrome]

Hospital Indicator for Physicians'
Orders
HIPPS
Health Insurance Prospective Payment
System
HiPRF
high pulse repetition frequency
HiPro, HiProt
high protein [diet] (*See also* HP)
HIR
head injury routine
hepatic ischemia and reperfusion
high irradiance response
HIRCAL
Hirji-Callander [grid]
HIRF
histamine inhibitory releasing factor
HIRO
hormonal imbalance related to ovulation
HIS
Hanover Intensive Score
Haptic Intelligence Scale
health information system
Health Intention Scale
Health Interview Survey
high index of suspicion (*See also*
HIOS)
high intermittent suction
Home Incapacity Scale
hospital information system
human immune system
hyperimmune serum
hyperimmunized suppressed
His
histidine (*See also* H)
His-
histidyl
-His
histidino
HISG, hISG
human immune serum globulin
HISMS
How I See Myself Scale [psychologic
test]
His-Pro-DKP
histidyl-proline-diketopiperazine
HISS
human immune status survey
HIST
hospital in-service training
hist
histidinemia
history (*See also* H, Hx, Hy)
HISTLINE
History of Medicine On-Line [obsolete]
HISTO
histoplasmosis

histo
histology
histoplasmin skin test
Histo-Dx
histologic diagnosis
histol
histologic
histology
HIT
hemagglutination inhibition test
heparin-induced thrombocytopenia
histamine inhalation test
histamine ion transfer
Holtzman Inkblot Technique
home infusion therapy
hypertrophic infiltrative tendinitis
hypertrophied inferior turbinate
HITB, HiTb
Haemophilus influenzae type b (*See also*
HIB)
HITS
high-intensity transient signal
HITT, HITTS
heparin-induced
thrombocytopenia-thrombosis
heparin-induced
thrombosis-thrombocytopenia syndrome
HiTT
high-dose thrombin time
high frequency induced thermal therapy
HIU
hyperplasia interstitialis uteri
HIV
human immunodeficiency virus
HIV-1
human immunodeficiency virus type 1
HIV-2
human immunodeficiency virus type 2
HIV-Ab
human immunodeficiency virus antibody
HIVAN
human immunodeficiency
virus-associated nephropathy
HIVAT
home intravenous antibiotic therapy
HIV-1C
human immunodeficiency virus-1
subtype C
HIV-D
human immunodeficiency virus dementia
HIVD
herniated intervertebral disc
HIV1E
human immunodeficiency virus type 1E
HIV-G
human immunodeficiency virus
gingivitis

H

HIVIg
anti-human immunodeficiency virus
immune serum globulin
human immunodeficiency virus
immunoglobulin

HiVit
high vitamin

HIVN
human immunodeficiency virus
nephropathy

HIV-NHL
human immunodeficiency
virus-associated non-Hodgkin
lymphoma

HIV-P
human immunodeficiency
virus-associated periodontitis
human immunodeficiency virus
periodontitis

HIV-PARSE
human immunodeficiency
virus-patient-reported status and
experience

HIV-QAM
human immunodeficiency virus quality
audit marker

HIV-QOL
human immunodeficiency virus quality
of life [questionnaire]

HIV-SGD
human immunodeficiency
virus-associated salivary gland disease

HIZ
high-intensity zone

HJ
Highlands J [virus]
Howell-Jolly [bodies]

HJA
hip joint angle

HJB
high jugular bulb
Howell-Jolly bodies

HJD
Hospital for Joint Disease

HJR
hepatojugular reflux

HJV
Highlands J virus

HK
hand-to-knee [test]
heat killed
heel-to-knee [test] (*See also* H-K, HTK)
hexokinase
human kidney [cell] (*See also* HKC)

H-K, H→K
hand-to-knee [test]
heel-to-knee [test] (*See also* HK, HTK)

HK1
hexokinase 1

hK2
human kallikrein 2

hK3
human kallikrein 3

HKA
hip-knee-ankle [orthosis]

HKAFO
hip-knee-ankle-foot orthosis

HKAO
hip-knee-ankle orthosis

HKC
human kidney cell (*See also* HK)

hKGK1
human kidney glandular kallikrein-1
gene

HKH
hyperkinetic heart syndrome

HKLM
heat-killed *Listeria monocytogenes*

HKMN
Hickman [catheter]

HKO
hip-knee orthosis

HKS
heel-knee-shin [test]
hyperkinesis syndrome

HKT
heterotopic kidney transplant(ation)

HL
hairline
hairy leukoplakia
half-life [element, pharmaceutical]
hallux limitus
harelip
hearing level
hearing loss
heart and lungs (*See also* H&L)
heavy lifting
heel lance
hemilaryngectomy
hemolysis (*See also* H, HEM, hem)
heparin lock (*See also* H/L,
hep lock)
hepatic lipase
Hickman line
histiocytic lymphoma
histocompatibility locus
Hodgkin lymphoma
human leukocyte
human lymphocyte
humerus length
hygienic laboratory
hyperlipidemia
hyperlipoproteinemia
hyperopia (hypermetropia), latent
(*See also* hL)
hyperreactio luteinalis
hypertrichosis lanuginosa
lateral habenular [nucleus]

H/L
　heparin lock (*See also* HL, hep lock)
H:L
　hydrophil to lipophil ratio
H&L
　heart and lung [machine]
　heart and lungs (*See also* HL)
HL7
　health level seven [physical
　　examination]
hL
　hectoliter
　hyperopia (hypermetropia), latent
　　(*See also* HL)
HLA
　heart, lungs, abdomen
　histocompatibility leukocyte antigen
　histocompatibility locus antigen
　homologous leukocyte antibody
　horizontal long axial
　human leukocyte antibody
　human leukocyte antigen (system)
　hypoplastic left atrium
hLA
　human leukocyte antigen [system, allele]
**HLA-A, HLA-B, HLA-C, HLA-D,
　HLA-DR**
　varieties of human leukocyte antigen
HLA-A24
　human leukocyte antigen-A24
HLA-B27
　human leukocyte antigen B27
HLA-B57
　human leukocyte antigen B57
　　[restriction element]
HLALD
　horse liver alcohol dehydrogenase
HLA-LD
　human lymphocyte antigen-lymphocyte
　　defined
HLA-SD
　human lymphocyte antigen-serologically
　　defined
HLB
　head, limbs, body
　hydrophilic-lipophilic balance
　hypotonic lysis buffer
HLBI
　human lymphoblastoid interferon
HLC
　heat loss center
HLCL
　human lymphoblastoid cell line
HLD
　hepatolenticular degeneration
　herniated lumbar disc
　high-level disinfection

high lipid disorder
　hypersensitivity lung disease
HLDH
　heat-stable lactic dehydrogenase
HLDP
　hypoglossia-limb deficiency phenotype
HLE
　human leukocyte elastase
HLEG
　hydrolysate lactalbumin Earle glucose
HLES
　hypertensive lower esophageal sphincter
HLF
　heat-labile factor
　hepatic leukemia factor
　high-level fluoroscopy
　human lung fibroblast
hLF
　human lung field
　human lung fluid
hL-FABP
　human liver-type fatty acid-binding
　　protein
HLFCB
　horizontal laminar flow clean benches
HLG
　hypertrophic lymphocytic gastritis
HLGBSP
　Healthy Lesbian, Gay, and Bisexual
　　Students Project
HLGR
　high-level gentamicin resistance
HLH
　helix-loop-helix
　hemophagocytic lymphohistiocytosis
　human luteinizing hormone (*See also*
　　hLH)
　hypoplastic left heart [syndrome]
　　(*See also* HLHS)
hLH
　heterodimeric luteinizing hormone
　human luteinizing hormone (*See also*
　　HLH)
HLHS
　hypoplastic left heart syndrome
　　(*See also* HLH)
HLI
　head lice infestation
　hemolysis inhibition
hLI
　human leukocyte (lymphocyte)
　　interferon
HLK, H-L-K
　heart, liver, kidneys
HLL
　hypoplasia of left heart
　hypoplastic left lung

H

HLM
heart-lung machine
hemosiderin-laden macrophage
HLN
hilar lymph node
hyperplastic liver nodule
hLN
human Lesch-Nyhan [cell]
H&L OK
heart and lungs normal
HLP
hepatic lipoperoxidation
hind leg paralysis
hyperkeratosis lenticularis perstans
hyperlipoproteinemia
HLR
heart to lung ratio
heart-lung resuscitation (resuscitator)
high-level resistance
HLS
Health Learning System
hLS
human lung surfactant
HLT
heart-lung transplant(ation)
high lateral tension
hLT
human lipotropin
human lymphocyte transformation
hlth
health
HLTK
holmium laser thermokeratoplasty
HLTx
heart-lung transplant(ation)
HLV
herpeslike virus
hypoplastic left ventricle
HLVS
hypoplastic left ventricular syndrome
HM
hand motion (movement)
harmonic mean
head movement
health maintenance
heart murmur
heavily muscled
heloma molle [soft corn]
hemifacial microsomia (*See also* HFM)
hemodynamic
hemodynamic monitoring
hepatic metabolism
high magnification
Holter monitor
home management
homosexual male
hospital management
human milk

humidity mask
hydatidiform mole
hyperimmune mouse
hyperopia (hypermetropia), manifest
(*See also* Hm)
hypoxic-metabolic
H:M
heart to mediastinum ratio [radiocontrast
uptake]
Hm
hyperopia (hypermetropia), manifest
(*See also* HM)
manifest hyperopia
hm
hectometer
HMA
hemorrhage and microaneurysm
heteroduplex mobility assay
h/ma
hemorrhage and microaneurysm
hMAM RNA
human mammaglobin ribonucleic acid
HMAS
hyperimmune mouse ascites [fluid]
HMB
beta-hydroxy-beta methylbutyrate
[leucine metabolite]
human menopausal gonadotropin
hydroxy beta methylbutyrate [leucine
metabolite]
HMBA
hexamethylene bisacetamide
HMBANA
Human Milk Bank Association of North
America
HMC
hand-mirror cell
health maintenance cooperative
heroin, morphine, cocaine [drugs of
abuse]
hospital management committee
hydroxymethyl cytosine
hypertelorism, microtia, clefting
[syndrome]
minor histocompatibility complex
hMCAF
human macrophage-monocyte
chemotactic and activating factor
HMCAS
hyperdense middle cerebral artery
sign
HMCCMP
human mammary carcinoma cell
membrane proteinase
HMCK
high molecular weight cytokeratin
HMD
head-mounted display
hyaline membrane disease

HMDP
hydroxymethylene diphosphonate
[radiopharmaceutical]
HMDS
hexamethyldislazane
HME
Health Media Education
heat, massage, and exercise (*See also*
HMX)
heat/moisture exchanger
hemimegalencephaly
hereditary multiple exostoses
home medical equipment
human monocytic ehrlichiosis
human monocytotropic ehrlichiosis
HMEC
human mammary epithelial cell
HMEF
heat and moisture exchanging filter
HMETSC
heavy metal screen
HMF
human milk fortifier
hydroxymethylfurfural
HMFG
human milk fat globule
HM/3ft
hand motion at 3 feet [vision test]
HMG
high mobility group
human menopausal gonadotropin
hydroxymethylglutaric (acid)
hydroxymethylglutaryl
hMG
human menopausal gonadotropin
HMG CoA, HMG-CoA
beta-hydroxy-beta-methylglutaryl-
coenzyme A
(beta-hydroxy-β-methylglutaryl-CoA)
HMG-CoA
3-hydroxy-3-methylglutaryl coenzyme A
(hydroxymethylglutaryl
coenzyme A)
HMI
healed myocardial infarction
history of medical illness
hypomelanosis of Ito
HMIS
hallux metatarsophalangeal
interphalangeal scale
hospital medical information system
HMK
high molecular weight kininogen
(*See also* HMWK)
homemaking
hML
human milk lysozyme

HM & LP
hand motion and light perception
[vision test]
HMM
heavy meromyosin [of muscle]
human malignant mesothelioma
HMMA
4-hydroxy-3-methoxymandelic acid
HMN
hereditary motor neuropathy
HMO
health maintenance organization
heart minute output
hypothetical mean organism
HMP
health maintenance plan
hexose monophosphate
hexose monophosphate pathway
hot moist pack
hydromotive pressure
HMPA
hexamethylphosphoramide
HMPAO
hexametazime
hexamethylpropyleneamine oxime
hexamethyl-propyleneamine oxime
HMPAO-SPECT
hexamethylpropylene amine oxime
single-photon emission computed
tomography
HMPG
hydroxymethoxyphenylglycol
HMPS
hexose monophosphate shunt (*See also*
HMS)
HMPT
hexamethylphosphoric triamide
HMR
histiocytic medullary reticulosis
Hoechst Marion Roussel [stain]
H-mRNA
H-chain messenger ribonucleic acid
1H-MRS
proton magnetic resonance spectroscopy
HMRT
hazardous materials response team
HMRTE
human milk reverse transcriptase
enzyme
HMRU
Hazardous Materials Response Unit
hazardous materials response unit
HMS
hexose monophosphate shunt (*See also*
HMPS)
high methacholine sensitivity
hyperactive malarial splenomegaly

H

HMS *(continued)*
hypermobility syndrome
hypothetic mean strain
HMSAS
hypertrophic muscular subaortic stenosis
hMSC
human mesenchymal stem cell
HMSN
hereditary motor-sensory neuropathy
[type IA, II, III–VII]
HMSR
high medical-social risk
HMSS
hyperactive malarial splenomegaly
syndrome
HMT
histamine methyltransferase
Hodkinson Mental Test
hospital management team
hMT
human molar thyrotropin
HMTV
human mammary tumor virus
HMV
hand-motion vision
HMVEC
human dermal microvascular endothelial
cell
HMW
high molecular weight
HMWC
high molecular weight component
HMW-CK
high molecular weight cytokeratin
HMWGP
high molecular weight glycoprotein
HMWK
high molecular weight kininogen
(*See also* HMK)
HMW-MAA
high molecular
weight-melanoma-associated antigen
HMWPE
high molecular weight polyethylene
HMX
heat, massage, exercise (*See also* HME)
HN
head and neck (*See also* H&N)
hemagglutinin neuraminidase
hematemesis neonatorum
hemorrhage of newborn
hereditary nephritis
high necrosis
high nitrogen
hilar node
histamine-containing neuron
home nursing
Huckman number [measure of brain at
lateral ventricle anterior horns]

hypertensive nephrosclerosis
hypertrophic neuropathy
NATO code for nitrogen mustard
HN1–HN3
NATO code for nitrogen mustard 1,
2, 3
H&N
head and neck (*See also* HN)
HNA
headache, nausea, anorexia
heparin-neutralizing activity
hereditary neuropathic amyloidosis
hypothalamoneurohypophysial axis
HNAC
Heymann nephritis antigenic complex
HNAD
hyperosmolar nonacidotic diabetes
HNB
human neuroblastoma
hydroxynitrobenzylbromide
HNBD
has not been drinking
HNC
head and neck cancer
human neutrophil collagenase
hypernephroma cell
hyperosmolar nonketotic coma
hyperoxic normocapnic
hypothalamoneurohypophyseal complex
hNC
human neutrophil collagenase
HNCa
head and neck cancer
HNCD
hereditary nonprogressive corneal
dystrophy
HNE
human neutrophil elastase
HNF
hepatocyte nuclear factor
HNF-1–HNF-6
hepatocyte nuclear factor 1–6
HNHL
hepatic non-Hodgkin lymphoma
HNI
hospitalization not indicated
HNID
Haemophilus-Neisseria identification
hNIS
human sodium/iodide symporter
HNK
human natural killer [cell]
HNKC
hyperosmolar nonketotic coma
HNKDC
hyperosmolar nonketotic diabetic
coma
HNKDS
hyperosmolar nonketotic diabetic state

HNL
 histiocytic necrotizing lymphadenitis
 human neutrophil lipocalin
HNLN
 hospitalization no longer necessary
HNMM
 head and neck mucosal melanoma
H&N mot
 head and neck motion
HNN
 hybrid neural network
HNP
 hereditary nephritic protein
 herniated nucleus pulposus
 human neurophysin
HNP-4
 human neutrophil peptide 4
HNPCC
 hereditary nonpolyposis colon cancer
  (carcinoma)
 hereditary nonpolyposis colorectal
  cancer (carcinoma)
HNPP
 hereditary neuropathy [with
  susceptibility to] pressure palsy
HNR
 head-neck [of femur] replacement
hnRNA
 heterogeneous nuclear ribonucleic acid
hnRNP
 heterogeneous nuclear ribonucleoprotein
HNS
 half-normal saline [0.45% sodium
  chloride]
 head, neck, shaft [of bone]
 head and neck surgery
HNSCC
 head and neck squamous cell carcinoma
HNSHA
 hereditary nonspherocytic hemolytic
  anemia
HNSN
 home, no services needed
HNT
 Hantaan (hantavirus) vaccine
 Hantaan virus (hantavirus)
HNTD
 highest nontoxic dose
HNTLA
 Hiskey-Nebraska Test of Learning
  Aptitude
HnTT
 heparin neutralized thrombin time
HNU
 human *neu* unit
HNV
 has not voided

HNWG
 has not worn glasses
HO
 hand orthosis
 hematology-oncology
 heme oxygenase
 hereditary ovalocytosis
 heterotopic ossification
 high oxygen
 hip orthosis
 hyperbaric oxygen
 hypertrophic ossification
HO1
 heme oxygenase 1
H$_2$O
 water
H$_2$O$_2$
 hydrogen peroxide
H/O, h/o
 history of
Ho
 holmium
 horse [slang for heroin] (*See also* H)
 horse [veterinary]
HOA
 hip osteoarthritis
 hypertrophic osteoarthritis
  (osteoarthropathy)
Ho antigen
 low-frequency blood group antigen
HoaRhLG
 horse anti-rhesus lymphocyte globulin
HoaTTG
 horse antitetanus toxoid globulin
HOB
 head of bed
HOBC
 hereditary ovarian/breast cancer
HOBr
 hypobromous acid
HOBT
 hyperbaric oxygen therapy
HOB UPSOB
 head of bed up for shortness of
  breath
HOC
 human ovarian cancer
 hydroxycorticoid (*See also* HC)
 hypertrophic obstructive cardiomyopathy
HOCA
 high-osmolar contrast agent
HOCl, HClO
 hypochlorous acid
HOCM
 high-osmolar contrast medium (*See also*
  HOM)
 hypertrophic obstructive cardiomyopathy

H

HO/CO
heme oxygenase/carbon monoxide
HOD
hereditary opalescent dentin
heroin overdose
hospital day (*See also* HD)
hyperbaric oxygen drenching
13-HODE
13-hydroxyoctadecadienoic acid
HOF, hof
height of fundus
hepatic outflow
human oviduct fluid
Hoff
Hoffmann [reflex] (*See also* H)
HOGA
hyperornithinemia with gyrate atrophy
HOH
hand-over-hand [suture, dressing]
hand over hand [exercise]
hard of hearing (*See also* HH)
HOI
hospital onset of infection
hypoiodous acid
HoIg
horse immunoglobulin
HOKPP
hypokalemic periodic paralysis
HOLD
hemostatic occlusive leverage device
HoLRP
holmium laser resection of prostate
HOM
high-osmolar [contrast] medium
(*See also* HOCM)
HOME
Home Observation for Measurement of
the Environment
Home-Oriented Maternity Experience
Homeo, Homeop
homeopathy
HOMER-D
home rehabilitation dialysis
HOMO
highest occupied molecular orbital
homolat
homolateral
HONC
hyperosmolar nonketotic coma
HONK
hyperosmolar nonketotic [state or
coma]
HOOD, HOODS
hereditary onychoosteodysplasia
(osteoonychodysplasia]
hereditary onychoosteodysplasia
syndrome
HOOE
heredopathia ophthalmootoencephalica

HOOI
Hall Occupational Orientation Inventory
HOP
high oxygen pressure
holoprosencephaly-polydactyly
[syndrome]
hourly output
hypothyroxinemia of prematurity
HOPA
hospital-based organ procurement
agency
HOPD
hospital outpatient department
HOPE
health-oriented physical education
high oxygen percentage
holistic orthogonal parameter estimation
HOPE-ROP
high oxygen percentage in retinopathy
of prematurity
HOPES
human immunodeficiency virus overview
of problems evaluation system
HOPI
history of present illness (*See also*
HPI)
HOPP
hepatic-occluded portal pressure
HOPT
hamster oocyte penetration test
hor, horiz
horizontal (*See also* H, h)
HORF
high-output renal failure
horm
hormone
HORS
Hemiballism/Hemichorea Outcome
Rating Score
HOS
human osteogenic sarcoma
(osteosarcoma)
hypoosmotic swelling
HoS
horse serum (*See also* HS)
HOSE
human ovarian surface epithelial
hosp
hospital (*See also* H)
hospitalization (*See also* H)
HOST
hypoosmotic shock treatment
HOT
home oxygen therapy
human old tuberculin
hyperbaric oxygen therapy
hypertension optimal treatment
HOTC
heterozygous ornithine transcarbamylase

HOTS
hypercalcemia, osteolysis, T-cell
   syndrome
HOW
hypothermia oxygen warmer
HOX
homeobox (gene)
Ho: YAG
holmium yttrium aluminum garnet laser
HP
Haemophilus pleuropneumoniae
halogen phosphorus
handicapped person
haptoglobin (*See also* HAPTO, Hp, Hpt)
Harding-Passey [melanoma]
hard palate
Harvard pump
hastening phenomenon
health professional
heater probe
heat production
heel-to-patella (*See also* H→P)
Helicobacter pylori
hemiparesis (*See also* hemi)
hemipelvectomy
hemiplegia (*See also* hemi)
hemoperfusion
herbal product
hereditary pancreatitis
herpetiform pemphigus
highly purified
high potency
high power
high pressure
high protein [diet] (*See also* HiPro)
Hodgen and Pearson [suspension
   traction] (*See also* H&P)
horizontal plane
horsepower
hospital participation
hot pack
hot pad
human pituitary
hybridoma product
Hydrocollator pack
hydrogen peroxide
hydrophilic petrolatum
hydrophobic protein
hydrostatic pressure
hydroxyproline (*See also* HYP)
hydroxypyruvate
hyperparathyroidism (*See also* HPT,
   HPTH, hyperpara)
hyperphoria (*See also* H)
hyperplastic polyp
hypersensitivity pneumonitis
hypertension plus proteinuria

hypoparathyroidism
hypopharynx
H&P
history and physical [examination]
   (*See also* HPE)
Hodgen and Pearson [suspension
   traction] (*See also* HP)
H→P
heel-to-patella (*See also* HP)
Hp
haptoglobin (*See also* HAPTO, HP, Hpt)
Helicobacter pylori
hematoporphyrin
hp
heaping
horsepower
HPA
alpha-haptoglobin
Helix pomatia agglutinin
hemagglutinating penicillin antibody
Hereford Parental Attitude (Survey)
Histoplasma capsulatum polysaccharide
   antigen
human pancreatic amylase
human platelet antigen
hybridization protection assay
hypothalamic-pituitary-adrenal [axis]
hypothalamic-pituitary axis
hypothalamopituitary adrenal
hypothalamic-pituitary-adrenocortical
   [system] (*See also* HPAC)
HPAA
hydroperoxyarachidonic acid
hydroxyphenylacetic acid
hydroxyphenylpyruvic acid
hypothalamic-pituitary-adrenal axis
HPAC
high-performance affinity
   chromatography
hypothalamic-pituitary-adrenocortical
   [system] (*See also* HPA)
HPAEPAD
high-pH anion exchange chromatography
   coupled with pulsed amperometric
   detection
HPAFT
hereditary persistence of alpha
   (α)-fetoprotein
HPAI
highly pathogenic avian influenza A
   virus
HPAL
Hamburg Pain Adjective List
hPASP
human pancreas-specific protein
HPAT
home parenteral antibiotic therapy

H

347

HPB
    hepatobiliary
HPBC
    hyperpolarizing bipolar cell
HPBF
    hepatotropic portal blood factor
HPBL
    human peripheral blood leukocyte
HPC
    hemangiopericytoma
    hematopoietic progenitor cell
    hereditary prostate cancer
    heterotopic plate count [bacteria]
    high-passage cell
    hippocampal pyramidal cell
    history of present complaint
    holoprosencephaly
    hydrophilic coated
    hydroxyphenylcinchoninic [acid]
    hydroxypropylcellulose
    hyperplastic-like mucosal change
HPC-1
    hereditary prostate cancer 1 locus
HPCD
    hemostatic puncture closure device
HPCE
    high-performance capillary
        electrophoresis
HPCF
    high-performance chromatofocusing
HPCL-R
    Hare Psychopathy Checklist-Revised
HPD
    hearing protection device
    hematoporphyrin derivative (*See also*
        HpD)
    hereditary progressive dystonia
    highly probably drunk
    high-protein diet
    home peritoneal dialysis
HP-D
    Hough-Powell digitizer
HpD
    hematoporphyrin derivative (*See also*
        HPD)
HPDR
    hypophosphatemic D-resistant rickets
HPE
    hemorrhage, papilledema, exudate
    hepatic portoenterostomy
    high permeability edema
    history and physical examination
        (*See also* H&P)
    holoprosencephaly
    hydrostatic pulmonary edema
HPET
    Helicobacter pylori eradication therapy
HPETE
    hydroperoxyeicosatetraenoic acid

5-HPETE
    5-hydroperoxyeicosatetraenoic acid
12-HPETE
    12-hydroperoxyeicosatetraenoic acid
HPF
    heparin-precipitable fraction
    hepatic plasma flow
    high-pass filter
    high-power field [microscope
        microscopy] (*See also* hpf)
    hypocaloric protein feeding
hpf
    high-power field [microscope
        microscopy] (*See also* HPF)
HPFH
    hereditary persistence of fetal
        hemoglobin
hPFSH, HPFSH
    human pituitary follicle-stimulating
        hormone
HPG
    hepatocyte growth factor (*See also*
        HGF)
    human pituitary gonadotropin
    hypothalamic-pituitary-gonadal
hPG
    human pituitary gonadotropin (*See also*
        HPG)
HPGe
    high-purity germanium
HPH
    halothane-percent-hour
    hypoxia-induced pulmonary
        hypertension
Hp-HB
    haptoglobin-hemoglobin complex
HPHO
    hyperplastic hyperostosis
HPI
    Haemophilus parainfluenzae
    hepatic perfusion index
    hepatocyte proliferation inhibitor
    Heston Personality Inventory (Index)
        [Test]
    history of present illness (*See also*
        HOPI)
HPIEC
    high-performance ion exchange
        chromatography
HPIP
    history, physical, impression, and plan
HPIV 1–4
    human parainfluenza virus 1–4
HPL
    human parotid lysozyme
    human peripheral lymphocyte
    human placental lactogen (*See also*
        hPL)
    hyperplexia

hPL
human placental lactogen (*See also* HPL)

HPLA
hydroxyphenyllactic acid

HPLAC
high-pressure liquid affinity chromatography

HPLC
high performance (pressure) (power) liquid chromatography

HPLH
hypoplastic left heart

HPLO
Helicobacter pylori-like organism

HPM
Harding-Passey melanoma
hemiplegic migraine

HPMC
high-performance membrane chromatography
human peripheral mononuclear cell
hydroxypropyl methylcellulose

HPN
home parenteral nutrition
hypertension (*See also* HT, HTN, hypn)

HP-NAP
neutrophil-activating protein of *Helicobacter pylori*

HPNI
hemodialysis prognostic nutrition index

HPNS
high-pressure neurologic (nervous) syndrome

HPNT
Hundred Pictures Naming Test

HPO
high-pressure oxygen
hydroperoxide
hydrophilic ointment
hypertrophic pulmonary osteoarthritis (osteoarthropathy)
hypothalamic-pituitary-ovarian [axis]

HPOA
hypertrophic pulmonary osteoarthropathy (*See also* HPO)

HPP
hereditary pyropoikilocytosis
history (of) presenting problems
hydroxyphenylpyruvate
hydroxypyrazolopyrimidine
hyperplastic periostosis

2HPP
two-hour postprandial [blood sugar]

hPP
human pancreatic polypeptide

HPPA
hydroxyphenylpyruvic acid

HPPH
hydroxyphenylphenylhydantoin

HPPM
hyperplastic persistent pupillary membrane

HPPO
high partial pressure of oxygen
hydroxyphenylpyruvate oxidase

HPP/SQ
Hilson Personnel Profile/Success Quotient

HPr, hPrL
human prolactin

hPR
human progesterone receptor

HPr
hospital peer review

HPRC
hereditary papillary renal [cell] carcinoma (cancer)

HPRI
Hopkins Pain Rating Instrument

hPRP
human platelet-rich plasma

HPRT
hot plate reaction time
hypoxanthine-guanine phosphoribosyltransferase
hypoxanthine phosphoribosyltransferase

HPS
hantavirus pulmonary syndrome
hematoxylin-phloxine-saffron [stain]
hemophagocytic syndrome
hepatopulmonary syndrome
high-protein supplement
His-Purkinje system
horizontal platform support
human platelet suspension
hypertrophic pyloric stenosis
hypothalamic pubertal syndrome

HpSA
Helicobacter pylori stool antigen

HPSEC
high-performance size-exclusion chromatography

HPT
heparin protamine titration
histamine provocation test
home pregnancy test
hot plate test
human placenta thyrotropin
hyperparathyroid(ism)
hypothalamic-pituitary-testicular [axis]
hypothalamic-pituitary-thyroid [axis]

H

Hpt
haptoglobin (*See also* HAPTO, HP, Hp)
hPT
human placental thyrotropin
human proximal tubule
HPTD
highly permeable transparent dressing
HPTH
hyperparathyroid(ism) (*See also* HP, HPT, hyperpara)
hPTH
human parathyroid hormone
hPTIN
human pancreatic trypsin inhibitor
HPTLC
high-performance thin-layer chromatography
HPTM
home prothrombin time monitoring
HPTX
hemopneumothorax
HPU
heater probe unit
HPUS
hydrogen peroxide ultrasound
HPV
Haemophilus pertussis vaccine
Hart Park virus
hepatic portal vein
human papillomavirus [1–30]
human parvovirus
hypoxic pulmonary vasoconstriction
HPVD
hypertensive pulmonary vascular disease
HPV-DE
high-passage virus-duck embryo [cell]
HPV-DK
high-passage virus-dog kidney [cell]
HPVG
hepatic portal venous gas
HPW
hypergammaglobulinemic purpura of Waldenström
HPX
high peroxidase content [cell]
hypophysectomized (*See also* HX, hypox)
partial hepatectomy
Hpx
hemopexin [serum protein]
H. pylori
Helicobacter pylori
HPZ
high-pressure zone
H₂Q
ubiquinol (*See also* Q-H₂)
HQL
health-related quality of life

H&R
hysterectomy and radiation
HR
hallux rigidus
Halstead-Reitan [battery] (*See also* HRB)
Harrington rod
hazard ratio
health related
heart rate (*See also* HRT)
hematopoietic reconstitution
hematopoietic resistance
hemorrhagic retinopathy
hepatorenal
heterosexual relations [scale]
higher rate
high resolution
high risk
histamine release
hormonal response
hospital record
hospital report
hour (*See also* H, h, hr)
human resources
hyperimmune reaction
hypertensive retinopathy
hypophosphatemic rickets
hypoxic reaction
hypoxic responder
2HR
two-hour [test]
H₂R
histamine-2 receptor
Hr -2
minus two hours [two hours prior to treatment]
hr
hour (*See also* H, h, HR)
hr 0
zero hour [when treatment starts]
HRA
health risk appraisal (assessment)
heart rate audiometry
hereditary renal adysplasia
high right atrial [pacing]
high right atrium
histamine-releasing activity
H2RA
histamine-2 receptor antagonist
HRAE
high right atrium electrocardiogram
HRANA
histone-reactive antinuclear antibody
HRARE
hybrid rapid acquisition with relaxation enhancement
HRB
Halstead-Reitan Battery (*See also* HR)
histamine release from basophils

HRBC
　high-risk breast cancer
　horse red blood cell
HRBCL
　histiocyte-rich B-cell lymphoma
HRC
　help-rejecting complainer
　high-resolution chromatography
　histidine-rich calcium-binding protein
　horse red cell
　human rights committee
HRCT
　high-resolution computed tomography
HRD
　human retroviral disease
　hypertensive renal disease
　hypoparathyroidism, retardation,
　　dysmorphism
HRE
　hair removal efficiency
　high-resolution electrocardiography
　high-resolution [protein] electrophoresis
　hormone-receptor enzyme
　hormone response element
HREC
　hepatic reticuloendothelial cell
HRECG
　high-resolution electrocardiography
HREH
　high-renin essential hypertension
HREM
　high-resolution electron microscopy
HRES
　high-resolution endoluminal
　　sonography
HRF
　Harris return flow
　health-related facility
　heartburn relief formula
　heart rate fluctuations
　high-resolution fingerprint
　histamine-releasing factor
　hypertensive renal failure
　hypoxic renal failure
HRH
　hypothalamic-releasing hormone
HR-HPV
　high-risk human papillomavirus
HRHS
　hypoplastic right heart syndrome
HRI
　Harrington rod instrumentation
　high-resolution infrared [imaging]
3H-RIA
　3H (tritium) radioimmunoassay
HRIF
　histamine release inhibitory factor

HRIG
　human rabies immune globulin
　　(immunoglobulin)
HRL
　head rotation to left
HRLA
　human reoviruslike agent
HRLM
　high-resolution light microscopy
hRLX-2
　synthetic human relaxin
HRM
　Halsted radical mastectomy
Hrmax
　maximal heart rate
HRMPC
　hormone-refractory metastatic prostate
　　cancer
HR-MR
　high-resolution magnetic resonance
HR-MRI
　high-resolution magnetic resonance
　　imaging
HRMS
　high-resolution mass spectrometry
　high-resolution multisweep
HRMTP
　high-risk model of threat perception
hRNA
　heterogeneous ribonucleic acid
HRNB
　Halstead-Reitan Neuropsychological Test
　　Battery
HRNES
　Halstead Russell Neuropsychological
　　Evaluation System
HRP
　high-pass resolution perimetry
　high right parasternal [view]
　high-risk pregnancy
　histidine-rich protein
　horseradish peroxidase
HRPBC
　high-risk primary breast cancer
HRPC
　hormone-refractory prostate
　　cancer
　hormone-resistant prostate cancer
HRPD
　Hamburg Rating Scale for Psychiatric
　　Disorders
hr-PET
　high-resolution positron emission
　　tomography
HRP-GD
　high-pass resolution perimetry global
　　deviation

H

351

HRP-II
histidine-rich protein II
HRP-LD
high-pass resolution perimetry local deviation
HRPT
hyperparathyoidism
HRQL, HRQOL
health-related quality of life
HRR
haplotype relative risk
Hardy-Rand-Ritter [color vision test kit]
head retraction reflex
head rotation to right
heart rate range
heart rate recovery
heart rate reserve
high-risk recipient
high-risk register
HRRI
heart rate retardation index
HRS
Hamilton Rating Scale
Hamman-Rich syndrome
Haw River syndrome
hepatorenal syndrome
Hodgkin-Reed-Sternberg [cells]
hormone receptor site
humeroradial synostosis
HRSA
Health Resources and Services Administration [U.S. Department of Health and Human Services]
heart rate power spectral analysis
HRS-D
Hamilton Rating Scale for Depression
HRSEM
high-resolution scanning electron microscopy
HRST
heat, reddening, swelling, tenderness
heavy resistance strength training
HRSUB
submaximal heart rate
HRSV
human respiratory syncytial virus
HRT
habit reversal training
half relaxation time
heart rate (See also HR)
heart rate turbulence
Heidelberg retina tomograph
heparin response test
high-risk transfer
hormone replacement therapy
hyperfractioned radiation [therapy]
HRTE
human reverse transcriptase enzyme

HRTEM
high-resolution transmission electron microscopy
HRT II
Heidelberg retina tomograph II
HRtV
human retrovirus
HRU
hormone response unit
HRV
heart rate variability
heterogeneous resistance to vancomycin
human reovirus
human rhinovirus
human rotavirus
HRV-A
human rhinovirus A
HRV-B
human rhinovirus B
HRVL
human reoviruslike
HRVLA
human retroviruslike agent
H/S
H:S helper to suppressor ratio
hysterosalpingograph(y) (hysterosalpingogram) (See also HS, HSG, HSP)
⚠ **HS**
at bedtime [L. *hora somni hour of sleep*] (See also h.s., QHS, q.h.s.) ⚠
half-scan
half strength ⚠
hamstrings (See also hams.)
hamstring sets
hand surgery
Hartmann-Shack [aberrometry]
Hartmann solution
Haynes-Stellite [alloy]
head sign
head sling
healthy subject
heart size
heart sounds
heat stable
heavy smoker
heel spur
heelstick (See also H)
heme synthetase
hemorrhagic septicemia (shock)
heparin sulfate
hereditary spherocytosis
herpes simplex
hidradenitis suppurativa
high school
hippocampal sclerosis
homologous serum
Hopelessness Scale
horizontally selective (visual cell)

horse serum (*See also* HoS)
hospital ship
hospital stay
hour of sleep (*See also* h.s., QHS,
   q.h.s.) ⚠
human serum
hypereosinophilic syndrome
hyperplastic synovium
hypersensitivity
hypertonic saline
hypertrophic scar
hypothalamic syndrome
hysterosalpingography (*See also* HSG,
   HSP, H/S)

H&S
hearing and speech
hemorrhage and shock
hysterectomy and sterilization

H→S
heel-to-shin [test] (*See also* HTS)

H:S
helper to suppressor [cell] ratio

H₂S
Hering law-EOM innervation, both eyes
Sherrington law-EOM innervation, one
   eye

Hs
hypochondriasis
hypochondriasis scale

⚠ **h.s.**
at bedtime [L. *hora somni hour of*
   sleep] (*See also* HS, QHS, q.h.s.) ⚠

HSA
Hazardous Substances Act
health service area
health systems agency
hereditary sideroblastic anemia
hourly scratching activity
human serum albumin (*See also* HuSA)
hypersomnia-sleep apnea [syndrome]

HSAG
hydroxyethylpiperazine ethanesulfonic
   acid-saline-albumin-gelatin [test
   reagent]

HSAN
head shaking after nystagmus
hereditary sensory and autonomic
   neuropathy [types I-IV]

HSAP
heat-stable alkaline phosphatase

HSAS
hereditary stenosis of aqueduct of
   Sylvius
hydrocephalus [due to congenital]
   stenosis of aqueduct of Sylvius
hypertrophic subaortic stenosis (*See also*
   HSS)

HSB
husband (*See also* H, husb)

HSBG
heel-stick blood gas

HSBS
evening blood sugar

HSC
health screening center
hematopoietic stem cell
hepatic stellate cell
horizontal semicircular canal
human skin collagenase

HSCAS
hemodynamically significant carotid
   artery stenosis

HSCCP
High School Career-Course Planner

HSCL
Hopkins Symptom Checklist

HSCL-90
Hopkins Symptom Checklist-90

HSCL-90 T
Hopkins Symptom Checklist-90 Total
   Score

HS-CoA
reduced coenzyme A

hs-CRP
high-sensitivity C-reactive protein
   [test]

HSCS
hematopoietic stem cell support

HSCSS
hypersensitive carotid sinus syndrome

HSCT
hematopoietic stem cell transplantation

HSD
Hill-Sachs defect [radial head]
honest significance difference
hydroxysteroid dehydrogenase
hypertonic saline and dextran
hypoactive sexual desire [disorder]

HSD2
hydroxysteroid dehydrogenase type 2

17β-HSD
17-beta-hydroixysteriod dehydrogenase

HSDA
high single dose alternate day

HSDD
hypoactive sexual desire disorder

HSDI
Health Self-Determination Index

HSE
hemorrhagic shock and encephalopathy
herpes simplex encephalitis
human serum esterase
human skin equivalent
hypertonic saline-epinephrine (solution)

H

Hse
homoserine
HSEP
heart synchronized evoked potential
HSES
hemorrhagic shock-encephalopathy
syndrome
HSF
heated soybean flower
heat shock factor
histamine-induced suppressor factor
histamine-sensitizing factor
hypothalamic secretory factor
HSF1
heat shock factor 1
HSG
herpes simplex genitalis
human salivary gland
hysterosalpingograph(y)
(hysterosalpingogram) (*See also* HS,
HSP, H/S)
hysterosonography
hSGF
human skeletal growth factor
hSGP
human sialoglycoprotein
HSGYV
heat, steam, gum, yawn, Valsalva
maneuver
HSH
hypomagnesemia with secondary
hypocalcemia
HSHC
hemisuccinate of hydrocortisone
HSI
heat stress index
human seminal [plasma] inhibitor
H-SIL, HSIL
high-grade squamous intraepithelial
lesion
HSIL/CA
high-grade squamous intraepithelial
lesion/cancer
HSJ
hepatic schistosomiasis japonica
HSK
herpes simplex keratitis
herpetic stromal keratitis
HSL
herpes simplex labialis
hormone sensitive lipase
H-SLAP
human stromelysin aggregated
proteoglycan
HSLC
high-speed liquid chromatography
HSM
heparin surface-modified intraocular
lens

hepatosplenomegaly
holosystolic murmur
HSM-IOL
heparin surface-modified intraocular
lens
HSMN I–III
hereditary sensory motor neuropathy
[type I–III]
HSN
Hansen-Street nail
heart sounds normal
hereditary sensory neuropathy
herpes simplex neonatorum
HSNC
human skin nurse cell
HSO
health services organization
hSOD
human superoxide dismutase
hSOSI
human son of sevenless [gene]
HSP
heat shock protein (*See also* hsp)
hemostatic screening profile
Henoch-Schönlein purpura
hereditary sclerosing poikiloderma
hereditary spastic paraplegia
human serum prealbumin
human serum protein
hypersensitivity pneumonitis panel
hysterosalpingography (*See also* HS,
HSG, H/S)
HSP47
heat shock protein 47
HSP70
heat shock protein 70
HSP90
heat shock protein 90
HSPC
hydrogenated soy phosphatidyl choline
HSPE
high-strength pancreatic enzymes
HSPG
[glycosylphosphatidylinositol-anchored]
heparan sulfate proteoglycan
H spike
His bundle electrogram deflection
HSPM
hippocampal synaptic plasma membrane
HSPN
Henoch-Schönlein purpura nephritis
HSPQ
High School Personality Questionnaire
HSQ
Health Status Questionnaire
home screening questionnaire
HSR
Harleco synthetic resin
heated serum reagent

homogeneous staining region [of chromosome]
hypersensitivity reaction
hypofractionated stereotactic radiotherapy
HSRA
high-speed rotational atherectomy
HSRCCT
high-spatial-resolution cine computed tomography
HSRD
hypertension secondary to renal disease
HS-RDEB
recessively inherited dystrophic epidermolysis bullosa of Hallopeau and Siemens
HSRS
Health-Sickness Rating Scale
Hess School Readiness Scale
HSS
half-strength saline [0.45% sodium chloride]
hepatic stimulatory substance
high-speed supernatant
Hospital for Special Surgery
hyperstimulation syndrome
hypertrophic subaortic stenosis (*See also* HSAS)
HSSCC
hereditary site-specific colon cancer
HSSE
high soapsuds enema
HSSG
hysterosalpingosonography
HST
health screening test
Hemoccult slide test
horseshoe tear
hst-1–hst-2
human stomach cancer-transforming factor 1–2
HSTF
human serum thymus factor
HSTS
human-specific thyroid stimulator
HSV
herpes simplex virus
highly selective vagotomy
hyperviscosity syndrome
HSV1, HSV2
herpes simplex virus 1, 2
HSVE
herpes simplex virus encephalitis
HSVtk
herpes simplex virus thymidine kinase
HSV1tk
herpes simplex virus type 1 thymidine kinase

HSyn
heme synthase
HT
hammertoe
hand test
Hand Test [psychologic test]
Hashimoto thyroiditis
head trauma
healing time
hearing test
hearing threshold
heart (*See also* H)
heart channel [acupuncture]
heart test
heart tone (*See also* ht)
heart transplant(ation)
hemagglutination titer
hemorrhagic transformation
heparin trap
hereditary tyrosinemia
high temperature
high tension (*See also* ht)
high threshold
histotechnology
home treatment
hormonotherapy
hospital treatment
Hough transform
House-Tree [Test]
Hubbard tank
Huhner test
human thrombin
hydrocortisone test
hydrotherapy (*See also* hydro)
5-hydroxytryptamine [serotonin] (*See also* 5-HT, 5HT, HTA)
hyperopia (hypermetropia), total (*See also* Ht)
hypertensive (hypertension)
hyperthermia
hyperthyroid(ism)
hypertransfusion
hypertropia
hypnotherapy
hypothalamus (*See also* H, HT, HTH, hyp)
hypothyroid(ism)
H-T
head-to-tail sperm agglutination
3-HT
3-hydroxytyramine [dopamine]
5-HT, 5HT
5-hydroxytryptamine [serotonin] (*See also* HT, HTA)
5-HT$_{2A}$
5-hydroxytryptamine 2A
H&T
hospitalization and treatment

H/T
　heel and toe [walking]
H(T)
　intermittent hypertropia
Ht
　heterozygote
　hyperopia (hypermetropia), total
　　(*See also* HT)
ht
　heat
　height (*See also* H, Hgt)
ht.
　draft, drink [L. *haustas*] (*See also* H,
　　haust.)
HTA
　heterophil transplant(ation) antigen
　human thymocyte antigen
　5-hydroxytryptamine [serotonin]
　　(*See also* HT, 5-HT, 5HT)
　hypertension artérielle [French for
　　arterial hypertension]
　hypophysiotropic area [of hypothalamus]
HTACS
　human thyroid adenylcyclase stimulator
ht aer
　heated aerosol (*See also* HA)
HTAT
　human tetanus antitoxin
HTB
　hot tub bath
　house tube [feeding] (*See also* HTF)
　human tumor bank
HTC
　heated tracheostomy collar
　hepatoma cell
　hepatoma tissue culture
　homozygous typing cell
　hypertensive crisis
HTCA
　human tumor colony assay
HTCP
　Hendler Test for Chronic Pain
HTCVD
　hypertensive cardiovascular disease
　　(*See also* HCVD)
HTD
　human therapeutic dose
HTDS
　high-throughput drug screening
HTDW
　heterosexual development of women
HTE
　horizontal toit externe [angle of hip]
　hypertensive encephalopathy
hTERT
　human telomerase reverse transcriptase
HTF
　heterothyrotropic factor
　house tube-feeding (*See also* HTB)

HTG
　high-tension glaucoma
　hypertriglyceridemia
hTg
　human thyroglobulin
HTGL
　hepatic triglyceride lipase
HTH
　helix-turn-helix
　homeostatic thymus hormone
　hypothalamus (*See also* H, HT, HTH,
　　hyp)
HTHD
　hypertensive heart disease (*See also*
　　HHD)
HTI
　hemisphere thrombotic infarction
　hepatic tumor index
　human tetanus immunoglobulin
hTIg
　homologous tetanus immune globulin
　human tetanus immune globulin
　　(immunoglobulin)
HTK
　heel-to-knee [test] (*See also* HK, H-K,
　　H→K)
HTL
　hamster tumor line
　hearing threshold level
　histologic technologist
　histotechnologist
　honey-thick liquid [diet consistency]
　human T-cell leukemia [virus]
　human T-cell lymphoma [virus]
　human thymic leukemia
HTLA
　high titer, low acidity
　human T-lymphocyte antigen
HTLV
　human T-cell leukemia-lymphoma virus
　human T-cell lymphotropic virus
HTLV-I
　human T-cell leukemia-lymphoma
　　virus I
　human T-lymphotropic virus I
HTLV-II
　human T-cell leukemia-lymphoma
　　virus II
　human T-lymphotropic virus II
HTLV-III
　human T-cell leukemia-lymphoma
　　virus III
　human T-lymphotropic virus III
HTLV-III/LAV
　human T-lymphotrophic virus type III
　lymphadenopathy associated virus
HTLV-MA
　human T-cell leukemia-lymphoma
　　virus-associated membrane antigen

HTM
Haemophilus test medium
high threshold mechanoceptors
HTML
hypertext markup language
HTN
hypertension (hypertensive)
hypertensive nephropathy
HTNV
Hantaan virus (hantavirus) (*See also* HV)
HTO
heterotropic ossification
high tibial osteotomy
hospital transfer order
HTOF
healthy tissue overdose factor [radiotherapy]
HTOH
hydroxytryptophol
HTP
House-Tree-Person [projective technique psychologic test]
hydroxytryptophan
hypothalamic, pituitary, thyroid
hypothromboplastinemia
5-HTP, 5HTP
5-hydroxytryptophan
5-hydroxy-L-tryptophan
HTPN
home total parenteral nutrition
HTR
hard tissue replacement
hemolytic transfusion react
hypermetropia, right
hTR
human telomerase ribonucleic acid [component]
human thyroid hormone receptor
HTRCCT
high temporal resolution cine computed tomography
HTR-MFI
hard tissue replacement malleable facial implant
HTR-PMI
hard tissue replacement patient matched implant
hTRT
human telomerase reverse transcriptase
HTS
hammertoe syndrome
head trauma syndrome
heel-to-shin [test] (*See also* H→S)
hemangioma-thrombocytopenia syndrome
Hematest stools
high-throughput screening

human thyroid-stimulating [hormone] (*See also* hTSH)
hypertonic saline [solution]
hTSAb
human thyroid-stimulating antibody
HTSCA
human tumor stem cell assay
hTSH
human thyroid-stimulating hormone (*See also* HTS)
HTST
high temperature-short time [pasteurization]
HTT
hand thrust test
HTP
hydroxyapatite/tricalcium phosphate
HTV
heat temperature vulcanized
herpes-type virus
HTVD
hypertensive vascular disease (*See also* HVD)
HTX
heart transplant(ation) (*See also* HT, HTx)
hemothorax
HTx
heart transplant(ation) (*See also* HT, HTX)
HU
head unit
heat unit
hemagglutinating unit
hemagglutinin unit
hemolytic unit
Hounsfield unit
human urinary
human urine
hydroxyurea (*See also* HUR, HYD)
hyperemia unit
hypertensive urgencies
H.U.
heat unit [American version of British thermal unit (Btu)]
human (*See also* H, h)
hU, hu
dihydrouridine (*See also* D)
HUAEC
human umbilical arterial endothelial cell
HUAM
home uterine activity monitor(ing)
HUAV
Huacho virus
HUC
hypouricemia

H

HW *(continued)*
   heparin well
   homework
   housewife *(See also* HWFE)
   hypertriglyceridemic waist
HWB, hwb
   hot water bottle
HWE
   hot water extract
HWFE
   housewife *(See also* HW)
HWG
   has worn glasses
HWH
   halfway house
HWOK
   heel walking normal (OK)
HWP
   hepatic wedge pressure
   hot wet pack
HWPG
   has worn prescription glasses
HWS
   hot water soluble
HWY
   hundred woman years [of
     exposure]
HX
   histiocytosis X
   hospital(ization) *(See also* H, hosp)
   hydrogen exchange
   hypophysectomized *(See also* HPX,
     hypox)
Hx
   history *(See also* H, hist, Hy)
   hypoxanthine *(See also* hyp)
2-HxG
   di(hydroxyethyl)glycine
HxGPRT
   hypoxanthine-guanine phosphoribosyl
     transferase
HXIS
   hard x-ray imaging spectrometer
Hx&Px
   history and physical
HXR
   hypoxanthine riboside
HY
   hypophysis *(See also* hyp)
Hy
   history *(See also* H, hist, Hx)
   hydraulics
   hydrostatics
   hyperopia (hypermetropia) *(See also*
     H, h)
   hyperopic *(See also* H)
   hypothenar
hy
   hysteria *(See also* hys, hyst)

HYCX
   hydrocephalus due to congenital stenosis
     of aqueduct of Sylvius
HYD
   hydrated to hydration
   hydroxyurea *(See also* HU, HUR)
Hyd
   hydrostatics
hydr
   hydraulic
hydrarg.
   mercury [L. *hydrargyrum* silver water]
     (See also Hg)
HYDRO
   hydronephrosis
hydro
   hydrotherapy *(See also* HT)
hydrox
   hydroxyline
hyd and tur
   hydration and turgor
hyg
   hygiene *(See also* H)
   hygienic *(See also* H)
HYL, Hyl
   hydroxylysine
5Hyl
   5-hydroxylysine
HYLL
   healthy years of life lost
Hyp
   hydroxyproline *(See also* HP, hypro)
   hypnosis *(See also* hypno)
3Hyp
   3-hydroxyproline
4Hyp
   4-hydroxyproline
hyp
   hypalgesia
   hyperresonance
   hypertrophy
   hypophysectomy *(See also* HE)
   hypophysis *(See also* HY)
   hypothalamus *(See also* H, HT, HTH)
HYPER
   above
   higher than
hyperal, hyper-al
   hyperalimentation *(See also* HA, HAL)
hyper-IgE
   hyperimmunoglobulin E
   hyperimmunoglobulinemia E
hyper K
   hyperkalemia
hyperpara
   hyperparathyroidism (See also HP, HPT,
     HPTH)
hyperstim
   hyperstimulation

hyper T&A
hypertrophy of tonsils and adenoids
hypes
hypesthesia
hypn
hypertension (*See also* HPN, HT, HTN)
hypno
hypnosis (*See also* HYP)
HYPO
below
lower than
%HYPO
percentage of hypochromic red cell
hypo
hypochromasia
hypochromia
hypodermic [injection] (*See also* H, (H))
hypo A
hypoactive
hypo K
hypokalemia
hypopit
hypopituitarism
hypox
hypophysectomized (*See also* HPX, HX)
HYPP
hypersegmented neutrophil

HypRF
hypothalamic-releasing factor
hypro
hydroxyproline (*See also* HP, HYP)
HYs
healthy years of life
hys, hyst
hysterectomy
hysteria (*See also* hy)
hysterical
HZ
herpes zoster
hypertrophic zone
Hz
hertz [SI unit of frequency]
HZD
herpes zoster dermatitis
HZFO
hamster zona-free ovum [test]
Hz/G
hertz/gauss [resonance]
HZI
hemizona assay index
HZO
herpes zoster ophthalmicus
HZV
herpes zoster virus

H

I

implant(ation) (*See also* IP)
impression (*See also* IMP)
inactive (*See also* inac)
incisal (*See also* INC)
incisor [deciduous, permanent]
incontinent (*See also* INC)
increase(d) (*See also* INC)
independent (*See also* IND, INDEP)
index (*See also* IND)
indicate(d) (*See also* IND, indic)
indirect treatment (*See also* IND)
induction (*See also* IND)
inhalation (*See also* INH, inhal)
inhibit(ing) (*See also* inhib)
inhibition (*See also* inhib)
inhibitor
initial
insoluble (*See also* insol)
inspiration (*See also* insp, inspir)
inspired [gas]
intact (*See also* INT, IT)
intake
intensity
intensity of magnetism
intermediate (*See also* INT, intmd)
intestine (*See also* intest)
iodine
ionic strength
iota [ninth letter of Greek alphabet uppercase]
iris
isochromosome
isoleucine (*See also* ILE)
isotope
isotropic [band, disc] (*See also* ISO)
moment of inertia
one [Roman numeral]
optically inactive [chemical]
radiant intensity [W X sr^{-1}]
vector cardiography electrode [right midaxillary line]

^{123}I

iodine-123

^{125}I

iodine-125

^{127}I

iodine-127

^{131}I

iodine-131

^{132}I

iodine-132

⚠ **i, ii, iii**

quantity of drug to be delivered (*See also* Ṫ, ṪṪ, ṪṪṪ) ⚠

IA

ibotenic acid (*See also* ibo)
ideational apraxia
idiopathic anaphylaxis
image amplification
immune adherence
immunobiologic activity
impedance angle
imperforate anus
inactive alcoholic
incidental appendectomy
incurred accidentally
indolaminergic-accumulating [cells]
indulin agar
infantile apnea
infantile autism
infected area
inferior angle
inferior apical
infrequent [episodic] asthma
inhibitory antigen
interbronchial angle
internal auditory [canal] (*See also* IAC)
intraalveolar
intraamniotic (*See also* IAM)
intraaortic
intraarterial
intraarticular
intraatrial
intraauricular
invasive aspergillosis
irradiation area
isonicotinic acid
isopropyl alcohol (*See also* IPA)

I&A

irrigating (irrigation) and aspirating (aspiration)

Ia

immune [region]-associated antigen

Ia+

immune-associated antigen-positive [macrophage]

IAA

ileoanal anastomosis
indoleacetic acid
infectious agent, arthritis
inhibitory amino acid
insulin autoantibody
interruption of (interrupted) aortic arch
intraabdominal abscess
iodoacetic acid
islet antigen autoantibody

I-3-AA

indole-3-acetic acid

IAAA
 inflammatory abdominal aortic abscess
 inflammatory abdominal aortic
  aneurysm

IA-A-F
 idiopathic anaphylaxis [or] angioedema,
  frequent

IA-A-I
 idiopathic anaphylaxis [or] angioedema,
  infrequent

IAAR
 imidazoleacetic acid ribonucleotide

IAAT
 Iowa Algebra Aptitude Test
 intraabdominal adipose tissue

IAB
 incomplete abortion
 induced abortion
 intermittent androgen blockade
 intraabdominal
 intraaortic balloon

IABA
 intraaortic balloon assistance

IABC
 intraaortic balloon catheter
 intraaortic balloon counterpulsation
  (*See also* IABCP, IBC)

IABCP
 intraaortic balloon counterpulsation
  (*See also* IABC, IBC)

IABM
 idiopathic aplastic bone marrow

IABP
 intraaortic balloon pulsation
 intraaortic balloon pump (pumping)
  (*See also* IBP)
 intraarterial blood pressure

IABPA
 intraaortic balloon pumping assistance

IAC
 image analysis cytometry
 immunoaffinity chromatography
 indwelling arterial catheter
 ineffective airway clearance
 interatrial communication
 internal auditory canal (*See also* IA)
 interposed abdominal compression
 intraarterial catheter
 intraarterial chemotherapy
 intraarticular calcification
 Inventory of Anger Communications
 isolated adrenal cell
 isolated angiitis of CNS (central
  nervous system)

IACA
 immediate active cutaneous
  anaphylaxis

IACB
 intraaortic counterpulsation balloon

IAC-CPR
 interposed abdominal compressions
  cardiopulmonary resuscitation

IACD
 implantable automatic
  cardioverter-defibrillator
 intraatrial conduction defect

IACG
 intermittent angle closure glaucoma

IACI
 idiopathic arterial calcification of
  infancy

IACNS
 isolated angiitis of central nervous
  system

IACOV
 Iaco virus

IACP
 intraaortic counterpulsation

IAD
 implantable atrial defibrillator
 inactivating dose
 inhibiting antibiotic dose
 instructional advance directive
 intermittent androgen deprivation
 internal absorbed dose
 intracranial atherosclerotic disease
 intractable atopic dermatitis
 intraoperative autologous [blood]
  donation

IADH
 inappropriate antidiuretic hormone

IADHS
 inappropriate antidiuretic hormone
  syndrome

IADL
 impairment of activities of daily living
 Instrumental Activities of Daily Living

IAds
 immunoadsorption

IADSA
 intraarterial digital subtraction
  angiograph(y) (angiogram)

IAE
 intraarterial electrocardiogram
 intraatrial electrocardiogram

IAF
 idiopathic alveolar fibrosis
 intraabdominal fat

IAFI
 infantile amaurotic familial idiocy

IAG
 indolyl-3-acryloylglycine

IA-G-F
 idiopathic anaphylaxis generalized
  frequent

IA-G-I
 idiopathic anaphylaxis generalized
  infrequent

IAGT
  indirect antiglobulin test (*See also* IAT, IDAT)
IAH
  idiopathic adrenal (adrenocortical) hyperplasia
  immune adherence hemagglutination
  implantable artificial heart
IAHA
  idiopathic autoimmune hemolytic anemia
  immune adherence hemagglutination assay
IAHC
  intraarterial hepatic chemotherapy
IAHD
  idiopathic acquired hemolytic disease
IAHS
  infection-associated hemophagocytic syndrome
IAI
  intraabdominal infection
  intraabdominal injury
  intraamniotic infection
IAIA
  immune adherence immunosorbent assay
IAIS
  insulin autoimmune syndrome
  intraamniotic infection syndrome
IAK
  islet after kidney [transplantation]
IALD
  instrumental activities of daily living
IAM
  intraamniotic (*See also* IA)
  internal auditory (acoustic) meatus
IAN
  idiopathic aseptic necrosis
  indinavir-associated nephrolithiasis
  inferior alveolar nerve
iANP
  immunoreactive atrial natriuretic peptide
IAO
  immediately after onset
  intermittent aortic occlusion
IAP
  idiopathic acute pancreatitis
  immunosuppressive acidic protein
  independent adjudicating panel
  innervated antral pouch
  inosinic acid pyrophosphorylase
  intermittent acute porphyria
  intraabdominal pressure
  intracarotid amobarbital procedure
  intrapartum antibiotic prophylaxis
  islet-activating protein
IAPG
  interatrial pressure gradient

IAPP
  islet amyloid polypeptide
IAPS
  3-[^{125}I] iodo-4-azidophenetylamido-7-O-succinyldeacetyl
IAPT
  idiopathic auricular paroxysmal tachycardia
IAPV
  intermittent abdominal pressure ventilation
IAQ
  indoor air quality
IA-Q
  idiopathic anaphylaxis questionable
IAR
  immediate asthmatic reaction
  inhibitory anal reflex
  instantaneous axis of rotation
  iodine-azide reaction
IARF
  ischemic acute renal failure
IARP
  Integrated Auricular Reconstruction Protocol
IARSA
  idiopathic acquired refractory sideroblastic anemia
IART
  intraatrial reentrant (reentry) tachycardia
IAS
  idiopathic ankylosing spondylitis
  illness attitude scale
  immunosuppressive acidic substance
  infant apnea syndrome
  Integrated Assessment System
  interatrial septum
  interatrial shunting
  intermittent androgen suppression
  internal anal sphincter
  intraabdominal sepsis
  intraamniotic saline [infusion]
  intraarterial secretin
IASA
  idiopathic acquired sideroblastic anemia
  interatrial septal aneurysm
IASD
  interatrial septal defect (*See also* ISD)
IASH
  isolated asymmetric septal hypertrophy
IAT
  immunoaugmentative therapy
  indirect antiglobulin test (*See also* IAGT, IDAT)
  instillation abortion time
  intracarotid amobarbital test
  intraoperative autologous transfusion
  invasive activity test
  iodine azide test
  Iowa Achievement Test

IATT
intraarterial thrombolytic therapy

IAV
interactive video
intermittent assisted ventilation
intraarterial vasopressin

IA-V
idiopathic anaphylaxis variant

IAVB
incomplete atrioventricular block

IAVC
intrinsic atrioventricular conduction

IAVI
International AIDS Vaccine Initiative

IAVM
intramedullary arteriovenous
malformation

IB
idiopathic blepharospasm
ileal bypass
immune balance
immune body
inclusion body (*See also* IncB)
index of body build
infantile botulism
infectious bronchitis
inferior basal
insulin receptor binding test
irradiated bone
isolation bed

I-B
interbody [vertebral]

IBA
isobutyric acid

IBAM
idiopathic bile acid malabsorption

I band
isotropic band [striated muscle fiber]
(*See also* I disc)

IBAT
intravascular bronchoalveolar tumor

IBAV
Ibaraki virus

IBB
intestinal brush border

IBBB
intra blood-brain barrier

IBBBB
incomplete bilateral bundle branch
block

IBC
Illness Behavior Checklist
inflammatory breast cancer (carcinoma)
intraaortic balloon counterpulsation
(*See also* IABC, IABCP)
invasive bladder cancer
iodine-binding capacity
iron-binding capacity
isobutyl cyanoacrylate (*See also* IBCA)

IBCA
isobutyl cyanoacrylate (*See also*
IBC)

IBD
identical by descent
infectious bowel disease
infectious bursal disease
inflammatory bowel disease
irritable bowel disease
ischemic bowel disease
isosulfan blue dye

IBDQ
Inflammatory Bowel Disease
Questionnaire

IBDV
infectious bursal disease virus

IBE
inclusion body encephalitis
individual bioequivalence

IB-EP
immunoreactive beta endomorphin

IBF
immature brown fat [cell]
immunoglobulin-binding factor
Insall-Burstein-Freeman [total knee
instrumentation]
intermittent biliary fever
intestinal blood flow

IBG
iliac bone graft
insoluble bone gelatin

IBI
intermittent bladder irrigation
internal borderzone infarct
ischemic brain infarction

ibid.
in the same place [L. *ibidem*]

IBIDS
ichthyosis, brittle [hair], [impaired]
intelligence, decreased [fertility], short
[stature] [syndrome]
ichthyosis plus BIDS [syndrome]

IBILI
indirect bilirubin

IBK
infectious bovine keratoconjunctivitis

IBL
immunoblastic lymphadenopathy
immunoblastic lymphoma

IBM
ideal body mass
inclusion body myositis
intact bridge mastectomy
isotonic-isometric brief maximum

IBMI
initial body mass index

IBMTR
International Bone Marrow Transplant
Registry

IBNR
  incurred but not reported
ibo
  ibotenic acid (*See also* IA)
IBOW
  intact bag of waters
IBP
  intraaortic balloon pump (pumping)
    (*See also* IABP)
  intrableb pigmentation
  invasive blood pressure
  iron-binding protein
IBPB
  interscalene brachial plexus block
IBPMS
  indirect blood pressure measuring
    system
IBPS
  Insall-Burstein posterior stabilizer
IBQ
  Illness Behavior Questionnaire
IBR
  immediate breast reconstruction
  Infant Behavior Record
  infectious bovine rhinotracheitis
IBRS
  Inpatient Behavior Rating Scale
IBRV
  infectious bovine rhinotracheitis virus
IBS
  ichthyosis bullosa of Siemens
  imidazole-buffered saline
  immunoblastic sarcoma
  inflammatory bowel syndrome
  inside bathing solution
  irritable bowel syndrome
  isobaric solution
IBSA, iBSA
  immunoreactive bovine serum albumin
  iodinated bovine serum albumin
IBSN
  infantile bilateral striatal necrosis
    [syndrome]
IBT
  immune-based therapy
  immunobead test
  inflatable bone tamp
  ink blot test [Rorschach test]
  interblinking time
  intracavitary brachytherapy
IBTR
  intrabreast tumor recurrence
  ipsilateral breast tumor recurrence
IBU
  international benzoate unit
IBV
  [avian] infectious bronchitis virus

  [avian] infectious bronchitis
    vaccine
IBW
  ideal body weight
IC
  between meals L. *inter cibos* (*See also*
    i.c.)
  icterus (icteric) (*See also* ICT)
  ileocecal
  iliac crest
  iliococcygeal
  iliocostal
  immune complex (*See also* ICX)
  immune cytotoxicity
  immunocompromised
  immunocytochemistry (*See also* ICC)
  impedance cardiograph(y) (cardiogram)
    (*See also* ICG)
  incipient cataract [grade 11 to 41]
  incomplete (*See also* INC, incomp,
    incompl)
  indeterminate colitis
  indirect calorimetry
  indirect Coombs [test] (*See also* ICT)
  individual counseling
  infection control
  inferior colliculus
  information content
  informed consent
  inhibitory concentration
  inner canthal [distance] (*See also* ICD)
  inorganic carbon
  inspiratory capacity
  inspiratory center
  institutional care
  integrated care
  integrated circuit
  integrated concentration
  intensive care (*See also* ICU)
  intercarpal
  intercostal [space] (*See also* ICS, IS)
  intercourse
  intermediate care
  intermittent catheterization (*See also*
    IMC)
  intermittent claudication
  internal capsule
  internal carotid
  internal cerebral
  internal conjugate [diameter]
  internal connection
  international classification
  interstitial cell (*See also* ISC)
  interstitial change
  interstitial cystitis
  intracameral
  intracapsular

IC *(continued)*
   intracardiac
   intracarotid
   intracavitary (*See also* ICAV)
   intracellular
   intracerebral
   intracisternal [injection] (*See also* ICI)
   intracoronary
   intracranial
   intracutaneous
   intraoperative cholangiography
   intrapleural catheter
   invalid chair
   invasive cancer
   ion chromatography
   irritable colon (*See also* ICS)
   Isaacson classification [gastric
     lymphoma]
   islet cell [of pancreas]
   isovolumic contraction (*See also* IVC)

I&C
   incision and curettage

IC$_{50}$
   concentration that inhibits 50%

i.c.
   between meals [L. *inter cibos*]
     (*See also* IC)

ICA
   ileocolic anastomosis
   immunocytochemical assay
   intercountry adoption
   intermediate care area
   internal carotid artery
   intracranial abscess
   intracranial anatomy
   intracranial aneurysm
   islet cell antibody (*See also* ICAb)
   islet cell antigen

iCa
   ionized calcium

ICAb
   islet cell antibody (*See also* ICA)

ICAF
   internal carotid artery flow

ICAM1–ICAM3
   intercellular adhesion molecule 1–3

ICAO
   internal carotid artery occlusion

ICAP
   intracisternal A particle

ICAS
   intermediate coronary artery syndrome

ICAT
   infant cardiac arrest tray
   intracoronary aspiration thrombectomy

ICAV
   intracavitary (*See also* IC)

ICB
   intracranial bleeding

ICBF
   inner cortical blood flow
   intramyocardial coronary blood flow

ICBG
   iliac crest bone graft

ICBN
   intercostobrachial nerve

ICBP
   intracellular binding protein

ICBT
   intercostobronchial trunk

ICC
   idiopathic chronic cough
   immunocompetent cell
   immunocytochemistry (*See also* IC)
   Indian childhood cirrhosis
   infection control committee
   intensive coronary care
   interchromosomal crossing-over
   intermediate cell column
   intermittent clean catheterization
   internal conversion coefficient
   interstitial cells of Cajal
   intraclass correlation coefficient
     [statistics]
   intracluster correlation coefficient
     [statistics]
   intracranial cavity
   intrahepatic cholangiocarcinoma
   invasive cervical cancer
   islet cell carcinoma

ICCD
   intensified charge-coupled device

ICCE
   intracapsular cataract extraction

ICCEc̄PI
   intracapsular cataract extraction with
     peripheral iridectomy

ICCM
   idiopathic congestive cardiomyopathy

ICD
   I-cell disease
   idiopathic cerebral dysfunction
   immune complex disease
   immune complex dissociation
   implantable cardioverter-defibrillator
   impulse control disorder
   inclusion cell disease
   indigocarmine dye
   induced circular dichroism
   informed consent document
   initial consonant deletion
   inner canthal distance (*See also* IC)
   instantaneous cardiac death
   intercanthal distance
   internal cardioverter-defibrillator
   internal cervical device
   International Classification of Diseases
     [World Health Organization]

intracardiac defibrillator
intracervical device
intrauterine contraceptive device
(*See also* IUCD, IUD)
Inventory for Counseling and
Development
irritant contact dermatitis
ischemic coronary disease
isocitrate dehydrogenase (*See also* IDH,
ICDH)
isolated conduction defect

ICD-9
International Classification of Diseases,
9th Edition

ICD-10
International Classification of Diseases
and Related Health Problems, 10th
Edition

ICDA
International Classification of Diseases,
Adapted [for use in United States]

ICDB
incomplete database
Interstitial Cystitis Data Base

ICDC
implantable cardioverter-defibrillator
catheter

ICDCD
International Classification of Diseases
and Causes of Death

ICD-CM
International Classification of Diseases
Clinical Modification

ICD-9-CM
International Classification of Diseases,
9th Edition, Clinical Modification

ICDH
isocitrate dehydrogenase (*See also* ICD,
IDH)
isocitric acid dehydrogenase

ICD-O
International Classification of Diseases
for Oncology

ICD p24
immune-complex dissociated p24
antigen

ICDS
Integrated Child Development Scheme

ICE
ice, compression, elevation
ichthyosis-cheek-eyebrow [syndrome]
immunoglobulin-complexed enzyme
individual career exploration
interleukin-1 alpha (α) converting
enzyme
interleukin-1 beta (β) converting
enzyme

intracardiac echocardiography
iridocorneal endothelial [syndrome]

+ice
add ice

ICED
index of coexistent disease

ICEDP
intraspinal epidural pressure

ICEEG
intracranial electroencephalography

ICEG
intracardiac electrocardiography

I-cell
inclusion cell

ICER
incremental cost-effectiveness ratio
inducible cyclic adenosine
monophosphate (cAMP) early
repressor

ICES
ice, compression, elevation, support

ICET
[Forty-Eight] Item Counseling
Evaluation Test
induced current electrical impedance
tomography

ICEUS
intracaval endovascular ultrasound
(ultrasonography)

ICF
immediate care facility
immunodeficiency, centromeric
instability, facial anomalies [syndrome]
indirect centrifugal flotation
intercellular fluorescence
interciliary fluid
intracellular fluid
intravascular coagulation and fibrinolysis
[syndrome]

ICFA
incomplete Freund adjuvant (*See also*
IFA)
induced complement-fixing antigen

ICFM
isolated congenital folate malabsorption

ICF-MR
intermediate-care facility for mentally
retarded

IC fx
intracapsular fracture

ICG
impedance cardiograph(y) (cardiogram)
(*See also* IC)
indocyanine green [dye]
isotope cisternography

ICGA
indocyanine green angiography

ICGN, IC-GN
immune complex glomerulonephritis
ICG-PDR
indocyanine green plasma disappearance
rate
ICH
idiopathic cortical hyperostosis
immunocompromised host
infantile cortical hyperostosis
infectious canine hepatitis
intracerebral hematoma
intracerebral hemorrhage
intracerebral hypertension
intracranial hemorrhage
intracranial hypertension
ICHD
ischemic coronary heart disease
ICHPPC
International Classification of Health
Problems in Primary Care
ICI
Interpersonal Communication Inventory
intracardiac injection
intracardiac infection
intracisternal injection (*See also* IC)
intracranial injury
IC-IC
intracranial to intracranial (anastomosis)
ICIDH
International Classification of
Impairments, Disabilities, and
Handicaps
ICIDH-2
International Classification of
Impairments, Activities, and
Participation
ICIS
imaging center information system
integrated clinical information system
ICISS
International Classification of Diseases
[9th Ed.] Injury Severity Score
ICIT
intensified conventional insulin
therapy
intracavernosal injection therapy
ICJ
ileocecal junction
ICK
infectious crystalline keratopathy
ICL
idiopathic CD4 (CD4+) T-cell
lymphocytopenia
implantable contact lens
intracorneal lens
intracorporeal laser lithotripsy
intracranial lesion
iris-clip lens
isocitrate lyase

I$_{Cl}$
chloride current
ICLE
intracapsular lens extraction
ICM
image cytometry
infracostal margin
inner cell mass
intelligent cardiovascular monitor
intercostal margin
intercostal muscle
interference-contrast microscopy
intracytoplasmic membrane
ion conductance modulator
ipsilateral competing message
ischemic cardiomyopathy
isolated cardiovascular malformation
ICMA
immunochemiluminescence assay
immunochemiluminescent assay
immunochemiluminometric assay
ICMI
Inventory of Childhood Memories and
Imaginings
ICN
inferior calcaneonavicular ligament
intercostal neuralgia
ICNC
intracerebellar nuclear cell
ICO
idiopathic cyclic oedema (edema)
[British]
impedance cardiac output
intracellular organism
ICOD
infectious cause of death
ICOS
inducible costimulatory [molecule]
ICOV
Icoaraci virus
ICP
incubation period (*See also* IP)
inductively coupled plasma
infantile cerebral palsy
infectious cell protein
inflammatory cloacogenic polyp
intercostal position [chest lead]
intermittent catheterization protocol
intracavernous pressure
intracranial pressure
intracytoplasmic
intrahepatic cholestasia (cholestasis) of
pregnancy
↑ICP
increased intracranial pressure (*See also*
IICP)
ICP-AES
inductively coupled plasma atomic
emission spectrometry

ICPC
intracranial pressure catheter
IC-PC
internal carotid and posterior
communicating [arteries]
ICPMM
incisors, canines, premolars, molars
[permanent dentition formula]
ICP-MS
inductively-coupled plasma-mass
spectrometer
ICP-OES
inductively-coupled plasma-optical
emission spectrometry
ICPP
intubated continuous positive-pressure
ICPS
Interpersonal Cognitive Problem Solving
[approach]
ICR
[distance between] iliac crests
intercostal retractions
intermittent catheter routine
international calibrated ratio
intracardiac catheter recording
intracavitary radium
intracorneal ring [implant]
intracranial reinforcement
intrastromal corneal ring
ion cyclotron resonance
I-CRF
immunoreactive corticotropin-releasing
factor
ICrH
intracranial hemorrhage
ICRS
Index Chemicus Registry System
intrastromal corneal ring segment
ICRT
Individualized Criterion Referenced
Testing
intracoronary radiation therapy
ICRTM
Individualized Criterion Reference
Testing Mathematics
ICRTR
Individualized Criterion Reference
Testing Reading
ICRU
International Commission on Radiation
Units [and Measurements]
ICS
ileocecal sphincter
immotile cilia syndrome
improved Chen-Smith [image coder]
impulse-conducting system
inferior capsular shift

inhaled corticosteroid
intensive care, surgical
intercellular space (*See also* IS)
intercostal space (*See also* IC, IS)
intermediate coronary syndrome
international compression system
intracellular cytokine staining
intracellular-like, calcium-bearing
crystalloid solution
intracranial stimulation
irritable colon syndrome (*See also* IC)
ICSA
islet cell surface antibody
ICSC
idiopathic central serous
chorioretinopathy
ICSD
*International Classification of Sleep
Disorders: Diagnostic and Coding
Manual*
ICSF
idiopathic calcium [renal] stone
formation
ICSH
interstitial cell-stimulating hormone
ICSHI
intracytoplasmic sperm head injection
ICSI
intracytoplasmic sperm injection
ICSK
intracoronary streptokinase
ICSO
intermittent coronary sinus occlusion
ICSPF
internal carotid systolic peak flow
ICSR
Individual Case Safety Reports
intercostal space retractions
ICSS
intracranial self-stimulation
ICT
icterus (icteric) (*See also* IC)
immunoglobulin consumption test
indirect Coombs test (titer) (*See also*
IC)
induction chemotherapy
inflammation of connective tissue
insulin coma (convulsive) therapy
intensive conventional therapy
intermittent cervical traction (*See also*
ICTX)
interstitial cell tumor
intracardiac thrombus
intracranial tumor
intracutaneous test
intradermal cancer test
intraoral cariogenicity test

ICT *(continued)*
islet cell transplant(ation)
isolated cortical tubule
isovolumic contraction time (*See also* IVCT)

ICt$_{50}$
incapacitating Ct$_{50}$ [concentration incapacitating to half a group]

iCT
immunoreactive calcitonin

ict ind
icterus index (*See also* II)

ICTP
carboxy terminal telopeptide of type 1 collagen

ICTS
idiopathic carpal tunnel syndrome

ICTX
intermittent cervical traction (*See also* ICT)

ICU
immunologic contact urticaria
intensive care unit (*See also* IC)

ICUS
intracoronary ultrasound

ICV
internal cerebral vein
intracellular volume
intracerebroventricular
into cerebral ventricles

ICVA
intracranial vertebral artery

ICVH
ischemic cerebrovascular headache

ICVM
intracerebroventricular administration of morphine

ICW
in connection with
intact canal wall
intercellular water
intracellular water
intracranial width

ICX
immune complex (*See also* IC)

ICXA
intermediate circumflex artery

ID
identify (identification)
idiotype
iditol dehydrogenase
ill-defined
immune deficiency (immunodeficiency)
immunodiffusion [test]
immunoglobulin deficiency
inappropriate disability
incapacitating dose
inclusion disease
index of discrimination

individual dose
induction delivery
infant death
infecting dose
infectious disease (*See also* INF, inf dis)
infective dose
inhibitory dose
inhomogeneous deposition
initial diagnosis
initial dose
initial dyskinesia
injected dose
inner diameter
inside diameter
insufficient data
intellectual disability
interdigitating
interhemispheric disconnection
internal derangement
internal diameter
interscan delay
interstitial disease
intradermal (*See also* i.d.)
intraduodenal

I-D
intensity-duration [curve]

I&D
incision and drainage
irrigation and debridement
irrigation and drainage

ID$_{50}$
median incapacitating dose [chemical]
median infective dose [microorganism]

Id
idiotypic
infradentale [craniometric]

i.d.
intradermal (*See also* ID)

id.
the same [L. *idem*]

IDA
iduronidase
idiopathic destructive arthritis
image display and analysis
iminodiacetic acid
insulin-degrading activity
iron deficiency anemia

IDAM
infant of drug abusing mother

IDAT
indirect antiglobulin test (*See also* IAGT, IAT)

IDAV
immunodeficiency-associated virus

IDB
incomplete database

IDBR
indirect bilirubin

IDBS
infantile diffuse brain sclerosis
IDC
idiopathic dilated cardiomyopathy
indwelling catheter
infiltrating ductal carcinoma
interdigitating cells
interdigitating dendritic cell
interlocking detachable coil
intervertebral disc calcification
intraductal carcinoma
invasive ductal carcinoma
IDCF
immunodiffusion complement fixation
immunodiffusion complement-fixing
IDCI
intradiplochromatid interchange
IDCM
idiopathic dilated cardiomyopathy
IDCN
intermediate dorsal cutaneous nerve
IDCS
diffuse cutaneous scleroderma
interdigitating dendritic cell sarcoma
IDD
insulin-dependent diabetes
intervertebral disc disease
intraluminal duodenal diverticulum
iodine-deficiency disorder
I/DD
intellectual and developmental
disabilities
IDDF
investigational drug data form
IDDM
insulin-dependent diabetes mellitus
IDDM-MED
insulin-dependent diabetes mellitus [and]
multiple epiphysial dysplasia
[syndrome]
IDDRT
Infectious Disease Death Review Team
IDDS
implantable drug delivery system
investigational drug data sheet
IDDT
immunodouble diffusion test
IDE
inner dental epithelium
insulin-degrading enzyme
Investigational Device Exemption
IDEA
Individuals with Disabilities Education
Act
IDEAS
Interest Determination, Exploration
Assessment System, (Enhanced
Version)

ID:ED
internal diameter to external diameter
ratio [cardiac valve replacement]
IDEM
ischemic, drug, electrolyte, metabolic
[effect]
IDET
intradiscal electrothermal therapy
(treatment)
IDF
inferior duodenal flexure
IDFC
immature dead female child
IDG
interdental groove
interdisciplinary group
intermediate dose group
IDGH
ischemic disease of growing hip
IDH
intradialytic hypotension
intramural duodenal hematoma
isocitrate dehydrogenase (*See also* ICD,
ICDH)
IDH1, IDH-S
isocitrate dehydrogenase, soluble
IDH2, IDH-M
isocitrate dehydrogenase, mitochondrial
IDI
immunologically detectable insulin
induction-delivery interval
Interpersonal Dependency Inventory
intractable diarrhea of infancy
intrathecal drug infusion
IDIS
intraarterial digital subtraction
intraoperative digital subtraction
[angiography]
IDISA
intraoperative digital subtraction
angiography
I disc
isotropic disc (striated muscle fiber)
(*See also* I band)
IDK
internal derangement of knee [joint]
IDL
Index to Dental Literature
intensity difference limen
intermediate-density lipoprotein
ischemic digital loss
IDL-C
intermediate-density lipoprotein-
cholesterol complex
IDLH
Immediately Dangerous to Life or
Health [classification of airborne
CBWs]

IDM
idiopathic disease of myocardium
immune defense mechanism
indirect method
infant of diabetic mother
intensive diabetes management

IDMC
immature dead male child
interdigestive motility (motor)
(myoelectric) complex (*See also*
IDMEC, IMC)

IDMEC
interdigestive motility (motor)
(myoelectric) complex (*See also*
IDMC, IMC)

ID-MS
isotope dilution-mass spectrometry

IDMS
isolated diffuse mesangial sclerosis

IDN
interdigital neuroma

IDNA
iron-deficient, not anemic

iDNA
intercalary deoxyribonucleic acid

IDO
indoleamine 2,3-dioxygenase

IDP
imidodiphosphonate
immunodiffusion procedure
initial dose period
initiate discharge planning
inosine diphosphatase
instantaneous diastolic pressure

IDPase
inosine diphosphatase (*See also*
IDP)

IDPH
idiopathic pulmonary hemosiderosis
(*See also* IPH)

IDPN
inflammatory demyelinating
polyneuropathy
intradialytic parenteral nutrition

IDR
idiosyncratic drug reaction
intradermal reaction

IDS
iduronate sulfatase [deficiency]
immune deficiency state
incremented dynamic scanning
inhibitor of DNA synthesis
integrated delivery system
intradermal smear
intraduodenal stimulation
investigational drug service

IDSA
intraoperative digital subtraction
angiography

IDSI
internodular difference in signal
intensity

IDST
intraductal secretin test

IDT
immune diffusion test
instillation delivery time
intensive diabetes treatment
interdisciplinary team
interdivision time
intradermal test
intradermal typhoid [and paratyphoid
vaccine]

IDTP
immunodiffusion tube precipitin

IDTS
Inventory Of Drug-Taking Situations

IDU
infectious disease unit
injecting drug user
injection drug use(r)
intravenous drug use(r)
iododeoxyuridine (5-iodo-2′-
deoxyuridine)
Ivy dog unit

IdUA
iduronic acid

IDUS
injecting drug user
intraductal ultrasound
(ultrasonography)

IDV
intermittent demand ventilation

IDVC
indwelling venous catheter

IDWG
interdialytic weight gain

Idx
cross-reactive idiotype

IE
immediate early
immunizing unit [Ger. *immunitäts
Einheit*] (*See also* IU, ImmU)
immunoelectrophoresis (*See also* IEP)
induced emesis
infectious (infective) endocarditis
inner ear
intake energy [unit of food]
internal ear
internal elastica
intraepithelial
introversion-extroversion [scale]
(*See also* IES)

I-E
internal versus external

I&E
ingress and egress
internal and external

I:E
> inspiratory to expiratory ratio

i.e.
> that is [L. *id est*]

IEA
> immediate early antigen
> immunoelectroadsorption
> immunoelectrophoretic analysis
> immunoenzyme assay
> infectious equine anemia
> inferior epigastric artery
> intravascular erythrocyte aggregation

IEB
> idiopathic erythroblastopenia

IEBD
> intraesophageal balloon distention

IEBI
> intereye blink interval

IEC
> injection electrode catheter
> inpatient exercise center
> intestinal epithelial cell
> intradiscal electrothermal coagulation
> intraepithelial carcinoma
> ion-exchange chromatography

IE Ca cx
> intraepithelial carcinoma of cervix

IECRT
> intraoperative endoscopic Congo red test

IED
> immune-enhancing diet
> improvised explosive device
> inherited epidermal dysplasia
> intermittent explosive disorder

IEE
> inner enamel epithelium

IEEG
> intracranial electroencephalography

IEF
> isoelectric focusing [electrophoresis]

IEF-PAGE
> isoelectric focusing electrophoresis in
>   polyacrylamide gel

IEGM
> intracardiac electrogram

IEHL
> intracorporeal electrohydraulic lithotripsy

IEI
> idiopathic environmental intolerance
> isoelectric interval

IEL
> intestinal epithelial cell
> internal elastic lamina
> intraepithelial leukocyte (lymphocyte)

IEM
> immune electron (immunoelectron)
>   microscopy
> inborn error of metabolism
> ineffective esophageal motility
> internal elastic membrane

IEMA
> immunoenzymatic assay

IEMG
> integrated electromyograph(y)
>   (electromyogram)

IEMR
> integrated electronic medical record

IEN
> intraepithelial neoplasia

IEOP
> immunoelectroosmophoresis

IEP
> idiopathic erythropoiesis
> immunoelectrophoresis (*See also* IE)
> individualized education program
> intraesophageal pressure

IEPA
> immunoelectrophoresis analysis

IER
> in expected range

IERIV
> Ieri virus

IERM
> idiopathic epiretinal membrane

IES
> Impact of Events Scale
> inferior esophageal sphincter
> ingressive-egressive sequence
> introversion-extroversion scale (*See also*
>   IE)

IET
> infantile esotropia
> intrauterine exchange transfusion

IETT
> immediate exercise treadmill testing

IEU
> idiopathic esophageal ulcer

IF
> idiopathic fibroplasia
> idiopathic flushing
> immersion foot
> immunofluorescence (immunofluorescent)
>   (*See also* IFL)
> index finger
> indirect fluorescence
> inferior facet
> infrared [light] (*See also* IFR, infra., IR)
> inhibiting factor
> initiation factor
> injury factor
> inspiratory force
> instantaneous flow
> interbody fusion
> interfollicular

IF *(continued)*
    interfrontal
    intermaxillary fixation (*See also* IMF)
    intermediate filament (*See also* IMF)
    intermediate frequency
    internal fixation
    internal friction
    interstitial fluid (*See also* ISF)
    intracellular fluid
    intrinsic factor
    involved field
    intensifying factor
IFA
    idiopathic fibrosing alveolitis
    immune fluorescent
        (immunofluorescence) antibody
    immunofluorescence (immunofluorescent)
        assay
    incomplete Freund adjuvant (*See also*
        ICFA)
    indirect fluorescent antibody
    indirect fluorescent assay
    indirect immunofluorescent antibody
IF-A
    inflammatory factor of anaphylaxis
I-FABP
    intestinal fatty acid-binding protein
IFAP
    ichthyosis, follicularis, atrichia (or
        alopecia), photophobia syndrome
IFAT
    immunofluorescence antibody
        test
    indirect fluorescent antibody test
IFC
    inspiratory flow cartridge
    interferential current
    interferential stimulation
    intermittent flow centrifugation
    intrinsic factor concentrate
IFCL
    intermittent flow centrifugation
        leukapheresis
IFCS
    inactivated fetal calf serum
IFDC
    infiltrating ductal carcinoma
IFDS
    isolated follicle-[stimulating hormone]
        deficiency syndrome
IFE
    immunofixation electrophoresis
    in-flight emergency
    interfollicular epidermis
IFEV
    Ife virus
IFF
    inner fracture face

IFG
    impaired fasting glucose
    inferior frontal gyrus
IFGS
    interstitial fluid and ground substance
IFI
    indirect immunofluorescence
    Institutional Functioning Inventory
        [psychologic test]
    intrafollicular insemination
IFIX
    immunofixation
IFL
    immunofluorescence (immunofluorescent)
        (*See also* IF)
    indolent follicular lymphoma
    inferior frontal lobe
IFM
    internal fetal monitoring
    intrafusal muscle
IFN
    immunoreactive fibronectin
    interferon [type I, II, III]
IFN alpha(α)–omega(ω)
    interferon type alpha (α), beta (β),
        gamma (γ), epsilon (ϵ), omega (ω)
If nec
    if necessary
IFO
    in front of
    implanted fertilized ovum
IFOBT
    immunological fecal occult blood test
IFP
    inflammatory fibroid polyp
    intermediate filament protein
    interstitial fluid pressure
    intimal fibrous proliferation
    intrapatellar fat pad
IFR
    infrared [light] (*See also* IF, infra., IR)
    inspiratory flow rate
IFRA
    indirect fluorescent rabies antibody
        [test]
IFROS
    ipsilateral frontal routing of signals
IFRT
    involved field radiotherapy
IFS
    interstitial fluid space
    intrinsic fluorescence spectroscopy
IFSA
    individualized functional status
        assessment
IFSAC
    Inventory of Functional Status After
        Childbirth

IFSE
internal fetal scalp electrode
IFSP
individual(ized) family service plan
IFT
immunofluorescence technique (test)
International Frequency Tables
inverse Fourier transform
IFU
interferon unit
IFV
interstitial fluid volume (*See also* ISFV)
intracellular fluid volume
IG
image guide
immature granule
immunology
intragastric
I-G
insulin-glucagon
Ig
immunoglobulin
iG
immunoreactive human gastrin
IGA
infantile genetic agranulocytosis
IgA
immunoglobulin A
IgA1
immunoglobulin A subclass 1
IgA2
immunoglobulin A subclass 2
IgA-IFA
IgA immunofluorescent antibody
IgA tTG
immunoglobulin A transglutaminase
antibody
IGBB
image-guided breast biopsy
IGC
intragastric cannula
IGCN
intratubular germ cell neoplasm
(*See also* ITGCN)
IGCNU
intratubular germ cell neoplasia,
unclassified type
IGCS
inpatient geriatric consultation services
IGD
idiopathic growth hormone deficiency
interglobal distance
isolated gonadotropin deficiency
IgD
immunoglobulin D
IgD1
immunoglobulin D subclass 1

IgD2
immunoglobulin D subclass 2
IGDE
idiopathic gait disorders of elderly
IGDM
infant of mother with gestational
diabetes mellitus
IGDR
interstitial granulomatous drug
reaction
IGE
impaired gas exchange
IgE
immunoglobulin E
IgE1
immunoglobulin E subclass 1
IGF
insulinlike growth factor (*See also*
ILGF)
IGF1
insulinlike growth factor 1
IGF2
insulinlike growth factor 2
IgF
immunoglobulin F
IGFA
indocyanine-green fundus angiography
IGFBP
insulinlike growth factor-binding
protein
IGFBP-1–IGFBP-6
insulinlike growth factor-binding protein
1–6
IG-FESS
image-guided functional endoscopic
sinus surgery
IGFET
insulated gate field effect transistor
IGF-1R
insulinlike growth factor 1 receptor
IGF-2R
insulinlike growth factor 2 receptor
IgG
immunoglobulin G
IgG1
immunoglobin G1
IgG2
immunoglobulin G2
IgG2a
immunoglobulin G2a
IgG4
immunoglobulin G4
IgG AGA
immunoglobulin G antigliadin
antibody
IgG RF
immunoglobulin G rheumatoid factor

IGH
idiopathic growth hormone
immunoreactive growth hormone
(*See also* IRGH)

IGHD I–III
isolated growth hormone deficiency 1–3

IGHD IB
isolated growth hormone deficiency type
IB

IGHL
inferior glenohumeral ligament

IGI
Image Guided Implantology
[system]
Institutional Goals Inventory

IgIM
immunoglobulin, intramuscular

IgIV
immunoglobulin, intravenous

IGLLC
inferior glenohumeral ligament labral
complex

IgM
immunoglobulin M

IgM1
immunoglobulin M subclass 1

IgM-IFA
IgM immunofluorescent antibody

IgM RF
immunoglobin M-rheumatoid factor

IGP
injection gold probe
interstitial glycoprotein
intestinal glycoprotein

IGPA
infragenicular popliteal artery

IGPD
inherited giant platelet disorder

IgQ
immunoglobulin quantitation

IGR
immediate generalized reaction
integrated gastrin response
intrauterine growth retardation

IGRT
image-guided radiation therapy
(radiotherapy)

IGS
image-guided surgery
implantable gastric stimulation
inappropriate gonadotropin secretion

IgSC
immunoglobulin-secreting cell

IGSS
immunogold-silver staining

IGT
impaired glucose tolerance
interpersonal group therapy
intragastric titration

IGTN
impaired glucose tolerance and
neuropathy
ingrown toenail

IGTT
intravenous glucose tolerance test

IGV
idiopathic genu valgum
intrathoracic gas volume (*See also*
ITGV)
isolated gastric varices [type 1, 2]

IH
in hospital
ichthyosis hystrix
idiopathic hirsutism
idiopathic hypercalciuria
immediate hypersensitivity
incomplete healing
indirect hemagglutination
industrial hygiene
infantile hydrocephalus
infectious hepatitis
inguinal hernia
inguinal herniorrhaphy
inhibiting hormone
in-house
inner half
inpatient hospital
intermittent heparinization
intimal hyperplasia
intracerebral hematoma
intracranial hypertension
intramural hematoma
intraretinal hemorrhage
iris hamartoma
iron hematoxylin

IHA
idiopathic hyperaldosteronism
immune hemolytic anemia
indirect hemagglutination antibody
[test]
indirect hemagglutination assay
indirect hemagglutinin assay
infusion hepatic arteriography
intrahepatic atresia

IHAC
intrahepatic artery chemotherapy

IHAS
idiopathic hypertrophic aortic stenosis

IHB
incomplete heart block

IHb
hemoglobin content index

IHBT
incompatible hemolytic blood
transfusion

IHBTD
incompatible hemolytic blood
transfusion disease

IHC
idiopathic hemochromatosis
idiopathic hypercalciuria
immobilization hypercalcemia
immunohistochemical
immunohistochemistry
infantile hydrocephalus
inner hair cell [of cochlea]
intrahepatic cholestasis (*See also* IHPC)
IHCA
isocapnic hyperventilation with cold air
IHCM
ichthyosis hystrix Curth-Macklin [type]
IHD
in-center hemodialysis
intermittent hemodialysis
intraheptic duct(ule)
ischemic heart disease
IHDI
ischemic heart disease index
IHDN
integrated health delivery network
IHES
idiopathic hypereosinophilic syndrome
IHF
interhemispheric fissure
IHG
ichthyosis hystrix gravior
IHGD
isolated human growth deficiency
IHH
idiopathic hypogonadotropic
hypogonadism
idiopathic hypothalamic hypogonadism
infectious human hepatitis
isolated hypogonadotropic hypogonadism
IHHE
infantile hepatic hemangioendothelioma
IHHS
idiopathic hyperkinetic heart syndrome
IHJ
intrahepatic jaundice
IHN
ischemic hemorrhagic necrosis
IHNV
infectious hematopoietic necrosis virus
IHO
idiopathic hypertrophic osteoarthropathy
IHP
idiopathic hypoparathyroidism
idiopathic hypopituitarism
inferior hypogastric plexus
interhospitalization period
inverted hand position
isolated hepatic perfusion
IHPC
intrahepatic cholestasis (*See also* IHC)

IHPH
intrahepatic portal hypertension
IHPS
infantile hypertrophic pyloric stenosis
IHR
inguinal hernia repair
intrahepatic resistance
intrinsic heart rate
IHRA
isocapnic hyperventilation with
room air
IHS
Idiopathic Headache Score
idiopathic hypereosinophilic syndrome
inactivated horse serum
Indian Health Service [U.S. Public
Health Service]
infrahyoid strap (*See also* IS)
integrated healthcare system
intracranial hypotension syndrome
IHSA
iodinated human serum albumin
IHSC
immunoreactive human skin collagenase
IHSS
idiopathic hypertrophic subaortic
sclerosis (stenosis)
in-home support services
IHT
insulin hypoglycemia test
insulin-induced hypoglycemic therapy
intravenous histamine test
ipsilateral head turning
I5HT
intraplatelet serotonin
IHU
inpatient hospice unit
IHW
inner heel wedge
II
icterus index (*See also* ict ind)
image intensifier (intensification)
insurance index
irradiated iodine
I or I
illness or injuries
I&I
illness and injuries
IIA
indirect immunofluorescence assay
internal iliac artery
IIBC
immunized bovine colostrum
IIBD
idiopathic inflammatory bowel disease
IIC
integrated ion current

IICP
    increased intracranial pressure (*See also* ↑ICP)

IID
    infectious intestinal disease
    insulin-independent diabetes

IIDM
    insulin-independent diabetes mellitus

IIE
    idiopathic ineffective erythropoiesis

IIED
    intention imprinted electronic device

IIEF
    International Index of Erectile Function

IIF
    immune interferon
    indirect immunofluorescence
        (immunofluorescent)
    isolated intraperitoneal fluid

IIFT
    intraoperative intraarterial fibrinolytic
        therapy

IIGR
    ipsilateral instinctive grasp reaction

IIH
    idiopathic infantile hypercalcemia
    idiopathic intracranial hypertension
    iodine-induced hyperthyroidism

IIHR
    insulin-induced hypoglycemic response

IIHT
    iodine-induced hyperthyroidism

IIIVC
    infrahepatic interruption of inferior vena
        cava

IIM
    idiopathic inflammatory myopathy
    intracortical interaction mapping

^{123}I-IMP
    iodine-123 isopropyl-iodoamphetamine

IINB
    ilioinguinal-iliohypogastric nerve block
    ilioinguinal nerve block

IIP
    idiopathic interstitial pneumonia
        (pneumonitis)
    idiopathic intestinal pseudo-obstruction
    increased intracranial pressure
    indirect immunoperoxidase
    Intra- and Interpersonal (Relations
        Scale)

IIPF
    idiopathic interstitial pulmonary fibrosis

^{123}I-IPPA
    iodine-123 iodophenyl pentadecanoic
        acid

IIQ-R
    Incontinence Impact
        Questionnaire-Revised

IIRS
    Illness Intrusiveness Rating Scale

IIS
    intensive immunosuppression
    intermittent infusion set

IIT
    ineffective iron turnover
    integrated isometric tension
    intensive insulin therapy

IITR
    International Islet Transplant Registry

IJ
    ileojejunal
    internal jugular [vein]
    intrajejunal
    intrajugular

IJC
    internal jugular catheter

IJD
    inflammatory joint disease

IJO
    idiopathic juvenile osteoporosis

IJP
    inhibitory junction potential
    internal jugular pressure

IJR
    idiojunctional rhythm

IJT
    idiojunctional tachycardia

IJV
    internal jugular vein

IK
    immobilized knee
    immune body [Ger. *Immunekörper*]
    immunoconglutinin
    infusoria killing [unit] (*See also* IKU)
    interstitial keratitis

IKDC
    International Knee Documentation
        Committee

IKE
    ion kinetic energy

IKI
    iodine potassium iodide [Lugol solution]

IKU
    infusoria killing unit (*See also* IK)

IL
    ileum [bowel]
    iliolumbar
    ilium [bone]
    immature lung
    incisolingual
    independent laboratory
    inguinal ligament
    insensible loss
    inspiratory loading
    intensity level
    interleukin
    intermediary letter

intestinal lymphocyte
intralesional
intralipid
intralumbar
intraocular lens (*See also* IOL)

IL 1–18
interleukin 1–18

I-L
intensity-latency

Il
ilinium [obsolete name for element 97, berkelium]

ILA
inferior lateral angle
insulinlike activity

IL 1 alpha (α)
interleukin 1 alpha (α)

IL 1 beta (β)
interleukin 1 beta (β)

ILa
incisolabial

131I-labeled MIBG
iodine-131 I-labeled metaiodobenzylguanidine

ILAP
interstitial laser ablation of prostate

ILB
incidental Lewy body
infant, low birth (weight) (*See also* ILBW)

ILBBB
incomplete left bundle-branch block

ILBW
infant, low birth weight (*See also* ILB)

ILC
ichthyosis linearis circumflexa
incipient lethal concentration
infiltrating lobular carcinoma
Integrated Light Control
interstitial laser coagulation
invasive lobular cancer

ILCP
interstitial laser coagulation of prostate

ILD
immature lung disease
indentation load deflection
intermediate density lipoproteins
interstitial lung disease
ischemic leg disease
ischemic limb disease
isolated lactase deficiency

ILDCSI
Individual Learning Disabilities Classroom Screening Instrument

ILDL
intermediate low-density lipoprotein

ILE
infantile lobar emphysema
involutional lateral entropion
isoleucine (*See also* I)

ILEAD
Instructional Leadership Evaluation and Development Program

ILEV
Ilesha virus

ILFC
immature living female child

ILGF
insulinlike growth factor (*See also* IGF)

ILHDL
isolated low high-density lipoprotein

ILHP
ipsilateral hemidiaphragmatic paresis

ILHV
Ilheus virus

ILI
influenzalike illness

ILL
inequality in leg length
intermediate lymphocytic lymphoma
intracorporeal laser lithotripsy

ILM
insulinlike material
internal limiting membrane

I-LMA, ILMA
intubating laryngeal mask airway

ILMC
immature living male child

ILMI
inferolateral myocardial infarct(ion)

ILNR
intralobar nephrogenic rest

ILo
iodine lotion

ILP
inadequate luteal phase
interstitial laser photocoagulation
interstitial lymphocytic pneumonia
intralesional laser photocoagulation
intraligamentary pregnancy
isolated limb perfusion

ILQTS
idiopathic long QT [interval] syndrome

ILR
implantable loop recorder
irreversible loss rate

IL-2R
interleukin-2 receptor

IL-4R
interleukin-4 receptor

IL-1RA
interleukin-1 receptor antagonist

IL-3Ra^{bright}
interleukin-3 receptor alpha (α) bright

ILS
idiopathic leucine sensitivity
idiopathic lymphadenopathy syndrome
increase in life span
infrared liver scanner
intralabyrinthine schwannoma
intralobular sequestration
intraluminal stapler

ILSA
Interpersonal Language Skills and
Assessment

ILSS
integrated life support system
intraluminal somatostatin

ILT
iliotibial tract
interstitial laser therapy

ILUS
intraluminal ultrasound

ILV
independent lung ventilation
instantaneous lung volume
[recording]

ILVEN
inflammatory linear verrucous epidermal
nevus

IM
ice massage
idiopathic myelofibrosis (See also IMF)
immunosuppression method
impaired mentation
Index Medicus (See also Ind Med)
industrial medicine (See also Ind Med,
IND, indust)
infection medium
infectious mononucleosis (See also
INFM, inf mono, mono)
inner membrane
innocent murmur
inspiratory muscle
intermediate megaloblast
intermetatarsal
intermuscular
internal malleolus
internal mammary [artery]
internal margin [imaging]
internal medicine (See also Int Med)
internal monitor
intestinal malrotation
intestinal mesenchyme
intestinal metaplasia
intracellular macroadenoma
intramedullary
intramuscular [injection] (See also i.m.)
invasive mole

i.m.
intramuscular (See also IM)

IMA
immunometric assay
inferior mesenteric artery
intermetatarsal angle
internal mammary artery (See also IM)
internal maxillary artery (See also
IMAX)

IMAA
iodinated macroaggregated albumin

IMAB
internal mammary artery bypass

IMAC
immobilized metal affinity
chromatography

IMAG
internal mammary artery graft

IMAI
internal mammary artery implant

IMARD
immunomodulating antirheumatic drug

IMAT
intensity-modulated arc therapy
[radiotherapy]

IMAX
internal maxillary artery (See also IMA)

IMB
intensity-modulated beam [radiotherapy]
intermenstrual bleeding

IMBC
indirect maximal breathing capacity
initially metastatic breast carcinoma

IMBP
immobilized mismatch binding protein

IMBT
intestinal mucinous borderline tumor

IMC
immunohistochemical
index of marrow conversion
information memory concentration
interdigestive migrating complex
interdigestive migrating contraction
interdigestive motility, (motor)
(myoelectric) complex (See also IDM,
IDMEC)
intermittent catheterization (See also IC)
internal mammary chain [lymph nodes]
intestinal mucosal mast cell
intramedullary catheter
irregular menstrual cycle

IMCA
intramural coronary artery

IMCD
inner medullary collecting duct

IMCE
intravenous myocardial contrast
echocardiography

IMCI
Integrated Management of Childhood
Illness

IMC-N
inframammary crease-to-nipple [distance]

IMD
immune-mediated diabetes
immunologically mediated disease
inherited metabolic disorder
intramammary distance

ImD$_{50}$
immunizing dose sufficient to protect
50% of subjects

IMDC
intramedullary metatarsal decompression

IMDD
idiopathic midline destructive disease

IME
important medical event
independent medical evaluation
independent medical examination
indirect medical education
isometric exercise

IMEHD
implantable middle ear hearing device

IMEM
improved minimal essential medium

IM/EM
intramedullary [and/or] extramedullary

IMEM-HS
improved minimal essential medium,
hormone supplemented

IMET
isometric endurance test (time)

IMEX
image segmentation [radiotherapy]

IMF
idiopathic mediastinal fibrosis
idiopathic myelofibrosis (*See also* IM)
immobilization of mandibular fracture
inframammary fold
intermaxillary fixation (*See also* IF)
intermediate filament (*See also* IF)

IMG
inferior mesenteric ganglion
internal mammary graft
international medical graduate

IMGG
intramuscular gamma globulin

IMGU
insulin-mediated glucose uptake

IMH
idiopathic myocardial hypertrophy
idiopathic myometrial hypertrophy
indirect microhemagglutination (test)
(*See also* IMHT)
intramural hemorrhage

IMHT
indirect microhemagglutination test
(*See also* IMH)

IMI
immunologically measurable insulin
Impact Message Inventory
impending myocardial infarct(ion)
indirect membrane immunofluorescence
inferior [wall] myocardial infarct(ion)
(*See also* Inf MI)
intermeal interval
intramuscular injection

^{123}I-MIBG
iodine-123 metaiodobenzylguanidine

^{125}I-MIBG
iodine-125 metaiodobenzylguanidine

^{131}I-MIBG
iodine-131 metaiodobenzylguanidine

IMIG
intramuscular immunoglobulin

IML
intermediolateral
intermetacarpal ligament
internal mammary lymphoscintigraphy

IMLA, IMLAD
intramural left anterior descending
[coronary artery]

IMLC
incomplete mitral leaflet closure
intramyocellular lipid content

IMLNS
idiopathic minimal lesion nephrotic
syndrome

ImLy
immune lysis

IMM
immobility
immune modulating nutrition
(immunonutrition)
immunization (*See also* immun)
immunology
inhibitor-containing minimal medium
internal medial malleolus

immat
immature
immaturity

IMMC
interdigestive migrating motor complex
intestinal mucosal mast cell

immed
immediately

immobil
immobilization
immobilize

ImmU
immunizing unit (*See also* IE, IU)

immun
immune
immunity
immunization (*See also* IMM)

immunol
immunology
IMN
idiopathic membranous nephropathy
immune modulating nutrition
internal mammary [lymph] node
intramammary [lymph] node
intramedullary nailing
ischemic muscular necrosis
IMO
idiopathic multicentric osteolysis
in my opinion
IMP
iatrogenic multiple pregnancy
idiopathic myeloid proliferation
impact(ed) (impaction) (*See also* impx)
important
impression (*See also* I)
improved
incomplete male pseudohermaphroditism
Innovative Medical Products
inosine monophosphate (inosine
5′-monophosphate)
Inpatient Multidimensional Psychiatric
[scale]
intramembranous particle
intramuscular [compartment] pressure
IMPA
incisal mandibular plane angle
IMPDH
inosine monophosphate dehydrogenase
imperf
imperfect
imperforate
IMPEX
immediate postexercise
IMPL
impulse
IMPS
Inpatient Multidimensional Psychiatric
Scale
IMPT
intensity-modulated proton therapy
impvt
improvement
impx
impact(ed) (impaction) (*See also* IMP)
IMR
individual medical record
infant mortality rate
infectious mononucleosis receptor
IMRA
immunoradiometric assay
IMRAD, IMRD
introduction, materials and methods,
results, and discussion [formal
structure of scientific article]
Imreg-1–Imreg-2
immunomodulator 1–2

IMRI, I-MRI, iMRI
interventional magnetic resonance
imaging
IMRS
intensity-modulated radiosurgery
IMRT
intensity-modulated radiation therapy
(radiotherapy)
IMS
incurred in military service
industrial methylated spirit
inframammary syndrome
integrated medical services
ion mobility spectrometry
IMSC
intramedullary supracondylar
IMSS
in-flight medical support system
IMT
implantable miniaturized telescope
induced muscular tension
inflammatory myofibroblastic tumor
inspiratory muscle training
integrated massage therapy
intimal-medial thickness
ImU
international milliunit
IMV
inferior mesenteric vein
intermittent mandatory ventilation
intermittent mechanical ventilation
IMVC, IMViC, imvic
indole, methyl red, Voges-Proskauer,
and citrate [test]
IMVP
idiopathic mitral valve prolapse
IMX
whole-body antibody technique
⚠ **IN**
icterus neonatorum
impetigo neonatorum
incidence
incompatibility number
infantile nephrotic [syndrome]
infundibular nucleus
intermediate nucleus
interneuron
interstitial nephritis
intranasal ⚠
In
indium
inion [craniometric]
inulin
in.
inch
in²
square inch
in³
cubic inch

I

^{111}In
    indium-111
^{113m}In
    indium-113m
INA
    infectious nucleic acid
    inferior nasal artery
I_{Na}
    sodium current
INAA
    instrumental neutron activation
        analysis
inac
    inactive (*See also* I)
INAD
    infantile neuroaxonal dystrophy
    investigational new animal drug
    in no apparent distress
INB
    intercostal nerve blockade
    internuclear bridging
    ischemic necrosis of bone
inbr
    inbreeding
INC
    illuminated near card
    image not clear
    incisal (*See also* I)
    incision(al)
    including (*See also* incl)
    incompatibility
    incomplete (*See also* IC, incomp,
        incompl)
    inconclusive
    incontinent (*See also* I)
    increase(d) (*See also* I, incr)
    increment (*See also* incr)
    incurred
    inside-the-needle catheter
    internodular cortex
    interstitial nucleus of Cajal
Inc.
    incorporated
INCA
    infant nasal cannula assembly
    infant nasal CPAP (continuous positive
        airway pressure) assembly
Inc Ab
    incomplete abortion
IncB
    inclusion body (*See also* IB)
INCD
    infantile nuclear cerebral degeneration
INCL
    infantile neuronal ceroid lipofuscinosis
incl
    including (*See also* INC)

IncO$_2$
    incubator oxygen
incomp, incompl
    incomplete (*See also* IC, INC)
incont
    incontinent
incr
    increase(d) (*See also* INC)
    increment
INCS
    incomplete resolution, scan [to]
        follow
incur
    incurable
IND
    independent (*See also* I, INDEP)
    index (*See also* I)
    indicate(d) (*See also* I, indic)
    indigent
    indigo
    indirect
    indirect treatment (*See also* I)
    induce(d)
    induction (*See also* I)
    industrial [medicine] (*See also* indust,
        IM, IND)
    internodal distance
    intestinal neuronal dysplasia
    investigational new drug
INDA
    Investigational New Drug
        Application
INDEP
    independent (*See also* I, IND)
indic
    indicate(d) (*See also* I, IND)
    indication
indig
    indigestion
INDIV
    individual
INDM
    infant of nondiabetic mother
Ind Med
    Index Medicus (*See also* IM)
Ind-Med
    industrial medicine (*See also* IM, IND,
        indust)
^{111}In-DTPA
    indium diethylenetriamene pentaacetic
        acid
indust
    industrial [medicine] (*See also* IM, IND,
        Ind Med)
INE
    infantile necrotizing
        encephalomyelopathy

INEX
    inexperienced
INF
    infancy
    infant
    infantile
    infarct(ion)
    infect(ed) (*See also* INFC, infect., infx)
    infection (*See also* INFC, infect., infx)
    infectious [disease] (*See also* ID, inf dis)
    infective (*See also* infect.)
    inferior (*See also* infer.)
    infirmary
    information
    infundibulum [of neurohypophysis]
    infuse(d)
    infusion (*See also* inf)
    intravenous nutritional fluid
    pour in [L. *infunde*] (*See also* inf.)
inf.
    pour in [L. *infunde*] (*See also* INF)
INFa
    influenza virus, attenuated live vaccine
INFC
    infect(ed) (*See also* INF, infect., infx)
    infection (*See also* INF, infect., infx)
InfCM
    inflammatory cardiomyopathy
inf dis
    infectious disease (*See also* ID, INF)
infect.
    infect(ed) (*See also* INF, INFC, infx)
    infection (*See also* INF, INFC, infx)
    infective (*See also* INF)
infer.
    inferior (*See also* INF)
INFH
    ischemic necrosis of femoral head
INFi
    influenza virus inactivated vaccine
infl
    inflam(ed)
    inflammation (*See also* inflamm)
    inflammatory (*See also* inflamm)
    influence
    influx
inflamm
    inflammation (*See also* infl)
    inflammatory (*See also* infl)
infl proc
    inflammatory process
INFM, inf mono
    infectious mononucleosis (*See also* IM, mono)
Inf MI
    inferior [wall] myocardial infarct(ion) (*See also* IMI)

info
    information
infra.
    infrared [light] (*See also* IF, IFR, IR)
INFs
    influenza virion vaccine, split virion
INFs-AB3
    influenza virus inactivated vaccine, split virion, types A and B, trivalent
INFw
    influenza virion vaccine, whole virion
infx
    infection (*See also* INF, INFC, infect.)
ING
    inguinal
    isotope nephrogram
INGAP
    islet-cell neogenesis-associated protein
INGV
    Ingwavuma virus
INH
    inhalation (*See also* I, inhal)
    inhaler
inhal
    inhalation (*See also* I, INH)
inhib
    inhibit(ing) (*See also* I)
    inhibition (*See also* I)
INI
    intranuclear inclusion [agent]
^{111}**In**
    indium-111
INIV
    Inini virus
inj
    inject(ion) (*See also* inject.)
    injure(d)
    injurious
    injury
inject.
    inject(ion) (*See also* inj)
INK
    injury not known
INKV
    Inkoo virus
inl
    inlay
INLSD
    ichthyosis and neutral lipid storage disease
INN
    International Nonproprietary Name
innerv
    innervate(d)
    innervation
INO
    infantile nephrotic [syndrome], other [type]
    inhaled nitrous oxide

internodal ophthalmoplegia
internuclear ophthalmoplegia
Ino
inosine
iNO
inhaled nitric oxide
INOC, inoc
inoculate(d)
inoculation
INOH
instantaneous orthostatic hypotension
inop
inoperable
inorg
inorganic
iNOS
inducible nitric oxide synthase
(synthetase)
Inox
inosine, oxidized
INP
idiopathic neutropenia
INPAV
intermittent negative pressure-assisted
ventilation (*See also* INPV)
INPC
International Neuroblastoma Pathology
Classification
INPRCNS, INPRONS
information processing in central
nervous system
IN-PT
inpatient
INPV
intermittent negative pressure-[assisted]
ventilation (*See also* INPAV)
INQ
inferior nasal quadrant
Inquiry Mode Questionnaire: A Measure
of How You Think and Make
Decisions
INR
immediate nasal response
international normalized ratio
INREM
internal radiation (roentgen) equivalent
man [radiation dose]
INS
idiopathic nephrotic syndrome
insert(ion)
inspection
insurance
insure(d)
INS Ab
insulin antibody
INS, ARG65HIS
hyperproinsulinemia, familial dbSNP

INS, ARG65LEU
hyperproinsulinemia, familial [proinsulin
Kyoto]
INS, ARG65PRO
hyperproinsulinemia, familial
insem
insemination
INS, HIS10ASP
hyperproinsulinemia, familial [proinsulin
Providence]
insid
insidious
INSK
interstitial nonsyphilitic keratitis
insol
insoluble (*See also* I)
insp
inspect(ion)
inspiration (*See also* I, inspir)
ins, PHE25LEU
insulin Chicago .0001
INS, PHE24SER
insulin Chicago .0002
inspir
inspiration (*See also* I, insp)
INSR
insulin receptor
INSS
International Neuroblastoma Staging
System
INST
instrumental [delivery]
inst
institute
instrument
instr
instruct
insuf, insuff
insufficiency
insufficient
insufflation
INS, VAL3LEU
insulin Wakayama [diabetes mellitus
with hyperinsulinemia]
INT
intact (*See also* I, IT)
integral
interest
intermediate (*See also* I, intmd)
intermittent (*See also* INTR)
intermittent needle therapy
intern
internal (*See also* intern.)
interval
intestinal (*See also* intest)
intestine (*See also* I, intest)
iodonitrotetrazolium

int2
> integration gene 2

INTEG
> integument

intern.
> internal (*See also* INT)

internat
> international

INTERP
> interpret(ation)

intertroch
> intertrochanteric

intest
> intestinal (*See also* INT)
> intestine (*See also* I, INT)

int/ext
> internal/external [rotation]

INTH
> intrathecal [anesthesia, injection]
> (*See also* IT, ITh, i-thec)

int hist
> interval history

intmd
> intermediate (*See also* I, INT)

Int Med
> internal medicine (*See also* IM)

int mon
> internal monitor

int obst
> intestinal obstruction (*See also* IO)

intol
> intolerance

INTOX
> intoxication

INTR
> intermittent (*See also* INT)

intraMLN
> intramammary lymph node

int-rot
> internal rotation (*See also* IR)

int trx
> intermittent traction (*See also* IT)

intub
> intubation

INV
> inferior nasal vein

inv
> invalid
> inverse
> inversion (*See also* inver)
> involuntary (*See also* invol)

inver
> inversion (*See also* inv)
> invert(ed)

invest.
> investigation

invet
> inveterate

inv/ev
> inversion/eversion

inv ins
> inverted insertion

INVM
> isolated noncompaction of ventricular myocardium

invol
> involuntary (*See also* inv)

involv
> involve(d)
> involvement

IO
> incisal opening
> inferior oblique [eye muscle]
> inferior olive
> initial opening [pressure]
> inoperable
> inside-out [vesicle]
> intensive observation
> internal os [cervix]
> intestinal obstruction (*See also* int obst)
> intraocular [pressure] (*See also* IOP)
> intra-Ommaya [reservoir]
> intraoperative
> intraosseous

I&O, I and O, I/O
> input/output
> intake and output
> in and out

IO$_2$
> inspired oxygen

Io
> ionium [former term for thorium-230]

IOA
> inner optic anlage
> intact on admission
> intraoral appliance

IOC
> intern on call
> intraoperative cholangiograph(y) (cholangiogram) (*See also* IOCG)
> in our culture

IOCG
> intraoperative cholangiograph(y) (cholangiogram) (*See also* IOC)

IOCM
> isosmolar contrast medium

IOD
> implant-supported overdenture
> injured on duty
> integrated optical density
> interorbital distance

IODM
> infant of diabetic mother

IOE
> intraoperative echocardiography
> intraoperative endoscopy
> intraoperative enteroscopy

IOEBT
  intraoperative electron beam therapy
IOECS
  intraoperative electrical cortical
    stimulation
IOERT
  intraoperative electron radiation therapy
IOF
  intraocular fluid
IOFB
  intraocular foreign body
IOFNA
  intraoperative fine-needle aspiration
IOFNM
  intraoperative facial nerve monitoring
IOH
  idiopathic orthostatic hypotension
IOHDR
  intraoperative high dose rate
IOHDRBT
  intraoperative high-dose-rate
    brachytherapy
IOI
  idiopathic orbital inflammation
  intraosseous infusion
IOIS
  idiopathic orbital inflammatory
    syndrome
IOL
  induction of labor
  intraocular lens (*See also* IL)
IOLI
  intraocular lens implantation
IOLM
  intraoperative lymphatic mapping
IOLP
  intraocular lens power
IOM
  infraorbital margin
  Institute of Medicine [of the National
    Academies]
  interosseous membrane
  intraocular muscle
  intraoperative neurophysiologic
    monitoring
IOML
  infraorbitomeatal line
ION
  ischemic optic neuropathy
IONIS
  indirect optic nerve injury syndrome
IONTO
  iontophoresis
IOOA
  inferior oblique overaction
IOP
  intraocular pressure (*See also* IO)
  intraosseous puncture

IOPC
  intraductal oncocytic papillary carcinoma
IOPN
  intraductal oncocytic papillary neoplasm
IOR
  ideas of reference
  immature oocyte retrieval
  index of response
  inferior oblique recession
  information outflow rate
IO-RB
  intraocular retinoblastoma
IORT
  intraoperative radiation therapy
    (radiotherapy)
IOS
  infant observation scale
  intraoperative sonography
IOSH
  Institute for Occupational Safety and
    Health [United Kingdom]
IOT
  intraocular tension
  intraocular transfer
  ipsilateral optic tectum
ι, iota
  iota [ninth letter of Greek alphabet
    lowercase]
IOTA
  information overload testing aid
IOTEE
  intraoperative transesophageal
    echocardiography
IOTT
  intensification of treatment trigger
    [criteria]
IOU
  international opacity unit
IOUS
  intraocular ultrasound
  intraoperative ultrasound
    (ultrasonography)
IOV
  initial office visit
  inside-out vesicle
IOVA
  intraocular vision aid
IOVP
  intraesophageal variceal pressure
IOWA
  inattention-overactivity with aggression
IP
  ice pack
  icterus praecox
  ileoproctostomy
  iliopsoas [muscle]
  imaging plate
  immune precipitate

IP *(continued)*
  immunoblastic plasma
  immunoperoxidase
  implant(ation) *(See also* I)
  inactivated pepsin
  incisoproximal
  incisopulpal
  incontinentia pigmenti
  incubation period *(See also* ICP)
  individualized plan
  induced potential
  induction period
  industrial population
  infection prevention
  inflation point
  infrapatellar
  infundibular process
  infundibulopelvic [ligament]
  infusion pump
  initial pressure
  inlet pouch
  inorganic phosphate
  inosine phosphorylase
  inositol phosphate
  inpatient
  instantaneous pressure
  International Pharmacopoeia
  interpeduncular [nucleus]
  interphalangeal [joint] *(See also* IPJ)
  interpharyngeal
  interpositus [nucleus]
  interpupillary
  interstitial pneumonia
  intervening peptide
  intestinal permeability
  intestinal pseudoobstruction
  intracellular proteolysis
  intraperitoneal *(See also* i.p.)
  invasive procedure
  inverted papilloma
  ionization potential
  in plaster
IP3, IP₃
  inositol triphosphate (inositol
    1,4,5-triphosphate)
IP-10
  interferon-inducible protein 10
I/P
  iris and pupil
I&P
  influenza and pneumonia
i.p.
  intraperitoneal *(See also* IP)
IPA
  idiopathic pulmonary arteriosclerosis
  immunoperoxidase assay
  incontinentia pigmenti achromians
  independent practice association
  indole pyruvic acid

infantile papular acrodermatitis
International Phonetic Alphabet
interpleural analgesia
intrapleural analgesia
intrapulmonary artery
invasive pulmonary aspergillosis
isopropyl alcohol *(See also* IA)
Ipa
  pulse average intensity
IPAA
  ileal pouch anal anastomosis
IPAO
  insulin-induced peak acid output
IPAP
  inspiratory positive airway pressure
IPAT
  [Cattell's] Institute for Personality and
    Ability Testing [Anxiety Scale]
  Iowa Pressure Articulation Test
iPAT
  integrated parallel acquisition technique
IPB
  infrapopliteal bypass
  intraperitoneal bleeding
IPBH
  intraparenchymal brain hemorrhage
IPC
  indirect pulp cavity
  intermediate posterior curve
  intermittent pneumatic compression
  interpeduncular cistern
  intraductal papillary carcinoma
  intraperitoneal chemotherapy
  ion-pair chromatography
  ischemic preconditioning
  isopropyl chlorophenyl
IPCD
  idiopathic paroxysmal cerebral
    dysrhythmia
  infantile polycystic [kidney] disease
    (See also IPCK)
IPCK
  infantile polycystic kidney [disease]
    (See also IPCD)
IPCS
  infrapatellar contracture syndrome
IPCT
  intraperitoneal chemotherapy
IPCV
  idiopathic polypoidal choroidal
    vasculopathy
IPD
  idiopathic Parkinson disease
  idiopathic protracted diarrhea
  immediate pigment darkening
  incomplete pancreas divisum
  increase in pupillary diameter
  incurable problem drinker
  inflammatory pelvic disease

intermittent peritoneal dialysis
intermittent pigment darkening
interpupillary distance
invasive pneumococcal disease
Inventory of Psychosocial Development
IPE
    individual protective equipment
    infectious porcine encephalomyelitis
    initial psychiatric development
    injury pulmonary edema
    interstitial pulmonary emphysema
    iris pigment epithelium
IPEC
    intragastral provocation under
      endoscopy
IPEH
    intravascular papillary endothelial
      hyperplasia
IPEUS
    intraportal endovascular ultrasonography
IPEX
    immune dysregulation,
      polyendocrinopathy, enteropathy,
      X-linked [syndrome]
IPF
    idiopathic pulmonary fibrosis
    infection-potentiating factor
    International Primary Factors [Test
      Battery]
    interstitial pulmonary fibrosis
    intramural protruding form
IPF-1
    insulin promoter factor 1
IPFC
    inflammatory polyp-fold complex
      [endoscopic/radiologic finding in
      children]
IPFD
    intrapartum fetal distress
IPFM
    integral pulse frequency modulation
IPFM/SDC
    integral pulse frequency
      modulation/Smith delay compensatory
IPG
    immobilized pH gradient
    impedance phlebograph
    impedance plethysmography
    implantable pulse generator
    individually polymerized grass
      [immunotherapy]
    inositolphosphoglycan
    inspiratory phase gas
iPGE
    immunoreactive prostaglandin E
IPGTT
    intraperitoneal glucose tolerance test

IPH
    idiopathic portal hypertension
    idiopathic pulmonary hemorrhage
    idiopathic pulmonary hemosiderosis
      (*See also* IDPH)
    infant passive hand [prosthesis]
    inflammatory papillary hyperplasia
    intraparenchymal hemorrhage
    intraperitoneal hemorrhage
    intraplaque hemorrhage
    isolated postchallenge hyperglycemia
IPHC
    intraperitoneal hyperthermic
      chemotherapy
IPHEP
    independent progressive home exercise
      program
IPHP
    inflammatory papillary hyperplasia of
      palate
    intraperitoneal hyperthermic perfusion
IPHR
    inverted polypoid hamartoma of rectum
IPI
    Imagined Process Inventory
    infertility perceptions inventory
    International Prognostic Index
    interphonemic interval
    interpulse interval
    intraperitoneal insemination
    Inwald Personality Inventory
IPIA
    immunoperoxidase infectivity assay
IPITx
    isolated pancreatic islet transplant(ation)
IPJ
    interphalangeal joint (*See also* IP)
IPK
    indurated plantar keratoma
    interphalangeal keratosis
    intractable plantar keratosis
IPKD
    infantile polycystic kidney disease
IPL
    inner plexiform layer
    intense pulsed light
    interpupillary line
    intrapleural
IPLS
    intense pulsed light source
IPLVAS
    implantable left ventricular assist system
IPM
    impulse per minute
    inch per minute
    infant passive mitt [hand prosthesis]
    inflammatory prostatic mass

IPM *(continued)*
  interventional pain management
  intranodal-palisaded myofibroblastoma
  intrapulmonary metastasis
  intrauterine pressure monitor
IPMI
  inferoposterior myocardial infarct(ion)
IPMN
  intraductal papillary mucinous neoplasm
IPMT
  intraductal papillary and mucinous
    tumor [of pancreas]
IPN
  infantile periarteritis nodosa
  infantile polyarteritis nodosa
  infected pancreatic necrosis
  interim progress note
  interpeduncular nucleus
  interpenetrating polymer network
  interstitial pneumonitis
IPn
  interstitial pneumonitis
IPNP
  intraductal papillary neoplasm of
    pancreas
IPNV
  infectious pancreatic necrosis virus
IPO
  improved pregnancy outcome
  initial planning option
IPOF
  immediate postoperative fitting
IPOM
  intraperitoneal onlay mesh [hernia
    repair]
IPOP
  immediate postoperative prosthesis
IPP
  independent practice plan
  inferior point of pubic [bone]
  inflatable penile prosthesis
  inorganic pyrophosphate (*See also* PPi,
    PP$_i$)
  inosine, pyruvate, phosphate [medium]
  inspiratory plateau pressure
  intermittent positive pressure
  intrahepatic portal pressure
  intrapericardial pressure
  intrapleural pressure
  intravesical protrusion of prostate
  isolated pelvic perfusion
Ipp
  interpulse potential
IPPA
  inspection, palpation, percussion,
    auscultation
  iodophenyl pentadecanoic acid
IPPB
  intermittent positive-pressure breathing

IPPB/I
  intermittent positive-pressure
    breathing/inspiratory
IP-PDT
  intraperitoneal photodynamic therapy
IPPF
  immediate postoperative prosthetic
    fitting
IPPI
  interruption of pregnancy for psychiatric
    indication
IPPO
  intermittent positive-pressure [inflation
    with] oxygen
IPPR
  integrated pancreatic polypeptide
    response
  intermittent positive-pressure
    respiration
IPPT
  Inter-Person Perception Test
IPPUAD
  immediate postprandial upper abdominal
    distress
IPPV
  intermittent positive-pressure ventilation
IPPYV
  Ippy virus
IPQ
  Intermediate Personality Questionnaire
    [for Indian Pupils]
  intimacy potential quotient
IPQ-R
  Illness Perceptions
    Questionnaire-Revised
IPR
  immediate phase reaction
  independent professional review
  insulin production rate
  interval patency rate
  intraparenchymal resistance
IP3R
  inositol 1,4-5-triphosphate receptor
i-Pr
  isopropyl- [prefix denoting 1-methylethyl
    group]
IPRL
  isolated perfused rabbit lung
  isolated perfused rat liver
IPRT
  interpersonal reaction test
IPS
  idiopathic pneumonia syndrome
  idiopathic postprandial syndrome
  immediate postoperative stability
  impulse per second
  inch per second
  infundibular pulmonary stenosis
  initial prognostic score

intermittent photic stimulation [electroencephalography]
Interpersonal Perception Scale
intraparietal sulcus
intraperitoneal shock
intraurethral prostaglandin suppository
Inventory of Perceptual Skills
ischiopubic synchondrosis

IPSAQ
Internal, Personal, And Situational Attributions Questionnaire

IPSB
intrapartum stillbirth

IPSC
inhibitory postsynaptic current
islet-producing stem cell

IPSC-E
Inventory of Psychic and Somatic Complaints in the Elderly

IPSF
immediate postsurgical fitting [of prosthesis]

IPSI
Iowa Structured Psychiatric Interview

IPSID
immunoproliferative small-intestine disease

IPSP
inhibitory postsynaptic potential
intrapixel sequential processing

IPSS
infantile partial striatal sclerosis
inferior petrosal sinus sampling
International Prostate Symptom Score

IPSTL
inferior parietal and superior temporal lobe

IPSY
intermediate psychiatry

IPT
idiopathic perifoveal telangiectasis
immunoperoxidase technique
immunoprecipitation
inflammatory pseudotumor
insulin potentiation therapy
intermittent pelvic traction (*See also* IPTX)
interpersonal psychotherapy
interpersonal therapy
intraductal papillary tumor

IPTA
Illinois Test of Psycholinguistic Abilities

IPTG, iPrSGal
isopropylthiogalactoside

iPTH
immunoassay for parathyroid hormone

immunoreactive parathyroid hormone
intact parathyroid hormone

IPTR
International Pancreas Transplant Registry

IPTX
intermittent pelvic traction (*See also* IPT)

IPU
inpatient unit

IPV
inactivated poliovirus vaccine
incompetent perforator vein
infectious pustular vulvovaginitis [of cattle]
intermittent percussive ventilation
interpersonal (intimate partner) violence
intrapulmonary percussive ventilation
intrapulmonary vein
inactivated polio vaccine

IPVC
interpolated premature ventricular contraction

IPVD
index of pulmonary vascular disease

IPW
interphalangeal width

IQ
intelligence quotient

IQR
interquartile range

IQ&S
iron, quinine, strychnine

I-R
Ito-Reenstierna [reaction, test]

IR
idiopathic rhinitis
ileal resection
immediate-release [tablets]
immune response
immunization rate
immunologic response
immunoreactive
immunoreagent
impedance rheography
incisal ridge
index of response
individual reaction
inferior rectus [muscle]
inflow resistance
infrared [light] (*See also* IF, infra., IFR)
infrarenal
inside radius
insoluble residue
inspiratory reserve
inspiratory resistance
insulin receptor

IR *(continued)*
- insulin requirement
- insulin resistance
- insulin response
- integer ratio
- intelligence ratio
- internal reduction
- internal resistance
- internal rotation (*See also* int-rot)
- interventional radiology
- intrarectal
- intrarenal
- intrastent restenosis
- inversion recovery
- inverted repeats [genetics]
- ionizing radiation
- irritant reaction
- ischemia and reperfusion
- isotonic reversal
- isovolumetric relaxation

I&R
- insertion and removal

Ir
- immune response [gene]
- iridium

^{192}Ir
- iridium-192

^{194}Ir
- iridium-194

IRA
- ileorectal anastomosis
- immunoradioassay
- immunoregulatory alpha (α-)globulin
- inactive renin activity
- infarct-related artery

IRAAF
- intraoperative radiofrequency ablation for chronic atrial fibrillation

IR-ACTH
- immunoreactive adrenocorticotropic hormone

IRA-EEA
- ileorectal anastomosis with end-to-end anastomosis

IRAK
- integrated reference air-kerma

IrANP
- immunoreactive atrial natriuretic peptide

IRAP
- insulin-responsive aminopeptidase
- interleukin-1 receptor antagonist protein

IR-AVP
- immunoreactive arginine-vasopressin

IRB
- institutional review board

IRBBB
- incomplete right bundle-branch block

IRBC
- immature red blood cell

- infected red blood cell
- irradiated red blood cells

IRBP
- implantable rotary blood pump
- interphotoreceptor retinoid-binding protein

IRC
- implant-related complication
- indirect radionuclide cystography
- infrared coagulator [photocoagulator]
- inspiratory reserve capacity
- instantaneous resonance curve
- institutional review committee
- instrument recirculation center

IRCA
- intravascular red cell aggregation

IRCM
- iodinated radiologic contrast medium

IRCRS
- infusion-related cytokine release syndrome

IRCS
- International Research Communications System

IRD
- immune renal disease
- infantile Refsum syndrome
- isorhythmic dissociation

IRDA
- intermittent rhythmic delta activity

IRDM
- insulin-resistant diabetes mellitus

IR-DRG
- International-Refined Diagnosis-Related Group

IRDS
- idiopathic respiratory distress syndrome
- infant respiratory distress syndrome

IRE
- Impact Of Race-Related Events
- inhibitory response element
- internal rotation in extension

IRED
- infrared emission detection

IR-EPI
- inversion recovery echo planar imaging

IRES
- internal ribosome entry site

IRF
- idiopathic retroperitoneal fibrosis
- inpatient rehabilitation facility
- interferon regulatory factor
- internal rotation in flexion

IRF-1
- interferon regulatory factor 1

IRF-2
- interferon regulatory factor 2

IRFPAI
Inpatient Rehabilitation Facility–Patient Assessment Instrument
IRG
immunoreactive gastrin
immunoreactive glucagon (*See also* IRGl)
immunoreactive glucose
IRGH
immunoreactive growth hormone (*See also* IGH)
IRGl
immunoreactive glucagon (*See also* IRG)
IRH
intraretinal hemorrhage
IRhC
immunoradioassayable human chorionic
IRhCG
immunoreactive human chorionic gonadotropin
IRhCS
immunoreactive human chorionic somatomammotropin
IRhGH
immunoreactive human growth hormone
IRhPL
immunoreactive human placental lactogen
IRI
immunoreactive insulin
insulin radioimmunoassay
insulin resistance index
IRIA
indirect radioimmunoassay
irid
iridescent
IRI:G
immunoreactive insulin to [serum or plasma] glucose ratio
IRIg
insulin-reactive immunoglobulin
IRIS
intensified radiographic imaging system
interleukin regulation of immune system
IRIV
immunopotentiating reconstituted influenza virosomes
Irituia virus
IRK
insulin receptor kinase
IRKO
insulin receptor knockout
IRLT
intraoperative red light therapy
intravascular red light therapy
IRM
idiopathic retractile mesenteritis

inherited releasing mechanism
innate releasing mechanism
intermediate restorative material
IRMA
Immediate Response Mobile Analysis
immunoradiometric analysis (assay)
intraretinal microangiopathy
intraretinal microvascular abnormality
IRME
immunoreactive methionine-enkephalin
IRMP
intersegmental range of motion palpation
IRMS
isotope ratio mass spectrometry
IRN
iterated rippled noise [acoustics, neurology]
iRNA
immune ribonucleic acid
informational ribonucleic acid
IRNS
intercostal repetitive nerve stimulation
IROS
ipsilateral routing of signal
IRP
idiopathic recurrent pancreatitis
immunoreactive plasma
immunoreactive proinsulin
incus replacement prosthesis
inhibitor of radical processes
insulin-releasing polypeptide
International Reference Preparation
interstitial radiation pneumonitis
interventional reference point
IR-PCR
inter-repeat polymerase chain reaction
IR-PEP
inspiratory resistance and positive expiratory pressure
IRPGN
idiopathic rapidly progressive glomerulonephritis
IRR
incidence rate ratio
infrared radiation
infrared refractometry
insulin receptor-related receptor
intrarenal reflux
irradiation
irregular rate and rhythm
irritation
irreg
irregular(ity)
IRR HYDRO
irreversible hydrocolloid

IRRIG, IRRG
irrigate
irrigation

IRS
idiopathic recurring stupor
immunoreactive secretin
impaired regeneration syndrome
India rubber skin
infrared spectrophotometry
insulin receptor species
insulin receptor substrate [protein]
insulin-resistance syndrome

IRS-1
insulin receptor substrate 1

IRS-2
insulin receptor substrate 2

IRSA
idiopathic refractory sideroblastic anemia
iodinated rat serum albumin

IRSB
intravenous regional sympathetic block

IRSE
inversion recovery spin-echo sequence

IRT
immunoreactive trypsin [test]
immunoreactive trypsinogen
incident response team
instrument retrieval container
interresponse time
interstitial radiation therapy
(radiotherapy)
intracoronary radiation therapy
isometric relaxation time
item response theory [psychologic
testing]

IRTK
insulin receptor tyrosine kinase

IRTO
immunoreactive trypsin output

IRTU
integrating regulatory transcription unit

IRU
interferon reference unit

IRV
inferior radicular vein
inspiratory reserve volume
inverse-ratio ventilation

IS
ileal segment [intestine]
ilial segment [bone]
iliosacral
immediate sensitivity
immune serum
immune suppressor (immunosuppressor)
immune suppression
(immunosuppression)
impingement syndrome
incentive spirometer
index of saponification

index of sexuality
induced sputum
infantile spasm
infant size
information system
infrahyoid strap (See also IHS)
initial segment
insertion sequence
insufficient signal
insulin secretion
intercellular space (See also ICS)
intercostal space (See also IC, ICS)
interictal spike [in
electroencephalography]
internal standard
international standard
interspace (See also ISP)
interstitial space
interventricular septum (See also IVS)
intracardial shunt
intraspinal
intrasplenic
intrastriatal
invalided from service
inventory of systems
Ionescu-Shiley [artificial cardiac valve]
(See also I-S)
ipecac syrup
ischemic score
island (See also is.)
in situ [in original place] [L. in situ]
(See also i.s.)

I-10-S
invert sugar (10%) in saline

I-S
incudostapedial [bone]
Ionescu-Shiley [artificial cardiac valve]
(See also IS)

I/S
instruct/supervise

is.
island (See also IS)
islet
isolation

i.s.
in situ [in original space] [L. in situ]
(See also IS)

ISA
ileosigmoid anastomosis
induced sputum analysis
intraoperative suture adjustment
intrinsic stimulating activity
intrinsic sympathomimetic activity
iodinated serum albumin
irregular spiking activity [in
electroencephalography]

I(sa)
spatial average intensity
[ultrasound]

ISA₅
  internal surface area [of lung at volume of] five [liters]

ISADH
  inappropriate secretion of antidiuretic hormone

ISAGA
  immunosorbent agglutination assay

ISAH
  isolated systolic arterial hypertension

ISAM
  infant of substance-abusing mother

I(sapa)
  spatial average pulse average [ultrasound]

I(sapt)
  spatial peak, temporal average intensity [ultrasound]

I(sata)
  spatial average, temporal average intensity [ultrasound]

ISB
  incentive spirometry breathing

ISBP
  interscalene brachial plexus

ISC
  immunoglobulin-secreting cell
  indwelling subclavian catheter
  infant servocontrol
  infant skin control
  insoluble collagen
  intensive supportive care
  intermittent self-catheterization
  intermittent straight catheterization
  International Statistical Classification
  intershift coordination
  interstitial cell (*See also* IC)
  intersystem crossing
  irreversible sickle cell
  irreversibly sickled cell
  Isolette servocontrol

ISCA
  Interview Schedule for Children and Adolescents

ISCC
  invasive squamous cell carcinoma

ISCCO
  intersternocostoclavicular ossification

ISCF
  interstitial cell fluid

ISCM
  intramedullary spinal cord metastasis

ISCN
  International System for Human Cytogenetic Nomenclature

ISCOM
  immune-stimulating (immunostimulating) complex

ISCP
  infection surveillance and control program

ISD
  immunosuppressive drug
  inhibited sexual desire
  initial sleep disturbance
  intensity [of service], severity [of illness], discharge [screens]
  interatrial septal defect (*See also* IASD)
  interspinous distance
  interventricular septal defect (*See also* IVSD)
  intrinsic sphincter deficiency
  intrinsic sphincter dysfunction

ISDB
  indirect self-destructive behavior

ISE
  inhibited sexual excitement
  integrated square error
  inversion spin-echo [pulse sequence]
  ion-selective electrode
  ion-sensitive electrode

ISED
  Interview Schedule for Events and Difficulties

ISEDP
  intraspinal epidural pressure

ISEL
  Interpersonal Support Evaluation List
  in situ end labeling

ISET
  isolation by size of epithelial tumor cells [assay]

ISF
  interstitial fluid (*See also* IF)

ISFET
  ion-specific field effect transducer

ISFV
  interstitial fluid volume (*See also* IFV)
  Isfahan virus

ISG
  immune serum globulin

ISH
  icteric serum hepatitis
  isocapnic hyperventilation
  isolated septal hypertrophy
  isolated systolic hypertension
  in situ hybridization

ISHH
  in situ hybridization histochemistry

ISHT
  isolated systolic hypertension

ISI
  infarct size index
  initial slope index
  injection scan interval
  injury severity index

ISI *(continued)*
  International Sensitivity Index
  International Slope Index
  interstimulus interval
ISIH
  interspike interval histogram
ISIS
  image-selected in vivo spectroscopy
  Infectious Disease Surveillance
    Information System
  integrated shape and imaging system
ISK
  immune stromal keratitis
  isokinetic
ISKD
  intramedullary skeletal kinetic distractor
ISKV
  Issyk-Kul virus
ISL
  interscapular line
  interspinous ligament
ISLE
  intraoperative sustained limited
    expansion
ISM
  intersegmental muscle
ISMA
  infantile spinal muscular atrophy
ISMLCSA
  intrastent minimal lumen cross-sectional
    area
IS-5-MN, Is-5-Mn
  isosorbide-5-mononitrate
ISNA
  iron-sufficient, not anemic
ISO
  International Standards Organization
  isocenter
  isodose
  isoenzyme
  Isolette (*See also* Isol)
  isotropic (*See also* I)
ISO$_2$
  oxygen saturation index [singular]
    (indices [plural])
ISO-30
  Inventory of Suicide Orientation 30
ISOK
  isokinetic
Isol
  Isolette (*See also* ISO)
isol
  isolate(d)
  isolation
Is of Lang
  islets of Langerhans
isom
  isometric
  isometropic

8-iso-PGF$_{2alpha}$
  8-iso-prostaglandin F2 alpha
IsoRAS
  isorenin-angiotensin system
ISP
  [distance between] iliac spines
  immunoreactive substance P
  immunosuppressed protocol
  inferior spermatic plexus
  input signal processor
  interspace (*See also* IS)
  interspinal
  interstitial pregnancy
  interstitial pressure
  intraspinal
I(sp)
  spatial peak intensity [ultrasound]
IS-PCR
  in situ polymerase chain reaction
ISPP
  individualized sleep promotion plan
I(sppa)
  spatial peak pulse average intensity
    [ultrasound]
ISPT
  interspecies [ovum] penetration test
isp-Tx
  intrasplenic transplant(ation)
ISPX
  Ionescu-Shiley pericardial xenograft
ISR
  immediate skin response
  information storage [and] retrieval
    (*See also* IS and R)
  injection site reaction
  in-stent restenosis
  insulin secretion rate
  insulin secretory response
  integrated secretory response
IS and R
  information storage and retrieval
    (*See also* ISR)
ISRE
  interferon-stimulated regulatory
    element
ISS
  idiopathic short stature
  immunostimulatory DNA sequence
  Individual Self-Rating Scale
  infantile sialic acid storage
    [disease]
  inferior sagittal sinus
  Injury Severity Scale (Score)
  integrated summary of safety
  invasive surgical staging
  ion-scattering spectroscopy
  ion surface scattering
  irritable stomach syndrome
  isotonic saline solution

IS10S
  10% invert sugar in 0.9% sodium
    chloride [saline] injection
ISSD
  infantile sialic acid storage disorder
ISSHL
  idiopathic sudden sensory hearing loss
ISSI
  interspinous segmental spinal
    instrument(ation) [technique]
  interspinous surgical staging
ISSLC
  International Staging System for Lung
    Cancer
ISSNHL
  idiopathic sudden sensorineural hearing
    loss
ISS-ODN
  immunostimulatory oligodeoxynucleotide
ISSP
  Infant Support Services Program
IST
  immunosuppressive therapy
  inappropriate sinus tachycardia
  injection sclerotherapy
  insulin sensitivity test
  insulin shock therapy
  interstitiospinal tract
  isometric systolic tension
ISTD
  insulin standard
ISUB
  immunosubtraction
I-sub
  inhibitor substance
ISVP
  infectious subviral particle
ISW
  interstitial water
IS10W
  10% invert sugar injection [in water]
ISWI
  incisional surgical wound infection
ISWL
  intracorporeal shock wave lithotripsy
ISWT
  incremental shuttle walking test
ISY
  intrasynovial
IT
  iliotibial
  immunity test
  immunologic test
  immunotherapy
  immunotoxin therapy
  implantation test
  incentive therapy

individual therapy
inferior temporal
inferior turbinate
information technology
inhalation test
inhalation therapy
injection time
inspiratory (inspiration) time (*See also*
  I-time)
insulin therapy
insulin treatment
intact (*See also* I, INT)
intensive therapy
intentional tremor
intermittent traction (*See also* int trx)
internal thoracic
interstitial tissue
intertrochanteric
intertuberous [pelvic diameter]
intimal thickening
intolerance and toxicity
intracellular tachyzoite
intradermal test
intratesticular
intrathecal [anesthesia, injection]
  (*See also* INTH, ITh, i-thec)
intrathoracic
intratracheal [tube] (*See also* ITR)
intratumoral (*See also* i-tumor)
ischial tuberosity
isomeric transition [of radioactive
  isotopes]
I/T
  intensity/time [duration of contractions]
ITA
  individual treatment assessment
  inferior temporal artery
  internal thoracic artery
  islet transplant(ation) alone
  itaconic acid
I(ta)
  temporal average intensity
    [ultrasound]
ITAG
  internal thoracic artery graft
ITAL
  intrathoracic artificial lung
ITAM
  immunoreceptor tyrosine [kinase]
    activation motif [protein]
ITAQ
  Insight and Treatment Attitudes
    Questionnaire
ITAS
  internal telomerase standard
ITAV
  Itaituba virus

ITB
iliotibial band
ITBC
intraluminal typical bronchial carcinoid
ITBFS
iliotibial band friction syndrome
ITBS
iliotibial band syndrome
Iowa Tests of Basic Skills
131I-TBS
iodine-131 total body scan
ITBV
intrathoracic blood volume
ITC
incontinence treatment center
inferior temporal cortex
infrared thermographic calorimetry
Interventional Therapeutics Corporation
in-the-canal [hearing aid]
isolated tumor cell
isothermal titration calorimetry
ITc
International Table calorie
ITCL
interosseous talocalcaneal ligament
ITCM
integral traditional Chinese medicine
ITCP
idiopathic thrombocytopenic purpura
(*See also* ITP)
ITCU
intensive thoracic cardiovascular unit
ITCVD
ischemic thrombotic cerebrovascular
disease
ITD
idiopathic torsion dystonia
insulin-treated diabetic
intensely transfused dialysis [patient]
iris transillumination defect
ITE
insufficient therapeutic effect
in-the-ear [hearing aid]
intrapulmonary interstitial emphysema
ITEA
intermittent thoracic epidural anesthesia
ITERS
Infant/Toddler Environment Rating
Scale
ITET
isotonic endurance test
ITF
inpatient treatment facility
ITFF
intertrochanteric femoral fracture
ITFS
iliotibial tract friction syndrome
incomplete testicular feminization
syndrome

ITFx
intertrochanteric fracture
ITG
immunotactoid glomerulopathy
ITGCN
intratubular germ cell neoplasm
(*See also* IGCN)
ITGV
intrathoracic gas volume (*See also* IGV)
ITH
immediate-type hypersensitivity
ITh, i-thec
intrathecal [anesthesia, injection]
(*See also* INTH, IT)
ITI
inter-alpha-trypsin inhibitor
intertrial interval
intratubal insemination
ITIM
immunoreceptor tyrosine inhibitory
motif
I-time
inspiratory (inspiration) time (*See also*
IT)
ITIV
Itimirim virus
ITL
inspiratory threshold load
ITLC
instant thin-layer chromatography
ITLC-SG
instant thin-layer chromatography-silica
gel
ITM
improved Thayer-Martin [medium]
ITN
idiopathic trigeminal neuralgia
ITOC
intratracheal oxygen catheter
ITOP
intentional termination of pregnancy
ITP
idiopathic thrombocytopenic purpura
(*See also* ITCP)
immune thrombocytopenic purpura
inosine triphosphate (inosine
5′-triphosphate)
interim treatment plan(ning)
inverse treatment plan(ning)
islet-cell tumor of pancreas
I(tp)
temporal peak intensity [ultrasound]
ITPA
Illinois Test of Psycholinguistic
Abilities
inosine triphosphatase (*See also* ITPase)
intrathecal *Treponema pallidum* antibody
ITPase
inosine triphosphatase (*See also* ITPA)

ITPV
intratracheal pulmonary ventilation
Itaporanga virus

ITQ
Infant Temperament Questionnaire
inferior temporal quadrant

ITQV
Itaqui virus

ITR
intraocular tension recorder
intratracheal [tube] (*See also* IT)
isotretinoin

I tracing
interrupted tracing

ITS
internal transcribed spacer
isometric trunk stabilization

ITSC
It Scale for Children [psychologic test]

ITSHD
isolated thyroid-stimulating hormone
deficiency

ITT
identical twins [raised] together
iliotibial tract
incremental treadmill test
insulin tolerance test
intention-to-treat [analysis]
internal tibial torsion
iron tolerance test

ITTP
idiopathic thrombocytopenic purpura

i-tumor
intratumoral (*See also* IT)

ITUV
Itupiranga virus

ITV
impedance threshold valve
infantile tibia vara
inferior temporal vein

ITVAD
indwelling transcutaneous vascular
access device

ITW
idiopathic toe-walker
idiopathic toe-walking

ITX
immunotoxin
intertriginous xanthoma

⚠ **IU**
immunizing unit (*See also* IE, ImmU)
infectious unit
International Unit ⚠
intrauterine
in utero

IUA
intrauterine adhesion

IUC
idiopathic ulcerative colitis
intrauterine catheter

IUCD
intrauterine contraceptive device
(*See also* ICD, IUD)

IUD
interuncal distance
intrauterine [contraceptive] device
(*See also* ICD, IUCD)
intrauterine death

IUDE
in utero drug exposure

IUF
isolated ultrafiltration

IUFB
intrauterine foreign body

IUFD
intrauterine fetal death (demise)
intrauterine fetal distress

IUFGR
intrauterine fetal growth retardation

IUFT
intrauterine fetal transfusion

IUG
infusion urogram
intrauterine gas
intrauterine gestation
intrauterine growth

IUGR
intrauterine growth rate
intrauterine growth restriction
(retardation)

IUH
initial urinary hesitancy

IUI
intrauterine infection
intrauterine insemination

⚠ **IU/L**
International Unit per liter ⚠

IULN
institutional upper limit of normal

IUM
internal urethral meatus
intrauterine [fetally] malnourished
intrauterine malnourishment
intrauterine malnutrition
intrauterine membrane

⚠ **IU/min**
International Unit per minute ⚠

IUMR
intrauterine myelomeningocele repair

IUP
intrauterine pregnancy
intrauterine pressure

IUPAT
intrauterine pregnancy at term

IUPC
intrauterine pressure catheter
IUPD
intrauterine pregnancy, delivered
IUPM
infectious units per million
IUPTB
intrauterine pregnancy, term birth
IUP,TBCS
intrauterine pregnancy, term birth,
cesarean section
IUP,TBLC
intrauterine pregnancy, term birth, living
child
IUP,TBLI
intrauterine pregnancy, term birth, living
infant
IUR
intrauterine retardation
IUT
intrauterine transfusion
IUTD
immunizations up-to-date
IV
ichthyosis vulgaris
immunodeficiency virus
interventricular
intervertebral
interview
intravaginal
intravascular
intravenous(ly) (*See also* I.V., i.v.)
intraventricular (*See also* IVT)
intravertebral
invasive
inversion
iodine value
in vitro
in vivo
I.V.
intravenous(ly) (*See also* IV, i.v.)
i.v.
intravenous(ly) (*See also* I.V., IV)
IVA
integrated visual and auditory
intraoperative vascular angiography
IVAC
intravascular accurate control
intravenous access
intravenous accurate control [device]
intravenous automated controller
IVAD
implantable vascular access device
implantable venous access device
implantable ventricular assist device
IVag
intravaginal
IVAP
in vitro antibody production [assay]

in vivo adhesive platelet [count]
intestinal and vascular access port
IVAR
insulin variable
IVAS
intracorporeal ventricular assist system
IVB
intravenous bolus
intraventricular block
intravitreal blood
IVBAT
intravascular bronchioalveolar tumor
IVBC
intravascular blood coagulation
IVBH
intraventricular brain hemorrhage
IVBT
intravaginal brachytherapy
IVC
individually viable cell
indwelling venous catheter
inferior vena cava
inferior venacavograph(y)
(venacavogram) (*See also* IVCV)
inspiratory vital capacity
inspired vital capacity
integrated vector control
intravascular coagulation
intravenous chemotherapy
intravenous cholangiograph(y)
(cholangiogram) (*See also* IVCh)
intraventricular catheter
intraventricular conduction
isovolumic contraction (*See also* IC)
IVCBO
inferior vena cava balloon occlusion
IVCC
intravascular consumption coagulopathy
IVCD
intraventricular conduction defect
intraventricular conduction delay
intraventricular conduction disease
IVCF
inferior vena cava filter
IVCh
intravenous cholangiograph(y)
(cholangiogram) (*See also* IVC)
IVCI
intravenous continuous infusion
IVC-LA
inferior vena cava and left atrium
IVCO
inferior vena cava occlusion
IVCR
inferior vena cava reconstruction
IVCT
inferior vena cava thrombosis
intravenously [enhanced] computed
tomography

isovolumic contraction time (*See also* ICT)

in vitro contracture test

IVCU
isotope voiding cystourethrography

IVCV
inferior venacavograph(y) (venacavogram) (*See also* IVC)

IVD
insufficient ventilatory drive
intervertebral disc
intravenous drip
in vitro diagnostic

IVDA
intravenous drug abuse (abuser)

IVDSA
intravenous digital subtraction angiography

IVDSI
intervertebral disc space infection

IVDU
intravenous drug use (user)

IVET
in vivo expression technology

IVF
interventricular foramen
intervertebral foramen
intravascular fluid
intravenous fluid
intravenous fluorescein
intravertebral foramen
in vitro fertilization
in vivo fertilization

IVFA
intravenous fluorescein angiography

IVFE
intravenous fat emulsion

IVF-ET
in vitro fertilization [and] embryo transfer

IVFT
intravenous fetal transfusion

IVG
isotopic ventriculogram

IVGG
intravenous gamma globulin

IVGTT
intravenous glucose tolerance test

IVH
integrated visual healing
intravenous hyperalimentation
intraventricular hemorrhage [grade 1–4]
in vitro hyperploidy

IVH2RA
intravenous H2 receptor antagonist

IVHT
intravenous histamine test

IVI
intravaginal insemination
intravenous injection

IVID
intravenous iron dextran

IVIg
intravenous immune globulin (immunoglobulin)

IVIM
intravoxel incoherent motion [MRI]

IVJC
intervertebral joint complex

IVL
indwelling venous line
intravascular lymphomatosis
intravenous leiomyomatosis
intravenous lock

IVLBW
infant of very low birth weight (*See also* VLBWI)

IVM
immediate visual memory
intracranial venous malformation
intravascular mass

IVN
intravenous nutrition

IVNC
isolated ventricular noncompaction

IVNF
intravitreal neovascular frond

IVNR
interventional neuroradiology

IVO
intraoral vertical osteotomy

IVOTTS
Irvine viable organ-tissue transport system

IVOX
intravascular oxygenator

IVP
intravascular pressure
intravenous push [dose] (*See also* IVp, IVPU)
intravenous pyelograph(y) (pyelogram)
intraventricular pressure
intravesical pressure

IVp, IVPU
intravenous push [dose] (*See also* IVP)

IVPB
intravenous piggyback [drug administration]

IVPD
in vitro protein digestibility

IVPF
isovolume pressure flow [curve]

IVR
idioventricular rhythm
interactive voice-response [system]
internal visual reference
intravaginal ring
intravenous retrograde
intravenous rider
isolated volume responder
isovolumic relaxation [time] (*See also* IVRT)

IVRA
intravenous regional anesthesia

IVRAP
intravenous retrograde access port

IVRF
incomplete vertical root fracture

IVRG
intravenous retrograde

IV-RNV
intravenous radionuclide venography

IVRO
intraoral vertical ramus osteotomy

IVRP
isovolumic (isovolumetric) relaxation period

IVRS
interactive voice response system

IVRT
isovolumic relaxation time (*See also* IVR)

IVS
inappropriate vasopressin secretion
intact ventricular septum
intervening sequence
interventricular septum (*See also* IS)
intervillous space
irritable voiding syndrome

IVSCT
in vitro skin corrosivity test

IVSD
interventricular septal defect (*See also* ISD)

IVSE
interventricular septal excursion

IVSO
intraoral vertical segmental osteotomy

IVST
interventricular septal thickness

IVT
idiopathic ventricular tachycardia
index of vertical transmission
interactive video technology
interventional video tomography

interventricular trigone
Intrasound vibration test
intrauterine fetal transfusion
intravenous transfusion
intraventricular (*See also* IV)
intravesical therapy
isovolumic (isovolumetric) time

IVTT
in vitro transcription/translation

IVTTT
intravenous tolbutamide tolerance test

IVU
intravenous urograph(y) (urogram)

IVUC
intravenous ultrasound catheter

IVUS
intracoronary vascular ultrasound
intravascular ultrasound

IVV
influenza virus vaccine

IW
ideal weight
inner wall
inspiratory wheeze

I-5-W
invert sugar 5% in water

IWB
indeterminate Western blot [test]
Index of Well-Being

IWD
individual with disability

IWI
inferior wall infarct(ion)
interwave interval

IWL
infant water loss
insensible water loss
inter-wave latency
involuntary weight loss

IWMI
inferior wall myocardial infarct(ion)

IWML
idiopathic white matter lesion

IWP
ischial weightbearing prosthesis

IWS
Index of Work Satisfaction

IWT
ice water test
impacted wisdom teeth
intimal wall thickness

IZ
infarction zone

J

jejunostomy
joule [SI unit of work or energy]
juvenile (*See also* juv)
juxtapulmonary-capillary [receptor]
magnetic polarization
polypeptide chain in polymeric
  immunoglobulins
reference point following QRS complex,
  at beginning of ST segment
sound intensity

J1–J16

Jaeger near acuity [lines of various
  type sizes, numbered 1 to 16]

JA

jet area
joint aspiration
juvenile arthritis
juvenile atrophy
juxtaarticular

Jab1

Jun activation domain binding
  protein 1

JABE

juxtaarticular bone erosion

Jack

jacknife [position]

JACV

Jacareacanga virus

JAFAR

Juvenile Arthritis Functional Assessment
  Report

JAG1

human jagged-1 gene

JAI

juvenile amaurotic idiocy

Jak

Janus kinase

Jak1–Jak2

Janus kinase 1–2

Jak/Stat

Janus kinase/signal transducer and
  activator of transcription

JAM

joint alignment and motion

JAMG

juvenile autoimmune myasthenia gravis

JAMV

Jamanxi virus

JAN

Japanese Accepted Name

JAPV

Japanaut virus

JAR

juvenile alveolar rhabdomyosarcoma

JARIV

Jari virus

JAS

Jenkins Activity Survey [psychologic
  test]
Job Attitude Scale
joint activated system
juvenile ankylosing spondylitis

jaund

jaundice (*See also* JD, jnd)

JAV

Johnson Atoll virus

JB

jugular bulb

JBC

Jesness Behavior Checklist

JBE

Japanese B encephalitis

JC

Jakob-Creutzfeldt [disease] (*See also*
  CJD)
Jamestown Canyon
joint contracture

J/C

joule per coulomb

jc

juice

JCA

juvenile chronic arthritis

JCAHO

Joint Commission on Accreditation of
  Healthcare Organizations [The Joint
  Commission]

JCC

Jackson cross cylinder [astigmatism
  test]

JCE

job capacity evaluation

JCF

juvenile calcaneal fracture

JCGC

Japanese Classification for Gastric
  Carcinoma

JCIH

Joint Committee on Infant Hearing

J/cm

joule per centimeter

J/cm²

joule per centimeter squared

JCMIH

Joint Commission on Mental Illness and
  Health

JCML

juvenile chronic myelocytic
  (myelogenous) leukemia

JCP
  juvenile chronic polyarthritis
JCQ
  Job Content Questionnaire
JCS
  joint coordinate system [anatomic joint relationship]
JCT
  juxtaglomerular cell tumor
jct
  junction (*See also* junct, Jx)
JCV
  Jamestown Canyon virus
JD
  jaundice (*See also* jaund, jnd)
  jejunal diverticulitis
  jugulodigastric [node] (*See also* JDG)
  juvenile delinquent
  juvenile-onset diabetes [mellitus]
    (*See also* JOD, JODM)
JDG
  jugulodigastric [node] (*See also* JD)
JDI
  Job Description Index
JDM
  juvenile dermatomyositis (*See also* JDMS)
  juvenile diabetes mellitus
JDMS
  juvenile dermatomyositis (*See also* JDM)
JDMS/PM
  juvenile dermatomyositis/polymyositis
JDV
  Juan Diaz virus
JE
  Japanese encephalitis
  junctional escape [rhythm] (*See also* JER)
JEB
  junctional epidermolysis bullosa
  junctional escape beat
JEB-PA
  junctional epidermolysis bullosa-pyloric atresia [syndrome]
JEE
  Japanese equine encephalitis
JEJ, jej
  jejunum
JEN
  Japanese encephalitis vaccine
JEPI
  Junior Eysenck Personality Inventory
JER
  Japanese erection ring
  junctional escape rhythm (*See also* JE)
JET
  jejunal extension tube
  junctional ectopic tachycardia

JETPEG
  jejunal tube through percutaneous endoscopic gastrostomy
JEV
  Japanese encephalitis virus
JE-VAX
  Japanese encephalitis virus vaccine
JF
  joint fluid
  jugular foramen
  junctional fold
JFET
  junction field-effect transistor
JFS
  jugular foramen syndrome
JG
  June grass [test]
  juxtaglomerular
jg, j-g
  jugular (*See also* jug.)
JGA
  juxtaglomerular apparatus
JGC
  juxtaglomerular cell
JGCT
  juvenile granulosa cell tumor
  juxtaglomerular cell tumor
JGI
  jejunogastric intussusception
  juxtaglomerular granulation index
  juxtaglomerular index
JGP
  juvenile general paralysis
JH
  Jarisch-Herxheimer [reaction] (*See also* JHR)
  juvenile hormone [of insects]
jH
  heat transfer factor
JHA
  juvenile hormone analog
JHMV
  J. Howard Mueller virus
JHR
  Jarisch-Herxheimer reaction (*See also* JH)
JI
  jejunoileal
  jejunoileitis
  jejunoileostomy
  Jesness Inventory
JIA
  juvenile idiopathic arthritis
JIB
  jejunoileal bypass
JIDC
  juvenile intervertebral disc calcification

JIH
joint interval histogram
JIRI
Johnston Informal Reading Inventory
JIS
juvenile idiopathic scoliosis
JJ
jaw jerk
jejunojejunostomy
J/kg
joule per kilogram
JKP
jackknife position
JKST
Johnson-Kenney Screening Test
[psychologic test]
JL
jet length
Judkins left [catheter]
JL4
Judkins left 4 [catheter]
JL5
Judkins left 5 [catheter]
JLO
Judgment of Line orientation
JLP
juvenile laryngeal papilloma(tosis)
JLVIA
Jacko Low Vision Interaction
Assessment
JM
jugomaxillary
juxtamembrane
*j*M
heat transfer factor, mass
JMC
Jansen metaphysial (metaphyseal)
chondrodysplasia
JMD
juvenile macular degeneration
JME
juvenile myoclonic epilepsy
JMH
John Milton Hagen [antibody]
JMML
juvenile myelomonocytic leukemia
JMR
Jones-Mote reactivity
JN
Jamaican neuropathy
JNA
juvenile nasopharyngeal angiofibroma
JNB
jaundice of newborn
JNCL
juvenile-onset neuronal ceroid
lipofuscinosis

JND
just noticeable difference
jnd
jaundice (*See also* jaund, JD)
JNK
Jun kinase
JNP
Jadassohn nevus phakomatosis
JNPA
juvenile nasopharyngeal
angiofibroma
jnt
joint (*See also* jt, Jx)
JNVD
jugular neck vein distention
JOAG
juvenile open-angle glaucoma
JOD, JODM
juvenile-onset diabetes mellitus (*See also*
JD)
JOF
juvenile ossifying fibroma
JOIV
Joinjakaka virus
JOMAC
judgment, orientation, memory,
abstraction, calculation
JOMACI
judgment, orientation, memory,
abstraction, calculation intact
JOMID
juvenile-onset multisystem inflammatory
disease
JOR
jaw-opening reflex (response)
JORRP
juvenile-onset recurrent respiratory
papilloma(tosis)
JOS
jaw osteosarcoma
jour
journal (*See also* jrnl, jrl)
JP
Jackson-Pratt [drain] (*See also* JPD)
Jobst pump
joint protection (*See also* JTP)
juvenile periodontitis
juvenile polyposis
JPA
juvenile paralysis agitans
juvenile pilocytic astrocytoma
JPB
junctional premature beat
JPBS
Jackson-Pratt to bulb suction
JPC
junctional premature contraction

J

JPD
Jackson-Pratt drain (*See also* JP)
juvenile plantar dermatitis (dermatosis)
juxtapapillary diverticulum

JPI
Jackson Personality Inventory
jejunal pouch interposition

JPS
joint position sense
juvenile polyposis syndrome

JR
jaw reflex
Jolly reaction
Judkins right [catheter]
junctional rhythm

JR4
Judkins right 4 [catheter]

JR5
Judkins right 5 [catheter]

JRA
juvenile rheumatoid arthritis
[type I, II]

Jr BF
junior baby food

JRC
joint replacement center

jrnl, jrl
journal (*See also* jour)

JROM
joint range of motion

JRT
junctional recovery time

JS
jejunal segment
joint space
junctional slowing
Junkman-Schoeller [unit of thyrotropin]
(*See also* JSU)

J/s
joule per second

JSATO₂
jugular vein oxygen saturation

JSF
Japanese spotted fever

JSI
Jansky Screening Index [psychologic
test]

JSMA
juvenile spinal muscular atrophy

JSRV
Jaagsiekte sheep retrovirus

JSU
Junkman-Schoeller unit [of thyrotropin]
(*See also* JS)

JSV
Jerry-Slough virus

JT
jejunostomy tube (*See also* J-tube)
junctional tachycardia

J/T
joule per tesla

jt
joint (*See also* jnt, Jx)

JTA
job task analysis
juvenile temporal arteritis

jt asp
joint aspiration

JTF
jejunostomy tube feeding

JTF-CS
Joint Task Force for Civil Support
[Department of Defense]

JTJ
jaw-to-jaw [position]

JTP
joint protection (*See also* JP)

JTPS
juvenile tropical pancreatitis syndrome

J-tube
jejunostomy tube (*See also* JT)

Ju
jugale [craniometric]

jug.
jugular (*See also* jg, j-g)

jug. comp.
jugular compression [test]

JUGV
Jugra virus

junct
junction (*See also* jct, Jx)

JUNV
Junin virus

JURV
Jurona virus

JUTV
Jutiapa virus

juv
juvenile (*See also* J)

juxt.
near [L. *juxta*]

JV
jugular vein
jugular venous [pressure, pulse]

JVBF
Jan van Breemen Function
[Questionnaire]

JVC
jugular venous catheter

JVD
jugular venous (jugulovenous) distention

JVI
jugular valve incompetence

JVIS
Jackson Vocational Interest Survey

JVP
jugular vein pulse
jugular venous pressure

jugular venous pulsation
jugular venous pulse
JVPT
jugular venous pulse tracing
JW
jump walker
JWHS
Juvenile Wellness and Health Survey

JW-NT
Jehovah's Witness - no transfusion
Jx
joint (*See also* jnt, jt)
junction (*See also* jct, junct)
JXG
juvenile xanthogranuloma
JXRS
juvenile X-linked retinoschisis

J

K

burst of diphasic slow waves in response to stimuli during sleep [in electroencephalography]
calix [Gr. *kalyx* cup]
capsular antigen [Ger. *Kapsel* capsule]
carrying capacity [genetics]
cathode (*See also* CA, C, cath)
coefficient [universal symbol] (*See also* C)
constant [universal symbol] (*See also* C)
cornea (*See also* C)
cornea curvature
cretaceous
K-electron capture
kappa [10th letter of Greek alphabet uppercase]
Kell blood group (system) (factor)
kelvin [SI fundamental unit of temperature]
keratometer
keratometric power
kerma
ketamine (Super K)
kidney (*See also* KID)
killer (cell)
kinetic energy (*See also* KE)
Kirschner [wire]
Klebsiella
knee (*See also* Kn)
kosher
Küntscher [nail or rod]
lysine (*See also* LYS)
modulus of compression
motor coordination [in General Aptitude Test Battery]
potassium [L. *kalium*] (*See also* kal, pot., potass)
ratio of curvature of flattest meridian of apical cornea [in fitting of contact lens]
thousand (*See also* thous.)
vitamin K

K₁

vitamin K_1 [phylloquinone, phytonadione]

K₂

vitamin K_2 [menatetrenone]

K₃

vitamin K_3 [menadione]

K4

fourth Korotkoff sound

K5

fifth Korotkoff sound

°K

degree kelvin

K⁺

potassium ion

³⁹K

potassium-39

⁴⁰K

potassium-40

⁴²K

potassium-42

⁴³K

potassium-43

k

Boltzmann constant
constant [universal symbol] (*See also* C, K)
kilo-

KA

kainic acid
kala-azar
keratoacanthoma
ketoacidosis
King-Armstrong [unit] (*See also* K-A, KAU)
kynurenic acid

K-A

King-Armstrong [unit] (*See also* KA, KAU)

K:A

ketogenic to antiketogenic ratio

Ka

dissociation constant of an acid (*See also* Kd)

kA

kiloampere

KAAD

kerosene, alcohol, acetic acid, dioxane [mixture]

KAB

knowledge, attitude, behavior

KABC

Kaufman Assessment Battery for Children

KABINS

knowledge, attitude, behavior, improvement in nutritional status

KAC

kidney adenocarcinoma

KACT

kaolin-activated clotting time

KADV

Kadam virus

KAF

conglutinogen-activating factor
kidney arteriovenous fistula

K

KAF *(continued)*
    killer-assisting factor
    kinase-activating factor
KAFO
    knee-ankle-foot orthosis
KAIT
    Kaufman Adolescent and Adult
    Intelligence Test
KAIV
    Kaikalur virus
kal
    potassium [L. *kalium*] (*See also* K, pot.,
    potass)
KALIG-1
    Kallmann syndrome interval gene 1
KALP
    Kallmann pseudogene
KAMV
    Kamese virus
KANV
    Kannamangalam virus
KAO
    knee-ankle orthosis
KAP
    knowledge, aptitudes, [and] practices
κ
    kappa [10th letter of Greek alphabet
    lowercase]
    magnetic susceptibility
    one of two immunoglobulin light chains
KAR
    killer-activating receptor
KAS
    Katz Adjustment Scales [psychologic
    test]
KASH
    knowledge, abilities, skills, [and] habits
KASS
    Kaneda anterior spinal/scoliosis system
KAST
    Kindergarten Auditory Screening Test
KASV
    Kasba virus
KAT
    kanamycin acetyltransferase
    kinesthetic ability trainer
kat
    katal [enzyme unit of measurement]
kat/L
    katal per liter
KATP
    potassium adenosine triphosphate
    [channel, channel blocker]
KAU
    King-Armstrong unit [catalytic amount
    of phosphate] (*See also* KA, K-A)
KB
    human oral epidermoid carcinoma
    cells

    ketone body
    knee-bearing
    knee brace
    knuckle-bender [splint]
    Kussmaul breathing
K-B
    Kleihauer-Betke [test or stain for fetal
    hemoglobin]
K$_b$, *K$_b$*
    base ionization constant
    dissociation constant of a base
kb
    kilobase
K-BIT
    Kaufman Brief Intelligence Test
kbp
    kilobase pair
kBq
    kilobecquerel
KBR
    ketone body ratio
    kidney length to body height
    ratio
KBr
    potassium bromide
KBV
    Kachemak Bay virus
KC
    kangaroo care
    katacalcin
    keratoconjunctivitis
    keratoconus
    knees to chest
    knuckle cracking
    Korean conflict
    Kupffer cell
kC
    kilocoulomb
kc
    kilocycle
kcal
    kilocalorie (kilogram calorie)
k$_{cat}$
    turnover number
KCC
    cathodal (kathodal) closing contraction
    [Ger. *Kathodenschlie
    βungs-Kontraktion*] (*See also* KSK)
    Kulchitsky cell carcinoma
KCCT
    kaolin-cephalin clotting time
KCD
    kinestatic charge detector
K cell
    killer cell
KCF
    key clinical findings
KCG
    kinetocardiogram

KChlPs
   potassium channel-interacting
      proteins
KCI
   Kolbe Conative Index
kCi
   kilocurie
KCl
   potassium chloride
KCN
   potassium cyanide
KCNJ1
   potassium inwardly-rectifying channel,
      subfamily J, member 1
K complex
   slow waves related to sleep arousal (in
      electroencephalography)
KCP
   knee-chest position
kcps
   kilocycle per second (*See also* kc/sec,
      kc/s)
KCS
   keratoconjunctivitis sicca
kc/sec, kc/s
   kilocycle per second (*See also* kcps)
KCT
   kaolin clotting time
KCV
   Kern Canyon virus
KD
   cathodal (kathodal) duration
   ketogenic diet
   kidney donor
   killed
   knee disarticulation
   knitted Dacron
   knowledge deficit
Kd
   dissociation constant (*See also* Ka)
K_d
   partition coefficient [radiation
      contamination equal to quantity of
      adsorbate adsorbed per mass of solid
      to amount of adsorbate remaining in
      solution at equilibrium]
kDa, kD
   kilodalton
KDA
   known drug allergies
KDD
   Kidney Disease Questionnaire
kDNA
   kinetoplast deoxyribonucleic acid
KDO
   ketodeoxyoctonic (acid)
KDP
   potassium dihydrogen phosphate

KDS
   Kaufman Development Scale
   Kupfer-Detre System [dialysis and renal
      transplantation QOL]
KDSS
   Kurtzke Disability Status Scale
KDT
   knee-drop test
KDU
   Kidney Dialysis Unit
kdyn
   kilodyne
KE
   first order elimination rate constant in
      hr.-1
   Kendall compound E (cortisone)
   kinetic energy (*See also* K)
K_e
   exchangeable body potassium
KEAT
   Kaprelian easy-access tweezers
KED
   Kendrick extrication device
K3 EDTA
   tripotassium ethylenediaminetetraacetate
kel
   elimination rate constant
KELS
   Kohlman Evaluation of Living
      Skills
kemo Tx
   chemical therapy (chemotherapy)
KEMV
   Kemerovo virus
KEP
   knee-elbow position
K_{eq}
   equilibrium constant
KER
   keratin
kera
   keratitis
kerma
   kinetic energy released in material
      (medium) [kinetic energy released per
      unit mass]
KET
   ketones
KETV
   Ketapang virus
KEUV
   Keuraliba virus
keV
   kiloelectron volt
KEVD
   Krupin eye valve with disc
KEYV
   Keystone virus

KF
 Kayser-Fleischer [ring]
 Kenner fecal [medium]
 kidney function (*See also* KFn)
kf
 flocculation rate in antigen-antibody
  reaction
KFA
 kinetic fibrinogen assay
KFAB, KFAb
 kidney-fixing antibody
K factor
 gamma-ray dose [roentgens per hour at
  1 cm from 1-mCi point source of
  radiation]
KFAO
 knee-foot-ankle orthosis
KFD
 Kinetic Family Drawings
 Kyasanur forest disease
KFE
 knee flexion and extension
KFn
 kidney function (*See also* KF)
KFR
 Kayser-Fleischer ring
KFSD
 keratosis follicularis spinulosa
  decalvans
K-G
 Kimray-Greenfield [filter]
KG
 ketoglutarate
KG-1
 Koeffler Golde 1 [cell line]
kG
 kilogauss
kg
 kilogram (*See also* kilo)
kg-cal
 kilogram-calorie
kg/cm²
 kilogram per square centimeter
KGDH
 ketoglutarate dehydrogenase
KGDHC
 ketoglutarate dehydrogenase
  complex
KGF
 keratinocyte growth factor
KGF-2
 keratinocyte growth factor 2
kgf
 kilogram-force
KGFR
 keratinocyte growth factor
  receptor
kg/L
 kilogram per liter

KGM
 ketoglutaramate
kg-m
 kilogram-meter
kg/m²
 kilogram per meter squared
kg-m/s²
 kilogram-meter per second squared
Kgn
 kininogen
KGS
 ketogenic steroid
17-KGS
 17-ketogenic steroid
kg/s
 kilogram per second
KGTI
 Kinetik great toe implant
KGy
 kiloGray
KH
 Krebs-Henseleit [cycle]
K24H
 potassium in 24-hour [urine]
 potassium [urine] 24-hour
KHB
 Krebs-Henseleit bicarbonate [buffer]
KHb
 potassium hemoglobinate
KHC
 kinetic hemolysis curve
 knot holding capacity
KHD
 kinky-hair disease
KHE
 kaposiform hemangioendothelioma
KHF
 Korean hemorrhagic fever
K6HF
 keratin 6HF [gene]
KHG
 ketotic hyperglycinemia
KHM
 keratoderma hereditaria mutilans
KHN
 Knoop hardness number [of
  solids]
KHS
 kinky-hair syndrome
 Krebs-Henseleit solution
kHz
 kilohertz
KI
 karyopyknotic index (*See also* KPI)
 kidney channel [acupuncture] (*See also*
  ki)
 knee immobilizer
 Krönig isthmus
 potassium iodide

K_I
dissociation of enzyme-inhibitor complex
inhibition constant

ki
kidney channel [acupuncture] (*See also* KI)

KIA
Kligler iron agar [medium]

KIC
ketoisocaproic [acid]

KICB
killed intracellular bacteria

KID
keratitis, ichthyosis, and deafness [syndrome]
kidney (*See also* K)

KIDDIE-SADS
Schedule for Affective Disorders and Schizophrenia for School-Age Children (*See also* K-SADS)

Kiddie-SADS-E
Kiddie Schedule For Affective Disorders And Schizophrenia (*See also* K-SADS-E)

KIDS
Kent Infant Development Scale

kilo
kilogram (*See also* kg)
kilometer (*See also* km)
one thousand (*See also* K)

KIMSV
Kirsten murine sarcoma virus

KIMV
Kimberley virus

KIN
kinetic

KIP
key intermediary protein
kinase inhibitory protein

KIPS
knowledge information processing system

KIR
killer [cell] inhibitor(y) receptor
killer immunoglobulin-like receptor

$K_{ir}6.2$
inward-rectifying K^+-channel 6.2

KIR-HLA
killer [cell] inhibitor receptor-human leukocyte antigen

KISCC
keratinizing invasive squamous cell carcinoma

KISS
key integrative social system
kidney internal splint/stent

potassium iodide, saturated solution (*See also* SSKI)

KISV
Kismayo virus

KIT
Kahn intelligence test
kinase tyrosine

KIU
kallikrein inactivating (inactivation) unit
kallikrein-inhibiting unit

KJ, kj
knee jerk

kJ
kilojoule

KJR
knee jerk reflex

KK
kallikrein-kinin
knee kick
knock-knee

kkat
kilokatal

KKESH
King Khaled Eye Specialist Hospital

KKS
kallikrein-kinin system

KKV
Kaeng Khoi virus

KL
kidney lobe
kit ligand
Klebs-Löffler [bacillus] (*See also* KLB)

K&L
Kellgren and Lawrence [scale for osteoarthritis assessment]

kL
kiloliter

kl
musical overtone [ringing, in acoustics] [Ger. *Klang*]

KLA
keratolimbal allograft

KLAV
Klamath virus

KLB
Klebsiella vaccine
Klebs-Loeffler bacillus (*See also* KL)

KL-BET
Kleihauer-Betke [test or stain for fetal hemoglobin] (*See also* K-B)

Kleb, Klebs
Klebsiella

K level
lowest level [of x-rays]

KLF6
Kruppel-like factor 6 [tumor suppressor protein]

K

KLH
keyhole-limpet hemocyanin
KLK1
kallikrein 1
KLS
kidneys, liver, spleen
KLST
Kindergarten Language Screening Test
KLT
Karhunen-Loéve transform
KM
κ-immunoglobulin [light chain]
keratomileusis
Km, K$_m$
Michaelis constant (Michaelis-Menten
dissociation constant)
km
kilometer (*See also* kilo)
km^2
square kilometer
KMA
kinetic motor aphasia
KMC
kangaroo mother care
kMc
kilomegacycle
K-MCM
potassium-containing minimal
capacitation medium
kMc/s, kMcps
kilomegacycle per second
KMDAT
Key Math Diagnostic Arithmetic Test
KMEF
keratin, myosin, epidermin, fibrin [class
of proteins]
KMFTR
Kotz modular femur and tibia resection
KMnO4
potassium permanganate
KMO
Kaiser-Meyer-Olkin [measure of
statistical sampling adequacy]
knee management orthosis
kmps, km/s
kilometer per second
KMPV
Kammavanpettai virus
KMS
Kabuki makeup syndrome
kwashiorkor-marasmus syndrome
KMSV
Kirsten murine sarcoma virus
KMV
killed measles virus (vaccine)
Kn
knee (*See also* K)
Knudsen number [low-pressure gas
flow]

kN
kilonewton
KNF
Koshland-Némethy-Filmer [model]
KNO
keep needle open
knork
knife and fork [physical medicine]
KNRK
Kirsten sarcoma virus in normal rat
kidney [cell]
KNSA
Kron Nutritive Sucking Apparatus
KO
keep on (continue) (*See also* K/O)
keep open (*See also* K/O)
killed organism
knee orthosis
knock(ed) out (*See also* KO'd)
K/O
keep on (continue) (*See also* KO)
keep open (*See also* KO)
KOC
cathodal (kathodal-obsolete) opening
contraction
KO'd
knocked out (*See also* KO)
KOH
potassium hydroxide [stain]
kOhm
kilohm [electrical impedance]
KOIS
Kuder Occupational Interest Survey
KOKV
Kokobera virus
KOLV
Kolongo virus
KOOV
Koongol virus
KOR
kappa opioid receptor
keep open rate
KOT
Knowledge of Occupations Test
KOTV
Kotonkan virus
KOUV
Koutango virus
KOWV
Kowanyama virus
KP
Kaufmann-Peterson [base]
keratic precipitate
keratitis punctata
keratoprecipitate
keratotic patch
kidney protein
kidney punch [trauma]
killed parenteral [vaccine]

kinetic perimetry
knowledge of performance
Köbner phenomenon
K-P
Kaiser Permanente
kp
kilopond [unit of force]
kPa
kilopascal
kPas/L
kilopascal-second per liter
KPB
kalium (potassium) phosphate buffer
KPE
Kelman phacoemulsification
KP-e
experimentally induced Köbner
phenomenon
KP-h
Köbner phenomenon by history
KPI
karyopyknotic index (*See also* KI)
kpm
kilopond-meter [unit of force]
KPR
key pulse rate
Kuder Preference Record
KPR-V
Kuder Preference Record—Vocational
KPS
Karnofsky performance score
(status)
KPT
kidney punch test [physical exam]
Kuder Performance Test
KPTI
Kunitz pancreatic trypsin inhibitor
KPTT
kaolin partial thromboplastin time
KPV
killed parenteral vaccine
killed polio vaccine
KQI
key quality indicator
KR
knowledge of result
Kopper Reppart [medium]
17-KR
17-ketosteroid reductase
Kr
krypton
81mKr
krypton-81m
85Kr
krypton-85
kR
kiloroentgen

KRB, KRBB
Krebs-Ringer bicarbonate (buffer)
KRBG
Krebs-Ringer bicarbonate (buffer) with
glucose
KRBS
Krebs-Ringer bicarbonate solution
KRD
kinetic rehab device
K readings
keratometric readings
KRIV
Kairi virus
KRP
Kolmer [test with] Reiter protein
[antigen]
Krebs-Ringer phosphate
KRPS
Krebs-Ringer phosphate solution
KRRS
kinetic resonance Raman spectroscopy
KRT
Kindergarten Readiness Test
kineradiotherapy
KS
Kabuki syndrome
Kaposi sarcoma
keratan sulfate
ketosteroid
kidney stone
Kveim-Siltzbach [sarcoidosis test]
kyphoscoliosis
17-KS
17-ketogenic steroid (17-ketosteroid)
ks
kilosecond
KSA
knowledge, skills, abilities
K-SADS
Schedule for Affective Disorders and
Schizophrenia for School-Age Children
(*See also* KIDDIE-SADS)
K-SADS-E
Schedule for Affective Disorders and
Schizophrenia for School-Age
Children-Epidemiologic Version
(*See also* KIDDIE-SADS-E)
K-SADS-P
Schedule for Affective Disorders and
Schizophrenia for School-Age
Children-Present Episode
KSBOP
Kaderavek-Sulzby Bookreading
Observational Protocol
KSCC
keratinizing squamous cell
carcinoma

K

KSE
knee sling exercises
K-SEALS
Kaufman Survey of Early Academic and Language Skills
KSHV
Kaposi sarcoma herpesvirus
KSIV
Karshi virus
KSK
cathodal closing contraction [Ger. *Kathodenschlie βungs-Kontraktion*] (*See also* KCC)
KS/OI
Kaposi sarcoma and opportunistic infections
KSOM
potassium simplex optimized medium
KSOV
Kaisodi virus
KSP
Karolinska Scale of Personality
kidney-specific protein
K$_{sp}$
potassium solubility product
KSU
Kent State University (Speech Discrimination Test)
KSV
Kao Shuan virus
KSW
knife stab wound
KT
kidney transplant(ation)
kidney treatment
kinesiotherapy
known to
Kuder test
kT
kiloton
KTA
kidney transplant(ation) alone
KTC
knee-to-chest
K-TEA
Kaufman Test of Educational Achievement
KTI
kallikrein-trypsin inhibitor
KTP
potassium titanyl phosphate [laser, crystal]
KTRP
Kolmer test with Reiter protein
KTS
kethoxal thiosemicarbazone
KTSA
Kahn Test of Symbol Arrangement

KTU
known to us
KTVS
Keystone Telebinocular Visual Survey
KTx
kidney transplant(ation)
KU
kallikrein unit
Karmen unit
Kimbrel unit
Ku
kurchatovium
KUB
kidneys, ureters, bladder [x-ray]
kidneys and urinary bladder
kidney ultrasound biopsy
KUF
ultrafiltration coefficient [kidney]
KUNV
Kunjin virus
KUS
kidneys, ureters, spleen [x-ray]
KV
kidney vacuolating virus
killed vaccine
kV
kilovolt (kilovoltage)
kVA
kilovolt-ampere
KVBA
kanamycin-vancomycin blood agar
kVcp
kilovolt constant potential
KVE
Kaposi varicelliform eruption
KVLB
kanamycin-vancomycin laked blood
KVLBA
kanamycin-vancomycin laked blood agar
KVO
keep vein open [IV lines]
KVO C D5W
keep vein open with 5% dextrose in water
kVp
kilovoltage peak
kilovoltage potential
KW
Keith-Wagener [classification of eye ground findings] (*See also* KWB)
kidney weight
Kruskal-Wallis [test, statistics]
K$_w$
dissociation constant of water
kW
kilowatt

KWAV
    Kwatta virus
KWB
    Keith-Wagener-Barker [classification
    of eye ground findings] (*See also*
    KW)

kWh, kW-hr
    kilowatt-hour
kyf, kyph
    kyphosis
KYZV
    Kyzylagach virus

K

L

angular momentum
Avogadro number (*See also* Λ, NA)
boundary [L. *limes*] (*See also* LIM)
fifty [Roman numeral]
inductance [electrical inductance]
Lactobacillus
lambert [CGS unit of luminance]
  (*See also* La, Lb)
latent heat [energy released or stored in
  phase change]
lateral (*See also* LAT)
latex (*See also* LX, Lx)
Latin
left (*See also* (L), LT, lt)
Legionella
Leishmania
length
lesser
let
lethal [Erlich's symbol for fatal]
leucine (*See also* Leu)
levorotatory
licensed [to practice]
ligament (ligamentum) [singular]
  (*See also* Lgt, lgt, lig)
light [chain of protein molecules]
  (*See also* LC, L chain)
lilac [indicator color]
limes [singular] (limites [plural])
  [limit, boundary, threshold]
lingual (*See also* ling)
linking number
liquor (*See also* liq., liqr)
Listeria
liter [always use capital L]
  (*See also* l)
liver (*See also* LIV)
living (*See also* LIV)
longitudinal
low (lower) (lowest) (*See also* LO)
lues [syphilis] (*See also* LI–LIII)
lumbar [nerve, spine, vertebra] (*See also*
  lum, lumb)
lung (*See also* LU)
lymph (*See also* LYM)
lymphocyte (*See also* lymph)
lysosome (*See also* LYS)
NATO code for lewisite
radiance [radiant flux or power
  W x sr^{-1} × cm^{-2}]
self-inductance [electrical current]

L0

no lymphatic invasion [TNM
  classification]

L$_0$

limes zero [neutralized toxin-antitoxin
  mixture] [L. *limes nul*]

L1

(See FAB L1)
lymphatic invasion [TNM classification]

L1–L5

lumbar nerve 1–5
lumbar vertebra 1–5

LI–LIII

stages of lues [syphilis] 1–3

L2

(See FAB L2)

L3

(See FAB L3)

L/3

lower third (of leg bone)

(L)

left (*See also* L, LT, lt)
lunch

L$_+$

limes tod [toxin-antitoxin mixture that
  contains one fatal dose in excess]

l

liter [official SI symbol; use L instead
  to avoid confusion with numeral 1]
  (*See also* L)
specific latent heat [energy released or
  stored in phase change]

l-

levorotatory

L-

sterically related to L-glyceraldehyde

LA

labial
lactic acid
language age
laparoscopic adrenalectomy
laparoscopic appendectomy (*See also*
  LAP-APPY)
large amount
laser angioplasty
late abortion
late antigen
lateral apical
latex agglutination [test] (*See also* LAT)
left angle
left angulation
left arm (*See also* LARM)
left atrial (atrium)
left auricle [obsolete in reference to
  heart]
leucine aminopeptidase (*See also*
  LAP)
leukemia antigen

L

LA *(continued)*
   leukoagglutinating
   leukoaraiosis
   levator ani [muscle]
   lichen amyloidosis
   light adaptation
   linguoaxial
   linoleic acid
   lobuloalveolar
   local anesthesia (anesthetic)
   long-acting [drug] *(See also* L.A.)
   long arm [cast] *(See also* LAC)
   Los Angeles
   low anxiety
   Ludwig angina
   lupus anticoagulant *(See also* LAC)
   lymphocyte antibody

LA$_{50}$
   lethal area 50 [total body surface area
   of burn that will kill 50% of
   patients]

L&A, L+A, l&a
   light and accommodation
   living and active [family history]

L.A.
   long acting [drug designation] *(See also*
   LA)

La
   lambert [CGS unit or luminance]
   (See also L, Lb)
   lanthanum

LAA
   left atrial abnormality
   left atrial appendage
   left atrial area
   left auricular appendage [obsolete]
   leukemia-associated antigen
   leukocyte ascorbic acid

LAAH
   laparoscopic-assisted abdominal
   hysterectomy

LAAL
   lower anterior axillary line

LAAO
   L-amino acid oxidase

LA:Ao, LA:A
   left atrial to aortic ratio

LA:AR
   left atrium to aortic root ratio

LAARD
   long-acting antirheumatic drug

LAB
   left abdomen
   Leisure Activities Blank [psychology]

lab
   laboratory *(See also* LB)

LABA
   laser-assisted balloon angioplasty
   (See also LBA)

LABBB
   left anterior bundle branch block

LABC
   locally advanced breast cancer

LABD
   linear IgA bullous dermatosis

LABR
   laparoscopic-assisted bowel resection

LABS
   laboratory admission baseline
   studies

LABV
   left atrial ball valve

LABVT
   left atrial ball-valve thrombus

LAC
   laceration
   lactose
   laparoscopic-assisted colectomy
   left antecubital
   left atrial catheter
   left atrial circumflex [branch of
   coronary artery]
   left atrial contraction
   linguoaxiocervical
   locally advanced cancer
   long arm cast *(See also* LA)
   low-amplitude contraction
   lung adenocarcinoma cell
   lupus anticoagulant *(See also* LA)

LaC
   labiocervical

lac
   lactate *(See also* lact)
   lactating (lactation) *(See also* lact)

LACC
   Life After Cancer Care
   locally advanced cervical carcinoma

lac & cont
   laceration and contusion

LACD
   left apexcardiogram, calibrated
   displacement

LACI
   lacunar circulation infarct
   lipoprotein-associated coagulation
   inhibitor

lacr
   lacrimal

LACS
   lacunar syndrome
   laser-assisted capsular shrinkage

LAC T
   lactose tolerance

LACT
   Lindamood Auditory Conceptualization
   Test [psychology]

lact
   lactate *(See also* lac)

lactating (lactation) (*See also* lac)
lactic

LACT-ART
lactate arterial

LACV
La Crosse virus

LAD
lactate (lactic acid) dehydrogenase
(*See also* LADH, LD, LDH)
language acquisition device
left anterior descending [coronary
artery] (*See also* LADA, LADCA)
left atrial defect
left atrial diameter
left atrial dimension
left axis deviation
ligament augmentation device
ligamentous anterior dislocation
linear [immunoglobulin] A disease
linoleic acid depression
lipoamide dehydrogenase
lymphocyte-activating determinant

LAD1–LAD4
leukocyte adhesion deficiency type 1–4

LADA
laboratory animal dander allergy
latent autoimmune diabetes of adults
left acromion dorsum anterior
(acromiodorsoanterior) [fetal position]
left anterior descending [coronary]
artery (*See also* LAD, LADCA)

LADB
left anterior descending branch [of
coronary artery]

LADCA
left anterior descending coronary artery
(*See also* LAD, LADA)

LADD
lacrimoauriculodentodigital [syndrome]
left anterior descending diagonal
[coronary artery]

LADH
lactate (lactic acid) dehydrogenase
(*See also* LAD, LD, LDH)
liver alcohol dehydrogenase

LADME
liberation, absorption, distribution,
metabolism, excretion

LAD-MIN
left axis deviation, minimal

LAD-NSCLC
locally advanced nonsmall-cell lung
cancer (*See also* LANSCLC)

LADP
left acromion dorsum posterior
(acromiodorsoposterior) [fetal
position]

left anterior descending [arterial]
pressure

LADPG
laparoscopically assisted distal partial
gastrectomy

LADu
lobuloalveolar-ductal

LAE
left atrial enlargement
long above-elbow [cast]

LAEC
locally advanced esophageal cancer

LAEDV
left atrial end-diastolic volume

LAEI
left atrial emptying index

LAER
late auditory evoked response

LAESV
left atrial end-systolic volume

LAF
laminar air flow (*See also* LAM)
Leisure Activities Finder
leukocyte-activating factor
low animal fat
lymphocyte-activating factor

LAFB
left anterior fascicular block

LAFF
lateral arm free flap

LAFM
locally acquired [*Plasmodium*]
falciparum malaria

LAFR
laminar air flow room

LAFS
long-axis fractional shortening

LAFU
laminar air flow unit

LAG
linguoaxiogingival
lymphangiograph(y) (lymphangiogram)

LaG
labiogingival

LAH
lactalbumin hydrolysate
laparoscopic-assisted hepatectomy
left anterior hemiblock (*See also* LAHB)
left atrial hypertrophy

LAHB
left anterior hemiblock (*See also* LAH)

LA-HFOV
liquid-assisted high-frequency oscillatory
ventilation

LAHNC
locally advanced head and neck
cancer

L

LAHT
 laser-assisted hair transplant(ation)
LAHV
 leukocyte-associated herpesvirus
LAI
 laboratory-acquired infection
 latex agglutination inhibition
 left atrial involvement
 left atrial isomerism
 leukocyte adherence inhibition
  (inhibitor)
LaI
 labioincisal
LAID
 left anterior internal diameter
LAIF
 leukocyte adherence inhibition
  factor
LAIT
 latex agglutination inhibition test
LAIV
 live attenuated influenza vaccine
LAK
 lymphokine-activated killer [cell]
  (*See also* LAKC)
LAKC
 lymphokine-activated killer cell (*See also*
  LAK)
LAL
 laser-adjustable lens
 left axillary line
 Limulus [horseshoe crab] amoebocyte
  lysate
 low air loss
LaL
 labiolingual
L-Ala
 L-alanine
LALB
 low air loss bed
LALI
 lymphocyte antibody lymphocytolytic
  interaction
LALL
 lymphomatous acute lymphoblastic
  leukemia
LALLS
 low-angle laser light scattering
LALT
 larynx-associated lymphoid tissue
 low air loss therapy
LALV
 lucerne Australian latent virus
LAM
 lactational anovulatory method [birth
  control]
 lactation amenorrhea method [birth
  control]
 laminar air flow (*See also* LAF)

laminectomy (*See also* lam)
laminogram
laparoscopic-assisted myomectomy
laser-assisted myringotomy
late ambulatory monitoring
left anterior measurement
left atrial myxoma
limb accurate measurement
lipoarabinomannan
lymphangioleiomyomatosis
lymphangiomyomatosis
LAM-1
 leukocyte adhesion molecule 1
lam
 lamina
 laminectomy (*See also* LAM)
 laminogram
LAMA
 laser-assisted microanastomosis
LA–MAX
 maximal left atrial [dimension]
LAM-B
 lipoarabinomannan B
LAMB
 lentigines, atrial myxomas, cutaneous
  papular myxomas, blue nevi
Λ
 Avogadro number (*See also* NA, L)
 lambda [11th letter of Greek alphabet
  uppercase]
 Ostwald solubility coefficient
 radioactive constant
λ
 decay constant
 junction of lambdoid and sagittal
  sutures (lambda) [craniometric]
 lambda [11th letter of Greek alphabet
  lowercase]
 mean free path
 one of two immunoglobulin light chains
 thermal conductivity (*See also* TC,
  TCD)
lam & fus
 laminectomy and fusion
lami
 laminotomy
LAMMA
 laser microprobe mass analyzer
LAMP
 lysosomal-associated membrane protein
LAN
 long-acting neuroleptic
 lymphadenopathy
LANA
 latency-associated nuclear antigen
LANC
 long arm navicular cast
lang
 language

LANSCLC
locally advanced nonsmall-cell lung
cancer (*See also* LAD-NSCLC)
L ANT
left anterior
LANV
left atrial neovascularization
LAO
left anterior oblique
left anterior occipital
left atrial overload(ing)
LAP
laparoscopy (*See also* lap., LSC)
laparotomy (*See also* lap., lapt)
laryngeal adductor paralysis
laser-assisted palatoplasty
latency-associated peptide
left abdominal pain
left arterial pressure
leucine aminopeptidase (*See also* LA)
leukemia-associated phenotype
leukocyte alkaline phosphatase (*See also*
LEUKAP)
liver-enriched activating protein
low atmospheric pressure
lower abdominal pain
lymphangiomatous polyp
lyophilized anterior pituitary [tissue]
LAP-1
Los Angeles preservation solution 1
lap.
laparoscopy (*See also* LAP)
laparotomy (*See also* LAP, lapt)
LAPA
leukocyte alkaline phosphatase activity
locally-advanced pancreatic
adenocarcinoma
LAP-APPY
laparoscopic appendectomy (*See also*
LA)
LAPC
locally advanced prostate cancer
LAP CHOLE
laparoscopic cholecystectomy (*See also*
LC, LCC)
LAPF
low-affinity platelet factor
LAPMS
long arm posterior-molded splint
lap Nissen
laparoscopic Nissen fundoplication
(*See also* LNF)
lapt
laparotomy (*See also* LAP, lap.)
lapUS
laparoscopic ultrasound
(ultrasonography) (*See also* LUS)

LAPW
left atrial posterior wall
LAQ
long arc quad
LAR
laryngeal adductor reflex
laryngology (*See also* Laryngol)
larynx (*See also* LX, Lx)
late asthmatic response
left arm, reclining [blood pressure,
pulse measurement]
left arm, recumbent [blood pressure,
pulse measurement]
leukocyte antigen-related
leukocyte automated recognition
long-acting release
low anterior resection
LARC
leukocyte automatic recognition
computer
locally advanced rectal cancer
LAR/CAA
low anterior resection in combination
with coloanal anastomosis
LARD
lacrimoauriculoradiodental
[syndrome]
LARIS
laser atomization resonance ionization
spectroscopy
LARM
left arm (*See also* LA)
LARS
Language-Structured Auditory Retention
Span [Test]
laparoscopic antireflux surgery
leucyl-transfer ribonucleic acid
synthetase
LARSI
lumbar anterior-root stimulator
implant
laryn
laryngeal
laryngitis
laryngoscopy
Laryngol
laryngology (*See also* LAR)
LAS
laboratory automation system
lactic acidosis syndrome
lateral amyotrophic sclerosis
laxative abuse syndrome
left anterior superior
left arm, sitting [blood pressure, pulse
measurement]
linear alkyl sulfonate
local adaptation syndrome

L

LAS *(continued)*
    long arm splint
    low-amplitude signal
    lower abdominal surgery
    lymphadenopathy syndrome
    lymphangioscintigraphy
LASA
    left anterior spinal artery
    Linear Analogue Self-Assessment
    [scales]
    lipid-associated sialic acid
    Lisfranc articular set angle
LASCC
    locally advanced squamous-cell
    carcinoma
LASE
    laser-assisted spinal endoscopy
LASEC
    left atrial spontaneous echo contrast [on
    TEE]
LASEK
    laser-assisted subepithelial (epithelial)
    keratomileusis (keratectomy)
LASFB
    left anterior-superior fascicular block
LASGB
    laser adjustable silicone gastric banding
LASH
    left anterior-superior (anterosuperior)
    hemiblock
LASIK
    laser-assisted intrastromal (in situ)
    keratomileusis
LASS
    labile aggregation stimulating substance
    Linguistic Analysis of Speech Samples
LASSI
    Learning and Study Strategies Inventory
LASSI-HS
    Learning and Study Strategies Inventory
    High School Version
LAST
    left anterior small thoracotomy
    leukocyte-antigen sensitivity testing
    limited anterior small thoracotomy
LASTAC
    laser transluminal angioplasty catheter
LASV
    Lassa virus
LAT
    lactic acidosis threshold
    latency-associated transcript
    latent
    lateral *(See also* L)
    lateral atrial tunnel
    latex agglutination test *(See also* LA)
    latissimus dorsi [muscle] *(See also* lats,
    LD)
    left anterior thigh

    left atrial thrombus
    limbal autograft transplant(ation)
    linker for activation of T cell [protein]
lat
    latitude
LAT-A
    latrunculin A
LAT-B
    latrunculin B
LATC
    lateral talocalcaneal
LATCH
    literature attached to charts
lat decub
    lateral decubitus
lat & loc
    lateralizing and localizing
L · atm
    liter-atmosphere
lat men
    lateral meniscectomy
LATP
    left atrial transmural pressure
LATPT
    left atrial transesophageal pacing test
lat Rin
    lactated Ringer [solution] *(See also* LR,
    LRS)
LATS
    long-acting thyroid-stimulating
    [hormone]
    long-acting thyroid stimulator
    long-acting transmural stimulator
lats
    latissimus dorsi [muscle] *(See also* LAT,
    LD)
LATS-P
    long-acting thyroid stimulator-protector
LATu
    lobuloalveolar tumor
LATV
    Latino virus
LAUP
    laser-assisted uvulopalatoplasty
LAUPPP
    laser-assisted uvulopalatopharyngoplasty
LAV
    left atrial volume
    lymphadenopathy-associated virus
LAVA
    laser-assisted vasal anastomosis
    liver acquisitions with volume
    acceleration [imaging]
LAVH
    laparoscopic-assisted vaginal
    hysterectomy (hysteroscopy)
LAVM
    laparoscopic-assisted vaginal
    myomectomy

LAW
    LDH (lactate dehydrogenase), AST (aspartate aminotransferase), WBC (white blood cells) [blood tests]
    left atrial wall
LAWER
    life-terminating acts without explicit request
LAX
    long axis
lax.
    laxative
    laxity
LAX-DSS
    long axis-discrete subaortic stenosis
LAY
    look after yourself
LAYH
    look after your heart
LB
    laboratory (*See also* lab)
    lamellar body
    large bowel
    laser bullectomy
    lateral basal
    lateral bending
    left breast
    left bronchus
    left bundle
    left buttock
    leiomyoblastoma (*See also* LMB)
    lipid body
    live birth (*See also* LIVB)
    liver biopsy
    living bank
    loose body
    low back [pain] (*See also* LBP)
    low breakage
    lung biopsy
    lymphoid body
Lb
    lambert [CGS unit of luminance] (*See also* L, La)
L-B
    Liebermann-Burchard [test for cholesterol]
L:B
    lesion to brain ratio
L&B
    left and below
lb.
    pound [singular] [L. *libra*] (*See also* lb. avdp, lbs.)
LBA
    laser balloon angioplasty (*See also* LABA)

left basal artery
    lower body adiposity
    lymphocyte blastogenesis assay
LBAII
    Leader Behavior Analysis II
lb. avdp
    avoirdupois pound [L. *libra avoirdupois*] (*See also* lb., lbs.)
LBB
    left breast biopsy
    left bundle branch
    long back board
    low back bend
LBBB
    left bundle branch block
LBBsB
    left bundle branch system block
LBBX
    left breast biopsy examination
LBC
    lamellar body count
    lidocaine blood concentration
    locoregional breast cancer
    lymphadenosis benigna cutis
LBCD
    left border of cardiac dullness (*See also* LBD)
LBCF
    Laboratory Branch Complement Fixation [test]
LBCL
    large B-cell lymphoma
L/B/Cr
    electrolytes, blood urea nitrogen, serum creatinine
LBD
    lamellar body density
    large bile duct
    left border of dullness [cardiac] (*See also* LBCD)
    left brain damage
    Lewy body dementia
    low back disability
    lower back disorder
    lumbar body density
LBDQ
    Leader Behavior Description Questionnaire
LBE
    line bisection error [neuropsychology]
    long below-elbow [cast]
LBF
    Lactobacillus bulgaricus factor [pantetheine]
    limb blood flow
    liver blood flow
    localized bone fibrosis

L

lbf
  pound-force
LBG
  light beam generator
LBH
  length, breadth, height
LBI
  low serum-bound iron
lbf/in²
  pound-force per square inch [non SI
    unit of pressure] (*See also* psi)
LBL
  labeled lymphoblast
  lymphoblastic lymphoma
LBM
  last bowel movement
  lean body mass
  little brown mushroom
  loose bowel movement
  lung basement membrane
LBMI
  last body mass index
LBNA
  lysis bladder neck adhesions
LBNP
  lower body negative pressure
LBO
  large-bowel obstruction
LBOTC
  laryngeal and base of tongue carcinoma
LBP
  lipopolysaccharide binding protein
  low back pain (*See also* LB)
  low blood pressure
  lumbar back pain
LBPF
  long bone or pelvic fracture
LBPP
  lower body positive pressure
LBPQ
  Low Back Pain Questionnaire
LBQC
  large base quad cane
LBRF
  louse-borne relapsing fever
LBS
  Lactobacillus selector [agar]
  Leisure Boredom Scale
  low back strain
  low back syndrome
  lumbar back strain
LBSA
  lipid-bound sialic acid (*See also* LSA)
lbs.
  pounds [plural] [L. *librae*] (*See also* lb.,
    lb. avdp)
LBT
  lactulose breath test
  loaded breathing test

low back tenderness
low back trouble
lupus band test
LBTI
  lima bean trypsin inhibitor
LBV
  Lagos bat virus
  left brachial vein
  low biological value
  lung blood volume
LB-V
  left bundle-ventricle
LBVO
  left brachial vein occlusion
LBVP
  luminal balloon valvuloplasty
LBW
  lean body weight
  low birth weight
LBWC
  limb-body wall complex
LBWI
  low-birth-weight infant (*See also* Low
    BI)
LBWR
  lung to body weight ratio
LC
  inductance-capacitance [meter, circuit]
  Laënnec cirrhosis
  lamina cortex
  Langerhans cell
  laparoscopic cholecystectomy (*See also*
    LCC, LAP CHOLE)
  large cell
  large chromophobe
  large cleaved [cell]
  late clamped [umbilical cord]
  lateral canthotomy
  lateral compression
  lateral projection
  lecithin cholesterol [acyltransferase]
    (*See also* LCAT)
  left circumflex [coronary artery]
    (*See also* LCA, LCC, LCCA, LCF,
    LCX, LCx)
  left [ear], cold [stimulus] [Bárány
    caloric test]
  leisure counseling
  lethal concentration (*See also* LCt)
  level of consciousness (*See also* LOC)
  life care
  light chain (*See also* L, L chain)
  light coagulation
  lingual cusp
  linguocervical
  lining cell
  lipid cytosome
  liquid chromatography
  liquid crystal

lithocholic [acid] (*See also* LCA)
liver cirrhosis
living children
locus caeruleus
long chain
longus capitis [muscle]
low calorie [diet] (*See also* lo cal)
low contrast
lung cancer
lung cell
lymphangitic carcinomatosis
lymph capillary
lymphocyte count
lymphocytic colitis
lymphocytotoxin (*See also* LCT, LT)
lymphoma culture

3LC
triple-lumen catheter

L&C
lids and conjunctivae

L:C
lesion to countersite ratio

LCA
latent class analysis
lateral cricoarytenoid
Leber congenital amaurosis
left carotid artery
left circumflex [coronary] artery
(*See also* LC, LCC, LCCA, LCF,
LCX, LCx)
left coronary angiography
left coronary artery (*See also* LCyA)
leukocyte common antigen
life cycle assessment
light contact assist
lithocholic acid (*See also* LC)
liver cell adenoma
lymphocyte chemoattractant activity
lymphocytotoxic antibody (*See also*
LCTA)

LCACoA
long chain acyl coenzyme A

LCAD
lipid coronary artery disease
long-chain acyl-coenzyme A
dehydrogenase

LCA:DCA
lithocholic acid to deoxycholic acid
ratio

LCAD:MCAD
long chain acyl-coenzyme A
dehydrogenase to medium-chain
acyl-coenzyme A dehydrogenase ratio

LCAH
life-care at home
lipoid congenital adrenal hyperplasia

LCAL
large-cell anaplastic lymphoma

LCAO
linear combination of atomic orbitals

LCAO MO
linear combination of atomic orbitals
molecular orbital

LCAR
late cutaneous anaphylactic reaction

LCAT
lecithin-cholesterol acyltransferase
(acetyltransferase) (*See also* LC)
limbal-conjunctival autograft
transplant(ation)

LCATA
lecithin-cholesterol acetyltransferase
alpha

LCB
left costal border
lymphomatosis cutis benigna

LCBF
local cerebral blood flow

LCC
lactose coliform count
laparoscopic cholecystectomy (*See also*
LC, LAP CHOLE)
large-cell change
left circumflex coronary [artery]
(*See also* LC, LCA, LCCA, LCF,
LCX, LCx)
left coronary cusp
light-cured composite [resin]
liver cell carcinoma
long calcaneocuboid

LCCA
late cortical cerebellar atrophy
left circumflex coronary artery (*See also*
LC, LCA, LCC, LCF, LCX, LCx)
left common carotid artery
leukocytoclastic angiitis

LCCE
length contraction compensation
element

LCCND
large-cell carcinoma [of lung] with
neuroendocrine differentiation

LCCNM
large-cell carcinoma [of lung] with
neuroendocrine morphology

LCCP
limited channel-capacity process

LCCS
lower cervical cesarean section

LCCSCT
large-cell calcifying Sertoli cell tumor

LCD
lattice corneal dystrophy type I, II, III,
IIIA
lipochondral degeneration
liquid crystal display

L

LCD *(continued)*
> liquor carbonis detergens [coal tar solution]
> localized collagen dystrophy
> low-calcium diet (*See also* LoCa, lo calc)

LC-DCP, LCDCP
> low-contact dynamic compression plate

LCDD
> light-chain deposition disease

LCDE
> laparoscopic common duct exploration

LCDV
> lymphocystic disease virus

LCDVA
> low-contrast distance visual acuity

LCE
> left carotid endarterectomy
> lower completely edentulous

LCED
> liquid chromatography with electrochemical detection

LC-EMR
> lift-and-cut endoscopic mucosal resection

LCF
> least common factor
> left circumflex [coronary artery] (*See also* LC, LCA, LCC, LCCA, LCX, LCx)
> left common femoral [artery]
> linear correction factor
> low-frequency current field
> lymphocyte chemoattractant factor
> lymphocyte culture fluid

LCFA
> long-chain fatty acid

LCFA-CoA
> long chain fatty acyl-coenzyme A

LCFAO
> long-chain fatty acid oxidation

LCFC
> linear combination of fragment configuration [chemistry]

LCFM
> laser cell and flare meter
> left circumflex marginal [coronary artery]

LCFU
> leukocyte colony-forming unit

LCG
> Langerhans cell granule
> Langerhans cell granulomatosis
> liquid chemical germicide

LCGL
> large-cell granulocytic leukemia

LCGU
> local cerebral glucose utilization

LCH
> Langerhans cell histiocytosis

LCHAD
> long-chain 3-hydroxyacyl coenzyme A dehydrogenase

L chain
> light chain [polypeptides with low molecular weight] (*See also* L, LC)

LCI
> length complexity index
> lung clearance index

LCIN
> low-grade cervical intraepithelial neoplasia

LCIS
> lobular carcinoma in situ

LCL
> large cell lymphoma
> lateral collateral ligament
> Levinthal-Coles-Lillie [cytoplasmic inclusion body]
> localized cutaneous leishmaniasis
> lower confidence limit
> lymphoblastoid cell line
> lymphocytic lymphosarcoma (*See also* LCLS)
> lymphoid cell line

LCLC
> large-cell lung carcinoma

LCLD
> low-calorie liquid diet

LCLS
> lymphocytic lymphosarcoma (*See also* LCL)

LCM
> laser-capture microdissection
> latent cardiomyopathy
> left costal margin
> leukocyte-conditioned medium
> lower costal margin
> lowest common multiple
> lymphocytic choriomeningitis [virus] (*See also* LCMV, LCV)

LCMG
> long-chain monoglyceride

L/cm H_2O
> liter per centimeter of water

LC/MS
> liquid chromatography/mass spectrometry

LC-MS-MS
> liquid chromatography coupled to tandem mass spectrometry

LCMV
> lymphocytic choriomeningitis virus (*See also* LCM, LCV)

LCN
> lateral cervical nucleus
> left caudate nucleus

LCNB
large-core needle biopsy
LCNEC
large-cell neuroendocrine carcinoma
LCNF
large-cell carcinoma with
neuroendocrine features
LCNHL
large-cell non-Hodgkin lymphoma
LCNST
late central nervous system toxicity
LCO
left coronary ostium
low cardiac output
LCOS
low cardiac output syndrome (See also
LOS)
LCP
leukocyte apheresis
long-chain polysaturated [fatty acid]
long, closed, posterior [cervix]
LCPUFA
long-chain polyunsaturated fatty acid
LCQG
left caudal quarter ganglion
LCR
laryngeal cough reflex [test]
late cortical response
late cutaneous reaction
ligamentous and capsular repair
ligase chain reaction
locus control region
LCRS
Living Conditions Rating Scale
LCS
laparoscopic coagulating shears
laser correlational spectroscopy
lateral crural steal
left coronary sinus
Leydig cell stimulation
lichen chronicus simplex
lids, conjunctivae, sclerae [plural]
life care service
liquor cerebrospinalis
low constant (continuous) suction
low-contact stress
Lung Cancer Subscale [Functional
Assessment of Cancer, FACT]
LCSG
left cardiac sympathetic ganglionectomy
LCSLC
Low-Contrast Sloan Letter Chart
LCSS
lethal congenital contracture syndrome
Lung Cancer Symptom Score
LCST
lateral corticospinal tract

LCWS
low continuous wall suction
LCT
Leydig cell tumor
liquid crystal thermography
Listening Comprehension Test
liver cell tumor
long-chain triglyceride
low cervical transverse
lung capillary time
Luscher Color Test
lymphocytotoxicity test
lymphocytotoxin (See also LC, LT)
LCt
lethal concentration (See also LC)
LCt$_{50}$
lethal concentration 50 [concentration
lethal to half a group]
LCTA
lungs clear to auscultation
lymphocytotoxic antibody (See also
LCA)
LCTCS
low cervical transverse cesarean section
LCTD
low-calcium test diet
LCU
laparoscopic contact ultrasonography
LCV
Lake Clarendon virus
lecithovitellin [test]
leukocytoclastic vasculitis
low cervical vertical [incision]
lymphocytic choriomeningitis virus
(See also LCM, LCMV)
LCVA
left hemisphere cerebrovasular accident
(stroke)
LCVP
laser coagulation vaporization procedure
LCWI
left cardiac work index
LCX, LCx
left circumflex [coronary artery]
(See also LC, LCA, LCC, LCCA,
LCF)
LCXB
left circumflex branch [of coronary
artery]
LCyA
left coronary artery (See also LCA)
LD
laboratory data
labor and delivery (See also L&D)
labyrinthine defect
lactate [lactic acid] dehydrogenase
(See also LAD, LADH, LDH)

L

LD *(continued)*
  laser Doppler
  last dose
  latissimus dorsi [muscle] *(See also* LAT, lats)
  learning disability (disabled)
  learning disorder
  left deltoid
  Legionnaires' disease
  Leishman-Donovan [body] *(See also* LDB)
  lethal dose
  leukodystrophy
  levodopa *(See also* L-dopa)
  lichenoid dysplasia
  light-dark
  light difference (differentiation)
  light duty
  limited disease
  linear dichroism
  linguodistal
  lipodystrophy
  lithium diluent
  lithium discontinuation
  liver disease
  living donor
  loading dose
  local deviation
  Lombard-Dowell [agar]
  long dwell [catheter]
  longitudinal diameter
  long [time] dialysis
  low density
  low dose
  lung destruction
  lymphocyte defined
  lymphocyte depletion
  lymphocytically determined
L&D
  labor and delivery *(See also* LD)
  light and distance [in ophthalmology]
L:D
  light to dark [amplitude] ratio
LD$_1$
  lactate dehydrogenase [heart, lungs, kidneys]
LD$_{2-3}$
  lactate dehydrogenase [lungs]
LD$_4$
  lactate dehydrogenase [liver]
LD$_5$
  lactate dehydrogenase [liver and muscles]
LD$_1$–LD$_5$
  lactate dehydrogenase fraction 1–5
LD$_{50}$
  median lethal dose [lethal for 50% of test subjects] *(See also* MLD)

LD$_{50/30}$
  lethal dose for 50% of test subjects within 30 days
LD$_{100}$
  lethal dose in all exposed subjects
LDA
  laser Doppler anemometry
  lateral disc attachment
  lateral divergence angle
  left descending artery
  left dorsum anterior (dorsoanterior) [fetal position]
  limiting dilution analysis
  linear discriminant analysis [statistics]
  linear displacement analysis
  low density area
  low-dose arm
  lymphocyte-dependent antibody
LDAR
  latex direct agglutination reaction
LDB
  lamb dysentery bacillus
  Legionnaires' disease bacillus
  Leishman-Donovan body *(See also* LD)
  ligand-binding domain
LDC
  lactose digestion capacity
  Langerhans dendritic cell
  leukocyte differential count
  lymphoid dendritic cell
LDCC
  lectin-dependent cellular cytotoxicity
LDCI
  low-dose continuous infusion
LDCOC
  low-dose combination oral contraceptive
LDCT
  late distal cortical tubule
LDD
  laser disc decompression
  late dedifferentiation
  Lee and Desus D [test]
  light-dark discrimination
  low drain [class] D [battery]
LDDE
  low-dose dobutamine echocardiogram
LDE
  Lateral Dominance Examination
LDEA
  left deviation of electrical axis
LDER
  lateral-view dual-energy radiography
LDES
  Learning Disability Evaluation Scale
LD-EYA
  Lombard-Dowell egg yolk agar

LDF
  laser Doppler flowmetry
  laser Doppler flux
  limit dilution factor
  lumbodorsal fascia
LDG
  lingual developmental groove
  long-distance group
  low-dose group
LDH
  lactate (lactic acid) dehydrogenase
    (*See also* LAD, LADH, LD)
  low-dose heparin
LDH$_1$–LDH$_5$
  lactate (lactic acid) dehydrogenase
    fraction 1 through 5 (*See also*
    LD$_1$–LD$_5$)
LDHA
  lactate (lactic acid) dehydrogenase A
LDHB
  lactate (lactic acid) dehydrogenase B
LDHD
  lymphocyte-depleted Hodgkin disease
LDHI
  lactate (lactic acid) dehydrogenase
    isoenzyme (*See also* LDISO)
LDHV
  lactic dehydrogenase virus (*See also*
    LDV)
LDIH
  left direct inguinal hernia
LDIR
  low-dose of ionizing radiation
LDISO
  lactate (lactic acid) dehydrogenase
    isoenzyme (*See also* LDHI)
LDI-TOF-MS
  laser desorption/ionization
    time-of-flight-mass spectrometer
LDL
  limitation of daily life
  loudness discomfort level
  low-density lipoprotein (*See also* LDLP)
  low-density lymphocyte
LDLA
  low-density lipoprotein apheresis
LDL-C
  low-density lipoprotein-cholesterol
    [complex]
LDL:HDL
  low-density lipoprotein to high-density
    lipoprotein ratio
LDLP
  low-density lipoprotein (*See also* LDL)
LDLR
  low-density lipoprotein receptor
    [gene]

LDLT
  living donor liver transplant(ation)
LDM
  lactate (lactic acid) dehydrogenase,
    muscle
  limited dorsal myeloschisis
LDMA
  lymphocyte detected membrane antigen
LDMCF, LDMF
  latissimus dorsi myocutaneous flap
LDMRT
  low-dose mediastinal radiation therapy
LDN
  laparoscopic donor nephrectomy
  living donor nephrectomy
LD-NEYA
  Lombard-Dowell neomycin egg yolk
    agar
LDNF
  lung-derived neurotrophic factor
L-dopa
  levodopa (*See also* LD)
LDP
  laparoscopic distal pancreatectomy
  late diastolic potential
  left dorsum posterior (dorsoposterior)
    [fetal position]
  lumbodorsal pain
LD-PCR
  limiting dilution polymerase chain
    reaction
  long-distance polymerase chain reaction
LDPM
  laser Doppler perfusion monitoring
LDR
  labor, delivery, recovery
  length to diameter ratio
  long-duration response
  low-dose rate
LDRP
  labor, delivery, recovery, postpartum
LDS
  late dumping syndrome
  ligate-divide-staple
  ligating and dividing stapler
  locked door seclusion
LDSST
  low-dose short synacthen test
LDT
  left dorsum transverse (dorsotransverse)
    [fetal position]
LD-T
  lactate (lactic acid) dehydrogenase total
LDU, LDUB
  long double upright [brace]
LDUH
  low-dose unfractionated heparin

L

LDV
    lactic dehydrogenase virus (*See also* LDHV)
    large dense-cored vesicle
    laser Doppler velocimetry
    lateral distant view
    Le Dantec virus

LE
    labor epidural
    left ear
    left eye
    lens extraction
    leucine enkephalin
    leukocyte esterase (*See also* LKESTR)
    leukoerythrogenic (leukoerythrogenetic)
    live embryo
    local excision
    Long Evans [rat]
    lower extremity (*See also* L ext, l/ext, LX, Lx)
    lupus erythematosus [cell]

Le
    Leonard [cathode ray unit]
    Lewis [blood group, gene]
    Lewis [number, diffusivity to diffusion coefficient of a fluid]

Le^a
    Lewis a antibody

LEA
    language experience approach
    lower extremity amputation
    lower extremity arterial
    lumbar epidural anesthesia

LEAD
    longitudinal expert evaluation using all available data
    lower extremity arterial disease

LEADS
    Leadership Evaluation and Development Scale

LEAP
    latex ELISA for antigen protein
    Lewis expandable adjustable prosthesis
    low-energy all-purpose [collimator]
    Lower Extremity Amputation Prevention [program for diabetes patients]

LEAS
    level of emotional awareness scale

Le^b
    Lewis b antibody

LEB
    lumbar epidural block
    lupus erythematosus body

LEBV
    Lebombo virus

LEC
    lens epithelial cell
    leukoencephalitis
    life events checklist

    Life Experiences Checklist
    low-energy cardioversion
    low-energy charged [particle]
    lower esophageal contractility
    lymphoepithelioma-like carcinoma

LECBD
    laparoscopic exploration of common bile duct

LECEMRA
    lower extremity contrast-enhanced magnetic resonance angiography

LECL
    lymphoepithelioid cell lymphoma

LECP
    low-energy charged particle

LE-CTV
    lower extremity computed tomography venography

LED
    light-emitting diode
    lowest effective dose
    lupus erythematosus disseminatus

LEDC
    low energy direct current

LEDS
    life events and difficulties schedule

LEDV
    Lednice virus

LEED
    low-energy electron diffraction

LEEDS
    low-energy electron diffraction spectroscopy

LEEP
    left end-expiratory pressure
    loop electrosurgical (electrocautery) excision procedure

LEER
    lower extremity equipment related [injury]

LEETZ
    loop electrosurgical excision of transformation zone

LEF
    leukokinesis-enhancing factor
    lower extremity fracture
    lupus erythematosus factor

LEFS
    Lower Extremity Functional Scale

leg.
    legal
    legislation (legislative)

leg. com
    legal commitment
    legally committed

LEH
    liposome-encapsulated hemoglobin

LEHPZ
    lower esophageal high-pressure zone

LeIF
: *Leishmania* elongation initiation factor
: leukocyte interferon

leio
: leiomyoma

LEIS
: low-energy ion scattering

LEJ
: ligation of esophagogastric junction

LEL
: low-energy laser
: lowest effect level [of toxicity]
: lymphoepithelial lesion

LELC
: lymphoepithelioma-like carcinoma

LEM
: lateral eye movement
: Leibovitz-Emory medium
: leukocyte endogenous mediator
: light electron microscope
: low-electrolyte meal

LEMA
: lower extremity mobility aid

LEMG
: laryngeal electromyography

LEMO
: lowest empty molecular orbital

LEMS
: Lambert-Eaton myasthenic
  syndrome

LENI
: lower extremity noninvasive

lenit.
: lenitive
: gently [L. *leniter*]

L-ent
: leucine-enkephalin

LENT
: late effects of normal tissue [scoring
  system]

⚠ **LEOD**
: lens extraction, oculus dexter ⚠

LEOPARD
: lentigines, electrocardiographic
  conduction abnormalities, ocular
  hypertelorism, pulmonary stenosis,
  abnormalities of genitalia, retardation
  of growth, sensorineural deafness
  [autosomal dominant syndrome]

⚠ **LEOS**
: lens extraction, oculus sinister ⚠

LEP
: leptospirosis
: lethal effective phase [leptospirosis]
: lipoprotein electrophoresis (*See also*
  LPE)
: longitudinal epiphysial bracket

: low egg passage [strain of virus]
: lower esophageal pressure
: lupus erythematosus preparation
  (*See also* LE$_{prep}$)

LEP2
: leptospirosis 2

L$_{EPN}$
: effective perceived noise level

LE$_{prep}$
: lupus erythematosus preparation
  (*See also* LEP)

LEPT
: leptocyte

LEPTOS
: leptospirosis agglutinins

Leq
: loudness equivalent

LER
: lysozymal enzyme release

LERG
: local electroretinogram

L-ERX
: leukoerythroblastic reaction

LES
: Lawrence Experimental Station [agar]
: lesser esophageal sphincter
: Life Experience Survey
: Liquid Embolic System
: local excitatory state
: Locke egg serum [medium]
: lower esophageal segment
: lower esophageal sphincter (*See also*
  LOS)
: lower esophageal stricture
: low excitatory state
: lumbar epidural steroid
: lupus erythematosus, systemic

les
: lesion
: low excitatory state

LESA
: liposomally entrapped second antibody

LESEP
: lower extremity somatosensory evoked
  potential

LESI
: lumbar epidural steroid injection

LESP
: lower esophageal sphincter pressure

LESR
: lower esophageal sphincter relaxation

LESS
: lateral electrical spine stimulation
: lateral electrical surface stimulation

LESSD
: lupus erythematosus-specific skin
  disease.

LET
    language enrichment therapy
    left esotropia
    leukocyte esterase test
    lidocaine, epinephrine, tetracaine [topical
        anesthetic]
    linear energy transfer
    low energy transfer
LETC
    lymphoepithelioma-like thymic
        carcinoma
LETD
    lowest effective toxic dose
LET-II
    Learning Efficiency Test II
LETS
    large external transformation-sensitive
        [protein]
LE-TUMT
    low-energy transurethral microwave
        thermotherapy
LETZ
    loop excision of transformation zone
LEU
    leukocyte equivalent unit
Leu
    leucine (See also L)
leu-CAM
    leukocyte cell adhesion molecule
LEUHR
    low-energy ultra-high resolution
leuk, leuko
    leukocyte
LEUKAP
    leukocyte alkaline phosphatase (See also
        LAP)
LEV
    levator [muscle]
    lower extremity venous
levit.
    lightly [L. leviter]
LEVT
    lower extremity venous tracing
LEW
    Lewis [rat]
LEX
    lactate extraction
L ext, l/ext
    lower extremity (See also LE, LX, Lx)
LeY
    Lewis Y [antigen]
LF
    labile factor
    laparoscopic fundoplication
    laryngofissure
    Lassa fever
    latex fixation
    lavage fluid
    leaflet

    left foot
    left forearm
    left frontal
    lethal factor
    leucine flux
    ligamentum flavum
    limit of flocculation (See also Lf)
    lingual fossa
    living female
    low-fat [diet]
    low forceps [delivery] (See also
        LFD)
    low frequency
    lymphatic filariasis
Lf
    limes flocculation [unit, dose of toxin
        per mL]
LFA
    left femoral artery
    left forearm
    left front anterior (frontoanterior) [fetal
        position] (See also FLA)
    leukocyte function-associated antigen
    leukotactic factor activity
    low friction arthroplasty
    lymphocyte function-associated
        antigen
LFA-1–LFA-3
    leukocyte (lymphocyte) function
        associated antigen 1–3
LFAC
    low frequency alternating current
LFB
    lingual-facial-buccal
    low-flow cardiopulmonary bypass
    low frequency band
LFBW
    lateral frontal bone window
LFC
    lateral femoral cutaneous
    left frontal craniotomy
    living female child
    low fat and cholesterol [diet]
LFCS
    low flap cesarean section
LFCT
    lung-to-finger circulation time
LFD
    lactose-free diet
    large for dates [fetus]
    late fetal death
    lateral facial dysplasia
    least fatal dose
    low-fat diet
    low-fiber diet
    low forceps delivery (See also LF)
    lunate fossa depression
LFECT
    loose fibroelastic connective tissue

LFER
  linear free-energy relationship
LFF
  low-filter frequency
LFGNR
  lactose fermenting gram-negative rod
LFH
  left femoral hernia
LFHL
  low-frequency hearing loss
LFI
  local-field irradiation
LFIT
  low-friction ion treatment
LFL
  left frontolateral [fetal position]
  leukocyte feeder layer
LFl
  latex flocculation [test] (*See also* LFT)
LFLA
  lactoferrin latex bead agglutination
LFM
  laser flare meter
  lateral force microscopy
LFN
  lactoferrin
LFOV
  large field of view
LFP
  left front posterior (frontoposterior) [fetal position] (*See also* FLP)
LFPPV
  low-frequency positive pressure ventilation
LFR
  lymphoid follicular reticulosis
LF-RF
  local-regional failure
LFR-TMS
  low-frequency right-sided repetitive transcranial magnetic stimulation
LFS
  lateral facet syndrome
  leukemia-free survival
  limbic forebrain structure
  liver function series
LFT
  lateral femoral torsion
  latex fixation test
  latex flocculation test (*See also* LFI)
  left front transverse (frontotransverse) [fetal position] (*See also* FLT)
  liver function test
  localized fibrous tumor
  low flap transverse
  low-frequency tetanic [stimulation]

low-frequency transduction
low-frequency transfer
lung function test
LFU
  limes flocculation unit
  lipid fluidity unit
  lost to follow-up (followup) (*See also* LTF)
LFUS
  low frequency ultrasound
LFV
  large field of view
  Lassa fever virus
  low-frequency ventilation
L fx
  linear fracture
LG
  lactoglobulin
  lamellar granule
  large (*See also* lge)
  laryngectomy
  lateral ground
  left gluteal
  left gluteus
  leg
  light guide
  lingual groove
  linguogingival
  lipoglycopeptide
  liver graft
  long
  low glucose
  lymph gland
  lymphocytic gastritis
  lymphography
L-G
  Lich-Gregoire [ureteroneocystostomy]
LGA
  large for gestational age
  left gastric artery
  localized granuloma annulare
  low-grade astrocytoma
LGB
  lateral geniculate body
  lazy gallbladder
LGBP/LC
  laparoscopic gastric bypass with laparoscopic cholecystectomy
LGBT
  lesbian, gay, bisexual, transsexual (*See also* GLBT)
LGC
  left giant cell
LGD
  Leaderless Group Discussion [situational test]
  low-grade dysplasia

L

LGd
  [dorsal] lateral geniculate [nucleus]
LGDA
  lichenoid and granulomatous dermatitis
    of AIDS
LGE
  Langat encephalitis (*See also* LGT)
  linear gingival erythema
lge
  large (*See also* LG)
LGESS
  low-grade endometrial stromal sarcoma
LGF
  lateral giant fiber
L-GG
  Lactobacillus rhamnosus strain GG
LGG
  low-grade glioma
LGH
  lactogenic hormone (*See also* LTH)
  little growth hormone
LGI
  large glucagon immunoreactivity
  lower gastrointestinal
LGIB
  lower gastrointestinal bleeding
LGIOS
  low-grade intraosseous-type
    osteosarcoma
LGL
  large granular leukocyte (lymphocyte)
  lobular glomerulonephritis
  low grade lymphoma
LGM
  left gluteus medius
LGMD
  limb-girdle muscular dystrophy
LGN
  lateral geniculate nucleus
  lobular glomerulonephritis
lg-NHL
  low-grade non-Hodgkin lymphoma
LGP
  labioglossopharyngeal
LGS
  large green soft [stool]
  limb-girdle syndrome
  low Gomco suction
LGSIL
  low-grade squamous intraepithelial
    lesion
LGT
  Langat encephalitis (*See also* LGE)
  late generalized tuberculosis
Lgt, lgt
  ligament (ligamentum) [singular]
    (*See also* L, lig)
LGTI
  lower genital tract infection

LGTV
  Langat virus
LGU
  leg glucose uptake
LGV
  large granular vesicle
  lymphogranuloma venereum
LGV-CFT
  lymphogranuloma venereum complement
    fixation test
LGVHD
  lethal graft-versus-host disease
LGV-TRIC
  lymphogranuloma venereum-trachoma
    inclusion conjunctivitis
LgX
  lymphogranulomatosis X
LH
  late healed
  lateral hypothalamic [syndrome]
  lateral hypothalamus
  learning handicap
  left hand(ed) (*See also* L+H)
  left heart
  left hemisphere
  left hyperphoria
  liver homogenate
  loop of Henle
  lower half
  lues hereditaria (hereditary syphilis)
  lung homogenate
  luteinizing hormone
  luteotropic hormone (*See also* LTH)
  lymphoid hyperplasia
  lymphocytic histiocytic
L/H
  lymphocytic/histiocytic [cell]
L:H
  lung to heart ratio
LHA
  lateral hypothalamic area
  left hepatic artery
LHB
  long head of biceps
LHb
  lateral habenular
LH-beta (β)
  luteinizing hormone beta (β)
LHBT
  lactose hydrogen breath test [lactose
    intolerance]
  lactulose hydrogen breath test [gastric
    emptying time]
  long head of biceps tendon
LHBV
  left heart blood volume
LHC
  left heart catheterization
  left hypochondrium

LHCG
    luteinizing hormone-chorionic
      gonadotropin [hormone]

LHD
    lateral head displacement
    left-hand dominant
    left hemisphere [brain] damage
    left hepatic duct

LHE
    light and heat energy
      [phototherapy]

LHF
    left heart failure
    ligament of head of femur

LHFA
    lung Hageman factor activator

LH-FSH
    luteinizing hormone-follicle-stimulating
      hormone

LH-FSH-RF
    luteinizing hormone-follicle-stimulating
      hormone-releasing factor

LHG
    left-hand grip
    localized hemolysis in gel

LHH
    left homonymous hemianopia

LH-hCG
    luteinizing hormone-human chorionic
      gonadotropin

LHI
    lipid hydrocarbon inclusion

LHL
    left hemisphere lesion
    left hepatic lobe

LHM
    lymphohistiocytoid mesothelioma

LHMP
    Life Health Monitoring Program

LHMT
    low-range heparin management test

LHN
    lateral hypothalamic nucleus

LHON
    Leber hereditary optic neuropathy

LHP
    lateral hypopharyngeal pouch
    left hemiparesis
    left hemiplegia

LHPC
    lipomatous hemangiopericytoma

LHPZ
    lower [esophageal] high-pressure zone

LHQ
    Life History Questionnaire

LHR
    legal health record
    leukocyte histamine release [test]
    liquid holding recovery
    [right] lung to head [circumference]
      ratio

LHRF, LH-RF
    luteinizing hormone releasing factor
      (*See also* LRF)

LHRH, LH-RH
    luteinizing hormone-releasing hormone
      (*See also* LRH)

LHRH-A
    luteinizing hormone-releasing hormone
      analogue

LHRT
    leukocyte histamine release test

LHS
    left-hand side
    left heart strain
    left heel strike
    long-handled sponge
    lymphatic and hematopoietic system

LHSH
    long-handled shoe horn

LHT
    left hypertropia

LHV
    left hepatic vein

LI
    labeling index
    lactose intolerance
    lacunar infarction
    lamellar ichthyosis
    language impairment
    large intestine
    large intestine channel [acupuncture]
      (*See also* li)
    laser iridotomy
    laterality index
    learning impaired
    left iliac
    left injured
    left involved
    life island
    linguoincisal
    lithogenic index
    liver involvement
    loop ileostomy
    low impulsiveness
    lumbar index

L&I
    liver and iron

Li
    labrale inferius [craniometric]
    lithium

li
    large intestine channel [acupuncture]
      (*See also* LI)

L

LIA
   laser interference acuity
   left iliac artery
   leukemia-associated inhibitory activity
   local infiltrative anesthesia
   lock-in amplifier
   lymphocyte-induced angiogenesis
   lysine-iron agar
LIAC
   light-induced absorbance change
LIAD
   low-impact aerobic dance
LIAF
   laser-induced arterial fluorescence
   lymphocyte-induced angiogenesis factor
LIAFI
   late infantile amaurotic familial idiocy
LIB
   left in bottle
LIBC
   latent iron-binding capacity
LIBS
   ligand-induced binding site
LIC
   left iliac crest
   left internal carotid
   left interventricular coronary [artery]
   leisure-interest class
   limiting isorrheic concentration
   local intravascular coagulation
LICA
   laser image custom arthroplasty
   left internal carotid artery
LICC
   lectin-induced cellular cytotoxicity
LICD
   lower intestinal Crohn disease
LICM
   left intercostal margin
LICS
   left intercostal space (See also LIS)
LICU
   laparoscopic intracorporeal ultrasound
   (ultrasonography)
LID
   late immunoglobulin deficiency
   levodopa-induced dyskinesia
   low-iron diamine
   lymphocytic infiltrative disease
LIDC
   low-intensity direct current
LIE
   labioincisal edge
   linguoincisal edge
LIF
   laser-induced fluorescence
   left iliac fossa
   left index finger
   leukemia-inhibiting [inhibitory] factor

leukocyte infiltration factor
   leukocyte inhibitory factor
   leukocytosis-inducing factor
   liver [migration] inhibitory factor
   local intraarterial fibrinolysis
LIFE
   laser-induced fluorescence emission
   laser-induced fluorescence endoscopy
   lifestyle intervention, food exercise
   program
   lung imaging fluorescence endoscope
   (endoscopy)
LIFEC
   lumbar intersomatic fusion expandable
   cage
L-IFN
   lymphoblastoid interferon
LIFS
   laser-induced fluorescence spectroscopy
LIFT
   laser-assisted internal fabrication
   technique
   lymphocyte immunofluorescence test
LIG
   lymphocyte immune globulin
lig
   ligament (ligamentum) [singular]
   (See also L, Lgt, lgt)
   ligate
   ligation
   ligature
ligg
   ligaments (ligamenta) [plural]
LIGHT
   homologous to lymphotoxin, exhibits
   inducible expression, competes with
   herpes simplex virus glycoprotein D
   for HVEM on T cells
LIGHTS
   phototherapy lights
LIH
   laparoscopic inguinal herniorrhaphy
   Lars Ingvar Hansson [hookpin]
   left inguinal hernia
LIHA
   low impulsiveness, high anxiety
LIhFE
   living with heart failure
   [questionnaire]
LIHPS
   local infusion of heparin prior to
   stenting
LII
   Leisure Interest Inventory
LIJ
   left internal jugular
LIKE
   Learning Inventory of Kindergarten
   Experiences

LILA
low impulsiveness, low anxiety
LILI
low-intensity laser irradiation
LILT
low-intensity laser therapy
LIM
boundary [L. *limes*] (*See also* L)
limit(ation)
limited toxicology screening
LIMA
left internal mammary artery [graft]
LIM [domain]
Lin11, Isl1, Mec3 genes
LIMM
lethal infantile mitochondrial myopathy
LIMS
laboratory information management
system
LIN
laryngeal intraepithelial neoplasia
lin
linear
liniment (*See also* Linim)
LINAC
linear accelerator
LINAC-RS
linear accelerator-based radiosurgery
LINCL
late infantile neural ceroid
lipofuscinosis
LINDI
lithium-induced nephrogenic diabetes
insipidus
LINE
long interspersed element [nucleotide]
ling
lingual (*See also* L)
lingular
Linim
liniment (*See also* lin)
LIO
laser-indirect ophthalmoscope
left inferior oblique [extraocular
muscle]
LIOU, LIOUS
laparoscopic intraoperative ultrasound
(ultrasonography)
LIP
lipoate (lipoic acid)
lipoid interstitial pneumonitis
lithium-induced polydipsia
liver-enriched inhibiting protein
lymphocytic interstitial pneumonia
(pneumonitis)
lymphoid interstitial pneumonia
(pneumonitis)

LIPA
line probe assay
lysosomal acid lipase A
LIPB
lysosomal acid lipase B
LIPHE
Life Interpersonal History Enquiry
lipoMM
lipomyelomeningocele
LIP P
lipid profile
LIP/PLH
lymphoid interstitial
pneumonia/pulmonary lymphoid
hyperplasia
LIPS
Leiter International Performance Scale
LIPT
Leiter International Performance Test
LIPV
left inferior pulmonary vein
Lipovnik virus
LIQ
lower inner quadrant
low inner quadrant
liq.
liquid [L. *liquidus*]
liquor (*See also* L, liqr)
liq dr
liquid dram
liq oz
liquid ounce
liq pt
liquid pint
liq qt
liquid quart
liqr
liquor [L. *liquor*] (*See also* L, liq.)
LIR
left iliac region
left inferior rectus [muscle]
LIRBM
liver, iron, red bone marrow
LIS
laboratory information system
late-onset idiopathic scoliosis
lateral intercellular space
left intercostal space (*See also* LICS)
lobular in situ [carcinoma]
locked-in syndrome
low-intensity stimulator
low intermittent suction
low ionic strength
lung injury score
LISL
laser-induced intracorporeal shock wave
lithotripsy

L

LISS
less invasive stabilization system
low ionic strength solution [medium]

LIT
literature
liver injury test

LITA
left internal thoracic artery

LITE
low-intensity treadmill exercise [protocol]

LITH
lithotomy

litho
lithotripsy

LITT
laser-induced interstitial thermotherapy

LITx
liver and intestinal transplant(ation)

LIV
law of initial value
left innominate vein
live
liver (*See also* L)
liver channel [acupuncture]
living (*See also* L)
louping ill virus

LIVB
live birth (*See also* LB)

LIV-BP
leucine, isoleucine, valine-binding protein

LIVC
left inferior vena cava

LIVEN
linear inflammatory verrucous epidermal nevus

LIVIM
lethal intestinal virus of infant mice

L-IVP
limited intravenous pyelograph(y) (pyelogram)

LIVPRO
liver profile

LIWS
low intermittent wall suction

LJ
left jugular
lockable joints
Löwenstein-Jensen [medium] (*See also* LJM)

LJAV
Landjia virus

LJL
lateral joint line

LJM
limited joint mobility
Löwenstein-Jensen medium (*See also* LJ)

LJP
localized juvenile periodontitis

LJV
La Joya virus

LK
lamellar keratoplasty (*See also* LKP)
left kidney (*See also* LKID)
lichenoid keratosis

LK⁺
low potassium ion

LKA
Lazare-Klerman-Armour [Personality Inventory]

LKESTR
leukocyte esterase (*See also* LE)

LKID
left kidney (*See also* LK)

LKKS
liver, kidneys, spleen (*See also* LKS)

LKM
liver-kidney microsome [antibody]

LKM-1
liver-kidney microsomal type 1 [antibody]

LKP
lamellar keratoplasty (*See also* LK)

LKPD
Lillehei-Kaster pivoting disc

LKS
liver, kidneys, spleen (*See also* LKKS)

LKSB
liver, kidneys, spleen, bladder

LKSNP, LKS non. pal.
liver, kidneys, spleen not palpable

LKT
liver and kidney transplant(ation)

LKV
laked kanamycin vancomycin [agar]
Lengyeh-Kerman-Vargar [rating]

LL
large local
large lymphocyte
laser lithotripsy
late latent
lateral lemniscus
left lateral (*See also* LLAT, L lat, lt lat)
left leg
left lower
left lung
lepromatous leprosy
lesion length
lid lag
lines [plural]
lingual lipase
lipoprotein lipase (*See also* LPL)
long leg
loudness level
lower (eye)lid

lower limb
lower lip
lower lobe
lumbar laminectomy (*See also* L lam)
lumbar length
lung length
lymphocytic lymphoma
lymphoid leukemia
lysolecithin (*See also* LLT)

LL2
limb lead two

L&L
lids and lashes

LLA
lids, lashes, adnexa
limulus lysate assay
lipid-lowering agent
lobar lung atrophy
lupuslike anticoagulant

L lam
lumbar laminectomy (*See also* LL)

LLAT
left lateral (*See also* LL, L lat, lt lat)
lysolecithin acyltransferase

L lat
left lateral (*See also* LL, LLAT, lt lat)

LLB
last living breath
left lateral bending
left lateral border
left lower border
long leg brace
lower lobe bronchus

LLBCD
left lower border of cardiac dullness

LLBP
long leg brace with pelvic [band]

LLC
labrum-ligament complex
laparoscopic laser cholecystectomy
laser laparoscopic cholecystectomy
Lewis lung carcinoma
liquid-liquid chromatography
long leg cast
lower level of care
lymphocytic leukemia, chronic

LLCC
long leg cylinder cast

LLD
Lactobacillus lactis Dorner (*See also* LLDF)
late life depression
lead locking device
left lateral decubitus [position]
leg length differential
leg length discrepancy
limb-length discrepancy
lipid-lowering drug

liquid-liquid distribution
long-lasting depolarization

LLDA
labial-lingual double articulation

LLDF
Lactobacillus lactis Dorner factor [vitamin B_{12}] (*See also* LLD)

LLDH
liver lactate dehydrogenase

LLDN
laparoscopic live donor nephrectomy

LLDP
left lateral decubitus position

LLE
left lower extremity (*See also* LLX)
Little League elbow

LLETZ
large loop excision of transformation zone

LLETZ/LEEP
large loop excision of transformation zone [and] loop electrosurgical excision procedure

LLF
Laki-Lorand factor [factor XIII]
late-life forgetfulness
left lateral femoral [site of injection]
left lateral flexion

LLFG
long leg fiberglass [cast]

LLG
left lateral gaze

LL-GXT
low-level graded exercise test

LLI
leg length inequality

LLL
left liver lobe
left long leg [brace]
left lower (eye)lid
left lower leg
left lower limb
left lower lobe [lung]
left lower lung
localized *Leishmania* lymphadenitis
lower fossa active, lateral knee pain, long leg on side ipsilateral to weak fossa [orthopedic evaluation]

LLLE
lower lid, left eye (*See also* LLOS)

LLLL
lids, lashes, lacrimals, lymphatics

LLLM
low liquid level monitor

LLLNR
left lower lobe, no rales

LLLT
low-level laser therapy

L

LLM
localized leukocyte mobilization
LLN
lower limit of normal
LLNA
local lymph-node assay
LLO
Legionella-like organism
lower limb orthosis
⚠ **LLOD**
lower lid, oculus dexter [right eye]
(*See also* LLRE) ⚠
lower limit of detection
⚠ **LLOS**
lower lid, oculus sinister [left eye]
(*See also* LLLE) ⚠
LLP
late luteal phase
long-lasting potentiation
long leg plaster (cast)
lower limb prosthesis
LLPDD
late luteal phase dysphoric disorder
LLPMS
long leg posterior molded splint
LLPS
low-load prolonged stress
low-load prolonged stretch
LLPV
left lower pulmonary vein
LLQ
Leatherman Leadership Questionnaire
left lower quadrant
LLR
large local reaction
left lateral rectus [eye muscle]
left lumbar region
LLRE
lower lid, right eye (*See also* LLOD)
LLS
lateral loop suspensor
lazy leukocyte syndrome
leaky lung syndrome
long leg splint
LLSB
left lower scapular border
left lower sternal border
LLSD
laser light scattering detector
LLSV
Llano Seco virus
LLT
left lateral thigh
lowest level term
lysolecithin (*See also* LL)
LLV
lymphatic leukemia virus
[Friend-associated] (*See also* LLV-F)
lymphoid leukosis virus [fowl]

LLV-F
lymphatic leukemia virus,
Friend-associated (*See also* LLV)
LLVP
left lateral ventricular preexcitation
LLW
low-level waste
LLWBC
long leg weightbearing cast
LLWC
long leg walking cast
LLX
left lower extremity (*See also* LLE)
LM
labiomental
lactic [acid] in mineral [medium]
lactose malabsorption
landmark
laryngeal mask
laryngeal melanosis
laryngeal muscle
lateral malleolus
left main
left marginal [coronary artery]
left median
legal medicine
lemniscus medialis
lentigo melanoma
leptomeningeal
leptomeningeal metastasis
light microscopy (microscope)
light minimum
lingual margin
linguomesial
lipid mobilization
liquid membrane
Listeria monocytogenes
living male
longitudinal muscle
lower motor [neuron] (*See also* LMN)
lung metastasis
lymphatic malformation
L/M
left message
liter per minute (*See also* L/min, Lpm)
lm
lumen [SI unit of luminous flux]
LMA
lactose malabsorption
laryngeal mask airway
left main [coronary] artery
left mentum anterior (mentoanterior)
[fetal position] (*See also* MLA)
limbic midbrain area
liver [cell] membrane autoantibody
liver membrane antibody
LMB
left mainstem bronchus
leiomyoblastoma (*See also* LB)

LMBD
   lingular mandibular bony defect
LMC
   large motile cell
   lateral motor column
   left main coronary [artery]
   left middle cerebral [artery]
   living male child
   lymphocyte-mediated cytolysis
   lymphocyte-mediated cytotoxic(ity)
   lymphocyte microcytotoxic(ity)
   lymphomyeloid complex
LMCA
   left main coronary artery
   left middle cerebral artery
LMCAD
   left main coronary artery disease
LMCAO
   left marginal coronary artery
      occlusion
LMCAT
   left middle cerebral artery thrombosis
LMCL
   left midclavicular line
   lower midclavicular line
LMCT
   ligand-to-metal charge transfer
LMD
   left main disease (cardiology)
   leptomeningeal disease
   lipid-moiety modified derivative
   local medical doctor
   low molecular [weight] dextran
      (*See also* LMDX, LMWD)
LMDF
   lupus miliaris disseminatus faciei
LMDS
   locally multiply damaged sites
LMDX
   low molecular [weight] dextran
      (*See also* LMD, LMWD)
LME
   left mediolateral episiotomy (*See also*
      LMLE)
   leukocyte migration enhancement
LMEE
   left middle ear exploration
LMF
   left middle finger
   lymphocyte mitogenic factor
lm/ft²
   lumen per square foot
LMG
   lethal midline granuloma
   low mobility group
LMH
   lipid-mobilizing hormone

lm h
   lumen hour [unit of quantity of
      light]
LMI
   large multivalent immunogen
   lateral medullary infarct(ion)
   lateral myocardial infarct(ion)
   leukocyte migration inhibition [assay]
LMIF
   leukocyte migration inhibition factor
L/min
   liter per minute (*See also* L/M, Lpm)
L/min/m²
   liter per minute per square meter
LMIR
   leukocyte migration inhibition
      reaction
LMIS
   [AOFAS] Lesser Metatarsophalangeal-
      Interphalangeal Scale
LMIT
   leukocyte migration inhibition test
LMJA
   longitudinal midtarsal joint axis
LML
   large and medium lymphocytes
   left mediolateral
   left middle lobe
   lower midline
LMLE
   left mediolateral episiotomy (*See also*
      LME)
LML scar w/h
   lower midline scar with hernia
LMM
   Lactobacillus maintenance medium
   laser microbeam microdissection
   lentigo maligna melanoma
   light molecular [weight] meromyosin
lm/m²
   lumen per square meter
LMMH
   low molecular mass heparin
LMN
   letter of medical necessity
   lower motor neuron (*See also* LM)
LMND
   lower motor neuron deficiency
LMNL
   lower motor neuron lesion
LMO
   localized molecular orbital
LMP
   last menstrual period
   latent membrane protein
   left mentum posterior (mentoposterior)
      [fetal position] (*See also* MLP)

L

LMP *(continued)*
    low malignant potential
    lumbar puncture (*See also* LP)
LMP 1
    latent membrane protein 1
LMPS
    lethal multiple pterygium syndrome
LMR
    left medial rectus [eye muscle]
    linguomandibular reflex
    localized magnetic resonance
    log magnitude ratio
    lymphocytic meningopolyradiculitis
LMRM
    left modified radical mastectomy
LMRP
    local medical review policy
LMS
    laser marker system
    lateral medullary syndrome
    left mainstem [bronchus]
    left main stem [coronary artery]
    leiomyosarcoma (*See also* LS)
lm s
    lumen second [unit of quantity of light]
LMS-CAD
    left main stem coronary artery disease
LMSV
    left maximal spatial voltage
LMT
    left main trunk
    left mentum transverse (mentotransverse)
    [fetal position]
    leukocyte migration technique
    light moving touch
    luteomammotrophic [hormone]
LMTA
    Language Modalities Test for
    Aphasia
LMV
    larva migrans visceralis
LMVD
    lymphatic microvessel density
LMW
    low molecular weight
lm/W
    lumen per watt
LMWD
    low molecular weight dextran (*See also*
    LMD, LMDX)
LMWH
    low molecular weight heparin
LMWP
    low molecular weight protein
LN
    labionasal
    laminin
    latent nystagmus
    later [onset] nephrotic [syndrome]

    left nostril (naris)
    lipoid nephrosis
    Lisch nodule
    lobular neoplasia
    lupus nephritis
    lymph node
L/N
    letter/numerical [system]
LN₂
    liquid nitrogen
ln
    logarithm, natural
LNA
    alpha linolenic acid (*See also* ALA)
    latent nuclear antigen
    linolenic acid
LNa
    low sodium (*See also* LoNa, LS)
LNAA
    large neutral amino acid
LNAB
    large-needle aspiration biopsy (*See also*
    LNB)
LNaCl
    low sodium chloride [salt]
L-NAME
    $N\Omega$-nitro-L-arginine methyl ester
    NG-nitro-L-arginine methyl ester
LNB
    large-needle [aspiration] biopsy (*See also*
    LNAB)
    Lyme neuroborreliosis
    lymph node biopsy
LNC
    large noncleaved
    lymph node cell
LND
    light-near dissociation
    lymph node dissection
LNE
    lymph node enlargement
    lymph node excision
LNF
    laparoscopic Nissen foundolication
    (*See also* lap Nissen)
LNG
    liquified natural gas
LNGFR
    low-affinity nerve growth factor
    receptor
LNH
    large number hypothesis
LNI
    logarithm neutralization index
LNKS
    low natural killer [cell] syndrome
LNL
    lower normal limit
    lymph node lymphocyte

LNLS
linear-nonlinear least squares [statistics]
LNM
lymph node metastasis (*See also* LN-met)
LNMC
lymph node mononuclear cells
LN-met
lymph node metastasis (*See also* LNM)
L-NMMA
NG-monomethyl-L-arginine
LNMP
last normal menstrual period
LNNB
Luria-Nebraska Neuropsychological Battery
LNP
large neuronal polypeptide
LNPF
lymph node permeability factor
LNR
lymph node region
LNRS
lymph node revealing solution
LNS
lateral nuclear stratum
localized nodular synovitis
lymph node sampling
lymph node seeking [spleen cells]
LNT
late neurological toxicity
LNV
last normal vertebra
LO
lateral oblique [x-ray view]
leave open
lesser omentum
leucine oxidation
linguo-occlusal
low (lower) (lowest) (*See also* L)
lumbar orthosis
5-LO
5-lipoxygenase
LOA
late-onset agammaglobulinemia
leave of absence
Leber optic atrophy
left occiput anterior (occipitoanterior) [fetal position] (*See also* OLA)
looseness (loosening) of associations
loss of attachment
lysis of adhesions
LOAD
late-onset Alzheimer disease
LOAEL
lowest observed adverse effect level
LOB
loss of balance

LOBC
large operable breast cancer
LOC
laxative of choice (*See also* LXC)
level of care
level of comfort
level of concern
level of consciousness (*See also* LC)
liquid organic compound
local(ized) (*See also* loc)
locus of control
loss of consciousness
loss of coordination
loc
local(ized) (*See also* LOC)
location
LOCA
low-osmolar contrast agent
LoCa, lo calc
low calcium [diet] (*See also* LCD)
lo cal
low-calorie [diet] (*See also* LC)
LOC-C
Locus of Control Chance
loc. cit.
in the place cited [L. *loco cilato*]
LOCD
local cementoosseous dysplasia
LOC-E
Locus of Control External
LOCF
last observation carried forward
LoCHO
low carbohydrate
LoChol, lo chol
low cholesterol
LOC-I
Locus of Control Internal
LOCM
low-osmolar contrast medium
LOC-PO
Locus of Control Powerful Others
LOCS
laryngoonychocutaneous syndrome
Lens Opacities Classification System
LOD
limit of detection
line of duty
logarithm of odds [method of genetics linkage analysis] (*See also* lod)
lod
logarithm of odds (*See also* LOD)
LOE
left otitis externa
LOF
leaking of fluid
leave on floor
low outlet forceps

L

LOFD
low outlet forceps delivery
LOFFLEX
low-fiber, fat-limited exclusion [diet]
log.
logarithm
LOGIC
laryngeal and ocular granulation tissue in children from Indian subcontinent
LOGL
lowest-observed-effect level
logMAR
logarithmic Minimum Angle of Resolution [visual acuity chart]
logP
partition [distribution] coefficient [differential solubility of compound in 2 solvents]
LOH
length of hospitalization
loop of Henle
loss of heterogeneity
loss of heterozygosity
LOHF
late onset hepatic failure
LOI
level of incompetence
level of injury
Leyton Obsessive Inventory
limit of impurities
loss of imprinting
LOIH
left oblique inguinal hernia
LOINC
Logical Observation Identifier Names and Codes
LoK
low kalium (potassium)
LOKV
Lokern virus
LOL
left occiput lateral (occipitolateral) [fetal position]
Lol p
Lolium perenne [perennial rye grass]
LOM
left otitis media
ligament of Marshall
limitation of motion (movement)
loss of motion (movement)
low-osmolar [contrast] medium
LOMPT
Lincoln-Oseretsky Motor Performance Test
LOMS
left otitis media, suppurative
LOMSA
left otitis media, suppurative, acute

LOMSC, LOMSCH
left otitis media, suppurative, chronic
LoNa
low sodium (*See also* LNa, LS)
long.
longitudinal
long-ETL FSE
long echo train length fast spin-echo [imaging]
LOO
length of operation
LOP
laparoscopic orchiopexy
leave on pass
left occiput posterior (occipitoposterior) [fetal position] (*See also* OLP)
level of pain
LoPro
low protein (*See also* LP)
LOPS
length of patient stay
loss of protective sensation
LOQ
Leadership Opinion Questionnaire
left outer quadrant
limit(s) of quantitation
lower outer quadrant
LOR
lack of response
line of response
loss of resistance
loss of righting [reflex]
lord.
lordosis
lordotic
LORETA
low-resolution electromagnetic tomography
LORS-1
Level of Rehabilitation Scale 1
LOS
length of stay (*See also* LS)
limits of stability
lipooligosaccharide
loss of sight
low [cardiac] output syndrome (*See also* LCOS)
lower oesophageal sphincter [British] (*See also* LES)
LOT
lateral olfactory tract
left occiput transverse (occipitotransverse) [fetal position]
lengthened off-time [audiometry]
lot.
lotion
LOTCA
Löwenstein Occupational Therapy Cognitive Assessment

LOTCA-G
Löwenstein Occupational Therapy Cognitive Assessment Geriatric

LOU
lower obstructive uropathy

LOV
large opaque vesicle
loss of vision

LOVA
loss of visual acuity

LOVE
laser office ventilation of ears

LOVE IT
laser office ventilation of ears with insertion of tubes

LOWBI
low-birth-weight infant (*See also* LBWI)

low-Mr PTP
low relative molecular mass protein-tyrosine phosphatase

LOX, lox.
liquid oxygen

LOZ
lozenge

LP
labile peptide
labile protein
laboratory procedure
lactic peroxidase
lamina propria
laryngopharyngeal
latency period
latent period
lateralis posterior [muscle]
lateral plantar
lateral pylorus
latex particle
leading pole
Legionella pneumophila
leukocyte poor
leukocytic pyrogen
levator palati [muscle]
levator palpebrae [muscle]
lichen planus
ligamentum patellae
lightly padded
light perception (*See also* LPerc)
linear prediction
linear programming
lingua plicata
linguopulpal
lipid panel
lipoprotein
liver-pancreas
liver plasma [concentration]
lost privileges
low potency

low power
low pressure
low protein (*See also* LoPro)
lumbar puncture (*See also* LMP)
lumboperitoneal
lung parenchyma
lung perfusion
lymphocyte predominant
lymphoid plasma
lymphoid predominance
lymphomatoid papulosis
lymphomatous polyposis
[nucleus] lateralis posterior

L:P
lactate to pyruvate ratio (*See also* LPR)
liver to plasma concentration ratio
lymphocyte to polymorph ratio
lymph to plasma ratio

LPA
larval photoreceptor axon
latex particle agglutination
left pulmonary artery
lipoprotein A
low physical activity
lymphocyte (lymphocytic) proliferation assay
lysophosphatidic acid

LPA%
left pulmonary artery oxygen saturation

LPAR
late-phase allergic reaction

LPB
lipoprotein B
low-profile bioprosthesis (*See also* LPBP)

LPBP
low-profile bioprosthesis (*See also* LPB)

LPC
laser photocoagulation
late positive component
leukocyte-poor cells
limiting precursor cell
localized prostate carcinoma
lysophosphatidyl choline

LPCB
lactophenol cotton blue [stain, test]

LPCh
lateral posterior choroidal

LPC-L
lymphoplasmacytoid lymphoma (*See also* LPL)

LPCM
low-placed conus medullaris

LPcP
light perception with projection

LPCR
late-phase cutaneous reaction

LPCT
late proximal cortical tubule
LPCV
laser photocoagulation of communicating vessel
LPD
leiomyomatosis peritonealis disseminata
lipoprotein deficiency
lower partial dentures
low potassium dextran
low-protein diet
luteal phase defect (deficiency)
lymphoproliferative disease
LPDA
left posterior descending artery
LPDF
lipoprotein-deficient fraction
LPE
lipoprotein electrophoresis (*See also* LEP)
lower partially edentulous
LPEP
left preejection period
LPerc
light perception (*See also* LP)
LPF
leg protection factor
leukocytosis-promoting factor
leukopenia factor
lipopolysaccharide factor
liver plasma flow
localized plaque formation
low-power field (*See also* lpf)
lymphocytosis-promoting factor
lpf
low-power field (*See also* LPF)
LPFB
left posterior fascicular block
LPFN
low pass filtered noise
LPFS
low pass filtered signal
LPG
lipophosphoglycan
liquified petroleum gas
LPH
lactase-phlorizin hydrolase
left posterior hemiblock (*See also* LPHB)
lipotropic pituitary hormone (lipotropin) (*See also* LPT)
lumbar puncture headache
LPHAS
limb and pelvis hypoplasia/aplasia syndrome
LPHB
left posterior hemiblock (*See also* LPH)

LPHC
low probability, high consequence event
LPHD
lymphocyte-predominant Hodgkin disease
LPHR
laparoscopic paraesophageal hernia repair
LPHS
loin pain hematuria syndrome
LPI
laser peripheral iridectomy
laser projection imaging
Leadership Practices Inventory
left posterior inferior (posteroinferior)
leukotriene pathway inhibitor
long process of incus
lysinuric protein intolerance
LPICA
left posterior internal carotid artery
LPIFB
left posterior inferior (posteroinferior) fascicular block
LPIH
left posterior inferior (posteroinferior) hemiblock
LPI/LRI
lymphocyte proliferation [and] lymphocyte regression index
LPK
liver pyruvate kinase
LPL
lamina propria lymphocyte
laparoscopic pelvic lymphadenectomy
left posterolateral
lichen planus-like lesion
lipoprotein lipase (*See also* LL)
local probability of lesion
long plantar ligament
lymphoplasmacytoid lymphoma (*See also* LPC-L)
LPLA
lipoprotein lipase activity
LPLC
low-pressure liquid chromatography
LPLND
laparoscopic pelvic lymph node dissection
LPM
latent primary malignancy
lateral pterygoid muscle
left posterior measurement
liver plasma membrane
localized pretibial myxedema
lymphoproliferative malignancy
Lpm
liter per minute (*See also* L/M, L/min)

LPME
    liquid-phase microextraction [test method]
Lpm/m²
    liter per minute per meter squared
LPN
    laparoscopic partial nephrectomy
LPO
    lateral preoptic [area]
    left posterior oblique
    left posterior occipital
    light perception only
    lobus parolfactorius
LPOA
    lateral preoptic area
L POST
    left posterior
LPP
    lateral pterygoid plate
    leak point pressure
    lichen planopilaris
LP&P
    light perception and projection
LPPC
    leukocyte-poor packed cells
LPPH
    late postpartum hemorrhage
LPPS
    low-pressure plasma-sprayed
LPR
    lactate to pyruvate ratio (*See also* L:P)
    laryngopharyngeal reflux
    late-phase reaction (response)
    late pulmonary response
    leprosy [Hansen disease] vaccine
LPRBC
    leukocyte-poor red blood cells
LProj
    light projection
LPS
    large particle sorting [module]
    last Pap smear
    late progressing stroke
    lateral pharyngeal space
    levator palpebrae superioris [muscle]
    linear profile scan
    lipase
    lipopolysaccharide
    London Psychogeriatric Scale
    lung perfusion scan
Lps
    liter per second
LPSA
    late postoperative suture adjustment
LP SHUNT
    lumboperitoneal shunt

LPSP
    light perception without projection
LPSR
    lipopolysaccharide receptor
LPSS
    laryngopharyngeal sensory stimulation
LPT
    Language Proficiency Test
    lateral position test
    leptospirosis vaccine
    lipotropin (lipotropic pituitary hormone) (*See also* LPH)
    lymphocyte-predominant thymoma
LPV
    left portal view
    left pulmonary vein(s)
    lymphopathia venereum
    lymphotropic papovavirus
LPVP
    left posterior ventricular preexcitation
LPW
    lateral pharyngeal wall
LPX
    lipoprotein X
LQ
    left quadrant
    linear-quadratic [function, dose]
    longevity quotient
    lordosis quotient
    lower quadrant
    lowest quadrant
LQT
    long QT [interval, syndrome] (*See also* LQTS)
LQT1
    long QT1 [interval]
LQT2
    long QT2 [interval]
LQTS
    long QT syndrome (*See also* LQT)
L-R, LR, L→R, L/R
    left to right
LR
    labeled release [experiment]
    laboratory reference
    laboratory report
    labor room
    lactated Ringer [solution] (*See also* lat Rin, LRS)
    large reticulocyte
    laser resection
    latency reaction
    latency relaxation
    lateral rectus [eye muscle]
    lateral retinaculum
    lateral rotation

L

LR *(continued)*
 left-right
 left rotation (*See also* Lrot)
 leishmaniasis recidivans
 ligand receptor
 light reaction
 light reflex
 likelihood ratio
 limit of reaction
 lingual ridge
 lingual root
 livedo reticularis
 local recurrence
 locoregional [disease]
 lymphatic reconstruction
 lymphocyte recruitment
L&R
 left and right
L:R
 left to right ratio
Lr
 lawrencium
 limes reacting [dose of diphtheria toxin]
LRA
 left radial artery
 left renal artery
 low right atrium
LRC
 locomotor-respiratory coupling
 locoregional control
 lower rib cage
LRCH
 lymphocyte-rich classic Hodgkin
lrCLAL
 living-related conjunctival limbal
  allograft
LRCM
 longitudinal random coefficient
  model
LRCP
 low-risk chest pain
LRD
 limb reduction defect
 limb reduction deformity
 living related donor
 living renal donor
LRDT
 living related donor transplant(ation)
LRE
 lamina rara externa
 least restrictive environment
 leukemic reticuloendotheliosis
 localization-related epilepsy
 lymphoreticuloendothelial
LREH
 low renin essential hypertension
LRF
 latex [with] resorcinol [and]
  formaldehyde

 left rectus femoris
 left ring finger
 leukoreduction filter
 liver residue factor
 local-regional (locoregional) failure
 luteinizing hormone-releasing factor
  (*See also* LHRF, LH-RF)
LRFFS
 locoregional failure-free survival
LRFS
 local recurrence-free survival
LRH
 luteinizing hormone-releasing hormone
  (*See also* LHRH, LH-RH)
LRHT
 living related hepatic transplant(ation)
LRI
 lamina rara interna
 limbal relaxing incision
 lower respiratory [tract] infection
  (illness) (*See also* LRTI)
 lymphocyte reactivity index
LRL
 long radiolunate
LRLT
 living related [donor] transplant(ation)
LRM
 left radical mastectomy
 local [and] regional metastases
LRMP
 last regular menstrual period
LRN
 Laboratory Response Network
 laparoscopic radical nephrectomy
 lateral reticular nucleus
LRNA
 low renin, normal aldosterone
LRND
 left radical neck dissection
LRO
 long range objective
LROP
 lower radicular obstetrical
  paralysis
Lrot
 left rotation (*See also* LR)
⚠ **LROU**
 lateral rectus both eyes ⚠
LRP
 laparoscopic radical prostatectomy
 low-density lipoprotein (LDL)
  receptor-related protein
 leukocyte common antigen-related
  phosphatase
 lichen ruber planus
 locking reconstruction plate
 long-range planning
 luciferase reporter mycobacteriophage
 lung resistance protein

Lr-PET
low-resolution positron emission tomography

LRPH
laparoscopic repair of paraesophageal hernia

LRQ
lower right quadrant

LRQG
left rostral quarter ganglion

LRR
labyrinthine righting reflex
leucine rich repeat [super family]
light reflection rheography
lymphatic return rate

LRRFS
locoregional recurrence-free survival

LRRT
locoregional radiotherapy

LRS
lactated Ringer solution (*See also* lat Rin, LR)
lateral recess stenosis
lateral recess syndrome
lumboradicular syndrome
lymphoreticular system

LRSF
lactating rat serum factor
liver regenerating serum factor

LR-SH
left to right shunt

LRSP
long-range systems planning

LRSS
late respiratory systemic syndrome

LRSx
lower respiratory [tract] symptom

LRT
living related transplant(ation)
living renal transplant(ation)
local radiation therapy
lower respiratory tract
low-risk tumor

LRTD
living relative transplant(ation) donor

LRTI
ligament reconstruction with tendon interposition
lower respiratory tract infection (illness) (*See also* LRI)

LRUT
locally made rapid urease test

LRV
Lato River virus
left renal vein
log reduction value

LRv
life review [process]

LS
lateral septal
lateral suspensor [ligament]
least squares [statistics] (*See also* LSQ)
left sacrum
left septum
left side
legally separated
leiomyosarcoma (*See also* LMS)
length of stay (*See also* LOS)
lesser sac
lichen sclerosus
life science
light sensitive (sensitivity)
light sleep
Likert scale [psychology]
limbic system
liminal sensation (sensitivity)
linear scleroderma
line scanning
lipid synthesis
liver scan
liver and spleen (*See also* L&S)
long seal
long stem
lower segment
low salt
low sodium (*See also* LNa, LoNa)
lumbar spine
lumbosacral
lung sounds
lung strip
lymphosarcoma (*See also* LSA)

L5-S1
lumbar fifth vertebra to sacral first vertebra

L:S
lactase to sucrase ratio
lecithin to sphingomyelin ratio
lipid to saccharide ratio
liver to spleen ratio

L&S
ligation and stripping
liver and spleen (*See also* LS)

LSA
Language Sampling Analysis
left sacrum anterior (sacroanterior) [fetal position] (*See also* SLA)
left subclavian artery
leukocyte-specific activity
lichen sclerosus et atrophicus (*See also* LS&A)
lipid-bound sialic acid (*See also* LBSA)
low-sedating antihistamine
lymphosarcoma (*See also* LS)

LS&A
lichen sclerosus et atrophicus (*See also* LSA)

LSAB
labeled streptavidin biotin
LSANA
leukocyte-specific antinuclear
antibody
LSAR
lymphosarcoma [cell]
LSA/RCS
lymphosarcoma [and] reticulum cell
sarcoma
LSAT
low [oxyhemoglobin] saturation
LSB
least significant bit [binary numbers]
left scapular border
left sternal border
local standby
long spike burst
lower sternal border
lumbar spinal block
lumbar sympathetic block
LSBE
long-segment Barrett esophagus
LS-BMD
lateral spine bone mineral density
LS BPS
laparoscopic bilateral partial
salpingectomy
LSC
laparoscopy (*See also* LAP, lap.)
laser scanning cytometry
last sexual contact
late systolic click
least significant change
left-sided colon [cancer]
left subclavian [artery]
lichen simplex chronicus
liquid scintillation counting
liquid-solid chromatography
lower segment cesarean [section]
(*See also* LSCS)
LScA
left scapula anterior (scapuloanterior)
[fetal position] (*See also* ScLA)
left subclavian artery
LSCC
laryngeal squamous cell carcinoma
LSCCB
limited-state small-cell cancer of bladder
LSCL
lymphosarcoma cell leukemia
LSCM
laser-scanning confocal microscopy
LScP
left scapula posterior (scapuloposterior)
[fetal position] (*See also* ScLP)
LSCS
lower segment cesarean section
(*See also* LSC)

LSCTS
long-segment congenital tracheal
stenosis
LSCV
left subclavian vein
LSCVP
left subclavian central venous pressure
LSD
least significant difference [statistics]
least significant digit [computers]
low-salt diet
low-sodium diet
lumbosacral derangement
lysergic acid diethylamide (*See also*
LSD-25)
lysosomal storage disease
LSD-25
lysergic acid diethylamide (*See also*
LSD)
LSE
left sternal edge
lifestyle education
living skin equivalent
local side effect
L/sec
liter per second
LSed
level of sedation
LSEP
left somatosensory evoked potential
LSES
Salamon-Conte Life Satisfaction in the
Elderly Scale
LSESR
lipidosterolic extract of *Serosa repens*
LSF
line spread function [microscopy,
radiography]
low saturated fat
lymphocyte-stimulating factor
LSFA
low-saturated fatty acid [diet]
LSG
labial salivary gland
low specific gravity
lymphoscintigraphy
LSGB
left stellate ganglionic blockade
LSH
laparoscopic supracervical hysterectomy
lutein-stimulating hormone
lymphocyte-stimulating hormone
Lsh
leishmaniasis gene
LSHG
leucine-sensitive hypoglycemia
LSI
large-scale integration
Life Satisfaction Index

light scattering index
Limb Salvage Index
lumbar spine index

LSIA
Life Satisfaction Index A

LSIB
Life Satisfaction Index B

LSIL, L-SIL
low-grade squamous intraepithelial
lesion

LSIZ
Life Satisfaction Index Z

LSK
liver, spleen, kidneys

LSKM
liver-spleen-kidney megaly

LSL
left sacrum lateral (sacrolateral) [fetal
position]
left short leg [brace]
lymphosarcoma [cell] leukemia

LSLF
low sodium, low fat [diet]

LSM
laser scanning microscope
late systolic murmur
least squares mean [statistics]
lifestyle modification
limited sampling model
liver [and] spleen masses
lymphocyte separation medium

LSMFT
liposclerosing myxofibrous tumor

LSMT
life-sustaining medical treatment

LSN
left substantia nigra
left sympathetic nerve

LSNRC
lower sacral nerve root compression

LSO
[cerium-doped] lutetium oxyorthosilicate
lateral superior olive [brain]
left salpingo-oophorectomy
left superior oblique
lumbosacral orthosis

LSP
Learning Style Profile
left sacrum posterior sacroposterior
[fetal position] (*See also* SLP)
liver-specific protein

LSp
life span

LSPA
left stenotic pulmonary artery

L-spine
lumbar spine

LSPV
left superior pulmonary vein

LSQ
least squares [statistics] (*See also* LS)
Life Situation Questionnaire

LSR
lanthanide shift reagent [magnetic
resonance imaging]
laser skin resurfacing
left superior rectus
Life Satisfaction Rating

LSRA
low septal right atrium

LSRT
lens-sparing [external beam] radiation
therapy

LSS
lexical-syntactic syndrome
Life Span Study
Life Study Sample
life support station
light-scattering spectroscopy
limb sparing surgery
liver-spleen scan
lumbar spinal stenosis
lumbosacral spine

LSSA
lipid-soluble secondary antioxidant

LSSCLC
limited-stage small-cell lung cancer

LSSS
Liverpool Seizure Severity Scale

LST
laser tomography scanner
lateral sinus thrombophlebitis
lateral spinothalamic tract
left sacrum transverse (sacrotransverse)
[fetal position] (*See also* SLT)
leptospirosis, spirochetosis,
toxoplasmosis
lysis, storage, transportation

LSTAT
life support for trauma and transport

LSTC
laparoscopic tubal cautery
(coagulation)

LSTL
laparoscopic tubal ligation (*See also*
LTL)

LSTM
lean soft tissue mass

Ls & Ts
lines and tubes

LSU
lactose-saccharose-urea [agar]
life support unit
Louisiana State University

L

LSUMC
Louisiana State University Medical Center

LSV
lateral sacral vein
left subclavian vein
lenticulostriate vasculopathy
lesser saphenous vein
Lone Star virus

LSV2
Vocational Learning Styles

LSVC
left superior vena cava

LSVT
left saphenous vein thrombophlebitis

LSW
left-sided weakness

LSWA
large amplitude, slow wave activity [electroencephalography]

LT
(heat-)labile toxin
lactate threshold
laminar tomography
left (*See also* L, (L), lt)
left thigh
left triceps
length-tension curve
less than
lethal time
lethal toxin
leukotriene
Levin tube
light (*See also* lt)
light touch
long term
low temperature
low tension
low transverse
lues test
lumbar traction
lung transplant(ation) (*See also* LTx)
lunotriquetral
lymphocyte transformation
lymphocyte transitional
lymphocytic thyroiditis
lymphocytotoxin (*See also* LC, LCT)
lymphotoxin

lt
left (*See also* L, (L), LT)
light (*See also* LT)
low tension

LTA
laryngeal tracheal (laryngotracheal) anesthesia
laryngotracheal applicator
laser thermal ablation
lateral thoracic arteries
leukotriene A

lipoate transacetylase
lipoteichoic acid
local tracheal anesthesia
lost-time accident
lymphocyte-transforming activity

LTA$_4$
leukotriene A$_4$

LTAC
long-term acute care

LTAF
local tissue advancement flap

LTalpha (α)
lymphotoxin alpha (α)

LTAR
low-temperature antigen retrieval

LTAS
lead tetraacetate Schiff [procedure, reaction]
left transatrial septal [approach]

LTB
laparoscopic tubal banding
laryngotracheobronchitis
leukotriene B
life-threatening behavior

LTB$_4$
leukotriene B4

LTbeta (β)
lymphotoxin beta (β)

LTBI
latent tuberculosis infection

LTC
large transformed cell
lateral talocalcaneal ligament
left to count
leukotriene C
lidocaine tissue concentration
long-term care
long thick closed
low transverse cesarean
lysed tumor cell

LTC$_4$
leukotriene C4

LTCBDE
laparoscopic transcystic common bile duct exploration

LTC-IC
long-term culture-initiating cell [assay]

LTCCS
low transverse cervical cesarean section

LTCF
long-term care facility

LTCL
laparoscopic transcystic lithotripsy

LTCP
levo-tryptophan-containing product
L-tryptophan-containing product

LTCR
long-term complete remission

LTCS
low transverse cervical [cesarean] section
LTD
largest tumor dimension
Laron-type dwarfism
leg transfer device
leukotriene D
limited
long-term depression
long-term disability
LTD₄
leukotriene D4
LTDA
limited amount [of substance for test]
LTE
laryngotracheoesophageal
less than effective
leukotriene E
LTE₄
leukotriene E4
LT-ECG
long-term electrocardiography
LTED
long-term estrogen deprivation
LTF
lipotropic factor
lost to follow-up (followup) (*See also* LFU)
lymphocyte-transforming factor
LTFU
long-term follow-up (followup)
LTG
long-term goal
low-tension glaucoma
LTGA
left transposition of the great arteries
LTH
lactogenic hormone (*See also* LGH)
left total hip [procedure]
lingual tonsil hyperplasia
local tumor hyperthermia
low-temperature holding [pasteurization]
luteotropic hormone (*See also* LH)
LtH
left-hand(ed) (*See also* LH)
LTHMAR
low-temperature, heat-mediated antigen retrieval
LTI
low temperature isotropic
lupus-type inclusion
LTK
laser thermal keratoplasty
LTL
laparoscopic tubal ligation (*See also* LSTL)
left temporal lobectomy

lt lat
left lateral (*See also* LL, LLAT, L lat)
LTM
long-term memory
long-term monitoring
LTN
lateral telangiectatic nevus
LTNP
long-term nonprogressor
LTO
laparoscopic total occlusion
LTOM
low turnover osteomalacia
LTOT
long-term oxygen therapy
LTP
laryngotracheoplasty
laser trabeculoplasty
lateral thigh perforator [flap]
leukocyte thromboplastin
long-term plan
long-term potentiation
L-Trp
L-tryptophan
LTPA
leisure time physical activity
LTPP
lipothiamide pyrophosphate [obsolete]
LTR
laryngotracheal reconstruction
local twitch response
long terminal repeat [sequence]
lower trunk rotation
lymphocyte transfer reaction
LTRA
leukotriene receptor antagonist
L-transposition
levotransposition
LTS
laparoscopic tubal sterilization
laryngotracheal stenosis
long-term storage
long-term survival
long-term surviving
long tract sign [neurology]
LTT
lactose tolerance test
lateral tibial torsion
leucine tolerance test
limited treadmill test
lymphoblastic transformation test
lymphocyte transformation test
LTUI
low transverse uterine incision
LTV
long-term variability
long-term ventilation

LTV *(continued)*
    Lucké tumor virus
    lung thermal volume
LTV0
    long-term variability absent
LTV+
    long-term variability average to
      moderate
LTVC
    long-term venous catheter
LTW
    Leydig-cell tumor in Wistar [rat]
LTWN
    long-term white noise
LTX
    lophotoxin [marine neurotoxin]
LTx
    lung transplant(ation) *(See also* LT)
LU
    left uninjured
    left uninvolved
    left upper
    left ureteral
    living unit
    loudness unit
    lung *(See also* L)
    lung channel [acupuncture] *(See also* lu)
    lytic unit
L&U
    lower and upper
Lu
    lutetium
¹⁷⁷Lu
    lutetium-177
lu
    lung channel [acupuncture] *(See also*
      LU)
LUA
    left upper arm
    Legionella urinary antigen
LUC
    large unstained cell
LUCL
    lateral ulnar collateral ligament
LUD
    left uterine displacement [device]
LUE
    left upper extremity *(See also* LUX)
LUF
    luteinized unruptured follicle
LUFF
    left upper [arm] free flap
LUFS
    luteinized unruptured follicle
      syndrome
LUIS
    low-dose urea in invert sugar
LUKV
    Lukuni virus

LUL
    left upper (eye)lid
    left upper limb
    left upper lobe [lung]
    left upper lung
lum, lumb
    lumbar [nerve, spine, vertebra]
      (See also L)
LUMD
    lowest usual maintenance dose
LUMO
    lowest unoccupied molecular orbital
LUNA
    laser uterosacral nerve ablation
LUO
    left ureteral orifice
LUOB
    left upper outer buttock
LUOQ
    left upper outer quadrant
LUP
    left ureteropelvic [junction]
    low urethral pressure
LUPP
    laser uvulopalatoplasty
LUPV
    left upper pulmonary vein
LUQ
    left upper quadrant
LURD
    living unrelated donor
LUS
    laparoscopic ultrasound
      (ultrasonography) *(See also* lapUS)
    lower uterine segment
LUSB
    left upper scapular border
    left upper sternal border
LUSLR
    laparoscopic resection of ureterosacral
      ligament
LUST
    lower uterine segment transverse
      [cesarean section]
LUT
    lower urinary tract
LUTD
    lower urinary tract dysfunction
LUTE
    long ultrashort T2-suppressed echo
      time
LUTO
    lower urinary tract obstruction
LUTS
    lower urinary tract symptom
LUTT
    lower urinary tract tumor
LUV
    large unilamellar vesicle

LUX
  left upper extremity (*See also* LUE)
LV
  Lactobacillus viridescens
  lactoovovegetarian
  laryngeal vestibule
  lateral ventricle
  left ventricle (ventricular)
  leukemia virus
  liquid ventilation
  live vaccine
  live virus
  low vertical
  low volume
  lumbar vertebra
  lung volume
lv
  leave
LVA
  left ventricular aneurysm(ectomy)
  left vertebral artery
  low vision aid
LVAD
  left ventricular assist device
LV Angio
  left ventricular angiogram
LVAS
  left ventricular assist system
LVAT
  left ventricular activation time
LVBBB
  left ventricular bundle branch block
LVBP
  left ventricle (ventricular) bypass
    pump
LVC
  laser vision correction
  low-viscosity cement
LVCS
  low vertical cesarean section
LVD
  left ventricular dimension
  left ventricular dysfunction
LVDD
  left ventricular diastolic dimension
LVDP
  left ventricular diastolic pressure
  left ventricle (ventricular) developed
    pressure
LVDs
  left ventricular systolic diameter
LVDT
  linear variable differential transformer
LVDV
  left ventricular diastolic volume
LVE
  left ventricular ejection
  left ventricular enlargement

LVECoG
  low-voltage electrocortical activity
LVED
  left ventricular end diastole
LVEDA
  left ventricular end-diastolic area
LVEDC
  left ventricular end-diastolic
    circumference
LVEDD
  left ventricular end-diastolic diameter
  left ventricular end-diastolic dimension
LVEDI
  left ventricular end-diastolic [volume]
    index
LVEDP
  left ventricular end-diastolic pressure
LVEDV
  left ventricular end-diastolic volume
LVEF
  left ventricular ejection fraction
LVEJT
  left ventricular ejection time
LVEndo
  left ventricular endocardial
LVES
  low-vision enhancement system
LVESA
  left ventricular end-systolic area
LVESD
  left ventricular end-systolic dimension
LVESV
  left ventricular end-systolic volume
LVESVI
  left ventricular end-systolic volume
    index
LVET
  left ventricular ejection time
LVETI
  left ventricular ejection time index
LVF
  left ventricular failure
  left ventricular function
  left visual field
  low-voltage fast
  low-voltage focus [singular] (foci
    [plural])
LVFA
  low-voltage fast activity
LVFP
  left ventricular filling pressure
LVFS
  left ventricular functional shortening
LVFSE
  Low Vision Functional Status
    Evaluation
LVFW
  left ventricular free wall

L

LVFWD
left ventricular free wall rupture
LVG
left ventriculogram
left ventrogluteal
low-voltage galvanism
LVH
large vessel hematocrit
left ventricular hypertrophy
LVHR
laparoscopic ventral hernia repair
LV-HRSEM
low-voltage high-resolution scanning
electron microscopy
LVI
large-vessel infarction
left ventricular insufficiency
left ventricular ischemia
lymph (lymphatic) vessel invasion
LVID
left ventricular internal diameter
left ventricular internal diastolic
left ventricular internal dimension
LVIDD
left ventricular internal diastolic
diameter
left ventricular internal diastolic
dimension
LVIDed
left ventricular internal diameter at end
diastole
LVIDes
left ventricular internal diameter at end
systole
LVIDP
left ventricular initial diastolic pressure
LVIDs
left ventricular internal dimension at
end systole
LVIV
left ventricular infarct volume
left ventricular inflow volume
LVL
large-volume leukapheresis
large-volume lipoplasty
left vastus lateralis [muscle]
LVLG
left ventrolateral gluteal [injection site]
LVM
lateral ventromedial [nucleus]
left ventricular mass
lymphatic-venous (lymphaticovenous)
malformation
LVMF
left ventricular minute flow
LVMI
left ventricular mass index
LVmid
midanterior left ventricle

LVMM
left ventricular muscle mass
LVN
lateral ventricular nerve
lateral vestibular nucleus
limiting viscosity number
LVO
left ventricular outflow [tract] (*See also*
LVOT)
LVOA
left ventricular overactivity
LVOH
left ventricular outflow [tract] height
LVOT
left ventricular outflow tract (*See also*
LVO)
LVOTG
left ventricular outflow tract gradient
LVOTO
left ventricular outflow tract obstruction
LVOV
left ventricular outflow volume
LVP
large-volume paracentesis
large-volume parenteral [infusion]
left ventricular pressure
levator veli palatini [muscle]
LVPC
localized vulvar pemphigoid of
childhood
LVPEP
left ventricular preejection period
LVPFR
left ventricular peak filling rate
LVPmax
maximum left ventricular pressure
LVPmin
minimum left ventricular pressure
LVPSP
left ventricular peak systolic
pressure
LVPVR
left ventricular pressure-volume
relationship
LVPW
left ventricular posterior wall
LVPWT
left ventricular posterior wall
thickness
LVQOL
Low Vision Quality of Life
[questionnaire] (*See also* LVQOLQ)
LVQOLQ
Low Vision Quality of Life
Questionnaire (*See also* LVQOL)
LVR
left ventricular reduction
limb vascular resistance
lung volume reduction

L$_2$VR
second lumbar ventral [nerve] root
L$_1$VR
first lumbar ventral [nerve] root
LVRD
left ventricular replacement device
LVRS
lung volume reduction surgery
LVRT
liver volume replaced by tumor
LVS
laryngeal videostroboscopy
lateral venous sinus
left ventricular strain
live vaccine strain
LVs
left ventricular systolic [pressure]
LVSB
leftward ventricular septal bowing
LVSD
left ventricular systolic dimension
left ventricular systolic dysfunction
LVSEMI
left ventricular subendocardial
myocardial ischemia
LVSF
left ventricular systolic function
LVSI
left ventricular systolic index
lymphovascular involvement
lymphovascular space invasion
LVSO
left ventricular systolic output
LV-SO
left ventricular site of origin
LVSP
left ventricular systolic pressure
LVST
lateral vestibulospinal tract
LVSV
left ventricular stroke volume
LVSVI
left ventricular stroke volume
index
LVSW
left ventricular septal wall
left ventricular stroke work
LVSWI
left ventricular stroke work index
LVT
left ventricular tension
lysine-vasotocin
LVV
left ventricular volume
LeVeen valve
live varicella vaccine
live varicella virus

LVW
lateral vaginal wall
lateral ventricular width
left ventricular wall
left ventricular work
LVW:HW
lateral ventricular width to hemispheric
width ratio
LVWI
left ventricular work index
LVWM
left ventricular wall motion
LVWMA
left ventricular wall motion
abnormality
LVWMI
left ventricular wall motion index
LVWT
left ventricular wall thickness
LW
lacerating wound
lateral wall
Lee-White [blood clotting method]
(*See also* LWCT)
left [ear], warm [stimulus] [Báráng
caloric test]
living will
lung weight
lung width
L-10-W
levulose (10%) in water
L&W
living and well
Lw
lawrencium
LWA
low weight for age
LWAQ
Living with Asthma Questionnaire
LWBS
left without being seen
LWC
leave without consent
LWCT
Lachar-Wrobel Critical Items
Lee-White clotting time (*See also*
LW)
left without completing treatment
LWD
Leri-Weill dyschondrosteosis
living with disease
LWK
large white kidney
LWOP
leave without pay
LWOT
left without treatment

L

LWP
    large whirlpool
    lateral wall pressure
LX, Lx
    larynx (*See also* LAR)
    latex (*See also* L)
    local irradiation
    lower extremity (*See also* LE, L ext, l/ext)
    lymphatic invasion cannot be assessed [TNM classification]
lx
    lux [SI unit for measuring illumination (illuminance) of surface]
LXC
    laxative of choice (*See also* LOC)
LXT
    left exotropia
LY
    lyophilization
LYCD
    live yeast cell derivative
LYDMA
    lymphocyte-detected membrane antigen
LYEL
    lost years of expected life
LYES
    liver yang exuberance syndrome
LYG
    lymphomatoid granulomatosis
LYM
    Lyme disease vaccine
    lymph (*See also* L)
    lymphoma
LYMPH%
    percentage of lymphocytes [in differential count]

lymph
    lymphocyte (*See also* L)
    lymphocytic
LyNeF
    lytic nephritic factor
lyo
    lyophilized
LYP
    lactose, yeast, peptone [agar]
    lower yield point
LyP, Lyp
    lymphomatoid papulosis
LYS
    large yellow soft [stools]
    life-year saved
    lysosome (*See also* L)
Lys
    lysine (*See also* K)
LySLk
    lymphoma syndrome leukemia
LYST
    lysosomal trafficking regulator [gene]
lytes
    electrolyte panel
    electrolytes
LYVE1
    lymphatic endothelial hyaluronan receptor
LZ
    landing zone
LZM, lzm
    lysozyme
LZRS
    Lazarus [vector]
LZT
    lead/zirconium/titanium [crystal, oxide]

M

blood factor in the MNS blood group system
chin [L. *mentum*]
death [L. *mors*]
dullness [of sound] [L. *mutitas*]
handful [L. *manipulus*] (*See also* man., manip.)
macroglobulin
male
malignant (malignancy) (*See also* MAL, malig)
manual
marital (*See also* MAR)
married
masculine (*See also* masc)
masked [audiology]
mass (*See also* m)
maternal contribution
matrix (*See also* MA, MX)
matte [dull, slightly granular, bacterial colonies]
mature (*See also* MAT, mat.)
maximum (*See also* max)
meatus
media
medial (*See also* MED)
median (*See also* md)
mediator [chemical released in the tissues]
medical (*See also* MED)
medicine (*See also* MED)
medium (*See also* MED)
mega-
membrane (*See also* memb)
memory (*See also* MEM)
mental
mesial (*See also* MES)
meta-
metabolite
metal
metastasis (*See also* MET)
methionine (*See also* Met)
method
microfold
mild
million
minimum (*See also* MIN)
minute (*See also* m, MIN, min)
mitochondria
mitosis
mitral (*See also* mit)
mix(ed) (mixture) (*See also* m., mix., mixt, mx)

modulus
molar [permanent tooth]
molar [concentration of solution mol/L] (*See also* molc, mol/L)
mole (*See also* mol)
molecular (*See also* mol)
Monday
monkey (*See also* Mk)
monoclonal (*See also* MO)
monocyte (*See also* mon, MONO, mono, monos)
month (*See also* MO, mo, mon)
morgan [unit of gene separation]
mother (*See also* MO, MOM, MTR)
motile (*See also* m)
mouse
mouth
movement [response to human figure] (*See also* MVMT, MVT, Mx)
mucoid [colony] (*See also* m)
mucous [adjective]
mucus [noun]
multipara
murmur (*See also* (m))
muscle (*See also* musc, m)
muscular [response to electrical stimulation of motor nerve]
mu [12th letter of Greek alphabet uppercase]
Mycobacterium
Mycoplasma
myopia (myopic) (*See also* My, myop)
myosin
noon [L. *meridiem*] (*See also* N)
soften [L. *macerare*] (*See also* mac.)
sample mean [statistics]
thousand [L. *mille*]

M0

(See FAB M0)
no evidence of distant metastases [TNM classification]

M1

(See FAB M1)
left mastoid
mitral component 1[slight dullness, first heart sound]
mitral first sound [slight dullness] (*See also* MFS)
myeloblast

MI

meiosis I

1M–5M

metatarsal 1–5

M2
  (See FAB M2)
  mitral component 2 [marked dullness,
    first heart sound]
  right mastoid
MII
  meiosis II
M3
  (See FAB M3)
  mitral component 3 [absolute dullness,
    first heart sound]
M4
  (See FAB M4)
M5
  (See FAB M5)
M5a
  [See FAB M5a]
M6
  (See FAB M6)
M7
  (See FAB M7)
M/3
  middle third [long bones]
M/10
  tenth molar solution
M/100
  hundredth molar solution
(m)
  by mouth (See also m, PO, p.o.)
  murmur (See also M)
m
  by mouth (See also (m), PO, p.o.)
  magnetic moment [magnetic dipole
    moment]
  mass (See also M)
  meter
  milli-
  minute (See also M, min, MIN)
  molality [concentration of solution
    mol/kg of solvent]
  molar [deciduous tooth]
  motile (See also M)
  mucoid (See also M)
  muscle [Singular] (See also M, mm)
  pole [magnet] strength [ampere-meter]
m.
  mix [L. misce]
  mixture [L. mistura]
  send [L. mitte]
m²
  meters squared
  square meter (See also sq m)
m³
  cubic meter (See also cu m)
MA
  machine
  main arteriole
  malignant arrhythmia
  manifest achievement

masseter
maternal age
maternal aunt
matrix (See also M, MX)
maximum amplitude
mean arterial
mechanically assisted
medical abbreviation
medical assistance
medical audit
medical authorization
megaampere
megaloblastic anemia
membrane antigen
menstrual age
mental age
mentum anterior (mentoanterior) [fetal
  position]
metabolic acidosis
metastatic adenocarcinoma
metatarsus adductus
microadenoma
microagglutination
microalbuminuria
microaneurysm
microcytotoxicity assay
microscopic agglutination
migraine with aura
Miller-Abbott [tube] (See also MAT)
mitochondrial antibody
mitogen activation
mitotic apparatus
mitral anulus (annulus)
mixed agglutination
mixed apnea
moderately advanced
monoamine
monoarthritis
monoclonal antibody (See also MAb,
  MoAb)
monomorphic adenoma
motor area
motorcycle accident (See also MCA)
movement artifact
multiple action
muscle actin
muscle activity
mutagenic activity
myelinated axon
myoclonic absence
M/A
  male altered [animal] (See also
    MALT)
  mood and/or affect
M&A
  myringotomy & aspiration
Ma
  mass of atom
  masurium [obsolete]

mA
 meter-angle
 milliampere [correct abbreviation]
 (*See also* mAMP [slang])

MAA
 macroaggregated albumin (*See also* MIAA)
 mandibular advancement appliance
 Medical Assistance for the Aged
 melanoma-associated antigen
 microphthalmia [or anophthalmos] with associated anomalies
 moderate aplastic anemia
 monoarticular arthritis

MAAAP
 macroaggregated albumin arterial perfusion

MAACL
 Multiple Affect Adjective Check List

MAAS
 Motor Activity Assessment Scale

MAAS-R
 Maastricht History and Advice Checklist Revised

MAB
 management of assaultive behavior
 maximal androgen blockade

MAb
 monoclonal antibody (*See also* MA, MoAb)

MABI
 Mother's Assessment of the Behavior of Her Infant

MAb-LA
 monoclonal antibody-based latex agglutination

MABP
 maltose-binding protein
 mean arterial blood pressure

MAC
 MacConkey [agar]
 macrocytic erythrocyte
 macrophage
 macula
 macule
 malignancy-associated change
 maximal acid concentration
 maximal allowable concentration
 maximum (maximal) allowable cost
 McAndrews Alcoholism Scale
 medial arterial calcification
 medical alert center
 membrane (membranolytic) attack complex
 Mental Adjustment to Cancer [scale]
 microcystic adnexal carcinoma
 midarm circumference
 minimum (minimal) anesthetic concentration
 minimum (minimal) antibiotic concentration
 minimum (minimal) alveolar concentration
 Minimum Auditory Capabilities Test
 mitral annular calcium
 mitral anulus calcification
 modulator of adenylate cyclase
 monitored anesthesia care (control)
 multiaccess catheter
 multidimensional actuarial classification
 Mycobacterium avium-intracellulare complex [dictated/printed Mycobacterium avium complex]
 (*See also* MAI, MAIC)

1-MAC
 1-minimum alveolar concentration

Mac
 MacIntosh [laryngoscope blade]
 (*See also* MAC)

mac.
 maceration (*See also* macer)
 soften [L. *macerare*] (*See also* M)

MAC AWAKE
 minimal alveolar [anesthetic] concentration [patient recovering from general anesthesia able to respond to instructions]

MACC
 macroovalocyte

MACE
 main (major) adverse coronary event
 Malone antegrade continent enema
 methylchloroform chloroacetophenone [tradename Mace]

MAC EIA
 immunoglobulin M antibody capture

macer
 maceration (*See also* mac.)

mAChR
 muscarinic acetylcholine receptor

MACI
 Millon Adolescent Clinical Inventory

MACIS
 metastasis, age, completeness [of resection], [local] invasion, tumor [size]

MACR
 macrocytosin
 mean axillary count rate

macro
 macrocyte (macrocytic)
 macroscopic

macro-EMG
 macroelectromyography

M

MACS
    magnetically activated cell sorter
    maximum aortic cusp separation
MACTAR
    McMaster-Toronto Arthritis Patient
      Reference [Disability Questionnaire]
MACV
    Machupo virus
MAD
    major affective disorder
    mandibular advancement device
    maximal allowable dose
    maximum accumulated dose
    maximum (maximal) acid determination
    mean axis direction
    methylandrostenediol [Methandrol]
      [anabolic steroid]
    mind-altering drug
    minimal average dose
    moderate atopic dermatitis
    mucosal atomization device
    multiple autoimmune disorder
    myoadenylate deaminase
mAD, MADA
    muscle adenylate deaminase
MadCAM-1
    mucosal addresin cell adhesion molecule
      1
MADD
    mixed anxiety depression disorder
    multiple acyl-coenzyme A
      dehydrogenase deficiency
MADL
    mobility activities of daily living
MADRS
    Montgomery-Åsberg Depression Rating
      Scale
MADV
    Madrid virus
MAE
    medical air evacuation
    moves all extremities
    Multilingual Aphasia Examination
mAECA
    monoclonal antiendothelial cell antibody
MAEEW
    moves all extremities equally well
MAES
    moves all extremities slowly
MAEW
    moves all extremities well
MAF
    macrophage-activating (activation) factor
    macrophage-agglutinating (agglutination)
      factor
    malignant ascites fluid
    master apical file
    maximum atrial fragmentation
    metabolic activity factor

    metanephric adenofibroma
    minimum acceptable field
    minimum (minimal) audible field
    mouse amniotic fluid
    movement after effect
MAFA
    midarm fat area
    movement-associated fetal [heart rate]
      accelerations
MAFH
    macroaggregated ferrous hydroxide
MAFO
    molded ankle-foot orthosis
MAFP
    maternal alpha fetoprotein
    methylarachidonyl fluorophosphonate
MAG
    large [L. *magnus*]
    magnify (magnification) (*See also*
      magnif)
    medication administration guideline
      [record]
    Minnesota antilymphocyte globulin
    multifocal atrophic gastritis
    myelin-associated glycoprotein
MAG-3
    [^{99m}TC] mercaptoacetyltriglycine
      [imaging contrast agent]
mag cit
    magnesium citrate
MAGE
    mean amplitude of glycemic excursions
    melanoma-associated gene
MAGF
    male accessory gland fluid
MAGIC
    microprobe analysis generalized intensity
      correction
magnif
    magnify (magnification) (*See also* MAG)
MAGP
    meatal advancement glans-phalloplasty
      (*See also* MAGPI)
    microfil-associated glycoprotein
MAGPI
    meatal advancement and glansplasty
      (*See also* MAGP)
    meatal advancement, glansplasty,
      penoscrotal junction meatotomy
      (*See also* MAGP)
MAGS
    microscopic angiogenesis grading
      system
    Multidimensional Assessment of Gains
      in School [psychologic test]
mag sulf
    magnesium sulfate (*See also* MgSO$_4$)
MAGV
    Maguari virus

MAH
    malignancy-associated hypercalcemia
    minimal acceptable height
    monocular asteroid hyalitis
mAh
    milliampere-hour
MAHA
    microangiopathic hemolytic anemia
    (*See also* MHA)
MAHH
    malignancy-associated humoral
    hypercalcemia
MAHI, MAHIV
    medically acquired human
    immunodeficiency virus
MAI
    magnetic-assisted intervention
    Marriage Adjustment Inventory
    maximal aggregation index
    Medication Appropriateness Index
    microscopic aggregation index
    minor acute illness
    mitotic activity index
    morbid anxiety inventory
    movement arousal index
    Movement Assessment of Infants
    Mycobacterium avium-intracellulare
    [complex] (*See also* MAC, MAIC)
mAi
    milliampere impulse
MAIC
    Mycobacterium avium-intracellulare
    complex (*See also* MAC, MAI)
MAIDS
    murine-acquired immunodeficiency
    syndrome
MAII
    Milwaukee Academic Interest
    Inventory
MAIN
    medication-induced, autoimmune,
    infectious, neoplastic [diseases
    associated with antiphospholipid
    antibodies]
MAINA
    monoclonal antibody immobilization of
    neutrophil antigen
MAIPA
    monoclonal antibody-specific
    immobilization of platelet antigen
MAIR
    metabolic acidosis-induced retinopathy
MAKA
    major karyotypic abnormality
MAL
    malaria vaccine
    malfunction

    malignant (malignancy) (*See also* M,
    malig)
    midaxillary line
    motor activity log
mal.
    ill [L. *malum*]
MALA
    malarial parasites
MALAR
    malaria
Mal-BSA
    maleated bovine serum albumin
MALDI
    matrix-assisted laser desorption
    ionization
MALDIMS
    matrix-assisted laser desorption
    ionization mass spectrometry
MALDI-TOF
    matrix-assisted laser desorption
    ionization time of flight
MALDI-TOFMS
    matrix-assisted laser desorption
    ionization time of flight mass
    spectrometry
MALG
    Minnesota antilymphoblast globulin
malig
    malignant (malignancy) (*See also* M,
    MAL)
MALIMET
    Master List of Medical (Indexing)
    Terms
MALL
    massive all layer liposuction
MALT
    male altered [animal] (*See also*
    M/A)
    mucosa-associated lymphoid tissue
    Munich Alcoholism Test
MALToma
    mucosa-associated lymphoid tissue
    lymphoma
MALV
    Malakal virus
MAM
    mammograph(y) (mammogram) (*See also*
    mammo, MMG)
    median age at menarche
    methylazoxymethanol
    monitored administration of
    medication
    Mycoplasma arthritidis mitogen
M+AM
    compound myopic astigmatism
mAm
    milliampere-minute

M

MAMA
    midarm muscle area
    monoclonal antimalignin antibody

MAMC
    mean arm muscle circumference
    midarm muscle circumference

MAmg
    medial amygdaloid [nucleus]

mammo
    mammography (mammogram) (*See also*
    MAM, MMG)

mAMP
    milliampere [slang] (*See also* mA)

MaMT
    Maudsley Mentation Test

MAMTT
    minimal active muscle tendon tension

MAN
    magnocellular nucleus [of anterior
    neostratum]
    malignancy-associated neutropenia
    mannose

Man
    mannose

man.
    handful [L. *manipulus*] (*See also* M,
    manip.)
    manipulate (manipulation) (*See also*
    manip.)
    morning [L. *mane*] (*See also* mng)

MANCOVA
    multivariate analysis of covariance
    [statistics]

mand
    mandible (mandibular) (*See also* MB,
    MD)

MANE
    Morrow Assessment of Nausea and
    Emesis

manif
    manifestation

manip.
    handful [L. *manipulus*] (*See also* M,
    man.)
    manipulate (manipulation) (*See also*
    man.)

MANOVA
    multivariate analysis of variance
    [statistics]

Man6P
    mannose-6-phosphate

MAO
    maximal acid output
    medical ankle orthosis
    monoamine oxidase

MAO-A
    monoamine oxidase type A

MAO-B
    monoamine oxidase type B

MAOI
    monoamine oxidase inhibitor

MAoP
    mean aortic pressure

MAP
    magnesium, ammonium, phosphate
    [struvite stones]
    malignant atrophic papulosis
    mandibular angle plane
    maximal aerobic power
    mean airways pressure
    mean aortic pressure
    mean arterial pressure
    megaloblastic anemia of pregnancy
    mercapturic acid pathway
    methyl acceptor protein
    methylaminopurine
    microlithiasis alveolarum pulmonum
    microtubule-associated protein
    Miller Assessment for Preschoolers [test
    for developmental delays]
    minimum (minimal) audible pressure
    mitogen-activated (activating) protein
    monophasic action potential
    morning after pill [oral contraceptives]
    mouse antibody production [test]
    multiantigenic peptide
    Multiaxial Assessment of Pain
    Muma Assessment Program [student
    assessment]
    muscle-action potential
    Musical Aptitude Profile
    Mycobacterium avium paratuberculosis

MAPA
    muscle adenosine phosphoric acid

MAPC
    migrating action potential complex

MAPCA
    major aortopulmonary collateral artery

MAPD
    monophasic action potential duration

MAPE
    Multidimensional Assessment of
    Philosophy of Education

MAPF
    microatomized protein food

MAPI
    microbial alkaline protease inhibitor
    Millon Adolescent Personality Inventory

MAPK
    mitogen-activated protein kinase

MAPS
    Make A Picture Story [test]

MAPs
    Making Action Plans

MAPSS
    multiangle polarized scatter separation

MAPV
    Mapputta virus

MAQOL
  Mini Asthma Quality of Life
MAR
  marasmus
  marital (*See also* M)
  marrow
  maximal aggregation ratio
  mean atrial rate
  medication administration record
  melanoma-associated retinopathy
  microanalytical reagent
  mineral apposition rate
  minimal angle resolution
  mixed agglutination reaction
  mixed antiglobulin reaction
mar22
  marker 22
mar
  marker [chromosome]
MARC
  Multicenter Airways Research
    Collaboration
  multifocal and recurrent choroidopathy
MARE
  manual active-resistive exercise
marg
  margin (*See also* MG)
MARIA
  macroaggregated radioiodinated albumin
MARS
  Mathematics Anxiety Rating Scale
  modular acetabular reconstruction
    system
  molecular adsorbent recirculating system
  motion artifact rejection system
  mouse antirat serum
MARS-A
  Mathematics Anxiety Rating Scale
    Adolescents
MARSA
  methicillin [and]
    aminoglycoside-resistant *Staphylococcus*
    aureus
MART, MART 1, MART 2
  melanoma antigen recognized by T cell
MARTI
  mobile advanced real-time image
MARV
  Marburg virus
  Marrakai virus
marX
  marker X
MAS
  MacAndrew Addiction Scale
  macrophage activation syndrome
  mammary aspiration specimen
  Management Appraisal Survey

  Manifest Anxiety Scale
  Maternal Attitude Scale
  mean allograft survival
  meconium aspiration syndrome
  medical advisory service
  Memory Assessment Scale
  mesoatrial shunt
  midaortic syndrome
  milk-alkali syndrome
  minimum-access surgery
  minor axis shortening [of left
    ventricle]
  mitral aortic septum
  mixed antiinflammatory syndrome
  mobile arm support
  modified Ashworth scale [muscle tone
    0-5]
  motion analysis system
  Motor Assessment Scale
  multiple anal sphincterotomies
  mycobacteria antibiotic supplement
  myoclonic astatic seizure
mAs, mA-s
  milliampere second
MASA
  mutant allele-specific amplification
masc
  masculine (*See also* M)
  mass concentration (*See also* massc)
MASCT
  mammary aspiration specimen cytology
    test
MAS-PCR
  multiple allele specific polymerase chain
    reaction
MASER
  microwave amplification by stimulated
    emission of radiation
MASF
  Melcher acid soluble fraction
MASH
  multiple automated sample harvester
Mash-2
  mammalian achaete-scute homologous
    protein 2
MASH POT
  mashed potatoes
MASP
  MBL (mannose binding
    lectin)-associated serine protease
MASS
  metastatic adenocarcinoma in serosal
    surfaces
  minimal access spine surgery
  mitral valve (prolapse), aortic
    (anomalies), skeletal (changes), and
    skin (changes)

M

mass
massage (*See also* MSS, mss)
massive
massc
mass concentration (*See also* masc)
MAST
medical antishock trousers
Michigan Abuse Screening Test
Michigan Alcoholism Screening Test
military antishock trousers
minimal access spine technology
motion artifact suppression technique
multiple antigen stimulation test
multithread allergosorbent test
mAST
mitochondrial aspartate aminotransferase
mast
mastectomy
mastoid
MAT
Manipulative Aptitude Test
manual arts therapist
maternal (*See also* mat.)
maternity (*See also* mat.)
mature (*See also* M, mat.)
mean absorption time
medication administration team
metabolic activation therapy
methionine adenosyltransferase
Metropolitan Achievement Test
microagglutination test
microscopic agglutination test
Miller-Abbott tube (*See also* MA)
Miller Analogies Test
motivation analysis test
multifocal atrial tachycardia
multiple agent therapy
Music Achievement Test [1-4]
MAT7
Metropolitan Achievement Test, Seventh
Edition
mat.
material
maternal (*See also* MAT)
maternity (*See also* MAT)
mature (*See also* M, MAT)
MATE
Marital Attitudes Evaluation
Maternal Attitudes Evaluation
MATHS
muscle [pain], allergy, tachycardia and
tiredness, headache syndrome
MATPP
Medical Audiologic Tinnitus Patient
Protocol
MATSA
Marek associated tumor-specific antigen
MATV
Matucare virus

MAU
microalbuminuria
MAV
mechanical auxiliary ventricle
minimal alveolar ventilation
minimal apparent viscosity
minute alveolar volume
movement arm vector
multinucleated atypia of vulva
myeloblastosis-associated virus
MAVA
multiple abstract variance analysis
MAVD
mixed aortic valve disease
MAVIS
mobile artery and vein imaging
system
MAVR
mitral and aortic valve replacement
max
maxilla
maxillary
maximal (maximum)
MAX A
maximum assistance (assist)
MAXCONT
maximum contrast method
max EP
maximal esophageal pressure
MAxL
midaxillary line
MAYO
mayonnaise
MAYV
Mayaro virus
MB
Mallory body
mammillary body
mandible
margin, buccal
Marsh-Bendall [factor]
maximum breathing
medical board
medulloblastoma
mercury bougie
mesiobuccal
methyl bromide
methylene blue (*See also* MBl, MeB)
microbiologic assay
microbiology
microbubble
muscle balance
muscle-brain
myocardial band (*See also* CPK-MB)
myocardial bridging
M5b
(See FAB M5b)
6MB
six-meal bland [diet]

M/B
mother/baby
Mb
mandible body
myoglobin (*See also* MYO,
MYOGLOB)
MBA
Maxwell-Brancheau arthroereisis
methylbenzyl alcohol
methylbovine albumin
MBAR
myocardial beta (β) adrenergic receptor
mbar
millibar
MBAS
methylene blue active substance
MBB
modified barbital buffer
MBC
bactericidal concentration
male breast cancer (carcinoma)
maximum bladder capacity
maximum breathing capacity
mesiobuccal cusp
metastatic breast cancer (carcinoma)
methylthymol blue complex
microcrystalline bovine collagen
minimal (minimum) bacterial
(bactericidal) concentration
MB CK, MB-CK
M and B isoenzyme (myocardial band)
of creatine kinase (*See also* CPK-MB)
MBCL
monocytoid B-cell lymphoma
MbCO
carbon monoxide myoglobin
MBCR
mesiobuccal cusp ridge
MBCU
metallic bead-chain cystourethrograph
MBD
maximum (maximal) bactericidal
dilution
metabolic bone disease
methylene blue dye
minimal brain damage
minimal brain dysfunction [syndrome]
MBDG
mesiobuccal developmental groove
MBE
may be elevated
medium below-elbow [amputation, cast]
MBEST
modulus blipped echo-planar
single-pulse technique
MBF
meat base formula
medullary blood flow
mesenteric blood flow
muscle blood flow
myocardial blood flow
MBFC
medial brachial fascial compartment
MBFLB
monaural bifrequency loudness balance
M-BFU-E
mature burst-forming unit erythroid
MBG
mean blood glucose
MBGS
Morphine-Benzedrine Group Scale
MBGV
Marburg virus
MBH
maximal benefit from hospitalization
medial basal hypothalamus
MBH$_2$
methylene blue, reduced (*See also*
MBR)
MBHI
Millon Behavioral Health Inventory
MBI
Maslach Burnout Inventory
methylene blue instillation
MBIP
model-based image processing
MBK
methyl butyl ketone
MBL
mannan-binding lectin
mannose-binding lectin
medium brown loose [stool]
menstrual blood loss
minimum (minimal) bactericidal level
MBl
methylene blue (*See also* MB, MeB)
MBLA
methylbenzyl linoleic acid
mouse-specific bone marrow-derived
lymphocyte antigen
MBM
mind-body medicine
mineral basal medium
mother's breast milk
MBNW
multiple-breath nitrogen washout
MBO
mesiobuccoocclusal
MbO$_2$
oxymyoglobin
MBOT
mucinous borderline ovarian tumors
MBP
major basic protein
malignant brachial plexopathy
maltose-binding protein

M

MBP *(continued)*
mannan-binding protein
mannose-binding protein
mean blood pressure
medullary bone pain
melitensis, bovine, porcine [antigen
from *Brucella melitensis, B. bovis* and
B. suis]
mesiobuccopulpal
modified Bagshawe protocol
myelin base (basic) protein

M2BP
Mac-2 binding protein

MBPA
malposition of branch pulmonary
artery

MBPM
modified backward Prony method
[spectral analysis]

MBPS
multigated [cardiac] blood pool
scanning

MBq
megabecquerel

MBR
major breakpoint region
mesiobuccal root
methylene blue, reduced *(See also*
MBH$_2$)

MbR
morbidity rate

MBRT
methylene blue reduction time

MBRVO
macular branch retinal vein occlusion

MBS
modified barium swallow
Multi Balance System

MBSA
methylated bovine serum albumin

MBSD
maple bark stripper's disease

MBS-MRA
minimum basis set magnetic resonance
angiography

MBSP
Monitoring Basic Skills Progress

MBSR
mindfulness-based stress reduction

MBT
maternal blood type
mercaptobenzothiazole
midbrain tremor
mixed bacterial toxin
mucinous borderline tumor
multiple blunt trauma

MBTI
Myers-Briggs Type Indicator
[psychologic test]

MBTS
modified Blalock-Taussig shunt

MBV
mitral balloon valvotomy

M-C
Magovern-Cromie [prosthesis]
mineralocorticoid *(See also* MC)

MC
macroglobulinemia
magnetocardiograph
male child
mass casualty
mast cell
maximal concentration
maximum (maximal) control
medium-chain [triglyceride]
medullary carcinoma
medullary cavity
medullary cystic [disease]
megacoulomb
megacycle
melanoma cell
meningeal carcinomatosis
Merkel cell
mesangial cell
mesenchymal chondrosarcoma
mesenteric collateral
mesiocervical
mesocaval [shunt]
metacarpal
metatarsocuneiform
methyl cellulose
methylcholanthrene *(See also* MCA)
microcephaly
microciliary clearance
microcirculation
microscopic colitis
midcapillary
midcarpal
mineralocorticoid *(See also* M-C)
minicatheterization
minilaparotomy cholecystectomy
minimal change
miscarriage
mitotic cycle
mitral commissurotomy
mixed cellularity
mixed cryoglobulinemia
molluscum contagiosum
monkey cell
mononuclear cell
Moraxella catarrhalis
mouth care
musculocutaneous
mycelial phase [of fungi]
myocardial channeling
myocarditis

MC-540
merocyanine 540 [dye]

M&C
morphine and cocaine
M/C
male castrated [animal]
Mc
mandible coronoid
mitral commissurotomy [closure]
mC
millicoulomb
MCA
main coronary artery
major coronary artery
medical care administration
mesial contact area
metacarpal amputation
methylcholanthrene (*See also* MC)
microcarcinoma
micrometastases clonogenic assay
middle cerebral aneurysm
middle cerebral artery (*See also* mCA)
middle colic artery
monocarboxylic acid
motorcycle accident (*See also* MA)
mucinlike carcinoma-associated antigen
multichannel analyzer
multiple congenital abnormalities
multiple congenital anomalies
2-MCA
2-methyl citric acid
mCA
middle cerebral artery (*See also* MCA)
MCAB, MC-Ab
Minnesota Clerical Assessment Battery
MCAD
medium-chain acyl-coenzyme A
dehydrogenase
MCAF
macrophage chemotactic and activating
factor
monocyte chemoattractant and activity
factor
monocyte chemotactic and activating
factor
MCAG
multiple colloid adenomatous goiter
MCA/MR
multiple congenital anomalies [and]
mental retardation [syndrome]
MCAO
middle cerebral artery occlusion
MCAP
middle cerebral artery pressure
MCAR
melanocortin receptor type 4
mixed cell agglutination reaction
MCAS
middle cerebral artery syndrome
modular clip application system

MCAT
Medical College Admission Test
middle cerebral artery thrombosis
Minnesota Clerical Aptitude Test
myocardial contrast appearance time
MCAV
Macaua virus
MCB
membranous cytoplasmic body
midcycle bleeding
middle chamber bubbling
monochlorobenzidine
McB
McBurney [point]
mCBF
mean cerebral blood flow
MCBM
muscle capillary basement membrane
MCBMT
muscle capillary basement membrane
thickening
MCBR
minimum (minimal) concentration of
bilirubin
MCC
marked cocontraction
mean corpuscular [hemoglobin]
concentration (*See also* MCHbC,
MCHC)
measure mucociliary clearance
medial cell column
Merkel cell carcinoma
metacarpocarpal [joint]
metacerebral cell
metastatic cord compression
microcalcification cluster
microcrystalline cellulose
microcrystalline collagen
midstream clean catch [urine]
minimum (minimal) complete-killing
concentration
mucociliary clearance
mucocutaneous candidiasis
mutated in colon cancer
mutated colorectal carcinoma
Mycobacterium cell wall complex
McC
McCarthy [panendoscope]
McCoy [antibody]
MCCD
minimum (minimal) cumulative
cardiotoxic dose
MCCN
mesangiocapillary glomerulonephritis
MCCS
Minnesota Cocaine Craving Scale
MCCU
mobile coronary care unit

M

MCD
magnetic circular dichroism
malformation of cortical development
marginal corneal dystrophy
margin crease distance
mast cell degranulation
mean cell diameter
mean central dose
mean consecutive difference
mean corpuscular diameter
medullary collecting duct
medullary cystic disease
metabolic coronary dilation
metacarpal cortical density
metaphysial chondrodysplasia
metastatic Crohn disease
minimal cerebral dysfunction
minimal change disease
molecular coincidence detection
molybdenum cofactor deficiency
multicentric Castleman disease
multicystic disease
multicystic dysplasia
multiple carboxylase deficiency
muscle carnitine deficiency

MCDD
multiple complex developmental disorder

MCDI
Minnesota Child Development Inventory

MCDK
multicystic dysplasia (dysplastic) kidney

MCDP
mast cell degranulating peptide

MCDT
mast cell degranulation test
multiple choice discrimination test

MCDU
mercaptolactate-cysteine disulfiduria

MCE
major coronary event
medical care evaluation
minimal cytotoxic epitope
multicystic encephalopathy
multiple cartilaginous exostosis
myocardial contrast echocardiography

MCES
multiple cholesterol emboli syndrome

MCF
macrophage chemotactic factor
macrophage cytotoxicity factor
median cleft face
medium corpuscular fragility
microcomplement fixation
monocyte chemotactic factor
mononuclear cell factor
most comfortable frequency
multicentric foci
myocardial contraction (contractile)
force

MCFA
medium-chain fatty acid
miniature centrifugal fast analyzer

MCFP
mean circulating filling pressure

MCFSR
mean circumferential fiber-shortening
rate

MCG
magnetocardiograph(y)
(magnetocardiogram)
membrane cell graft
membrane coating granule
mesencephalic central gray
monoclonal gammopathy (*See also* MG)

mcg
microgram (*See also* μg)

MCGC
metacerebral giant cell

MCGF
mast cell growth factor

mcg/kg min
microgram per kilogram per minute

MCGN
mesangiocapillary glomerulonephritis
minimal-change glomerulonephritis
mixed cryoglobulinemia with
glomerulonephritis

MCGNX
mesangiocapillary glomerulonephritis
X-linked

MCH
maternal and child health
mean cell hemoglobin
mean corpuscular hemoglobin (*See also*
MCHb)
melanin-concentrating hormone
methacholine
microfibrillar collagen hemostat
mucous cell hyperplasia
muscle contraction headache

MCHA
microsome antibody

MCHb
mean corpuscular hemoglobin (*See also*
MCH)

MCHbC
mean corpuscular hemoglobin
concentration (*See also* MCC, MCHC)
mean corpuscular hemoglobin count

MCHC
maternal and child health care
mean corpuscular hemoglobin
concentration (*See also* MCC,
MCHbC)
microcrystalline calcium hydroxyapatite
complex

MCHD
mixed-cellularity Hodgkin disease

MCHS
  maternal and child health service
MCI
  mass casualty incident
  mean cardiac index
  midcarpal instability
  mild cognitive impairment
  mucociliary insufficiency
  multiple casualty (multicasualty)
    incident
  muscle contraction interference
MCi
  megacurie
mCi
  millicurie
MCID
  minimum clinically important
    difference(s)
mCid
  millicurie destroyed
mCi-hr
  millicurie-hour
MCINS
  minimal change idiopathic nephrotic
    syndrome
MCK
  multicystic kidney
mckat
  microkatal (*See also* μkat)
MCKD
  multicystic kidney disease
MCL
  mantle cell lymphoma
  maximal comfort level
  maximal containment laboratory
  medial collateral ligament
  midclavicular line
  midcostal line
  minimal change lesion
  mixed culture, leukocyte
  modified chest lead
  most comfortable level
  most comfortable loudness
  mucocutaneous leishmaniasis
  multiple cutaneous leiomyomata
MCL-1
  myeloid-cell leukemia
mcL
  microliter [1/1,000 of an mL] (*See also*
    μL)
MCLC
  medial collateral ligament complex
MCLL
  most comfortable listening level
  most comfortable loudness level
MCL-N
  midclavicular line to nipple

MCLNS, MCLS
  mucocutaneous lymph node
    syndrome
MCLR
  most comfortable loudness range
MCMI-I–MCMI-III
  Millon Clinical Multiaxial
    Inventory I–III [psychiatric
    battery]
mcmol
  micromole (*See also* μmol)
M-CMTC
  macrocephaly, cutis marmorata,
    telangiectatica congenita
MCN
  minimal-change nephropathy
  mixed cell nodular [lymphoma]
  mucinous cystic neoplasm
MCNS
  minimal-change nephrotic syndrome
mCNV
  myopic choroidal neovascularization
MCO
  managed (medical) care organization
  marked corneal opacity
MCOV
  Marco virus
MCP
  maximum contraction pattern
  maximum (maximal) closure pressure
  mean carotid pressure
  melanosis circumscripta precancerosa
  membrane cofactor protein
  metacarpophalangeal [joint] (*See also*
    MP, MCPJ)
  methyl-accepting chemotaxis protein
  mitotic control protein
  monocyte chemoattractant (chemotactic)
    protein
  mucin clot prevention [test]
  mucopolysaccharidoses [plural]
  mucosal carrier protein
  multifocal choroiditis with panuveitis
MCP-1
  monocyte chemoattractant (chemotactic)
    protein 1
  mucosal carrier protein 1
MCPJ
  metacarpophalangeal joint (*See also*
    MCP, MP)
MCPP
  metacarpophalangeal profile
MCPS
  Missouri Children's Picture Series
    [psychologic test]
Mcps
  megacycle per second (*See also* Mc/s)

M

MCPT
  Macular Computerized Psychophysical Test
  Monte Carlo photon transport
MCQ
  multiple choice question
MCR
  mesial cusp ridge
  message competition ratio
  metabolic clearance rate
  midcarpal radial
  minor cluster region
  mother-child relationship
  mutation cluster region
  myocardial revascularization
  myotonia congenita recessive
  metabolic clearance rate
MC=R
  moderately constricted and equally reactive [pupils]
MC2-R–MC4-R
  melanocortin 2 melanocortin–4 receptor
MCRC
  metastatic colorectal cancer
MCRD
  monolithic controlled release device [cardiac pacing]
MCRE
  Mother-Child Relationship Evaluation
MCRI
  multifactorial cardiac risk index
MCS
  magnetic control suturing
  malignant carcinoid syndrome
  Marlow-Crowne Scale [psychology]
  massage of carotid sinus
  Mental Component Summary
  mesocaval shunt
  methylcholanthrene [-induced] sarcoma
  microculture and sensitivity
  middle coronary sinus
  moderate constant suction
  multiple chemical sensitivity
  multiple combined sclerosis
  myocardial contractile state
MC&S
  microscopy, culture, sensitivity
Mc/s
  megacycle per second (See also Mcps)
MCSA
  McCarthy Scales of Children's Ability
  minimal cross-sectional area
  Moloney cell surface antigen
MCSDS
  Marlowe-Crown Social Desirability Scale
M-CSF
  macrophage colony-stimulating factor
  monocyte colony-stimulating factor

MC-SR
  moderately constricted and slightly reactive [pupils]
MCSS
  multiple chemical sensitivity syndrome
MCT
  manual cervical traction
  mast cell tryptase-positive chymase-negative
  mean cell thickness
  mean cell threshold
  mean circulation time
  mean colonic transit
  mean corpuscular thickness
  medial canthal tendon
  medium-chain triglyceride
  medullary carcinoma of thyroid
  medullary collecting tubule
  methylcholine challenge testing
  microwave coagulation therapy
  microwave computed tomography
  Minnesota Clerical Test
  monocarboxylate/proton cotransporter [family]
  monocrotaline
  motor coordination test
  mucinous cystic tumor
  mucociliary transport
  multiple compressed tablet
MCTC
  mast cell tryptase- and chymase-positive
  metrizamide computed tomography (tomographic) cisternography
MCTD
  mixed connective-tissue disease
MCTF
  mononuclear cell tissue factor
MCTT
  mucociliary clearance time
MCU
  malaria control unit
  maximal care unit
  micturating cystourethrograph(y) (cystourethrogram)
  midcarpal ulnar
  motor cortex unit
MCUG
  micturating urogram
MCV
  mean cell volume
  mean clinical value
  mean corpuscular volume
  measles-containing vaccine
  melanoma whole-cell vaccine
  molluscum contagiosum virus
  motor conduction velocity
  myelocytomatosis virus
MCVr
  mean corpuscular volume reticulocyte

MCVRI
  minimal coronary vascular resistance
    index
MCW
  mass-casualty weapon
MCYLS
  marginal cost per year of life saved
MD
  macula densa
  macular degeneration
  magnesium deficiency
  main duct
  maintenance dialysis
  maintenance dose
  major depression
  malate (malic) dehydrogenase
  malrotation of duodenum
  mammary dysplasia
  mandibular
  manic depression
  manic-depressive
  Mantoux diameter
  Marek disease [avian]
  maternal deprivation
  maximal dose
  mean deviation
  mean diastolic
  measurable disease
  Meckel diverticulum
  medialis dorsalis [nucleus]
  mediastinal disease
  medical department
  mediodorsal
  medium dosage
  meningococcal disease
  mental deficiency
  mental depression
  mentally deficient
  mesiodistal
  methyldichloroarsine [chemical weapon]
  microtube dilution
  minimum (minimal) dosage
  mitral disease
  mixed diet
  moderate disability
  moderately differentiated
  monocular deprivation
  movement disorder
  multiple deficiency
  multiple dose
  muscular dystrophy
  myeloproliferative disease
  myocardial damage
  myocardial disease
  myotonic dystrophy
Md
  mendelevium (*See also* Mv)

md
  median (*See also* M, mdn)
MDA
  malondialdehyde
  malonyldialdehyde
  manual dilatation of anus
  mass drug administration
  methylenedioxyamphetamine
  micrometastases detection assay
  monodehydroascorbate
  motor discriminative acuity
  multiple displacement amplification
  multivariant discriminant analysis
  right mentum anterior mentoanterior
    [fetal position] [L. *mento-dextra
    anterior*] (*See also* RMA)
mda1–mda9
  melanoma differentiation-associated gene
    1–9
MDAC
  multidose activated charcoal
  multiple-dose activated charcoal
  multiplying digital-to-analog converter
MDAD
  mineral dust airway disease
MDA-LDL, MDALDL
  malondialdehyde [conjugated, modified]
    low-density lipoprotein
MDAP
  Machover Draw-A-Person (Test)
MDASI
  MD Anderson Symptom Inventory
MDB
  medulloblastoma
  Mental Deterioration Battery
MDBK
  Madin-Darby bovine kidney [cell]
MDBP
  mean resting diastolic blood pressure
MDC
  macrophage-derived chemokine
  major diagnostic category
  medial dorsal cutaneous [nerve]
  minimum (minimal) detectable
    concentration
MDCA
  mean distal contraction amplitude
MDCK
  Madin-Darby canine kidney [cell]
MDCM
  mildly dilated congestive
    cardiomyopathy
MDCN
  medial dorsal cutaneous nerve
MDCT
  multidetector (multidetector-row)
    computed tomography

M

MDCV
Mojui Dos Campos virus
MDD
major depressive disorder
manic-depressive disorder
mean daily dose
mesial developmental depression
MDDA
Minnesota Differential Diagnosis of
Aphasia
MDDC
monocyte-derived dendritic cell
MDE
major depressive episode
minimum defibrillation energy
mucinous ductal ectasia
MDEA
N-ethyl-3,4-methylenedioxyamphetamine
(*See also* MDMA)
MDEBP
mean daily erect blood pressure
MDF
map-dot-fingerprint [dystrophy]
mean dominant frequency
myocardial depressant factor
MDFR
midexpiratory dynamic flow rate
MDG
mean diastolic gradient
Millennium Development Goals [United
Nations]
MDGF
macrophage-derived growth factor
MDGI
mammary-derived growth inhibitor
MDH
malate dehydrogenase
medullary dorsal horn
MDHR
maximum determined heart rate
MDHV
Marek herpesvirus disease
MDI
manic-depressive illness
mental development index
metered-dose inhaler
methylenedioxyindenes
methylene diphenyl diisocyanate
Michelson Doppler imager
multidirectional instability
multiple daily injection
multiple dose injection
Multiscore Depression Inventory
MDIA
Mental Development Index,
Adjusted
MDI-DED
metered-dose inhaler with delivery
enhancement device

MDII
multiple daily insulin injection
MDIS
metered-dose inhaler-spacer (device)
MDIT
mean disintegration time
MDK
multicystic dysplastic kidney
MDL
master drug list
MD-LKP
maximum depth lamellar keratoplasty
MDLS
Miller-Dieker lissencephaly syndrome
MDLVP
mean diastolic left ventricular pressure
MDM
medical decision-making
middiastolic murmur
minor determinant mix [skin test for
penicillin]
MDMA
N-ethyl-3,4-methylenedioxyamphetamine
(*See also* MDEA)
methylenedioxymethamphetamine
MDMQ
Menstrual Distress Management
Questionnaire (*See also* MDQ)
MDMS
methylene dimethane sulfonate
mdn
median (*See also* M, md)
mDNA
mitochondrial deoxyribonucleic acid
MDNB
mean daily nitrogen balance
metadinitrobenzene
methylene diphosphate
MDNCF
monocyte-derived neutrophil chemotactic
factor
MDNT
midnight
MDO
mentally disordered offender
mesiodistocclusal
MDOT
modified directly observed therapy
modified double-opposing tab
MDOV
Monte Dourado virus
MDP
mandibular dysostosis and peromelia
manic-depressive psychosis
maximum diastolic potential
maximum digital pulse
maximum (maximal) deliverable
pressure
methylene diphosphate [imaging agent]

methylene diphosphonate [imaging
agent]
minimum distending pressure
muramyldipeptide
muscular dystrophy, progressive
right mentum posterior (mentoposterior)
[fetal position] [L. *mento-dextra
posterior*] (*See also* RMP)
MDPD
maximum dose permissible dose
MDPI
maximal daily permissible intake
MDQ
memory deviation quotient
Menstrual Distress Questionnaire
(*See also* MDMQ)
minimal detectable quantity
minimum (minimal) deductible quantity
MDR
mammalian diving response
median duration of response
Medical Device Reporting (regulation)
minimal daily requirement
minimum daily requirement
multidrug resistance
multidrug-resistant
multiple drug resistance
multiple drug-resistant
MD=R
moderately dilated and equally reactive
[pupils]
MDR-1
multidrug resistance gene
MDR1
multidrug resistance 1
MDRD
modification of diet in renal disease
MDRE
multiple drug-resistant enterococci
MDREF
multidrug resistant enteric fever
MDRH
multidisciplinary rehabilitation hospital
MDRO
multidrug-resistant organism
MDRS
Mattis Dementia Rating Scale
MDRSP
multidrug-resistant *Streptococcus
pneumoniae*
MDRT
multiple-drug rescue therapy
MDR-TB, MDRTB
multidrug-resistant tuberculosis
multiple-drug resistant tuberculosis
MDS
maternal deprivation syndrome

medical data screen
medical data system
membrane-spanning domain
microdebrider system
microdilution system
microsurgical drill system
milk drinker's syndrome
minimum data set
multidimensional scaling
myelodysplastic syndrome
myocardial depressant substance
MDS/AML
myelodysplastic syndrome and acute
myeloblastic leukemia
MDSBP
mean daily supine blood pressure
MDSO
mentally disordered sex offender
MD-SR
moderately dilated and slightly reactive
[pupils]
MDSU
medical day stay unit
MDT
maggot débridement therapy
mast (cell) degeneration test
mean dissolution time
median detection threshold
minimal deformation target
motion detection threshold
multidisciplinary team
multidrug therapy
right mentum transverse
(mentotransverse) (fetal position)
[L. *mento-dextra transversa*]
MDTA
McDonald Deep Test of Articulation
MDTM
multidisciplinary team meeting
MDTP
multidisciplinary treatment plan
MDTR
mean diameter-thickness ratio
MDU
microvascular Doppler ultrasonography
MDUO
myocardial disease of unknown
origin
MDV
Main Drain virus
Marek disease virus
mucosal disease virus
multiple dose vial
myocardial Doppler velocity
M-DVPA
Modified Dynamic Visual Processing
Assessment

M

MDW
monophasic defibrillation waveform
MDY
month, date, year
Mdyn
megadyne
ME
macular edema
magnitude estimation
male equivalent
male escutcheon
malic enzyme
manic episode
marginal excision
maximum (maximal) effort
median eminence
medical education
medical events
medical evidence
medical examiner
meningoencephalitis
mercaptoethanol
metabolic and electrolyte
[disorder]
metabolic energy
metabolic equivalent
metabolism
metabolizable energy
metamyelocyte
methionine enkephalin
methyleugenol
microembolism
microembolization
middle ear
mouse embryo
mouse epithelial [cell]
muscle energy
muscle examination
myalgic encephalomyelitis
myoclonic epilepsy
myoepithelial [cell]
M & E
mucositis and enteritis
me
electron rest mass
M:E
metabolic to endocrine ratio
myeloid to erythroid ratio
ME$_{50}$
50% maximal effect
Me
menton [craniometric]
methyl (See also meth)
MEA
measles virus vaccine
mercaptoethylamine
microwave endometrial ablation
multiple endocrine abnormalities
(adenomatosis) (adenopathies)

MEAI–MEAII
multiple endocrine adenomatosis type
I–II
mEAD
monophasic action potential early
afterdepolarization
MeAIB
methylaminoisobutyric acid
MEAMS
Middlesex Elderly Assessment of
Mental state
MEANS
modular electrocardiogram analysis
system
MEAP
Multiphasic Environmental Assessment
Procedure
meas
measurement
MEAT
Minnesota Engineering Analogies Test
MEAV
Meaban virus
MEB
medical evaluation board
muscle-eye-brain [disease]
MeB
methylene blue (See also MB, MBI)
MEBMM
mixed epithelial papillary cystadenoma
of borderline malignancy of müllerian
type
MEBS
muscle-eye-brain syndrome
MeBSA
methylated bovine serum albumin
MEBV
Mount Elgon bat virus
MEC
mammary epithelial cell
meconium
median effective concentration
middle ear canal
middle ear cell
minimum effective concentration
moderately emetogenic chemotherapy
mucoepidermoid carcinoma
myoepithelial cell
5-MeC
5-methylcytosine
MECA
Methods for Epidemiology of Child and
Adolescent Mental Disorders
MECC
micellar electrokinetic capillary
chromatography
MECG
maternal electrocardiogram
mixed essential cryoglobulinemia

mech
mechanical
MeCP2
methyl-CpG-binding protein 2
MECT
maximal extrapolated clotting time
MECTA
mobile electroconvulsive therapy
apparatus
MED
male erectile dysfunction
maximum economic dose
medial (*See also* M)
median erythrocyte diameter
medical (*See also* M)
medication
medicine (*See also* M)
medium (*See also* M)
medulloblastoma
minimum (minimal) effective diameter
minimal erythema dose
minimum (minimal) effective dose
multiple epiphysial dysplasia
MEDAC
multiple endocrine deficiency, Addison
disease, candidiasis [syndrome]
multiple endocrine deficiency [and]
autoimmune candidiasis
MED-ART
Medical Automated Records Technology
MedDRA
Medical Dictionary for Regulatory
Activities
MEDEX, Medex
medication administration record
military medical corpsmen [Fr. *medicin
exension*]
MEDICS
meat, eggs, dairy, invisible fat,
condiments, snacks
Medical Examination and Diagnostic
Coding System
MED-IDDM
multiple epiphysial dysplasia [and] early
onset diabetes mellitus syndrome
MEDLARS
Medical Literature Analysis and
Retrieval System
MEDLINE
MEDLARS On-Line
MEDLS
Milwaukee Evaluation of Daily Living
Skills
med men
medial meniscectomy
medial meniscus
MED NEC
medically necessary

MEDPAR
Medical Provider Analysis and Review
MEdREP
Medical Education Reinforcement and
Enrichment Program
MEDS
medications
microsurgical extraction of ductal sperm
med stern
medial sternotomy
MedSurg
medicine and surgery
Med Tech
medical technology
MEE
maintenance energy expenditure
measured energy expenditure
methylethyl ether
middle ear effusion
multilocus enzyme electrophoresis
M-EEG
magnetoencephalograph(y)
(magnetoencephalogram)
MEF
maximum (maximal) expiratory flow
middle ear fluid
midexpiratory flow
migration enhancement factor
mouse embryo fibroblast
MEF$_{50}$
maximum expiratory flow at 50% vital
capacity
mean maximal expiratory flow
MEFR
maximum (maximal) expiratory flow
rate
midexpiratory flow rate
MEFSR
maximum (maximal) expiratory
flow-static recoil (curve)
MEFV
maximum (maximal) expiratory flow
volume
MEFVC
maximum (maximal) expiratory flow
volume curve
mechanical expiratory flow volume
curve
MEG
magnetoencephalograph(y)
(magnetoencephalogram)
megakaryocyte
metabolic, endocrine, gastrointestinal
multifocal eosinophilic granuloma
MEG3
maternally expressed gene 3
MEG-CSF
megakaryocyte colony-stimulating factor

M

MEGD
minimal euthyroid Graves disease
mEGF
mouse epidermal growth factor
MEGX
monoethylglycinexylidide
MeHg
methylmercury
MEI
magnetic endoscopic imaging
maximally exposed individual
medical economic index
metastatic efficiency index
middle ear implantable
middle ear infection
MEIA
microparticle (microparticulate) enzyme
immunoassay
MEK
mitogen activated protein (MAP)/
extracellular signal-related kinase
(ERK) kinase
methyl ethyl ketone (methylethylketone)
MEKC
micellar electrokinetic chromatography
MEKK
mitogen activated kinase (MEK)
kinase
MEKS
Mediterranean Kaposi sarcoma
MEL
maximum exposure limit
melatonin
metabolic equivalent level
mouse (murine) erythroleukemia
mel
melanoma
melena
mel 1–3
Meleagris adenovirus 1-3
MELAN
melanin
MELAS
(mitochondrial) myopathy,
encephalopathy, lactic acidosis, and
strokelike episodes syndrome
MELC
murine erythroleukemia cell
Mel-CAM
melanoma cell adhesion molecule
MELD
Model for End-Stage Liver Disease
[score]
MELDOS
meliodosis
MELI
metenkephalinlike immunoreactivity
MELV
Melao virus

MEM
[Eagle] minimum essential medium
macrophage electrophoretic migration
(mobility)
malignant epithelioid mesothelioma
memory (*See also* M)
monocular estimate method
MEMA
methyl methacrylate (*See also* MMA)
MEMB
modified eosin-methylene blue [agar]
memb
membrane (*See also* M)
MEMP
multiecho multiplane
MEMPHIS
Memphis Educational Model Providing
Handicapped Infant Services
MEMR
multiple exostoses-mental retardation
[syndrome]
MEMS
medication event monitoring system
MEN
meningococcal (*Neisseria meningitidis*)
(serogroups unspecified) vaccine
methylethylnitrosamine
multiple endocrine neoplasia
(neoplasms)
MEN1–MEN3
multiple endocrine neoplasia type 1–3
MEN2a–MEN2b
multiple endocrine neoplasia type
2A–2B
men.
meningeal
meninges
meningitis
MenCon
meningococcal conjugate
MEND
Medical Education for National
Defense
MENG
magnetoenterograph(y)
(magnetoenterogram)
MENS
microamperage electrical nerve
stimulation
microcurrent electrical neuromuscular
stimulation (stimulator)
minielectrical nerve stimulator
multiple endocrine neoplasia syndrome
menst
menstrual
menstruate
menstruating
MEO
malignant external otitis

ME/OC
  middle ear exploration with ossicular chain [reconstruction]
MeOH
  methyl alcohol
MEOS
  microsomal ethanol oxidizing system
MEP
  maximum (maximal) expiratory pressure
  mean effective pressure
  mitochondrial encephalopathy
  motor end plate
  motor evoked potential
  mucoid exopolysaccharide
  multimodality evoked potential
MEPC
  miniature endplate current
MEPOP
  mitochondrial encephalomyopathy with sensorimotor polyneuropathy, ophthalmoplegia, paralysis
MEPP
  miniature endplate potential
MEPS
  means-end problem solving
mEq
  milliequivalent
mEq/24 H
  milliequivalent per 24 hours
mEq/L
  milliequivalent per liter
MER
  mean ejection rate
  medical evidence of record
  mersalyl (acid)
  methanol extraction residue
  methanol-extruded residue
  molar esterification rate
  motor-evoked response
  multimodality-evoked response
  murmur to energy ratio
MERAC
  musculoskeletal evaluation, rehabilitation and conditioning
MERB
  metenkephalin receptor binding
MERCI
  mechanical embolus removal in cerebral ischemia [system]
MERG
  macular electroretinographc(y) (electroretinogram)
MERRF
  myoclonic epilepsy with ragged red fibers
MERV
  Mermet virus

MES
  maintenance electrolyte solution
  maximal electroshock seizure
  medical equipment set
  mesial (*See also* M)
  Metrazol-electroshock seizure
  microcurrent electrical stimulator
  microembolic signal
  morpholinoethanesulfonic acid
  mucosal electrosensitivity
  multiple endocrine syndrome
  muscle in elongated state
  myoelectric signal
Mes
  mesencephalic
  mesencephalon
MESA
  microsurgical epididymal sperm aspiration
  myoepithelial sialadenitis
mesc
  mescaline
MESCH
  Multi-Environment Scheme
MESF
  molecule of equivalent soluble fluorochrome
MESGN
  mesangial glomerulonephritis
MeSH
  Medical Subject Heading [in MEDLARS]
MESI
  mangled extremity syndrome index
MESOR
  midline estimating statistic of rhythm [cardiology]
MESP
  maximal exercise systolic pressure
MesPGN
  mesangial proliferative glomerulonephritis
MESS
  Mangled Extremity Severity Score
  multiple echo single shot
mESS
  meridional end-systolic stress
MESSIER
  Matson Evaluation of Social Skills in Individuals with Severe Retardation
MEST
  mesodermal specific transcript
MET
  maximal exercise test
  medical emergency treatment
  metabolic (*See also* metab)
  metabolic equivalent

M

MET *(continued)*
metabolic equivalent task
metamyelocyte
metastasis [singular] *(See also* M*)*
metastatic *(See also* M*)*
metallic [chest sounds]
metastasize [metastasizing]
midexpiratory time
minimum elicitation threshold
Minimum Essentials Test
multistage exercise test
muscle energy technique
Met
methionine *(See also* M*)*
META
metamyelocyte
methacryloxyethyl trimellitic
(methacryloxyethyltrimellitic) anhydride
meta
metacarpal
metatarsal
metab
metabolic *(See also* MET*)*
metabolism *(See also* ME*)*
metas
metamyelocytes [CBC differential]
met-enkephalin
methionine-enkephalin
Meth
methamphetamine
methedrine
meth
methyl *(See also* Me*)*
MetHb
methemoglobin *(See also* HbMet*)*
MeTHF
methyltetrahydrofolic acid
MetMb
metmyoglobin
MET-PET
methionine positron emission
tomography
METS
metastases [plural]
METT
maximum (maximal) exercise tolerance
test
metz
Metzenbaum [scissors]
MEV
maximal exercise ventilation
murine erythroblastosis virus
MeV
megaelectron volt (million)
MEWDS
multiple evanescent white dot syndrome
MF
magnification factor
Malassezia folliculitis

Malassezia furfur
march [stress] fracture
masculinity/femininity
mass fragmentography
meat free
median frequency
medium frequency
megafarad
melamine-formaldehyde [resin]
merthiolate [and] formaldehyde
[solution] *(See also* MFS*)*
mesial facial [surface]
methanol Formaldehyde
microfibrile
microfilament
microfilia
microscopic factor
midcavity forceps [obstetrics]
middle finger
midforceps [delivery]
Millipore filter
mitogenic factor
mitotic figure
mossy fiber
mucosal fluid
multifactorial
multiplication factor
mutation frequency
mutton fat
mycosis fungoides
myelin figure
myelofibrosis
myocardial fibrosis
myofibrillar
M:F
male to female ratio
moment to force ratio
M&F
male and female
mother and father
Mf
maxillofrontal [craniometric]
microfilaria
mF
millifarad
MFA
malaise, fatigue, anorexia
methyl fluoracetate
monofluoroacetate [poisoning]
multifocal functional autonomy
multifunctional acrylic
multiple factor analysis
Musculoskeletal Function Assessment
MFAT
multifocal atrial tachycardia
MFB
medial forebrain bundle
metallic foreign body
multiple-frequency bioimpedance

MFC
    mean frequency of compensation
    medial femoral condyle
    minimal fungicidal concentration
    multifocal choroiditis
m-FC
    membrane focal coli [broth]
MFCV
    muscle fiber conduction velocity
MFD
    mandibulofacial dysostosis
    Memory for Designs [test]
    midforceps delivery
    milk-free diet
    minimal fatal dose
    monorhythmic frontal delta (EEG)
    multiple fractions per day [radiotherapy]
MFE
    multifocal electroretinography
MFEL
    medical free electron laser
MFEM
    maximal forced expiratory maneuver
MFF
    Matching Familiar Figures [test]
      (*See also* MFFT)
    metal fume fever
MFFT
    Matching Familiar Figures Test
      (*See also* MFF)
MFG
    magnetic field gradient
    manofluorography
    middle frontal gyrus
    milk fat globule
    modified heat-degraded gelatin
MFGM
    milk fat globule membrane
MFH
    malignant fibrous histiocytoma
      (fibrohistiocytoma)
    membrane-free hemolysate
MFH-B
    malignant fibrous histiocytoma of bone
MFI
    malleable facial implant
    mean fluorescent intensity
    Multidimensional Fatigue Index
      (Inventory)
MFID
    multielectrode flame ionization detector
M-FISH
    multispectral fluorescent in situ
      hybridization
mFISP
    mirrored fast imaging with steady-state
      precession

MFLB
    macrofollicular lymphoblastoma
MFM
    magnetic force microscope (microscopy)
    maternal fetal medicine
    Millipore filter method
    multifidus muscle
MFMN
    multifocal motor neuropathy
MFO
    mixed function oxidase
MFP
    monofluorophosphate
    myofascial pain
MFPR
    multifetal pregnancy reduction
MFPS
    myofascial pain syndrome
MFPVC
    multifocal premature ventricular
      contraction
MFR
    mean flow rate
    midexpiratory flow rate
    midforceps rotation
    mucus flow rate
    myofascial release
MFRL
    maximal force at rest length
MFS
    maternal-fetal surgery
    maxillofacial surgery
    medical fear survey
    medical fee schedule
    merthiolate formaldehyde solution
      (*See also* MF)
    metastasis-free survival
    mitral first sound (*See also* M1)
    monofixation syndrome
MFSR
    maximum expiratory airflow-static lung
      elastic recoil pressure
MF/SS
    mycosis fungoides [and] Sézary
      syndrome
MFT
    medial femoral torsion
    multifocal atrial tachycardia
    muscle function test
MFU
    medical followup
MFVD
    midforceps vaginal delivery
MFVL
    maximum (maximal) flow-volume loop
MFVNS
    middle fossa vestibular nerve section

M

MFVPT
  Motor-Free Visual Perception Test
    (*See also* MVPT)
MFVR
  minimal forearm vascular resistance
MFW
  multiple fragment wounds
MG
  Marcus Gunn [pupil] (*See also* MGP)
  margin (*See also* marg)
  mean gradient
  medial gastrocnemius [muscle]
  membranous glomerulonephritis
    (*See also* MGN)
  membranous glomerulopathy
  menopausal gonadotropin
  mesiogingival
  methylglucoside
  methylguanidine
  Michaelis-Gutmann [body]
  Miller-Galante [total knee arthroplasty]
  minigastrin
  monoclonal gammopathy (*See also*
    MCG)
  monoglyceride
  mucigen granule
  mucous granule
  muscle group
  myasthenia gravis (*See also* MyG)
  myoglobin
M&G
  myringotomy and grommets
Mg
  magnesium
mG
  milligauss
mg
  milligram
mg%
  milligram percent
MGA
  malposition of the great arteries
  medical gas analyzer
MGAB
  mucous gland adenoma of bronchus
MGB
  medial geniculate body
Mgb
  myoglobulin
MGC
  megacolon
  minimal glomerular change
  multinucleated giant cell
MgC
  magnocellular neuroendocrine cell
MGCE
  multifocal giant cell encephalitis
MgCO₃
  magnesium carbonate

MGCT
  malignant giant cell tumor
  malignant glandular cell tumor
  mixed germ cell tumor
MGD
  maximal glucose disposal
  meibomian gland dysfunction
  mixed gonadal dysgenesis
  multiglandular disease
MGDF
  megakaryocyte growth and development
    factor
mg/dL
  milligram per deciliter
mg-el
  milligram-element
MGES
  multiple gated equilibrium scintigraphy
MGF
  macrophage growth factor
  mast cell growth factor
  maternal grandfather
MGG
  May-Grünwald-Giemsa [staining]
  molecular and general genetics
  mouse gamma globulin
  multinucleated giant cell
MGGM
  maternal great grandmother
MGH
  microglandular hyperplasia
  monoglyceride hydrolase
mg/h, mg-hr
  milligram per hour
MGHL
  middle glenohumeral ligament
MGI
  macrophage and granulocyte inducer
MGIT
  Mycobacteria growth indicator tube
MGJ
  mucogingival junction
mg/kg
  milligram per kilogram
mg/kg d
  milligram per kilogram per day
mg/kg hr
  milligram per kilogram per hour
MGL
  minor glomerular lesion
mg/L
  milligram per liter
MGM
  maternal grandmother
  meningioma
MGN
  medial geniculate nucleus
  membranous glomerulonephritis
    (*See also* MG)

MgO
magnesium oxide
MG/OL
molecular genetics/oncology laboratory
MGP
Marcus Gunn pupil (*See also* MG)
marginal (marginated) granulocyte pool
matrix Gla protein
medical group practice
membranous glomerulonephropathy
methyl green pyronin [dye]
mucinglycoprotein
mucous glycoprotein
MGPS
Marcus Gunn pupil sign
MGR
modified gain ratio
multiple gas rebreathing
murmurs, gallops, rubs
MGS
magnetic guidance system
malignant glandular schwannoma
metric gravitational system
MGSA
melanoma growth-stimulating
(stimulatory) activity
MGSD
mean gestational sac diameter
⚠ **MgSO₄**
magnesium sulfate [Epsom salt]
(*See also* mag sulf) ⚠
MGT
malignant glomus tumor
management
mgtis
meningitis
mgtt
minidrop [60 minidrops = 1 mL]
MGUS
monoclonal gammopathy of
undetermined (unknown)
significance
MGW
magnesium sulfate, glycerin, water
[enema]
multiple gunshot wounds
MGXT
multistage graded exercise test
mGy
milligray
MH
macular hemorrhage
macular hole
maintenance hemodialysis
maleic hydrazide
malignant histiocytosis
malignant hyperpyrexia

malignant hypertension
malignant hyperthermia
mammotropic hormone
mannoheptulose
marital history
medial hypothalamus
medical history
Medtronic-Hall [prosthesis]
melanophore-stimulating hormone
(*See also* MSH)
menstrual history
mental health
mental hygiene
mesothelial hyperplasia
moist heat
monosymptomatic hypochondriasis
multiple handicapped
murine hepatitis
mutant hybrid
Mycobacterium haemophilum
myohyoid
M-H
Mueller-Hinton [agar] (*See also*
MHA)
M/H
microcytic hypochromic [anemia]
Mh
mandible head
mH
millihenry
m/h
midbrain-hindbrain
MHA
major histocompatibility antigen
May-Hegglin anomaly
methemalbumin
microangiopathic hemolytic anemia
(*See also* MAHA)
microhemagglutination assay
middle hepatic artery
migraine headache
mixed hemadsorption
Mueller-Hinton agar (*See also* M-H)
MHAQ
Modified Health Assessment
Questionnaire
MHA-TP
microhemagglutination assay [for
antibodies to] *Treponema pallidum*
MHB
maximum (maximal) hospital benefit
mental health (insurance) benefit
MHb
medial habenular
myohemoglobin
MHBSS
modified Hanks balanced salt solution

M

MHC
major histocompatibility complex
maximal (maximum) hip circumference
mental health care
minor histocompatibility complex
multiphase (multiphasic) health checkup
myosin heavy chain

MHC I–II
major histocompatibility complex class
I–II

mhcp
mean horizontal candle power

m/hct
microhematocrit

MHD
maintenance hemodialysis
maximum (maximal) heart distance
maximum (maximal) human dose
mean hemolytic dose
minimum (minimal) hemolytic dilution
minimum (minimal) hemolytic dose

MHE
multiple hereditary exostosis

MHH
mental health hold

MHHP
Minnesota Heart Health Program

MHI
malignant histiocytosis of intestine
Mental Health Index
mild head injury

MHK
metaherpetic keratitis

MHL
maximum (maximal) heart length
moist heat pack

MHLC
Multidimensional Health Locus of
Control [scale]

MHLS
metabolic heat load stimulator

MH/MR
mental health and mental retardation

MHN
massive hepatic necrosis
Mohs hardness number
morbus hemolyticus neonatorum

MHNTG
multiheteronodular toxic goiter

MHO
microsomal heme oxygenase

mho
siemens [inverse of ohm]

MHOCE
multiple hereditary osteochondral
exostosis

MHP
hyperphenylalaninemia
maternal health program
monosymptomatic hypochondriacal
psychosis

MHPA
mild hyperphenylalaninemia
Minnesota-Hartford Personality Assay

M-HPC
meningeal hemangiopericytoma

MHPG
3-methoxy-4-hydroxyphenylglycol

MHR
major histocompatibility region
malignant hyperthermia resistance
maternal heart rate
maximum (maximal) heart rate
methemoglobin reductase (*See also* MR)

MHS
major histocompatibility system
malignant hyperthermia syndrome
malignant hypothermia susceptibility
monomethyl hydrogen sulfate
multiple health screening

MHSA
microaggregated human serum albumin

MHSC
multipotential (multipotent) hemopoietic
stem cell

MHST
multiphasic health screen test

MHT
malignant hypertension
meningohypophysial trunk
multiphasic health testing

MHTI
minor hypertensive infant

MHV
magnetic heart vector
Mahogany Hammock virus
mechanical heart valve
middle hepatic vein
minimal height velocity
mouse hepatitis virus

MHVD
Marek herpesvirus disease

MHW
medial heel wedge
metatarsal head width

MHx
medical history

MhxR
medical history review

MHz
megahertz

MI
magnetic-guided intubation
maturation index
meconium ileus
medical inspection
melanophore index
membrane intact

menstruation induction
mental illness
mental institution
mentally impaired
mesenteric ischemia
mesioincisal
metabolic index
methyl indole
microsatellite instability
migration index
migration inhibition
mild irritant
mitotic index
mitral incompetence
mitral insufficiency
mononucleosis infectiosa
morphology index
motility index
myocardial infarction
myocardial ischemia
myoinositol

M&I
maternal and infant [care]

mi
mile

MIA
medically indigent adult
melanoma inhibitory activity
missing in action
multiinstitutional arrangement
multiple intracranial aneurysms

MIAA
microaggregated albumin (*See also* MAA)

MIAD
mild idiopathic adulthood biliary ductopenia

MIAP
modified innervated antral pouch

MIB
minimally invasive biopsy

MIBB
minimally invasive breast biopsy

MIBE
measles inclusion body encephalitis

MIBG, mIBG
metaiodobenzylguanidine
metaiodobenzyl-guanidine

MIBI
methoxyisobutyl isonitrile

MIBI-SPECT
methoxyisobutyl isonitrile single-photon emission computed tomography

MIBK
methylisobutyl ketone

MIC
maternal and infant care

mean intercriterion correlation [statistics]
medical intensive care
methacholine inhalation challenge
microcytic erythrocyte
microinvasive carcinoma
microscope (microscopic)
minimal isorrheic concentration
minimum (minimal) inhibitory concentration
mobile intensive care
model immune complex

MICA
mentally ill chemical abuser
microinvasive cervical cancer
mirror-image complementary antibody

MICAB
minimally invasive coronary artery bypass

MICABG
minimally invasive coronary bypass grafting

MICE
mesothelial/monocytic incidental cardiac excrescence

MICG
macromolecular insoluble cold globulin

MICR
methacholine inhalation challenge response

Mi:Cr
myoinositol to creatine ratio

micro
microcyte
microcytic
microscopic [findings]

⚠ **μ**

chemical potential
dynamic viscosity
electrophoretic mobility
heavy chain of immunoglobulin M
micro- ⚠
micron
mutation rate
mu [12th letter of Greek alphabet lowercase] ⚠
permeability [magnetism]
population mean [statistics]

⚠ **μA**
microampere ⚠

micro-AVM
cerebral microarteriovenous malformation

μB
Bohr magneton

⚠ **μbar**
microbar ⚠

microbiol
microbiological
microbiology
⚠ **μC**
microcoulomb ⚠
⚠ **μCi**
microcurie ⚠
⚠ **μCi-hr**
microcurie-hour ⚠
microCT
micro computerized tomography
⚠ **μEq**
microequivalent ⚠
⚠ **μF**
microfarad ⚠
⚠ **μg**
microgram (*See also* mcg) ⚠
⚠ **μγ**
microgamma ⚠
⚠ **μg/kg**
microgram per kilogram ⚠
⚠ **μg/L**
microgram per liter ⚠
⚠ **μGy**
microgray ⚠
⚠ **μH**
microhenry ⚠
⚠ **μin**
microinch ⚠
⚠ **μIU**
one-millionth International Unit ⚠
⚠ **μkat**
microkatal [micromole per second]
(*See also* mcKat) ⚠
⚠ **μL**
microliter (*See also* λmcL) ⚠
⚠ **μM**
micromolar [concetration of solution
micromole per liter] (*See also*
μmol/L) ⚠
⚠ **μm**
micrometer ⚠
micromilli- ⚠
⚠ **μm³**
cubic micrometer ⚠
⚠ **μmg**
micromilligram [nanogram] (*See also*
ng) ⚠
⚠ **μmHg**
micrometer of mercury ⚠
⚠ **μμ**
micromicro- ⚠
micromicron ⚠
⚠ **μmm**
micromillimeter [nanometer] ⚠
⚠ **μμCi**
micromicrocurie [picocurie] (*See also*
pCi) ⚠

⚠ **μμF**
micromicrofarad [picofarad] (*See also*
pF) ⚠
⚠ **μμg**
micromicrogram [picogram] (*See also*
pg) ⚠
⚠ **μmol**
micromole (*See also* mcmol) ⚠
⚠ **μmol/L**
micromole per liter (*See also* μM) ⚠
⚠ **μN**
micronewton (*See also* mN) ⚠
⚠ **μΩ**
microhm ⚠
⚠ **μOsm**
micro-osmolar ⚠
⚠ **μR**
microroentgen ⚠
⚠ **μs**
microsecond (*See also* μsec) ⚠
⚠ **μsec**
microsecond (*See also* μs) ⚠
⚠ **μU**
microunit ⚠
⚠ **μV**
microvolt ⚠
⚠ **μW**
microwatt ⚠
MICS
microincision cataract surgery
minimally invasive cardiac surgery
Mother/Infant Communication
Screening
MID
maximum (maximal) inhibiting dilution
maximum (maximal) inhibiting duration
maximum (maximal) interincisal
distance
mesioincisodistal
microvillus inclusion disease
midinfarct dementia
minimum (minimal) infecting dose
minimum (minimal) infective dose
minimum (minimal) inhibitory dilution
minimum (minimal) inhibitory dose
minimum (minimal) irradiation dose
Modular Internal Distraction
[orthopedics]
multiinfarct dementia
multiple ion detection
mid
middle
midposition
mid/3
middle third [of long bone]
MIDA
mass isotopomer distribution analysis
myocardial ischemia dynamic analysis

MIDAS
microphthalmia, dermal aplasia, sclerocornea syndrome
Migraine Disability Assessment Scale
MIDCAB
minimally invasive direct coronary artery bypass
MIDCABG
minimally invasive direct coronary artery bypass graft
MIDD
maternally inherited diabetes and deafness
MID EPIS
midline episiotomy
MIDI
Microbial Identification System
Mid I
middle insomnia
midsag
midsagittal
MIE
maximim inspiratory effort
meconium ileus equivalent
medical improvement expected
methyl isoeugenol
MIEI
medication-induced esophageal injury
MIF
macrophage-inhibiting factor
maximum inspiratory flow
mean inspiratory flow
melanocyte-inhibiting factor
melanocyte[-stimulating hormone] inhibiting factor
merthiolate, iodine, formaldehyde [method]
merthiolate, iodine, formalin [solution]
methylene, iodine, formalin [solution]
microimmunofluorescence [test]
midinspiratory flow
migration-inhibiting (inhibition) (inhibitory) factor
mixed immunofluorescence
müllerian-inhibiting factor
MIFC
merthiolate, iodine, formaldehyde concentration
minimally invasive follicular carcinoma
MIFR
maximal inspiratory flow rate
midinspiratory flow rate
MIFT
merthiolate, iodine, formaldehyde technique
MIF 50%VC
midinspiratory flow at 50% of vital capacity

MIg
malaria immunoglobulin
measles immunoglobulin
membrane immunoglobulin
MIGET
multiple inert gas elimination technique
MIGW
maximal increment in growth and weight
MIH
medication-induced headache
melanotropin release-inhibiting hormone
migraine with interparoxysmal headache
minimal intermittent [dosage of] heparin
monoiodohistidine
müllerian-inhibiting (inhibitory) hormone
myointimal hyperplasia
MIHR
magnetically influenced homeopathic remedy
MII
McDowell Impairment Index
Mobile Image Intensifier
MIIO
minimally invasive intraoperative osteosynthesis
Mik
Mikulicz [disease, clamp]
MIKA
minor karyotype abnormality
MIKE
mass-analyzed ion kinetic energy
MIL
mesial incisal lingual [surface]
military
mother-in-law (See also M/L)
MiLIF
minimally invasive lumbar interbody fusion
MILMD
Management Inventory on Leadership, Motivation and Decision-Making
MILP
mitogen-induced lymphocyte proliferation
MILS
medication information leaflet for seniors
MILTA
mucosal intact laser tonsillar ablation
MIM
Mendelian Inheritance in Man
MIMCOM
multimode imaging confocal optical microscope
MIME
mean indices of meal excursions

MIMIC
multivane intensity modulation compensator
MIMS
Medical Information Management System
Medical Inventory Management System
MIMV
Maferr Inventory of Masculine Values
MIMyCA
maternally inherited myopathy and cardiomyopathy
MIN
mammary intraepithelial neoplasia
medial interlaminar nucleus
melanocytic intraepidermal neoplasia
microsatellite instability
mineral
minimal
minimum (*See also* M)
minor
minute (*See also* min, M, m)
multiple intestinal neoplasia
min
minim (pharmacology)
minute (*See also* MIN, M, m)
MINA
monoisonitrosoacetone
MIN A
minimal assistance (assist)
Mincep
Minnesota Comprehensive Epilepsy Program
MINE
medical improvement not expected
MINI
Mini International Neuropsychiatric Interview
MINIA
monkey intranuclear inclusion agent
mini-allo
mini allographic stem cell transplant(ation)
mini-FES
mini functional endoscopic sinus
minilap, mini-lap
minilaparotomy
mini-MUD
mini matched unrelated donor [stem cell transplant(ation)]
minIP
minimal intensity projection
MINV
Minnal virus
MIO
minimal identifiable odor
monocular indirect ophthalmoscopy
MION
monocrystalline iron oxide

MIOP
magnetic iron oxide particle
MIP
macrophage inflammatory protein
maximum (maximal) inspiratory pressure
maximum-intensity pixel
maximum-intensity projection [radiology]
mean intrathoracic pressure
mean intravascular pressure
medical improvement possible
megameatus intact prepuce
membrane integral protein
metacarpointerphalangeal
middle interphalangeal [joint]
minimal inspiratory pressure
minimally invasive procedure
MIP-1
macrophage inflammatory protein 1
MIP-1 alpha (α)
macrophage inflammatory protein 1 alpha (α)
MIP-1 beta (β)
macrophage inflammatory protein 1 beta (β)
MIP-2
macrophage inflammatory protein 2
mip
macrophage infectivity potentiator
MIPcor
coronal maximum-intensity projection
MIPI
mean interpotential interval
MIPO
minimally invasive plate osteosynthesis
MIPS
myocardial isotopic perfusion scan
MIQ
Minnesota Importance Questionnaire
MIR
mastectomy with immediate reconstruction
middle infrared
multiple isomorphous replacement
MIRBI
Mini Inventory of Right Brain Injury
MIRD
medical internal radiation dose (dosimetry)
MIRF
macrophage immunogenic antigen-recruiting factor
MIRI
myocardial infarction recovery index
MIRP
myocardial infarction rehabilitation program
MIRS
Medical Improvement Review Standard

MIRU
 myocardial infarction research unit
MIRV
 Mirim virus
MIS
 macrophage inflammatory protein
 management information system
 Medical Information Service
 meiosis-inducing substance
 melanoma in situ
 microbial identification system
 minimally invasive surgery
 minimum incision surgery
 miscarriage
 mitral insufficiency
 moderate intermittent suction
 müllerian-inhibiting substance
MISA
 mentally ill and substance abusing
misc
 miscarriage
 miscellaneous
M Isch
 myocardial ischemia
MISG
 modified immune serum globulin
MISH
 multiple in situ hybridization
MISHAP
 microphallus, imperforate [anus],
 syndactyly, hamartoblastoma, abnormal
 [lung lobulation] polydactyly
MISS
 minimally invasive spine surgery
 modified injury severity score [scale]
MIST
 Medical Information Service by
 Telephone
 minimally invasive surgical technique
MIT
 magnetic induction tomography
 male impotence test
 marrow iron turnover
 mean input time
 meconium in trachea
 melodic intonation therapy
 metabolic intolerance test
 metabolism inhibition test
 migration inhibition test
 miracidial immobilization test
 monoiodinated tyrosine
 (monoiodotyrosine)
 Motor Impersistence Test
 multiple injection therapy [of
 insulin]
mit
 mitral

MITF
 microphthalmia-associated transcription
 factor
MITF-M
 melanocyte specific
 microphthalmia-associated transcription
 factor (MITF)
MITGCN
 malignant intratubular germ-cell
 neoplasia
MITI
 myocardial infarction triage and
 intervention
mit insuf
 mitral insufficiency
MITT
 minimally invasive thermal therapy
MIU
 million International Units
mIU
 milli-International Unit [one-thousandth
 of an International Unit]
MIV
 major injury vector
MIVAP
 minimally invasive video-assisted
 parathyroidectomy
MIVE
 Maastricht Interview on Vital
 Exhaustion
 maximum isometric voluntary exercise
MIVF
 maximum isometric voluntary flexion
MIVOD
 mesenteric inflammatory venoocclusive
 disease
MIVP
 mean intravascular pressure
MIVR
 minimally invasive valve repair
 (replacement)
MIW
 mental inquest warrant
MIX
 methylisobutylxanthine
mix.
 mixture (*See also* M, m., mixt, mx)
mix. mon
 mixed monitor
mixt
 mixture (*See also* M, m., mix., mx)
MJ
 marijuana (*See also* POT)
 medial joint
 megajoule
mJ
 millijoule

M

MJA
mechanical joint apparatus
MJAD
Machado-Joseph Azorean disease
MJDQ
Minnesota Job Description Questionnaire
MJI
mid-joint injury
MJL
medial joint line
MJS
medial joint space
MJT
Mead Johnson tube
Mowlem-Jackson technique
MK
marked
menaquinone [vitamin K_2] (*See also* MQ)
monkey kidney (*See also* MkK)
myokinase
M-K
McCarey-Kaufman [medium]
Mk
monkey (*See also* M)
MKAB
may keep at bedside
MKAS
Meyer-Kendall Assessment Survey
mkat
millikatal
mkat/L
millikatal per liter
MKB
married, keeping baby
megakaryoblast
MKC
monkey kidney cell
MK-CSF
megakaryocyte colony-stimulating factor
mkg
meter-kilogram
MKHS
Menkes kinky hair syndrome
MKI
mitosis-karyorrhexis index
MkK
monkey kidney (*See also* MK)
MKM
myopic keratomileusis
MKP
monobasic potassium phosphate
MKP-1
mitogen-activated protein kinase phosphatase 1
mks
meter-kilogram-second [system of measurement]

MKSAP
Medical Knowledge Self-Assessment Program
MKTC
monkey kidney tissue culture
MKV
killed measles vaccine
M-L
Martin-Lewis [medium]
ML
main line [intravenous]
malignant lymphoma
marked latency
maximal left
mediolateral
meningeal leukemia
mesiolingual
middle lobe
midline
molecular layer
monocytoid lymphocyte
motor latency
mucolipidosis
mucosal leishmaniasis
multiple lentiginosis
muscular layer
myeloid leukemia
ML I–IV
mucolipidosis type I–IV
M:L
maltase to lactase ratio
monocyte to lymphocyte ratio
mL
millilambert
milliliter (*See also* mLa, mLb)
ml
midline
MLA
left mentum anterior [mentoanterior] [fetal position] [L. *mento-laeva anterior*] (*See also* LMA)
medical laboratory assay
medium long-acting
mesenteric lymphadenitis
monocytic leukemia, acute
multilanguage aphasia
MLa
mesiolabial (*See also* MLA)
mLa
millilumbert (*See also* mL, mLb)
MLAB
Multilingual Aphasia Battery
MLAC
minimum local analgesic concentration
MLAEP
middle latency (midlatency) auditory evoked potential
MLAER
middle latency auditory evoked response

MLaI
mesiolabioincisal
MLAP
mean left atrial pressure
MLaP
mesiolabiopulpal
MLB
midline bar
monaural loudness balance [test]
MLb
macrolymphoblast
mLb
millilumbert (*See also* mL, mLa)
MLBP
mechanical low back pain
MLBW
moderately low birth weight
MLC
chronic myelomonocytic leukemia
Marginal Line Calculus (Index)
mesiolingual cusp
metastatic liver cancer
minimum (minimal) lethal concentration
mixed leukocyte (lymphocyte) concentration
mixed leukocyte (lymphocyte) culture
mixed ligand chelate
morphinelike compound
multilamellar cytosome
multileaf collimator
multilevel care
multilumen catheter
myosin light chain
MLCI
marginal line calculus index
MLCK
myosin light chain kinase
MLCN
multilocular cystic nephroma
MLCP
myosin light chain phosphatase
MLCR
mesiolingual cusp ridge
mixed lymphocyte culture reaction
MLCT
metal-to-ligand charge transfer
ML-CVP
multilumen central venous pressure
MLCW
mixed lymphocyte culture, weak
MLD
manual lymph drainage
masking level difference
mean luminal diameter
median lethal dose (*See also* LD$_{50}$)
melioidosis [*Pseudomonas pseudomallei*] vaccine

metachromatic leukodystrophy
microlumbar discectomy
microsurgical lumbar discectomy
minimal lesion disease
minimum (minimal) lethal dose
minimum (minimal) lumen (luminal) diameter
MLDG
mesiolingual developmental groove
mL/dL
milliliter per deciliter
MLE
maximal likelihood estimation
midline episiotomy (*See also* MLEpis)
MLEE
multilocus enzyme electrophoresis
MLEpis
mediolateral episiotomy
midline episiotomy (*See also* MLE)
MLF
medial longitudinal fasciculus
mesiolingual fossa
morphinelike factor
MLG
membranous lupus glomerulonephritis
mesiolingual groove
mitochondria lipid glucogen
MLGN
minimal lesion glomerulonephritis
MLH
malignant lymphoma, histiocytic
multiple lobar hemorrhage
MLH1
human mismatch-repair protein MutL homolog
MLI
mesiolinguoincisal
mixed lymphocyte interaction
motilin-like immunoreactivity
mL/kg
milliliter per kilogram
MLL
malignant lymphoma, lymphoblastic (type)
mixed lineage leukemia
mL/L
milliliter per liter
mL/min
milliliter per minute
MLN
manifest latent nystagmus
mediastinal lymph node
membranous lupus nephropathy
mesenteric lymph node
mucocutaneous lymph node

M

MLNS
 minimal lesions nephrotic syndrome
 mucocutaneous lymph node syndrome
MLO
 mediolateral oblique
 mesiolinguo-occlusal
MLP
 left mentum posterior (mentoposterior)
 [fetal position] [L. *mento-laeva*
 posterior] (*See also* LMP)
 mesiolinguopulpal
 microsomal lipoprotein
 midlevel provider
 multiple lymphomatous polyposis
ML-PCR
 mixed-linker polymerase chain reaction
MLPD
 malignant lymphocytic proliferation
 disease
MLPP
 maximum loose-packed position
MLQ
 Multifactor Leadership Questionnaire
MLR
 major liver resection
 mean length of response
 middle latency response
 mixed leukocyte (lymphocyte) reaction
 mixed leukocyte (lymphocyte) response
 multiple logistic regression
 myocardial laser revascularization
MLRA
 multiple linear regression analysis
mlRNA
 messenger-like ribonucleic acid
MLS
 macrolides, lincosamides, streptogramins
 [resistance to]
 maxillary lymphosarcoma
 maximum likelihood score
 mean life span
 median life span
 median longitudinal section
 mediastinal B-cell lymphoma with
 sclerosis
 microphthalmia with linear skin defects
 middle lobe syndrome
 mini lag screw system
 multiple line scan
mL/sec
 milliliter per second
MLSI
 multiple line-scan imaging
MLST
 multilocus sequence typing
MLT
 mean latency time
 median lethal time
 melatonin

MLTC
 mixed leukocyte-trophoblast culture
 mixed lymphocyte-tumor culture
MLTI
 mixed lymphocyte target interaction
MLU
 mean length of utterance
MLUm
 mean length of utterance in morphemes
MLV
 monitored live voice
 Mono Lake virus
 multilaminar vesicle
 murine leukemia virus
MLVA
 multilocus variable number tandem
 repeat [VNTR] analysis
MLVDP
 maximal left ventricular developed
 pressure
MLWHF
 Minnesota Living with Heart Failure
 [questionnaire]
mlx
 millilux
MM
 macromolecule
 major medical [insurance]
 malignant melanoma
 malignant mesothelioma
 malignant myeloma
 manubrium of malleus
 Marshall-Marchetti [procedure for
 urinary incontinence]
 measuring-mounting
 medial malleolus
 mediastinal mass
 megamitochondria
 melanoma metastasis
 member months
 meningococcic meningitis
 metastatic melanoma
 methadone maintenance
 micrometastases
 middle molecule
 milk and molasses (*See also* M&M)
 minimal medium
 mismatch
 mist mask
 modified Miller maneuver
 [skull base]
 morbidity and mortality (*See also*
 M&M)
 motor meal
 mucous membrane
 Muller maneuver [airway]
 multiple myeloma
 muscle movement
 muscularis mucosae

myeloid metaplasia
myelomeningocele

MMI

maternal meiosis I

MMII

maternal meiosis II

M&M

Magenstrasse and Mill [operation for
obesity]
milk and molasses (*See also* MM)
morbidity and mortality (*See also* MM)

mM

millimolar [millimole per liter] [non-SI]
(*See also* mmol/L)

mm

methylmalonyl
millimeter
mucous membrane
murmur
muscles [plural] (*See also* ms)

mm²

square millimeter (*See also* sq mm)

mm³

cubic millimeter (*See also*
cmm, cu mm)

MMA

mastitis, metritis, agalactia [syndrome]
maxillomandibular advancement
medical materials account
methylmalonic acid(uria)
methylmercuric acetate
methyl methacrylate (*See also* MEMA)
middle meningeal artery
monocyte monolayer assay
monomethylarsonic acid

MMAA

mini-microaggregated albumin colloid

MMAD

mass median aerodynamic diameter

MMAP

Maine Medical Assessment Program
mean maternal arterial blood pressure

MMAT

Minnesota Mechanical Assembly Test

MMATP

methadone maintenance and aftercare
treatment program

MMC

mechanical myocardial channeling
migrating motor complex
migrating myoelectric complex
minimal medullary concentration
mucosal mast cell
murine mesangial cell
myelomeningocele

mMCAI

malignant middle cerebral artery
infarct(ion)

MMCM

macromolecular contrast medium

MMD

intramural microvessel density
malignant metastatic disease
mass median diameter [of particles]
mean marrow dose
minimal morbidostatic dose
moyamoya disease
mucous membranes dry
myotonic muscular dystrophy (*See also*
MyMD)

MMDA

5-methoxy-3,4-
methylenedioxyamphetamine
methyoxymethylene dioxyamphetamine

MMDG

mesial marginal developmental groove

MME

malignant myoepithelioma
membrane metalloendopeptidase
M-mode echocardiography
mouse mammary epithelium

MMECT

multiple monitored (multimonitored)
electroconvulsive therapy

MMEF

maximum midexpiratory flow (*See also*
MMF)

MMEFR

maximal midexpiratory flow rate
(*See also* MMFR)

MMEP

microcephaly, microphthalmia,
ectrodactyly, prognathism [syndrome]

MMF

mandibulomaxillary fixation
maxillomandibular fixation
maximal midexpiratory flow (*See also*
MMEF)
mean maximal flow

MMFG

mouse milk fat globule

MMFR

maximum (maximal) midexpiratory flow
rate (*See also* MMEFR)

MMFV

maximum (maximal) midexpiratory flow
volume

MMG

mammograph(y) (mammogram) (*See also*
MAM, mammo)
mean maternal glucose
mechanomyography

MMH

Marino and Muller-Hermelink [thymic
tumor classification]
monomethylhydrazine

M

mmHg
millimeter of mercury
mmH₂O
millimeter of water

$$mmH_2O$$

MMI
macrophage migration index
macrophage migration inhibition
maximal medical improvement
maximum medical improvement
medial medullary infarction
methylmercaptoimidazole

⚠ **mμ**
millimicron [obsolete] ⚠

MMIF
macrophage migration inhibition
(inhibitory) factor

MMIH
megacystis, microcolon, intestinal
hypoperistalsis

MMIHS
megacystis, microcolon, intestinal
hypoperistalsis syndrome

MMK
Marshall-Marchetti-Krantz
[cystourethropexy]

MML
minimum masking level
monomethyllysine

MMLV
Montana myotis leukoencephalitis
virus

MMM
metastatic malignant melanoma
microsome-mediated mutagenesis
mucous membranes moist
myelofibrosis with myeloid metaplasia
myeloid metaplasia with myelofibrosis
myelosclerosis with myeloid
metaplasia

MMMF
man-made mineral fiber

MMMM
megalocornea, macrocephaly, mental
motor retardation syndrome

mMMSE
modified version of mini mental status
examination

MMMT
malignant mixed mesodermal
tumor
malignant mixed müllerian tumor
metastatic mixed müllerian tumor

MMN
mismatch negativity
morbus maculosus neonatorum
multifocal motor neuropathy
multiple mucosal neuroma

MMNC
marrow mononuclear cell

MMO
maxillomandibular osteotomy
maximal mouth opening
methane monooxygenase

MMOA
maxillary mandibular odentectomy
alveolectomy

M-mode
time-motion mode [ultrasound]

mmol
millimole

mmol/L
millimole per liter [millimolar] (*See also*
mM)

MMP
matrix metalloprotease
(metalloproteinase)
maximum maintained pressure
multiple medical problems
multiplexed molecular profiling

MMP-1–MMP-28
matrix metalloproteinase 1–28

MMPC
metastatic malignant pheochromocytoma

MMPI
matrix metalloproteinase inhibitor
McGill-Melzack Pain Index
Minnesota Multiphasic Personality
Inventory

MMPI-2
Minnesota Multiphasic Personality
Inventory, Second Edition

MMPI-A
Minnesota Multiphasic Personality
Inventory Adolescent

MMPI-D
Minnesota Multiphasic Personality
Inventory Depression [Scale]

mmpp
millimeter [of] partial pressure

mm-PTH
midmolecule parathyroid hormone

MMR
masseter muscle rigidity
mass miniature radiography
(roentgenography)
maternal mortality rate
measles, mumps, rubella [vaccine]
megalocornea-mental retardation
syndrome
meningitis [or encephalitis] metabolic,
Reye [syndrome]
mesial marginal ridge
midline malignant reticulosis
mild mental retardation
mismatch repair
mobile mass x-ray
mortality rate ratio
mouth-to-mouth resuscitation

mutation mismatch repair
myocardial metabolic rate
MMRS
metropolitan medical response system
MMRSA
mupirocin-resistant, methicillin-resistant
Staphylococcus aureus
MMR-VAR
measles, mumps, rubella, varicella
vaccine
MMS
Maloney murine sarcoma
methyl methanesulfonate
Mini-Mental State [examination]
mixed mesodermal sarcoma
Mohs micrographic surgery
MMSE
Mini Mental State Examination
mm/sec
millimeter per second
MMSP
malignant melanoma of soft parts
mm st
muscles [plural] strength
MMT
malignant mesenchymal tumor
malignant mixed tumor
manual muscle test(ing)
meal tolerance test
medial meniscal tear
methadone maintenance treatment
microcephaly, mesobrachyphalangy,
tracheoesophageal fistula [syndrome]
Mini-Mental Test
mixed müllerian tumor
mouse mammary tumor
MMTC
mitomycin C trabeculectomy
MMTIC
Murphy-Meisgeier Type Indicator for
Children
MMTP
methadone maintenance treatment
program
MMTT
Multicenter Myocarditis Treatment Trial
MMTV
malignant mesothelioma of tunica
vaginalis
monomorphic ventricular tachycardia
mouse mammary tumor virus
MMUA
macromolecular uronate
⚠ **mμc**
millimicrocurie [obsolete, use nano-] ⚠
⚠ **mμg**
millimicrogram [obsolete, use nano-] ⚠

MMUS
multiple medically unexplained
symptoms
⚠ **mμs**
millimicrosecond [obsolete, use nano-] ⚠
MMV
mandatory minute ventilation
mandatory minute volume
MMVD
mixed mitral valve disease
MMVF
manmade vitreous fiber
MMVT
monomorphic ventricular tachycardia
MMWR
Morbidity and Mortality Weekly
Report
MMY
Mental Measurements Yearbook
MN
blood group in MNS blood group
system
malignant nephrosclerosis
median nerve
meganewton
melanocytic nevus
melena neonatorum
membranous nephropathy
membranous neuropathy
mesenteric node
metanephrine
micronucleated (micronucleus)
midnight (*See also* M/N)
mononuclear
motor neuron
mucosal neurolysis
multinodular
myoneural
M/N
macrocytic/normochromic [anemia]
microcytic/normochromic [anemia]
midnight (*See also* MN)
M&N
morning and night
Mn
manganese
mN
millinormal
MNA
maximal noise area
mean nuclear area
MNAP
mixed nerve action potential
MNB
monomicrobial nonneutrocytic
bacterascites
murine neuroblastoma

M

MNBCC
  multiple nevoid-basal cell carcinoma
MNC
  monomicrobial necrotizing cellulitis
  mononuclear cell
MNCV
  motor nerve conduction velocity
MND
  maxillonasal dysplasia
  minimal necrosing dose
  minimum (minimal) necrotizing dose
  minor neurologic dysfunction
  modified neck dissection
  motor neuron disease
MnDPDP
  mangafodipir trisodium [imaging agent]
MNE
  monosymptomatic nocturnal enuresis
MNF
  myelinated nerve fiber
MNG
  multinodular goiter
mng
  morning (*See also* man.)
MNG/CRD/DA
  multinodular goiter, cystic renal disease,
  digital anomalies [syndrome]
MNGIE
  mitochondrial neurogastrointestinal
  encephalomyopathy
  myoneuro-gastrointestinal encephalopathy
MNHL
  mixed large- and small-cell
  non-Hodgkin lymphoma
MNJ
  myoneural junction
MNL
  maximal number of lamellae
  mononuclear leukocyte (*See also* MNC)
MNM
  mononeuritis multiplex
MN/m²
  meganewton per square meter
MNMCB
  motor neuropathy with multifocal
  conduction block
MNMK
  maximal number of microbes killed
MNMS
  myonephropathic metabolic syndrome
MNNB
  Monas-Nitz Neuropsychological Battery
MNOE
  malignant necrotizing otitis externa
MNP
  malignant neoplasm
  mononuclear phagocyte
MNPA
  methoxynaphthyl propionic acid

MNPRT
  mixed neutron and photon radiotherapy
MNPV
  multiple nucleopolyhedrovirus
MNR
  marrow neutrophil reserve
MNRH
  may not require hospitalization
MNS
  blood group system consisting of
  groups M, N, and MN
  mean nocturnal saturation
  medial nuclear stratum
  microamperage neural stimulation
MNSER
  mean normalized systolic ejection
  rate
Mn-SOD
  manganese superoxide dismutase
MnSSEP
  median nerve somatosensory evoked
  potential
MNTB
  medial nucleus of trapezoid body
MNTBV
  Manitoba virus
MNTD
  maximum nontoxic dose
MNTI
  melanotic neuroectodermal tumor of
  infancy
Mn-TPPS₄
  manganese tetrasodium-meso-tetra
MNTV
  Minatitlan virus
MNX
  meniscectomy
MO
  manually operated
  medial oblique [x-ray view]
  menhaden oil
  mesioocclusal
  mineral oil
  minute output
  mitral orifice (opening)
  mode
  molecular orbital
  monoclonal (*See also* M)
  monooxygenase
  month (*See also* M, mo, mon)
  months old (*See also* mo)
  morbidly obese
  morbid obesity
  mother (*See also* M, MOM, MTR)
  myositis ossificans
M/O
  morning of
MO₂
  myocardial oxygen [consumption]

Mo
Moloney [strain]
molybdenum
⁹⁹Mo
molybdenum-99
mo
mode
month (*See also* M, MO, mon)
months old (*See also* MO)
MOA
mechanism of action
monoamine oxidase
MoAb
monoclonal antibody (*See also* MA, MAb)
MOAHI
mixed obstructive apnea and hypopnea index
MOAS
modified overt aggression scale
mob, mobil
mobility
mobilization
MOBV
Mobala virus
MOC
maximum (maximal) oxygen concentration
medial olivocochlear
mother of child
multiple ocular colobomas
multiple osteochondromatosis
MOCI
Maudsley Obsessional Compulsive Inventory
MoCM
molybdenum-conditioned medium
MOCNI
method of collection not indicated
MOCS-III
Minnesota Occupational Classification System III
MOD
maturity-onset diabetes (*See also* MODM)
mean optical density
mesial, occlusal, distal (mesioocclusodistal)
mode of death
moderate (*See also* mod)
moment of death
Multi-Operatory Dentalaser
multiple organ (multiorgan) dysfunction
mod
moderate (*See also* MOD)
moderation
modification

modify (modified)
modulation
module
MOD A
moderate assistance (assist)
ModAMeX
modified acetone methylbenzoate xylene
MODED
microcephaly, oculodigital, esophageal, duodenal syndrome
MODEMS
Musculoskeletal Outcomes Data Evaluation and Management Scale
MODI
modified independent [atom molecule]
MODM
maturity-onset diabetes mellitus (*See also* MOD)
MODS
multiple organ (multiorgan) dysfunction syndrome
MODV
Modoc virus
MODY
mature-onset diabetes of young (youth)
MOE
movement of extremities
MOEM
microoptoelectromechanical system
MOF
marine oxidation/fermentation
mesial occlusal facial
multiple (multiorgan) organ failure
MOFE
multiple organ failure in elderly
MOFS
multiple organ failure syndrome
MOG
myelin-oligodendrocyte glycoprotein
MOH
medication overuse headache
MOI
maximal oxygen intake
mechanism of injury
medical optimal imaging
multiplicities of infection
MOIOD
medial osseous interorbital distance
MOIVC
membranous obstruction of inferior vena cava
MOJAC
mood, orientation, judgment, affect, content
MOJUV
Moju virus

M

MOKV
Mokola virus
MOL
method of limits [perception test]
molecular layer
mol
mole [SI base unit of amount of
substance] (*See also* M)
molecular (*See also* M)
molecule
molc
molar concentration [mol/L, molar]
(*See also* M, mol/L)
MOLDR
mathematical optimization and logical
dimensioning for radiotherapy
molfr
mole fraction
mol/kg
mole per kilogram (molality)
mol/L
mole per liter (molar) (*See also* M,
molc)
mol/m³
mole per cubic meter
mol/s
mole per second
mol wt
molecular weight
MOM
milk of magnesia
modifier of Min [locus]
mother (*See also* M, MO, MTR)
mucoid otitis media
multiples of median [gestational
age]
MOMA
methoxyhydroxymandelic acid
MOMO
macrosomia, obesity, macrocephaly,
ocular abnormality [syndrome]
Mo-Mo
molybdenum-molybdenum [target filter
combination]
MoMLV
Moloney murine leukemia virus
MO-MOM
mineral oil and milk of magnesia
MOMP
major outer membrane protein
MOMS
multiple organ malrotation
syndrome
MOMSV
Moloney murine sarcoma virus
MOMX
macroorchidism marker X
MON
maximum observation nursery

Mongolian [gerbil]
monitor
mon
monocyte (*See also* M, MONO, mono,
monos)
month (*See also* M, MO, mo)
MONO, mono
monocyte (*See also* M, monos)
[infectious] mononucleosis (*See also* IM,
INFM, inf mono)
mono, di
monochorionic, diamniotic [twins]
mono, mono
monochorionic, monoamniotic (twins)
monos
monocytes (*See also* M, mon, MONO,
mono)
MOP
major organ profile
medical outpatient
medical outpatient program
MOPP
minimum mission-oriented protective
posture
MOPV
monovalent oral polio vaccine
MORA
mandibular orthopedic repositioning
appliance
MORD
magnetic optical rotatory dispersion
MORFAN
mental [retardation], overgrowth,
remarkable face, acanthosis nigrans
Mo-Rh
molybdenum-rhodium [target filter
combination]
morph
morphine
morphologic(al) (morphology) (*See also*
morphol)
morphol
morphologic(al) (morphology) (*See also*
morph)
mortal.
mortality
MORV
Moriche virus
MOS
medial orbital sulcus
medical optical spectroscopy
medical outcomes study
metal oxide semiconductor
mirror optical system
missed ostium sequence
mitral opening snap
myelofibrosis osteosclerosis
mos
months [plural]

MOSD
multiple organ [multiorgan] system dysfunction

MOSES
Multidimensional Observational Scale for Elderly Subjects

MOSF
multiple (multiorgan) organ system failure

MOSFET
metal oxide semiconductor field effect transistor

mOsm
milliosmole

mOsm/kg
milliosmole per kilogram

MOSP
myelin/oligodendrocyte-specific protein

MOSS
moral objections to suicide scale

MOST
manual organ stimulation technique
Modern Occupational Skills Test

MOSV
Mossuril virus

MOT
mini object test
motility
mouse ovarian tumor

MOTA
Manitoba oculotrichoanal [syndrome]

MOTS
mucosal oral therapeutic system

MOTSA
multiple overlapped thin slab acquisition

MOTT
mycobacteria other than tubercle (*Mycobacterium tuberculosis*)

MOU
memorandum of understanding

MOV
minimum obstructive volume
multiple oral vitamin

MOVC
membranous obstruction [of inferior] vena cava

MOW
Meals on Wheels

MP
machine preservation
macrophage
magnetization prepared
malignant pyoderma
matrix protein
mean pressure
mechanical percussion (percussor)

medial plantar
melting point
membrane potential
menstrual period
mentum posterior (mentoposterior) [fetal position]
mesenteric panniculitis
mesial pit
mesiopulpal
metacarpophalangeal [joint] (*See also* MCP, MCPJ, MPJ)
metatarsophalangeal [joint] (*See also* MPJ, MTP, MTPJ)
Mibelli porokeratosis
microfibrillar protein
middle phalanx
minimal pigment
minipool
modulator protein
moist pack
monitor pattern
monophasic
monophosphate
motor potential
mouthpiece
mouth pressure
mucopolysaccharide (*See also* MPS)
multiparous (*See also* multip)
multiprogrammable pacemaker
muscle potential
mycoplasmal pneumonia
myocardial perfusion

mp
melting point
millipond [metric unit of force]

MPA
main pulmonary artery
mean pulmonary arterial [pressure]
medial preoptic area
metatarsus primus adductus
microscopic polyangiitis
microstomia prevention appliance
minor physical anomaly
multiple progressive angioma

MPa
megapascal [metric unit of pressure or stress]

MPAA
male pattern androgenetic alopecia

MPAC
Memorial Pain Assessment Card

MPAI-3
Mayo-Portland Adaptability Inventory 3

MPAP
mean pulmonary artery pressure
multipurpose access port

M

MPAPC
mucus-producing adenopapillary carcinoma
MPAQ
McGill Pain Assessment Questionnaire
MPAWP
mean pulmonary artery wedge pressure
MPB
male pattern baldness
modified piggyback
MPBFV
mean pulmonary-blood-flow velocity
MPBNS
modified Peyronie bladder neck suspension
MPC
marine protein concentrate
marker for prostatic cancer
maximum (maximal) permissible concentration
membrane peeler cutter
metallophthalocyanine
micropapillary component
minimum (minimal) protozoacidal concentration
Mooney Problem Checklist
mucopurulent cervicitis
myeloblast-promyelocyte compartment
MPCD
metaphysial chondrodysplasia
minimal perceptible color difference
MPCh
medial posterior choroidal artery [ophthalmology]
MPCN
microscopically positive, culturally negative
MPCO
micropolycystic ovary [syndrome]
MPCP
mean pulmonary capillary pressure
M-PCR
multiplex polymerase chain reaction
MPCUR
maximal permissible concentration of unidentified radionuclides
MPCWP
mean pulmonary capillary wedge pressure
MPD
main pancreatic duct
main papillary duct
matched peripheral dose
maximum (maximal) permissible dose
mean population doubling
Measures of Psychosocial Development
membrane potential difference
minimum (minimal) perceptible difference

minimum (minimal) peripheral dose
minimum (minimal) phototoxic dose
minimum (minimal) popular dose
minimum (minimal) port diameter
Minnesota Percepto-Diagnostic [Test] (*See also* MPDT)
moisture permeable dressing
multiplanar display
multiple personality disorder
myeloproliferative disease
myofascial pain-dysfunction
MPDE
maximum (maximal) permissible dose equivalent
MPDS
mandibular pain dysfunction syndrome
myofascial pain dysfunction syndrome
MPDT
Minnesota Percepto-Diagnostic Test (*See also* MPD)
MPDW
mean percentage of desirable weight
MPE
malignant pleural effusion
malignant proliferation of eosinophils
massive pulmonary embolism
maximum (maximal) possible effect
maximum (maximal) possible error
maximum (maximal) permissible exposure
mean prediction error
multiphoton excitation
MPEAK
multipeak
MPEC
monopolar electrocoagulation
multipolar electrocoagulation
MPED
minimal phototoxic erythema dose
MPF
major proglucagon fragment
maturation-promoting factor
mean power frequency
methylparaben free
mitosis-promoting factor
MPFBT
Minnesota Paper Form Board Test
MPFF
micronized purified flavonoid fraction
MPFL
medial patellofemoral ligament
MPFM
mini-Wright peak flow meter
MPG
magnetopneumography
malignant paraganglioma
MPGM
monophosphoglycerate mutase

MPGN
    membranoproliferative glomerulonephritis
    [type I, II]
    mesangiocapillary glomerulonephritis
    [type I, II]
MPGR
    multiplanar gradient recall(ed) [magnetic
    resonance]
MP-H
    mandibular plane to hyoid
    [craniometric]
MPH
    macular pseudohole
    male pseudohermaphroditism
    massive pulmonary hemorrhage
    micronodular pneumocyte hyperplasia
    midparental height
    milk protein hydrolysate
mph
    mile per hour
M phase
    phase of mitosis in cell growth cycle
MPHD
    methoxy hydroxyphenol glycerol
    multiple pituitary hormone deficiencies
MPHR
    maximum (maximal) predicted heart
    rate
MPI
    mannose phosphate isomerase
    master patient index
    Maudsley Personality Inventory
    maximum (maximal) permitted intake
    maximum (maximal) point of impulse
    milk product intolerance
    Multidimensional Pain Inventory
    Multiphasic Personality Inventory
    Multivariate Personality Inventory
    myocardial perfusion imaging
MPIAS
    multiparameter intraarterial sensor
MPIF
    myeloid progenitor inhibitory factor
MPIF-1
    myeloid progenitor inhibitory factor 1
M6P/IGF-2R
    mannose-6-phosphate/IGF-2 receptor
MPI/MRI
    myelofibrosis proliferation/regression
    index
MPJ
    metacarpophalangeal joint (*See also* MP,
    MCP, MCPJ)
    metatarsophalangeal joint (*See also* MP,
    MTP, MTPJ)
MPKV
    Maprik virus

MPL
    maximum (maximal) permissible level
    mesiopulpolingual
MP-L
    midpapillary longitudinal
MPLa
    mesiopulpolabial
MPLC
    medium pressure liquid chromatography
MPM
    malignant papillary mesothelioma
    malignant peritoneal mesothelioma
    malignant pleural mesothelioma
    medial pterygoid muscle
    minor psychiatric morbidity
    Mortality Probability Model
    multiple primary malignancy
    multiple primary melanoma
    multipurpose meal
MPMT
    Murphy punch maneuver test
MPMV
    Mason-Pfizer monkey virus
MPN
    monthly progress note
    most probable number
    multiple primary neoplasms
MPNST
    malignant peripheral nerve sheath
    tumor
MPO
    male pattern obesity
    maximum (maximal) power output
    maximum minimal perceptible odor
    myeloperoxidase [bone marrow stain]
MPOA
    medial preoptic area
MPOS
    myeloperoxidase system
MPP
    massive periretinal proliferation
    maximum (maximal) perfusion pressure
    maximum (maximal) pressure picture
    medial pterygoid plate
    metacarpophalangeal profile
    multiple presentation phenotype
MPPC
    malignant primary pheochromocytoma
mppcf
    million particles per cubic foot [of air]
MPPG
    microphotoelectric plethysmography
MPPN
    malignant persistent positional
    nystagmus
MPPS
    modality performed procedure step

M

MPPT
methylprednisolone pulse therapy
mucin-producing pancreatic tumor
MPPv
main portal vein peak velocity
MPQ
McGill Pain Questionnaire
Multidimensional Personality
Questionnaire
MPR
mannose-6-phosphate receptor
marrow production rate
massive preretinal retraction
maximum (maximal) pulse rate
multiplanar reconstruction
multiplanar reformation (reformatting)
myeloproliferative reaction
myocardial perfusion reserve
MP-RAGE
magnetization-prepared rapid acquisition
gradient echo
MP-RAGE-WE
magnetization-prepared rapid gradient
echo-water excitation
MPRE
minimal pure radium equivalent
MPRV
Mapuera virus
MPS
macular photocoagulation study
Management Philosophies Scale [I-V]
Maternal Perinatal Scale
mean particle size
meconium plug syndrome
Michigan Picture Stories
microbial profile system
mononuclear phagocyte system
Montreal platelet syndrome
movement-produced stimulus
mucopolysaccharide (*See also* MP)
mucopolysaccharidoses [plural]
mucopolysaccharidosis [singular]
multiphasic screening
myocardial perfusion scintigraphy
myocardial protection system
myofascial pain syndrome
mps
meter per second
MPS-I
mucopolysaccharidosis I
MPS-IH
mucopolysaccharidosis type I Hurler
MPS-IHS
mucopolysaccharidosis type I
Hurler-Scheie
MPS-IS
mucopolysaccharidosis type I Scheie
MPS-II
mucopolysaccharidosis type II Hunter

MPS-IIIA
mucopolysaccharidosis type III
Sanfilippo A
MPS-IIIB
mucopolysaccharidosis type III
Sanfilippo B
MPS-IIIC
mucopolysaccharidosis type III
Sanfilippo C
MPS-IV
mucopolysaccharidosis type IV Morquio
MPS-VI
mucopolysaccharidosis type VI
Maroteaux-Lamy
MPS-VII
mucopolysaccharidosis type VII Sly, Di
Ferrante
MPSC
micropapillary serous carcinoma
MPSMT
Merrill-Palmer Scale of Mental Tests
MPSRT
matched pairs signed rank test
[statistics]
MPSS
massively parallel signature sequencing
Mood and Physical Symptoms Scale
MPT
maximum (maximal) predicted
phonation time
Michigan Picture Test
multidisciplinary pain treatment
multiple-parameter telemetry
multiple puncture (multipuncture) test
MP-T
midpapillary transverse [view]
MPTAH
Mallory phosphotungstic acid
hemotoxylin [stain]
MPTh
mechanical pain threshold
MPTP
N-methyl-4-phenyl-1,2,3,6-
tetrahydropyridine
MPTR
motor, pain, touch, reflex [deficit]
MPT-R
Michigan Picture Test, Revised
MPTRD
motor, pain, touch, reflex deficit
MPTS
minocycline periodontal therapeutic
system
MPU
maternal pediatric unit
MPV
main portal vein
mean plasma volume
mean platelet volume

metatarsus primus varus
mitral valve prolapse
MPVA
metatarsus primus varus angle
MPVP
mean pulmonary venous pressure
MPVR
multiplanar volume reformation
mpz
millipièze [metric unit of pressure]
MQ
Maastricht questionnaire
memory quotient
menaquinone [vitamin K_2] (*See also*
MK)
MQC
microbiologic quality control
MQOL
McGill Quality of Life [questionnaire]
MQOL-HIV
multidimensional quality of life
[questionnaire for person with] human
immunodeficiency virus
MQOV
Mosqueiro virus
MQSA
Mammography Quality Standards Act
MR
Maddox rod
magnetic resonance
malar rash
mandibular reflex
manifest refraction
mannose-resistant
maximal right
may repeat
measles-rubella [vaccine]
medial rectus [muscle]
medial rotation
median raphe
medical record
medical rehabilitation
medication responder
medium range
megaroentgen
menstrual regulation
mentally retarded
mental retardation
mesencephalic raphe
metabolic rate
methemoglobin reductase (*See also*
MHR)
methyl red
milk ring
mineralocorticoid receptor
mitral reflux
mitral regurgitation

mixed respiratory
moderate resistance
modulation rate
Moro reflex
mortality rate
mortality ratio
motivation research
multicentric reticulohistiocytosis
multiplication rate
multiplicity reactivation
muscle receptor
muscle relaxant
myocardial revascularization
myotactic reflex
M&R
measure and record
Mr
mandible ramus
relative molecular mass
mR
milliroentgen
MRA
magnetic resonance angiograph(y)
(angiogram)
magnetic resonance arteriograph(y)
(arteriogrem)
main renal artery
marrow repopulation activity
midright atrium
multivariate regression analysis
[statistics]
mrad
millirad
MRAP
maximum (maximal) resting anal
pressure
mean right atrial pressure
MRAr
magnetic resonance arthrograph(y)
(arthrogram)
MRAS
main renal artery stenosis
MRB
multiply resistant bacteria
MRBC
monkey red blood cell
mouse red blood cell
MRBF
mean renal blood flow
MRC
magnetic resonance cholangiograph(y)
(cholangiogram)
magnetic resonance colonograph(y)
maximum (maximal) recycling capacity
medullary renal carcinoma
methylrosaniline chloride [gentian violet,
crystal violet]

M

MRCA
magnetic resonance coronary angiograph(y) (angiogram)

MRCC
metastatic renal cell carcinoma

MRCD
mitochondrial respiratory chain disorder

MRCL
Medical Research Council Laboratories

MRCNS
methicillin-resistant coagulase-negative *Staphylococcus*

MRCP
magnetic resonance cholangiopancreatograph(y)
mental retardation, cerebral palsy
movement-related cortical potential

MRD
margin (marginal) reflex distance
matched related donor
mean reference diameter
method of rapid determination
minimal reacting dose (*See also* mrd)
Minimal Record of Disability
minimum (minimal) renal disease
minimum (minimal) residual disease
minimum (minimal) reacting dose

mRd
millirutherford

MRDD
maximum recommended daily dose
mentally retarded and developmentally disabled
Mental Retardation and Development Disabilities [Department of Human Services]

MRDM
malnutrition-related diabetes mellitus

MRDSA
magnetic resonance digital subtraction angiography

MR-DTI
magnetic resonance diffusion tensor imaging

MRE
magnetic resonance elastograph(y) (elastogram)
manual resistance exercise
maximum (maximal) risk estimate
maximum (maximal) restrictive exercise
most recent episode

MREI
mean rate ejection index

MRELD
mixed receptive-expressive language disorder

mrem
millirem (milliroentgen equivalent man)

mrep
millirep (milliroentgen equivalent physical) [obsolete]

MRF
magnetic resonance flowmetry
medical record file
melanocyte-releasing factor
melanocyte-[stimulating hormone]-releasing factor
mesencephalic reticular formation
midbrain reticular formation
mitral regurgitant flow
moderate renal failure
monoclonal rheumatoid factor
müllerian regression factor

MRFC
mouse rosette-forming cell

MRFT
modified rapid fermentation test

MRG
mean rejection grading
mean residual gap
median rhomboid glossitis
mortality reference group
murmurs, rubs, gallops

MRGT
magnetic resonance guided therapy

MRH
Maddox rod hyperphoria
melanocyte-releasing hormone
melanocyte[-stimulating hormone]-releasing hormone
melanotropin-releasing hormone

MRHA
mannose-resistant hemagglutination

MRHD
maximum (maximal) recommended human dose

mrhm
milliroentgen per hour at one meter

MRHT
modified rhyme hearing test

MRI
machine-readable identifier
magnetic resonance imaging
medical records information
moderate renal insufficiency

MRIF
melanocyte release-inhibiting factor

MRIH
melanocyte release-inhibiting hormone

M&R I&O, M&R/I&O
measure and record input and output

MRL
medical research laboratory
minimal response level
moderate rubra lochia

MRLT
mesalamine-related lung toxicity

MRLVD
maximum residue limits of veterinary drugs

MRM
magnetic resonance mammography
modified radical mastectomy

MRMT
Minnesota Rate of Manipulation test

MRN
magnetic resonance neurography
malignant renal neoplasm
medical record number

mRNA
messenger ribonucleic acid

mRNP
messenger ribonucleoprotein

MRO
minimal recognizable odor
multidrug-resistant organism
muscle receptor organ

MROC
malrotation of colon

△ **MROU**
medial rectus, both eyes △

MRP
magnetic resonance pancreatography
mandibular reconstruction plate
maximum (maximal) response plateau
maximum (maximal) reimbursement point
maximum (maximal) resting pressure
mean resting potential
medical reimbursement plan
medication-related problem
multidrug resistance protein

MRP2
multidrug resistance protein 2

MRPAH
mixed reverse passive antiglobulin hemagglutination

MRR
marrow release rate
maximum (maximal) relaxation rate
medical record review

MRS
magnetic resonance spectroscopy
mania rating scale
median range score
medical receiving station
mental retardation syndrome
methicillin-resistant *Stapylococcus*
microaggregate recipient set

MRSA
methicillin-resistant *Staphylococcus aureus*

MRSD
mental retardation, skeletal dysplasia, abducens palsy [syndrome]

MRSE
methicillin-resistant *Staphylococcus epidermidis*

MRSI
magnetic resonance spectroscopic imaging

MRSS
methicillin-resistant *Staphylococcus species*
modified Rodman skin thickness score

MRT
magnetic resonance tomograph(y) (tomogram)
major role therapy
malignant rhabdoid tumor
mean residence time
mean resistance time
mean response time
median reaction time
median recognition threshold
median relapse time
Metropolitan Readiness Test
microreflux test
microwave resonance therapy
milk ring test
modified rhyme test
muscle response test

MRTA
magnetic resonance tomographic angiograph(y) (angiogram)

MRTK
malignant rhabdoid tumor of kidney

MRTS
malignant rhabdoid tumor of soft tissue

MRU
magnetic resonance urograph(y) (urogram)
mass radiography unit
mean relational utterance
measure of resource use
medical resource utilization
minimum (minimal) reproductive unit
molecular recognition unit

MRUI
Magnetic Resonance User Interface

MRUS
maximum (maximal) rate of urea synthesis

MRV
magnetic resonance venograph(y) (venogram)
mammalian orthoreovirus
minute respiratory volume
Mitchell River virus
mixed respiratory vaccine
mononuclear Reed-variant [cell]

MR-VAX
measles and rubella virus vaccine

M

MRVP
    mean right ventricular pressure
    methyl red, Voges-Proskauer [medium] ⚠ **ms**
MRX
    Moraxella catarrhalis vaccine
MRx1
    may repeat times one (once)
MRXA
    X-linked mental retardation-aphasia
    syndrome
MRXS1–MRXS6
    X-linked mental retardation syndrome
    1–6
MRZ
    measles, rubella, zoster
⚠ **MS**
    main scale
    maladjustment score
    mannose-sensitive
    mass spectrometry
    mass spectrophotometer
    maxillary sinus
    mean score
    mechanical stimulation
    Meckel syndrome
    median sternotomy
    medical services
    medical supply
    medical-surgical
    medical survey
    melanonychia striata
    menopausal syndrome
    mental status
    metabolic syndrome
    microscope slide
    milkshake
    minimal support
    mitral sound
    mitral stenosis
    mobile surgical [unit]
    modal sensitivity
    moderately susceptible
    molar solution
    mongolian spot
    morning stiffness
    morphine sulfate (*See also* ms, MSO4) ⚠ **MSAO**
    motile sperm
    mucosubstance
    multilaminated structure
    multiple sclerosis
    muscle shortening
    muscle spasm
    muscle strength
    musculoskeletal (*See also* MSK)
    myasthenic syndrome
    myeloid sarcoma
3MS
    Modified Mini-Mental Status
    (examination)

M&S
    microculture and sensitivity
ms
    manuscript
    millisecond (*See also* msec)
    morphine sulfate (*See also* MS,
    MSO4) ⚠
    murmurs [plural] (*See also* mm)
m/s
    meter per second (*See also* m/sec)
m/s²
    meter per second squared
MSA
    major serologic antigen
    male specific antigen
    mammary serum antigen
    mannitol salt agar
    Marriage Skills Analysis
    Medical Savings Accounts
    membrane stabilizing action
    membrane-stabilizing activity
    methanesulfonic acid
    metropolitan statistical area
    microsomal autoantibody
    mitotic spindle apparatus
    mixed sleep apnea
    mouse serum albumin
    multichannel signed averager
    Multidimensional Scalogram Analysis
    multiple system atrophy
    multiplication-stimulating activity
    muscle-specific actin
    muscle sympathetic activity
    myositis-specific autoantibody
MSAA
    multiple sclerosis-associated agent
MSAD
    maximum short-axis diameter
    multiple scan average dose
MSAF
    meconium-stained amniotic fluid
MSAFP
    maternal serum alpha fetoprotein
mSAH
    monosymptomatic adult hysteria
MSAO
    meal-stimulated acid output
MSAP
    mean systemic arterial pressure
MSAS
    Mandel Social Adjustment Scale
    Memorial Symptom Assessment
    Scale
MSAS-P
    Memorial Symptom Assessment Scale
    Physical
MSAS-Psych
    Memorial Symptom Assessment Scale
    Psychological

MSAS-SF
Memorial Symptom Assessment Scale short form
MSAT
Minnesota Scholastic Aptitude Test
MSB
mainstem bronchus
martius scarlet blue
mediastinal shed blood
mid small-bowel
most significant bit
MSBC
maximal specific binding capacity
MSBLA
mouse-specific B-lymphocyte antigen
MSBOS
maximal surgical blood order schedule
MSBP
mandibular staple bone plate
Münchausen syndrome by proxy
(See also MSP)
MSC
major symptom complex
mesenchymal stem cell
mesenchymal stromal cell
midsystolic click
multiple sibling case
MSCA
McCarthy Scales of Children's Abilities
MSCC
malignant spinal cord compression
midstream clean-catch [urine]
MSCE
monitored self-care evaluation
MSCHN
metastatic squamous carcinoma of head and neck
MSCL
mean sleep cycle length
MSCLC
mouse stem cell-like cell
MSCNS
methicillin-susceptible coagulase-negative *Staphylococcus*
mscp
mean spherical candle power [obsolete]
MSCS
Multidimensional Self Concept Scale
MSCT
multislice computed tomography
multislice spiral computed tomography
MSCTA
multislice computed tomographic angiography
MSCV
multislice cardiovolume

MSCWP
musculoskeletal chest wall pain
MSD
male sexual dysfunction
matched sibling donor
mean sac diameter
mean sorted difference [statistics]
mean square deviation [statistics]
metabolic screening disorder
microsurgical discectomy
midsagittal diameter
midsleep disturbance
mild sickle [cell] disease
most significant digit [statistics]
multiple sulfatase deficiency
musculoskeletal disorder
MSDBP
mean sitting diastolic blood pressure
MSDI
Martin Suicide Depression Inventory
multigated spectral Doppler imaging
MSDS
material safety data sheet
MSE
mean spherical equivalent
medical support equipment
mental status examination
muscle-specific enolase
3MSE
Modified Mini-Mental State Examination
(See also 3Ms)
mse
mean square error [statistics]
msec
millisecond (See also ms)
m/sec
meter per second (See also m/s)
MSEL
Mullen Scales of Early Learning
myasthenic syndrome of Eaton-Lambert
mSENSE
modified sensitivity encoding (SENSE)
MS-EPI
multishot echo-planar imaging
MSER
mean systolic ejection rate
Mental Status Examination Record (report)
MSES
medical school environmental stress
MSET
multistage exercise test
MSEV
microsurgical epididymovasostomy
MSF
macrophage slowing factor
macrophage spreading factor

M

MSF *(continued)*
  meconium-stained fluid
  Mediterranean spotted fever
  megakaryocyte-stimulating factor
  migration-stimulating factor
  modified sham feeding
MSFC
  Multiple Sclerosis Functional Composite
MSG
  massage
  monosodium glutamate
MSH
  medical self-help
  melanocyte-stimulating hormone
  melanophore-stimulating hormone
    (*See also* MH)
  minimally symptomatic
    hypothyroidism
MSHA
  mannose-sensitive hemagglutination
MSH-IF
  melanocyte-stimulating
    hormone-inhibiting factor
MSHRF
  melanocyte-stimulating
    hormone-releasing factor
MSHSC
  multiple self-healing squamous
    carcinoma
MSI
  magnetic source imaging
  mass sociogenic illness
  medium-scale integration
  metered solution inhaler
  microsatellite instability
  microstructured implant
  motor-sensory impairment
  multiple subcortical infarct(ion)
  musculoskeletal impairment
MSIA
  mass spectrometric immunoassay
MSIS
  Multiple Severity of Illness System
  multistate information system
MSK
  medullary sponge kidney
  musculoskeletal (*See also* MS)
MSKP
  Medical Sciences Knowledge Profile
MSL
  mean sentence length
  menopause symptom list
  midsternal line
  multiple symmetric lipomatosis
MSLA
  mouse-specific lymphocyte antigen
  multisample Luer adapter
MSLR
  mixed skin [cell] leukocyte reaction

MSLSS
  Multidimensional Student Life
    Satisfaction Scale
MSLT
  Multiple Sleep Latency Test
MSM
  magnetic starch microsphere
  men [who have] sex with men
  methylsulfonylmethane
  midsystolic murmur
  mineral salts medium
MSN
  medial septal nucleus
  mildly subnormal
MSNA
  muscle sympathetic nerve activity
MSO
  managed services organization
  medial superior olive
  mentally stable and oriented
  mental status, oriented
  most significant other
⚠ **MSO4**
  morphine sulfate (*See also* MS, ms) ⚠
MSOD
  multiple-system (multisystem) organ
    dysfunction
MSOF
  multiple system (multisystem) organ
    failure
MSP
  maximum (maximal) squeeze pressure
  mouse serum protein
  multiple sexual partners
  Münchausen syndrome by proxy
    (*See also* MSBP)
MS-PCR
  methylation-specific polymerase chain
    reaction
MSPECT
  myocardial single photon emission
    tomography
MSPGN
  mesangial proliferative
    glomerulonephritis
MSPQ
  modified somatic perception
    questionnaire
MSPS
  musculoskeletal pain syndrome
  myocardial stress perfusion
    scintigraphy
MSPSS
  Multidimensional Scale of Perceived
    Social Support
MSPv
  midshunt peak velocity
MSQ
  Managerial Style Questionnaire

mental status questionnaire
Minnesota Satisfaction Questionnaire
MSQLI
Multiple Sclerosis Quality of Life
Inventory
MSR
mitral stenoregurgitation
monosynaptic reflex
muscle stretch reflex
MSRA
maximal static response assay
MSRPP
Multidimensional Scale for Rating
Psychiatric Patients
MSRT
Minnesota Spatial Relations Test
MSS
Marital Satisfaction Scale
massage (*See also* mass, mss)
mean sac size
mental status schedule
microsatellite stable
Minnesota Satisfaction Scale
monophasic synovial sarcoma
motion sickness susceptibility
mucus-stimulating substance
multiple sclerosis susceptibility
muscular subaortic stenosis
mss
massage (*See also* mass, MSS)
MSSA
methicillin-susceptible *Staphylococcus
aureus*
MSSB
MacArthur Story Stem Battery
MSS-CR
mean sac size and crown-rump length
MSSG
multiple sclerosis susceptibility gene
MSSST
Meeting Street School Screening
Test
MSSU
midstream specimen of urine
MST
maladies sexuellement transmissible
[French for sexually transmitted
disease]
malignant salivary gland tumor
maximum stimulation test
mean survival time
mean swell time [botulism test]
medial superior temporal
median survival time
mental stress test
multiple subpial transections
multisystemic therapy

M&ST
menthol and salicylamide tests
MSTA
mumps skin test antigen
MSTh
mesothorium [disintegration product of
thorium]
MSTI
multiple soft tissue injuries
MSU
maple syrup urine
memory for symbolic unit
midstream specimen of urine
midstream urine [specimen]
monosodium urate
myocardial substrate uptake
MSUA
midstream urinalysis
MSUD
maple syrup urine disease
MSUM
monosodium urate monohydrate
MSUS
musculoskeletal ultrasound
MSV
maximal sustained [level of] ventilation
mean scale value
mSv
millisievert [radiation dose unit]
MSVC
maximal sustained (sustainable)
ventilatory capacity
MSVL
maximal spatial vector to left
MSW
multiple stab wounds
MSWYE
modified sea water yeast extract [agar]
MSYN
monophasic synovial sarcoma
MT
empty
macroglobulin-trypsin [complex]
macular target
maggot therapy
magnetization transfer
maintenance therapy
malaria therapy
malignant teratoma
mammary tumor
Martin-Thayer [plate, medium]
massage therapy
mastoid tip
maximal therapy
maximal toleration
medial temporal
medial thalamus

M

MT *(continued)*
    medial thickening
    mediastinal tube
    medical treatment
    melatonin
    membrana tympani
    membrane thickness
    membrane type [1–6]
    mesangial thickening
    metallothionein
    metatarsal
    methyltyrosine
    microtome
    microtubule
    middle temporal
    middle turbinate
    midtrachea
    milieu therapy [psychology]
    minimal threshold
    Monroe tidal drainage (*See also* MTD)
    more than
    mucosal thickening
    multiple tics
    multitest [plate]
    mural thrombus (thrombosis)
    muscle and tendon (*See also* M&T)
    muscle test(ing)
    muscle tone
    music therapy
    myringotomy tube

M/T
    masses [or] tenderness
    masses [or] tumors
    myringotomy [with] tubes

M&T
    myringotomy and tubes
    Monilia and *Trichomonas*
    muscle and tendon (*See also* MT)

MTA
    malignant teratoma, anaplastic
    mammary tumor agent
    Management Transactions Audit
    medullary-type adenocarcinoma
    metatarsal adduction
    metatarsus adductus
    mineral trioxide aggregate
    moving time average
    multitargeted antifolate
    myoclonic twitch activity

MTAC
    mass transfer area coefficient

⚠ **MTAD**
    tympanic membrane of right ear [L.
    membrana tympana auris dextrae] ⚠

MTAI
    Minnesota Teacher Attitude
    Inventory

MT/AK
    music therapy [and] audiokinetics

MTAL
    medullary thick ascending limb

⚠ **MTAS**
    Maternal Trait Anxiety Score
    tympanic membrane of left ear [L.
    membrana tympana auris sinistrae] ⚠

⚠ **MTAU**
    tympanic membranes of both ears [L.
    membranae tympani aures unitae] ⚠

MTB
    methylthymol blue
    Mycobacterium tuberculosis

MTBE
    meningeal tick-borne encephalitis
    methyl tertiary butyl ether

MTBF
    mean time between (before) failures

mTBI
    mild traumatic brain injury

MTBV
    Marituba virus

MTC
    magnetization transfer contrast
    [radiology]
    mass transfer coefficient
    maximum (maximal) tolerated
    concentration
    maximum (maximal) toxic
    concentration
    medical test cabinet
    medullary thyroid cancer (carcinoma)
    metatarsocuneiform
    multilocular thymic cyst

mtCK
    mitochondrial creatine kinase

MTCSA
    midthigh muscle cross-sectional area

MTCT
    mother-to-child transmission

MTD
    maximum (maximal) tolerated dose
    mean total dose
    mean tubular diameter
    metastatic trophoblastic disease
    minimum (minimal) toxic dose
    Monroe tidal drainage (*See also* MT)
    multiple tic disorder
    Mycobacterium tuberculosis direct [test]
    (*See also* MTDT)

MTDDA
    Minnesota Test for Differential
    Diagnosis of Aphasia

MTDI
    maximal tolerable daily intake

MT-DN
    multitest, dermatophytes, *Nocardia*
    [plate]

mtDNA
    mitochondrial deoxyribonucleic acid

MTDT
 modified tone decay test
 Mycobacterium tuberculosis direct test
 (*See also* MTD)
MTE
 main timing event
 medical toxic environment
 mesenteric thromboembolism
 multiple trace elements
MTET
 modified treadmill exercise test(ing)
MTF
 maximum (maximal) terminal flow
 medical treatment facility
 mesial triangular fossa
 modulation transfer factor (function)
 Musculoskeletal Transplant Foundation
MTG
 middle temporal gyrus
 midthigh girth
MTg
 mouse thyroglobulin
MTHFR
 methylene tetrahydrofolate reductase
 [gene]
MTI
 magnetization transfer imaging
 malignant teratoma, intermediate
 minimum (minimal) time interval
MTJ
 midtarsal joint
MTL
 Marco trial lens
 Metropolitan Life Table [for desirable
 weight]
 middle temporal lobe
MTLE
 medial (mesial) temporal-lobe epilepsy
MTLP
 metabolic toxemia of late pregnancy
MTM
 mouth-to-mouth [resuscitation]
 modified Thayer-Martin [agar]
MT-M
 multitest, mycology [plate]
MT-MMP
 matrix membrane-type metalloproteinase
mtMRI
 magnetization transfer magnetic
 resonance imaging
MTMT
 maximum tolerated medical therapy
MTMX
 X-linked myotubular myopathy
MTOC
 microtubule organizing center
 mitotic organizing center

mTOR
 mammalian target of rapamycin
MTP
 master treatment plan
 maximal tolerated pressure
 medial tibial plateau
 medical termination of pregnancy
 mesencephalic tegmental paralysis
 metatarsal periostitis
 metatarsophalangeal [joint] (*See also*
 MP, MPJ, MTPJ)
 microsomal triglyceride transfer protein
 microtubule protein
 multidisciplinary treatment plan
MTPI
 metatarsophalangeal implant
MTPJ
 metatarsophalangeal joint (*See also* MP,
 MPJ, MTP)
MTPT
 1-methyl-4-phenyl-1,2,3,6-
 tetrahydropyridine
MTQ
 methaqualone [drug of abuse]
MTR
 magnetization transfer ratio
 mass, tenderness, rebound [abdominal
 examination]
 Meinicke turbidity reaction
 mental treatment rules
 mother (*See also* M, MO, MOM)
MTR-0
 no masses, tenderness, rebound
 [abdominal examination]
M-tropic
 macrophage tropic
MTRV
 Matruh virus
MTS
 medial tibial syndrome
 mesial temporal sclerosis
 mitochondrial targeting sequence
 moderate tactile stimulus
 multicellular tumor spheroid
MTSA
 multiple thin slab acquisition
MTSI
 macular translocation with scleral
 infolding
MTSS
 medial tibial stress syndrome
 menstrual toxic shock syndrome
MTST
 maximal treadmill stress test
MTT
 malignant triton tumor
 malignant trophoblastic teratoma

M

MTT (*continued*)
    mammillothalamic tract
    maximum (maximal) treadmill testing
    meal tolerance test
    mean pulmonary transit time
    mean transit time
    medial tibial torsion
    methylthiotetrazole
    monotetrazolium

MTU
    malignant teratoma, undifferentiated

M-TURP
    minimal transurethral resection of
      prostate

MTV
    maximum (maximal) tolerable
      (toleration) volume
    metatarsus varus

MT-Y
    multitest yeast [plate]

MU
    maternal uncle
    megaunit
    mescaline unit
    million units
    monitor unit
    Montevideo unit
    motor unit
    mouse unit
    Murphy unit

Mu
    Mache unit [measurement of
      concentration in radioactive
      material]

mU
    milliunit

mu
    millimass unit [SI unit of mass (symbol
      mmu obsolete)]

MUA
    manipulation under anesthesia
    middle uterine artery
    multiple unit activity

MUAC
    middle upper arm circumference

MUAP
    motor unit action potential

MUC
    maximum (maximal) urinary
      concentration
    mucosal ulcerative colitis

muc
    mucilage

MUCL
    medial ulnar collateral ligament

MUCP
    maximum urethral closure pressure

MUCV
    Mucambo virus

MUD
    matched unrelated donor
    minimal urticarial dose

MUDV
    Munguba virus

MUE
    medication use evaluation

MUFA
    monounsaturated fatty acid

MUFR
    maximal urinary flow rate

MUGA
    multigated angiogram
    multiple gated (multigated) acquisition

MUGEx
    multigated [blood pool scan during]
      exercise (*See also* MUGX)

MUGR
    multigated [blood pool image at] rest

MUGS
    monoclonal gammopathy of
      undetermined undetermined (unknown)
      significance

MUGUS
    monoclonal gammopathy of (unknown)
      significance

MUGX
    multigated [blood pool image during]
      exercise (*See also* MUGEx)

mu (μ)-HCD
    mu (μ)-heavy-chain disease

MULE
    microcomputer upper limb exerciser

mulibrey
    muscle, liver, brain, eye [disease]

mult
    multiple
    multiplication

multi-CSF
    multicolony-stimulating factor

multip
    multiparous (*See also* MP)

MUMPS
    Massachusetts General Hospital Utility
      Multi-Programming System

MUNSH
    Memorial University of Newfoundland
      Scale of Happiness

MUNV
    Munguba virus

MUN(WI)
    Munich Wistar [rat]

MUO
    metastasis of unknown origin
    myocardiopathy of unknown origin

MΩ
    megohm

mΩ
    milliohm

MUP
major urinary protein
maximal urethral pressure
4-methylumbelliferyl phosphate
motor unit potential
mouse urine protein

MUPAT
multiple-site perineal applicator
technique

MUPIT
Martinez universal Perineal interstitial
template

Mur
muramic acid

MURC
measurable undesirable respiratory
contaminant

MURCS
müllerian, renal, cervicothoracic, somite
abnormalities

MURD
matched unrelated donor

MurNAc
N-acetylmuramate

MURV
Murutucu virus

musc
muscle
muscular
musculature

MUSICA
multiscale image detail contrast
amplification

mus-lig
musculoligamentous

MUST
medical unit, self-contained and
transportable

MUSTPAC
medical ultrasound 3D portable, with
advanced communication

mut.
mutation

MUU
mouse uterine unit

mUW
modified University of Wisconsin
[solution]

MUWU
mouse uterine weight unit

MV
main venule
manual ventilation
maternal venous
maximal ventilation
measles virus
mechanical ventilation

megavolt
mesenteric vasculitis
microvillus [singular] (microvilli
[plural])
midventricular
minute ventilation
minute volume
mitral valve
mixed venous
multivesicular
multivessel

Mv
mendelevium [obsolete symbol, use Md]
(*See also* Md)

mV
millivolt

MVA
malignant ventricular arrhythmia
manual vacuum aspiration
mechanical ventricular assistance
mevalonic acid
microvascular angiopathy
microvillus atrophy
mitral valve area
modified vaccinia virus Ankara
motor vehicle accident

MV · A
megavolt-ampere

mV · A
millivolt-ampere

MVAD
mechanical ventricular assist device

MVB
manual ventilation bag
microvascular bleeding
mixed venous blood
multivesicular body

MVC
maximum (maximal) vital capacity
maximum (maximal) voluntary contraction
microvessel count
minute virus of canines
motor vehicle collision (crash)
myocardial vascular capacity

MVc
mitral valve closure

MV(c)ELISA
measles virus competitive enzyme-linked
immunosorbent assay

MVD
Marburg virus disease
microvascular decompression
microvessel density
mitral valve disease
mouse vas deferens
multivessel [coronary] disease
myocardial vasodilation

M

MVE
 maximum (maximal) voluntary effort
 mitral valve echo
 mitral valve excursion [echocardiogram]
 Murray Valley encephalitis [virus]
MVF
 mitral valve flow
MVFE
 Mediterranean fever [gene]
MVG, MVgrad
 mitral valve gradient
MVH
 massive variceal hemorrhage
 massive vitreous hemorrhage
MVI
 malignant vascular injury
 mitral valve insufficiency
 motor vehicle injury
 multiple vitamin injection
 multivalvular involvement
 multivitamin infusion
MVIC
 maximum voluntary isometric
  contraction
MVID
 microvillus inclusion disease
MVII
 Minnesota Vocational Interest Inventory
MVK
 Massachusetts Vision Kit
MVL
 mitral valve leaflet
MVLS
 mandibular vestibulolingual sulcoplasty
 Mecham Verbal Language Scale
 modified varicellalike syndrome
MVM
 Maharishi Vedic medicine
 medullary venous malformation
 microvillous membrane
 minute virus of mice
MVMT
 movement (*See also* M, MVT, Mx)
MVN
 medial ventromedial nucleus
 medial vestibular nucleus
MVO
 maximum (maximal) venous outflow
 mean venous outflow
 mitral valve orifice (opening)
 mixed venous oxygen
MVO$_2$
 mixed venous oxyhemoglobin
  saturation
 oxygen content of mixed venous blood
 myocardial volume oxygen
  consumption
MVOA
 mitral valve orifice area

MVP
 maximum vasal pressure
 mean platelet volume
 mean venous pressure
 microvascular pressure
 mitral valve prolapse
 moisture vapor permeable
MVPA
 moderate to vigorous physical activity
MVPS
 mitral valve prolapse syndrome
MVP-SC
 mitral valve prolapse [and] systolic
  click
MVPT
 Mertens Visual Perception Test
 Motor-Free Visual Perception Test
  (*See also* MFVPT)
MVR
 massive vitreous retraction
 massive vitreous retractor [blade]
 maximum (maximal) ventilation rate
 microvitreoretinal
 minimum (minimal) vascular resistance
 mitral valve regurgitation
 mitral valve replacement
MVS
 Massachusetts XII Vitrectomy System
 microvitrectomy system
 mitral valve stenosis
 motor, vascular, sensory
MVSD
 muscular ventricular septal defect
mV-sec
 millivolt-second
MVT
 maximal ventilation time
 mesenteric vein thrombosis
 monomorphic ventricular tachycardia
 movement (*See also* M, MVMT, Mx)
 multiform ventricular tachycardia
 multivitamin
 music vibration table
MV-T
 mitral valve-transverse
MVTR
 moisture vapor transmission rate
MVU
 Montevideo unit [labor]
MVV
 maximum (maximal) ventilatory volume
 maximum (maximal) voluntary
  ventilation
 mixed vespid venom
MVVT
 Maharishi Vedic vibration technology
MW
 mean weight
 megawatt

microwave
Munich Wistar (rat)
muscle wasting

M-W
men and women

6-MW
6-minute walk

12-MW
12-minute walk

mW
milliwatt

MWAV
Manawa virus

MWB
mild wheezy bronchitis
minimal weight bearing

mWb
milliweber

MWC
major wound complications
Monod-Wyman-Changeux [allostery model]

MWCB
manufacturer's working cell bank

MWCO
molecular weight cutoff

MWD
maximum walking distance
microwave diathermy
molecular weight distribution

6-MWD
6-minute walking distance

MWF
metal working fluid

M-W-F
Monday-Wednesday-Friday

MWLT
Modified Word Learning Test

MWMT
Monotic Word Memory Test

MwoA
migraine without aura

MWP
mean wedge pressure

MWPC
multiwire proportional chamber

MWT
maintenance of wakefulness test
Mallory-Weiss tear
malpositioned wisdom teeth
maximum walking time
myocardial wall thickness

6-MWT
6-minute walking test

MX
matrix (See also M, MA)

Mx
manifest refraction
mastectomy
maxillary
maxwell [CGS unit of magnetic flux]
MEDEX [physician assistant training program]
movement (See also M, MVMT, MVT)
multiple
myringotomy (See also MYR)

mx
mixture (See also M, m., mix., mixt)

M$_{xy}$
transverse magnetization

My
myopia (myopic) (See also M, myop)
myxedematous

MyBP-C
myosin-binding protein C

Mycol
mycology

MYD
mydriatic

MyD
myotonic (muscular) dystrophy (See also MMD, MyMD)

MYEL
multiple myeloma

myel
myelin(ated)
myelocyte

myelo
myelocyte
myelograph(y) (myelogram)

MyG
myasthenia gravis (See also MG)

myg
myriagram [obsolete metric unit of mass]

MYH9
myosin heavy chain 9

MYHC
heavy chain cardiac myosin

MYHCA
myosin heavy chain alpha (α)

MYKV
Mykines virus

myL
myrialiter [obsolete]

mym
myriameter [obsolete metric unit of distance]

MyMD
myotonic muscular dystrophy (See also MMD, MyD)

MYO
myoglobin (See also MB, MYOGLB)

M

myo
   myocardial
   myocardium
MYOC
   myocilin [glaucoma gene]
MyoD
   myogenic regulatory protein [family of
   genes]
MYOGLB
   myoglobin (*See also* MB, MYO)
myop
   myopia (myopic) (*See also* M,
   My)
MYR
   myringotomy (*See also* Mx)
MYS
   medium yellow soft [stools]
   myasthenia syndrome
MYST
   mediastinal yolk sac tumor

MYTGC
   Miller-Yoder Test of Grammatical
   Comprehension
MZ
   mantle zone
   marginal zone
   monozygotic [twin]
M_z
   longitudinal magnetization
m:z
   mass to charge ratio
MZA
   monozygotic [twins raised] apart
MZBCL, MZBL
   marginal zone B-cell lymphoma
MZL
   marginal zone B lymphocyte
   marginal zone lymphoma
MZT
   monozygotic [twins raised] together

N

asparagine (*See also* Asn)
blood factor in MNS blood group
nasal (*See also* NAS)
nasion [carniometric]
nausea
negative (*See also* neg)
Neisseria
neural
neuraminidase (*See also* NA)
neutron number [number of neutrons in an atom]
never
newton [SI unit of force]
nicotinamide (*See also* NA)
nitrogen (*See also* N_2)
no
node (nodal)
nodule
none
Nonne [globulin test]
noon (*See also* M)
nor (*See also* n)
normal [concentration]
normality [equivalent/liter]
north
not
notified
noun
nucleoside (*See also* Nuc)
nucleus (*See also* Nu, nucl)
number (*See also* n, NO, no.)
number in sample
number of observations [in statistics]
numerical aptitude [General Aptitude Test Battery]
nu [13th letter of Greek alphabet uppercase]
sample size (*See also* n)
spin density

0.02N

fiftieth-normal [solution] (*See also* N/50)

0.1N

tenth-normal [solution] (*See also* N/10)

0.5N

half-normal [solution] (*See also* N/2)

N0

no lymph nodes containing cancer cells [TNM classification]

N1

regional lymph node metastases [TNM classification]

N=1

number equal to one [single patient in clinical trial]

2N

double-normal [solution]

N_2

nitrogen

N/2

half-normal [solution] (*See also* 0.5N)
seminormal

5'-N

5'-nucleotidase

N-9

nonoxynol-9

N/10

tenth-normal [solution] (*See also* 0.1N)

^{13}N

nitrogen-13

^{14}N

nitrogen-14

^{15}N

nitrogen-15

N/50

fiftieth-normal [solution] (*See also* 0.02N)

n

haploid chromosome number
nano- (prefix)
nervus (nerve) [singular]
neutron [dosage unit]
number (*See also* N, NO, no.)
principal quantum number
refractive index (*See also* RI, RI)
rotational frequency
sample size (*See also* N)

$\bar{n}$

mean value of n for a number of observations [statistics]

n.

born [L. *natus*]
nostril [L. *naris*]

n_0

Loschmidt number

2n

diploid chromosome number

3n

triploid chromosome number

4n

tetraploid chromosome number

NA

nalidixic acid
Narcotics Anonymous
nasopharyngeal angiofibroma
needle aspiration
neuraminidase
nephrogenic adenoma
neurologic age
neuropathic arthropathy

N

NA *(continued)*
neutralizing antibody (*See also* NAb)
neutrophil antibody
new admission
nicotinamide (*See also* N)
nicotinic acid
no abnormality
nodular amyloidoma
Nomina Anatomica
nonadherent
non-A [hepatitis]
nonalcoholic
nonamniotic (nonamnionic)
nonmyelinated axon
normal axis
nosocomially acquired
not admitted
not antagonized
not applicable (*See also* N/A)
not attempted
not available
nuclear antibody (antigen)
nucleic acid
nucleus accumbens
nucleus ambiguus
numeric aperture

N/A
no alternative
not applicable (*See also* NA)

N&A
normal and active

Na
sodium [L. *natrium*] (*See also* sod.)

²³Na
sodium-23

²⁴Na
sodium-24

nA
nanoampere

NAA
N-acetylaspartate
naphthalene acetic acid
neutral amino acid
neutron activation analysis
neutrophil aggregation activity
nicotinic acid amide
no apparent abnormalities
nucleic acid amplification

NAAC
no apparent anesthetic complication

NAACP
neoplasia, allergy, Addison [disease], collagen [vascular disease], and parasites

NAA:Cr
N-acetylaspartate to creatine ratio

NAAD
neoadjuvant androgen deprivation

NAAG
N-acetylaspartylglutamate

NAAK
nerve agent antidote kit

NAAP
N-acetyl-4-amino-phenazone
National Arthritis Action Plan

NAAT
nucleic acid amplification techniques (testing) (*See also* NAT)

NAATPT
not available at the present time

NAB
nocturnal acid breakthrough
not at bedside
novarsenobenzene [neoarsphenamine]

NAb
neutralizing antibody (*See also* NA)

NABS
normal abdominal bowel sounds
normoactive bowel sounds

NABT
normal-appearing brain tissue

NABX
needle aspiration biopsy

NAC
nasal allergen challenge
neoadjuvant chemotherapy (*See also* NACT, NCT)
nerve-approximating clamp
nipple-areola complex
no acute changes
no anesthesia complications
nonadherent cell

NACD
no anatomical cause of death
not acidified

NAC-EDTA
N-acetyl-ʟ-cysteine ethylenediamine-tetraacetic acid

n-Ach
achievement need [in psychology]

NaCl
sodium chloride [salt]

NaCMC
sodium carboxymethyl cellulose

NaCN
sodium cyanide

NACS
neonate adaptive capacity to stimulus
Neurologic and Adaptive Capacity Score

NACT
neoadjuvant chemotherapy (*See also* NAC, NCT)

NAD
nevus with architectural disorder
new antigenic determinant
nicotinamide adenine dinucleotide

nicotinic acid dehydrogenase
no abnormal discovery
no abnormality demonstrable
no active disease
no acute disease
no acute distress
no apparent distress
no appreciable disease
normal axis deviation
nothing abnormal detected (discovered)

NAD$^+$
oxidized form of nicotinamide adenine
dinucleotide

NaD
sodium dialysate

NADA
New Animal Drug Application

NADase
nicotinamide adenine dinucleotidase

NADG
nicotinamide adenine dinucleotide
glycohydrolase

NADH
nicotinamide adenine dinucleotide
[reduced form]

NaDodSO$_4$
sodium dodecyl sulfate (*See also* SDS)

NADP$^+$
nicotinamide adenine dinucleotide
phosphate positive [oxidized form]

NADPH, NADP
nicotinamide adenine dinucleotide
phosphate

NADSIC
no apparent disease seen in chest

NAE
net acid excretion

Na$_e$
exchangeable body sodium (natrium)

NAEL
no adverse effect level

NAEP
National Asthma Education Program

NAEPP
National Asthma Education and
Prevention Program [Guidelines]

NAET
Nambudripad allergy elimination
technique

NAF
net acid flux
neutrophil-activating factor
nipple aspirate (aspiration) fluid
normal adult female
Notice of Adverse Findings [FDA
post-audit letter]

NaF
sodium fluoride

NAFD
Nager acrofacial dysostosis

NaFl
sodium fluorescein

NAFLD
nonalcoholic fatty liver disease

NAG
N-acetyl-beta (β) glucosaminidase
N-acetylglutamate
narrow-angle glaucoma
nonagglutinable
nonagglutinating

NAGO
neuraminidase and galactose oxidase

NAGS
natural apophysial glides

NAH
neonatal adrenal hemorrhage

NaHCO$_3$
sodium bicarbonate

NAHI
nonaccidental head injury

NAHV
non-A hepatitis virus

NAI
net acid input [urinary]
neuraminidase inhibition (*See also* NI)
no accidental injury
no action indicated
no acute inflammation
nonaccidental injury
nonadherence index
Nuremberg Aging Inventory

NaI
sodium iodide

NAIM
nonvasculitic autoimmune inflammatory
meningoencephalitis

NAION
nonarteritic anterior ischemic optic
neuropathy
nonarteritic ischemic optic
neuropathy

NAIR
nonadrenergic inhibitory response

NAIT
neonatal alloimmune thrombocytopenia

NaI(Tl)
thallium-activated sodium iodide crystal
[in gamma ray detectors]

Na&K
sodium and potassium

Na$^+$-K$^+$
sodium-potassium

NaK-ATPase
sodium-potassium adenosine
triphosphatase [sodium-potassium
pump]

N

Na&KSP
sodium and potassium spot [urine test]
NAL
nasal angiocentric lymphoma
nonadherent leukocyte
NALC
N-acetyl-L-cysteine-sodium hydroxide
[test]
NALD
neonatal adrenoleukodystrophy
NALL
null [cell line of] acute lymphocytic
leukemia
NALP
neuroadenolysis of pituitary
NALS
neonatal adjuvant life support
NALT
nasopharyngeal-associated lymphoid
tissue
nose-associated lymphoid tissue
NAM
nail-apparatus melanoma
natural actomyosin
no abnormal mass
normal adult male
nAMD
neovascular age-related macular
degeneration
NAME
nevi, atrial myxomas, myxoid
neurofibromas, ephelides [syndrome]
NAMN
nicotinic acid mononucleotide
NAMSD
neuropathy, axonal, motor-sensory with
deafness and mental retardation
[Cowchock syndrome]
NAN
neurasthenic neurosis
NANA
N-acetylneuraminic acid
NANB, NANBH
non-A, non-B (hepatitis) [hepatitis C]
NANBNC, NANBNCH
non-A, non-B, non-C hepatitis
NANBV
non-A, non-B [hepatitis] virus
NANC
nonadrenergic noncholinergic
noncholinergic [neuron]
NANIPER
nonallergic noninfectious perennial
rhinitis
NANSAID
nonaspirin nonsteroidal antiinflammatory
drugs
NaOCl
sodium hypochlorite [household bleach]

NaOH
sodium hydroxide
NAP
narrative, assessment, and plan
nasion-pogonion [craniometrics]
nerve action potential
neutrophil-activating protein
neutrophil alkaline phosphatase
p-nitro-alpha-acetylamino-beta-
hydroxypropiophenone
nodular adrenocortical pathology
nonacute profile
nosocomial acquired pneumonia
nucleic acid panel
nucleic acid phosphatase
8NAP
eighth nerve action potential
NaP
sodium phosphate
NAPA
N-acetyl procainamide
NAPD
no active pulmonary disease
NAPH
naphthyl
NAPI
Neurodevelopmental Assessment
[Procedure] for Preterm Infants
NAPP
nerve agent pyridostigmine
pretreatment
NAPQI
N-acetyl-p-benzoquinoneimine
NAPS
nurse-administered propofol sedation
N$_{aqs}$
number of planar acquisitions
NAR
nasal airway resistance
no action required
no adverse reaction
nonambulatory restraint
nonanaphylactic reaction
nonarticular rheumatism
not at risk
NARA
Narcotics Addict Rehabilitation Act
NARC, narc
narcotic (*See also* narco)
narcotics [hospital, officer, treatment
center] (*See also* narco)
Narc
nucleus arcuatus (nucleus infundibularis)
narco
narcolepsy
narcotic (*See also* NARC, narc)
narcotic addict
narcotics [hospital, officer, treatment
center] (*See also* NARC, narc)

Na/reab
  sodium reabsorption rate
NARES
  nonallergic rhinitis with eosinophilia
  syndrome
NaRI
  noradrenaline reuptake inhibitor
NARL
  no adverse response level
NARMS
  National Antimicrobial Resistance
  Monitoring System
NARP
  neuropathy, ataxia, retinitis pigmentosa
  [syndrome]
NARS
  neuropsychiatric AIDS (acquired
  immunodeficiency syndrome) rating
  scale
NART
  National Adult Reading Test [United
  Kingdom]
NAS
  nasal (*See also* N)
  Nasoule virus
  Neonatal Abstinence Score
  neonatal abstinence syndrome
  neonatal air leak syndrome
  neuroallergic syndrome
  neurobehavioral assessment scale
  [sedation scoring]
  no abnormality seen
  no added salt
  normalized alignment score
NASA
  not a surgical abdomen
NASBA
  nucleic acid sequence based
  amplification (analysis)
NaSCN
  sodium thiocyanate
NASDCA
  naphthol AS-D chloracetate [Leder
  stain]
NASDCE
  naphthol-AS-D-chloracetate esterase
  [stain]
NASH
  nonalcoholic steatohepatitis
Na-Spt
  sodium spot [urine test]
NASS
  Neonatal Abstinence Scoring
  System
NaSSA
  noradrenergic and specific serotonergic
  antidepressant

NASTT
  nonspecific abnormality of ST segment
  and T wave
NAT
  N-acetyltransferase
  natal
  National Attention Test
  neonatal alloimmune thrombocytopenia
  no action taken
  no acute trauma
  nonaccidental trauma
  nonspecific abnormality of T wave
  Nonverbal Ability Test
  not adequately treated
  nucleic acid amplification test (*See also*
  NAAT)
  nucleic acid test (testing)
  Numerical Attention Test
nat
  national
  native
  natural
  nature
NATB
  Non-Reading Aptitude Test Battery
NATL
  nasal angiocentric T-cell lymphoma
NATO
  North Atlantic Treaty Organization
NATP
  neonatal alloimmune thrombocytopenic
  purpura
NAUC
  normalized area under curve
NAUTI
  nosocomially-associated urinary tract
  infection
NAVEL
  nerve, artery, vein, empty space,
  lymphatics
NAVV
  Navarro virus
NAW
  nasal antral window
NAWM
  normal-appearing white matter
NB
  nail bed
  needle biopsy
  Negri bodies
  nervus buccalis
  neuroblast(oma) (*See also* NBL)
  neurometric (test) battery
  newborn
  nitrogen balance
  nitrous oxide-barbiturate [anesthesia]
  non-B [hepatitis]

N

NB *(continued)*
normoblast (*See also* nbl)
nuclear bag [certain intrafusal muscle
fiber nuclei of a neuromuscular
spindle]
nutrient broth

N:B
neopterin to biopterin ratio

Nb
niobium

n.b.
note well [L. *nota bene*]

NBAS
Neonatal Behavioral Assessment Scale

NBAS-K
Neonatal Behavioral Assessment Scale
with Kansas Supplements

NBC
nasobiliary catheter
nephroblastomatosis complex
newborn center
nonbacterial cystitis
nonbattle casualty
nonbed care
nuclear, biological, chemical [weapon,
warfare]

NBCA, N-BCA
N-butyl cyanoacrylate

NBCC
nevoid basal cell carcinoma

NBCCS
nevoid basal cell carcinoma syndrome

NBCIE
nonbullous congenital ichthyosiform
erythroderma

NBD
nasobiliary drain
necrotizing bowel disease
neurogenic (neurologic) bladder
dysfunction
no brain damage
nucleotide-binding domain

NB-DNJ
N-butyldeoxynojirimycin

NBE
northern bean extract

NBEI
nonbutanol-extractable iodine

NBF
not breastfed

NBH
new bag (bottle) hung

NBHH
newborn helpful hints

NBI
neutrophil bactericidal index
no bone injury
nonbattle injury
nosocomial bacterial infection

NBIL
neonatal bilirubin

nBiPAP
nasal bilevel (biphasic) positive airway
pressure

NBL
neuroblast(oma) (*See also* NB)

nbl
normoblast (*See also* NB)

NBL/OM
neuroblastoma and opsoclonus-
myoclonus

NBM
no bowel movement
normal bone marrow
normal bowel movement
nothing by mouth (*See also* NPO,
n.p.o.)
nucleus basalis of Meynert

nbM
newborn mouse

nbMb
newborn mouse brain

NBME
normal bone marrow extract

NBN
narrow band noise

NBNC CLD
non-B, non-C chronic liver disease

NBO
nonbed occupancy

NBP
National Biomonitoring Program
needle biopsy of prostate
neoplastic brachial plexopathy
no bone pathology
nonbacterial prostatitis

NBQC
narrow-base quad cane

NBR
no blood return

NBRS
Nursery Neurobiological Risk
Score

NBS
neonatal Bartter syndrome
neuroblastoma suppressor
nevoid basal [cell carcinoma]
syndrome
New Ballard Score
newborn screen [serum thyroxine and
phenylketonuria]
Nijmegen breakage syndrome
no bacteria seen
normal blood serum
normal bowel sounds
normal brain stem
normal burro serum
nystagmus blockage syndrome

NBT
nasobiliary tube
nitroblue tetrazolium [test]
normal breast tissue
NBTE
nonbacterial thrombotic endocarditis
NBTG
nitrobenzylthioguanosine
NBTNF
newborn, term, normal, female
NBTNM
newborn, term, normal, male
NBT-PABA
nitroblue tetrazolium-paraaminobenzoic
acid
NBTV
nonbacterial thrombotic vegetation
NBUVB
narrowband ultraviolet B
NBV
Nelson Bay orthoreovirus
NBVV
nonbleeding visible vessel
NBW
normal birth weight
NC
nabothian cyst
nasal cannula
nasal clearance
natural cytotoxicity
neck complaint
neonatal cholestasis
nephrocalcin
nerve conduction
neural crest
neurocirculatory
neurogenic claudication
neurologic check
neurologic control
nevus comedonicus
nitrocellulose
no caffeine
no casualty
no change
no charge
no complaints
noise criterion
noncardiac
noncirrhotic
noncompliant
noncontributory
normal control
normocephalic
nose clamp (clip)
nose cone
not classified
not completed

not cultured
nucleocapsid
nursing coordination
N&C
nerves and circulation
N:C
nuclear to cytoplasmic ratio (*See also*
NCR)
N/C
neurocirculatory
nC
nanocoulomb
NCA
neurocirculatory asthenia
neutrophil chemotactic activity
no congenital abnormalities
nodulocystic acne
noncontractile area
nonspecific cross-reacting antigen
normal coronary arteries
nuclear cerebral angiogram
n-CAD
negative coronoradiographic
documentation
NCAH
nonclassical adrenal hyperplasia
NCAM, N-CAM
nerve (neural) cell adhesion molecule
NcAMP
nephrogenous cyclic adenosine
monophosphate
N/CAN
nasal cannula
NCAP
nasal continuous airway pressure
NCAT, NC/AT
normocephalic and atraumatic
NCB
natural childbirth
needle core biopsy
no code blue
NCC
nasal conditioning capacity
neurocysticercosis
no concentrated carbohydrates
noncoronary cusp
nucleus caudalis centralis
nursing care card
nursing care continuity
NCCA
noncontact corneal aesthesiometer
NC-CAH
nonclassic congenital adrenal hyperplasia
NCCP
noncardiac chest pain
NCCT
noncontrast computed tomography

N

NCD
  neck to [hip] capsule distance
  neurocirculatory dystonia
  nitrogen clearance delay
  no congenital deformities
  noncommunicable disease
  normal childhood diseases (disorders)
  not considered disabling
  not considered disqualifying
  Nursing-Care Dependency [scale]
NCDB
  National Cancer Data Base
NCDV
  Nebraska calf diarrhea virus
NCE
  negative-contrast echocardiography
  new chemical entity
  nonconvulsive epilepsy
  normochromatic erythrocyte
NCEP
  National Cholesterol Education Program
NCF
  neutrophil chemotactic factor
  night care facility
  no cold fluids
NCF(C)
  neutrophil chemotactic factor
  (complement)
NCGL
  nucleus corporis geniculati lateralis
NCGN
  necrotizing crescentic glomerulonephritis
NCHCT
  noncontrast helical computed
  tomography
NCHS
  National Center for Health Statistics
  [CDC]
NCI
  naphthalene, creosote, iodoform
  [obsolete]
  National Cancer Institute
  nuclear contour index
  nucleus colliculi inferioris
  nursing care integration
nCi
  nanocurie
NCI-CTC
  National Cancer Institute Common
  Toxicity Criteria
NCIS
  nursing care information sheet
NCIT
  Nursing Care Intervention Tool
NCJ
  needle catheter jejunostomy
NCL
  neuronal ceroid lipofuscinosis
  no cautionary label

noncoronary leaflet
  nuclear cardiology laboratory
NCLD
  neonatal chronic lung disease
NCM
  nailfold capillary microscope
N/cm^2
  newton per square centimeter
NCMC
  natural cell-mediated cytotoxicity
NCNC
  normochromic, normocytic [anemia or
  erythrocyte] (*See also* NCNCA, N/N,
  NNA)
NCNCA
  normochromic normocytic anemia
  (*See also* NCNC, N/N, NNA)
NCO
  no complaints offered
N-CoR
  nuclear receptor corepressor
NCP
  no caffeine or pepper
  nonclonogenic proliferating [cells]
  noncollagen protein
  noncontrast phase
  normal chromosomal pattern
  nursing care plan
NCPAP, n-CPAP
  nasal continuous positive airway
  pressure
NC-PAS
  noncontact photoacoustic spectroscopy
NCPB
  neurolytic celiac plexus block
NCPE
  noncardiac (noncardiogenic) pulmonary
  edema
NCPF
  noncirrhotic portal fibrosis
NCPG
  nonchromaffin paraganglioma
NcpPCu
  nonceruloplasmin plasma copper
NCPR
  no cardiopulmonary resuscitation
NCQA
  National Committee for Quality
  Assurance
NCR
  neurologic, circulatory, range [of
  motion]
  neutrophil chemotactic response
  nuclear to cytoplasmic ratio (*See also*
  N:C)
nCR
  nodular complete response
NCRC
  nonchild-resistant container

NCRLM
noncolorectal liver metastasis
NCS
nasal congestion score
nerve conduction study
neurocutaneous syndrome
newborn calf serum
no concentrated sweets
noncircumferential stenosis
noncontact supervision
noncoronary sinus
noncured sarcoidosis
noncurrent serum
not clinically significant
numb chin syndrome
nystagmus compensation syndrome
NCSD
National Cardiac Surgery Database
NCSE
nonconvulsive status epilepticus
NCT
neoadjuvant chemotherapy (*See also* NAC, NACT)
nerve compression test
nerve conduction test
neural crest tumor
neutron capture therapy
noncontact tonometer (tonometry)
number connection test
NCV
nerve conduction velocity
no commercial value
noncholera *Vibrio*
nuclear venogram
NCVS
nerve conduction velocity study
ND
nasal decongestant
nasal deformity
nasal discharge
nasoduodenal
nasolacrimal duct
natural death
neck dissection
neonatal death (*See also* NND)
neoplastic disease
nerve deafness
nervous debility
neurologic development
neuropsychologic deficit
neurotic depression
neutral density
Newcastle disease [avian]
new drug
no data
no date
no disease

nondetectable
nondetermined
nondiabetic
nondiagnostic (NDx)
nondirective
nondisabling
nondistended
none detectable (detected) (*See also* NOND)
normal delivery
normal deposition
normal development
normal dose
nose drops
not detectable (detected)
not determined
not diagnosed
not done
nothing done
not nondetectable
nucleus of Darkschewitsch
nurse's diagnosis
nutritionally deprived
N&D
nodular and diffuse [lymphoma]
N/D
no defects
Nd
neodymium
number of dissimilar [matches]
NDA
New Drug Application [FDA]
no data available
no demonstrable antibodies
no detectable activity
no detectable antibody
NDC
National Drug Code [FDA]
nondifferentiated cell
nuclear dehydrogenating clostridia
NDD
no-dialysis days
NDDH
neutrophilic dermatosis of dorsal hand
NDE
near-death experience
nondiabetic extremity
NDEA
no deviation of electrical axis
NDEV
Ndelle virus
NDF
neu [gene] differentiation factor
neutral density filter [test]
neutral detergent fiber
neutrophil diffraction factor
new differentiation factor

N

NDF *(continued)*
new dosage form
no disease found
NDFP
nodular and diffuse fibrous proliferation
NDH
neurogenic dysplasia of hip
NDI
naphthalene diisocyanate
National Death Index
Nepean Dyspepsia Index
nephrogenic diabetes insipidus
NDIR
nondispersive infrared
NDIRS
nondispersive infrared spectrometer
NDM
neonatal diabetes mellitus
NDMA
nitrosodimethylamine
NDN
nondysplastic nevus
nDNA
native deoxyribonucleic acid
N/D NHL
nodular/diffuse non-Hodgkin lymphoma
Nd/NT
nondistended/nontender
NDO
neurogenic detrusor overactivity
nondigestible oligosaccharide
NDP
net dietary protein
nucleoside diphosphate
NDP-K
nucleoside diphosphate kinase
NDR
neonatal death rate
neurotic depressive reaction
normal detrusor reflex
nucleus dorsalis raphe
NDS
Neurologic Disability Score
New Drug Submission [FDA]
normal dog serum
NDSA
nondermatomal sensory abnormality
NDSO
nasolacrimal drainage system obstruction
NDST
neurodevelopmental screening test
NDT
nasal duodenostomy tube
neurodevelopmental treatment
(technique) [physical therapy]
noise detection threshold
nondestructive testing
NDUV
Ndumu virus

NDV
Newcastle disease virus
Nyando virus
NDW
number of different words
NDx
nondiagnostic (*See also* ND)
Nd:YAG
neodymium:yttrium-aluminum-garnet
[surgical laser]
Nd:YLF
neodymium:yttrium-lithium-fluoride
[laser]
NE
nasoenteric
national emergency
nausea and emesis
necrotic enteritis
neonatal encephalopathy
nephropathia epidemica
nerve ending
nerve excitability [test]
neural excitation
neuroendocrine
neuroendocrinology
neuroepithelium
neurologic examination
neutropenic enterocolitis
neutrophil elastase
never exposed
no ectopia
no effect
no enlargement
nonelastic
nonendogenous
norepinephrine (*See also* NOR-EPI)
not elevated
not enlarged
not equal
not evaluated
not examined
not exposed
nutcracker esophagus
Ne
neon
NEA
neoplasm embryonic antigen
no evidence of abnormality
NEAA
nonessential amino acid
NEAD
nonepileptic attack disorder
NEAT
nonexercise activity thermogenesis
Norris Educational Achievement
Test
NEB
nebulizer [treatments]
neuroendocrine body

nebul.
nebula
NEC
necrotizing enterocolitis
nephrogenic erythrocyte
neuroemotional complex
neuroendocrine carcinoma
neuroendocrine cell
Neurological Examination for Children
no essential change
noise effective count
noise equivalent count
nonesterified cholesterol
not elsewhere classifiable (classified)
not elsewhere coded
not enough cells
nec
necessary
NECT
nonenhanced computed tomography
NED
no evidence of disease
no expiration date
normal equivalent deviation
NEDEL
no epidemiologically detectable exposure
level
NED-SD
no evidence of disease stationary
disease
NEDSS
National Electronic Disease Surveillance
System
NEE
neonatal epileptic encephalopathy
NEEE
Near East equine encephalomyelitis
NEEG
neoelectroencephalography
normal electroencephalogram
NEEP
negative end-expiratory pressure
NEF
negative expiratory force
negative factor
nephritic factor (*See also* NF)
NEFA
nonesterified fatty acid
NEFG
normal external female genitalia
NEG
neglect
nonenzymatic glycation
neg
negative (*See also* N)
NEH
neutrophilic eccrine hidradenitis

NEI-VFQ
National Eye Institute Visual Function
Questionnaire
NEJ
neuroeffector junction
NEM
N-ethylmaleimide
neurotrophic enhancing molecule
no evidence of malignancy
nonspecific esophageal motility
[disorder]
nem
nutritional milk unit [Ger. *Nährungs
Einheit Milch*]
nema
nematode [threadworm]
NEMD
nonexudative macular degeneration
nonspecific esophageal motility
disorder
nonspecific esophageal motor
dysfunction
NENAR
noneosinophilic nonallergic rhinitis
NEO
necrotizing external otitis
Neuroticism, Extroversion, and
Openness [test]
neo
neonatal (*See also* neonat, NN)
neovascularity
NEOB
New England Organ Bank
NEOH
neonatal/high [risk]
NEOM
neonatal/medium [risk]
neonat
neonatal (*See also* neo, NN)
NEOPO
Northeast Organ Procurement
Organization
NEP
needle-exchange program
negative expiratory pressure
nephrology (*See also* NEPH)
neutral endopeptidase
no evidence of pathology
noise equivalent power
nep
nephrectomy (*See also* NX)
NEPD
no evidence of pulmonary disease
NEPH
nephrology (*See also* NEP)
neph
nephritis

N

NEPHGE
nonequilibrium pH gradient [gel] electrophoresis

NEPHRO
nephrograph(y) (nephrogram)

NEP-I
neutral endopeptidase inhibition

NEPPK
nonepidermolytic palmoplantar keratoderma

NEPV
Nepuyo virus

NEQ
Needs Evaluation Questionnaire

NER
no evidence of recurrence
nonionizing electromagnetic radiation
nucleotide excision repair [DNA mechanism]

NERD
no evidence of recurrent disease
nonerosive reflux disease

NERDS
nodules, eosinophilia, rheumatism, dermatitis, swelling

NERO
noninvasive evaluation of radiation output

nerv, ner
nervous(ness)

NES
nonepileptic seizure
nonstandard electrolyte solution
norepinephrine-selective
not elsewhere specified

NESP
novel erythropoiesis-stimulating protein

NESP55
neuroendocrine secretory protein 55

NET
nasoendotracheal tube (See also NETT)
nerve excitability test
neuroectodermal tumor
neuroemotional technique
neuroendocrine tumor
norepinephrine transporter

net
Internet

NETI
nasotracheal endotracheal intubation

NETT
nasal endotracheal tube (See also NET)

NETZ
needle [diathermy] excision of transformation zone

neu
neurilemma

NeuAc
N-acetylneuraminic acid

neur, neuro, neurol
neurologic
neurology (See also N, NRO)

NEUROD1
neurogenic differentiation 1 [gene]

neuropath
neuropathology (See also NP)

neurosurg
neurosurgery (See also NS, NSurg)

neut
neuter
neutral
neutralize (neutralizing) (neutralization) (See also NT)
neutrophil

NEV
noninvasive extrathoracic ventilator

NEVA
nocturnal electrobioimpedance volumetric assessment

NEX
nose to ear to xiphoid [measurement for NG tube length]
number of excitations [radiology]

NEY, NEYA
neomycin egg yolk [agar]

NF
nasopharyngeal fibroma
National Formulary
necrotizing fasciitis
nephritic factor (See also NEF)
neurofibromatosis (See also NFM)
neurofilament
neutral fraction
night frequency [of voiding]
Nissen fundoplication
nitrofurazone Foley [catheter]
no fracture
noise factor
none found
nonfasting (See also NONF)
nonfiltered
nonfluent
nonfront
nonfunction
nonwhite female
normal flow
not filtered
not found
nursed fair
nursing facility
nylon fiber

NF 1–2
neurofibromatosis type 1–2

nF
nanofarad

NFA
near-fatal asthma

NFA-1–NFA-2
normal fecal antigen 1–2
NFAP
nursing facility-acquired pneumonia
NFAR
no further action required
NFAT
nuclear factor of activated T cell
NFB
nonfermentative [gram-negative]
bacillus
nonfermenting bacteria
NFC
not favorably considered
NFCD
nonfatal coronary disease
NFCE
near-fatal choking episode
NFCS
neonatal facial coding system
NFD
neurofibrillary degeneration
no family doctor
NFDR
neurofacial-digitorenal
(neurofaciodigitorenal) [syndrome]
NFE
nonferrous extract
NFFD
not fit for duty
NFH
nonfamilial hematuria
NFI
nerve-function impairment
Neurobehavioral Functioning Inventory
no-fault insurance
no further information
normal female infant
NF-KB, NF-kappa-B
nuclear factor kappa (κ) B
NFL
nerve fiber layer
NFLD
nerve fiber layer defect
NFM
neurofibromatosis (*See also* NF)
northern fowl mite
NF-NS, NFNS
neurofibromatosis-Noonan syndrome
NFP
natural family planning
neurofilament protein
neurofilament [triplet] polypeptide
no family physician
not for publication
NFPA
nonfunctioning pituitary adenoma

NFPI
Neonatal Facial Pain Inventory
NFS
neural foraminal stenosis
no free sugar
nonfire setter
NFSA
nonfamilial splenic anemia
NFT
neurofibrillary tangle
Nitrazine fern test
no further treatment
NFTD
normal full-term delivery
NFTE
not found this examination
NFTSD
normal full-term spontaneous
delivery
NFTT
neurogenic failure to thrive
nonorganic failure to thrive
NFW
nursed fairly well
N-G
nasogastric (*See also* NG)
NG
nasogastric (*See also* N-G)
new growth
night guard
nodose ganglion
no good
no growth
nongenetic
nongroupable
not given (*See also* n giv)
Ng
Neisseria gonorrhoeae
ng
nanogram (*See also* μmg)
NGA
nutrient gelatin agar
NGAV
Ngaingan virus
NGB
neurogenic bladder
NGC
nongynecologic cytopathology
nucleus [reticularis] gigantocellularis
N-Ger
neurologic geriatrics
NGF
nerve growth factor
NG fdgs
nasogastric feedings
NGFR
nerve (neural) growth factor receptor

N

NiCr
nickel-chromium
NICS
noninvasive carotid studies
NICTH
nonislet-cell tumor hypoglycemia
NICU
neonatal intensive care unit
nonimmunologic contact urticaria
NID
no identifiable disease
not in distress
NIDA
National Institute on Drug Abuse [NIH]
NIDCR
National Institute of Dental and
Craniofacial Research
NIDD
noninsulin-dependent diabetes
NIDDK
National Institute of Diabetes, Digestive
and Kidney Disease
NIDDM
noninsulin-dependent diabetes mellitus
NIDDY
noninsulin-dependent diabetes of young
NIDJD
noninflammatory degenerative joint
disease
NIDS
nonionic detergent soluble
NIEPS
noninvasive electrophysiological study
NIF
negative inspiratory force (*See also* NiF)
neutrophil-immobilizing factor
nonintestinal fibroblast
not in file
NiF
negative inspiratory force (*See also* NIF)
nif
nitrogen fixation [gene]
NIFID
neuronal intermediate filament inclusion
disease
NIFS
noninvasive flow study
nIg
nonimmunoglobulin
nig.
black [L. *niger*]
NIH
National Institutes of Health
[Department of Health and Human
Services]
neointimal hyperplasia
NIH-CPSI
National Institutes of Health Chronic
Prostatitis Symptom Index

NIHD
noise-induced hearing damage
NIHF
nonimmune hydrops fetalis
NIHL
noise-induced hearing loss
NIHSS
National Institutes of Health Stroke
Scale
NIID
neuronal intranuclear inclusion disease
NIL
noise interference level
nothing in light
not in labor
nil.
nothing [L. *nihil*]
NIMA
noninherited maternal antigen
N-IMF
nipple-to-inframammary fold [distance]
NIMH-DIS
National Institute of Mental Health
Diagnostic Interview Schedule
NIMH-ECA
National Institute of Mental
Health-Epidemiologic Catchment Area
NIMH-OC
National Institute of Mental
Health-Global Obsessive Compulsive
Scale
NIMV
noninvasive motion ventilation
NIN
nucleotide-excision repair instability
NINDB
National Institute of Neurologic
Diseases and Blindness
NINDS
National Institutes of Neurological
Disorders and Stroke
NI-NR
no infection no rejection
NINVS
noninvasive neurovascular studies
NIOPCs
no intraoperative complications
NIOSH
National Institute for Occupational
Safety and Health
NIP
catnip
National Immunization Program
negative inspiratory pressure
nipple
nitroiodophenyl
no infection present
no inflammation present
nonimmigrant patient

nonspecific [chronic] interstitial
pneumonitis (pneumonia)
nonspecific interstitial pneumonia
(pneumonitis)

NIPA
noninherited paternal antigen

NIPD
nightly intermittent peritoneal dialysis

NIPH
no improvement with pinhole

NIPPV
noninvasive positive pressure ventilation

NIPS
Neonatal Infant Pain Scale
noninvasive programmed stimulation
noninvolved psoriatic skin

NIPSV
noninvasive pressure-support ventilation

NIPTS
noise-induced permanent threshold
shift

NIQV
Nique virus

NIR
near infrared
near-infrared interactance (interactant)
nitroprusside-induced relaxation
nonidentified risks
noninfectious rhinitis

nirA
nitrite reductase gene

NIRCA
nonisotopic RNase cleavage assay

NIRD
nonimmune renal disease

NIRP
near infrared photoplethysmography

NIRR
noninsulin-requiring remission

NIRS
near-infrared spectroscopy (See also
NIS)
normal inactivated rabbit serum

NIS
near-infrared spectroscopy (See also
NIRS)
no impact sports
no inflammatory signs
nonimmune sheep [serum]
sodium-iodide symporter [gene]

NISD
neonatal iron-storage disease

NISH
nonisotopic in situ hybridization
nonradioactive in situ hybridization

NISM
nucleus of stria medullaris

NISS
New Injury Severity Score

NIST
nucleus of stria terminalis
National Institute of Standards and
Technology

NISV
nonionic surfactant vesicle

NIT
nasointestinal tube
neonatal isoimmune thrombocytopenia

NITD
neuroleptic-induced tardive dyskinesia
noninsulin-treated disease

NiTi
nickel-titanium

nit. ox.
nitric oxide (See also NO)

NITTS
noise-induced temporary threshold
shift

NIV
nodule-inducing virus
noninvasive
noninvasive ventilation

NIVA
noninvasive vascular assessment

NIVLS
noninvasive vascular laboratory
studies

NIVS
noninvasive ventilatory support

nixie
numeric indicator experimental [tube
displaying numerals]

NIZ
noninfarct zone

NJ
nasojejunal

nJ
nanojoule

NJF
nasojejunal feeding

NJLV
Naranjal virus

NK
natural killer [cell]
not known

NK1
neurokinin 1

N.K.
Nomenklatur Kommission

NKA
neurokinin A
no known allergies

nkat
nanokatal

NKB
neurokinin B
no known basis
not keeping baby
NKC
natural killer cell
nonketotic coma
NKCC2
sodium-potassium chloride cotransporter 2 [protein]
NKD
no known diseases
NKDA
no known drug allergies
NKDC
nonketotic diabetic coma
NKE
needle-knife electrocautery
NKECN
nonkeratinizing epidermoid carcinoma
NKF
needle-knife fistulotomy
NKFA
no known food allergies
NKH
nonketotic hyperglycemia (*See also* NKHG)
nonketotic hyperglycinemia
nonketotic hyperosmolar
NKHA
nonketotic hyperosmolar acidosis
NKHG
nonketotic hyperglycemia (*See also* NKH)
nonketotic hyperglycinemia
NKHHC
nonketotic hyperglycemic-hyperosmolar coma
NKHOC
nonketotic hyperosmolar coma
NKHS
nonketotic hyperosmolar syndrome
normal Krebs-Henseleit solution
NKMA
no known medication allergies
NKOV
Nkolbisson virus
NKP
needle-knife papillotomy
NKPP
needle-knife precut papillotomy
NKSF
natural killer [cell]-stimulating factor
NKT
natural killer T [cell]
NKTS
natural killer target structure
NL
nasolacrimal

neural lobe
neutral lipid
nodular lymphoma
nonlatex
normal (*See also* NOR, norm, NR)
normal libido
normal limits
normolipemic
nL
nanoliter
NLA
naphthoxylactic acid
neuroleptanalgesia
neuroleptanesthesia
normal lactase activity
NLAL
nodule-like alveolar lesion
NLB
needle liver biopsy
NLBB
needle-localized breast biopsy
NLC
nasolabial crease
nocturnal leg cramps
NL ClCl, NLC&C, NL C/CI
normal libido, coitus, climax
NLD
nasolacrimal duct
necrobiosis lipoidica diabeticorum
no local doctor
NLDL
normal low-density lipoprotein
n-LDL
native low-density lipoprotein
NLDO
nasolacrimal duct obstruction
NLE
neonatal lupus erythematosus
normal life expectancy
nurse's late entry
Nle
norleucine
NLEA
Nutrition Labeling and Education Act of 1990
NLF
nasolabial fold
neonatal lung fibroblast
nonlactose fermentation
NLFGNR
nonlactose fermenting gram-negative rod
NLGCLS
Noonan-like giant cell lesion syndrome
NLH
nodular lymphoid hyperplasia
NLHEP
National Lung Health Education Program

NLL
  nonleukemic lymphoma
  nonlymphoblastic leukemia
NLM
  National Library of Medicine [NIH]
  noise level monitor
  no limitation of motion
NLMC
  nocturnal leg muscle cramp
NLN
  no longer needed
NLO
  nasolacrimal occlusion
NLOB
  needle-localized open biopsy
NLP
  natural language processing
  neurolinguistic programming
  nodular liquefying panniculitis
  no light perception
  normal light perception
  normal luteal phase
NLPD
  nodular-lymphocytic, poorly
    differentiated
NLS
  neonatal lupus syndrome
  nonlinear least squares [statistics]
  normal lymphocyte supernatant
  nuclear localization signal [motif]
NLSD
  normal life span for dogs
NLT
  Names Learning Test
  normal lymphocyte transfer (test)
  not later than
  not less than
  nucleus lateralis tuberis
NLV
  Norwalk-like virus
NLX
  nephrolithiasis, X-linked
NM
  neuromedical
  neuromuscular
  neuronal microdysgenesis
  nevomelanocytic
  nictitating membrane [L. *nictitare* to
    wink]
  night and morning (*See also* N&M,
    n.m.)
  nocturnal myoclonus
  nodular melanoma
  nodular mixed [lymphoma] (*See also*
    NML)
  nonmalignant
  nonmotile [bacteria]
  nonwhite male

normetadrenaline
normetanephrine (*See also* NMN,
  normet)
not measurable (measured)
not mentioned
not motile
nuclear matrix
nuclear medicine
nuclear membrane
N&M
  nerve and muscle
  night and morning (*See also* NM, n.m.)
N/m
  newton per meter
N/m²
  newton per square meter
nM
  nanomolar
n.m.
  night and morning [L. *nocte et mane*]
    (*See also* N&M, NM)
nm
  nanometer
  nonmetallic
  nux moschata [nutmeg, homeopathic]
NMA
  neurogenic muscular atrophy
NMATWT
  New Mexico Attitude Toward Work
    Test
NMB
  neuromuscular blockade
  neuromuscular blocker (blocking) [drug,
    agent]
NMBA
  neuromuscular blocking agent
  nitrosomethylbenzylamine
NMC
  neuromuscular control
  nodular mixed cell [lymphoma]
  no malignant cells
  nucleus [reticularis] magnocellularis
NMCD
  nephrophthisis-medullary cystic
    disease
NMCPT
  New Mexico Career Planning Test
NMD
  neuromuscular disorder
  neuromyodysplasia
  neuronal migration disorder
  normal mental development
  normal muscle development
NMDA
  N-methyl-D-aspartate
NMDP
  National Marrow Donor Pool
  National Marrow Donor Program

N

NME
    necrolytic migratory erythema
    neuromyeloencephalopathy
    new molecular entity
NMEP
    neurogenic motor evoked potential
NMES
    neuromuscular electrical stimulation
    (stimulator)
NMF
    neuromuscular facilitation
    nonmigrating fraction [of spermatozoa]
NMG
    N-methyl-D-glucamide
    no Marcus Gunn [pupil]
NMGTD
    nonmetastatic gestational trophoblastic
    disease
NMH
    neurally mediated hypotension
NMHH
    no medical health history
NMI
    no manifest improvement
    no mental illness
    no middle initial
    no more information
    normal male infant
NMID
    N-terminal midfragment
NMIS
    nuclear medicine information system
NMJ
    neuromuscular junction
NMJAPT
    New Mexico Job Application
    Procedures Test
NMKB
    not married, keeping baby
NMKOT
    New Mexico Knowledge of Occupations
    Test
NML
    nodular mixed lymphoma (*See also*
    NM)
NMM
    nevoid malignant melanoma
    nodular malignant melanoma
NMN
    neurotized melanocytic nevus
    nicotinamide mononucleotide
    N1-methylnicotinamide
    no middle name
    normetanephrine (*See also* NM, normet)
    Novy-McNeal-Nicolle [medium, culture]
    (*See also* NNM)
NMN+
    nicotinamide mononucleotide [reduced
    form]

NMNKB
    not married, not keeping baby
NMO
    nitrogen mustard oxide
NMOH
    no medical ocular history
nmol
    nanomole
nmol/L
    nanomole per liter
NMOS
    N-type metal oxide semiconductor
NMP
    nail matrix phenolization
    neuromuscular pacification
    neutral metallopeptidase
    normal menstrual period
    nuclear matrix protein
    nucleoside 5′-monophosphate
NMPCA
    nonmetric principal component analysis
NMR
    Neill-Mooser reaction
    neonatal mortality rate (risk)
    nictitating membrane response
    nuclear magnetic resonance
NMRI
    nuclear magnetic resonance imaging
NMRL
    normal-mode ruby laser
NMRS
    nuclear magnetic resonance spectroscopy
NMRT
    National Medical Response Team
NMS
    neurally mediated syncope
    neuroleptic malignant syndrome
    neuromuscular spindle
    N-methylspiroperidol
    normal mouse serum
N · m/s
    newton times meter per second
NMSC
    nonmelanoma skin cancer
NMSE
    normalized mean square root [statistics]
NMSIDS
    near-miss sudden infant death syndrome
NMT
    nebulized mist treatment
    neuromuscular tension
    neuromuscular therapy
    neuromuscular transmission
    no more than
    nuclear medicine technology
NMTB
    neuromuscular transmission blockade
NMTD
    nonmetastatic trophoblastic disease

NMTS
 neuromuscular tension state
NMTSS
 nonmenstrual toxic shock syndrome
NMU
 neuromuscular unit
NMUT
 nitrosomethylurethane
NMV
 New Minto virus
NMVS
 neurally mediated vasovagal
  syncope
NN
 narrative notes
 Navajo neuropathy
 nearest neighbor
 neonatal (*See also* neo, neonat)
 neural network
 nevocellular nevus
 normally nourished
 normal to normal
 nurse's notes (*See also* N/N)
N/N
 negative/negative
 normocytic/normochromic [anemia]
  (*See also* NNA, NCNC, NCNCA)
 nurse's notes (*See also* NN)
N-N
 nurse-to-nurse [orders]
N:N
 azo group [chemical group with two
  nitrogen atoms]
N&N
 nephritis and nephrosis
n.n.
 new name [L. *nomen novum*] (*See also*
  n. nov., nom. nov., nov. n.)
nn
 nervi (nerves) [plural]
NNA
 nonneuronopathic amyloidosis
 normochromic normocytic anemia
  (*See also* N/N, NCNC, NCNCA)
NNAS
 neonatal narcotic abstinence syndrome
NNB
 normal newborn
NNBC
 node-negative breast cancer
NND
 neonatal death (*See also* ND)
 New and Nonofficial Drugs
 nonspecific nonerosive duodenitis
NNDSS
 National Notifiable Diseases
  Surveillance System [CDC]

NNE
 neonatal necrotizing enterocolitis
 nonneuronal enolase
NNG
 nonspecific nonerosive gastritis
NNH
 number needed to harm
  [epidemiology]
NNI
 noise and number index
NNIS
 National Nosocomial Infectious
  Surveillance [CDC]
NNJ
 neonatal jaundice
NNL
 no new laboratory [test orders]
NNM
 neonatal mortality
 Nicolle-Novy-MacNeal [medium,
  culture] (*See also* NMN)
NNN
 nitrosonornicotine
NNO
 no new orders
n. nov.
 new name [L. *nomen novum*] (*See also*
  n.n., nom. nov., nov. n.)
NNP
 nerve net pulse
 nonnociceptive pain
N:NPK
 nitrogen to nonprotein kilocalories
  ratio
NNR
 New and Nonofficial Remedies
 not necessary to return
NNRTI
 nonnucleoside reverse transcriptase
  inhibitor
NNS
 nasal nicotine spray
 neonatal screen [hematocrit, total
  bilirubin, total protein]
 nicotine nasal spray
 nonneoplastic syndrome
 nonnutritive sucking
 number needed to screen [clinical trial
  statistic]
NNT
 neonatally tolerant
 neonatology
 number needed to treat [clinical trial
  statistic]
NNTB
 number needed to treat to benefit
  [clinical trial statistic]

N

NNTH
number needed to treat to harm
[clinical trial statistic]
NNU
net nitrogen utilization
NNV
nasal nocturnal ventilation
NNWI
Neonatal Narcotic Withdrawal Index
NNWT
noncontact normothermic wound therapy
NO
nasal oxygen
nitric oxide
nitroso-
none obtained
nonobese
not operable
number (*See also* N, n, no.)
N₂O
nitrous oxide
NO₂
nitrogen dioxide
No
nobelium
no.
number [L. *numero*] (*See also* N, n,
NO)
NOA
nitric oxide analyzer
notice of admission
NOABX
no antibiotic
NOAEL
no observed adverse effect level
NOAR
Norfolk Arthritis Register
NOBT
nonoperative biopsy technique
NOC
N-nitroso compound
nonorgan confined
nursing outcome classification
noc, noct
at night
nocturia
nocturnal [L. *noctis*]
NO-CCE
no clubbing, cyanosis, or edema
NOD
nodular [melanoma]
nondefinitive [pattern]
nonobese diabetic
notice of disagreement
notify of death
NOE
nasoorbitoethmoid
no observable effect
nuclear Overhauser effect

NOEC
no observed effect concentration
NOED
no observed effect dose
NOEL
no observed effect level [of
toxin]
no ess abn
no essential abnormalities
NOF
nonossifying fibroma
N/OFQ
nociceptin/orphanin FQ [peptide]
NOFT
nonorganic failure to thrive
NOFTT
nonorganic failure to thrive
NOGM
no gammopathy
nonoxidative glucose metabolism
NOH
neurogenic orthostatic hypotension
NOHSS
National Oral Health Surveillance
System
NOI
nature of illness
NOII
nonocclusive intestinal ischemia
NOK
next of kin
NOL
not on label
NOLAV
Nola virus
NOM
nonoperative management
nonsuppurative otitis media
normal ocular movements
nom. dub.
a doubtful name [L. *nomen dubium*]
NOMI
nonocclusive mesenteric infarct(ion)
nonocclusive mesenteric ischemia
NOMID
neonatal-onset multisystem inflammatory
disease
nom. nov.
new name [L. *nomen novum*] (*See also*
n.n., n. nov., nov. n.)
nom. nud.
name without designation [L. *nomen
nudum*]
NOMS
not on my shift
NON
nape of neck
NO/N₂
nitric oxide/nitrogen

NOND
none detectable (detected) (*See also* ND)
NONF
nonfasting (*See also* NF)
non-FCC
nonfollicular center cell
non-MALT
nonmucosa-associated lymphoid tissue
NONMEM
nonlinear mixed-effects model (modeling)
non pal
not palpable
non-Q MI
non-Q wave myocardial infarct(ion) (*See also* NQMI, NQWMI)
non reb
nonrebreathing [mask] (*See also* NR, NRB, NRM)
nonREM, non-REM
nonrapid eye movement (*See also* NREM)
non rep
do not repeat (*See also* NR, n.r.)
NONS
nonspecific (*See also* NS)
NO-NSAID
nitric oxide-releasing nonsteroidal antiinflammatory agent (NSAID)
nonseg
nonsegmented [neutrophil]
non-SSM
nonskin-sparing mastectomy
non-STEMI
non-ST segment elevation myocardial infarction
nonvis, nonviz
nonvisualized
N₂O:O₂
nitrous oxide to oxygen ratio
NOOB
not out of bed
N₂O-O₂-opioid
nitrous oxide-oxygen-opioid [anesthetic technique]
NOP
national outpatient profile
not on patient
not otherwise provided [for] (*See also* NP)
4NOQ
4-nitroquinoline-1-oxide-induced tumor
NOR
noradrenaline (*See also* Noradr)
normal (*See also* NL, norm, NR)
nucleolar (nucleolus) organizing region [cytogenetics]

Noradr
noradrenaline (*See also* NOR)
NORC
normal curve
NOR-EPI
norepinephrine (*See also* NE)
norleu
norleucine
norm
normal (*See also* NL, NOR, NR)
normet
normetanephrine (*See also* NM, NMN)
NORV
Northway virus
NOS
network operating system
new-onset seizures
nitric oxide synthase
nitrous oxide synthase
nonorgan-specific
no organisms seen
not on staff
not otherwise specified
NOS1
nitric oxide synthase 1 [gene]
nos
numbers [plural]
NOSAC
nonsteroidal antiinflammatory compound
NOSE
normal ovarian surface epithelium
NOSI
nitric oxide synthase inhibitor
NOSIE
Nurses' Observation Scale for Inpatient Evaluation
NoSOS
no surgery on site
NOT
nocturnal oxygen therapy
nucleus of optic tract
NOTT
nocturnal oxygen therapy trial
nov.
new [L. *novam*]
nov. n.
new name [L. *nomen novum*] (*See also* n.n., n. nov., nom. nov.)
nov. sp.
new species [L. *novam species*]
NOW
negotiable order of withdrawal
NOX
number of excitations [radiology]
NP
nasal polyp
nasal prongs

N

NP *(continued)*
  nasopharyngeal
  nasopharynx *(See also* NPhx)
  natriuretic peptide
  near point [ophthalmology]
  necrotizing pancreatitis
  neonatal-perinatal
  nephrographic phase
  nerve palsy
  neuritic plaque
  neuropathic pain
  neuropathology *(See also*
    neuropath)
  neuropeptide
  neuropsychiatric
  neuropsychiatry
  neutrogenic precautions
  newly presented
  new patient
  Niemann-Pick [disease]
  nitrogen-phosphorus [detector in gas
    chromatography]
  nitrophenol
  nodular paragranuloma
  nonpalpable
  nonpathologic
  nonpaying
  nonphagocytic
  nonpracticing
  nonproducer [cell]
  no pain
  no phone
  no progress
  no progression
  normal plasma
  normal pressure
  nosocomial pneumonia
  not [otherwise] provided [for] *(See also*
    NOP)
  not palpable
  not perceptible
  not performed
  not practiced
  not pregnant
  not present
  not protected
  nuclear pharmacy
  nucleoplasmic [index]
  nucleoprotein
  nucleoside phosphorylase
  nursed poorly
  nursing practice (procedure)
  proper name [L. *nomen proprium*]
    (See also n.p.)
3NP
  3-nitropropionic acid
N-P
  need-persistence

Np
  neper (napier) [unit expressing ratio of
    2 numbers as natural logarithm]
  neptunium
  neurophysin
n.p.
  proper name [L. *nomen proprium*]
    (See also NP)
np
  nucleotide pair
NPA
  nasopharyngeal airway
  nasopharyngeal aspirate
  near point of accommodation
  Niemann-Pick disease type A [classical
    infantile]
  no previous admission
  nucleus of pretectal area
NPa
  nail patella [syndrome]
NPAT
  nonparoxysmal atrial tachycardia
Np-AVP
  neurophysin associated with
    vasopressin
NPB
  Nellcor Puritan Bennett
    [instrumentation]
  Niemann-Pick disease type B [visceral
    form]
  nodal premature beat
  nonprotein bound
NPBC
  node-positive breast cancer
NPBF
  nonplacental blood flow
NPBV
  negative pressure body ventilator
NPC
  nasopharyngeal cancer (carcinoma)
  near point of convergence
  negative peritoneal cytology
  nephrogenic polycythemia
  Niemann-Pick disease type C [subacute
    or juvenile]
  nodal premature contractions
  nonparenchymal (liver) cell
  nonpatient contact
  nonproductive cough
  nonprotein calorie
  no prenatal care *(See also* NPNC)
  no previous complaint
  nucleus of posterior commissure
NPC1
  Niemann-Pick disease type C1 gene
NPCa
  nasopharyngeal cancer (carcinoma)
    (See also NPC)

NPCC
nonprotein carbohydrate calories
NPCIS
nasopharyngeal carcinoma in situ
NP-CPAP, NPCPAP
nasal prong continuous positive airway pressure
NPCR
normalized protein catabolic rate
NPD
narcissistic personality disorder
natriuretic plasma dialysate
negative pressure device
Niemann-Pick disease type D [Nova Scotian type]
nitrogen-phosphorus detector
nonpathologic diagnosis
nonprescription drug
no pathologic diagnosis
normal protein diet
NPDDP
National Preventive Dentistry Demonstration Program
NPDL
nodular poorly differentiated lymphocytic (lymphoma)
NPDR
nonproliferative diabetic retinopathy
NPE
neurogenic pulmonary edema
neuropsychologic examination
nonpulmonary route of elimination
no palpable enlargement
normal pelvic examination
NPEM
nocturnal penile erection monitoring
NPEV
nonpolio enterovirus
NPF
nasopharyngeal fiberscope
no predisposing factor
normal pelvic findings
NPFS
nonpenetrating filtering surgery
NPFT
Neurotic Personality Factor Test
NPG
nonpregnant
NPGS
neopentyl glycol succinate
NPH
nephronophthisis
no previous history
normal-pressure hydrocephalus
nucleus pulposus herniation
NPH1
nephronophthisis type 1

NPhx
nasopharynx (*See also* NP)
NPI
Narcissistic Personality Inventory
National Provider Identifier [Department of Health and Human Services]
neonatal perception inventory
Neuropsychiatric Inventory
no present illness
Nottingham Prognostic Index
nucleoplasmic index
NPIC
neurogenic peripheral intermittent claudication
NPII
Neonatal Pulmonary Insufficiency Index
NPIS
Numeric Pain Intensity Scale
NPJT
nonparoxysmal [atrioventricular] junctional tachycardia
NPK
nonprotein kilocalories
NPL
nasopharyngolaryngoscopy
neoproteolipid
nodular poorly differentiated lymphoma
no perception of light
NPLEx
Naturopathic Physicians Licensing Examination
NPLSM
neoplasm
NPM
neonatal-perinatal medicine
nonpacemaker
nothing per mouth (*See also* NPO, n.p.o.)
NPN
necrotic pseudoxanthomatous nodule
nonprotein nitrogen
nPNA
normalized protein nitrogen appearance
NPNC
no prenatal care (*See also* NPC)
NPNT
nonpalpable, nontender
NPO
nothing by mouth [L. *nil per os*] (*See also* NBM)
nucleus preopticus
n.p.o.
nothing by mouth [L. *nil per os*] (*See also* NPO, NBM)
NPOC
nonpurgeable organic carbon

N

NPO/HS
nothing by mouth at bedtime [L. *nil per os hora somni*]
NPOS
nitrite positive
NPOT
narrow pulmonary outflow tract
Np-OT
oxytocin-associated neurophysin
NPOW
not prisoner of war
NPP
nitrophenylphosphate
normally progressing pregnancy
normal pooled plasma
normal postpartum
NPPB
normal perfusion pressure breakthrough
NPPE
negative pressure pulmonary edema
NPPI
nonpeptidic protease inhibitor
NPPNG
nonpenicillinase-producing *Neisseria gonorrheae*
NP polio
nonparalytic poliomyelitis
NPPV
nasal positive pressure ventilation
noninvasive positive-pressure ventilation
NPR
nasopharyngeal reflux
natriuretic peptide receptor
net protein ratio
normal pulse rate
nothing per rectum
nucleoside phosphoribosyl
nPR
nodular partial remission
NPRL
normal pupillary reaction to light
NPRM
notice of proposed rulemaking
NPRS
numerical pain rating scale
NPS
nail-patella syndrome
nasopharyngeal secretion
nasopharyngeal stenosis
National Pharmaceutical Stockpile
neonatal progeroid syndrome
new patient set-up
Nps
nitrophenylsulfenyl
NPSA
normal pilosebaceous apparatus
NPSD
nonpotassium-sparing diuretic

NPSG
nocturnal polysomnograph(y) (polysomnogram)
NPSH
nonprotein sulfhydryl [group]
NP-SLE, NPSLE
neuropsychiatric systemic lupus erythematosus
NPT
nasal provocation test
near patient test
neoprecipitin test
neuropsychological test
nocturnal penile tumescence
no prior tracings
normal pressure and temperature
NPTS
nocturnal painful tonic spasm
NPU
net protein utilization
NPV
negative predictive value
negative pressure ventilation
nothing per vagina
nuclear polyhidrosis virus
nucleus paraventricularis
NPY
neuropeptide Y
NPZ
neuropsychological test Z score
NQA
nursing quality assurance
NQMI
non-Q wave myocardial infarct(ion) (*See also* non-Q MI, NQWMI)
NQR
nuclear quadruple resonance
NQWMI
non-Q wave myocardial infarct(ion) (*See also* non-Q MI, NQMI)
NR
do not repeat [L. *non repetatur*] (*See also* non rep, n.r.)
nephrogenic rest
nerve root
neural retina
neutral red
newly reformulated
noise reduction
none reported
nonreactive
nonrebreather (nonrebreathing) [mask] (*See also* NRB, non reb, NRM)
nonreimbursable
nonresponder
no radiation
no reaction
no recurrence
no refill

no rehearsal
no rejection
no report
no respiration
no response
no result
no return
normal (*See also* NL, NOR, norm)
normal range
normal reaction
normal record
normotensive rat (*See also* NTR)
not reached
not reacting
not readable
not recorded
not reported
not resolved
nuclear radiology
nuclear receptor
nucleotide residue
number
nutrition ratio

N/R
not remarkable

n.r.
do not repeat [L. *non repetatur*]
(*See also* non rep, NR)

nr
near

NRA
nitrate reductase activity
nucleus retroambigualis

NRAF
nonrheumatic atrial fibrillation

NRAM
neuroretinal angiomatosis

Nramp
natural resistance macrophage-associated
protein

NRB
nonrebreather [oxygen mask] (*See also*
non reb, NR, NRM)
nonrejoining [DNA strand] break
nonreportable birth

NRBA
neutrophil respiratory burst
activity

NRBC, NRbc
normal red blood cell
nucleated red blood cell

NRBS
nonrebreathing system

NRC
noise reduction coefficient
normal retinal correspondence
not routine care

NRCL
nonrenal clearance

NRD
nonrenal death

NRDS
neonate respiratory distress
syndrome

NRE
nonregulatory element

NREH
normal renin essential hypertension

NREM, NREMS
nonrapid eye movement [sleep]
(*See also* nonREM, non-REM)

NRF
normal renal function

NRFC
nonrosette-forming cell

NRFHR
nonreassuring fetal heart rate

NRG
neuregulin

NRGC
nucleus reticularis gigantocellularis

NRG1–NRG4
neuregulin 1–4 [protein]

NRH
nodular regenerative hyperplasia [of
liver]

NRI
nerve root involvement
nerve root irritation
neutral regular insulin
nonrespiratory infection
no recent illnesses
norepinephrine reuptake inhibitor

NRIT
Non-Reading Intelligence Test, Levels
1-3

NRIV
Ngari virus

NRK
normal rat kidney

NRL
normal rubber latex
nucleus reticularis lateralis

N-RLX
nonrelaxed

NRM
nonrebreathing mask (*See also* non reb,
NR, NRB)
no regular medicines
normal retinal movement
normal range [of] motion (*See also*
NROM)
nucleus raphe magnus
nucleus reticularis magnocellularis

N

NRMI
National Registry of Myocardial Infarction

NRN
no return necessary

nRNA
nuclear ribonucleic acid

nRNP
nuclear ribonucleoprotein

NRNST
nonreassuring nonstress test

NRO
neurology (*See also* N, neur, neuro, neurol)

NROM
normal range of motion (*See also* NRM)

NRP
neonatal resuscitation program
nonreassuring pattern
nucleus reticularis parvocellularis

NRPAT
net revenue, patient

NRPC
nucleus reticularis pontis caudalis

NRPG
nucleus reticularis paragigantocellularis

NRPR
nonbreathing pressure relieving

NRR
net reproduction rate
Noise Reduction Rating
note, record, report

NRS
Neurobehavioral Rating Scale
nonimmunized rabbit serum
normal rabbit serum
normal reference serum
numeric rating scale

nrsng
nursing (*See also* NSG, nsg)

NRSTS
nonrhabdomyosarcoma soft tissue sarcoma

NRT
neuromuscular reeducation technique
nicotine replacement therapy
nitron radical trap

NRTI
nucleoside [analog] reverse transcriptase inhibitor

NRTOT
net revenue, total

NRTP
nucleus reticularis tegmenti pontis

NRV
Neckar river virus
nucleus reticularis ventralis

NS
nasal spray
nasal steroid
natural science
needle shower
nephrosclerosis
nephrotic syndrome
nerve sheath
nervous system
neurologic sign
neurologic surgery
neurologic survey
neurosarcoidosis
neurosecretory
neurosurgery (*See also* neurosurg, NSurg)
neurosyphilis
neurotic score
nevus sebaceus
nipple stimulation
nodular sclerosis
nodus sinuatrialis
nonsmoker (*See also* NSM)
nonsnorer
nonspecific (*See also* NONS)
nonstimulation
nonstructural [protein]
nonstutterer
nonsymptomatic
normal saline (*See also* N/S)
normal serum
normal sodium (diet)
normal study
normospermic
Norwegian scabies
no sample
no sequela [singular] (sequelae [plural])
no-show
nosocomial sinusitis
no specimen
not seen
not significant
not specified (*See also* NSP)
not stated
not sufficient
not symptomatic
novelty speaking
nuclear sclerosis (sclerotic)
nursing services
nutritive sucking
nylon suture (*See also* ns)

N/S
normal saline (*See also* NS)

N:S
noise to signal ratio

Ns
nasopinale [craniometric]

ns
nanosecond (*See also* nsec)

NSA
> neck-shaft angle [femur]
> nonspecific arrhythmia
> normal serum albumin
> no salt added
> no serious abnormality
> no significant abnormality
> no significant anomaly
> number of signals averaged [magnetic resonance]
> nutritional status assessment

NSAA
> nonsteroidal antiandrogen

NSAD
> no signs of acute disease

NSAE
> nonserious adverse event
> nonsupported arm exercise

NSAIA
> nonsteroidal antiinflammatory agent

NSAID
> nonsteroidal antiinflammatory drug

NSAP
> nonspecific abdominal pain

NSB
> nonspecific binding

NSBC
> nonskull base chordoma

NSBGP
> nonspecific bowel gas pattern

NSBR
> nonspecific bronchial reactivity
> Nottingham modification of Scarff-Bloom-Richardson grading

NSC
> neurosecretory cell
> nonservice connected [death or disability] (*See also* NSCD)
> nonspecific suppressor cell
> no significant change

NSCC
> nonsmall-cell cancer
> nonsmall-cell carcinoma

NSCD
> nonservice connected death (disability) (*See also* NSC)

NSCFPT
> no significant change from previous tracing

NSCLC
> nonsmall-cell lung cancer (carcinoma)

NSCLC-ND
> nonsmall-cell lung carcinoma with neuroendocrine differentiation

NS/CST
> nipple stimulation/contraction stress test

NSD
> N-acetylneuraminic acid storage disease
> Nairobi sheep disease
> nasal septal deviation
> neonatal staphylococcal disease
> neurosecretory dysfunction
> neurosensory deficit
> night sleep deprivation
> nitrogen-specific detector
> nominal single dose
> nominal standard dose
> normal single dose
> normal spontaneous delivery
> normal standard dose
> no significant defect
> no significant deficiency
> no significant deviation
> no significant difference
> no significant disease

NSDA
> nonsteroid-dependent asthmatic

NSDV
> Nairobi sheep disease virus

NSE
> neuron-specific enolase
> nonspecific esterase
> normal saline enema

NS̄E
> nausea without emesis [Fr. *sans*]

NSEACS
> non-ST elevation acute coronary syndrome

nsec
> nanosecond (*See also* ns)

NSED
> nonsurgeon, emergency department

NSF
> N-ethylmaleimide-sensitive-factor
> nodular subepidermal fibrosis
> no significant findings

NSFTD
> normal spontaneous full-term delivery

NSG
> necrotizing sarcoid granulomatosis
> neurosecretory granule
> nursing (*See also* nrsng, nsg)

nsg
> nursing (*See also* nrsng, NSG)

NSGCT
> nonseminomatous germ [cell] tumor (*See also* NSGT)

NSGCTT
> nonseminomatous germ cell testicular tumor

NSTGCT
> nonseminomatous testicular germ cell tumor

N

NSGI
nonspecific genital infection
NSGO
nonspecific granulomatous orchitis
NSG STA
nursing station
NSGT
nonseminomatous germ [cell] tumor
(*See also* NSGCT)
NSH
normal scalp hair
NSHC
no self-harm contract
NSHD
nodular sclerosing Hodgkin disease
NSHL
nonsyndromic hearing loss
NSHPT
neonatal severe hyperparathyroidism
NSI
needlestick injury
negative self-image
neurosensory impairment
nonsyncytium-inducing [virus]
no sign of infection
no sign of inflammation
NSIDS
near-sudden infant death syndrome
NSILA
nonsuppressible insulinlike activity
NSILP
nonsuppressible insulinlike protein
NSIP
nonspecific interstitial pneumonia
(pneumonitis)
NSIS
nonsulfonylurea insulin secretagogue
NSIVCD
nonspecific intraventricular conduction
delay
NSJ
nevus sebaceus of Jadassohn
NSK
nonsquamous keratin
NSL
nonsalt loser
NSLF
normal sheep lung fibroblast
NSLN
nonsentinel lymph node
NSM
nerve sheath myxoma
neurosecretory material
neurosecretory motor neuron
nonantigenic specific mediator
nonsmoker (*See also* NS)
nutrient sporulation medium
N · s/m²
newton times second per square meter

NSMMVT
nonsustained monomorphic ventricular
tachycardia
NSN
nephrotoxic serum nephritis
nicotine-stimulated neurophysin
nonsentinel [lymph] node
nonspecific neurotic [syndrome]
number of similar negatives
NSND
nonsymptomatic, nondisabling
NSO
nonnutritive sucking opportunity
nucleus supraopticus
NSol
nerve to soleus
NSOM
near field scanning optical
microscope
nonsuppurative osteomyelitis
NSOP
no soft organs palpable
NSP
nasal speech pattern
neck and shoulder pain
neuron-specific protein
neurotoxic shellfish poisoning
nonstarch polysaccharide
not specified (*See also* NS)
number of similar positives
NSP1–NSP5
nonstructural protein 1–5
NSPE
no specimen [obtainable]
NSPVT
nonsustained polymorphic ventricular
tachycardia
NSQ
Neuroticism Scale Questionnaire
not sufficient quantity
NSR
nasoseptal reconstruction
nasoseptal repair
nonspecific reaction
nonsystemic reaction
normal sinus rhythm
not seen regularly
nSRBC
normal sheep red blood cell
NSR/M
no sign of recurrence or metastasis
NSRP
nerve-sparing radical prostatectomy
NSRR
normal sinus rate and rhythm
NSRRL
neutral, sidebent right, rotated left
NSRT
nonsurgical septal reduction therapy

NSS
    nasal symptom score
    nephron-sparing surgery
    neurological signs stable
    neuropathy symptom score
    normal saline solution
    normal size and shape
    not statistically significant
NSSC
    normal size, shape, consistency
NSSL
    normal size, shape, location
NSSP
    normal size, shape, position
NSSPAVAF
    normal size, shape, position, anteverted,
      anteflexed (uterus)
NSST
    nonspecific ST [wave segment changes
      on electroencephalogram]
    Northwestern Syntax Screening Test
NSSTT
    nonspecific ST and T [wave changes
      on electrocardiogram]
NSST-TWC
    nonspecific ST and T wave change
NST
    neospinothalamic [tract]
    neostigmine test
    nerve stimulation therapy
    neurostructural integration technique
    nonmyeloablative stem cell
      transplant
    Nonsense Syllable Test
    nonshivering thermogenesis
    nonstress test [fetal monitoring]
    normal sphincter tone
    no specific type
    not sooner than
    nutritional status type
NSTD
    nonsexually transmitted disease
NSTEMI
    non-ST segment elevation myocardial
      infarct(ion)
NSTEP
    National Spit Tobacco Education
      Program
NSTI
    necrotizing soft-tissue infection
NSTT
    nonseminomatous testicular tumor
NSU
    necrotizing sclerocorneal ulceration
    nonspecific urethritis
NSurg
    neurosurgery (*See also* neurosurg, NS)

NSV
    nonspecific vaginitis
NSVD
    nonstructural valve deterioration
    normal spontaneous vaginal delivery
NSVR
    normalized systemic vascular resistance
NSVT
    nonsustained ventricular tachycardia
NSX
    neurosurgical examination
NSY
    nursery
N-T, N&T
    nose and throat
NT
    nasotracheal
    neurofeedback training
    neurotensin
    neurotoxin
    neutralization technique
    neutralization test
    neutralize (neutralizing) (neutralization)
      (*See also* neut)
    next time
    nontender
    nontypeable
    normal temperature
    normal tissue
    normotensive
    no test
    not tender
    not tested
    nourishment taken
    N-telopeptide
    nucleation time
    numbness and tingling
NT-1–NT-5
    neurotrophin-1–5
5′-NT
    5′-nucleotidase
N:T
    neck to thigh ratio
Nt
    amino terminal
NTA
    natural thymocytotoxic autoantibody
    nitrilotriacetic acid
    Nurse Training Act
NTAB
    nephrotoxic antibody
N Tachy
    nodal tachycardia
NT-ANP
    N-terminal atrial natriuretic peptide
NTAV
    Ntaya virus

N

NTB
  necrotizing tracheobronchitis
  nontumor-bearing
N/TBC
  nontuberculous
NTBR
  not to be resuscitated
NTC
  neurotrauma center
NTCC
  National Type Culture Collection
NTCP
  noninvasive transcutaneous cardiac
    pacing
NTCS
  no tumor cells seen
NTD
  negative to date
  neural tube defect
  nitroblue tetrazolium dye
  noise tone difference
NTE
  neuropathy target esterase
  neurotoxic esterase
  neutral thermal environment
  nontest ear
  not to exceed
  nuclear track emulsion
NTED
  neonatal toxic [shock syndromelike]
    exanthematous disease
NTF
  nasogastric tube feeding
  neurotrophic factor
  normal throat flora
NTG
  nitroglycerin (See also NTZ)
  nontoxic goiter
  nontreatment group
  normal-tension glaucoma
  normal triglyceridemia
NTHH
  nontumorous hypergastrinemic
    hyperchlorhydria
NTHI
  native tissue harmonic imaging
  nontypeable *Haemophilus influenzae*
NTI
  narrow therapeutic index
  nasotracheal intubation
  nonthyroid illness
  nonthyroid index
  no treatment indicated
NTL
  near-total laryngectomy
  nectar-thick liquid [diet consistency]
  no time limit
NTLE
  neocortical temporal lobe epilepsy

NTLI
  neurotensinlike immunoreactivity
NTM
  Neuman-Tytell medium
  nocturnal tumescence monitor
  nontuberculous mycobacteria (See also
    NTMB)
NTMB
  nontuberculous mycobacteria (See also
    NTM)
NTMI
  nontransmural myocardial infarction
NTMNG
  nontoxic multinodular goiter
NTN
  nephrotoxic nephritis
  neurturin
NTND
  not tender, not distended [abdomen]
NTNG
  nontoxic nodular goiter
NTOM
  nerve territory oriented macrodactyly
NTP
  narcotic treatment program
  nonthrombocytopenic preterm [infant]
  normal temperature and pressure
  nucleoside triphosphate
NT&P
  normal temperature and pressure
NTPD
  nocturnal tidal peritoneal dialysis
NTPPH, NTPPPH
  nucleoside triphosphate
    pyrophosphohydrolase
NT-proBNP
  N-terminal prohormone brain natriuretic
    peptide
NTR
  negative therapeutic reaction
  normotensive rat (See also NR)
  nutrition
NTR1–NTR3
  neurotensin receptor type 1–3
NTRK1
  neurotrophic tyrosine kinase receptor,
    type 1
NTS
  nasotracheal suction
  nephrotoxic serum
  nicotine transdermal system
  nontropical sprue
  nonturning [against] self [psychology]
  nontyphi (nontyphoidal) *Salmonella*
  nucleus tractus solitarius
NTSN
  nephrotoxic serum nephritis
NTT
  nasotracheal tube

nearly total thyroidectomy
nonthrombocytopenic term
 [infant]
nontreponemal test
nuchal translucency thickness
NTTP
no tenderness to palpation
NTU
nephelometric turbidity unit
N-TUL
internal tumescent ultrasound
 liposculpture
NTV
nervous tissue vaccine
NTVR
normal transvalvular
 regurgitation
NTx
N-telopeptide
NTZ
nitroglycerin (*See also* NTG)
normal transformation zone
 [colposcopy]
v
dispersiveness of lens or prism
 [constringence]
kinematic viscosity (*See also* v)
number of digrees of freedom
 [statistics]
nu [13th letter of Greek alphabet,
 lowercase]
photon [light energy]
NU
name unknown
Nu
nucleolus
nucleus (*See also* N, nucl)
nU
nanounit
nu
neurilemma
neutrino
nude (mouse)
NUC
nuclear (*See also* nucl)
nuclear medicine
Nuc
nucleoside (*See also* N)
nuc
nucleated
NU-CHIPS
Northwestern University Children's
 Perception of Speech test
nucl
nuclear (*See also* NUC)
nucleus (*See also* N, Nu)
NUD
nonulcer (nonulcerous) dyspepsia

NUG
necrotizing ulcerating (ulcerative)
 gingivitis
NUGV
Nugget virus
NUI
number user identification
nullip
nulliparous
num
numerator
NuMA
nuclear mitotic apparatus
numc
number concentration
NUN
nonurea nitrogen
NUP
necrotizing ulcerating (ulcerative)
 periodontitis
NURB
Neville upper reservoir buffer
NURD
nonuniform rotational defect
NUV
near-ultraviolet
negative ulnar variance
NV
naked vision (*See also* Nv, Nv.)
nausea and vomiting (*See also* N/V,
 N&V)
near vision
negative variation
neovascularization
neurovascular
new vessel
next visit
nodular vasculitis
nonvaccinated
nonvegetarian
nonvenereal
nonveteran
nonvolatile
normal value
normal volunteer
normovolemic
Norwalk virus
not vaccinated
not venereal
not verified
not volatile
N/V, N&V
nausea and vomiting (*See also* NV)
Nv, Nv.
naked vision (*See also* NV)
NVA
near visual acuity
normal visual acuity

Nva
norvaline
NVAF
nonvalvular atrial fibrillation
NVB
neurovascular bundle
NVBG
nonvascularized bone graft
NVC
neurovascular checks
nonvalved conduit
normal vital capacity
NVCC
neurovascular cross compression
nvCJD
new variant Creutzfeldt-Jakob disease
NVD
nausea, vomiting, diarrhea
neck vein distention
neovascularization of [optic] disc
neurovesicle dysfunction
Newcastle virus disease [chickens]
nonvalvular [heart] disease
normal vaginal delivery
no venereal disease
no venous distention
N/V/D/
nausea, vomiting, diarrhea
NVDC
nausea, vomiting, diarrhea,
constipation
NVE
native
native valve endocarditis
neovascular edema
neovascularization (new vessels)
elsewhere [on retina]
NVFS
nuclear ventricular function study
NVG
neovascular glaucoma
neoviridogrisein
nonventilated group
NVI
neovascularization of iris
NVL
neurovascular laboratory
neurovisceral lipidosis
no visible lesion
NVLD
nonverbal learning disability
NVM
neovascular membrane
nonvolatile matter
NVP
nausea and vomiting of pregnancy
near visual point
NVR
no [radiographically] visible recurrence

NVS
nasal vestibular stenosis
neurologic vital signs
neurovascular status
nonvaccine serotype
nutritionally variant streptococcus
NVSS
normal variant short stature
NVT
nerve, vein, tendon
NW
naked weight
nasal wash
nicotine withdrawal
nonwithdrawn
not weighed
nursed well
NWB
nonweight-bearing
no weightbearing
NWBL
nonweightbearing, left
NWBR
nonweightbearing, right
NWC
number of words chosen
NWCL
New World cutaneous
leishmaniasis
NWD
neuroleptic withdrawal
normal well-developed
NWF
new working formulation
NWI
Neonatal Withdrawal Inventory
notch width index
NWm
nitrogen washout, multiple [breath]
NWR
normotensive Wistar rat
NWS
New World screwworm (*Cochliomyia
hominivorax* [Coquerel])
NWs
nitrogen washout, single [breath]
NWSM
Nocardia water-soluble nitrogen
Nx
nephrectomy (*See also* nep)
nourishment
regional lymph nodes cannot be
assessed [TNM classification]
NXG
necrobiotic xanthogranuloma
N x m
newton by meter
NYC
New York City [medium]

NYD
> not yet diagnosed
> not yet discovered

NYHA
> New York Heart Association
> [classification]

NYHAFC
> New York Heart Association Functional
> Class

NYP
> not yet published

nyst
> nystagmus

NYV
> New York virus

NYVAC-Pf7
> New York vaccinia virus [malaria
> vaccine]

NZ
> enzyme
> neutral zone
> normal zone

NZB
> New Zealand black [mouse]

NZGLM
> New Zealand green-lipped
> mussel

NZO
> New Zealand obese [mouse]

NZR
> New Zealand red [rabbit]

NZV
> New Zealand virus

NZW
> New Zealand white
> [mouse]

N

O

blood type in ABO blood group

eye [L. *oculus*]

no special preparation necessary [for test]

obese (obesity) (*See also* OB)

object(ive) (*See also* obj)

observation (*See also* OBS)

obstetrics (*See also* OB, OBS)

obvious

occiput (occipital) (*See also* OCC, occip)

occlusal (*See also* OCC)

often

old

open(ing) (*See also* OP, opg)

operon [genetics]

opium

oral(ly) (*See also* (O))

orange [indicator color]

orbit

orotidine (*See also* Ord)

osteocyte

output

oxidative

oxygen (*See also* O_2, Ox, OXY, oxy)

respirations [on anesthesia chart]

somatic antigen test [nonmotile strain of organism]

$1O_2$

singlet oxygen

O_2

oxygen [symbol for diatomic gas]

O_2-

superoxide

O2

both eyes (*See also* O.U.)

O_3

ozone

^{15}O

oxygen-15

^{16}O

oxygen-16

^{17}O

oxygen-17

^{18}O

oxygen-18

(O)

oral(ly) (*See also* O)

O+

blood type O positive

O−

blood type O negative

o-

ortho- [chemical symbol]

O-A

Objective-Analytic [Anxiety Battery]

OA

[Wechster Adult Intelligence Scale] Object Assembly [subtest]

obstructive apnea

occipital artery

occipitoatlantal

occiput anterior (occipitoanterior) [fetal position]

occupational asthma

ocular albinism

old age

oleic acid

on admission

on arrival

open adrenalectomy

open appendectomy

ophthalmic artery

opiate analgesia

opioid antagonist

opsonic activity

optic atrophy

oral airway (*See also* OAW)

oral alimentation

oral appliance

orotic acid (*See also* Oro)

orthophonic acid

osteoarthritis (*See also* osteo)

osteoid area

ovalbumin (*See also* OV)

ovarian ablation

ovarian artery

overall assessment

Overeaters Anonymous

oxalic acid

oxolinic acid

O&A

observation and assessment

odontectomy and alveoloplasty

O/A

on or about

O_2a

oxygen availability

OAA

Old Age Assistance

optic atrophy ataxia

oxaloacetic acid [test]

OAAD

ovarian ascorbic acid depletion [test]

OAAS, OAA/S

Observer Assessment of Alertness and Sedation

O

OAB
old age benefits
overactive bladder
OABP
organic anion-binding protein
OAC
oral anticoagulant
overaction
OAD
obstructive airways disease
occlusive arterial disease
organic anionic dye
overall diameter [contact lens]
overanxious disorder
OADC
oleic acid, albumin, dextrose, and
catalase [medium]
OADMT
Oliphant Auditory Discrimination
Memory Test
OADP-CDS
Oregon Adolescent Depression
Project-Conduct Disorder
Screener
OAdV 1–6
ovine adenovirus 1–6
OAE
open-access endoscopy
otoacoustic emission [test]
OAF
off-axis factor
open air factor
osteoclast-activating factor
osteocyte activation factor
OAG
open-angle glaucoma
OAH
ovarian androgenic hyperfunction
OAI
Ostomy Assessment Inventory
OAJ
open apophysial joint
OAK
Kjer optic atrophy
OALF
organic acid [and] labile fluoride
OALL
ossification of anterior longitudinal
ligament
OAM
Office of Alternative Medicine
[NCCAM NIH]
outer acrosomal membrane
oxyacetate malonate
OAO
ophthalmic artery occlusion
OAP
old age pension(er)
ophthalmic artery pressure

osteoarthropathy
oxygen at atmospheric pressure
OAPs
Occupational Ability Patterns
[psychologic test]
OAR
off-axis ratio
organs at risk
orientation/alertness remediation
other administrative reasons
Ottawa Ankle Rules
OARS
Older Americans Resources and
Services
OARSA
oxacillin- and aminoglycoside-resistant
Staphylococcus aureus
OAS
old age security
Older Adult Services
oral allergy syndrome
Oral Analogue Scale
orbital apex syndrome
organic anxiety syndrome
osmotically active substance
overall survival
Overt Aggression Scale
OASD
ocular albinism-sensorineural deafness
[syndrome]
OASH
obstructive asymmetrical septal
hypertrophy
OASIS
osteotomy analysis simulation software
Outcomes and Assessment Information
Set
OASO
overactive superior oblique
OASP
organic acid-soluble phosphorus
OASR
overactive superior rectus
OASS
Overt Agitation Severity Scale
OAST
Oliphant Auditory Synthesizing Test
OAT
ornithine aminotransferase
OATP
organic anion-transporting
polypeptide
OATS
oligoasthenoteratozoospermia syndrome
osteochondral autograft transfer
system
OAV
oculoauriculovertebral [dysplasia,
syndrome] (*See also* OAVD, OAVS)

OAVD
  oculoauriculovertebral dysplasia
  (*See also* OAV)
OAVS
  oculoauriculovertebral spectrum (*See also*
  OAV)
OAW
  oral airway (*See also* OA)
OAWO
  opening abductory wedge osteotomy
OB
  obese (obesity) (*See also* O)
  objective benefit
  obliterative bronchiolitis
  obstetric(s) (*See also* O, OBS, obstet)
  occult bacteremia
  occult blood (bleeding)
  olfactory bulb (*See also* OLB)
  oligoclonal band
  open biopsy
  osteoblast(oma)
OB+
  occult blood positive
O&B
  opium and belladonna
OBA
  office-based anesthesia
  oral bile acid
OB-A
  obstetrics aborted
OBAD
  optimal biologically active dose
OBB
  own bed bath
OBC
  operable breast cancer
OBD
  optimum biologic dose
  organic brain disease (disorder)
OB-Del
  obstetrics delivered
OBE
  out-of-body experience
OBE-CALP
  placebo capsule [or tablet]
OBF
  ocular blood flow
  organ blood flow
OB-GYN, OB/GYN
  obstetrics and gynecology (*See also* OG,
  O&G)
obj
  object(ive) (*See also* O)
OBK
  obstructed kidney
  ocular band keratitis
obl
  oblique

OBLA
  onset of blood lactate accumulation
OB marg
  obtuse marginal (*See also* OM-1, OM-2,
  OMB$_1$, OMB$_2$)
OBN
  occult-blood negative
OB-ND
  obstetrics not delivered
OBOV
  Obodhiang virus
OBP
  occult-blood positive
  office blood pressure
  ova, blood, parasites [stool exam]
OBS
  observation
  observe(d) (*See also* obsd)
  obsolete
  obstetric(s) (*See also* O, OB,
  obstet)
  organic brain syndrome
obsd
  observed (*See also* OBS)
obst
  obstipation
  obstruct(ed) (obstruction)
obstet
  obstetric(s) (*See also* O, OB, OBS)
OBT
  occult blood test
  Olivier-Bertrand-Tipal [stereotactic
  frame]
obt
  obtain(ed)
OB-US
  obstetrical ultrasound
OBW
  open bed warmer
OC
  observed cases
  obstetrical conjugate
  occlusocervical
  office call
  oleoresin capsicum
  on call
  oncoming [fetal head]
  only child
  open cholecystectomy
  open colectomy
  open crib
  operative cholangiography
  optical chromatography
  optic chiasm (*See also* OX)
  oral care
  oral cavity
  oral contraceptive
  orbicularis oculi [muscle]

OC *(continued)*
    organ confined
    organ culture
    original claim
    osteocalcin
    osteoclast
    ostomy care
    outer canthal [distance]
    ovarian cancer (carcinoma)
    oxygen consumed
O-C, O&C
    onset and course [of disease]
Oc
    ochre suppressor [genetic mutation]
OCA
    oculocutaneous albinism
    olivopontocerebellar atrophy (*See also*
      OPCA)
    open care area
    operant conditioning audiometry
    oral contraceptive agent
OCA1
    oculocutaneous albinism [type 1A]
OCAD
    occlusive carotid artery disease
OCAIRS
    Occupational Circumstances
      Assessment-Interview Rating Scale
O₂ cap.
    oxygen capacity
OCB
    obsessive-compulsive behavior
    obstructive chronic bronchitis
    olivocochlear bundle
OCBF
    outer cortical blood flow
OCC
    occasional(ly)
    occiput (occipital) (*See also* O, occip)
    occlusal (*See also* O)
    occlusion (*See also* occl)
    occlusive
    occupation(al) (*See also* occup)
    occur(rence)
    oculocerebrocutaneous
    old chart called
    oral cavity cancer
    oral cholecystograph(y) (cholecystogram)
      (*See also* OCG)
OCCC
    open-chest cardiac compression
    ovarian clear-cell carcinoma
occip
    occiput (occipital) (*See also* OCC, O)
occip F
    occipitofrontal (*See also* OF)
occip-F HA
    occipitofrontal headache (*See also*
      OF-HA)

occl
    occlusion (*See also* OCC)
OCCM
    open-chest cardiac massage
OCCPR
    open-chest cardiopulmonary
      resuscitation
OccTh
    occupational therapy (*See also* Occup
      Rx, OT)
occup
    occupation(al) (*See also* OCC)
    occupy(ing) (occupies)
Occup Rx
    occupational therapy (*See also* OccTh,
      OT)
OCD
    obsessive-compulsive disorder
    osteochondral defect
    osteochondritis dissecans
    ovarian cholesterol depletion [test]
OCDM
    oculocranioorbital dysraphia-meningocele
OCDS
    Obsessive-Compulsive Drinking Scale
OCF
    osteopathy in cranial field
OCFS
    ovarian cancer family syndrome
OCG
    omnicardiogram
    oral cholecystograph(y) (cholecystogram)
      (*See also* OCC)
OCH
    oral contraceptive hormone
OCHP
    oculocutaneous hyperpigmentation
OCI
    Obsessive-Compulsive Inventory
    Ophthalmic Confidence Index
    Organizational Culture Inventory
OCIF
    osteoclastogenesis inhibitory factor
OCL
    Occupational Check List [psychologic
      test]
    oral colonic lavage
    Orthopedic Casting Lab [splint]
OCLG
    osteoclastlike giant [cell]
OCLM
    oculomedin [gene]
OCM
    Odorant Confusion Matrix
    oral contraceptive medication
OCN
    obsessive-compulsive neurosis
OCNS
    Obsessive-Compulsive Neurosis Scale

O-CNV
occult choroidal neovascularization
OCOR
on-call to operating room
OCP
octacalcium phosphate
ocular cicatricial pemphigoid
Onchocerciasis Control Program
oral contraceptive pill
ova, cysts, parasites [stool exam]
(*See also* OC&P)
OC&P
ova, cysts, parasites [stool exam]
(*See also* OCP)
OCPC
orthocresolphthalein complex
OCPD
obsessive-compulsive personality
disorder
occult constrictive pericardial disease
OCR
ocular counterrolling
ocular countertorsion reflex
oculocardiac reflex
oculocephalic reflux
oculocerebrorenal (*See also* OCRL)
off-center ratio
optical character recognition
oCRF
ovine corticotropin-releasing factor
OCRG
oxycardiorespirography
OCRL
oculocerebrorenal (*See also* OCR,
OCRS)
OCRS
oculocerebrorenal syndrome (*See also*
OCR, OCRL)
OCS
Obsessive-Compulsive Scale
Ondine's curse syndrome
open canalicular system [of platelets,
porcine]
oral cancer screening
oral contraceptive steroid
oxycorticosteroid
11-OCS
11-oxycorticosteroid
OCSD
oculocraniosomatic disease
O-CT
ortho-computed tomography
OCT
Object Classification Test
optical coherence tomography
optimal cutting temperature
[of medium]

oral cavity tumor
oral contraceptive therapy
ornithine carbamoyltransferase
orthotopic cardiac transplant(ation)
osseous coagulum trap
outer canthal distance
oxytocin challenge test
O₂CT
oxygen content
Oct-1
octamer-binding
OCTD
ornithine carbamoyltransferase deficiency
OCTR
open carpal tunnel release
OCTT
orocecal transit time
OCV
ordinary conversational voice
OCVM
occult cerebral vascular
(cerebrovascular) malformation
oculocerebrovasculometer
OCWO
oblique closing wedge osteotomy
OCX
oral cancer examination
O-D
obstacle-dominance
original-derived
⚠ **OD**
occipital dysplasia
occupational dermatitis
occupational disease
oculus dexter [right eye] [L. *oculus
dexter*] (*See also* o.d., RE) ⚠
oligodendroglial
once daily (*See also* od) ⚠
on duty
oocyte donation
open drop [anesthesia]
open duct
optical density
optic disc
optimal dose
oral-duodenal
organization development
originally derived
osteochondritis dissecans
outdoor
outer diameter
out-of-date
outside diameter
ovarian dysgerminoma
[drug] overdose (overdosage)
⚠ **od**
once daily (every day) (*See also* OD) ⚠

⚠ **o.d.**

oculus dexter [right eye] [L. *oculus dexter*] (*See also* OD, RE) ⚠

ODA

once-daily aminoglycoside

osmotic driving agent

right occiput anterior (occipitoanterior) [fetal position] [L. *occipitodextra anterior*] (*See also* ORA)

ODAC

on-demand analgesia computer

ODAT

one day at a time

ODB

opiate-directed behavior

ODC

oral disease control

ornithine decarboxylase

orotidylate decarboxylase

oxygen dissociation curve

ODCH

ordinary disease of childhood

ODD

oculodentodigital [dysplasia, syndrome]

once-daily dosing

oppositional defiant disorder

osteodental dysplasia

OD'd

overdosed [drug]

ODED

oculodigitoesophagoduodenal

ODF

osteoclast differentiation factor

ODI

oxygen desaturation index

ODM

occlusion dose monitor

ophthalmodynamometer (ophthalmodynamometry)

opponens digiti minimi [muscle] (*See also* OPM)

ODMP

ongoing data management plan

ODN

oligodeoxynucleotide

ODOD

oculodentoosseous dysplasia

Odont

odontology

odont

odontogenic

ODP

offspring of diabetic parents

right occiput posterior (occipitoposterior) [fetal position] [L. *occipitodextra posterior*] (*See also* ORP)

⚠ **OD/P**

right eye patched ⚠

ODQ

on direct questioning

opponens digiti quinti [muscle]

Oswestry Disability Questionnaire

ODRV

Odrenisrou virus

ODS

Operation Desert Storm

organized delivery system

osmotic demyelination syndrome

oxygen desaturation

ODSG

ophthalmic Doppler sonogram

ODT

oculodynamic test

optical Doppler tomography

orally disintegrating tablet

right occiput transverse (occipitotransverse) [fetal position] [L. *occipitodextra transversa*]

ODTS

organic dust toxic syndrome

ODU

optical density unit

OE

on examination (*See also* O/E)

orthopedic examination (*See also* OX)

otitis externa

O-E

standard observed minus expected [statistics]

O&E

observation and examination

O/E

on examination (*See also* OE)

O:E

observed to expected ratio

Oe

oersted [CGS unit of magnetic field strength]

OEC

olfactory ensheathment cell

outer ear canal

ovarian epithelial cancer

OEE

osmotic erythrocyte enrichment

outer enamel epithelium

OEF

oxygen extraction fraction

OEI

opioid escalation index

O$_2$EI

oxygen extraction index

OEIS

omphalocele, exstrophy [of the bladder], imperforate [anus], and spinal [abnormalities]

OEL

occupational exposure level (limit)

OELM
optimal external laryngeal manipulation

OEM
occupational and environmental medicine
open-end marriage
opposite ear masked

OENT
oral endotracheal tube (*See also* OET, OETT)

OEP
oil of evening primrose (evening primrose oil)

OER
osmotic erythrocyte [enrichment]
oxygen enhancement ratio
oxygen extraction rate (ratio)

O₂ER
oxygen extraction (rate) ratio (*See also* OER)

OERP
odor event-related potential

OERR
order entry/results reporting

OES
Olympus endoscopy system
optical emission spectroscopy
oral esophageal stethoscope

oesoph
oesophagus [British] (*See also* E, ES, ESO, esoph)

OESP
orthopedic examination, special

OET
open epicutaneous test
oral endotracheal tube (*See also* OENT, OETT)
oral esophageal tube

OETT
oral endotracheal tube (*See also* OENT, OET)

OF
occipital-frontal (occipitofrontal) (*See also* occip F)
opacity factor
open field [test]
optic fundus [singular] (optic fundi [plural])
orbital fracture
orbitofrontal
osmotic fragility (test)
osteitis fibrosa
outlet forceps [delivery]
Ovenstone factor [amniotic fluid analysis]
oxidation-fermentation [medium] (*See also* O-F, O/F)

O-F, O/F
oxidation-fermentation [medium] (*See also* OF)

OFA
oncofetal antigen

OFB
oval fat body

OFBM
oxidation-fermentation basal medium

OFC
occipital-frontal (occipitofrontal) circumference
open food challenge
oral food challenge
orbitofacial cleft
osteitis fibrosa cystica

ofc
office (*See also* off.)

OFCD
oculofaciocardiodental

OFCTAD
occipito-faciocervico-thoraco-abdomino-digital [dysplasia]

OFD
object-film distance [radiology]
occipital frontal (occipitofrontal) diameter
oral-facial-digital (orofaciodigital) [dysostosis, syndrome]

OFE
ovarian fibroepithelioma

off.
office (*See also* ofc)
official

OFG
orofacial granulomatosis

OF-HA
occipital-frontal (occipitofrontal) headache (*See also* occip-F HA)

OFI
other febrile illness

OFM
open face mask
oral focal mucinosis
orofacial malformation
orofacial movement

OFNE
oxygenated fluorocarbon nutrient emulsion

OFPF
optic fundi and peripheral fields

OFR
oxygen free radical

OF rad
occipital-frontal (occipitofrontal) radiation

OFTT
organic failure to thrive

O

OFx
open fracture
OG
obstetrics and gynecology (*See also* OB-GYN, OB/GYN, O&G)
occlusogingival
oligodendrocyte
optic ganglion
optic glioma
oral gastric (orogastric)
orange green [stain]
outcome goal [long-term goal]
O&G
obstetrics and gynecology (*See also* OB-GYN, OB/GYN, OG)
OGA
orogastric gonococcal aspirate
OGC
oculogyric crisis
OGCT
oral glucose challenge test
ovarian germ cell tumor
OGD
old granulomatous disease
OGF
opioid growth factor
ovarian growth factor
oxygen gain factor
OGH
ovine growth hormone
OGI
osteogenesis imperfecta
OGIMD
oculogastrointestinal muscular dystrophy
OGM
outgrowth medium
OGR
Orlon graft replacement [obsolete]
OGS
oxygenic steroid
OGT
oral glucose tolerance (*See also* OGTT)
orogastric tube
OGTT
oral glucose tolerance test(ing) (*See also* OGT)
OH
hydroxycorticosteroid (*See also* HCS, OHCS)
hydroxyl group
hydroxyl radical
obstructive hypopnea
occipital horn
occupational health
occupational history
ocular history
on hand
open-heart [surgery]

oral herpes
oral hygiene
orthostatic hypotension
out of hospital
outpatient hospital
17-OH, 17-OHCS
17-hydroxycorticosteroid
OHA
oral hypoglycemic agent
OHAHA
ophthalmoplegia-hypotonia-ataxia-hypacusis-athetosis [syndrome]
24-OHase
vitamin D 24-hydroxylase
Ohase
hydroxylase
OHB$_{12}$
hydroxocobalamin (vitamin B$_{12}$) (*See also* OH-Cbl)
O$_2$Hb
oxyhemoglobin
OHC
hydroxycholecalciferol
obstructive hypertrophic cardiomyopathy
outer hair cell
OHCA, OOH/CA
out [of hospital] cardiac arrest
OH-Cbl
hydroxocobalamin (*See also* OHB$_{12}$)
OHCS
hydroxycorticosteroid (*See also* HCS, OH)
OHD
hydroxy vitamin D
organic heart disease
25-OH-D3, 1,25(OH)2 D3, 25(OH)D3
1,25-dihydroxyvitamin D3
OHDA
hydroxydopamine (*See also* HD, HDA)
OHDC
oxyhemoglobin dissociation curve
OH-DOC
hydroxydeoxycorticosterone
OHF
old healed fracture
Omsk hemorrhagic fever
overhead frame
OHFA
hydroxy fatty acid
OHFT
overhead frame trapeze
OHFV
Omsk hemorrhagic fever virus
OHG
oral hypoglycemic
OHI
ocular hypertension indicator
operative hypertension indicator

Oral Hygiene Index
oral hygiene instructions

OH-IAA
hydroxyindoleacetic acid (*See also* HIAA)

OHIO
only handle it once

OHI-S
Oral Hygiene Index Simplified

OHL
hydroxylysine (*See also* HYL, Hyl)
oral hairy leukoplakia

ohm-cm
ohm-centimeter

OHN
optical nerve head

OHNS
otolaryngology, head, neck
surgery

OHP
hydroxyproline (*See also* HP, Hyp, hypro)
obese hypertensive patient
orthogonal-hole test pattern
oxygen under high pressure
oxygen under hyperbaric pressure

17-OHP
17-hydroxyprogesterone

OHRP
open-heart rehabilitation program

OHRR
open heart recovery room

OHS
obesity hypoventilation syndrome
occupational health and safety
ocular histoplasmosis syndrome
ocular hypoperfusion syndrome
open heart surgery
ovarian hyperstimulation syndrome
(*See also* OHSS)
Overcontrolled Hostility Scale

OHSS
ovarian hyperstimulation syndrome
(*See also* OHS)

OHT
ocular hypertension (*See also* OHTN)
ocular hypertensive [glaucoma suspect]
orthotopic heart transplant(ation)
(*See also* OHTx)
overhead trapeze

OHTN
ocular hypertension (*See also* OHT)

OHTx
orthotopic heart transplant(ation)
(*See also* OHT)

OHU
hydroxyurea

OI
objective improvement
obturator internus
occipitoiliacus
oligoclonal immunoglobulin
opportunistic illness
opportunistic infection
opsonic index
orgasmic impairment
Orientation Inventory [psychologic test]
orthoiodohippurate (*See also* OIH)
osteogenesis imperfecta [type I–IV]
otitis interna
ouabain insensitive
oxygenation index
oxygen income
oxygen intake

O-I
outer-to-inner

oi
orbitale inferius [craniometric]

OIA
optical immunoassay
osmotically induced asthma

OIC
osteogenesis imperfecta congenita

OID
ocular inflammatory disease
optimal immunomodulating dose
organism identification [number]

OIE
Occupational Interests Explorer

OIF
observed intrinsic frequency
oil immersion field [microscopy]
open internal fixation

OIH
orthoiodohippurate (*See also* OI)
ovulation-inducing hormone

OIHA
orthoiodohippuric acid

OI&I
occupational injury and illness

OILD
occupational immunologic lung
disease

OIM
optical immunoassay

oint
ointment

OIP
ophthalmomyiasis interna posterior
organizing interstitial pneumonia

OIR
oxygen-induced retinopathy

OIRD
object-to-image receptor distance

O

OIRDA
occipital intermittent rhythmic delta activity

OIS
Occupational Interests Surveyor
ocular ischemic syndrome
optical intrinsic signal [imaging]
optimum information size
Organ Injury Scaling [committee]

OIT
Organic Integrity Test [psychiatry]
osteogenesis imperfecta tarda
ovarian immature teratoma

OIU
optical internal urethrotomy

⚠ **OJ, oj**
orange juice (See also OrJ) ⚠
Orthoplast jacket

OK, ok
all right
approved
correct

OKAN
optokinetic after nystagmus

OKC
odontogenic keratocyst
open kinetic chain

OKCE
open kinetic chain exercises

OKHV
Okhotskiy virus

OKN
optokinetic nystagmus

OKOV
Okola virus

OKQ
Osteoporosis Knowledge Questionnaire

OKR
optokinetic response

OKS
optokinetic stimulus

OKT
ornithine-ketoacid transaminase
Ortho-Kung T [cell]

⚠ **OL**
left eye [L. *oculus laevus*] (See also LE, o.l. OS) ⚠
open label(ed) [study, trial]
other location
otolaryngology

⚠ **o.l.**
left eye [L. *oculus laevus*] (See also LE, OL, OS) ⚠

ol.
oil [L. *oleum*]

ol
orbitale laterale [craniometric]

OLA
left occiput anterior (occipitoanterior) [fetal position] [L. *occipitolaeva anterior*] (See also LOA)

OLAP
on-line analytical processing

OLB
olfactory bulb (See also OB)
open liver biopsy
open lung biopsy

OLBI
overlapping biphasic impulse

OLBPQ
Oswestry Low Back Pain Questionnaire

OLC
oligodendroglialike cell
ouabainlike compound

OLD
obstructive lung disease
occupational lung disease
orthochromatic leukodystrophy

OLE
olive leaf extract

OLF
ouabainlike factor

OLH, oLH
ovine lactogenic hormone
ovine leuteinizing hormone

OLIB
osmiophilic lamellar inclusion body

OLIDS
open-loop insulin delivery system

oligo
oligohydramnios

OLIV
Olifantsvlei virus

OLM
ocular larva migrans
ophthalmic laser microendoscope

OLMAT
Otis-Lennon Mental Ability Test

OLNM
occult lymph node metastasis

OLP
abnormal lipoprotein
left occiput posterior (occipitoposterior) [fetal position] [L. *occipitolaeva posterior*] (See also LOP)

OLR
optic labyrinthine righting
otology, laryngology, rhinology

ol res
oleoresin

OLS
ordinary least squares [statistics]
ouabainlike substance

OLSID, OLSIDI
Oral Language Sentence Imitation Diagnostic Inventory
OLSIST
Oral Language Sentence Imitation Screening Test
OLT
left occiput transverse (occipitotransverse) [fetal position]
orthotopic liver transplant(ation) (*See also* OLTx)
osteochondral lesion of talus
OLTP
online transaction processing
OLTx
orthotopic liver transplant(ation) (*See also* OLT)
OLULA
office laparoscopy under local anesthesia
OLV
one-lung ventilation
OM
occipitomental
occupational medicine
ocular melanoma
ocular movement
oculomotor
oncostatin M (*See also* OSM)
operating microscope
oral motor
oral mucositis
orbitomeatal
organomegaly
Osborn-Mendel [rat]
osteomalacia
osteomyelitis (*See also* osteo)
osteopathic manipulation
osteopathic manipulative [medicine]
otitis media
outer membrane
ovulation method [birth control]
oxygen mask
OM-1–OM-2
[first, second] obtuse marginal [artery] (*See also* OMA, OMB_1, OMB_2, OB marg)
O2M
oxygen mask
om
every morning
OMA
obtuse marginal artery (*See also* OM-1, OM-2, OMB_1, OMB_2, OB marg)
oculomotor apraxia
older maternal age

OMAC
otitis media, acute, catarrhal (*See also* OMCA)
OMAS
occupational maladjustment syndrome
Olerud-Molander Ankle Score
otitis media, acute, suppurating (*See also* OMSA)
OMB_1–OMB_2
[first, second] obtuse marginal [artery] branch (*See also* OM-1, OM-2, OMA, OB marg)
OMC
open mitral commissurotomy
ostiomeatal complex [sinuses]
short orientation-memory-concentration test
OMCA
otitis media, catarrhal, acute (*See also* OMAC)
OMCC, OMCCH
otitis media, catarrhal, chronic
OMChS
otitis media, chronic, suppurating (*See also* OMSC)
OMD
ocular muscle (muscular) dystrophy
oculomandibulodyscephaly
organic mental disorder
oromandibular dystonia (dysostosis)
OME
otitis media with effusion
Ω, omega
ohm
omega [24th and last letter of Greek alphabet uppercase]
ω, omega
angular frequency
angular velocity [speed]
carbon atom farthest from principal functioning group
omega [24th and last letter of Greek alphabet lowercase]
OMENS
orbital, mandibular, ear, neural, soft tissue [syndrome]
OMF
oculomandibulofacial (syndrome)
OMFAQ
Older Americans Resources and Services (OARS) Multidimensional Functional Assessment Questionnaire
OMFS
oral and maxillofacial surgery (*See also* OMS)
OMG
ocular myasthenia gravis

O

OMI
old myocardial infarct(ion)
oocyte maturation inhibitor

Θ, omicron
omicron [15th letter of Greek alphabet uppercase]

o, omicron
omicron [15th letter of Greek alphabet lowercase]

OMIEI
oral medication-induced esophageal injury

OMIM
Online Mendelian Inheritance in Man

OMJA
oblique midtarsal joint axis

OML
orbitomeatal line

OMM
oculomandibulomelic [dysplasia, syndrome]
ophthalmomandibulomelic [dysplasia, syndrome]
outer mitochondrial membrane

OMN
oculomotor nerve
oculomotor nucleus

OMOV
Omo virus

OMP
oculomotor [third nerve] palsy
olfactory marker protein
orotidine 5′-monophosphate
orotidylate
orotidylic acid pyrophosphorylase
outer membrane protein

OMPA
octamethyl pyrophosphoramide
otitis media, purulent, acute

OMPC, OMPCh
otitis media, purulent, chronic

OMR
operative mortality rate

OMS
offshore medical school
opsoclonus-myoclonus syndrome
oral and maxillofacial surgery (*See also* OMFS)
organic mental syndrome
organic mood syndrome
otomandibular syndrome

OM&S
osteopathic medicine and surgery

OMSA
otitis media, suppurative, acute (*See also* OMAS)

OMSC
otitis media, secretory, chronic

OMSCh
otitis media, suppurative, chronic (*See also* OMChS)

OMT, OM/T
oral mucosal transudate
osteomanipulative therapy
osteopathic manipulative treatment (therapy) (technique)
ovarian mucinous tumor

OMU
ostiomeatal unit

OMVAT
Ocular Microcirculation View Analysis Treatment

OMVC
open mitral valve commissurotomy

OMVD
optimized microvessel density [analysis]

OMVI
operating motor vehicle [while] intoxicated

ON
occipitonuchal
oncology
onlay
ophthalmia neonatorum
optic nerve
optic neuritis
optic neuropathy
oronasal
osteonecrosis
overnight

ONB
olfactory neuroblast

ONC
oncology (*See also* onco, oncol)
over-the-needle catheter

onco, oncol
oncology (*See also* ONC)

ONCORNA
oncogene ribonucleic acid

OND
orbitonasal dislocation
other neurologic disease (disorder)

ONDS
Oriental nocturnal death syndrome

ONDST
overnight high-dose dexamethasone suppression test

ONF
open Nissen fundoplication

ONG
optic nerve glioma

ONH
optic nerve head
optic nerve hypoplasia

ONHD
optic nerve head drusen

ONI
old nerve injury
ONL
olfactory nerve layer
ONM
ocular neuromyotonia
ONMRS
onychotrichodysplasia-neutropenia-mental retardation syndrome
ONNV
O'nyong-nyong virus
ONP
operating nursing procedure
osteoplastic nasal periostitis
ONPG, ONP-GAL
omicron(*o*)-nitrophenyl-beta(β)-galactosidase
ON RR
overnight recovery room
ONS
Office of National Statistics
ONSD
optic nerve sheath decompression
ONSF
optic nerve sheath fenestration
ONSM
optic nerve sheath meningioma
ONTD
open neural tube defect
ONTR
orders not to resuscitate
OO
oophorectomy
ophthalmic ointment
oral order
orbicularis oculi [muscle]
osteoid osteoma
out of
O-O
outer-to-outer
O&O
off and on
o/o
on account of
OOA
outer optic anlage
OOB
out of bed
out-of-body [experience]
OOBBRP
out of bed [with] bathroom privileges
OOBL
out of bilirubin lights
OOC
onset of contractions
orthokeratinized odontogenic cyst
out of cast
out of control

OOD
out of doors
outer orbital diameter
OOF
out of facility
OOG
optic oculography
OOH
out of hospital
OOH/CA
out-of-hospital cardiac arrest
OOH&NS
ophthalmology, otorhinolaryngology, head and neck surgery
OOH-SCD
out-of-hospital sudden cardiac death
OOI
out of Isolette
OOL
onset of labor
OOLR
ophthalmology, otology, laryngology, rhinology
OOM
onset of menarche
OOP
out on pass
out of pelvis
out of plaster [cast]
OOPS
out of program status
OOR
out of room
OORR
orbicularis oculi reflex response
OORW
out of radiant warmer
OOS
out of sequence
out of specification [deviation from standard]
out of splint
out of stock
OOT
out of town
OOW
out of wedlock
out of work
OP
oblique presentation
occipitoparietal
occiput posterior (occipitoposterior) [fetal position]
old patient [previously seen]
olfactory peduncle
open(ing) (*See also* O, opg)
opening pressure
operation

O

OP *(continued)*
operative
operative procedure
ophthalmology
opponens pollicis [muscle]
oral and pharyngeal mucositis
organophosphorous
original package
oropharynx
orthostatic proteinuria
oscillatory potential
osmotic pressure
osteoporosis
other [than] psychotic
outpatient (*See also* O/P, OPT)
overpressure
overproof
ovine prolactin
OP-1
osteogenic protein 1
O/P
outpatient (*See also* OP, OPT)
O&P
ova and parasites [stool exam]
Op
opisthocranion [craniometric]
OPA
oral pharyngeal airway
organ procurement agency
outpatient anesthesia
OPAC
opacity (opacification)
OPAT
outpatient parenteral antibiotic
therapy
OPB
outpatient basis
OPC
oculopalatocerebral [syndrome]
oligomeric proanthocyanidin
operable pancreatic carcinoma
oropharyngeal candidiasis
outpatient care
outpatient catheterization
oxypneumocardiogram
OPCA
olivopontocerebellar atrophy (*See also*
OCA)
[X-linked] olivopontocerebellar
ataxia
OPCAB
off-pump coronary artery bypass
OPCD
olivopontocerebellar degeneration
op. cit.
in the work cited [L. *opere citato*]
OPCOS
oligomenorrheic polycystic ovary
syndrome

OPCS-4
Classification of Surgical Operations
and Procedures 4th revision
OPD
obstetric prediabetes
obstructive pulmonary disease
optical path difference
optical penetration depth
oropharyngeal dysphagia
otopalatodigital [syndrome]
outpatient dispensary
OpDent
operative dentistry
OPDG
ocular plethysmodynamography
OPDS
otopalatodigital syndrome
OPDUR
on-line prospective drug utilization
review
OPE
oral peripheral examination
outpatient evaluation
OPERA
outpatient endometrial resection [and]
ablation
OPES
oropharyngoesophageal scintigraphy
OPG
oculoplethysmograph(y) (ocular
plethysmograph(y)) (*See also* OPPG)
oculopneumoplethysmograph(y) (ocular
pneumoplethysmograph(y))
ophthalmoplethysmograph(y)
orthopantomograph(y)
(orthopantomogram)
osteoprotegerin
oxypolygelatin [plasma volume
extender]
opg
opening (*See also* O, OP)
OPG/CPA
oculoplethysmography/carotid
phonoangiography
OPGF
osteoprotegerin factor
OPGL
osteoprotegerin ligand
OPH, Oph
obliterative pulmonary
hypertension
ophthalmia (ophthalmic)
ophthalmologic
ophthalmology (*See also* Ophth)
ophthalmoscope (ophthalmoscopy)
(*See also* Ophth)
OPHI-II
Occupational Performance History
Interview-Second Version

OphSeg
ophthalmic segment
Ophth
ophthalmology (*See also* OPH, Oph)
ophthalmoscope (ophthalmoscopy)
(*See also* OPH, Oph)
OPI
oculoparalytic illusion
Omnibus Personality Inventory
OPIDN
organophosphate-induced delayed
neuropathy
OPIDP
organophosphate-induced delayed
polyneuropathy
OPIM
other potentially infectious material
OPK
optokinetic
OPL
oral premalignant lesion
osmotic pressure [of proteins in]
lymph
other party liability
outer plexiform layer
ovine placental lactogen
OPLL
ossification of posterior longitudinal
ligament
OPLS
osteopathic lumbosciatalgia
OPM
occult primary malignancy
ophthalmoplegic migraine
opponens digiti minimi [muscle]
(*See also* ODM)
OPMD
oculopharyngeal muscular
dystrophy
OpMNPV
Orgyia pseudotsugata MNPV [virus]
OPN
osteopontin
OPO
optical parametric oscillator
organ procurement organization
overnight pulse oximetry
OPP
ocular perfusion pressure
opposing
opposite
osmotic pressure of plasma
ovine pancreatic polypeptide
oxygen partial pressure
OPPES
oil-associated pneumoparalytic
eosinophilic syndrome

OPPG
oculopneumoplethysmography (ocular
pneumoplethysmography) (*See also*
OPG)
OPPOS
opposition
OPPS
Outpatient Prospective Payment System
OPR
orbicularis pupillary reflex
OPRDU
outpatient renal dialysis unit
op reg
operative region
oprg
operating
OPRT
orotate phosphoribosyl transferase
OPS
Objective Pain Scores
operations [plural]
operations [military]
optical position sensor
Orpington prognostic scale
orthogonal polarization spectral
osteoporosis-pseudoglioma syndrome
outpatient service
outpatient surgery
overnight polysomnography
OPSA
ovarian papillary serous adenocarcinoma
OpScan
optical scan(ning)
OPSI
overwhelming postsplenectomy infection
OPSU
oblique partial sit-up
O PSY
open psychiatry
OPT
Ohio pediatric tent
optional
optimum (optimal)
orbital pseudotumor
outpatient (*See also* OP, O/P)
outpatient treatment
opt.
best [L. *optimus*]
optical
optician
optics [noun]
optometrist
OPT c̄ CA
Ohio pediatric tent with compressed
air
OPT c̄ O₂
Ohio pediatric tent with oxygen

O

OPTHD
optimal hemodialysis
OPTN
Organ Procurement and Transplantation Network
OPT-NSC
outpatient treatment, nonservice-connected
OPT-SC
outpatient treatment, service-connected
OPV
oral polio vaccine
outpatient visit
OPW, OPWL
opiate withdrawal
OQ
Occupational Questionnaire
OQSMAT
Otis Quick Scoring Mental Abilities Test
OR
oblique ridge
odds ratio
oil retention [enema] (*See also* ORE, OR en)
open reduction
operating room
operations research
optic radiation
oral rehydration
orbicularis oris [muscle]
organ recovery
orienting reflex (response)
orthopedic (*See also* Orth, ortho)
orthopedic research
ovary reserve
overrefraction
own recognizance
oxidized-reduced
O-R
oxidation-reduction [system]
Or
outflow rate
ORA
occiput right anterior [fetal position] (*See also* ODA)
opiate (opioid) receptor agonist
ORBC
ox red blood cell
ORC
oculorenocerebellar [syndrome]
order/results communication
ox red [blood] cell
ORCA
optimized robot for chemical analysis
ORCH
orchiectomy
orch
orchitis

ORD
optical rotary (rotatory) dispersion
oral radiation death
Ord
orotidine
ord
ordinate
ORE, OR en
oil-retention enema (*See also* OR)
OREF
open reduction and external fixation
ORF
open reading frame
OR&F
open reduction and fixation
org
organ
organic
organism
ORIF
open reduction and internal fixation
orig
origin
original
ORIV
Oriboca virus
OrJ
orange juice (*See also* OJ, oj)
ORL
oblique retinacular ligament
otorhinolaryngology
ORLAU
Orthotic Research and Locomotor Assessment Unit
ORMF
open reduction metallic fixation
ORN
osteoradionecrosis
Orn
ornithine
ORO
oil red O
Oro
orotate
orotic acid (*See also* OA)
OROS
oral osmotic [drug delivery]
osmotic release oral system
OROV
Oropouche virus
ORP
occiput right posterior [fetal position] (*See also* ODP)
oxidation-reduction potential (*See also* Eh, E_o+, E^0)
ORPM
orthorhythmic pacemaker
ORQ
Occupational Roles Questionnaire

ORR
  otolith-righting reflex
  overall response rate
ORS
  oculorespiratory syndrome
  olfactory reference syndrome
  oral rehydration salts
  oral rehydration solution
  oral surgery (*See also* OS)
  orthopedic surgery (*See also* OS)
ORSA
  oxacillin-resistant *Staphylococcus*
    aureus
ORSP
  optochin-resistant *Streptococcus*
    pneumoniae
O-R system
  oxidation-reduction system
ORT
  ocular radiation therapy
  oestrogen replacement therapy [British]
    (*See also* ERT)
  Operation Restore Trust [Department of
    Health and Human Services]
  oral rehydration therapy
  orthodromic reciprocating tachycardia
Orth, ortho
  orthopedic (*See also* OR)
  orthopedics
orthot
  orthotonus
ORUV
  Orungo virus
ORX
  orexin
ORx
  oriented
ORx1
  oriented to time
ORx2
  oriented to time and place (*See also*
    Ox2)
ORx3
  oriented to time, place, person (*See also*
    Ox3)
ORx4
  oriented to time, place, person, objects
    [watch, pen, book] (*See also* Ox4)
ORXV
  Oriximina virus
⚠ **OS**
  left eye [L. *oculus sinister*] (*See also*
    LE, O.L.) ⚠
  occiput-sacrum (occipitosacral) [fetal
    position]
  occupational safety
  oligospermic

  opening snap [heart sound]
  open splenectomy
  open surgery
  ophthalmic solution
  oral surgery (*See also* ORS)
  orbitale superius
  orthopedic surgery (*See also* ORS)
  osteogenic sarcoma
  osteoid surface
  osteosarcoma
  osteosclerosis
  ouabain sensitive
  overall survival
  oxidative stress
  oxygen saturation (*See also* O_2 sat.,
    SaO_2, SO_2)
⚠ **o.s.**
  left eye [L. *oculus sinister*] (*See also*
    LE, O.L.) ⚠
Os
  osmium
OSA
  obstructive sleep apnea
  off-site anesthesia
  optic system assessment
  osteosarcoma
OSAAD
  Objective Severity Assessment of
    Atopic dermatitis
OSA/H
  obstructive sleep apnea/hypoventilation
OSA/HS
  obstructive sleep apnea/hypopnea
    syndrome
OSAI
  organism-specific antibody index
OSAP
  Office Sterilization and Asepsis
    Procedures Research
OSAS
  obstructive sleep apnea syndrome
O_2 sat.
  oxygen saturation (*See also* OS, SaO_2,
    SO_2)
OSBCL
  Ottawa School Behavior Checklist
OSBT
  ovarian serous borderline tumor
OSC
  oral self-care
osc
  oscillate
OSCAR
  On-line Survey Certification and
    Reporting
OSCC
  oral squamous cell carcinoma

O

OSCE
  objective structural clinical
      examination
OSCJ
  original squamocolumnar junction
OSCM
  oil-soluble contrast medium
OS-CS
  osteopathia striata with cranial sclerosis
      [syndrome]
OSD
  obstructive sleep disorder
  ocular surface disease
  outside doctor
  overseas duty
  overside drainage
OSD-6
  Obstructive Sleep Disorders 6 [item
      test]
OSE
  ovarian surface epithelium
OSEM
  ordered subset expectation maximization
      [SPECT]
OSESC
  opening snap ejection systolic click
OSF
  outer spiral fibers [of cochlea]
  outlet strut fracture
  overgrowth-stimulating factor
OSFI
  organ system failure index
OSFT
  outstretched fingertips
OSG
  osteosonograph(y) (osteosonogram)
OSH
  oral surgery handpiece
  outside hospital
OSHA
  Occupational Safety and Health Act
      (Administration)
OSHN
  osteosarcoma of head and neck
OSI
  Occupational Stress Indicator
  optical surface imaging
OSIQ
  Offer Self-Image Questionnaire (for
      Adolescents)
OSL
  Osgood-Schlatter lesion
OSM
  oncostatin M (*See also* OM)
  osmolality
  ovine submaxillary mucin
  oxygen saturation meter
Osm
  osmole

osM
  osmolar
osm
  osmosis
  osmotic
OSMED
  otospondylometaphysial
      (otospondylometaphyseal) dysplasia
OSMF
  oral submucous fibrosis
Osm/kg
  osmolality [osmole of solute per
      kilogram of solvent]
Osm/L, Osm/l
  osmolarity [osmole of solute per liter
      of solution]
OSM S
  osmolality serum
OSM U
  osmolality urine
OSN
  off-service note
OSNP
  one-step nested polymerase chain
      reaction
OSP
  oncocytic schneiderian papilloma
  output signal processor
  outside pass
⚠ **OS/P**
  left eye patched ⚠
OsP
  osmotic pressure
osp
  outer surface protein
ospA–ospC
  outer surface protein A–C
OSPL
  output sound pressure level
OSS
  Object Sorting Scales [psychologic test]
  occupational stress syndrome
  osseous
  over-shoulder strap
OSSAV
  Ossa virus
OSSI
  orthognathic surgery simulating
      instrument
OS-SPT
  osmolality urine spot [test]
OST
  Object Sorting Test
  occipitosubtemporal [approach]
  optimal sampling theory
ost
  osteotomy
osteo
  osteoarthritis (*See also* OA)

osteomyelitis (*See also* OM)
osteopathology
osteopathy
osteocart
osteocartilaginous
osteopath
osteopathology (*See also* osteo)
OT
objective test
object test
oblique talus
occiput transverse (occipitotransverse)
[fetal position]
occlusion time
occupational therapy
ocular tension
office treatment
old terminology [anatomy]
olfactory threshold
olfactory tubercle (*See also* OTU)
on treatment
optic tract
oral temperature
oral thrush
oral transmucosal
orientation test
original (old) tuberculin [Koch]
orotracheal [tube]
orthopedic treatment
otolaryngology (*See also* OL, OTO, Oto,
Otolar)
otology (*See also* OTO, Oto)
outer table
outlier threshold
oxytocin (*See also* OX, OXT, OXY,
oxy)
OTA
oligoteratoasthenozoospermia
open to air
Opinions toward Adolescents
[psychologic test]
ornithine transaminase
orthotoluidine arsenite
OTADL
Occupational Therapy Activities of
Daily Living
OTAPS
Ohio Tests of Articulation and
Perception of Sounds
OTBA
open transaxillary breast
augmentation
OTC
occult tumor cell
ornithine transcarbamoylase
oval target cell
over the counter

OTc
heart rate-corrected T interval
OTCD
ornithine transcarbamylase deficiency
OTC Rx
over-the-counter prescription
OTD
optimal therapeutic dose
oral temperature device
organ tolerance dose
out the door
OTE
[McMaster] Overall Treatment
Evaluation
optically transparent electrode
OTF
oral transfer factor
OTH
other
OTHA
ocular total higher-order aberration
OTI
ovomucoid trypsin inhibitor
OTJ
on the job
OTO, Oto
one-time only
otolaryngology (*See also* OL, OT,
Otolar)
otology (*See also* OT)
Otolar
otolaryngology (*See also* OL, OT OTO,
Oto)
OTPT
oral triphasic tablets [contraceptive]
OT/PT
occupational therapy and physical
therapy
OTR
ocular tilt reaction
Ovarian Tumor Registry
OT/RT
occupational therapy and recreational
therapy
OTS
occipital temporal sulcus
orotracheal suction
OTT, OT(T)
orotracheal tube
overall treatment time
OTU
olfactory tubercle (*See also* OT)
operational taxonomic unit
OTW
off the wall
over the wire (over-the-wire catheter or
method)

O

⚠ **OU**
   both eyes [together] [L. *oculi unitas*] ⚠
   each eye [L. *oculi uterque*] ⚠

⚠ **o.u.**
   both eyes [together] [L. *oculi unitas*] ⚠
   each eye [L. *oculi uterque*] ⚠

OUAV
   Ouango virus

OUBIV
   Oubi virus

OUES
   oxygen uptake efficiency slope

OULQ
   outer upper left quadrant

OU/P
   both eyes patched

OURQ
   outer upper right quadrant

OUS
   obstetric ultrasound
   overuse syndrome

OUTI
   other urinary tract infection

oUW
   original University of Wisconsin
      [solution]

OV
   oculovestibular
   office visit
   osteoid volume
   outflow volume
   ovalbumin (*See also* OA)
   ovarian
   ovary
   overventilation
   ovulate (ovulation) (ovulating)
   ovum
   oyster virus

O₂V
   oxygen ventilation equivalent

Oᵥ
   outflow volume

OVAL
   ovalocyte

OVAR
   off-vertical axis rotation

OVAS
   ocular vergance and accommodation
      sensor

OVC, OVCA
   ovarian cancer (carcinoma)

OVD
   occlusal vertical dimension
   oculovertebral dysplasia
   ophthalmological viscosurgical
      device
   opticovestibular disturbance

OvDF
   ovarian dysfunction

OVDQ
   Organizational Value Dimensions
      Questionnaire

OVEM
   ovarian epithelial [cancer] metastasis

OVET
   ovarian epithelial tumor

OVF
   Octopus visual field [analyzer]

OVI
   overvalued ideation

OVIS
   Ohio Vocational Interest Survey

OVIT
   Oral Verbal Intelligence Test

OVLP
   overlap myositis

OVLT
   organum vasculosum laminae terminalis
      (vascular organ of lamina terminalis)

OVRV
   Oak-Vale virus

OVS
   obstructive voiding symptom

OVT
   ovarian vein thrombosis

OVX
   ovariectomized
   ovariectomy

OW
   off work
   once weekly
   open wedge [osteotomy]
   open wound
   ordinary warfare
   outer wall
   oval window
   ova weight

O/W
   oil in water [emulsion]

O:W
   oil to water ratio

o/w
   otherwise

OWA
   organics-in-water [analyzer]

OWCL
   Old World cutaneous leishmaniasis

OWL
   Old World leishmaniasis
   out of wedlock

OWNK
   out of wedlock and not keeping [child]

OWR
   ovarian wedge resection

OWS
   overwear syndrome

OWVI
   Ohio Work Values Inventory

OX

optic chiasm (*See also* OC)
orthopedic examination (*See also* OE)
oximeter (oximetry) (*See also* oxi)
oxytocin (*See also* OT, OXT, OXY, oxy)

Ox

oxygen (*See also* O_2, OXY, oxy)

Ox1

oriented to time (*See also* ORx1)

Ox2

oriented to time and place (*See also* ORx2)

Ox3

oriented to time, place, person (*See also* ORx3)

Ox4

oriented to time, place, person, objects [watch, pen, book] (*See also* ORx4)

OXA

oxacillinase

oxi

oximeter (oximetry) (*See also* OX)

oxid

oxidize(d)

OXK

Proteus mirabilis serogroup

OX40

tumor necrosis factor receptor superfamily member 4 [CD134]

OX40L

tumor necrosis factor receptor superfamily member 4 [CD134] ligand

OXLAT

oxalate

Ox-LDL, oxLDL, OxLDL

oxidized low-density lipoprotein

OXM

pulse oximeter

OXP

oxypressin

OXPHOS

oxidative phosphorylation

OXT

oxytocin (*See also* OT, OX, OXY, oxy)

OXY, oxy

oxygen (*See also* O_2, Ox)
oxytocin (*See also* OT, OX, OXT)

OYE

old yellow enzyme

OZ

optical zone

oz, oz.

ounce

oz ap

apothecary's ounce

oz t

troy ounce

O

P

after [L. *post*]
by weight [L. *pondere*]
face of polyhedron
father [L. *pater*] (*See also* F)
form perception [in General Aptitude
  Test Battery]
handful [L. *pugillus*]
near [L. *proximum*]
near point [of vision] [L. *punctum
  proximum*] (*See also* PP, p.p.)
[optic] papilla (*See also* p, pap.)
page (*See also* pg)
para (parity) (parous) (*See also* para)
parent
parenteral (*See also* parent.)
parietal [electrode placement in
  electroencephalography]
part
partial pressure (*See also* p, PP)
passive (*See also* pass.)
Pasteurella
paternal
paternally contributing [strain, genetics]
  (*See also* pat.)
patient (*See also* PAT, PT)
per
percentile
perceptual speed
percussion (*See also* percus)
peripheral
permeability [constant]
peta-
peyote
phenolphthalein
phon [unit of perceived loudness level]
phosphate [DNA/RNA group]
phosphorus (*See also* phos)
physiology (*See also* PHY, phy, PHYS,
  physiol)
pin
pink [indicator color]
placebo (*See also* OBE-CALP, PBO,
  PCB, PL, PLB, PLBO)
plan
plasma (*See also* Pl)
Plasmodium
Pneumocystis
poise [CGS unit of dynamic viscosity]
  (*See also* Po, Ps)
poison(ing) (poisoned) (*See also* pois)
polarity
polarization
pole
pons

poor
popular response
population (*See also* Pop.)
porcelain
porcine
porphyrin (*See also* porph)
position (*See also* pos)
positive (*See also* POS, pos)
posterior (*See also* PO, post, post.)
power
precipitin
pressure (*See also* PR, press.)
primary
primipara (*See also* I-para, para 1
  primip, PRIMP)
primitive
private [patient, room]
probability (*See also* prob)
probable error [statistics]
product(ion) (*See also* prod.)
proline (*See also* Pro)
properdin
Proteus
proximal (*See also* prox)
Pseudomonas
psoralen (*See also* PSOR)
psychiatry (*See also* PS, PSY, Psy,
  psych, psychiat)
psychosis
pulse
pupil
rho [17th letter of Greek alphabet
  uppercase]
significance probability [value, statistics]
wave corresponding to wave of
  depolarization crossing atria [EKG]
weight [L. *pondus*]

P1, P$_1$
orthophosphate
first parental generation

P2, P$_2$
pulmonic second heart sound

P-3
Pain Patient Profile

P/3
proximal third [of bone]

^{31}P
phosphorus 31

^{32}P
phosphorus-32

^{33}P
phosphorus-33

P-50
oxygen half-saturation pressure of
  hemoglobin

P

P53
    tumor suppressive gene [tumor protein 53]

/P
    partial lower denture

P/
    partial upper denture

p
    atomic orbital with angular momentum quantum number 1
    cleaved polyprotein precursor molecule product
    frequency of more common allele of pair
    [optic] papilla (*See also* P, pap.)
    partial [pressure] (*See also* P, PP)
    phosphate (*See also* phos)
    pico-
    pond [metric unit of gravitational force on 1-gram mass]
    proton
    sample proportion [statistics]
    short arm of chromosome
    sound pressure

p̄
    after [L. *post*]
    mean pressure [gas]

p-
    para- [chemical prefix for two symmetrical substitutions in benzene ring]

PA
    alveolar partial pressure
    panic attack
    pantothenic acid [vitamin B_5]
    paralysis agitans
    paranoia (paranoid) (*See also* Par)
    parietal [cell] antibody
    partial pressure of arterial (alveolar) fluid
    passive aggressive
    paternal aunt
    pathologic (pathology) (*See also* PATH, path., PTH)
    peak amplitude
    peanut allergy
    pentanoic acid
    periapical
    periarteritis
    peridural artery
    periodic acid
    periodontal abscess
    permeability area
    pernicious anemia
    peroxidatic activity
    persistent asthma
    phakic-aphakic
    phenol alcohol
    phenylacetate

phosphatidic acid
phosphoarginine
photo allergy
phthalic anhydride
physical activity
physical assistance
Picture Arrangement [psychology]
pineapple [test for butyric acid in stomach]
pituitary adenoma
pituitary-adrenal
plasma aldosterone
plasminogen activator
platelet adhesiveness
platelet aggregation
platelet associated
pleomorphic adenoma
polyacrylamide (*See also* PAA)
polyarteritis (*See also* PAr)
polyarthritis
postaural
posterior-anterior (posteroanterior)
prealbumin (*See also* PAB)
predictive accuracy
pregnancy associated
premature adrenarche
presents again
pressure, alveolar (*See also* Paiv)
pressure, atrial
pressure augmentation
primary aldosteronism
primary amenorrhea
primary anemia
prior to admission (*See also* PTA)
proactivator
proanthocyanidin
professional association
proinsulin antibody
prolonged action
prophylactic antibiotic
propionic acid
prostate antigen
protective antigen
proteolytic activity
prothrombin activity (*See also* PTA)
protrusio acetabuli
pseudoaneurysm (*See also* PSA)
Pseudomonas aeruginosa (*See also* PSAG)
psychoanalysis (*See also* PSAn, psychoan, PYA)
psychogenic aspermia
psychosocial assessment
pubic arch
pulmonary angiography (*See also* PAG)
pulmonary artery (arterial) (*See also* Ppa)
pulmonary atresia
pulmonary autograft

pulpoaxial
pulsus alternans
puromycin aminonucleoside
pyrophosphate arthropathy
pyrrolizidine alkaloid
yearly [L. *per annum*]

P/A

percussion [and] auscultation (*See also* P&A)
position [and] alignment (*See also* P&A)

P&A

percussion and auscultation (*See also* P/A)
position and alignment (*See also* P/A)
present and active [reflex]
protection and advocacy

P:A

perimeter to area ratio

P₂ = A₂

pulmonic second heart sound equal to aortic second heart sound

⚠ **P₂ > A₂**

pulmonic second heart sound greater than aortic second heart sound ⚠

⚠ **P₂ < A₂**

pulmonic heart sound less than aortic second heart sound ⚠

Pa

pascal [standard atmospheric pressure unit]
protactinium

pA

picoampere

pA₂

affinity constant [binding drug to drug receptor]

PAA

partial agonist activity
periampullary adenoma
phenylacetic acid
physical abilities analysis
plasma angiotensinase activity
polyacrylamide (*See also* PA)
polyacrylic acid
polyamino acid
postantalgic atrophy
pyridine acetic acid

PAAA

paraanastomotic aneurysm of aorta

PAAD

permanently and acutely disabled

P(A-aDO₂)

alveolar-arterial oxygen tension difference

PAAF

pancreatitis-associated ascites fluid

p(A-a)O₂

alveolar-arterial pressure difference

PAAP

percutaneous alcohol ablation of parathyroid gland

PAAS

panic and anticipatory anxiety scale
Pediatric Acute Admission Severity

PAAT

Parent as a Teacher Inventory

pAAT

plasma alpha 1 antitrypsin

PAB

para-aminobenzoic acid (*para*-amino benzoic acid) (*See also* PABA)
performance assessment battery
peripheral androgen blockade
pharmacologic autonomic block
polyacrylamide bead
positive attention behavior
posterior axillary boost [radiotherapy]
prealbumin (*See also* PA)
premature atrial beat
pulmonary artery banding
purple agar base [medium]

PAb

protein antibody

PABA

paraaminobenzoic acid (*para*-aminobenzoic acid) (*See also* PAB)

PABD

preoperative autologous blood donation

PABM

peak adult bone mass

PABP

postalcoholic behavior pattern
pulmonary artery balloon pump

PABV

percutaneous aortic balloon valvuloplasty

PAC

pancreatic adenocarcinoma
papular acrodermatitis of childhood
para-aminoclonidine
parent-adult-child [in transactional analysis]
pericarditis, arthropathy, camptodactyly
Physical Assessment Center
picture archiving communication [system] (*See also* PACS)
plasma aldosterone concentration
Port-A-Cath
preadmission certification
premature atrial contraction
premature auricular contraction [obsolete]
pressure-assist control
Progress Assessment Chart [of Social and Personal Development]

P

PAC *(continued)*
    prophylactic anticonvulsant
    pulmonary artery catheter(ization)
    (*See also* PACATH)
PACAP
    pituitary adenylate cyclase activating
    polypeptide
PACATH
    pulmonary artery catheter(ization)
    (*See also* PAC)
PACC
    protein A [immobilized in] collodion
    charcoal
PACD
    photoallergic contact dermatitis
PACE
    performance and cost efficiency
    Personal Assessment for Continuing
    Education
    personalized aerobics for cardiovascular
    enhancement
    population-adjusted clinical epidemiology
    Professional and Administrative Career
    Examination
    promoting aphasic's communicative
    effectiveness
    prospective acquisition correction
    Psychosocial Assessment of Childhood
    Experiences
    pulmonary angiotensin I converting
    enzyme
PACG
    Prevocational Assessment and
    Curriculum Guide
    primary angle-closure glaucoma
PACH
    Piper [forceps] to aftercoming head
    [delivery]
PACI
    partial anterior cerebral infarct(ion)
    partial anterior circulation
    infarct(ion)
PACL
    Personality Adjective Check List
PACNS
    primary angiitis of central nervous
    system (CNS)
PaCO2, Pa$_{CO2}$, PaCO$_2$
    arterial carbon dioxide pressure
    [tension]
    partial arterial gas pressure [tension] of
    carbon dioxide
PACONA
    periodic acid-concanavalin A
PACP
    pulmonary artery counterpulsation
PAC/PRA
    plasma aldosterone concentration/plasma
    renin activity

PACS
    partial anterior circulation syndrome
    picture archival communication system
    (*See also* PAC)
PACSRO
    picture archiving and communications
    systems in radiation oncology
PACT
    papillary carcinoma of thyroid
    precordial acceleration tracing
    Prescription Analyses and Cost [national
    data collection]
    prism and alternate cover test
    program of assertive community
    treatment
PACU
    postanesthesia care unit
PACV
    Pacui virus
PACWP
    pulmonary arterial capillary wedge
    pressure
PAD
    pain and distress
    pelvic adhesive disease
    per adjusted discharge
    percutaneous abscess drainage
    peripheral arterial disease
    persistently and acutely disabled
    pharmacologic atrial defibrillator
    phonologic-acquisition device
    photon absorption densitometry
    physician-assisted death
    Pick arteriopathic dementia
    practical approach design
    pre-aid to the disabled
    preliminary anatomic diagnosis
    preoperative autologous donation
    pressure applied dressing
    primary affective disorder
    psychoaffective disorder
    public access [to] defibrillator
    (defibrillation)
    pulmonary artery diastolic (*See also*
    PAd)
    pulsatile assist device
PAd
    pulmonary artery diastolic (*See also*
    PAD)
PADCAB
    perfusion-assisted direct coronary artery
    bypass
PADDS
    photon-activated drug delivery
    system
PADI
    posterior atlantodental interval
PADL
    personal activities of daily living

PADP
  pulmonary artery (arterial) diastolic pressure
PADP-PAWP
  pulmonary artery diastolic and wedge pressure
PADPRP
  poly adenosine diphosphate-ribose polymerase
PADS
  pain-associated disability syndrome
  Post Anesthesia Discharge Scoring System
PAE
  paradoxical air embolism
  percutaneous angiographic embolization
  postanoxic encephalopathy
  postantibiotic effect
  progressive assistive exercise
  Pygeum africanum extract
PA&E
  present, active, equal
PAEC
  pig aortic endothelial cell
paed
  paediatrics [British] (*See also* PD, PED, Peds)
PAEDP
  pulmonary artery end-diastolic pressure
PAEE
  physical activity energy expenditure
PAF
  paroxysmal atrial fibrillation (*See also* PAFIB)
  paroxysmal auricular fibrillation [obsolete]
  phosphodiesterase-activating factor
  platelet activating factor
  platelet aggregating factor (*See also* PAgF)
  pollen adherence factor
  posterior auricular flap
  premenstrual assessment form
  pseudoamniotic fluid
  pulmonary arteriovenous fistula
PA&F
  percussion, auscultation, fremitus
PAF-A
  platelet-activating factor of anaphylaxis
PAF-AH
  platelet-activating factor acetylhydrolase
PAFD
  percutaneous abscess and fluid drainage
  pulmonary artery filling defect
PAFE
  postantifungal effect

PAFG
  picric acid formaldehyde-glutaraldehyde
PAFI
  platelet-aggregating factor inhibitor
PAFIB
  paroxysmal atrial fibrillation (*See also* PAF)
PAFP
  pre-Achilles fat pad
PAG
  periaqueductal gray [matter]
  phenylacetylglutamine
  pictorial anticipatory guidance
  pineal antigonadotropin
  polyacrylamide gel
  pregnancy-associated globulin
  pulmonary angiography (*See also* PA)
pAg
  protein A-gold [technique]
PAGA
  premature appropriate for gestational age
PAGE
  perfluorocarbon-associated gas exchange
  polyacrylamide gel electrophoresis
PAGE-SS
  polyacrylamide gel electrophoresis with silver stain
PAgF
  platelet-aggregating factor (*See also* PAF)
PAGIF
  polyacrylamide gel isoelectric focusing (*See also* PIEF)
PAGMK
  primary African green monkey kidney
PAGOD
  pulmonary [hypoplasia], [hypoplasia of pulmonary] artery, agonadism, omphalocele/diaphragmatic [defect], dextrocardia [syndrome]
PAG/PVG
  periaqueductal gray [matter] [and] periventricular gray [matter]
PAH
  paraaminohippurate (*para*-aminohippurate)
  paraaminohippuric acid (*para*-aminohippuric acid) (*See also* PAHA)
  partial abdominal hysterectomy
  phenylalanine hydroxylase (*See also* PH)
  polycyclic aromatic hydrocarbon
  polynuclear aromatic hydrocarbon (*See also* PNAH)
  postatrophic hyperplasia
  prealbumin-associated hyperthyroxinemia

P

PAH *(continued)*
   predicted adult height
   primary adrenal hyperplasia
   pulmonary alveolar hypoventilation
   pulmonary artery (arterial) hypertension
   pulmonary artery hypotension
PAHA
   paraaminohippuric acid (*See also*
   PAH)
PAHV
   Pahayokee virus
PAHVC
   pulmonary alveolar hypoxic
   vasoconstrictor (vasoconstriction)
PAI
   pain appraisal (assessment) inventory
   Pair Attraction Inventory
   partial [incomplete] androgen
   insensitivity
   patient assessment instrument
   penetrating abdominal injury
   perforating arterial (artery) infarct(ion)
   Personality Assessment Inventory
   plasminogen activator inhibitor
   platelet accumulation index
PAI-1–PAI-2
   plasminogen activator inhibitor 1–2
PAIC
   procedures, alternatives, indications
   complications
PAIDS
   pediatric acquired immunodeficiency
   syndrome
PAIg
   platelet-associated immunoglobulin
PAIgG
   platelet-associated immunoglobulin G
PAIN
   pyoderma gangrenosum, aphthous
   stomatitis, inflammatory eye disease,
   erythema nodosum [disorders
   associated with inflammatory bowel
   disease]
PAIR
   percutaneous aspiration, instillation of
   hypertonic saline, reaspiration
   Personal Assessment of Intimacy in
   Relationships
   puncture, aspiration, injection,
   reaspiration
PAIS
   partial androgen insensitivity
   syndrome
   Psychosocial Adjustment to Illness
   Scale
   punctate area of increased signal
PAIVMs
   passive accessory intervertebral
   movements

PAIVS
   pulmonary atresia with intact ventricular
   septum
PAJ
   paralysis agitans juvenilis
PAJB
   primary antecubital jump bypass
PAK
   pancreas after kidney [transplant(ation)]
   pancreas and kidney
   percutaneous access kit
PAKY
   percutaneous access to kidney
PAL
   pacifier activated lullaby
   pathology laboratory
   peptidyl-alpha-hydroxyglycine
   alpha-amidating lyase
   peripheral arterial line
   phenylalanine ammonia lyase
   physical activity level
   posterior assisted levitation [cataract
   surgery]
   posterior axillary line
   posteroanterior and lateral (*See also*
   PA&Lat)
   power-assisted lipoplasty
   powered air loss
   product of activated lymphocyte
   Profile of Adaptation to Life
   pyogenic abscess of liver
pal.
   palate
PALA
   N-phosphonoacetyl-L-aspartic acid
PA&Lat
   posteroanterior and lateral (*See also*
   PAL)
PALE
   postantibiotic leukocyte enhancement
Pa Line
   pulmonary artery line
PALM
   premature accelerated lung maturation
PALN
   paraaortic lymph node
PALP
   placental alkaline phosphatase (*See also*
   PAP, PLAP)
palp
   palpable
   palpate
   palpation
   palpitation (*See also* palpit)
palpit
   palpitation (*See also* palp)
PALS
   Paired Associate Learning Subtest
   pediatric advanced life support

periarterial lymphatic sheath
periarteriolar lymphocyte sheath
prison-acquired lymphoproliferative
syndrome
PALS-ID
pernicious anemialike syndrome and
immunoglobulin deficiency
PALST
Picture Articulation and Language
Screening Test
PALT
Paired Associate Learning Task
PALV
Palyam virus
Palv
alveolar pressure (*See also* PA)
PAM
pancreatic acinar mass (metaplasia)
partial allosteric modulator
peptidylglycine alpha-amidating
monooxygenase
potential acuity meter
primary acquired melanosis
primary amebic meningoencephalitis
(*See also* PAME)
pulmonary alveolar macrophage
pulmonary alveolar microlithiasis
pulmonary artery mean pressure
(*See also* PAMP)
pulse amplitude modulation
pyridine aldoxime methiodide
PAMBA
paraaminomethylbenzoic acid
PAMC
pterygoarthromyodysplasia, congenital
PAMD
primary adrenocortical micronodular
dysplasia
PAME
primary amebic meningoencephalitis
(*See also* PAM)
PAMP
pathogen-associated molecular pattern
proadrenomedullin N-20 terminal
peptide
pulmonary artery mean pressure
(*See also* PAM)
PAN
pancreas (*See also* pan.)
panoral x-ray examination [Panorex]
(*See also* PanX, PRX)
periarteritis nodosa (*See also* PN)
periodic alternating nystagmus
peroxyacetyl nitrate
polyacrylonitrile
polyarteritis nodosa (*See also* PN)
polyomavirus-associated neuropathy

positional alcohol nystagmus
posterior ampullary nerve
primary afferent nociceptor neuron
puromycin aminonucleoside nephropathy
(nephrosis)
pan.
pancreas (*See also* PAN)
pancreatectomy (*See also* PX)
pancreatic
PANAS
Positive and Negative Affect Scale
P-ANCA, p-ANCA, pANCA
perinuclear antineutrophil cytoplasmic
antibody
PANCH
pituitary adenoma-adenohypophysial
neuronal choristoma
PAND
primary adrenocortical nodular
dysplasia
PANDA
Prevent Abuse and Neglect through
Dental Awareness
PANDAS
pediatric autoimmune neuropsychiatric
disorders associated with streptococcus
infections
PANDO
primary acquired nasolacrimal duct
obstruction
PANESS
physical and neurologic examination for
soft signs
PanIn-1
pancreatic intraepithelial neoplasm [low
grade]
PanIn-2
pancreatic intraepithelial neoplasm
[moderate grade]
PanIn-3
pancreatic intraepithelial neoplasm [high
grade]
PANP
pelvic autonomic nerve preservation
PANSS
Positive and Negative Stroke Scale
Positive and Negative Syndrome Scale
PanX
panoral x-ray examination [Panorex]
(*See also* PAN, PRX)
PAO
peak acid output
peripheral airway obstruction
peripheral arterial occlusion
plasma amine oxidase
polyamine oxidase
pulmonary artery occlusion

P

PAO₂, PaO₂
partial pressure alveolar oxygen
partial pressure arterial oxygen

P_ao
airway opening pressure

Pao
ascending aortic pressure

PAO₂–PaO₂
partial pressure of oxygen in
alveolar-arterial difference

PAOD
peripheral arterial (artery) occlusive
disease
peripheral arteriosclerotic
(atherosclerotic) occlusive disease

PAOGRP
peak acid output after gastrin-releasing
peptide

PAOI
peak acid output insulin-induced

PAOP
pulmonary artery occluded (occlusion)
pressure

PAOPg
peak acid output after pentagastrin
stimulation

PAOx
phenylacetone oxime

PAP
pancreatitis-associated protein
Papanicolaou [smear, test] (*See also*
Pap)
papaverine
papillary
papilloma
para-aminophenol
passive-aggressive personality
patient assessment program
patient assistance program
peak airway pressure
peroxidase antibody to peroxidase
peroxidase-antiperoxidase [technique,
complex]
3'-phosphoadenosine 5'-phosphate
placental alkaline phosphatase (*See also*
PALP, PLAP)
pokeweed antiviral protein
positive airway pressure
preoperative antimicrobial prophylaxis
primary atypical pneumonia
prostatic acid phosphatase
pulmonary alveolar proteinosis
pulmonary artery pressure
purified alternate pathway

Pap
Papanicolaou [smear, test] (*See also*
PAP)

pap.
papilla (*See also* P, p)

PAPA
preschool-age psychiatric assessment
pyogenic sterile arthritis, pyoderma
gangrenosum, acne

PAPase
phosphatidate phosphohydrolase
phosphatidic acid phosphohydrolase

PAPF
platelet adhesiveness plasma factor

PAPI
peroxidase-antiperoxidase
immunoperoxidase

pap. in. canthus
papilloma, inner canthus

PAPm
mean pulmonary artery pressure
(*See also* MPAP)

papova
papilloma virus, polyoma virus,
vacuolative virus

PAPP
para-aminopropiophenone
Pappenheimer bodies
pregnancy-associated plasma
protein

PAPP-A–PAPP-C
pregnancy-associated plasma protein
A–C

PAPS
adenosine 3'-phosphate 5'-phosphosulfate
3'-phosphoadenosine 5'-phosphosulfate
primary antiphospholipid antibody
syndrome

PA/PS
pulmonary atresia/pulmonary stenosis

PAPUFA
physiologically active polyunsaturated
fatty acid

PAPV
partial anomalous pulmonary vein
(venous)
peak hyperemic average velocity
positive airway pressure ventilation

Pa-Pv, pa-pv
pulmonary arterial pressure [and]
pulmonary venous pressure

PAPVC
partial anomalous pulmonary venous
connection

PAPVD
partial anomalous pulmonary venous
drainage

PAPVR
partial anomalous pulmonary venous
return

PAPW
posterior aspect pharyngeal wall

PAQ
Personal Attributes Questionnaire

Position Analysis Questionnaire [job analysis]

PAQLQ
Pediatric Asthma Quality of Life Questionnaire

PAR
paraffin
parainfluenza vaccine
parallel
passive avoidance reaction
percent(age) abnormal results
perennial allergic rhinitis
pharyngeal acid reflux
photosynthetically active radiation
physiologic aging rate
plain abdominal radiography
plasma appearance rate
platelet aggregate ratio
population attributable risks
positive attention received
possible allergic reaction
postanesthesia recovery
posterior apical radius
posterior wall of aortic root
primary angioplasty research
probable allergic rhinitis
problem-analysis report
procedures, alternatives, risks
Proficiency Assessment Report
protease-activated receptor
proximal alveolar region
pseudoallergic reaction
pulmonary arteriolar resistance
pulmonary artery resistance
pulse amplitude ratio

PAr
polyarteritis (*See also* PA)

Par
paranoia (paranoid) (*See also* PA)

para
number of pregnancies producing viable offspring
paraparesis
paraplegia (paraplegic)
parathyroid hormone (parathormone) (*See also* PH, PT, PTH)
parathyroidectomy (*See also* PTx)
woman who has given birth [parous]

para 0
nullipara [no child borne]

para 1, I-para
primipara [first pregnancy] (*See also* P, primip, PRIMP)
unipara [having borne one child]

para 2, II-para
bipara [having borne two children]
secundipara [second pregnancy]

para 3, III-para
tertipara [third pregnancy]
tripara [having borne three children]

para 4
quadripara [having borne four children]

para C, para c
paracervical (*See also* PCX)

par aff, par. aff.
[apply to] part affected

paraflu
parainfluenza [virus] (*See also* PF1–PF4, PI, PIV)

para L
paralumbar

parapsych
parapsychology

PARAS
postauricular and retroauricular scalping [flap]

parasit
parasite
parasitic
parasitology

parasym
parasympathetic [division of autonomic nervous system] (*See also* PNS, PS, PSNS)

para T
parathoracic

PARC
perennial allergic rhinoconjunctivitis

parent.
parenteral(ly) (*See also* P)

PARH
plasminogen activator-releasing hormone

PARK
photoastigmatic refractive keratectomy

PAROM
passive assistance range of motion

parox
paroxysm(al)

PARP
poly adenosine diphosphate (ADP)-ribose polymerase [autoantibody]

PAR-Q
Physical Activity Readiness Questionnaire

PARS
Personal Adjustment and Role Skills [Scale]
Personal and Role Skills
postanesthesia recovery score

PaRS
pararectal space

P

part.
of a part [L. *partis*]
partly [L. *partim*]
parturition

part. aeq.
in equal parts

PARTS
pain, asymmetry, range, tone, special [test]

PARV
Paraná virus

PAS
paraaminosalicylic acid (*para*-aminosalicylic acid) (*See also* PASA)
Parent Attitude Scale
patient appointments and scheduling
periodic acid-Schiff [stain]
peripheral access system
peripheral anterior synechia
persistent atrial standstill
personality assessment system
phosphatase acid serum
photoacoustic spectroscopy
physician-assisted suicide
pneumatic antiembolic stocking
postanesthesia score
posterior airway space
preadmission screening
pregnancy advisory service
premature atrial stimulus
premature auricular systole [obsolete]
progressive accumulated stress
pseudoachievement syndrome
pulmonary artery (arterial) stenosis
pulmonary artery systolic
pulsatile antiembolism system

Pa·s
pascal-second (*See also* Pa x s)

PASA
para-aminosalicylic acid (*See also* PAS)
primary acquired sideroblastic anemia
proximal articular set angle

PAS-AB
periodic acid Schiff-Alcian blue [stain]

PASAT
Paced Auditory Serial Addition Test

PaSat
saturation of oxygen in arterial blood (*See also* pSO$_2$)

PAS-C
para-aminosalicylic acid crystallized [with ascorbic acid]

PASCC
pseudovascular adenoid squamous cell carcinoma

PASCCL
pseudovascular adenoid squamous cell carcinoma of lung

PASCET
primary and secondary control enhancement training

PA/S/D
pulmonary artery systolic/diastolic

PASE
Physical Activity Scale for the Elderly

P'ase
alkaline phosphatase (*See also* alk phos, alk p'tase, ALP, AlPase, AP)

PASES
Performance Assessment of Syntax Elicited and Spontaneous [test]

Pas Ex
passive exercise

PASG
pneumatic antishock garment

PASH
periodic acid-Schiff hematoxylin [stain]
pseudoangiomatous stromal hyperplasia

PASI
psoriasis area sensitivity index

PASK
peripheral anterior stent keratopathy

PASM
periodic acid-silver methenamine [stain]

PASO
primitive aggressive self-organization

PASP
pulmonary artery systolic pressure

PASS
Pain Anxiety Symptoms Scale
Parent Awareness Skills Survey
Perception of Ability Scale for Students
polyaxial spine system

pass.
here and there [L. *passim*]
passive (*See also* P)

PAST
periodic acid-Schiff technique

PASTA
polarity-altered spectral selective acquisition [magnetic resonance]

PASV
pressure-activated safety valve

PASVR
pulmonary anomalous superior venous return

PAT
Pain Apperception Test
paroxysmal atrial tachycardia (*See also* PXAT)
passive alloimmune thrombocytopenia
patella
patient (*See also* P, PT)
percent(age) of acceleration time
percutaneous aspiration thromboembolectomy
peripheral arterial tone

Photo Articulation Test [psychology]
Physical Ability Test
picric acid turbidity
plasma antithrombin
platelet aggregation test
polyamine acetyltransferase
preadmission testing
Predictive Ability Test [psychology]
pregnancy at term
preventive allergy treatment
prism adaptation test
prophylactic antibiotic treatment
psychoacoustic test(ing)
pulmonary artery trunk
putative anion transporter

pat.
patent
paternal origin (*See also* P)
PAT1
putative anion transporter 1 (*See also* PAT)
PATAV
Pata virus
PATCH
Planned Approach to Community Health
PATE
prolonged acute tissue expansion
psychodynamic and therapeutic education
pulmonary artery thromboembolism
pulmonary artery thromboendarterectomy
PATEO
periarticular thenar erythema and onycholysis
PATH
pathologic (pathology) (*See also* PA, path., PTH)
pituitary adrenotropic hormone
Planning Alternative Tomorrows with Hope
path.
pathogen (pathogenesis) (pathogenic)
pathologic (pathology) (*See also* PA, PATH, PTH)
path. fx
pathologic fracture
PATI
Penetrating Abdominal Trauma Index
PATLC
Progressive Achievement Tests of Listening Comprehension
pat. med.
patent medicine
PATP
preadmission testing program
PATS
payment at time of service

PA-T-SP
periodic acid-thiocarbohydrazide-silver proteinate [stain]
pat. T
patellar tenderness
PAT/TM
patient's time
PATV
Patois virus
PAU
penetrating aortic ulcer
penetrating atherosclerotic (arteriosclerotic) ulcer
PAV
partial atrioventricular
percutaneous aortic valvuloplasty
poikiloderma atrophicans vasculare
posterior arch vein
preadmission visit
proportional assist ventilation (ventilator)
Pa Va Ex, pavex
passive vascular (venoarterial) exercise
PAVF, PA-VF
pulmonary arteriovenous fistula
PAVM
pulmonary arteriovenous malformation
PAVN
paraventricular nucleus
PAVNRT
paroxysmal atrioventricular nodal reciprocal tachycardia
pAVP
plasma arginine vasopressin
PAVSD
pulmonary atresia with ventricular septal defect
PAW
peak airway pressure
peripheral airway
primary affective witzelsucht [inappropriate humor, psychology]
pulmonary artery wedge
Paw
mean airway pressure
Pawo
pressure at airway opening
PAWP
pulmonary artery wedge pressure (*See also* Ppaw)
PAX
periapical x-ray
PAX3
paired box homeotic 3 [gene]
PAX6
paired box homeotic 6 [gene]
PAX8
paired box homeotic 8 (gene)

P

Pa × s
    pascal per second (*See also* Pa · s)
PB
    barometric pressure
    British Pharmacopoeia [*Pharmacopoeia Britannica*] (*See also* BP)
    pancreaticobiliary
    paraffin bath
    Paul-Bunnell [antibody, test] (*See also* PBT)
    perineal body
    periodic breathing
    peripheral blood
    peroneus brevis [muscle]
    phenylbutyrate
    phonetically balanced [word, lists]
    piggyback
    pinch biopsy
    pinealoblastoma
    posterior baffle
    powder bed (board)
    power building
    premature beat
    pressure balanced
    pressure breathing
    protein bound (binding)
    pudendal block
    punch biopsy
PB%
    phonetically balanced percentage [of word lists]
P & B
    Papanicolaou and breast [examination]
P&B
    pain and burning
P/B
    parallel bars
P$_B$
    barometric pressure
Pb
    lead [L. *plumbum*] (*See also* plumb.)
    presbyopia (*See also* PR)
p/b
    postburn
PBA
    percutaneous bladder aspiration
    percutaneous breathing assister
    polyclonal B-cell activity
    pressure breathing assister
    prolactin-binding assay
    prune belly anomaly
    pulpobuccoaxial
P$_{BA}$
    brachial arterial pressure
PBAL
    protected bronchoalveolar lavage
P-BAP
    Behavioral Assessment of Pain Questionnaire

PBAV
    percutaneous balloon aortic valvuloplasty
PBB
    polybrominated (polybromated) biphenyl
Pb-B
    lead level in blood
PBC
    perfusion balloon catheter
    periodic breathing cycle
    peripheral blood cell
    plasma bilirubin concentration
    point of basal convergence
    prebed care
    pregnancy and birth complication
    primary biliary cirrhosis
    progestin-binding complement
    protected brush catheter
PBCL
    parafollicular B-cell lymphoma
PBD
    percutaneous biliary drainage
    postburn day
    proliferating bile ductules
    proliferative breast disease
    psychotic and behavioral disturbances
PBE
    partial breech extraction
    population bioequivalence
    power building exercise
PBF
    pencil beam function [radiotherapy]
    percent(age) body fat
    peripheral blood flow
    phosphate-buffered formalin
    placental blood flow
    pulmonary blood flow (*See also* Qp)
PB-Fe
    protein-bound iron
PBFS
    penile blood flow study
PBG
    Penassay broth plus glucose
    poor breastfeed
    porphobilinogen
    pupillary block glaucoma
PBG-D
    porphobilinogen deaminase
PBGM
    Penassay broth plus glucose plus menadione
PBG-S
    porphobilinogen synthase
PBH
    pulling-boat hands
PBHA
    porous block hydroxyapatite
PBI
    parental bonding instrument

partial bony impaction
penile-brachial index
phenformin
protein-bound iodine

PbI

lead intoxication

PBK

Phonetically Balanced Kindergarten
phosphorylase *b* kinase
pseudophakic bullous keratopathy

PBL

peripheral blood leukocyte (lymphocyte)
primary bone lymphoma
primary brain lymphoma
primary breast lymphoma
problem-based learning

PBLC

premature birth live child

PBLI

premature birth live infant

PBLT

peripheral blood lymphocyte
transformation

PBM

peripheral basement membrane
peripheral blood monocyte
peripheral blood mononuclear [cell]
(*See also* PBMC, PBMNC)
pharmacy benefit management

PBMA

polybutylmethacrylate

PBMC, PBMNC

peripheral blood mononuclear cell
(*See also* PBM)

PBMTx

porcine bone marrow transplant(ation)

PBMV

pulmonary blood mixing volume

PBN

papillary breast neoplasm
paralytic brachial neuritis
peripheral benign neoplasm

PBNA

partial body neutron activation

PB:ND

problem: nursing diagnosis

PBNS

percutaneous bladder neck stabilization
percutaneous bladder neck suspension

PBO

placebo (*See also* OBE-CALP, P, PCB,
PL, PLB, PLBO)

PbO

lead monoxide

PBP

peak blood pressure
penicillin-binding protein

percutaneous balloon pericardiotomy
phantom breast pain
porphyrin biosynthetic pathway
progressive bulbar palsy
prostate-binding protein
protein-bound polysaccharide
pseudobulbar palsy
pulsatile bypass pump
purified *Brucella* protein

PBPC

peripheral blood progenitor cell

PBPCT

peripheral blood progenitor cell
transplant(ation)

PBPD

pediatric bipolar disorder

PBPF

primary bronchopulmonary fibrosarcoma

PBPI

penile-brachial pressure (pulse) index

PBPND

progressive bulbar palsy with neural
deafness

PBPV

percutaneous balloon pulmonary
valvuloplasty

PBQ

Preschool Behavior Questionnaire

PBR

peripheral-type benzodiazepine receptor

PBRT

phonetically balanced rhyme test

PBRVO

peripheral branch retinal vein occlusion

PBS

Pediatric Behavior Scale
peripheral-blood smear
peroneus brevis split
phosphate-buffered saline (sodium)
planar bone scan
protected brush specimen
prune belly syndrome
pulmonary branch stenosis

PBSC

peripheral blood stem cell

PBSCR

peripheral blood stem cell reserve

PBSCT

peripheral blood stem cell
transplant(ation)

PBSP

prognostically bad signs during
pregnancy

PBT

Paul-Bunnell [antibody, test] (*See also*
PB)
phenacetin breath test

P

PBT *(continued)*
    piebald trait
    primary brain tumor
    profile-based therapy
    pulmonary barotrauma
PBT4, PBT$_4$
    protein-bound thyroxine
PBTE
    percutaneous transhepatic liver biopsy
    with tract embolization
PbtO$_2$
    brain tissue partial pressure of
    oxygen
PBV
    percutaneous balloon valvuloplasty
    predicted blood volume
    pulmonary balloon valvuloplasty
    pulmonary blood volume
PbV
    Penicillium brevicompactum virus
PBVI
    pulmonary blood volume index
PBW
    posterior bite wing
    present breast width
PC
    avoirdupois weight [L. *pondus civile*]
    packed cells
    palliative care
    palmitoylcarnitine
    pancreatic cancer (carcinoma) (*See also*
    PCA)
    paper chromatography
    parent cell
    parent to child
    particulate component
    pathologic consultation
    peak clipping
    pelvic cramp
    penile carcinoma
    pentose cycle
    pericardium channel [acupuncture]
    peritoneal cell
    persistent condition
    pharmacology
    phase contrast
    pheochromocytoma (*See also* PCC,
    pheo)
    phosphate cycle
    phosphatidylcholine [lecithin]
    phosphocreatine
    phosphorylcholine
    photocoagulation
    photoconductive
    phrase construction
    picryl chloride
    picture completion
    pill counter
    pilomatrix carcinoma

    piriform cortex
    placebo-controlled [study]
    plasma cell
    plasma concentration
    plasma cortisol
    plasmacytoma
    platelet count
    Pneumocystis carinii [renamed
    Pneumocystis jiroveci]
    pneumotaxic center
    politically correct
    polycentric
    polyposis coli
    poor condition
    popliteal cyst
    portacaval [shunt]
    portal cirrhosis
    postcoital
    posterior canal
    posterior cervical
    posterior chamber
    posterior circulation
    posterior circumflex [artery]
    posterior column
    posterior commissure
    posterior cortex
    precordial
    premature contractions
    prepiriform cortex
    present complaint
    pressure control
    primary cleavage
    primary closure
    principal cell
    printed circuit
    procollagen
    producing cell
    productive cough
    professional corporation
    proliferative capacity
    proprotein convertase
    prostate (prostatic) cancer (carcinoma)
    (*See also* PCA, PCa, PcA)
    provisional cortex
    proximal colon
    pseudocyst
    Psychodevelopment Checklist
    pubococcygeus [muscle] (*See also* PCG,
    PCM)
    pulmonary capillary
    pulmonary circulation
    pulmonary compliance
    pulmonic closure
    pulp canal
    Purkinje cell (*See also* P-cell)
    pyloric canal
    pyruvate carboxylase
P-C
    phlogistic corticoid

PC1–PC3
 prohormone convertase 1–3
P&C
 prism and cover test [crossover test,
  screen and cover test in ophthalmology]
p.c.
 after a meal [L. *post cibum*]
 post cibum (after meals)
pc
 parsec
 percent(age)
pc1
 platelet count pretransfusion
pc2
 platelet count posttransfusion
PCA
 pancreatic cancer (carcinoma) (*See also*
  PC)
 para-chloramphetamine
 parenteral controlled analgesia
 parietal cell antibody
 passive cutaneous anaphylaxis
 patient-controlled analgesia (analgesic)
  (anesthesia) (anesthetic)
 perchloric acid
 percutaneous carotid angiography
  (angioplasty)
 percutaneous carotid arteriogram
 phenylcarboxylic acid
 photocontact allergic (allergy)
 plasma catecholamines
 porous-coated anatomic [prosthesis]
 portacaval anastomosis
 postcardiac arrest
 postciliary artery
 postconceptional age
 postcoronary arrest
 posterior cerebral artery
 posterior communicating [artery]
  aneurysm
 posterior communicating artery (*See also*
  PCoA, PCom, PComA)
 posterior cricoarytenoid
 precoronary care area
 prehospital cardiac arrest
 principal-components analysis
 procoagulant activity
 prostate (prostatic) cancer (carcinoma)
  (*See also* PC, PCa, PcA, PrCa)
 protected catheter aspirate
 pyrrolidone carboxylic acid
PCa, PcA
 prostate (prostatic) cancer (carcinoma)
  (*See also* PC, PCA, PrCa)
 prostatic adenocarcinoma
PCAD
 progression of coronary artery disease

PCAR
 presumed circle area ratio
PCAS
 Psychotherapy Competence Assessment
  Schedule
PCASSO
 patient-centered access to secure
  systems online
PCAV
 Pacora virus
PCAVC
 persistent complete atrioventricular canal
PCB
 paracervical block
 percutaneous biopsy
 placebo (*See also* OBE-CALP, P, PBO,
  PL, PLB, PLBO)
 polychlorinated biphenyl
  (polychlorobiphenyl)
 portacaval bypass
 postcoital bleeding
 prepared childbirth
 protected catheter brushing
 proximal communicating branch
 Pseudomonas cepacia bacteremia
PcB, Pcb
 near point of convergence to
  intercentral baseline [L. *punctum
  convergens basalis*]
PCBH
 personal care boarding home
PCBM
 particulate cancellous bone and marrow
PCBMN
 palmar cutaneous branch of median
  nerve
PC-BMP
 phosphorylcholine-binding myeloma
  protein
PCBS
 percutaneous cardiopulmonary bypass
  support
PCBUN
 palmar cutaneous branch of ulnar nerve
PCC
 Pasteur Culture Collection
 percutaneous catheter cecostomy
 percutaneous cecostomy
 percutaneous cervical cordotomy
 peripheral cholangiocarcinoma
 petrous carotid canal
 pheochromocytoma (*See also* PC, pheo)
 phosphate carrier compound
 plasma catecholamine concentration
 pneumatosis cystoides coli
 Poison Control Center
 postcoital contraception

P

PCC *(continued)*
  posterior central curve
  precipitated calcium carbonate
  precoronary care
  premature chromosome condensation
  propagating clustered contraction
  prothrombin-complex concentration
PCc
  periscopic concave [lens]
PCCI
  penetrating craniocerebral injury
PCCL
  percutaneous cholecystolithotomy
PCCP
  percutaneous cord cyst puncture
PCC-R
  Percentage of Consonants
    Correct-Revised
PCCS
  parent-child communication schedule
PCCTEA
  patient-controlled continuous thoracic
    epidural anesthesia
PCD
  pacer-cardioverter-defibrillator
  papillary collecting duct
  paraneoplastic cerebellar degeneration
  paroxysmal cerebral dysrhythmia
  percutaneous catheter drainage
  phosphate-citrate-dextrose [anticoagulant]
  phototoxic contact dermatitis
  plasma cell dyscrasia
  pneumatic compression device
  polycystic disease
  postcoital depression
  posterior capsular distance
  posterior corneal deposit
  postmortem cesarean delivery
  postparacentesis circulatory dysfunction
  precancerous dermatosis
  primary ciliary dyskinesia
  programmable cardioverter-defibrillator
  programmed cell death
  prolonged contractile duration
  pulmonary clearance delay
PCDAI
  Paediatric Crohn Disease Activity Index
    [British]
PCDC
  plasma clot diffusion chamber
PCDF
  polychlorinated dibenzofuran
PCDUS
  plasma cell dyscrasia of unknown
    significance
PCE
  physical capacity evaluation
  potentially compensable event
  precaliceal canalicular ectasia

pseudocholinesterase (*See also* PCHE,
    PsChE)
  pseudophakic corneal edema
  pulmocutaneous exchange
  Smith physical capacities evaluation
PCEA
  patient-controlled epidural analgesia
    (*See also* PEA)
pCEA
  polyclonal carcinoembryonic antigen
PCEC
  purified chick embryo cell [culture]
PCECV
  purified chick embryo cell vaccine
P-cell
  Purkinje cell (*See also* PC)
PCF
  partial conjunctival flap
  peak cough flow
  peripheral circulatory failure
  pharyngoconjunctival fever
  posterior cranial fossa
  prothrombin conversion factor
pcf
  pound per cubic foot
PCFIA
  particle concentration fluorescence
    immunoassay
PCFL
  primary cutaneous follicular lymphoma
PCFT
  platelet complement fixation test
Pc-fV
  Penicillium cyaneo-fulvum virus
PCG
  paracervical ganglion
  phonocardiogram
  Planning Career Goals [psychologic
    test]
  plasma cell granuloma
  pneumcardiograph(y)
    (pneumocardiogram)
  primary congenital glaucoma
  primate chorionic gonadotropin
  pubococcygeus [muscle] (*See also* PC,
    PCM)
PCGG
  percutaneous coagulation of gasserian
    ganglion
PCGLV
  poorly contractile globular left ventricle
PCH
  palpebral conjunctival hue
  paroxysmal cold hemoglobinuria
  periocular capillary hemangioma
  personal care home
  plasma cell hepatitis
  polycyclic hydrocarbon
  pseudochromhydrosis

pulmonary capillary hemangiomatosis
pulp chamber
PCHE
pseudocholinesterase (*See also* PCE,
PsChE)
PCHI
permanent childhood hearing impairment
PCHL
permanent childhood hearing loss
PC&HS
after meals and at bedtime
PCI
partial coherence interferometry
percutaneous coronary intervention
pneumatosis cystoides intestinalis
posterior curve intermediate [cornea]
Premarital Communication Inventory
prophylactic cranial irradiation
prothrombin consumption index
pCi
picocurie
pCi/L
picocurie per liter
PCINA
patient-controlled intranasal analgesia
PCIOL, PC-IOL
posterior chamber intraocular lens
PCIRF
radiologic contrast-induced renal failure
PCIRV, PC-IRV
pressure control (pressure-controlled)
inverse ratio ventilation
PCIS
Patient Care Information System
postcardiac injury syndrome
PCK
polycystic kidney
PCKD
polycystic kidney disease
PCL
pacing cycle length
persistent corpus luteum
plasma cell leukemia
polycation liposome
posterior chamber lens
posterior collagenous layer
posterior cruciate ligament
proximal collateral ligament
pubococcygeal line
PCLBCL
primary cutaneous large B-cell
lymphoma
PCLC
Paneth cell-like change
PCLD
polycystic liver disease (*See also*
PLD)

PCLI
plasma cell labeling index
posterior chamber lens implant
PCLR
paid claims loss ratio
PCLS
precision-cut lung slices [method]
PCM
paracoccidioidomycosis
pericellular matrix
pharmaceutical care management
phase contrast microscopy
primary cutaneous melanoma
prophylactic contralateral mastectomy
protein-calorie malnutrition
protein carboxymethylase
pubococcygeus muscle (*See also* PC,
PCG)
pulse code modulation
PCMB, p-CMB
parachloromercuribenzoate
(*para*-chloromercuribenzine)
PCMBSA
para-chloromercuribenzine sulfonic
acid
PCMD
pellucid corneal marginal degeneration
PCMF
perceptual cognitive motor function
PC-MRA
phase contrast magnetic resonance
angiography
PC-MRI
phase-contrast magnetic resonance
imaging
PCMT
pacemaker circus-movement tachycardia
PCMX
parachlorometaxylenol
(*para*–chloro-*m*-xylenol)
PCN
percutaneous nephrostomy
(nephrolithotomy)
PCNA
proliferating cell nuclear antigen
PCNA-LI
proliferating cell nuclear antigen
(PCNA) labeling index
PCNB
pentachloronitrobenzene
PCNHL
primary cerebral non-Hodgkin
lymphoma
PCNL
percutaneous nephrolithotomy
(nephrostolithotomy) (*See also* PNL)
percutaneous nephrolithotripsy

P

PCNS
primary central nervous system
PCNs
posterior cervical nodes
PCNSL
primary central nervous system
lymphoma
PCNT
percutaneous nephrostomy tube
PCNV
postchemotherapy nausea and vomiting
PCO
partial pressure of carbon monoxide
patient complains of
polycystic ovary
posterior capsule (capsular) opacification
predicted cardiac output
procyanidol oligomer
PCO$_2$, PCO2, P$_{CO2}$, P$co2$
partial pressure of carbon dioxide
PCoA
posterior communicating artery (*See also*
PCA, PCom, PComA)
PCOD
polycystic ovary (ovarian) disease
(*See also* POD)
PCOE
prescriber (physician) computer order
entry
PCom, PComA
posterior communicating artery (*See also*
PCA, PCoA)
PCOS
polycystic ovary (ovarian) syndrome
(*See also* POS)
PCP
palliative care program
parachlorophenate
patient care plan
pentachlorophenol
peripheral coronary pressure
persistent cough and phlegm
phencyclidine
pneumocystic pneumonia
Pneumocystis jiroveci pneumonia
[formerly *Pneumocystis carinii*]
pollen-coat protein
postoperative constrictive pericarditis
primary care physician (provider)
procollagen peptide
pulmonary capillary pressure
pulse cytophotometry
PCPA
parachlorophenylalanine
(*para*-chlorophenylalanine)
postcatheterization pseudoaneurysm
PCPB
percutaneous cardiopulmonary bypass
procarboxypeptidase B

PCPL
pulmonary capillary protein leakage
PC-PLD
phosphatidylcholine-specific
phospholipase D
pcpn
precipitation (*See also* pcpt, ppt, pptn,
precip)
PCPS
percutaneous cardiopulmonary
support
peroral cholangiopancreatoscopy
phosphatidylcholine-phosphatidylserine
pcpt
perception
precipitate(d) (*See also* ppt, pptd,
precip)
precipitation (*See also* pcpn, ppt, pptn,
precip)
PCPV
pseudocowpox virus
PCQ
Pain Coping Questionnaire
PCR
pathologically confirmed complete
remission
patient care report
patient contact record
percutaneous coronary
revascularization
photoconvulsive response
plasma clearance rate
polymerase chain reaction
postcompression remodeling
probable causal relationship
progressive condylar resorption
protein catabolic rate
PCr
phosphocreatine
PCRA
patient-controlled regional analgesia
percutaneous coronary rotational
atherectomy
pure red [blood] cell aplasia
PCRC
primary colorectal cancer
PCR-ISH
polymerase chain reaction in situ
hybridization
PCR/PSA
polymerase chain reaction analysis of
prostate-specific antigen
PCR-RFLP
polymerase chain reaction-restriction
fragment length polymorphism
PCR-SSCP
polymerase chain reaction-based
single-stranded conformation
polymorphism

PCR-SSOP
  polymerase chain reaction-sequence
    specific oligonucleotide probe
PCS
  Pain Catastrophizing Scale
  patient care system
  patient-controlled sedation
  pelvic congestion syndrome
  peroral cholangioscopy
  pharmacogenic confusional syndrome
  photon correlation spectroscopy
  Physical Component Summary
  portable cervical spine
  portacaval shunt
  postcardiac surgery
  postcardiotomy syndrome
  postcholecystectomy syndrome
  postconcussion syndrome
  precordial stethoscope
  primary cancer site
  primary cesarean section (*See also*
    P c/s)
  Priority Counseling Survey
  prolonged crush syndrome
  proportional counter spectrometry
  proximal coronary sinus
  pseudoclaudication syndrome
  pseudotumor cerebri syndrome
  pulp canal sealer
P c/s
  primary cesarean section (*See also* PCS)
pcs
  preconscious
PCSD
  prone cranial support device
PCSM
  percutaneous stone manipulation
PCT
  paracentesis
  parasite clearance time
  Physiognomic Cue Test [psychology]
  plasma clotting time
  plasmacrit test [for syphilis]
  plasmacytoma
  platelet hematocrit
  poker chip tool [pediatric pain
    assessment]
  polychlorinated triphenyl
  porcine calcitonin
  porphyria cutanea tarda
  portacaval transportation
  portacaval transposition
  positron computed tomography
  postcoital test
  posterior chest tube
  primary chemotherapy
  prism cover test

  procalcitonin
  progesterone challenge test
  progestin challenge test
  prothrombin consumption time
  proximal convoluted tubule
pct
  percent(age)
PCTA
  percutaneous coronary transluminal
    angioplasty
PC/TC
  power cut/tungsten carbide
PCTCL
  percutaneous transhepatic
    cholecystolithotomy
PCTI
  penetrating cardiac trauma index
PCU
  protein-calorie undernutrition
p cut
  percutaneous
PCV
  packed cell volume
  parietal cell vagotomy
  polycythemia vera (*See also* PV)
  porcine circovirus
  postcapillary venule
  pressure-control (pressure-controlled)
    ventilation
PCV7
  pneumococcal 7-valent conjugate
    vaccine
PCV23
  pneumococcal vaccine polyvalent
PcV
  Penicillium chrysogenum virus
PCVC
  percutaneous central venous catheter
PCVD
  pulmonary collagen vascular disease
PCV-M
  polycythemia vera [with myeloid]
    metaplasia
PCW
  pulmonary capillary wedge [pressure]
    (*See also* PCWP)
  purified cell walls
PCWP
  pulmonary capillary wedge pressure
    (*See also* PCW)
PCX
  paracervical (*See also* para C,
    para c)
PCx
  periscopic convex
PCXR
  portable chest radiograph (x-ray)

P

PD

(inter)pupillary distance
pancreas divisum
pancreatic duct
pancreatoduodenectomy
  (pancreaticoduodenectomy)
panic disorder
papilla diameter
paralyzing dose
Parkinson disease
parkinsonian dementia
paroxysmal discharge
pars distalis [pituitary]
patent ductus
patient day
patient demonstration
pediatric dose
pediatrics (*See also* paed, PED, Peds)
percutaneous discectomy
percutaneous drain
peritoneal dialysis
personality disorder
pharmacodynamics
phenyldichloroarsine
  (phenyldichlorarsine) [poison gas]
phosphate dehydrogenase
photosensitivity dermatitis
physical diagnosis
plasma defect
pocket depth
poorly differentiated
porphobilinogen deaminase
postdischarge
posterior descending [coronary artery]
posterior division
postnasal drainage
postural drainage
potential difference
present disease
pressor dose
pressure dressing
primary dendrite
prism diopter (*See also* p.d.)
probing depth
problem drinker
process diagnostic
progression [of] disease
progressive disease
prostatodynia
protein degradation
protein deprived
protein diet
provocation dose
psychopathic deviate
psychotic dementia
psychotic depression
pulmonary disease (*See also* PUD, PuD)
pulpodistal
pulsed diastolic

pulsed Doppler [wave]
pulse duration
pupil diameter
pupillary distance
pure dysarthria
pyloric dilator

2PD

two-point discrimination

PD$_{50}$

median paralyzing dose

P/D, p/d

packs per day [cigarettes] (*See also* PPD)
proximal to distal

P(D+)

probability of having disease

P(D−)

probability of not having disease

Pd

palladium

^{103}Pd

palladium 103

pd

period (*See also* PER)

p.d.

by the day [L. *per diem*]
prism diopter (*See also* PD)

PDA

parenteral drug abuser
patent ductus arteriosus
pathological demand avoidance
patient distress alarm
pediatric allergy
pericardial diaphragmatic adhesion
personal digital assistant
plantar digital artery
polymorphic delta activity
poorly differentiated adenocarcinoma
posterior descending [coronary] artery
predialyzed human albumin
property damage accident
pulmonary disease anemia

PDAB

para-dimethylaminobenzaldehyde

PD-AB-SAAP

pulsed diastolic autologous blood
  selective aortic arch perfusion

PDAC

pancreatic ductal adenocarcinoma

PDAD

photodiode array detector

PDAF

platelet-derived angiogenesis factor

PDAI

Perianal Crohn Disease Activity
  Index
Pouchitis Disease Activity Index

PDAK

partial depth astigmatic keratotomy

PDAP
peritoneal dialysis-associated peritonitis
PD/AR
photosensitivity dermatitis and actinic reticuloid syndrome
PDB
Paget disease of bone
para-dichlorobenzene (*See also* PDCB)
phosphorus-dissolving bacteria
preperitoneal dilator (distention) balloon
preventive dental [health] behavior
PDC
pancreatic duct-cell carcinoma
parkinsonism-dementia complex
patient denies complaints
pediatric cardiology
pentadecylcatechol
peritoneal dialysis catheter
physical dependence capacity
plasma digoxin concentration
plasma disappearance curve
poorly differentiated carcinoma
postdecapitation convulsion
prolonged detention center
property damage collision (crash)
pyruvate dehydrogenase complex (*See also* PDHC)
PD&C
postural drainage and clapping
PdC
pediatric cardiology
PDCA
Plan-Do-Check-Act [process improvement]
PDCB
para-dichlorobenzene (*See also* PDB)
PDCD
primary degenerative cerebral disease
PDCD4
programmed cell death 4 [gene]
PDCE
precaliceal diffuse canalicular dysplasia
PD-CSE
pulsed Doppler cross-sectional echocardiography
PDD
Parkinson disease with dementia
percent(age) depth dose
pervasive developmental disorder
premenstrual dysphoric disorder
primary degenerative dementia (disorder)
progressive diaphysial dysplasia
pyridoxine-deficient diet
PDDAT
primary degenerative dementia of Alzheimer type

PDDB
phenododecinium bromide
PDD-NOS
pervasive developmental disorder not otherwise specified
PDE
paroxysmal dyspnea on exertion
pediatric endocrinology
peritoneal dialysis effluent
personality disorder examination
phosphodiesterase (*See also* PDIE)
progressive dialysis encephalopathy
pulsed Doppler echocardiography
PDE5, PDE 5
phosphodiesterase 5
PdE
pediatric endocrinology
PDEC
poorly differentiated endocrine carcinoma
PD-ECGF
platelet-derived endothelial cell growth factor
PDEGF
platelet-derived epidermal growth factor
PDE-I
phosphodiesterase inhibitor (*See also* PDI)
PDE3I
phosphodiesterase 3 inhibitor
PDE5I
phosphodiesterase 5 inhibitor
PDET
poorly differentiated embryonal cell tumor
pDEXA
peripheral dual-energy x-ray absorptiometry (*See also* pDXA)
PDF
parameterized diastolic filling
peritoneal dialysis fluid
Portable Document Format
probability density function
PDFC
premature dead female child
PDG
parkinsonism dementia [complex of] Guam
phosphate-dependent glutaminase
PDGA
pteroyldiglutamic acid
PDGF
platelet-derived growth factor
PDGF-A
platelet-derived growth factor A
PDGF-B
platelet-derived growth factor B

P

PDGS
> partial form of DiGeorge syndrome

PD-GXT, PDGXT
> postdischarge (predischarge) graded-exercise test

PDH
> past dental history
> phosphate dehydrogenase
> progressive disseminated histoplasmosis
> pyruvate dehydrogenase

PDHC
> pyruvate dehydrogenase complex (*See also* PDC)

PdHO
> pediatric hematology-oncology

PDHRF
> platelet-derived histamine-releasing factor

PDI
> Pain Disability Index
> Periodontal Disease Index
> phasic detrusor instability
> phosphodiesterase inhibitor (*See also* PDE-I)
> plan-do integration
> power Doppler imaging
> protein disulfide isomerase
> psychiatric diagnostic interview
> Psychomotor Development Index

Pdi
> transdiaphragmatic pressure

PDIE
> phosphodiesterase (*See also* PDE)

PDIg
> platelet-directed immune globulin (immunglobulin)

PDIGC
> patient dismissed in good condition

P-diol
> pregnanediol

Pdisniff
> maximal sniff-induced transdiaphragmatic pressure

PDK
> phosphoinositide-dependent protein kinase

PDL
> periodontal ligament
> polycystic disease of liver
> poorly differentiated lymphocyte
> population doubling level
> postures of daily living
> preferred drug list
> primary dysfunctional labor
> progressively diffused leukoencephalopathy
> pulsed-dye laser [therapy]

Pdl
> pudendal (*See also* PUD)

pdl, pl
> poundal [British unit of force, engineering]

PDLC
> poorly differentiated lung cancer

PDLD
> poorly differentiated lymphocytic–diffuse

PDLL
> poorly differentiated lymphocytic lymphoma

PDLN
> poorly differentiated (lymphocytic) lymphoma–nodular

PDLP
> predigested liquid protein

PDLS
> physical daily living skills

PDM
> polydimethylsiloxane (*See also* PDMS)
> polymyositis and dermatomyositis (*See also* PM-DM, PM/DM)
> predentin matrix

PDMC
> premature dead male child

PDMS
> Patient Data Management Systems
> Peabody Developmental Motor Scale
> pharmacokinetic drug-monitoring service
> polydimethylsiloxane (*See also* PDM)

PDN
> Paget disease of nipple
> painful diabetic neuropathy (nephropathy)
> prosthetic disc nucleus

PDNE
> poorly differentiated neuroendocrine [carcinoma]

PdNEO
> pediatric neonatology

PdNEP
> pediatric nephrology

PDO
> pyknodysostosis

PDP
> pachydermoperiostosis
> pancreatic duct pressure
> papular dermatitis of pregnancy
> passive-dependent personality
> pattern disruption point
> peak diastolic pressure
> piperidinopyrimidine
> platelet-depleted plasma
> positive distending pressure
> primer-dependent deoxynucleic acid polymerase
> product development protocol

PD&P
> postural drainage and percussion

PDPD
  prolonged-dwell peritoneal dialysis
PDPDM
  protein-deficient pancreatic diabetes
    mellitus
PDPH
  postdural puncture headache
PDPI
  primer-dependent deoxynucleic acid
    polymerase index
PDPV
  postural drainage, percussion, vibration
PDQ
  parental development questionnaire
  Personality Diagnostic Questionnaire
  Physician Data Query
  Premenstrual Distress Questionnaire
  Prescreening Development Questionnaire
  pretty damn quick
  protocol data query
PDQ-39
  Parkinson Disease Questionnaire
PDQ-R
  Personality Diagnostic Questionnaire
    Revised
PDR
  pandevelopmental retardation
  pediatric radiology
  peripheral diabetic retinopathy
  Physician's Desk Reference
  pleiotropic drug resistance
  point of decreasing response
  postdelivery room
  primary drug resistance
  proliferative diabetic retinopathy
  prospective drug review
  pulsed dose rate
PdR
  pediatric radiology
pdr
  powder (*See also* powd, pwd)
PDRB
  Permanent Disability Rating Board
PDRčVH
  proliferative diabetic retinopathy with
    vitreous hemorrhage
PDRP
  proliferative diabetic retinopathy
PDS
  pain-dysfunction syndrome
  pancreatic duct sphincter
  paroxysmal depolarization (depolarizing)
    shift
  patient data system
  pediatric surgery (*See also* PdS, PS)
  penile Doppler study
  peritoneal dialysis system

persistent developmental stuttering
  pigment dispersion syndrome
  plasma-derived serum
  polydioxanone suture
  postdiphtheritic stenosis
  power Doppler sonography
  predialyzed [human] serum
  primary dependence study
  Progressive Deterioration Scale
PdS
  pediatric surgery (*See also* PDS, PS)
  psychiatric deviate, subtle
PDSG
  pigment dispersion syndrome
    glaucoma
PDSS
  panic disorder severity scale
  Postpartum Depression Screening Scale
PDT
  percutaneous dilational (dilatational)
    tracheostomy (tracheotomy)
  photodynamic therapy
  population doubling time
  postdisaster trauma
  provocative dose test
PDTC
  pyrrolidine dithiocarbamate
PDTP
  pharmacist directed therapy program
PDU
  pulsed Doppler ultrasonography
PDUF
  pulsed Doppler ultrasonic flowmeter
PDUFA
  Prescription Drug User Fee Act [1992]
PDUR
  postdialysis urea rebound
  Predischarge Utilization Review
  prospective drug utilization review
PDV
  peak diastolic velocity
PDVP
  permanent demand ventricular
    pacemaker
PDVR
  proliferative diabetic vitreoretinopathy
PDVT
  proximal deep vein thrombosis
PDW
  platelet distribution width
PDWHF
  platelet-derived wound healing factor
PDWI
  proton density-weighted image
PDx
  principal diagnosis
  probable diagnosis

P

pDXA
peripheral dual-energy x-ray absorptiometry (*See also* pDEXA)

PE
expiratory pressure (*See also* P_E)
pancreatic extract
panendoscopy
paper electrophoresis
parallel elastic [component of muscle]
partial epilepsy
pedal edema (*See also* ped ed)
pelvic examination (*See also* PvE)
penile erection
percutaneous endoscopic
pericardial effusion
peritoneal exudate
phacoemulsification (*See also* PHACO)
pharyngoesophageal
phase encoding
phosphatidylethanolamine
photographic effect
phycoerythrin
physical education (*See also* P Ed, Phys Ed)
physical evaluation
physical examination (*See also* PEx, Px)
physical exercise
physiologic ecology
pigment(ed) epithelium
plasma exchange (*See also* PEX#)
plating efficiency
pleiotropic functional defect
pleural effusion
pneumatic equalization
point of entry
polyethylene
polynuclear eosinophil
portal embolization
potential energy
powdered extract
preeclampsia
preexcitation
premature ejaculation
prescription error
present examination
pressure equalization
prior to exposure
probable error
probe excision
protein excretion
Pseudomonas exotoxin
psychotic event
pulmonary edema
pulmonary embolus (embolism)
pulmonary emphysema
pyramidal eminence
pyroelectric
pyrogenic exotoxin

P-E
portal [venous and] enteric [drainage technique]

PE2
secondary plating efficiency

P&E
prep and enema

P_E
expiratory pressure (*See also* PE)

Pe
Péclet number [measure of relative importance of advection of turbulent diffusion]
perylene
pressure on expiration

PEA
patient-controlled epidural analgesia (*See also* PCEA)
pelvic examination under anesthesia (*See also* PE↓A)
phenylethyl alcohol [agar]
phenylethylamine
polysaccharide egg antigen
preemptive analgesia
pulseless electrical activity

PE↓A
pelvic examination under anesthesia (*See also* PEA)

PEACH
Preschool Evaluation and Assessment for Children with Handicaps

PEAK
pulsed electron avalanche knife

PEAO
phenylethylamine oxidase

PEAP
positive end-airway pressure

PEAQ
Personal Experience and Attitude Questionnaire

PEARL
physiologic endometrial ablation/resection loop
pupils equal to accommodation, reactive to light (*See also* PERL, PERLA, PEARLA)

PEBB
percutaneous excisional breast biopsy

PEBD
partial external biliary diversion

PEBG
phenethylbiguanide

PEC
parallel elastic component
pectoralis [muscle]
peduncle of cerebrum
peritoneal exudate cell
perivascular epithelioid cell
politico-economic conservatism

protein-induced eosinophilic colitis
pulmonary ejection click
pyrogenic exotoxin C
PECAM-1
platelet endothelial cell adhesion
molecule 1
PECCE
planned extracapsular cataract extraction
PECHO, Pecho
prostatic echogram
PECHR
peripheral exudative choroidal
hemorrhagic retinopathy
PECO$_2$
mixed expired carbon dioxide tension
PEComa
perivascular epithelioid cell tumor
(*See also* PECT)
PECT
perivascular epithelioid cell tumor
(*See also* PEComa)
positron emission computed tomography
PED
palmoplantar ectodermal dysplasia
paroxysmal exertion-induced dyskinesia
pediatric emergency department
pediatrics (*See also* paed, PD, Peds)
peduncle [cerebral]
percutaneous external drainage
pharyngoesophageal diverticulum
pigment(ed) epithelial detachment
pollution and environmental degradation
postentry day
postexertional dyspnea
preexisting disease
prenatally exposed to drugs
progressive exertional dyspnea
P Ed
physical education (*See also* PE, Phys
ED)
ped
pedestrian
PEDD
proton-electron dipole-dipole
ped ed
pedal edema (*See also* PE)
PEDF
pigment epithelium-derived factor
PEDI
Pediatric Evaluation of Disability
Inventory
PEDI-DEG
pediatric deglycerolized red blood cells
PED/MV
pedestrian hit by motor vehicle
PEDRI
proton-electron double-resonance
imaging

PeDS
Pediatric Drug Surveillance
Peds
pediatrics (*See also* paed, PD, PED)
PEE
parallel elastic element
punctate epithelial erosion
PEEK
polyethylethylketone [bone cage]
PEEP
peak end-expiratory pressure
positive end-expiratory pressure
PEEP/CPAP
positive end-expiratory
pressure/continuous positive airway
pressure
PEEPi
intrinsic positive end-expiratory
pressure
PEER
Pediatric Examination of Educational
Readiness
primary emotional energy recovery
pronation eversion external rotation
PEET
Pediatric Extended Examination at
Three
PEEX
Pediatric Early Elemental Examination
PEF
parietal eye field
peak expiratory flow [rate] (*See also*
PEFR)
pharyngoepiglottic fold
Psychiatric Evaluation Form
pulmonary edema fluid
%PEF
percent predicted peak expiratory
flow
PEFR
peak expiratory flow rate (*See also*
PEF)
PEFSR
partial expiratory flow-static recoil
(curve)
PEFT
peak expiratory flow time
PEFV
partial expiratory flow volume
PEG
Patient Evaluation Grid
pegylated
percutaneous endoluminal gastrostomy
percutaneous endoscopic gastrostomy
pericyte edema generation
pneumonencephalograph(y)
(pneumoencephalogram)
polyethylene glycol

P

PEG-ADA
polyethylene glycol-modified [bovine] adenosine deaminase
PEG-ELS
polyethylene glycol electrolyte lavage solution
PEGG
Parent Education and Guidance Group
PEG-IL-2
polyethylene glycol-modified interleukin 2
PEG-J
percutaneous endoscopic gastrojejunostomy
PEG-JET
percutaneous endoscopic gastrostomy with jejunal extension tube
PEG-L-ASP, PEG-*l*-ASP
polyethylene glycol-conjugated *l*-asparaginase
PEG-SOD
polyethylene glycol-conjugated superoxide dismutase
PEH
palmoplantar eccrine hidradenitis
papillary endothelial hyperplasia
postexercise hypotension
PEHO
progressive encephalopathy, edema, hypsarrhythmia, optic atrophy
PEI
patient enablement instrument
percutaneous ethanol injection
phosphate excretion index
phosphorus excretion index
physical efficiency index
polyethylenimine
postexercise index
PEIT
percutaneous ethanol injection therapy
PEITC
phenethyl isothiocyanate
PEJ
percutaneous endoscopic jejunostomy
PEK
punctate epithelial keratopathy
PEL
peritoneal exudate lymphocyte
permissible exposure limit
primary effusion lymphoma
Pel
elastic recoil pressure of lung
PELA
peripheral excimer laser angioplasty
PELCA
percutaneous excimer laser coronary angioplasty
PELD
pediatric endstage liver disease

percutaneous endoscopic lumbar discectomy
PELISA
paper enzyme-linked immunosorbent assay
PELOD
pediatric logistic organ dysfunction [score]
PELV
pelvimetry
Pel-V
elastic pressure-volume
PEM
pediatric emergency medicine
peritoneal exudate macrophage
polymorphic epithelial mucin
positron emission mammography
precordial electrocardiographic mapping
prescription event monitoring
primary enrichment medium
probable error of measurement [statistics]
protein-energy malnutrition
pulmonary endothelial membrane
PEMA
phenylethylmalonamide
P_{Emax}
maximal expiratory mouth pressure
PEME
pulsed electromagnetic energy
PEMF
pulsed (pulsating) electromagnetic field
PEMS
physical, emotional, mental, safety
pulsed electromagnetic stimulator
PEN
palisaded encapsulated neuroma
pancreatic endocrine neoplasm
parenteral and enteral nutrition
Pharmacy Equivalent Name
pen.
penetrating
PENG
photoelectric nystagmography (photoelectronystagmography)
PENL
primary extranodal lymphoma
PENS
percutaneous electrical nerve stimulation
percutaneous epidural nerve (neurostimulator) stimulator
PEO
progressive external ophthalmoparesis
progressive external ophthalmoplegia
PEP
patient education program
peptidase
performance evaluation procedure
pharmacologic erection program

phosphoenolpyruvate
pigmentation, edema, plasma-cell
   dyscrasia [syndrome]
polyestradiol phosphate
positive expiratory pressure
postencephalitic parkinsonism
postendoscopic retrograde
   cholangiopancreatography (ERCP)
   pancreatitis
postexposure prevention
postexposure prophylaxis
preejection period
progestogen-dependent endometrial
   protein
protein electrophoresis (*See also* Pro
   EL)
Psychiatric Evaluation Profile
Psychoeducational Profile
Psycho-Epistemological Profile
pudendal evoked potential

PEPA
peptidase A
protected environment prophylactic
   antibiotics

PEPC
peptidase C

PEPc
corrected preejection period

PEPCK, PEPK
phosphoenolpyruvate carboxykinase

PEPD
peptidase D

PEP:ET
preejection period to ejection time ratio

PEPI
preejection period index

PEP:LVET
preejection period to left ventricular
   ejection time ratio

PEPP
payment error prevention program
positive expiratory pressure plateau

PEPR
precision encoder and pattern
   recognizer

PEP-R
psychoeducational profile-revised

PEPS
peptidase S
peroral electronic pancreatoscope
   (system)

PER
peak ejection rate
pediatric emergency room
perineal
period (*See also* pd)
periodic evaluation record

periodic (periodicity)
person
pertussis [whooping cough] vaccine,
   antigens not otherwise specified
protein efficiency ratio
pudendal evoked response

P-ER
pronation-external rotation

PERa
pertussis, acellular antigen(s), vaccine

PERC
panendoscopic recanalization
perceptual
potential erythropoietin-responsive
   cell

percus
percussion

PERD
photoelectric registration device

perf
perfect
perforation
perform(ed)

PERG
pattern-evoked electroretinogram

PERI
peritoneal fluid

peri
perineal

periap
periapical

peri-care
perineum care

perim
perimeter

PERIO
periodontal care
periodontal disease

Perio
periodontics

peri-pads, per pad
perineal pads

periph vasc
peripheral vascular

PERK
prospective evaluation of radial
   keratotomy

PERL
pupils equal and react(ive) to light
   (*See also* PEARL, PEARLA, PERLA)

PERLA, PEARLA
pupils equal and react(ive) to light and
   accommodation (*See also* PEARL,
   PERL)

PERM
progressive encephalomyelitis with
   rigidity and myoclonus

P

⚠ **perm**
permanent
permutation ⚠

⚠ **per os**
by mouth (*See also* m, (m), OS, PO, p.o.) ⚠

perp
perpendicular

PerQ SANS
Percutaneous Stoller Afferent Nerve Stimulation System

PERR
pattern evoked retinal response

PERRL
pupils equal, round, react(ive) to light

PERRLA
pupils equal, round, react(ive) to light and accommodation

PERR-LADC
pupils equal, round, react(ive) to light and accommodation directly and consensually

PERRRLA
pupils equal, round, regular, react(ive) to light and accommodation

PERS
patient evaluation rating scale
personal emergency response system

pers
personal

PERT
pancreatic enzyme replacement therapy
product-enhanced reverse transcriptase
program evaluation and review technique

PERV
Perinet virus
porcine endogenous retrovirus

PERw
pertussis, whole-cell antigens, vaccine

PES
pacing esophageal stethoscope
papillary fibroelastoma
photoelectron spectroscopy
plastic endosurgical system
Pleasant Events Schedule
polyethersulfone
postextrasystolic
preepiglottic space
preexcitation syndrome
primary empty sella [syndrome]
programmed electrical stimulation
pseudoepileptic seizure
pseudoexfoliation syndrome (*See also* PXS)

PESA
percutaneous epididymal sperm aspiration

PESDA
perfluorocarbon-exposed sonicated dextrose albumin

Pesend
end-expiratory esophageal pressure

PESP
postextrasystolic potentiation

pe SPL
peak equivalent sound pressure level

PESQ
Personal Experience Screening Questionnaire

PESS
powered endoscopic sinus surgery
primary empty sella syndrome

Pess
pessary

Pessniff
maximal sniff-induced esophageal pressure

PESST
Patterned Elicitation Syntax Screening Test

PEST
point estimation by sequential testing

PET
paraffin-embedded tissue
Parent Effectiveness Training
peak ejection time
pear-shaped extension tube
peritoneal equilibration test
polyethylene terephthalate
polyethylene tube
poor exercise tolerance
positron emission tomography
postexposure treatment
predominantly epithelial thymoma
preeclamptic toxemia
pressure equalization (equalizing) tube
problem elicitation technique
Professional Employment Test
progressive exercise test
pulmonary endodermal tumor

PETA
pentaerythritol triacrylate

PETCO$_2$
partial pressure of end-tidal carbon dioxide

PET-FDG
positron emission tomography with [^{18}F]-labeled fluorodeoxyglucose

PETFx
proximal end tibial fracture

PETG
polyethylene terephthalate

PETH
pink-eyed, tan-hooded [rat]

PETINIA
  particle-enhanced turbidimetric inhibition
    immunoassay
PETN
  pentaerythritol tetranitrate
petr
  petroleum
PETT
  pendular eye-tracking test
  phenethylthiazolethiourea
  positron emission transaxial
    tomography
  positron emission transverse
    tomography
PEU
  plasma equivalent unit
  polyether urethane
PEV
  pulmonary extravascular [fluid] volume
PeV
  peripheral vein (See also PV)
peV
  peak electron volt
PEVN
  periventricular nucleus
PEWV
  pulmonary extravascular water volume
PEx
  physical examination (See also PE, Px)
PEX#
  plasma exchange [followed by numeral]
    (See also PE)
PEXG
  pseudoexfoliative glaucoma
PF
  parafascicular [nucleus]
  parallel fiber
  parenteral feeding
  parotid fluid
  pars flaccida
  partially follicular
  patellofemoral [joint]
  peak flow
  pemphigus foliaceus
  pericardial fluid
  perifollicular
  perifolliculitis
  peripheral field
  peritoneal fluid
  permeability factor
  personality factor
  phenol formaldehyde
  physicians' forum
  picture-frustration [study, test] (See also
    P-F)
  plantar flexion
  plasma factor

plasma fibronectin
platelet factor (See also PF1–PF4)
pleural fluid
Pontiac fever [mild form of
  Legionnaires' disease]
port film
power factor
precursor fluid
preservative free
proflavin
prostatic fluid
protection factor
pterygoid fossa
pulmonary factor
pulmonary fibrosis
pulmonary function
Purkinje fiber
purpura fulminans
push fluids
P-F
  picture-frustration [study, test] (See also
    PF)
PF1–PF4
  parainfluenza virus 1–4 (See also
    paraflu, PI, PIV)
  platelet factor 1–4 (See also PF)
16 PF, 16PF
  16 Personality Factor Questionnaire
  The Sixteen Personality Factors test
P/F
  pass/fail [system]
pF
  picofarad
PFA
  phosphonoformic acid
  platelet function analysis (analyzer)
  profunda femoris artery
  psychological first aid
  pure free acid
PFAGH
  penalty, frustration, anxiety, guilt,
    hostility
PFAMC
  psychological factors affecting medical
    condition
PFAPA
  periodic fever, aphthous stomatitis,
    pharyngitis, cervical adenitis
PFAPE
  perfluoroalkylpolyether
PFAS
  performic acid-Schiff [reaction, stain]
PFB
  potential for breakdown
  present from birth
  properdin factor B
  pseudofolliculitis barbae

P

PFC
pancreatic fluid collection
patient-focused care
pelvic flexion contracture
perfluorocarbon
perfluorochemical
pericardial fluid culture
permanent flexure contracture
persistent fetal circulation
plaque-forming cell
prefrontal cortex
Press-Fit component
prolonged febrile convulsions
purified fibrillar collagen

pFc
noncovalently bonded dimer of
C-terminal immunoglobulin of Fc
fragment

PFCPH
persistent fetal circulation with
pulmonary hypertension

PFD
pancreatic functioning diagnostant
patellofemoral dysfunction
polyostotic fibrous dysplasia
polyurethane foam dressing
primary flash distillate

PFE
pelvic floor exercise

PFEAAC
posterior fossa extraaxial arachnoid
cyst

PFeeds
post [after] feedings

PfEMP-1
Plasmodium falciparum erythrocyte
membrane protein 1

PFF
perifollicular fibroma
polymer fume fever

PFFD
proximal (femur) femoral focal
deficiency
proximal focal femoral deficiency

PFFFP
Pall filtered fresh frozen plasma

PFG
patellofemoral grind
peak-flow gauge
pelvic fat girdle
percutaneous fluoroscopic gastrostomy
porcelain fused to gold
proximal femur geometry
pulsed-field gradient

PFGC
pseudofollicular growth center

PFGE
pulsed-field gel electrophoresis
pulsed-field gradient electrophoresis

PfHRP-2
Plasmodium falciparum histidine-rich
protein 2

PFHx
positive family history

PFI
percutaneous flank incision
pill-free interval
progression-free interval

PFIB
perfluoroisobutylene

PFIC
progressive familial intrahepatic
cholestasia (cholestasis)

PFJ
patellofemoral joint

PFJS
patellofemoral joint syndrome

PFK
periodically fluctuating protein
kinase
phosphofructoaldolase
phosphofructokinase
photorefractive keratectomy

PFKL
phosphofructokinase, liver (type)

PFKM
phosphofructokinase, muscle (type)

PFKP
phosphofructokinase, platelet (type)

PFL
profibrinolysin

PFLAG
Parents, Families And Friends Of
Lesbians And Gays

PFM
peak flow meter (flowmeter)
porcelain fused to metal
primary fibromyalgia

PFME
pelvic floor muscle exercise

PFN
partially functional neutrophil

PFNA
percutaneous fine-needle aspiration

PFNAB
percutaneous fine-needle aspiration
biopsy

PFNEI
percutaneous fine-needle ethanol
injection

PFNP
peripheral facial nerve palsy

PFO
patent foramen ovale
perfluoro-N-octane
plantar fasciitis orthosis

PFOB
perfluorooctyl bromide

PFOE
peripheral fractional oxygen extraction
PFP
patellofemoral pain
pentafluoropropionic anhydride
pentafluoropropionyl
platelet-free plasma
preceding foreperiod
progression-free probability
proinsulin fusion protein
purified fusion protein
PFPC
Pall-filtered packed cells
PFPS
patellofemoral pain syndrome
PFQ
personality factor questionnaire
PFR
parotid flow rate
peak filling rate
peak flow rate
pericardial friction rub
pleural friction rub
PFRC
plasma-free red cell
predicted functional residual capacity
PFROM
pain-free range of motion
PFS
patellar femoral syndrome
patient and family services
pelvic floor [electrical] stimulation
penile flow study
picture frustration study
prefilled syringe
preservative-free solution [system]
pressure-flow study
primary fibromyalgia syndrome
progression-free survival
protein-free supernatant
pulmonary function study (score)
P&FS
pit and fissure sealant [dental]
PFSDQ
Pulmonary Functional Status and
Dyspnea Questionnaire
PFSH
past, family, social history
PFST
positional feedback stimulation trainer
PFT
pancreatic function test
parafascicular thalamotomy
placentofetal transfusion
posterior fossa tumor
postoperative flexor tendon
pulmonary function test

PFT$_4$
proportion free thyroxine
PFTBE
progressive form of tick-borne
encephalitis
PFTC
primary fallopian tube carcinoma
PFU
plaque-forming unit
pock-forming unit
PFUO
prolonged fever of unknown origin
PFV
physiologic full value
portal-vein blood flow velocity
PFW
peak flow whistle
PFWB
Pall-filtered whole blood
PFWD
pain-free walking distance
PFWT
pain-free walking time
PG
parapsoriasis guttata
paregoric
parotid gland
partial gastrectomy
pathological gambling
pepsinogen
peptidoglycan
percutaneous gastrostomy
Pharmacopoeia Germanica (*See also*
PhG)
phosphate glutamate
phosphatidylglycerol
phosphatidyl glycine
phosphogluconate
phosphoglycerate
pigment granule
pituitary gonadotropin
placental grade [biophysical profile]
plasma gastrin
plasma glucose
plasma triglyceride
polygalacturonate
postgraduate
postgraft
postprandial glucose
pregnant (*See also* PR, preg,
pregn)
propylene glycol
prostaglandin
proteoglycan
pyoderma gangrenosum
PG1–PG3
prostaglandin 1–3

P

PG1–PG5
pepsinogen 1–5
Pg
gastric pressure
nasopharyngeal electrode placement in
electroencephalography
pogonion [craniometric]
pg
page (*See also* P)
picogram
PGA
pancreaticogastrostomy anastomosis
phosphoglyceric acid
polyglandular autoimmune [syndrome]
(*See also* PGAS)
polyglycolic acid
pteroylglutamic acid
PGAC
phenylglycine acid chloride
PGA I–II
polyglandular autoimmune syndrome,
type I–II
PGA–PGY
prostaglandin A–X
PGA-PLA
polyglycolic acid-polylactic acid
[copolymer]
PGAS
persisting galactorrhea-amenorrhea
syndrome
polyglandular autoimmune syndrome
(*See also* PGA)
Pgasniff
maximal sniff-induced gastric
pressure
PGAV
Pongola virus
PGC
percent(age) of goblet cells
pontine gaze center
primordial germ cell
PGCH
postinfantile giant-cell hepatitis
PGCMS
Philadelphia Geriatric Center Morale
Scale
PGCR
pharyngoglottal closure reflex
PGD
pathologic gambling disorder
phosphoglyceraldehyde dehydrogenase
preimplantation genetic diagnosis
pure gonadal dysgenesis
PGD2, PGD$_2$
prostaglandin D2
PGDH
phosphogluconate dehydrogenase
PGDR
plasma glucose disappearance rate

PGE
partial generalized epilepsy
percutaneous gastroenterostomy
platelet granule extract
posterior gastroenterostomy
primary generalized epilepsy
proximal gastric exclusion
PGE1, PGE$_1$
prostaglandin E1
PGE2, PGE$_2$
prostaglandin E2
PGEM
prostaglandin E metabolite
PGF
paternal grandfather
placental growth factor
primary graft failure
PGF2-alpha (α)
prostaglandin F2-alpha
PGF2, PGF$_2$
prostaglandin F2
PGG
polyclonal gamma globulin
PGG$_{II}$
prostaglandin G$_{II}$
PGGF
paternal great-grandfather
PGGM
paternal great-grandmother
pGGO
pure ground glass opacity
PGG-Q
porphobilinogen—quantitative
PGH
pituitary growth hormone
placental growth hormone
plasma growth hormone
porcine growth hormone
PGH2, PGH$_2$
prostaglandin H2
PGHS1–PGHS2
prostaglandin H synthase 1–2
PGI
peripheral glycerol injection
phosphoglucose isomerase
potassium, glucose, and insulin
PGI2, PGI$_2$
prostaglandin I2
PGID
postoperative gastrointestinal tract
dysfunction
PGK
phosphoglycerate kinase [gene]
phosphoglycerokinase [gene]
PGL
persistent generalized lymphadenopathy
phosphoglycolipid
primary gastric [non-Hodgkin]
lymphoma

PGLN
periglandular lymph node
PGlyM
phosphoglyceromutase
PGM
paternal grandmother
phosphoglucomutase
PGMA
polyglycerol methacrylate
PGN
proliferative glomerulonephritis
PGO
pontogeniculooccipital [spike or wave on EEG/PSG]
PGP
paternal grandparent
postgamma proteinuria
prepaid group practice
protein gene product
Pgp, P-gp
P-glycoprotein
Pg-Ppl
gastric-intrapleural pressure
PGR
pelvic girdle relaxation
percutaneous glycerol rhizolysis
progesterone receptor (*See also* PR)
psychogalvanic reflex (response)
pulse-generated runoff
P-graph
penile plethysmograph
1,3-P$_2$Gri
1,3-diphosphoglycerate
2,3-P$_2$Gri
2,3-diphosphoglycerate
P-GRN
progranulocyte
PGS
Persian Gulf syndrome
persistent gross splenomegaly
pineal gonadal syndrome
plant growth substance
posterior glottic stenosis
postsurgical gastroparesis syndrome
primary generalized seizure
prolapse gastropathy syndrome
prostaglandin synthetase
proteoglycan subunit
PGSE
pulsed-gradient spin echo
PGSI
prostaglandin synthetase inhibitor
PGSR
psychogalvanic skin resistance (response)
PGSRA
psychogalvanic skin response audiometry

PGT
play group therapy
PGTC
partial seizures with or without generalized tonic-clonic seizures
pGTD
persistent gestational trophoblastic disease
PGTP
primary glaucoma triple procedure
PGTR
plasma glucose tolerance rate
PGTT
prednisolone glucose tolerance test
PGU
peripheral glucose uptake
peripheral glucose utilization
postgonococcal urethritis
PGUT
phosphogalactose uridyl transferase
PGV
proximal gastric vagotomy
PGVS
postganglionic vagal stimulation
PGW
person gametocyte week
PGWB
Psychological General Well-Being [Scale]
PGWBI
Psychological General Well Being Index
PGY
postgraduate year
PGYE
peptone, glucose, yeast extract [medium]
PH
parathyroid (parathormone) hormone (*See also* para, PH, PT, PTH)
parenchymal hematoma
parenchymal hemorrhage
partial hepatectomy
partial hysterectomy
passive hemagglutination
past history (*See also* PHx, Px)
peliosis hepatitis
perianal herpes
persistent hepatitis
personal history
pharmacopeia (*See also* PHAR, phar, PHARM, pharm)
phenylalanine hydroxylase (*See also* PAH)
pinhole
polycythemia hypertonica
poor health
porphyria hepatica
posterior hypothalamus

P

PH *(continued)*
   previous history
   primary hyperparathyroidism
   primary hypogonadism
   prolylhydroxylase
   prostatic hypertrophy
   pseudohermaphroditism
   pubic hair
   public health
   pulmonary hypertension (*See also* PHT, PHTN)
   pulp horn
   punctate hemorrhage
PH-I–PH-II
   primary hyperoxaluria type I–II
PH-1
   primary hyperoxaluria type 1
P & H
   physical and history
Ph
   phenanthrene
   phenyl (*See also* Φ)
Ph1
   Philadelphia chromosome
Ph1⁻
   Philadelphia chromosome negative (*See also* Ph1-negative)
Ph1+
   Philadelphia chromosome positive (*See also* Ph1-positive)
pH
   hydrogen ion concentration [power of hydrogen]
pH$_{im}$
   intramucosal pH
ph
   phase
   phial
   phote [CGS unit of illuminance or illumination]
PHA
   passive hemagglutination
   paternal history of alcoholism
   peripheral hyperalimentation
   photometer
   phytohemagglutinin
   phytohemagglutinin activation
   phytohemagglutinin antigen
   polyhydroxy acid
   posterior hypothalamic area
   postoperative holding area
   proper hepatic artery
   pseudohypoaldosteronism
   pulse-height analyzer
pH$_A$, pHa
   arterial blood hydrogen ion concentration
PHA I–II
   pseudohypoaldosteronism type I–II

PHACE
   posterior [fossa malformation], [large facial] hemangiomas, [coarctation of] aorta, cardiac [defects], arterial [abnormalities], eye [abnormalities]
PHACES
   posterior [fossa malformation], [large facial] hemangiomas, [coarctation of] aorta, cardiac [defects], arterial [abnormalities], eye [abnormalities], sternal clefting [or supraumbilical raphe]
PHACO
   phacoemulsification (*See also* PE)
⚠ **PHACO OD**
   phacoemulsification of right eye ⚠
⚠ **PHACO OS**
   phacoemulsification of left eye ⚠
PHA-E
   Phaseolus vulgaris erythroglutinin
PHAL
   peripheral hyperalimentation
   phytohemagglutinin-stimulated lymphocyte
phal
   phalanx [singular] (phalanges [plural])
PHAlb
   polymerized human albumin
PHA-m
   phytohemagglutinin-mucopolysaccharide [fraction]
PHA-p
   phytohemagglutinin-protein [fraction]
PHAR, phar
   pharmaceutical
   pharmacopeia (*See also* PH, PHARM, pharm)
   pharmacy (*See also* PHARM, pharm)
   pharynx (*See also* Phx)
PHARM, pharm
   pharmacopeia (*See also* PH, PHAR, phar)
   pharmacy (*See also* PHAR, Phar)
PHAT
   pleomorphic hyalinizing angiectatic tumor
PHB
   preventive health behavior
PHb
   pyridoxalated hemoglobin
PHBB
   propylhydroxybenzyl benzimidazole
PHBD
   predominant hyperparathyroid bone disease
PHC
   permissive hypercapnia
   personal health cost
   posthospital care

premolar hypodontia, hyperhidrosis,
  canities prematura [Böök syndrome]
primary health care
primary hepatic carcinoma
primary hepatocellular carcinoma
proliferative helper cell
PHCA
profound hypothermia circulatory arrest
profoundly hypothermic circulatory
  arrest
PHCC
primary hepatocellular carcinoma
Ph1-CML
Philadelphia chromosome-positive
  chronic myelogenous leukemia
PHCO₃
plasma bicarbonate
PHD
paroxysmal hypnogenic dyskinesia
pathological habit disorder
personal heart device
photoelectron diffraction
potentially harmful drug
pulmonary heart disease
PHDD
personal history of depressive disorders
PHDPE
porous high-density polyethylene
PHE
periodic health examination
postheparin esterase
proliferative hemorrhagic enteropathy
Phe
phenylalanine (*See also* F)
PhEEM
photoemission electron microscopy
PHEMA
polyhydroxyethylmethacrylate
PHEN
pigmented hairy epidermal nevus
PHEN-FEN, phen-fen
phentermine and fenfluramine
phenom
phenomenon [singular] (phenomena
  [plural])
pheo
pheochromocytoma (*See also* PCC, PC)
PHEP
progressive home exercise program
PHEX
phosphate-regulating endopeptidase
  homolog X-linked
PHF
paired helical filaments
personal hygiene facility
PHFG
primary human fetal glia

PHG
portal hypertensive gastropathy
pulmonary hyalinizing granuloma
PhG
Pharmacopoeia Germanica (*See also*
  PG)
PHGG
polyclonal hypergammaglobulinemia
phgly
phenylglycine
PHH
paraesophageal hiatus hernia
posthemorrhagic hydrocephalus
PHHI
persistent hyperinsulinemic
  hypoglycemia of infancy
Φ, phi
phenyl (*See also* Ph)
phi [21st letter of Greek alphabet
  uppercase]
radiant flux [power, in watts]
φ, phi
ability continuum
osmotic coefficient
phi coefficient [statistics]
phi [21st letter of Greek alphabet
  lowercase]
quantum yield
PHI
passive hemagglutination inhibition
patient health information
peptide histidine isoleucine
phosphohexose isomerase
physiologic hyaluronidase inhibitor
pontine hyperintensity
prehospital index
protected health information
PhI
Pharmacopoeia Internationalis
pHi
intracellular hydrogen ion
  concentration
PHIM
posthypoxic intention myoclonus
PHIP
pleckstrin homology (PH) domain
  interacting protein
PHIQ
Philadelphia Head Injury Questionnaire
PHIS
post head injury syndrome
PHIV
portal hypertensive intestinal
  vasculopathy
PHK
platelet phosphohexokinase
postmortem human kidney

P

PHKC
  postmortem human kidney cell
PHL
  permanent hearing loss
PHLA
  postheparin lipolytic activity
PHM
  partial hydatidiform mole
  peptide histidine methionine
  peptidylglycine alpha-hydroxylating
    monooxygenase
  posterior hyaloid membrane
  preventive health maintenance
  Preventive Health Model
  psyllium hydrophilic mucilloid
PHM-27
  peptide hystidyl-methionine 27
PhM
  pharyngeal musculature
PHMB
  polyhexamethylene biguanine
    [ophthalmologic antiinfective]
PHMD
  pseudohypertrophic muscular dystrophy
PHN
  passive Heymann nephritis
  postherpetic neuralgia
  Puritan heated nebulizer
PH1-negative
  Philadelphia chromosome-negative
    (*See also* Ph1⁻)
PHNI
  pinhole no improvement
PHO
  pediatric hematology/oncology
  periarticular heterotopic ossification
  public health official
PH₂O
  partial pressure of water vapor
PHOB
  phobic anxiety
phos
  phosphatase
  phosphate (*See also* P)
  phosphorous (*See also* P)
PHP
  panhypopituitarism
  partial hospitalization program
  passive hyperpolarizing potential
  persistent hyperphenylalaninemia
  pooled human plasma
  postheparin phospholipase
  postheparin plasma
  prehospital program
  primary hyperparathyroidism
  pseudohypoparathyroidism (*See also* PHPT)
  pyridoxalated
    hemoglobin-polyoxyethylene

Ph1-positive
  Philadelphia chromosome positive
    (*See also* PH1+)
PHPP, *p*-HPPO
  p-hydroxyphenyl pyruvate
PHPPA
  parahydroxyphenylpyruvic acid
PHPPO
  Public Health Practice Program
    Office
PHPT
  primary hyperparathyroidism
  pseudohypoparathyroidism (*See also* PHP)
pHPT
  primary hyperparathyroidism
PHPV
  persistent hyperplasia of primary
    vitreous
  persistent hyperplastic (hypertrophic)
    primary vitreous
PHR
  peak heart rate
  personal health record
  photoreactivity
PHS
  phenylalanine hydroxylase stimulator
  pooled human serum
  posthypnotic suggestion
  pseudoprogeria/Hallermann-Streiff
PHSC
  pluripotent(ial) hemopoietic stem cell
PHSL
  primary hepatosplenic lymphoma
PHSQ
  Psychosocial History Screening
    Questionnaire
PHST
  Psychosocial History Screening Test
pH-stat
  apparatus for maintaining pH of
    solution
PHT
  passive hyperimmune therapy
  peroxide hemolysis test
  portal hypertension (*See also* PHTN)
  posterior hyaloid traction
  postmenopausal hormone therapy
  primary hyperthyroidism
  pulmonary hypertension (*See also* PH, PHTN)
PHTC
  pulmonary hypertensive crisis
PHTLS
  prehospital trauma life support
PHTN
  portal hypertension (*See also* PHT)
  pulmonary hypertension (*See also* PH, PHT)

PHV
  peak height velocity
  persistent hypertrophic vitreous
  Prospect Hill virus
PHVA
  pinhole visual acuity
pHVA
  plasma homovanillic acid
PHVD
  posthemorrhagic ventricular dilatation
  (dilation)
PHVE
  partial hepatic vascular exclusion
PHVM
  posthemorrhagic ventriculomegaly
PHx
  past history (*See also* PH, Px)
Phx
  pharynx (*See also* PHAR, phar)
PHY, phy
  pharyngitis
  physical
  physiology (*See also* P, PHYS, Physiol)
PhyO
  physician's orders
PHYS
  physiology (*See also* P, PHY, Physiol)
PhyS
  physiologic saline [solution]
phys dis
  physical disability
Phys Ed
  physical education (*See also* PE, PED,
  P ED)
physio
  physiologic
  physiotherapy
Physiol
  physiology (*See also* P, PHY, phy,
  PHYS)
Phys Med
  physical medicine
Phys Ther
  physical therapy (physiotherapy)
  (*See also* PT)
π, pi
  pi [16th letter of Greek alphabet
  lowercase]
  ratio of circumference to diameter of
  circle [3.1415926536]
PI
  international protocol
  pacing impulse
  package insert
  pallidal index
  pancreatic insufficiency
  paradoxical intention

parainfluenza [virus] (*See also* paraflu,
  PF1–PF4, PIV)
pars intermedia
paternity index
patient's interest
Pearl Index [effectiveness of birth
  control method]
percutaneous injury
performance improvement
performance index
performance intensity
perinatal injury
Periodontal Index
peripheral iridectomy
permanent incidence
permeability index
persistent illness
personal injury
Personality Index
personality inventory
phagocytic index
phosphatidylinositol (*See also* PtdIns)
physically impaired
pineal body
plaque index
pneumatosis intestinalis
poison ivy
polyphosphoinositide
ponderal index
pontine infarct
posteroinferior (posterior-inferior)
postictal immobility
postincident
postinfection
postinjury
postinoculation
preinduction [examination]
premature infant
prematurity index
preparatory interval
present illness
pressure on inspiration
primary immunodeficiency (immune
  deficiency)
primary infarct(ion)
primary infection
principal investigator
proactive inhibition
proactive interference
programmed instruction
proinsulin
prolactin inhibitor
proliferative index
propidium iodine
protease inhibitor
proximal intestine
pulmonary incompetence

P

615

PI *(continued)*
  pulmonary infarction
  pulmonic insufficiency
  pulsatility index
P of I
  proof of illness
PI3
  phosphoinositol-3
P$_i$
  inorganic orthophosphate
Pi
  inorganic phosphate
  pressure in inspiration
pI
  platelet count increment
p*I*
  isolectric point
PIA
  peripheral interface adapter
  personal injury accident
  phenylisopropyladenosine
  photoelectronic intravenous angiography
  plasma insulin activity
  polysaccharide intercellular adhesin
  porcine intestinal adenomatosis
  preinfarction angina
  purinergic agonist
PIAD
  papular infantile acrodermatitis
PIAPACS
  psychological information, acquisition,
    processing, control system
PIAT
  Peabody Individual Achievement Test
PIAV
  Picola virus
PIAVA
  polydactyly, imperforate anus, vertebral
    anomalies (syndrome)
PIB
  partial ileal bypass
  periinfarction block
  professional information brochure
PIBC
  percutaneous intraaortic balloon
    counterpulsation
PIBD
  paucity of interlobular bile ducts
PIBF
  progesterone-induced blocking factor
PIBIDS
  photosensitivity, ichthyosis, brittle hair,
    impaired intelligence, decreased
    fertility, short stature
PIC
  penicillin-inhibitor combinations
  peripherally inserted catheter
  personal injury collision (crash)
  Personality Inventory for Children

plasmin-inhibitor complex
polysaccharide-iron complex
posterior intermediate curve
postinflammatory corticoid
postintercourse
preinitiation complex
preinvasive cancer
punctate inner choroidopathy
PICA
  Pictorial Instrument for Children and
    Adolescents
  Porch Index of Communicative Abilities
  posterior inferior (posteroinferior)
    cerebellar artery
  posterior inferior (posteroinferior)
    communicating artery
PICAC
  Porch Index of Communicative Abilities
    in Children
PICC
  peripherally inserted central catheter
PICD
  periinfarction conduction defect
  photoirritant contact dermatitis
  primary irritant contact dermatitis
PICFS
  postinfective chronic fatigue syndrome
PICH
  primary intracerebral hemorrhage
PICHI
  pulse-inversion contrast harmonic
    imaging
PiCO$_2$
  partial pressure of intramuscular carbon
    dioxide
PICP
  carboxyterminal propeptide of type 1
    procollagen
PICS
  Parent Interview for Child Syndrome
  Patterns of Individual Change Scale
PICSES
  pancreatic islet cell-specific enhancer
    sequence
PICSI
  Picture Identification for
    Children-Standardized Index
PICSO
  pressure-controlled intermittent coronary
    sinus occlusion
PICSYMS
  picture symbols
PICT
  pancreatic islet cell transplant(ation)
PICV
  Pichinde virus
PICVA
  percutaneous in situ coronary venous
    arterialization

PICVC
peripherally inserted central venous catheter

PID
pain intensity difference [score]
pelvic inflammatory disease
photoionization detector
plasma iron disappearance
position-indicating device [dentistry]
post-inertia dyskinesia
preimplantation diagnosis
primary immunodeficiency (immune deficiency)
prolapsed intervertebral disc
proportional-integral-derivative
protruded intervertebral disc

PIDDST
pediatric infectious disease developmental screening test

PIDRA
portable insulin dosage-regulating apparatus

PIDS
primary immunodeficiency (immune deficiency) syndrome (*See also* PIS)

PIDT
plasma iron disappearance time

PIE
postinfectious encephalomyelitis (*See also* PIEM)
preimplantation embryo
prosthetic infectious endocarditis
pulmonary infiltrate (infiltration) with eosinophilia
pulmonary interstitial edema (emphysema)

PIEE
pulsed irrigation for enhanced evacuation

PIEF
isoelectric focusing in polyacrylamide (*See also* PAGIF)

PIEM
postinfectious encephalomyelitis (*See also* PIE)

PIES
Picture Interest Exploration Survey

PIEx
posteroinferior external

PIF
peak inspiratory flow
pigment inspiratory factor
point of identical flow
premorbid inferiority feeling
proinsulin-free
prolactin-inhibiting factor
proliferation-inhibiting (inhibitory) factor
prostatic interstitial fluid

PIFG
poor intrauterine fetal growth

PIFR
peak inspiratory flow rate

PIFT
platelet immunofluorescence test

PIG
pertussis immune globulin
phosphate-independent glutaminase
phosphatidylinositol glycan linkage

PIGI
pregnancy-induced glucose intolerance

pigm
pigment(ed)

PIGN
postinfectious glomerulonephritis

PIGPA
pyruvate, inosine, glucose phosphate, adenine

pIgR
polyimmunoglobulin receptor

PIH
pregnancy-induced hypertension
preventricular intraventricular hemorrhage
primary intracerebral hemorrhage
prolactin inhibiting (inhibitory) hormone
pseudointimal hyperplasia

PIHH
postinfluenza-like hyposmia and hypogeusia

PIHI
pulse-inversion harmonic imaging

PII
plasma inorganic iodine
primary irritation index

PIIID
peripheral indwelling intermediate infusion device

PIIn
posteroinferior internal

PIIP
portable insulin infusion pump

PIIS
posterior inferior iliac spine

PI3K
phosphatidylinositol 3′-kinase

PIL
patient information leaflet
primary intestinal lymphangiectasia
purpose in life

PILBD
paucity of interlobular bile ducts

PIM
penicillamine-induced myasthenia
pulse-inversion mode [ultrasound]

P_{Imax}
maximal inspiratory mouth pressure

P

PIMI
predictive index for myocardial infarction

PIMIA
potentiometric ionophore mediated immunoassay

PIMS
programmable implantable medication system

psychological irritable bowel/migraine syndrome

PIN
personal identification number

positive-intrinsic-negative [diode]

posterior interosseous nerve

prostatic intraepithelial neoplasia

PIN-1
prostatic intraepithelial neoplasia, mild dysplasia or low grade

PIN-2
prostatic intraepithelial neoplasia, moderate dysplasia or high grade

PIN-3
prostatic intraepithelial neoplasia, severe dysplasia or high grade

pin1
peptidyl-prolyl isomerase nucleoprotein

PIND
progressive intellectual and neurological deterioration

PINN
proposed international nonproprietary name

PINS
person in need of supervision

progressive inhibition of neuromuscular structures technique

PINV
postimperative negative variation

PIO$_2$
intraalveolar oxygen tension

partial pressure of inspiratory oxygen

PION
posterior interosseous nerve

posterior ischemic optic neuropathy

PIP
paraffin immunoperoxidase

paralytic infantile paralysis

peak inflation pressure

peak inspiratory pressure

personal injury protection

plasma cell interstitial pneumonitis

positive inspiratory pressure

posterior interphalangeal

postictal psychosis

postinflammatory polyposis

postinfusion phlebitis

postinspiratory pressure

pressure inversion point

probable intrauterine pregnancy

prolactin inducible protein

proximal interphalangeal [joint] (*See also* PIPJ)

psychosis, intermittent hyponatremia, polydipsia (syndrome)

Psychotic Inpatient Profile

pulmonary immaturity of prematurity

pulmonary insufficiency of the premature

PIP3
phosphatidylinositol 4,5-triphosphate

PI4P
phosphatidylinositol 4-phosphate

PI4,5P2
phosphatidylinositol 4,5-bisphosphate

PIPA
platelet ^{125}I-labeled [staphylococcal] protein A

PI-PB
performance versus intensity function for phonetically balanced words

PIP/DIP
proximal interphalangeal/distal interphalangeal [joints]

PIPE
persistent interstitial pulmonary emphysema

pharmacologically induced penile erection

PIPES
piperazine diethanesulfonic acid

PIPIDA
para-isopropyl-iminodiacetic acid (paraisopropyliminodiacetic acid) [scan]

PIPIS
Rhode Island Pupil Identification Scale

PIPJ
proximal interphalangeal joint (*See also* PIP)

PIPP
Premature Infant Pain Profile

PIQ
Performance Intelligence Quotient

PIR
piriform (pyriform)

postinhibition rebound

pressure increment rate

P-IRI
plasma immunoreactive insulin

PIRS
plasma immunoreactive secretion

postinfarct risk stratification

PIRYV
Piry virus

PIS
preinfarction syndrome

primary immunodeficiency (immune deficiency) syndrome (*See also* PIDS)

Provisional International Standard
pulmonary intimal sarcoma

PISA
phase-invariant signature algorithm
proximal isovelocity surface area
[echocardiography]

PISCES
percutaneously inserted spinal cord
electrical stimulation

PIT
pacing-induced tachycardia
patella (patellar) inhibition test
peak isometric torque
perceived illness threat
pericranial injection therapy
Picture Identification Test
pin-in-tube
plasma iron turnover
pulsed inotrope therapy

Pit-1
pituitary-specific transcription
factor 1

pit.
pituitary

PITC
phenylisothiocyanate

PITP
pseudoidiopathic thrombocytopenic
purpura

PITR
plasma iron turnover rate

PITS
parent-infant traumatic stress

PIU
polymerase-inducing unit

PI-urea
phosphate ion-urea

PIV
parainfluenza virus (*See also* paraflu,
PF1–PF4, PI, PIV)
peripheral intravenous
polydactyly, imperforate anus, vertebral
anomalies [syndrome]
Puffin Island virus

PIVD
protruded intervertebral disc

PIVH
peripheral intravenous hyperalimentation
periventricular-intraventricular
hemorrhage

PIVKA-II
prothrombin induced by vitamin K
absence or antagonist II

PIVM
passive intervertebral motion

PIVR
pacemaker-induced ventricular rate

PIW
proposed ideal weight

PIWT
partially impacted wisdom teeth

PIXE, PIXIE
particle-induced x-ray emission
proton-induced x-ray emission

pixel
picture element

PIXI
peripheral instantaneous x-ray
imaging

PIXV
Pixuna virus

PJ
pancreatic juice
patellar jerk
porcelain jacket [crown]

PJA
pancreaticojejunostomy anastomosis

PJB
premature junctional beat

PJC
premature junctional contraction

PJI
prosthetic joint infection

PJM
positive joint mobilization

PJP
pancreatic juice protein

PJRT
permanent junctional reciprocating
tachycardia

PJS
peritoneojugular shunt

PJT
paroxysmal junctional tachycardia

PJVT
paroxysmal junctional ventricular
tachycardia

PK
pack [cigarette]
penetrating keratoplasty (*See also*
PKP)
pericardial knock
pharmacokinetic
pig kidney
plasma potassium (*See also* P_K)
Prausnitz-Küstner [antibodies, reaction
test] (*See also* PKT)
protein kinase
psychokinesis (psychokinetic)
pyruvate kinase

P_K
plasma potassium (*See also* PK)

pK
ionization constant of acid

P

pK_a
negative logarithm of acid ionization constant [measure of acid strength]

pk
peck [unit of dry volume]

PKA
prekallikrein activator
prokininogenase
protein kinase A

PKAR
protein kinase activation ratio

PKase
protein kinase

pkat
picokatal

PKB
prone knee bend
protein kinase B

PKC
protein kinase C

PKD
paroxysmal kinesigenic dyskinesia
polycystic kidney disease
proliferative kidney disease
proteinase K digestion

PKDL
post-kala azar dermal leishmaniasis

PKF
phagocytosis and killing function

PKG
protein kinase G

PKI
potato kallikrein inhibitor

PKK
plasma prekallikrein
prekallikrein

PKN
parkinsonism

PKP
penetrating keratoplasty (*See also* PK)

PK/PD
pharmacokinetic/pharmacodynamic

PKPG
penetrating keratoplasty and glaucoma

PKR
phased knee rehabilitation
protein double-stranded RNA-activated

PKRS
Phelps Kindergarten Readiness Scale

PKS
pulmonary Kaposi sarcoma

PKSAP
Psychiatric Knowledge and Skills Self-Assessment Program

PKT
Prausnitz-Küstner test (*See also* PK)

PKU
phenylketonuria

PKV
killed poliomyelitis vaccine

pkV
peak kilovoltage

pkyrs
pack-year of smoking [2 packs a day for 20 years would be 40 pack-years] (*See also* PY, P/Y)

PL
palmaris longus
pancreatic lipase
perception of light
peroneus longus [muscle]
pharyngolaryngectomy
phospholipase
phospholipid (*See also* PPL)
photoluminescence
place
placebo (*See also* OBE-CALP, P, PBO, PCB, PLB, PLBO)
placental lactogen
plantar
plasmalemma
platelet (*See also* plat, PLT)
platelet lactogen
pleural (*See also* PLEU)
polymer of lactic [acid]
posterior lip [of acetabulum]
preferential looking
premalignant lesion
premature labor
problem list
proboscis lateralis
procaine and lactic acid
psychosocial-labile
pulpolingual
Purkinje layer
pyridoxal

P_L
transpulmonary pressure

Pl
plasma (*See also* P)
pleural pressure
Poiseuille [law, space]

pL
picoliter

pl
plural

PLA
peripheral laser angioplasty
peroxidase-labeled antibodies [test]
phospholipase A
platelet antigen
polylactic acid
posterolateral [coronary] artery
potentially lethal arrhythmia
Product License Application
pulpolinguoaxial

PLA2, PLA₂
  phospholipase A2
PLa
  pulpolabial
Pla
  left atrial pressure
PLAD
  proximal left anterior descending
    [artery]
PL-ADOS
  prelinguistic autism diagnostic
    observation
plague
  bubonic plague
PLAI
  Preschool Language Assessment
    Instrument
Plan B
  progestogen emergency contraceptive
PLAP
  placental alkaline phosphatase (*See also*
    PALP, PAP)
  polyclonal antiplacental alkaline
    phosphatase
plat
  platelet (*See also* PL, PLT)
PLAT C
  platelet concentration
PLAT P
  platelet pheresis
PLAV
  Playas virus
PLAX
  parasternal long axis
PLB
  parietal lobe battery [language function
    test]
  percutaneous liver biopsy
  phospholamban
  phospholipase B
  placebo (*See also* OBE-CALP, P, PBO,
    PCB, PL, PLBO)
  porous layer bead
  posterolateral branch
  primary [non-Hodgkin] lymphoma of
    bone
PLBO
  placebo (*See also* OBE-CALP, P, PBO,
    PCB, PL, PLB)
PLC
  peripheral lymphocyte (leukocyte) count
  personal locus of control
  phospholipase C
  pityriasis lichenoides chronica
  pleomorphic lobular carcinoma
  primary liver cell
  proinsulinlike component

protein-lipid complex
  pseudolymphocytic choriomeningitis
PLCC
  primary liver cell cancer
PLCH
  pulmonary Langerhans cell histiocytosis
PLCIS
  pleomorphic lobular carcinoma in situ
    [breast]
PLCL
  polyclonal gammopathy identified
PL-CLP
  platelet clump
PLCO
  postoperative low cardiac output
PLD
  partial lower denture
  percutaneous laser discectomy
  peripheral light detection
  phospholipase D
  platelet defect
  polycystic liver disease (*See also* PCLD)
  posterior latissimus dorsi [muscle]
  postlaser day
  potentially lethal damage
  pregnancy, labor, delivery
PLDD
  percutaneous laser disc decompression
  poorly differentiated lymphoma, diffuse
PLDH
  plasma lactic dehydrogenase
PLDR
  potentially lethal damage repair
PLE
  panlobular emphysema
  paraneoplastic limbic encephalopathy
  pleura [singular] (pleurae [plural])
  polymorphous light eruption (*See also*
    PMLE)
  protein-losing enteropathy
  pseudolupus erythematosus [syndrome]
PLED
  periodic lateralizing epileptiform
    discharge
PLES
  parallel line equal spacing
PLET
  polymyxin, lysozyme, EDTA, and
    thallous acetate [heart infusion agar]
PLEU
  pleural (*See also* PL)
PLEVA
  pityriasis lichenoides et varioliformis
    acuta
PLF
  perilymphatic fistula
  prior level of function

P

PLFC
premature living female child
PLFD
perilunate fracture-dislocation
PLFS
perilymphatic fistula syndrome
PLG
photoablative laser goniotomy
plague [*Yersinia pestis*] [la Peste]
vaccine
plasminogen
PLGA
polymorphous low-grade
adenocarcinoma
PlGF
placental growth factor
P-LGV
psittacosis lymphogranuloma venereum
PLH
paroxysmal localized hyperhidrosis
placental lactogenic hormone
pulmonary lymphoid hyperplasia
PLHB
percutaneous left heart bypass
PLIC
posterior limb of internal capsule
PLIF
posterior lumbar interbody fusion
posterolateral interbody fusion
PLIL
partial laryngectomy with imbrication
laryngoplasty
PLISSIT
permission, limited information, specific
suggestions, intensive therapy
PLK
pololike kinase
PLL
peripheral light loss
poly-L-lysine
posterior longitudinal ligament
pressure length loop
prolymphocytic leukemia
PLLA
poly-L-lactic acid
PLM
partial lateral meniscectomy
percent(age) of labeled mitoses
periodic leg (limb) movement
plasma level monitoring
polarized light microscopy (microscope)
precise lesion measuring
PLMC
premature living male child
PLMD
periodic leg (limb) movement disorder
PLMS
periodic leg (limb) movements during
sleep

PLMT
plasmacytoid lymphocyte
PLMV
posterior leaf mitral valve
PLN
pelvic lymph node
peripheral lymph node
popliteal lymph node
posterior lip nerve
PLNA
percutaneous lung needle aspiration
PLND
pelvic lymph node dissection
PLNR
perilobar nephrogenic rest
PLO
pluronic lecithin organogels
polycystic lipomembranous
osteodysplasia
PLOF
previous level of functioning
PLOM
papillomatosis of lips and oral
mucosa
PLOP
partial laryngopharyngectomy
PLOSA
physiologic low stress angioplasty
PLP
paraformaldehyde-lysine-periodate
parathyroid hormonelike protein
partial laryngopharyngectomy
phantom limb pain
pharyngolaryngeal paralysis
plasma leukapheresis
polystyrene latex particle
proteolipid protein
pyridoxal phosphate (pyridoxal
5'-phosphate)
PLPD
pseudoperiodic lateralized paroxysmal
discharge
PLPH
postlumbar puncture headache
PLR
persistent reactivity to light
pronation-lateral rotation [fracture]
pupillary light reflex
PLS
plastic leaf spring
plastic surgery (*See also* PLSURG, PS,
PSurg, P-surg)
point locator stimulator
preleukemic syndrome
Preschool Language Scale
primary lateral sclerosis
prostaglandin-like substance
pls
please

PLSA
　posterolateral spinal artery
PLSD
　protected least significant difference
　　[statistics]
PLSI
　Psoriasis Life Stress Inventory
PLSO
　posterior leaf spring orthosis
PLST
　progressively lowered stress threshold
PLSURG
　plastic surgery (*See also* PLS, PS,
　　PSurg, P-surg)
PLSV
　Palestina virus
PLT
　pancreatic lymphocytic infiltration
　peroneus longus tendinopathy
　platelet (*See also* PL, plat)
　primed lymphocyte test
　primed lymphocyte typing
　psittacosis, lymphogranuloma venereum,
　　trachoma
PLT EST
　platelet estimate
PLTF
　plaintiff
PLT-G
　giant platelet
PLTSS
　Pediatric Liver Transplant-Specific Scale
PLUG
　plug the lung until it grows [procedure]
plumb.
　lead [L. *plumbum*] (*See also* Pb)
PLUT
　Plutchnik [geriatric rating scale]
PLV
　panleukopenia virus
　partial liquid ventilation
　poliomyelitis live vaccine
　posterior left ventricular
plx
　plexus
PLYM
　prolymphocyte
PLYO
　plyometric
PLZF
　promyelocytic leukemia zinc finger
　　[protein]
PM
　after death [L. *post martem*]
　afternoon (evening) [L. *post meridiem*]
　　(*See also* p.m.)
　pacemaker

pagetoid melanocytosis
papillae mammae
papillary muscle
papular mucinosis
paraspinal mapping
partially muscular
partial meniscectomy
particulate matter
pectoralis major
perinatal mortality (morbidity)
periodontal membrane
peritoneal macrophage
petit mal [epilepsy]
photomultiplier
physical medicine
plasma membrane
platelet membrane
platelet microsome
pneumomediastinum
poliomyelitis (*See also* polio)
polymorphic
polymorphonuclear (*See also* PMN,
　poly)
polymyositis
poor metabolizer
porokeratosis of Mibelli
posterior mitral
postmenopausal
post meridiem [afternoon]
postmortem (*See also* post, post.)
premamillary nucleus
premolar
presents mainly
presystolic murmur
pretibial myxedema
preventive medicine (*See also* PRM,
　PrM, PVMed)
primary motivation
prostatic massage
protein methylesterase
psammomatous meningioma
pterygoid muscle
puberal macromastia
pulmonary macrophage
pulpomesial
PM I
　paternal meiosis I
PM II
　paternal meiosis II
PM10
　particulate matter less than 10
　　micrometers diameter
P:M
　parent to metabolite ratio
Pm
　promethium
　Plasmodium malariae

P

pM
    picomolar
p.m.
    afternoon [L. *post meridiem*] (*See also*
    PM)
pm
    picometer
PMA
    papillary, marginal, attached [gingiva]
    para-methoxyamphetamine
    peroneal muscular atrophy
    phenylmercuric acetate
    phorbolmyristate acetate (phorbol
      myristate acetate)
    phosphomolybdic acid
    positive mental attitude
    premenstrual asthma
    premenstrual exacerbation of asthma
    primary meningococcal arthritis
    primary mental abilities
    Prinzmetal angina
    progressive muscular atrophy
    progressive myoclonic ataxia
    psychomotor agitation
    pyridylmercuric acetate
PMAA
    Premarket Approval Application
    [medical devices FDA]
PMAC
    phenylmercuric acetate
Pmaip1
    phorbol-12-myristate-13-acetate-induced
      protein 1
PMAT
    Primary Mental Abilities Test
PMB
    papillomacular bundle
    para-hydroxymercuribenzoate
    polychrome methylene blue [stain]
    polymorphonuclear basophil
    postmenopausal bleeding
PMBC
    percutaneous mitral balloon
      commissurotomy
PMBV
    percutaneous mitral balloon valvotomy
      (valvuloplasty)
PMC
    papillary microcarcinoma
    percutaneous mitral commissurotomy
    peripheral multifocal chorioretinitis
    peritoneal mucinous carcinoma
    phenylmercuric chloride
    pleural mesothelial cell
    pontine micturition center
    premature mitral closure
    premotor cortex
    primary motor cortex
    pseudomembranous colitis

PMCP
    para-monochlorophenol
    perinatal mortality counseling program
PMCT
    percutaneous microwave coagulation
      therapy
    postmortem computed tomography
PMD
    papillary muscle dysfunction
    perceptual motor development
    piecemeal degranulation
    posterior mandibular depth
    primary myocardial disease
    private medical doctor
    programmed multiple development
    progressive muscular dystrophy
PMDD
    premenstrual dysphoric disorder
pMDI
    pressurized metered-dose inhaler
PM-DM, PM/DM
    polymyositis-dermatomyositis (*See also*
      PDM)
PMDS
    persistent müllerian duct syndrome
    premenstrual dysphoric syndrome
    primary myelodysplastic syndrome
PME
    peak of maximum enhancement
    pelvic muscle exercise
    phosphomonoester
    polymorphonuclear eosinophil
    postmenopausal estrogen
    progressive myoclonus epilepsy
PMEALS
    post [after] meals
PMEC
    pseudomembranous enterocolitis
PMEOAT
    Photo-Mask-and Etch-on-a-Tube
PMF, pmf
    peptide mass fingerprinting
    progressive massive fibrosis
    proton motive force
    pterygomaxillary fossa
    pupils mid-position, fixed
PMFBW
    paramedian frontal bone window
PMGCT
    primary malignant giant-cell tumor
    primary mediastinal germ-cell tumor
PMH
    past medical history (*See also* PMHx)
    posteromedial hypothalamus
    postmenopausal hormone
    programmed medical history
    pure motor hemiparesis
PMHR
    predicted maximal heart rate

PMHx
  past medical history (*See also* PMH)
PMI
  Pain Management Index
  past medical illness
  patient medical (medicine) (medication) instruction
  perioperative myocardial infarct(ion)
  petition of mental illness
  phosphomannose isomerase
  plea of mental incompetence
  point of maximal (maximum) impulse (intensity)
  posterior myocardial infarct(ion)
  postmortem interval
  postmyocardial infarct(ion)
  present medical illness
  previous medical illness
PMID
  painful minor intervertebral dysfunction
  PubMED Unique Identifier [National Library of Medicine]
PMIS
  postmyocardial infarction syndrome
PMJ
  progressive multifocal leuko-J encephalopathy
PMK
  pacemaker
  primary monkey kidney
PML
  peripheral motor latency
  polymorphonuclear leukocyte (*See also* PMN, PMNL, POLY, poly)
  posterior mitral leaflet (*See also* pML)
  premature labor
  progressive multifocal leukodystrophy
  progressive multifocal leukoencephalopathy
  prolapsing mitral leaflet
  promyelocytic leukemia
  pulmonary microlithiasis
pML
  posterior mitral leaflet (*See also* PML)
PMLCL
  primary mediastinal large-cell lymphoma
PMLE
  polymorphous light eruption (*See also* PLE)
PMLS
  primary mediastinal large cell lymphoma with sclerosis
PMM
  perilacunar mineral matrix
  protoplast maintenance medium

PMMA
  polymethyl methacrylate (polymethylmethacrylate)
PMME
  primary malignant melanoma of esophagus
PMMF
  pectoralis major myocutaneous flap
PMN
  polymodal nociceptor
  polymorphonuclear
  polymorphonuclear [leukocyte neutrophil] (*See also* POLY, poly)
  Premarket Notification [medical devices FDA]
PMNC
  percent(age) of multinucleated cells
  peripheral [blood] mononuclear cell
PMNG
  polymorphonuclear granulocyte
PMNL
  polymorphonuclear leukocyte (*See also* PML, PMN, POLY, poly)
PMNN
  polymorphonuclear neutrophil
PMNR
  periadenitis mucosa necrotica recurrens
PMNS
  postmalarial neurological syndrome
PMO
  postmenopausal osteoporosis
pmol
  picomole
PMP
  pain management program
  past menstrual period
  patient management problem
  patient medication profile
  peripheral myelin protein
  persistent mentum posterior (mentoposterior) [fetal position]
  previous menstrual period
  psychotropic medication plan
PMP22
  peripheral myelin protein 22
PMPM
  per member per month
PMPO
  postmenopausal palpable ovary
PMPS
  postmastectomy pain syndrome
PMPY
  per member per year
PMQ
  phytylmenaquinone [vitamin K1]

P

PMR
pacemaker rhythm
papillary muscle rupture
percutaneous (trans)myocardial revascularization
perinatal morbidity (mortality) rate
periodic medical review
physical medicine and rehabilitation
polymorphic reticulosis
polymyalgia rheumatica
posteromedial release
premedication regimen
prior medical record
progressive muscle relaxation
proportional (proportionate) morbidity (mortality) ratio
proton magnetic resonance
psychomotor retardation

PM&R
physical medicine and rehabilitation

PMRA
pulmonary magnetic resonance angiography

PMRB
postmenopausal recurrent bleeding

PMRP
portable monitor of respiratory parameters

31P-MRS
phosphorus-31 magnetic resonance spectroscopy

PMRT
postmastectomy radiation therapy

PMRV
Paramushir virus

PMS
patient management system
pectoralis major syndrome
performance measurement system
perimenstrual syndrome
periodic movements [during, of] sleep
peripheral muscle strength
poor miserable soul
postmarketing surveillance [FDA CDER]
postmenopausal syndrome
postmenstrual stress
postmitochondrial supernatant
pregnant mare serum
premenstrual syndrome
progressive multiple sclerosis
psychotic motor syndrome
pulse, motor, sensory
pureed, mechanical, soft [diet]

PMSC
pluripotent(ial) myeloid stem cell

PM-Scl
polymyositis-scleroderma

PMSG
pregnant mare serum gonadotropin

PMT
pacemaker-mediated (modulated) tachycardia
percutaneous mechanical thrombectomy
photoelectric multiplier tube
photomultiplier tube
point of maximum tenderness
Porteus maze test
postmenstrual tension
premenstrual tension
pseudosarcomatous myofibroblastic tumor

PMTH
premenstrual tension headache

PMTS
premenstrual tension syndrome

PMTT
pulmonary mean transit time

PMV
paralyzed and mechanically ventilated
Passy-Muir valve
percutaneous mitral valvuloplasty (valvotomy)
prolapsed (prolapse of) mitral valve

PMV 1–9
avian paramyxovirus virus 1–9

PmvCO$_2$
partial pressure of mesenteric venous carbon dioxide

PMVL
polymorphic ventricular tachycardia
posterior mitral valve leaflet

PMVP
pulmonary microvascular permeability to protein

PMW
pacemaker wire
progressive muscle weakness
proximal muscle wasting

PMZ
postmenopausal zest

PN
nightmare [L. *pavor nocturnus*]
papillary necrosis
parenteral nutrition
perceived noise
percussion note
percutaneous nephrosonogram (nephrostogram)
percutaneous nucleotomy
periarteritis nodosa (*See also* PAN)
peripheral nerve
peripheral neuropathy (*See also* PNP)
peripheral node
phrenic nerve
plaque neutralization
pneumonia (*See also* pneu, PNM)
polyarteritis nodosa (*See also* PAN)
polyneuritis

pontine nucleus
poorly nourished
positional nystagmus
posterior nares
postnasal
postnatal
predicted normal
premie nipple
progress note
pronucleus
psychiatry-neurology
psychoneurology
psychoneurotic
pyelonephritis
pyridine nucleotide
pyrrolnitrin
P&N
pins and needles
psychiatry and neurology
P:N
positive to negative ratio
pN0
no regional lymph node metastases
histologically [TNM pathology
classification]
pN1–pN3
increasing involvement of regional
lymph nodes histologically [TNM
pathology classification]
PN$_2$, P$_{N2}$, P$_{n2}$
nitrogen partial pressure
partial pressure of nitrogen
PNA
Paris Nomina Anatomica
peanut agglutinin
pentose nucleic acid
peptide nucleic acid
perinatal assessment
polynitroxyl albumin
P$_{Na}$
plasma sodium
PNAB
percutaneous needle aspiration biopsy
PNAC
parenteral nutrition-associated cholestatic
PNAD
pigmented nodular adrenocortical
disease
PNAH
polynuclear aromatic hydrocarbon
(*See also* PAH)
PNAR
perennial nonallergic rhinitis
PNAS
prudent no-salt-added [diet]
PNAvQ
positive-negative ambivalent quotient

PNB
percutaneous needle biopsy
popliteal nerve block
premature newborn
premature nodal beat
prostatic needle biopsy
PNBT
para-nitroblue tetrazolium
PNC
paranasal cancer
peripheral nerve conduction
peripheral nucleated cell
pneumotaxic center
postnecrotic cirrhosis
premature nodal contraction
prenatal care (course)
purine nucleotide cycle
PNCS
primary neuroendocrine carcinoma of
skin
PnCV
nonvalent pneumococcal conjugate
vaccine
PND
paroxysmal nocturnal dyspnea
partial neck dissection
pelvic node dissection
postnasal drainage (drip)
postnatal depression
postneonatal death
pregnancy, not delivered
purulent nasal drainage
PNdB
perceived noise level
PND-Rh
postnasal drainage (drip) due to
rhinitis
PNDS
postnasal drainage (drip) syndrome
PND-Si
postnasal drainage (drip) due to
sinusitis
PNE
percutaneous nerve evaluation
peripheral nerve evaluation
peripheral neuroepithelioma
plasma norepinephrine
pneumoencephalography
primary nocturnal enuresis
pseudomembranous necrotizing
enterocolitis
PNEC
pulmonary neuroendocrine cell
PNEE
pulmonary neuroepithelial endocrine
PNEM
paraneoplastic encephalomyelitis

PNET
peripheral neuroectodermal tumor
primary neuroectodermal tumor
primitive neuroectodermal tumor

PNET-MB
primitive neuroectodermal
tumor-medulloblastoma

pneu
pneumonia (*See also* PN, PNM)

PNEUMO
pneumothorax (*See also* pnthx, pnx, PT,
PTX, Px)

PNF
prenatal fluoride
primary nonfunction
proprioceptive neuromuscular facilitation
[flexibility training]

PNFA
progressive nonfluent aphasia

PNG
pneumogram

PNH
paroxysmal nocturnal hemoglobinuria
polynitroxyl-hemoglobin

PNI
perineural invasion
peripheral nerve injury
postnatal infection
prognostic nutritional index
pseudoneointimal
psychoneuroimmunology

PNID
Peer Nomination Inventory for
Depression

PNIF
peak nasal inspiratory flow

PNK
polynucleotide kinase

PNKD
paroxysmal nonkinesigenic
dyskinesia

PNL
percutaneous nephrolithotomy
(nephrostolithotomy) (*See also* PCNL)
peripheral nerve lesion
polymorphonuclear neutrophilic
leukocyte
posterior nipple line [mammography]

PNLA
percutaneous needle lung aspiration

PNLB
percutaneous needle liver biopsy

PNM
perinatal mortality (morbidity)
peripheral dysostosis, nail hypoplasia,
mental retardation
peripheral nerve myelin
pneumonia (*See also* PN, pneu)
postneonatal mortality [syndrome]

PNMA
progressive neuromuscular atrophy

PNMG
persistent neonatal myasthenia gravis

PNMR
perinatal mortality rate

PNMT
phenylethanolamine N-methyltransferase

PNN
probabilistic neural network

PNP
paraneoplastic pemphigus
para-nitrophenol
peak negative pressure
peripheral neuropathy (*See also* PN)
platelet neutralization procedure
polyneuropathy
polynucleoside phosphorylase
progressive nuclear palsy
psychogenic nocturnal polydipsia
purine nucleoside phosphorylase

PNPase
purine nucleoside phosphorylase

PNPB
positive-negative pressure breathing

PNPG
p-nitrophenylglycerol
para-nitrophenyl beta (β) galactoside

pNPP, *p*NPP
para-nitrophenylphosphate

PNPR
positive-negative pressure respiration

PNPS
para-nitrophenylsulfate

PNR
perineural fibroma
physician's nutritional recommendation

PNRB
partial nonrebreather [oxygen mask]

PNS
paraneoplastic syndrome
parasympathetic nervous system
(*See also* parasym, PS, PSNS)
paretic neurosyphilis
partial nonprogressive stroke
peripheral nervous stimulator
peripheral nervous system
posterior nasal spine

PNSH
perimesencephalic nonaneurysmal
subarachnoid hemorrhage

PNSP
penicillin-nonsusceptible *Streptococcus
pneumoniae*
posterior nasal spine to soft palate
[soft palate length]

PNSS
Pediatric Nutrition Surveillance
System

PNST
peripheral nerve sheath tumor
PNT
paroxysmal nodal tachycardia
partial nodular transformation
percutaneous nephrostomy tube
percutaneous neuromodulatory therapy
pnthx
pneumothorax (*See also* PNEUMO, pnx,
PT, PTX, Px)
PNTML
pudendal-nerve terminal motor latency
PNU
pneumococcal [*Streptococcus
pneumoniae*] vaccine, not otherwise
specified
protein nitrogen unit
PNUcn
pneumococcal [*Streptococcus
pneumoniae*] conjugate vaccine
PNUps
pneumococcal [*Streptococcus
pneumoniae*] polysaccharide
[vaccine]
PNV
postoperative nausea and vomiting
prenatal vitamins
pNX
regional lymph nodes cannot be
assessed histologically [TNM
pathology classification]
pnx
pneumonectomy
pneumothorax (*See also* PNEUMO,
pnthx, pnx, PT, PTX, Px)
PNZ
posterior necrotic zone
PO
by mouth [L. *per os*] (*See also* p.o., m,
(m), per os]
parapineal organ
parietal operculum
parietooccipital
perceptual organization
period of onset
perioperative
periosteum
per os
phone order
physician only
posterior
postoperative(ly) (*See also* POP, postop,
post-op)
predominating organism
prophylactic oophorectomy
pulse oximeter (oximetry)
punctal occlusion

P:O
oxidative phosphorylation ratio
protein to osmolar ratio
ratio of number of ATPs produced to
number of atmospheric oxygen
molecules converted to water
[glycolysis]
P&O
parasites and ova
prosthesis and orthosis
prosthetic and orthotic
PO$_2$, P$_{O2}$, P$_{o2}$
partial pressure of oxygen
pressure of oxygen
PO$_4$
phosphate
Po
opening pressure
Plasmodium ovale
polonium
porion [craniometric]
poise [CGS unit of dynamic viscosity]
(*See also* P, Ps)
p.o.
by mouth, orally [L. *per os*] (*See also*
m, (m), per os, PO)
POA
pancreatic oncofetal antigen
phalangeal osteoarthritis
point of application
power of attorney
preoptic area [of hypothalamus]
present on arrival
primary optic atrophy
POAD
peripheral occlusive arterial disease
POADS
postaxial acrofacial dysostosis syndrome
POAG
primary open-angle glaucoma
POAH
posterior occipitoatlantal hypermobility
POA-HA
preoptic anterior hypothalamic area
POB
place of birth
POBA
plain old balloon angioplasty
POBC
primary operable breast cancer
POBE
Profile of Out-of-Body Experiences
POBS
passage of bloody stool
POC
particulate organic carbon
plan of care

P

POC *(continued)*
point of care
polyolefin copolymer
position of comfort
postoperative care
postoperative check
presurgical orthopedic correction
products of conception
proximal occlusion catheter
POCAAN
People of Color Against AIDS Network
Po/C
ocular pressure
POCD
postoperative cognitive dysfunction
POCI
posterior circulation infarct
POCS
posterior circulation syndrome
POCT
point-of-care testing (therapy)
POCY
postoperative chronologic year
POD
pacing on demand
peroxidase
place of death
podiatry
polycystic ovary (ovarian) disease
(*See also* PCOD)
postoperative day
postovulatory day
pouch of Douglas
POD1
first postoperative day (day 1)
POD2
second postoperative day (day 2)
PODCO
power-oriented depth controlled
osteotomy cutter
PODQ
Perceptual Organization Deviation
Quotient
PODS
passage of dark stool
PODVT
postoperative deep venous
thrombosis
PODx
preoperative diagnosis
POE
patient-oriented evidence
pediatric orthopedic examination
periorbital edema
point of entry
port of entry
position of ease
postoperative endophthalmitis
postoperative exercise

prone on elbows [position]
proof of eligibility
provider order entry
POEMS
polyneuropathy, organomegaly,
endocrinopathy, M protein, and skin
lesions [syndrome]
POEMs
Patient-Oriented Evidence that
Matters
POES
polyoxyethylene stearate [pesticide]
POET
pulse oximeter/end tidal [carbon
dioxide]
POEx
point of exit (*See also* POX)
postoperative exercise
POF
physician's order form
position of function
premature ovarian failure
primary ovarian failure
pyruvate oxidation factor
POFO
passage of foreign object
POG
polymyositis ossificans generalisata
products of gestation
POGO
percent(age) of glottic opening
POGTD
primary ovarian gestational trophoblastic
disease
POH
past ocular history
perillyl alcohol
personal oral hygiene
postoperative hemorrhage
presumed ocular histoplasmosis
progressive osseous heteroplasia
prone on hands [position]
pOH
negative logarithm of hydroxide ion
concentration
hydroxyl permeability
POHI
physically or otherwise health-impaired
⚠ **POHS**
by mouth at bedtime ⚠
presumed (pseudo) ocular histoplasmosis
syndrome
POI
Personal Orientation Inventory
point of insertion
postoperative ileus
postoperative instructions
POIB
place outpatient in inpatient bed

POIK, poik
poikilocyte
poikilocytosis

point-EXACCT
point mutation detection using exonuclease amplification couple capture technique [for mutation detection]

pois
poison(ing) (poisoned) (*See also* P)

POL
physician's office laboratory
poliovirus vaccine, not otherwise specified
posterior oblique ligament
premature onset of labor

pol
polish(ing)

POLAR
posterior oblique lumbar arthrodesis

polio
poliomyelitis (*See also* PM)

POLIP
polyneuropathy, ophthalmoplegia, leukoencephalopathy, intestinal pseudoobstruction

poll.
pollicis

POLPSA
posterior labrocapsular periosteal sleeve avulsion

POLS
passage of light stool
postoperative length of stay

POLY
polychromic erythrocyte
polymorphonuclear neutrophilic leukocyte (*See also* PML, PMN, PMNL, poly)

poly
polydipsia
polyhydramnios
polymorphonuclear neutrophilic leukocyte (*See also* PML, PMN, PMNL, POLY)
polyphagia
polyuria

poly-A
polyadenylic acid

poly-C
polycytidylic acid

POLY-CHR
polychromatophilia

poly-G
polyguanylic acid

poly-HEMA
poly-(2-hydroxyethyl methacrylate)

poly-I
polyinosinic acid

poly-LC
copolymer of polyinosinic and polycytidylic acids

% POLYS
percent(age) of polymorphonuclear leukocytes

poly-T
polythymidylic acid

polytef
polytetrafluoroethylene (*See also* PTFE)

poly-U
polyuridylic acid

POM
pain on motion
peripheral osteoma of mandible
prescription-only medicine
pulse oximetry monitoring
purulent otitis media

POMA
Performance-Oriented Mobility Assessment

POMC
proopiomelanocortin

POMES
prospective outcomes monitoring evaluation system

POMP
phase-offset multiplanar [imaging]
phase-ordered multiplanar [imaging]
principal outer material protein

POMR
problem-oriented medical record (*See also* POR)

POMS
Profile of Mood States

POMS-FI
Profile of Mood States, Fatigue-Inertia [subscale]

PON
paraxonase
particulate organic nitrogen
postoperative note

PONI
postoperative narcotic infusion

PONS
Profile of Nonverbal Sensitivity

PONV
postoperative nausea and vomiting

POO
prostatic outlet obstruction

POOH
postoperative open heart [surgery]

POOL
premature onset of labor

P

POP
diphosphate group
pain on palpation
paroxypropione
posterior collateral ligament
(PCL)-oriented placement
persistent occipat posterior
(occipitoposterior) [fetal position]
persistent organic pollutant
pituitary opioid peptide
plasma oncotic pressure
plasma osmotic pressure
plaster of Paris (*See also* PP)
polymyositis ossificans progressiva
popliteal (*See also* poplit)
posterior oropharynx
postoperative(ly) (*See also* PO, postop,
post-op)
progestin-only pill

Pop.
population (*See also* P)

POPC
Pediatric Overall Performance Category
[scale]

poplit
popliteal (*See also* POP)

POPP
psoriatic onychopachydermoperiostitis

POP-Q
Pelvic Organ Prolapse-Quantified system

POPS
peroral pancreatoscopy

POR
physician of record
postocclusive oscillatory response
problem-oriented [medical] record
(*See also* POMR)

PORD
posterior reduction device

PORH
postocclusive reactive hyperemia
postoperative reactive hyperemia

PORN
progressive outer retinal necrosis

PORP
partial ossicular reconstruction
(replacement) prosthesis
prosthetic ossicular reconstruction
procedure

porph
porphyrin (*See also* P)

PORT
Perception of Relationships Test
perioperative respiratory therapy
postoperative radiation therapy
(radiotherapy)
postoperative respiratory therapy

port
portable

POS
paraosteal osteosarcoma
physician's order sheet
point of service
polycystic ovary (ovarian) syndrome
(*See also* PCOS)
positive (*See also* P, pos)
psychoorganic syndrome

pos
position (*See also* P)
positive (*See also* P, POS)

POSC
problem-oriented system (of) charting

POSIT
Problem-Oriented Screening Instrument
for Teenagers

POSM
patient-operated selector mechanism
plasma osmolality

pos pr
positive pressure (*See also* PP)

POSS
percutaneous on-surface stimulation
proximal over-shoulder strap

poss
possible

POST
peritoneal oocyte and sperm transfer
Police Officer Selection Test

post, post.
posterior (*See also* P, PO)
postmortem (*See also* PM)

PostC
posterior chamber

POST-CABG
post coronary artery bypass graft

PostCap
posterior capsule

postgangl
postganglionic

Post-M
post [after] prostate massage urine
specimen

postop, post-op
postoperative(ly) (*See also* PO, POP)

post prand.
post [after] dinner [L. *post prandium*]

POSTS
positive occipital sharp transients of
sleep

post sag D
posterior sagittal diameter

post tib
posterial tibial

PostVD
posterior vitreous detachment

POSYC
Pain Observation Scale for Young
Children

POT
  peak occupancy time
  periostitis ossificans toxica
  plans of treatment
  postoperative treatment
  primary orthostatic tumor
pot
  marijuana (*See also* MJ)
pot.
  a drink [L. *potus*]
  potash
  potential (*See also* poten)
  potion
PotAGT
  potential abnormality of glucose
    tolerance
Potass
  potassium (*See also* K, kal)
poten
  potential (*See also* pot.)
POTF
  preocular tear film
POTS
  postural orthostatic tachycardia
    syndrome
POU
  placenta, ovary, uterus
POV
  privately owned vehicle
PoV
  portal vein
POVT
  pelvic ovarian vein thrombosis
  puerperal ovarian vein thrombophlebitis
  puerperal ovarian vein thrombosis
POW
  Powassan [encephalitis]
  prisoner of war
powd
  powder (*See also* pdr, pwd)
POWSBP
  pulse oximetry waveform systolic blood
    pressure
POWV
  Powassan virus
POX
  point of exit (*See also* POEx)
  pulse oximeter (oximetry)
POZ
  posterior optical zone
P-P
  probability-probability [plots]
PP
  diphosphate group
  near point of accommodation [L.
    punctum proximum] (*See also* P, p.p.)
  pacesetter potential (*See also* PSP)

palmoplantar
pancreatic polypeptide
pancreatic pseudocyst
paradoxic pulse (pulsus paradoxus)
parietal pericardium
parietal pleura
partial pressure (*See also* P, p)
partial upper and lower dentures
pathology point
pedal pulse
pellagra preventive [niacin]
pentose pathway
perfusion pressure
periodontal pocket
peripheral pulse
peritoneal pseudomyxoma
permanent partial
per protocol
persisting proteinuria
Peyer patch
phosphorylase phosphatase
photoplethysmography
pink puffer (sign of emphysema)
pinpoint
pinprick
placental protein
plane polarization
Planned Parenthood
plasma pepsinogen
plasmapheresis
plasma protein
plaster of Paris (*See also* POP)
polypeptide
polyphosphate
polystyrene agglutination plate
poor person
population planning
porcine pancreatic
positive pressure (*See also* pos pr)
posterior papillary
posterior pituitary
postpartum
postpill (amenorrhea)
postprandial (*See also* $\overline{pp}$, PPD)
precocious pubarche
preferred provider
presenting part
private patient
private practice
prophylactics
prothrombin-proconvertin (*See also* PTP)
protoporphyria
proximal phalanx
pseudomyxoma peritonei
pterygoid process
pulmonary pressure
pulse pressure

P

PP (*continued*)
>pulsus paradoxus (paradoxic pulse)
>punctum proximum [near point of accomodation] (*See also* p.p.)
>purulent pericarditis
>push pills
>pyrophosphate (*See also* PYP, Pyro)

PP₁
>free pyrophosphate

PP I–X
>protoporphyrin [1–10]

PIIIP
>procollagen type 3 aminoterminal peptide

PP5
>placental protein 5

³²P
>phosphorus 32

P&P
>pins and plaster
>policy and procedure
>prothrombin and proconvertin (test)

p.p.
>punctum proximum [near point of accommodation] (*See also* PP)

p̄p̄
>after meals [L. *post prandial*] (*See also* pp, post prand.)

PPA
>palpation, percussion, auscultation (*See also* PP&A, pp&a)
>pelvic phased-array coil
>pepsin A
>phenylpyruvic acid
>Pittsburgh pneumonia agent
>plasmid pattern analysis
>polyphosphoric acid
>postpartum amenorrhea
>postpill amenorrhea
>primary progressive aphasia
>primary pulmonary adenoma
>pure pulmonary atresia
>pyrophosphate arthritis-pseudogout

PP&A, pp&a
>palpation, percussion, and auscultation (*See also* PPA)

Ppa
>pulmonary artery (arterial) (*See also* PA)

PPACK
>D-Phe-L-Pro-L-Arg-chloromethyl ketone (D-phenylalanyl-L-prolyl-L-arginine-chloromethyl ketone)

PPAF
>progressive perivenular alcoholic fibrosis

PPAR
>peroxisome proliferator-activated receptor

PPAR-alpha (α)
>peroxisome proliferator activated receptor alpha (α)

PPAR-delta (δ)
>peroxisome proliferator activated receptor delta (δ)

PPAR-gamma (γ)
>peroxisome-proliferator-activated receptor gamma (γ)

PPAR-gamma 2 (γ2)
>peroxisome proliferator activated receptor gamma (γ2)

PPAS
>peripheral pulmonary artery stenosis
>postpolio atrophy syndrome

Ppaw
>pulmonary artery wedge pressure (*See also* PAWP)

PPB, ppb
>part per billion
>platelet-poor blood
>pleuropulmonary blastoma
>pneumococcal pneumonia and bacteremia
>positive pressure breathing
>prepatellar bursitis
>prostate puncture biopsy

PPBE
>postpartum breast engorgement
>proteose-peptone beef extract

PPBS
>postprandial blood sugar

PPBTL
>postpartum bilateral tubal ligation

PPBV
>Phnom Penh bat virus

PPC
>pelvic and periaortic control
>pentose phosphate cycle
>peripheral posterior curve
>Personal Problems Checklist
>plasma prothrombin conversion
>plaster of Paris cast
>pneumopericardium
>pooled platelet concentrate
>positive peritoneal cytology
>posterior peripheral curve
>primary peritoneal carcinoma
>progressive patient care
>prostatic pressure coefficient
>proximal palmar crease
>pseudopurulent conjunctivitis

PP&C
>prefabricated post and core [prosthetic dentistry]

PPCA
>percent peripheral ciliary activity
>proserum prothrombin conversion accelerator [factor VIII]

PPC-A
>Personal Problems Checklist for Adolescents

PPCD
> posterior polymorphous corneal dystrophy

PPCF
> peripartum cardiac failure
> plasmin prothrombin conversion factor [factor V]

PPCH
> piperazinylmethyl cyclohexanone

PPCID
> pneumatic peripheral circulation improvement device

PPCM
> postpartum cardiomyopathy

PPCP
> Parent Perception of Child Profile

PPD
> packs per day [cigarettes] (See also P/D, p/d)
> paraphenylenediamine
> percussion and postural drainage (See also P and PD, P&PD)
> permanent partial disability
> photodynamic diagnosis
> pinch-point density
> posterior polymorphous dystrophy
> postpartum day
> postpartum depression
> postprandial (See also PP, $\overline{pp}$)
> primary peritoneal drainage
> primary physical dependence
> probing pocket depth [dental]
> progressive perceptive deafness
> progressive pulmonary dystrophy
> purified protein derivative [tuberculin, test]
> pylorus-sparing pancreaticoduodenectomy

P and PD, P&PD
> percussion and postural drainage (See also PPD)

ppd
> prepared (See also prepd, prepped)

PPDA
> paraphenylenediamine

PPD-B
> purified protein derivative–Battey

pp'-DDE
> pp'-dichlorodiphenyldichloroethane

PPDR
> preproliferative diabetic retinopathy

PPD-S
> purified protein derivative–standard

PPDS
> phonologic programming deficit syndrome

PPE
> palmoplantar erythrodysesthesia
> partial plasma exchange
> permeability pulmonary edema
> personal protective equipment
> polyphosphoric ester
> porcine pancreatic elastase
> postpartum endometritis
> professional performance evaluation
> programmed physical examination
> pruritic papular eruption

Ppeak
> peak airway pressure

PPED
> palmar-plantar erythrodysesthesia

PPEM
> potentially pathogenic environmental mycobacteria

PPES
> palmar-plantar erythrodysesthesia syndrome
> pedal pulses equal and strong

PPF
> palmoplantar fibromatosis
> pellagra preventive factor [niacin]
> percutaneous plantar fasciotomy
> phagocytosis promoting factor
> plasma protein fraction
> postprandial fullness

PPG
> pediatric pneumogram
> phalloplethysmography
> photoplethysmography
> polypropylene glycol
> polyurethane-polyvinyl graphite
> portal pressure gradient
> postpartum galactorrhea
> postprandial glucose
> pretragal parotid gland
> pylorus-preserving gastrectomy

ppg
> picopicogram

PPGA
> postpill galactorrhea/amenorrhea

PPG-AFO
> polypropylene glycol ankle-foot orthosis

PPGF
> polypeptide growth factor

PPGI
> psychophysiologic gastrointestinal [reaction]

PPGSS
> papular pruritic glove and socks syndrome

PPG-TLSO
> polypropylene glycol thoracolumbosacral orthosis

P

PPH
past pertinent history
persistent postdrainage hypotony
persistent pulmonary hypertension
postpartum hemorrhage
prepubertal panhypopituitarism
primary postpartum hemorrhage
primary pulmonary hypertension
procedure for prolapse and hemorrhoids
protocollagen proline hydroxylase

pphm
part per hundred million

PPHN
persistent pulmonary hypertension of
newborn

PPHP
pseudopseudohypoparathyroidism

PPHT
primary plexogenic hypertension

ppht
part per hundred thousand

PPHTN
portopulmonary hypertension

PPHx
previous psychiatric history

PPI
partial permanent impairment
patient package insert
permanent pacemaker insertion
Plan-Position-Indication
post pacing interval
preceding preparatory interval
prepulse inhibition
present pain intensity
proton pump inhibitor
Psychopathic Personality Inventory

PPi, PP$_i$
inorganic pyrophosphate (*See also* IPP)

PPIA
parental presence [during] induction of
anesthesia

PPID
peak pain intensity difference [score]

PPIE
prolonged postictal encephalopathy

PPIM
postperinatal infant mortality

PPIVM
passive physiological intervertebral
movement

PPJ
pure pancreatic juice

PPK
palmoplantar keratoderma (keratosis)
partial penetrating keratoplasty
population pharmacokinetics

PPL
pars plana lensectomy

penicilloyl-polylysine
(penicilloylpolylysine)
phospholipid (*See also* PL)
posterior pulmonary leaflet
postprandial lipemia
primary pituitary lymphoma
primary pulmonary non-Hodgkin
lymphoma
protein polysaccharide

Ppl
intrapleural pressure
pleural pressure

PPLF
postperfusion low flow

PPLO
pleuropneumonialike organisms

PPLOV
painless progressive loss of vision

PPM
permanent pacemaker
persistent pupillary membrane
phosphopentomutase
phosphopeptidomannan
physician practice management
pigmented pupillary membrane
posterior papillary muscle
potentially pathogenic microorganism

ppm
part per million
pulse per minute

PPMA
postpoliomyelitis muscular atrophy
progressive postmyelitis muscular
atrophy

PPMD
posterior polymorphic dystrophy [of
cornea]

PPMM
postpolycythemia myeloid metaplasia

PPMS
primary-progressive multiple sclerosis
psychophysiologic musculoskeletal
[reaction]
Purdue Perceptual-Motor Survey

PPN
partial parenteral nutrition
pedunculopontine nucleus
peripheral parenteral nutrition

PPNA
peak phrenic nerve activity

PPNAD
primary pigmented nodular
adrenocortical disease

PPNET
peripheral primitive neuroectodermal
tumor

PPNG
penicillinase-producing *Neisseria
gonorrhoeae*

PPO
diphenyloxazole (2,5-diphenyloxazole)
passive prehension orthosis
peak pepsin output
permanent punctal occlusion
platelet peroxidase
preferred provider organization
prepatient periods to oocyst
pump-prime only [aprotinin dose]

PPOB
postpartum obstetrics

PPO-HSA
penicillin-penicilloyl human serum
albumin

PPoma
pancreatic polypeptide-secreting tumor
pancreatic polypeptidoma

PPP
Pain Perception Profile
palatopharyngoplasty
palmoplantar pustulosis
passage, power, passenger [progress of
labor]
patient prepped and positioned
pearly penile papules
pedal pulse present
pentose phosphate pathway
peripheral pulse palpable
Pickford Projectives Picture
plasma protamine precipitating
platelet-poor plasma
point-to-point protocol
polyglactin 910-polydioxanon [patch]
poor platelet plasma
porcine pancreatic polypeptide
postnatal penicillin prophylaxis
postpartum psychosis
posttraumatic persistent pneumothorax
preferred practice patterns
proportional pulse pressure [systolic
minus diastolic divided by systolic]
protamine paracoagulation phenomenon
purified placental protein
pustulosis palmaris et plantaris

PP&P
posterior pole and periphery [eye]

PPPBL
peripheral pulses palpable both legs

PPPD
pylorus-preserving
pancreatoduodenectomy

PPPE
prolonged postpeel erythema

PPPG
postprandial plasma glucose

PPPH
purified placental protein, human

PPPM
Parents' Postoperative Pain Measure
per patient per month

PPPMA
progressive postpolio muscle atrophy

PPPPP
pain, pallor, pulse loss, paresthesia,
paralysis

PPPPPP
pain, pallor, paraesthesia, pulselessness,
paralysis, prostration

PPPY
per patient per year

PPQ
Postoperative Pain Questionnaire

PPR
patient-physician relationship
patient progress record
per patient's request
photopalpebral reflex
physiologic pattern release
pitch period perturbation
poor partial response
posterior primary ramus
Price precipitation reaction

PPr
paraprosthetic
periodontal prophylaxis

PPRC
physician payment review commission

PPRE
peroxisome proliferator response element

PPRF
paramedian pontine reticular formation
postpartum renal failure

PP-ribose-P
phosphoribosylpyrophosphate

PPRibp
5-phospho-α(alpha)-D-ribosyl-1-
pyrophosphate (*See also* PRPP)
phosphoribosyl pyrophosphate (*See also*
PRPP)

PPROM
preterm premature rupture of
membranes
prolonged premature rupture of
membranes

PPRST
Printing Performance School Readiness
Test

PPRWP
poor precordial R-wave progression

PPS
Pap plus speculoscopy
parapharyngeal space
patellofemoral pain syndrome
pepsin

P

PPS *(continued)*
peripheral pulmonary stenosis
personal portable stimulator
Personal Preference Scale
phosphoribosylpyrophosphate synthetase
point-prevalent survey
polyvalent pneumococcal polysaccharide [vaccine]
popliteal pterygium syndrome
postpartum sterilization
postperfusion syndrome
postpericardiotomy syndrome
postphlebitic syndrome
postpolio (postpoliomyelitis) syndrome
postpump syndrome
Prausnitz-Küstner sclerosis
presurgical psychological screening
primary acquired preleukemic syndrome
prospective payment (pricing) system
protein plasma substitute
pulse per second

PPSEQ
Postpartum Self-Evaluation Questionnaire

PPSH
pseudovaginal perineoscrotal hypospadias

PPSS
peripheral protein sparing solution

PPT
parietal pleural tissue
partial prothrombin time
peak-to-peak threshold
person, place, and time
Physical Performance Test
plant protease test
pneumonia prevention therapy
posterior pelvic tilt
postpartum thyroiditis
potassium phosphotungstate
pressure pain threshold
professional protective technology
pulmonary physical therapy
pulmonary platelet trapping

ppt
part per trillion
precipitate(d) (*See also* pcpt, pptd, precip)
precipitation (*See also* pcpn, pcpt, pptn, precip)

pPTCA
primary percutaneous transluminal coronary angioplasty

PPTD
postpartum thyroid disease

pptd
precipitate(d) (*See also* pcpt, ppt, precip)

PPTL
postpartum tubal ligation
pressure pain tolerance level

pptn
precipitation (*See also* pcpn, pcpt, ppt, precip)

PPTR
pulsed photothermal radiometry

PPTT
postpartum painless thyroiditis (with transient) thyrotoxicosis
prepubertal testicular tumor

PPU
perforated peptic ulcer

PPUG
positive-pressure urethrography

PPV
pars plana vitrectomy
patent processus vaginalis
percutaneous polymethylmethacrylate vertebroplasty
phacomatosis (phakomatosis) pigmentovascularis
pneumococcal polysaccharide vaccine
porcine parvovirus
positive predictive value
positive-pressure ventilation
Precarious Point virus
progressive pneumonia virus
pulmonary plasma volume

Ppv
pulmonary vein (*See also* PV)

PPVD
perifoveal posterior vitreous detachment

PPVT
Peabody Picture Vocabulary Test

PPVT-R
Peabody Picture Vocabulary Test Revised

PPW
patient protective wrap
plantar puncture wound
premature P-wave
pylorus-preserving Whipple modification

Ppw
pulmonary wedge pressure (*See also* PWP)

PPY
packs per year [cigarettes]

PPZSO
perphenazine sulfoxide

PQ
paraquat
permeability quotient
plastoquinone
pronator quadratus

pQCT
peripheral quantitative computed tomography

PQNS
protein, quantity not sufficient

PQOCN
Psychiatric Questionnaire
Obsessive-Compulsive Neurosis
PQOL
perceived quality of life
P:QRS
P wave to QRS wave ratio
PQRST
palliation, quality, radiation, severity,
time
position, quality, radiation, severity,
time
PR
punctum remotum [far point of
accommodation] [L. *punctum remotum*]
(*See also* p.r.)
pack removal
palindromic rheumatism
Panama red [variety of marijuana]
panic reaction
parallax [and] refraction
pars recta
partial reinforcement
partial remission
partial response
particulate respirator
patient relations
peer review
pelvic rock
percentile rank
perennial rhinitis
perfusion rate
peripheral resistance
per rectum
phenol red
photoreaction (photoreactivation)
physical rehabilitation
physician reviewer
pityriasis rosea
polymyalgia rheumatica
posterior root
postural reflex
potency ratio
potential relation
preference record
pregnancy (*See also* preg, pregn)
pregnancy rate
premature (*See also* prem, preemie,
premie)
presbyopia (*See also* Pb)
pressoreceptor
pressure (*See also* P, press.)
prevention (*See also* prev)
Preyer reflex [startle response to
auditory stimuli]
proctology
production rate

professional relations
profile
progesterone receptor (*See also* PGR)
progressive relaxation
progressive resistive (resistance) exercise
(*See also* PRE)
prolactin (*See also* PRL, Prl)
prolonged remission
prone
prosthion [craniometric]
protease
protein (*See also* PRO, prot)
psychotherapy responder
public relations
pulmonary regurgitation
pulmonary rehabilitation
pulmonic [valve] regurgitation
pulse rate
pulse repetition
pyramidal response
onset of ventricular depolarization [PR
interval on EKG]
P=R
pupils equal in size and reaction
PR3
proteinase 3
P–R
time between P wave and beginning of
QRS complex in electrocardiography
P:R
productivity to respiration ratio
P&R
pelvic and rectal [examination]
pulse and respiration
Pr
praseodymium
p.r.
punctum remotum [far point of
accommodation] [L. *punctum remotum*]
(*See also* PR)
PRA
panel reactive antibody
pendulous reference axis
phonation, respiration,
articulation-resonance
phosphoribosylamine
plasma renin activity
progesterone receptor assay
proximal reference axis
prac, pract
practice
practitioner
PRAFO
pressure-relief ankle-foot orthosis
(orthotic)
PrA-HPA
protein A hemolytic plaque assay

P

639

PRAMS
Pregnancy Risk Monitoring System
prand.
dinner [L. *prandium*]
PRAS
Patient Rated Anxiety Scale
prereduced anaerobically sterilized
[medium]
pseudo renal artery syndrome
PRAT
platelet radioactive antiglobulin test
PRB
partial rebreathing (rebreather) [mask]
pRb
retinoblastoma protein
PRBC
packed red blood cells (*See also* PRC)
PRBV
placental residual blood volume
PRC
packed red [blood] cells (*See also* PRBC)
peer review committee
phase response curve
plasma renin concentration
PRCA
pure red [blood] cell agenesis
pure red [blood] cell aplasia
PrCa
prostate cancer (carcinoma) (*See also*
PC, PCA, PCa, PcA)
PRCC
papillary renal cell carcinoma
PRD
partial reaction of degeneration
phosphate restricted diet
polycystic renal disease
postradiation dysplasia
PRDF
progressive recurrent
dermatofibrosarcoma
PRDX
postradiation dysplasia
PRE
Parkland Rapid Exam
partial-reinforcement effect
passive resistance exercise
photoreacting (photoreactivating) enzyme
physical reconditioning exercise
Picture Reasoning Test
pigmented retina epithelial [cell]
primary resection
progressive resistance (resistive) exercise
(*See also* PR)
proton relaxation enhancement
pre
preliminary
pre-AIDS
pre-acquired immune deficiency
syndrome

PREB
Pupil Record of Education Behavior
preChx
preoperative chemotherapy
precip
precipitate(d) (*See also* pcpt, ppt, pptd)
precipitation (*See also* pcpn, pcpt, ppt,
pptn)
pred
predict(ed) (predictive)
PREE
partial reinforcement extinction effect
preE
preeclampsia
preemie, premie
premature
premature infant
Pref-1
preadipocyte factor 1
pref
preference
prefd
preferred
PREG
pregnenolone
preg, pregn
pregnancy (*See also* PR)
pregnant (*See also* PG, PR)
pregang
preganglionic
PRELEX
presbyopic lens exchange
prelim
preliminary
PREM
Prematurity Risk Evaluation Measure
Pre-M
urine specimen before prostate massage
prem
premature (*See also* PR, preemie,
premie)
prematurity
premed
premedication
preop, pre-op
preoperative(ly)
prep
prepare (preparation)
prepare (for surgery) (*See also* prepd,
prepped)
preposition
prepd, prepped
prepared (for surgery) (*See also* ppd,
prep)
preproGRP
preprogastrin-releasing peptide
PRERLA
pupils round, equal, react to light and
accommodation

preRx
preoperative radiotherapy
PRES
posterior reversible encephalopathy syndrome
preserv
preservation
preserve
PRESS
point-resolved spectroscopy sequence
Pre-Reading Expectancy Screening Scale
press.
pressure (*See also* P, PR)
PREV
Pretoria virus
prev
prevent
prevention (*See also* PR)
preventive
previous
PrevAGT
previous abnormality of glucose tolerance
PREZ
posterior root entry zone
PRF
partial reinforcement
patient report form
peak repetition frequency
peptide regulatory factor
percutaneous radiofrequency rhizolysis
Personality Research Form
plasma-resistant fiber oxygenator
pontine reticular formation
progressive renal failure
prolactin-releasing factor
pulse repetition frequency
pyrogen-releasing factor
pRF
polyclonal rheumatoid factor
PRFA
plasma-recognition-factor activity
PRFD
percutaneous radiofrequency denervation
PRFM
premature rupture of fetal membranes (*See also* PROM)
prolonged rupture of fetal membranes (*See also* PROM)
PRFN
percutaneous radiofrequency
PRFNB
percutaneous radiofrequency facet nerve block
PRFR
pressure-retaining flow-relieving

PRFT
partially relaxed Fourier transform
PRG
phleborheograph(y) (phleborheogram)
purge
PRGI
percutaneous retrogasserian glycerol injection
PRH
past relevant history
postocclusive reactive hyperemia
preretinal hemorrhage
prolactin-releasing hormone
PRHBF
peak reactive hyperemia blood flow
PrHPT
primary hyperparathyroidism
PRI
Pain Rating Index
Partner Relationship Inventory
Patient Review Instrument
Personal Relationship Inventory
phosphate reabsorption index
phosphoribose isomerase
plexus rectales inferiores [venous plexus] (*See also* vvRI)
Prescriptive Reading Inventory
PRIAS
Packard radioimmunoassay system
PRICE
protection, restricted activity, ice, compression, elevation
PRICES
protection, rest, ice, compression, elevation, support [first aid]
PRIH
prolactin release-inhibiting hormone
prim
primary
PRIME
preinversion multiecho
PRIME-MD
Primary Care Evaluation of Mental Disorders
primip, PRIMP
primipara (*See also* para 1, I-para, P)
princ
principal
principle
PRIND
prolonged reversible ischemic neurologic deficit
PRINS
primed in situ labeling
PRISM
Pediatric Risk of Mortality (Score)

PRIST
    paper radioimmunosorbent technique
    (test)
PRIT
    pretargeted radioimmunotherapy
priv
    private
    privilege
PRK
    photorefractive keratectomy
    (keratoplasty)
    primary rabbit kidney
PRL, Prl
    preferred retinal locus
    prolactin (*See also* P, PR)
PRLA
    pupils react to light and accommodation
PRM
    partial rebreathing (rebreather) mask
    passive range of motion (*See also*
    PROM)
    phosphoribomutase
    photoreceptor membrane
    prematurely ruptured membrane
    preventive medicine (*See also* PM, PrM,
    PVMed)
    Primary Reference Material
PrM
    preventive medicine (*See also* PM,
    PRM, PVMed)
PRMF
    preretinal macular fibrosis
P-RMS
    paratesticular rhabdomyosarcoma
PRN, p.r.n.
    as needed [L. *pro re nata*]
PRNF
    primary nonfunction
PRNS
    phrenic repetitive nerve stimulation
PRO
    peer review organization
    Professional Review Organization
    projection
    prolapse
    pronation (*See also* pron)
    protein (*See also* PR, prot)
Pro
    proline (*See also* P)
proANF
    proatrial natriuretic factor
prob
    probability (*See also* P)
    probable
    problem
PROBE
    proton brain examination
PROBE-SV
    proton brain exam single voxel

proBNP
    prohormone B-type natriuretic
    peptide
proc
    procedure
    proceeding
    process
proct, PROCTO, procto
    proctology
    proctoscopy (proctoscopic)
prod.
    product(ion) (*See also* P)
PROEF
    postoperative regimen for oral early
    feeding
Pro El
    protein electrophoresis (*See also* PEP)
prof
    profession(al)
PROG
    progesterone
    prognathism
    program
    progress(ive) (*See also* progr)
prog, progn
    prognosis (*See also* Prx, Px)
progr
    progress(ive) (*See also* PROG)
proj
    project
prolong.
    prolongation
    prolong(ed)
PROM
    passive range of motion (*See also*
    PRM)
    prelabor rupture of membranes
    premature rupture of [fetal] membranes
    (*See also* PRFM)
    prolonged rupture of [fetal] membranes
    (*See also* PRFM)
prom.
    prominent
PROMIN
    programmable multiple ion monitor
PROMM
    passive range of motion machine
    proximal myotonic myopathy
Promy, PROMYEO
    promyelocyte
pron
    pronation (*See also* PRO)
    pronator
PROP1, PROP-1
    prophet of Pit1 [gene]
PROPELLER
    periodically rotated overlapping parallel
    lines with enhanced reconstruction
    [MRI technique]

proph, prop., prophy
prophylactic
prophylaxis (*See also* Px)
proPLA
prophospholipase A
proPTH
proparathyroid hormone
pros
prostate (*See also* prost)
prostatic
PROSE
prostate spectroscopy and imaging
examination
PROSO
protamine sulfate
PROST
pronuclear stage transfer
prost
prostate (*See also* pros)
PROSTALAC
prosthetic antibiotic-loaded acrylic
cement
prosth, PROS
prosthesis
prosthetic
prot
protein (*See also* PR, PRO)
protime, pro time, pro-time
prothrombin time (*See also* PT, PROX)
PROTO 1–10
protoporphyrin [1–10] (*See also* PP I–X)
PROT REL
protrusive relationship
prov
provisional [diagnosis]
PROVIMI
proteins, vitamins, minerals
PROX
prothrombin time (*See also* protime, pro
time, pro-time, PT)
prox
proximal
PRP
panretinal photocoagulation
patient recovery plan
penicillinase-resistant penicillin
penicillin-resistant pneumococcus
physiologic rest position
pityriasis rubra pilaris
platelet-rich plasma
polymer of ribose phosphate
polyribophosphate
polyribosyl ribitol phosphate
(polyribosylribitol phosphate)
poor R wave progression
postreplication repair
postural rest position

premenopausal hormone receptor
positive
pressure rate product
primary Raynaud phenomenon
problem reporting program
progressive rubella panencephalitis
proliferative retinopathy
photocoagulation
Psychotic Reaction Profile
PrP
prion protein
PrP^{Sc}
prion protein scrapie isoform
PrP^c
prion protein normal isoform
PRP-D
polyribosylribitol phosphate-diphtheria
toxoid conjugate
PRPG
platelet-rich plasma gel
PRPP
5-phospho-α(alpha)-D-ribosyl-1-
pyrophosphate (*See also* PPRibp)
phosphoribosyl pyrophosphate (*See also*
PPRibp)
PRP-T
polysaccharide tetanus conjugate vaccine
PRQ
Personal Resource Questionnaire
PRR
pattern recognition receptor
preventive resin restoration
proportional reporting ratio [vaccine
adverse events]
proton relaxation rate
pulmonary reimplantation response
PRRE
pupils round, regular, equal (*See also*
PERRL)
PRRERLA
pupils round, regular, equal; react(ive)
to light and accommodation (*See also*
PEARLA, PERRLA)
PR-RSV
Prague Rous sarcoma virus
PRS
parent's rating scale
Personality Rating Scale
photon radiosurgery system
photon-radiosurgical [therapy]
plasma renin substrate
positive rolandic spike
postradiation sarcoma
prolonged respiratory support
pupil rating scale
PRSA
plasma renin substrate activity

P

PRSL
potential renal solute load
PRSM
peripheral smear
PRSP
penicillin-resistant *Streptococcus pneumoniae*
PRSs
positive rolandic spikes
PRST
blood pressure, heart rate, sweating, tears [level of consciousness scale]
PRSv
postrecurrence survival
PRSW
preload recruitable stroke work
PRT
Pantomime Recognition Test
pelvic radiation therapy
Penicillium roqueforti toxin
percutaneous rotational thrombectomy
pharmaceutical research and testing
phosphoribosyl transferase (phosphoribosyltransferase) (*See also* PRTase)
photoradiation therapy
photostress recovery time
physiologic reflux test
Picture Reasoning Test
postoperative respiratory treatment (therapy)
progressive relaxation training
protamine response test
PRt
prospective randomized trial
PRTase
phosphoribosyl transferase (phosphoribosyltransferase) (*See also* PRT)
PRTCA
percutaneous rotational transluminal coronary angioplasty
PRTH
pituitary resistance to thyroid hormone
PRTH-C
prothrombin time control (*See also* PT-C, PT-CT)
PRU
percent(age) reduction in urea
peripheral resistance unit
PRUJ
proximal radioulnar joint
PRV
Paroo River virus
polycythemia rubra vera
pseudorabies virus
PRVA
peripheral vein renin activity

PRVC
pressure-regulated volume control
PRVEP
pattern reversal visual evoked potential
PRVR
peak to resting velocity ratio
PrVS
prevesical space
PRW
past relevant work
polymerized ragweed
PRWP
poor R-wave progression [electrocardiogram]
PRX
panoramic x-ray [Panorex] (*See also* PAN, PanX)
Prx
prognosis (*See also* prog, progn, Px)
PS
pacemaker syndrome
paired stimulation
Palmaz-Schatz [stent] (*See also* PSS)
pancreas sufficient
paradoxical sleep
paralaryngeal space
paranoid schizophrenia
paraseptal
paraspinal
parasternal
parasympathetic [division of autonomic nervous system] (*See also* parasym, PNS, PSNS)
parotid sialography
partial saturation
partial seizure
partial shoulder
pathologic stage
patient's serum
pediatric surgery (*See also* PDS, PdS)
performance status
performing scale [IQ]
periodic syndrome
peripheral smear
permeability surface
phosphate saline [buffer]
phosphatidylserine
photosensitivity
photosynthesis
phrenic [nerve] stimulation
physical status
phytosterol
pigeon serum
plastic surgery (*See also* PLS, PLSURG, PSurg, P-surg)
pleural space
point of symmetry
polysaccharide
polystyrene

polysulfone [filter]
population sample
Porter-Silber [chromogen or reaction]
postcardiotomy shock
posterior synechiae
posterior synechiotomy
postmaturity syndrome
pregnancy serum
prescription (*See also* Rx)
pressure sore
pressure support
prestimulus
primary stem
principal sulcus
prognostic score
programmed symbols
prostatic secretion
protective services
protein synthesis
psychiatric (*See also* psychiat)
pulmonary sequestration
pulmonary stenosis
pulmonic [valvular] stenosis
pulse sequence
pyloric stenosis

P-S

pancreozymin-secretin
pyramid surface

P:S

polyunsaturated to saturated fatty acids
ratio

P/S

polisher-stimulator

P&S

pain and suffering
paracentesis and suction
permanent and stationary

Ps

pseudocyst
poise [CGS unit of dynamic viscosity]
(*See also* P, Po)

ps

per second
picosecond (*See also* psec)

PS I

[American Society of Anesthesiologists
physical status] patient with stable
systemic disease and no other medical
problem

PS II

[American Society of Anesthesiologists
rating] patient with mild to moderate
systemic disease

PS III

[American Society of Anesthesiologists
physical status] patient with severe

systemic disease limiting activity but
not incapacitating

PS IV

[American Society of Anesthesiologists
physical status] patient with
incapacitating systemic disease

PS V

[American Society of Anesthesiologists
physical status] moribund patient not
expected to live

PSA

pacemaker system analysis
pathologic spontaneous activity
persistent sciatic artery
picryl sulfonic acid
Pisum sativum agglutinin
polyethylene sulfonic acid
polysubstance abuse
posterior spinal artery
power spectral analysis
procedural sedation and analgesia
product selection allowed
progressive spinal ataxia
prolonged sleep apnea
proportion of survivors affected
prostate-specific antigen
pseudoaneurysm (*See also* PA)
psoriatic arthritis
public service announcement

Psa

systemic arterial [blood] pressure

PSA-ACT

prostate-specific antigen bound to
alpha-1 antichymotrypsin

PSAD

prostate-specific antigen density
psychoactive substance abuse and
dependence

PSADT

prostate-specific antigen doubling
time

PSAG

pelvic sonoangiography
Pseudomonas aeruginosa (*See also* PA)

PSAGN

poststreptococcal acute
glomerulonephritis

PSAn

psychoanalysis (*See also* PA, psychoan,
PYA)
psychoanalytic(al) (*See also* psychoan)

PSAP

peak systolic aortic pressure
prostate-specific acid phosphatase

PSATZ, PSA-TZ

prostate-specific antigen density of
transition zone

P

PSAV
> prostate-specific antigen velocity

PSAX
> parasternal short axis

PSB
> patellar stabilizing brace
> protected specimen brush(ing)

PSBO
> partial small-bowel obstruction

PSC
> partial subligamentous calcification
> patient services coordination
> Pediatric Symptom Checklist
> percutaneous suprapubic cystostomy
> physiologic squamocolumnar
> pigmented spindle cell
> pluripotent(ial) stem cell
> Porter-Silber chromogen
> posterior semicircular canal
> posterior subcapsular cataract (*See also* PSCC, PSC Cat)
> primary sclerosing cholangitis
> pronation spring control
> propagated sensation along channel [acupuncture]
> pubosacrococcygeal [diameter]
> pulse-synchronized contractions

PSCA
> prostate stem cell antigen
> proximal subcontact area

PSCC
> posterior subcapsular cataract (*See also* PSC, PSC Cat)

PSC Cat
> posterior subcapsular cataract (*See also* PSC, PSCC)

PSCE
> presurgical coagulation evaluation

PS-CF
> pancreatic-sufficient cystic fibrosis

PSCH
> peripheral stem cell harvest

PsChE
> pseudocholinesterase (*See also* PCE, PCHE)

PSCI
> Primary Self-Concept Inventory

Psci
> pressure at slow component intercept

PSCM
> pokeweed activated spleen conditioned medium

PSCN
> plexiform spindle cell nevus

P/score
> pressure score

PSCP
> papillary serous carcinoma of peritoneum

posterior subcapsular cataractous plaque
posterior subcapsular precipitates

PSCT
> peripheral stem-cell transplant(ation)

PSD
> partial sleep deprivation
> particle size distribution
> pattern standard deviation
> peak skin dose
> pediatric spectrum of disease
> peptone-starch-dextrose [broth]
> percutaneous stricture dilatation
> periodic synchronous discharge
> phosphate supplemental diet
> photon-stimulated desorption
> pilonidal sinus disease
> pituitary stalk distortion
> pneumosinus dilatans
> posterior sagittal diameter
> post-stenosis (poststenotic) dilation (dilatation)
> poststroke depression
> postsynaptic density
> power spectral density
> presenile dementia
> psychosomatic disease

PSDA
> Patient Self-Determination Act

PSDES
> primary symptomatic diffuse esophageal spasm

PSDI
> Positive Symptom Distress Index

PSDK
> poststatic dyskinesia

PSDS
> palmar surface desensitization

PSE
> paradoxical systolic expansion
> partial splenic embolization
> penicillin-sensitive enzyme
> Pidgin Sign English
> point of subjective equality
> portal-systemic (portosystemic) encephalopathy
> postshunt encephalopathy
> preparticipation sports examination
> Present State Examination
> purified spleen extract

PSEC
> poststress ethanol consumption

psec
> picosecond (*See also* ps)

PSEK
> progressive symmetric erythrokeratodermia

PSF
> peak scatter factor
> point spread function [light microscopy]

posterior spinal (spine) fusion
prestress fracture
prostacyclin-stimulating factor
pseudosarcomatous fasciitis
psf
pound per square foot
PSFMT
pseudosarcomatous fibromyxoid tumor
PSFR
pancreatic secretory flow rate
peak secretory flow rate
PSG
peak systolic gradient
phosphate, saline, glucose
polysomnograph(y) (polysomnogram)
portosystemic gradient
presenile gangrene
presystolic gallop
PSGN
poststreptococcal glomerulonephritis
PSH
past social history
past surgical history (*See also* PSHx)
postspinal [anesthetic] headache
P&SH
personal and social history
PsHD
pseudoheart disease
PSHV
pulmonary syndrome hantavirus
PSHx
past surgical history (*See also* PSH)
Ψ, psi
pseudouridine (*See also* Q)
psi [23rd letter of Greek alphabet uppercase]
psychology (*See also* PSY, psy, psych, psychol)
ψ, psi
psi [23rd letter of Greek alphabet lowercase]
PSI
[auto accident with] passenger space intrusion
Parental (Parenting) Stress Index
patient state index
Pediatric Speech Intelligibility Test
pelvic support index
personal security index
Personal Style Inventory
physiologic stability index
pneumatically stented implant
Pneumonia Severity Index
portal shunt index
posterior sagittal index
posterior superior iliac [spine] (*See also* PSIS)

postponing sexual involvement
Predictive Salvage Index
problem solving information
prostaglandin synthetic inhibitor
Psychological Screening Inventory
psychosomatic inventory
punctate subepithelial infiltrate
psi, p.s.i.
pound per square inch (*See also* lbf/in^2)
psia
pound per square inch absolute
pSIDS
partially unexplained sudden infant death syndrome
PSIF
reverse fast imaging with steady-state free precession
PSIFT
platelet suspension immunofluorescence test
psig
pound per square inch gauge
PSIL
percent(age) signal intensity loss
preferred frequency speech interference level
P-SIMV
pressure synchronized intermittent mandatory ventilation
PSIS
posterior sacroiliac spine
posterior superior iliac spine (*See also* PSI)
PSK
polysaccharide Kreha
PSL
parasternal line
percent stroke length
pigmented skin lesion
potassium, sodium chloride, sodium lactate [solution]
PSLL
pancreatoscopic laser lithotripsy
PSLT
Picture Story Language Test
PSM
patient self-management
polysomnograph(y) (polysomnogram)
presystolic murmur
propagated sensation along meridian [acupunture]
prostate-specific membrane
PSMA
personal self-maintenance activities
progressive spinal muscular atrophy
prostate-specific membrane antigen
proximal spinal muscular atrophy

P

PSMed
>   psychosomatic medicine (*See also* PsychosMed)

PSMF
>   protein-sparing modified fast

PSM-R
>   Optimism-Pessimism Scale, revised

PSMS
>   Physical Self Maintenance Scale

PSN
>   pontosubicular neuron necrosis

PSNP
>   placental site nodule and plaque
>   progressive supranuclear palsy

PSNS
>   parasympathetic nervous system (*See also* parasym, PNS, PS)

PSO
>   pelvic stabilization orthosis
>   physician supplemental order
>   progressive supranuclear ophthalmoplegia
>   proximal subungual onychomycosis

pSO₂
>   arterial oxygen saturation (*See also* PaSat)

PsoE
>   erythrodermic psoriasis

Psol
>   partly soluble

PSOR
>   psoralen (*See also* P)

P/sore
>   pressure sore

PSP
>   pacesetter potential (*See also* PP)
>   pancreatic spasmolytic peptide
>   pancreatic stone protein
>   paralytic shellfish poisoning
>   parathyroid secretory protein
>   peak systolic pressure
>   periodic short pulse
>   persephin
>   Personnel Security Preview
>   phenolsulfonphthalein (phenol red)
>   photostimulable phosphor dental radiography
>   pigeon serum protein
>   positive spike pattern
>   postoperative survival probability
>   post space preparation
>   postsynaptic potential
>   primary spontaneous pneumothorax
>   professional simulated patient
>   progressive supranuclear palsy
>   pseudopregnancy

psp
>   posterior subcapsular plaque

PspA
>   pneumococcal surface protein A

PSPDV
>   posterior superior pancreaticoduodenal vein

PSPF
>   prostacyclin synthesis-stimulating plasma factor

PSPUMP
>   prostatic stromal proliferation of uncertain malignant potential

PSQ
>   Parent Symptom Questionnaire
>   patient satisfaction questionnaire
>   Personal Strain Questionnaire

PSQI
>   Pittsburgh Sleep Quality Index

PSR
>   [extrahepatic] portal-systemic resistance
>   pain sensitivity range
>   percutaneous stereotactic radiofrequency [rhizotomy]
>   Periodontal Screening Record (Recording)
>   phase sampling ratio
>   posthumous sperm retrieval
>   problem status report
>   proliferative sickle retinopathy
>   Psychiatric Status Rating [scale]
>   pulmonary stretch receptor

PSRA
>   poststreptococcal reactive arthritis (*See also* PSReA)
>   pressure sore risk assessment

PSRBOW
>   premature spontaneous rupture of bag of waters

PSReA
>   poststreptococcal reactive arthritis (*See also* PSRA)

PSRI
>   Professional Sexual Role Inventory

PSRO
>   Professional Standards Review Organization

PSROM
>   preterm spontaneous rupture of membranes

PSRS
>   Process Skills Rating Scale

PSRT
>   photostress recovery test

PSS
>   painful shoulder syndrome
>   pain sensation score
>   Palmaz-Schatz stent (*See also* PS)
>   partial striatal sclerosis
>   Perceived Stress Scale
>   Peritonitis Severity Score
>   physiologic saline (salt) solution
>   porcine stress syndrome

portosystemic shunting
primary Sjögren syndrome
progressive symptoms sclerosis
progressive systemic scleroderma
progressive systemic sclerosis
psoriasis severity scale
Psychiatric Status Schedule
pure sensory stroke
pure sensory syndrome

PSSE
partial saturation spin echo

PSS-HN
performance status scale for head and
neck [cancer]

PSS:NICU
Parental Stressor Scale: Neonatal
Intensive Care Unit

PSSP
penicillin-sensitive *Streptococcus
pneumoniae*

PST
pancreatic suppression test
paroxysmal supraventricular tachycardia
(*See also* PSVT)
patient self-testing
perceptual span time
peristimulus time
phenolsulfotransferase
phonemic segmentation test
platelet survival time
positive symptom total
poststenotic
poststimulus time
postural stimulation test
postural stress test
potassium sensitivity test
prefrontal sonic treatment
presenile tumor
promontory stimulation test
protein-sparing therapy
proximal straight tubule

PSTH
poststimulus time histogram (histograph)

PSTI
pancreatic secretory trypsin inhibitor

PSTO
Purdue Student-Teacher Opinionnaire

PSTP
pentasodium triphosphate

PSTT
placental site trophoblastic tumor

PSTV
potato spindle tuber viroid

PSU
photosynthetic unit
primary sampling unit
pseudomonas (*P. aeruginosa*) vaccine

PSUD
psychoactive substance use disorder

PSUR
periodic safety update reporting

PSurg, P-Surg
plastic surgery (*See also* PLS, PLSURG,
PS)

PSV
peak systolic velocity
persistent sciatic vein
positive-support ventilator
pressure-supported ventilation
pressure-support ventilation
primary systemic vasculitis [singular]
primary systemic vasculitides [plural]
psychological, social, vocational
[adjustment factors]
Punta Salinas virus

PSVER
pattern-shift visual-evoked response

PsV-F
Penicillium stoloniferum F virus

PsV-S
Penicillium stoloniferum S virus

PSVT
paroxysmal supraventricular tachycardia
(*See also* PVT)

PSW
past sleepwalker

PSWC
periodic sharp wave complex

PSWF
positive sharp wave fibrillations
[electromyograph]

PSWL
peroral shock wave lithotripsy

PSX
pseudoexfoliation (*See also* PXF)

PSY, Psy
presexual youth
psychiatry (*See also* P, psych, psychiat)
psychology (*See also* Ψ, psych, psychol)

psych
psychiatry (*See also* P, psychiat)
psychologic (*See also* psychol)
psychology (*See also* Ψ, psychol, PSY)

psychiat
psychiatric (*See also* PS)
psychiatry (*See also* P, PSY, Psy,
psych)

psychoan
psychoanalysis (*See also* PA, PSAn,
PYA)
psychoanalytic(al) (*See also* PSAn)

psychol
psychologic
psychology (*See also* Ψ, PSY, psych)

P

psychopath.
  psychopathic (*See also* psy-path)
  psychopathologic
  psychopathology
PsychosMed
  psychosomatic medicine (*See also* PSMed)
psychother
  psychotherapeutic
  psychotherapy
psy-path
  psychopathic (*See also* psychopath.)
PSZ
  pseudoseizure
ps-ZES
  pseudo-Zollinger-Ellison syndrome
PT
  parathyroid hormone (parathormone) (*See also* para, PH, PTH)
  paroxysmal tachycardia
  part (*See also* P)
  patient (*See also* P, PAT)
  pericardial tamponade
  permanent and total
  pertussis toxin
  pertussis toxoid [vaccine]
  phacotrabeculectomy
  phage type
  pharmacy and therapeutics
  phonation time
  phosphotransferase
  photophobia
  phototoxicity
  physical therapy (physiotherapy) (*See also* Phys Ther)
  physical training
  pine tar
  plasma thromboplastin
  pluridirectional tomography
  pneumothorax (*See also* PNEUMO, pnx, pnthx, PTX, Px)
  point
  polyvalent tolerance
  posterior tibial
  posttransplant(ation)
  preterm
  primary thrombocythemia
  process tomography
  pronator teres
  prothrombin time (*See also* protime, pro time, pro-time, PT, PROX)
  proximal tubule
  pseudotumor
  psychasthenia
  pulmonary thrombosis
  pulmonary toilet
  pulmonary trunk
  pulmonary tuberculosis (*See also* PTB)

  pure tone [audiometry]
  pyramidal tract
  temporal plane
P1/2T
  pressure half time
P/T
  pain and tenderness
P&T
  paracentesis and tubing [of ears]
  peak and trough
  permanent and total
  pharmacy and therapeutics
P$_T$
  total pressure
Pt
  platinum
pT0
  no histological evidence of primary tumor [TNM pathologic classification]
pT1–pT4
  increase in size and/or local extent of primary tumor histologically [TNM pathologic classification]
pt
  pint
PTA
  pancreas (pancreatic) transplant(ation) alone
  parathyroid adenoma
  parathyroid thymic aplasia
  patellar tendon autograft
  peak twitch amplitude
  percutaneous transluminal angioplasty
  peritonsillar abscess
  persistent trigeminal artery
  persistent truncus arteriosus
  phosphotungstic acid
  plasma thromboplastin antecedent
  posterior tibial artery
  posttraumatic amnesia
  pretreatment anxiety
  primitive trigeminal artery
  prior to admission (*See also* PA)
  prior to arrival
  prothrombin activity (*See also* PA)
  pure tone acuity
  pure tone average (*See also* PT(A))
PT(A)
  pure tone average (*See also* PTA)
PTAB
  popliteal-tibial artery bypass
  pterygoalar bar
PTAF
  policy target adjustment factor
P-TAG
  target-attaching globulin precursor
PTAH
  phosphotungstic acid-hematoxylin [stain]

PTAP
>purified [diphtheria] toxoid [precipitated by] aluminum phosphate

PTARF
>posttraumatic acute renal failure

PTAS
>percutaneous transluminal angioplasty with stent

PTAV
>percutaneous transluminal aortic valvuloplasty

PTB
>patellar tendon-bearing [cast prosthesis]
>phosphotyrosine binding [domain]
>pretibial bearing
>pretibial buttress
>prior to birth
>pulmonary tuberculosis (*See also* PT)

PTBA
>percutaneous transluminal balloon angioplasty

PTBD
>percutaneous transhepatic (transluminal) balloon dilatation (dilation)
>percutaneous transhepatic biliary drainage (*See also* PTHBD)

PTBD-EF
>percutaneous transhepatic biliary drainage-enteric feeding

PTBE
>pyretic tick-borne encephalitis

PTBNA
>protected transbronchial needle aspirate

PTBO
>patellar tendon-bearing orthosis

PTBP
>*para*-tertiary butylphenol

PTBPD
>posttraumatic borderline personality disorder

PTBS
>patellar tendon-bearing suspension
>posttraumatic brain syndrome

PTB-SC-SP
>patellar tendon-bearing–supracondylar-suprapatellar [prosthesis]

PT-C
>prothrombin time control (*See also* PRTH-C, PT-CT)

PTC
>papillary thyroid carcinoma
>patched gene
>patient to call
>percutaneous transhepatic cholangiograph(y) (cholangiogram)
>peritubular capillary

>phase transfer catalyst
>phenylthiocarbamide
>phenylthiocarbamoyl
>pheochromocytoma, thyroid carcinoma [syndrome]
>plasma thromboplastin component
>post-tetanic count
>premature tricuspid closure
>primary thymic carcinoma
>prior to conception
>prothrombin complex
>pseudotumor cerebri
>pulmonary tissue concentration

PTCA
>parent to child aggression
>percutaneous transhepatic cholangiograph(y) (cholangiogram) (*See also* PTC, PTHC)
>percutaneous transluminal coronary angioplasty (arteriography)

PTCC
>percutaneous transhepatic cholecystoscopy

PtcCO$_2$
>transcutaneous carbon dioxide tension

PTCD
>percutaneous transhepatic cholangial drainage (cholangiodrainage)

PTCDLF
>pregnancy, term, complicated delivered, living female

PTCDLM
>pregnancy, term, complicated delivered, living male

PTCH
>patched hedgehog [protein, gene]

PTCL
>peripheral T-cell lymphoma
>postthymic T-cell lymphoma

PTCP
>pseudothrombocytopenia

PTCR
>percutaneous transluminal coronary recanalization (revascularization)

PTCRA
>percutaneous transluminal coronary rotational ablation (atherectomy)

PTCS
>percutaneous transhepatic cholangioscopy
>Primary Test of Cognitive Skills

PTCSL
>percutaneous transhepatic cholangioscopic lithotomy

PT-CT
>prothrombin time control (*See also* PRTH-C, PT-C)

P

PTD
   para-toluenediamine
   percutaneous thrombolytic device
   percutaneous transhepatic drain(age)
   percutaneous transluminal dilatation
     (dilatation)
   percutaneous transpedicular discectomy
   period to discharge
   permanent total disability
   persistent trophoblastic disease
   personality trait disorder
   pharmacy to dose
   pharyngotracheal duct
   preterm delivery
   prevention and treatment of
     depression
   prior to delivery
   prior to discharge
   psychotropic drug

Ptd
   phosphatidyl

PtdCho
   phosphatidylcholine

PtdEth, PtdEtn
   phosphatidylethanolamine

PtdIns
   phosphatidylinositol (*See also* PI)

PtdIns(4,5)P$_2$
   phosphatidylinositol 4,5-bisphosphate

PTDM
   posttransplant(ation) diabetes
     mellitus

PTDP
   permanent transvenous demand
     pacemaker

PtdSer
   phosphatidylserine

PTE
   parathyroid extract
   peritumoral edema
   posttraumatic endophthalmitis
   posttraumatic epilepsy
   pretibial edema
   proximal tibial epiphysis
   pulmonary thromboembolectomy
   pulmonary thromboembolism
   pulmonary thromboendarterectomy

PTEC
   proximal tubular epithelial cells

PTED
   pulmonary thromboembolic disease

PTEF
   peak tidal expiratory flow
   time to peak tidal expiratory flow

PteGlu
   pteroylglutamic [acid]

PTEN
   phosphatase and tensin homologue
     [gene]

PTER
   percutaneous transluminal
     endomyocardial revascularization

pter
   end of short arm of chromosome

PTF
   parathyroid fever
   patient transfer form
   patient treatment file
   plasma thromboplastin factor
   posterior talofibular
   posttetanic facilitation
   posttransfusion fever

PTF1
   pancreatic transcription factor 1

PTFA
   prothrombin time fixing agent

PTFE
   polytetrafluoroethylene (*See also*
     polytef)

PTFL
   posterior talofibular ligament

PTFNA
   percutaneous transthoracic fine-needle
     aspiration

PTFS
   posttraumatic fibromyalgia syndrome

PTG
   parathyroid gland

PTGA
   pteroyltriglutamic acid

PTGBD
   percutaneous transhepatic gallbladder
     drain(age)

PTGC
   progressive transformation of germinal
     center

PTGDS
   patellar tendon graft donor site

PTH
   parathyroid hormone (parathormone)
     (*See also* para, PH, PT)
   pathologic (pathology) (*See also* PA,
     PATH, path.)
   plasma parathyroid hormone
   plasma thromboplastin [component]
   posttransfusion hepatitis
   prior to hospitalization

PTh
   primary thrombocythemia

Pth
   chest wall elastic recoil pressure

PTHBD
   percutaneous transhepatic biliary
     drain(age) (*See also* PTBD)

PTHC
   percutaneous transhepatic
     cholangiograph(y) (cholangiogram)
     (*See also* PTC, PTCA)

PTH-LP
parathyroid hormonelike polypeptide
PTHR, PThHR
pituitary thyroid hormone resistance
PTHRP, PTH-rP, PTHrP
parathyroid hormone-related peptide (protein)
PTHS
parathyroid hormone secretion [rate]
posttraumatic hyperirritability syndrome
PTHV
Pathum Thani virus
PTI
pancreatic trypsin inhibitor
persistent tolerant infection
Personnel Tests for Industry
Pictorial Test of Intelligence
pressure-time index (integral)
PTIF
peak tidal inspiratory flow
pTis
carcinoma in situ [TNM pathologic classification]
PTJV
percutaneous transtracheal jet ventilation
PTK
phototherapeutic keratectomy
posttraumatic keratitis
protein tyrosine kinase
PTL
perinatal telencephalic leukoencephalopathy
peripheral T-cell lymphoma
pharyngotracheal lumen [airway]
posterior tricuspid [valve] leaflet
preterm labor
pudding-thick liquid [diet consistency]
pTL
percutaneous transhepatic lymphography
PTLA
pharyngeal tracheal lumen airway
PTLC
precipitation thin-layer chromatography
PTLD, PTLPD, PT-LPD
posttransplant(ation) lymphoproliferative disorder (disease)
prescribed tumor lethal dose
PTLR
percutaneous transmyocardial laser revascularization
PTM
patient monitored
posterior trabecular meshwork
posttransfusion mononucleosis
posttraumatic meningitis
pressure time per minute
preterm milk
pretibial myxedema

Ptm
pterygomaxillary [fissure]
transmural pressure [airway, blood vessel]
PTMA
phenyltrimethylammonium
PTMC
percutaneous transvenous mitral commissurotomy
PTMDF
pupils, tension, media, disc, fundus
PTMR
percutaneous transluminal myocardial revascularization
percutaneous transmyocardial revascularization
PTN
pain transmission neuron
posterior tibial nerve
proximal tibial nail
PT-NANB, PT-NANBH
posttransfusion non-A, non-B [hepatitis]
PTNB
percutaneous transthoracic needle biopsy
preterm newborn
pTNM
pathologic tumor, nodes, metastases [TNM pathologic classification]
PTN/MK
pleiotrophin/midkine [growth enhancer]
PTNS
percutaneous tibial nerve stimulation
PTO
Klemperer tuberculin [Ger. *Perlsucht Tuberculin Original*]
part-time occlusion [eye patch]
percutaneous transhepatic obliteration
personal time off
please turn [the patient] over
proximal tubal obstruction
Purdue Teacher Opinionnaire
P to P
point to point
PTP
percutaneous transhepatic portography
periodic thyrotoxic paralysis
phonation threshold pressure
Physical Tolerance Profile
posterior tibial pulse
posttetanic potentiation
posttransfusion purpura
pressure time product
previously treated patient
prior to program
prothrombin-proconvertin (*See also* PP)
proximal tubular pressure
pseudothrombophlebitis

P

Ptp
transpulmonary pressure
PTPase
tyrosine specific protein phosphatase
PTP1B
tyrosine specific protein phosphatase 1B
PTPI
posttraumatic pulmonary insufficiency
PTPM
posttraumatic progressive myelopathy
PTPN
peripheral [vein] total parenteral
nutrition
PTPS
postthrombophlebitis syndrome
PT-PTT
prothrombin time and partial
thromboplastin time
PTQ
Parent-Teacher Questionnaire
Purdue Teacher Questionnaire
PTR
paratesticular rhabdomyosarcoma
patella tendon reflex
patient to return
patient termination record
peripheral total resistance
plasma transfusion reaction
pressure transmission ratio
prothrombin time ratio
psychotherapy research
psychotic trigger reaction
tuberculin *Mycobacterium tuberculosis
bovis* [Ger. *Perlsucht Tuberculin Rest*]
PTr
porcine trypsin
PTRA
percutaneous transluminal rotational
atherectomy
percutaneous transluminal (transfemoral)
renal angioplasty
PTRIA
polystyrene-tube radioimmunoassay
PTR-MS
proton transfer reaction-mass
spectrometry
PTRTH
peripheral tissue resistance to thyroid
hormone
Ptrx
pelvic traction
PTS
painful tonic seizure
para-toluenesulfonic [acid]
patella (patellar) tendon socket
patellar tendon stabilization
patellar tendon suspension
Pediatric Trauma Scale (Score)
permanent threshold shift

phosphotransferase system
postthrombotic syndrome
posttraumatic syndrome
prior to surgery
6-PTS
6-pyruvoyltetrahydropterin synthase
[enzyme]
pts
patients [plural]
PTSD
posttraumatic stress disorder
PTSMA
percutaneous transluminal septal
myocardial ablation
PTSS
posttraumatic signs or symptoms
posttraumatic stress syndrome
PTT
partial thromboplastin time
particle transport time
patellar tendon transfer
pharyngeal transit time
platelet transfusion therapy
posterior tibial tendinitis
posterior tibial tendon
posterior tibial transfer
protein truncation test(ing)
pulmonary transit time
pulse transit (transmission) time
pure tone threshold
PTT-C, PTT-CT
partial thromboplastin time control
PTTD
posterior tibial tendon dysfunction
PTTG
pituitary tumor transforming gene
PTTH
prothoracotropic hormone [insects]
PTTI
penetrating thoracic trauma index
PTT-LA
partial thromboplastin time lupus
anticoagulant
PTTW
patient tolerated traction well
PTU
pregnancy, term, uncomplicated
PTUCA
percutaneous transluminal ultrasonic
coronary angioplasty
PTUDLF
pregnancy, term, uncomplicated
delivered, living female
PTUDLM
pregnancy, term, uncomplicated
delivered, living male
P-TUMT
periurethral transurethral microwave
thermotherapy

PTV
patient-triggered ventilation
percutaneous transtracheal jet ventilation
planning target volume
posterior temporal vertical
posterior terminal vein
posterior tibial vein
Punta Toro virus
PtVP
portal venous pressure
PTVV
Ponteves virus
PTWTKG
patient's weight in kilograms
PTX
pancreas transplant(ation)
phototherapy
phototoxic reaction
picrotoxinin
pneumothorax (*See also* PNEUMO, pnx, pnthx, PT, Px)
PTx
parathyroidectomy (*See also* para)
pelvic traction
pTX
primary tumor cannot be assessed histologically [TNM pathologic classification]
PTXA
parathyroidectomy and autotransplant(ation)
PTZ
pentylenetetrazol
PU
passed urine
paternal uncle
pelvicureteric (pelvic-ureteric)
pelviureteral
pepsin unit
peptic ulcer
polyurethane
posterior urethra
precursor uptake
pregnancy urine
prostatic urethra
by way of urethra [L. *pr urethra*]
Pu
plutonium
PUA
pelvic [examination] under anesthesia
plasma uric acid
PUB
percutaneous umbilical blood
pubic
pub, publ
public

PUBS
percutaneous umbilical blood sampling (sample)
purple urine bag syndrome
PUC
pediatric urine collector
PUCV
Puchong virus
PUD
partial upper denture
peptic ulcer disease
percutaneous ureteral dilatation
pudendal (*See also* Pdl)
pulmonary disease (*See also* PD, PuD)
PuD
pulmonary disease (*See also* PD, PUD)
PUE
pyrexia of unknown etiology
PUF
polyurethane film (foam)
pure ultrafiltration
PUFA
polyunsaturated fatty acid
PUFFA
polyunsaturated free fatty acid
PUH
pregnancy urine hormone
PUI
posterior urethral injury
PUJ
pelviureteral (pelviureteric) junction
PUJO
pelviureteric junction obstruction
PUK
peripheral ulcerative keratitis
PUL, pul
percutaneous ultrasonic lithotripsy
pubourethral ligament
pulmonary (*See also* P, pulm)
pulm
gruel [L. pulmentum]
pulmonary (*See also* P, PUL, pul)
pulmonic
PULP
pulpotomy
Pulse A
pulse apical
PULSE OX, pulsox
pulse oximeter cooximetry
Pulse R
pulse radial
PULSES
physical condition, upper limb function, lower limb function, sensory component, excretory function, support function [physical profile]

P

PUN
 plasma urea nitrogen
PUND
 pregnancy, uterine, not delivered
 (undelivered)
PUNL
 percutaneous ultrasonic nephrolithotripsy
PUNLMP
 papillary urothelial neoplasm of low
 malignant potential
PUO
 pyrexia of undetermined (unknown)
 origin
PUP
 percutaneous ultrasonic pyelolithotomy
 previously untreated patient
PU-PC
 polyunsaturated phosphatidylcholine
PU/PL
 partial upper and partial lower
 [dentures]
PUPP
 pruritic urticarial papules and
 plaques
PUPPP
 pruritic urticarial papules and plaques
 of pregnancy
PUR
 polyurethane
Pur
 purine
 purple
purg
 purgative
PURV
 Purus virus
PUS
 percutaneous ureteral stent
 preoperative ultrasound
PUSH
 Pressure Ulcer Scale for Healing
PUT
 provocative use test
 putamen
 putrescine
PUU
 Puumala hantavirus
PUUV
 Puumala virus
PUV
 positive ulnar variance
 posterior urethral valve
 [type I–IV]
PUVA
 [oral administration of] psoralens plus
 ultraviolet A [long wavelength
 radiation] [phototherapy]
 posterior urethrovesical angle
 pulsed ultraviolet actinotherapy

PUVA/UVB
 psoralens plus ultraviolet A [long
 wavelength radiation] and ultraviolet B
 [short wavelength radiation]
 [phototherapy]
PUVD
 pulsed ultrasonic [blood] velocity
 detector
PUVT
 paraumbilical vein tumor
PUW
 pick-up walker
PV
 pancreatic vein
 papilla of Vater
 papillomavirus
 paraventricular
 partial volume
 parvovirus
 pemphigus vulgaris
 peripheral vascular
 peripheral vein (*See also* PeV)
 peripheral vessel
 per vagina
 phonation volume
 photovoltaic
 picornavirus
 pinocytotic vesicle
 pityriasis versicolor
 plasma viscosity
 plasma volume
 pneumococcus vaccine
 pneumonia virus
 polio vaccine
 polycythemia vera (*See also*
 PCV)
 polyoma virus
 polyvinyl
 popliteal vein
 portal vein
 postvasectomy
 postvoiding
 predictive value
 prenatal vitamins
 pressure-volume
 projectile vomiting
 pulmonary vein (*See also* Ppv)
 pulmonic valve
 pure vegetarian
 by way of vagina [L. *per
 vaginam*]
P-V
 Paton-Valentine [leukocidin]
P:V
 pressure to volume (ratio)
P&V
 peak and valley
 percuss and vibrate
 pyloroplasty and vagotomy

Pv
  Plasmodium vivax
  Proteus vulgaris
  venous pressure (*See also* VP)
PVA
  partial villous atrophy
  peripheral venous alimentation
  Personal Values Abstract
  polyvinyl alcohol [fixative]
  polyvinyl alcohol [foam]
  Prinzmetal variant angina
  ventricular pseudoaneurysm
PVAB
  postventricular atrial blanking
PVAc
  polyvinyl acetate
PVAD
  prolonged venous access devices
PVAM
  potential visual acuity meter
PVAR
  pulmonary vein atrial reversal
PVARP
  postventricular atrial refractory period
PVAS
  postvasectomy
PVB
  paravertebral block
  pigmented villonodular bundle
  polyvinyl butyral [resin]
  porcelain veneer bridge
  premature ventricular beat
PVBS
  possible vertebrobasilar system
PVC
  peripheral venous catheterization
  persistent vaginal cornification
  polyethylene vacuum cup
  polyvinyl chloride
  porcelain veneer crown
  postvoiding cystogram
  predicted vital capacity
  premature ventricular complex
  premature ventricular contraction
  primary visual cortex
  pulmonary venous capillary
  pulmonary venous congestion
PVCI
  portal vein congestive index
PVCM
  paradoxical vocal cord motion
Pvco2, Pv$_{co2}$
  partial pressure [tension] of carbon
    dioxide, vein or venous blood
PVD
  patient very disturbed
  percussion, vibration, drainage

  peripheral vascular disease
  peripheral vestibular deficit
  portal vein dilation
  posterior vitreal (vitreous) detachment
  postural vertical dimension
  postvagotomy diarrhea
  premature ventricular depolarization
  pulmonary valve dysplasia
  pulmonary vascular disease
PVDF
  polyvinylidene difluoride
PVE
  perivenous encephalomyelitis
  periventricular echogenicity
  portal vein embolization
  premature ventricular event
  premature ventricular extrasystole
  prosthetic valve endocarditis
PvE
  pelvic examination (*See also* PE)
PV:ECF
  plasma volume to extracellular fluid
    ratio
PVEL
  periventricular echolucency
PVEM
  postvaccination (postvaccinal)
    encephalomyelitis
PVEP
  pattern visual evoked potential
PVER
  pattern visual evoked response
P vera
  polycythemia vera
PVF
  peripheral visual field
  portal venous flow
  primary ventricular fibrillation
  pulmonary venous flow
PVFD
  paradoxical vocal fold dysfunction
PVFS
  postviral fatigue syndrome
PVG
  periventricular gray matter
  pulmonary valve gradient
PVGM
  perifoveolar vitreoglial membrane
PVH
  perivascular hemorrhage
  periventricular hemorrhage
  periventricular hyperintensity
  persistent viral hepatitis
  pulmonary vascular hypertension
  pulmonary venous hypertension
PVH-B
  persistent viral hepatitis, type B

P

PVH-NANB
persistent viral hepatitis, non-A, non-B
PVI
pelvic venous incompetence
peripheral vascular insufficiency
perivascular infiltration
periventricular inhibitor
Personal Values Inventory
portal vein infusion
protracted venous infusion
pulmonary valve insufficiency
PV-IVH
periventricular and intraventricular
hemorrhage
PVL
peripheral vascular laboratory
perivalvular leakage
periventricular leukomalacia
periventricular radiolucency
permanent vision loss
plasma viral load
proliferative verrucous leukoplakia
P-VL
Panton-Valentine leukocidin
PVM
parallel virtual machine
paravertebral muscle
pneumonia virus of mice
proteins, vitamins, minerals
PVMed
preventive medicine (*See also* PM,
PRM, PrM)
PVMS
paravertebral muscle spasm
PVMT
Primary Visual Motor Test
PVN
paraventricular nucleus
peripheral venous nutrition
predictive value of a negative
[test]
PVNPS
post-Vietnam psychiatric syndrome
PVNS
pigmented villonodular synovitis
pigmented villonodular tenovagosynovitis
PVO
peripheral vascular occlusion
portal vein obstruction (occlusion)
pulmonary vascular obstruction
pulmonary venous obstruction
(occlusion)
PVo
pulmonary valve opening
PvO2, Pvo2, Pv$_{O2}$
partial oxygen pressure [tension] in
mixed venous blood
PVOD
peripheral vascular occlusive disease

pulmonary vascular obstructive disease
pulmonary venoocclusive disease
PVP
peripheral vein plasma
peripheral venous pressure
photoselective vaporization of prostate
polyvinylpyrrolidone (povidone)
portal venous [-dominant] phase
portal venous pressure
posteroventral pallidotomy
predictive value of a positive [test]
pulmonary venous pressure
PVPG
paravertebral paraganglioma
PVPI
polyvinylpyrrolidone (povidone)–iodine
PVR
paraventricular nuclear stratum
peripheral vascular resistance
perspective volume rendering
postvoid(ing) residual
proliferative vitreoretinopathy
prosthetic valve regurgitation
pulmonary valve replacement
pulmonary vascular resistance
pulmonary venous redistribution
pulse value recording
pulse volume recorder (recording)
pVR
perspective volume rendering
PVRI
peripheral vascular resistance index
pulmonary vascular resistance
index
PVS
Beery Picture Vocabulary Screening
paravesical space
percussion, vibration, suction
peripheral vascular surgery
peripheral vascular system
peritoneovenous shunt
persistent vegetative state
persistent viral syndrome
pigmented villonodular synovitis
poliovirus sensitivity (susceptibility)
polyvinyl sponge
portal venous sampling
premature ventricular systole
preventricular stenosis
programmed ventricular stimulation
prosthetic valve stenosis
pulmonary vein stenosis
pulmonic valve stenosis
PVST
prevertebral soft tissue
PVT
paraventricular thalamic nucleus
paroxysmal ventricular tachycardia
Peabody Vocabulary Test

physical volume test
portal vein thrombosis
pressure, volume, temperature
previous trouble
primary ventricular tachycardia
private [patient]
proximal vein thrombosis

PVTT
portal vein tumor thrombus
tumor thrombus in the portal vein

PVV
persistent varicose veins
portal venous velocity

PVW
posterior vaginal wall

PW
pacing wire
patient waiting
peristaltic wave
plantar wart
posterior wall
pressure wave
psychological warfare
pulmonary wedge [pressure]
pulsed wave
pulse width
puncture wound

P&W
pressure and wave

Pw
progesterone withdrawal

PWA
person with acquired immunodeficiency
syndrome (AIDS)
P-wave axis

PWACR
Prader-Willi/Angelman critical region
[gene locus]

PWARC
person with AIDS-related complex

PWB
partial weightbearing
Positive Well-being [scale]
psychologic well-being
Puno-Winter-Byrd [transpedicular spine
fixation system]

PWBC
peripheral white blood cell

PWBL
partial weight bearing, left

PWBR
partial weight bearing, right

PWBRT
prophylactic whole brain radiation
therapy

PWBT
partial weightbearing therapy

PWC
peak work capacity
physical work capacity
powered wheelchair

PWCA
personal watercraft accident

PWCT
perfusion-weighted computed
tomography

PWD
person with diabetes
person with a disability
precipitated withdrawal diarrhea
pulsed-wave Doppler

pwd
powder (*See also* pdr, powd)

PWDS
postweaning diarrhea syndrome

PWE
person with epilepsy
posterior wall excursion

PWH
progressive weakness and hypotonia

PWI
pediatric walk-in clinic
perfusion-weighted [magnetic resonance]
imaging
posterior wall infarct

PWLV
posterior wall of left ventricle

PWM
pokeweed mitogen

PWMI
posterior wall myocardial infarction

PWO
persistent withdrawal occlusion

PWOS
postworkout syncope

PWP
Parents Without Partners
pulmonary wedge pressure (*See also*
Ppw)

PWS
plagiocephaly without synostosis
port-wine stain
pulse-wave speed

PWT
pad weight test
posterior wall thickness
primary writing tremor

PWTD
pulsed-wave tissue Doppler

PWTd
posterior wall thickness at
end-diastole

PWTT
pulse wave transit time

P

PWV

    peak weight velocity
    Polistes wasp venom
    posterior wall velocity
    pulse wave velocity

PX

    pancreatectomized
    pancreatectomy (*See also* pan.)
    peroxidase

Px

    past history (*See also* PH, PHx)
    physical examination (*See also* PE, PEx)
    pneumothorax (*See also* PNEUMO, pnx,
      pnthx, PT, PTX)
    prognosis (*See also* prog, progn, Prx)
    prophylaxis (*See also* proph, prop.,
      prophy)

PXA

    pleomorphic xanthoastrocytoma

PXAT

    paroxysmal atrial tachycardia (*See also*
      PAT)

PXE

    pseudoxanthoma elasticum

PXF

    pseudoexfoliation (*See also* PSX)

PXM

    projection x-ray microscopy

PXS

    dental prophylaxis [cleaning]
    pseudoexfoliation syndrome (*See also*
      PES)

PY, P/Y

    pack-year [cigarettes] (*See also* pkyrs)
    person-year

Py

    phosphopyridoxal
    pyrene
    pyridine

PYA

    psychoanalysis (*See also* PA, PSAn,
      psychoan)

PyC

    pyogenic culture
    pyrolytic carbon

PYD

    pyridinium
    pyridinoline

PYE

    peptone and yeast extract [medium]
    person-years of exposure

PYG

    peptone-yeast [extract]-glucose [broth]

PYGM

    peptone-yeast-glucose-maltose [broth]

PYHx

    pack per year history

PYLL

    potential years of life lost

PYM

    psychosomatic [medicine]

PYME

    pyloric metaplasia

PYP

    pyrophosphate (*See also* PP, Pyro)

PYR

    person-year rad
    pyrrolidonyl arylamidase

PyR

    L-pyrrolidonyl-beta-naphthylamide

Pyr

    pyridine
    pyrimidine
    pyroglutamic acid
    pyruvate

Pyro

    pyrophosphate (*See also* PP, PYP)

pyro-Glu-His-Pro-amide

    pyroglutamyl-histidyl-proline amide

PyrP

    pyridoxal phosphate

PYS

    pyriform (piriform) sinus

PYY

    peptide YY

PZ

    pancreozymin
    peripheral zone
    prazosin
    pregnancy zone
    proliferative zone

Pz

    parietal midline [zero] electrode
      placement [electroencephalography]

pz

    piéze [metric unit of pressure]

PzB

    parenzyme, buccal

PZ-CCK

    pancreozymin-cholecystokinin

PZD

    partial zona dissection (drilling)

PZE

    piezoelectric

Pzf

    zero-flow pressure

PZI

    protamine zinc insulin

PZM

    pressure zone microphone

PZP

    pregnancy zone protein

PZR

    posterior zygomatic root

Q

blood flow (*See also* BF, Q_B)
cardiac output (*See also* CO)
clerical perception [General Aptitude Test Battery]
electrocardiographic wave
1,4-glucan branching enzyme
flow volume
flow rate
glutamine (*See also* Gln)
perfusion [flow]
Quaalude
quadriceps (*See also* quad)
quantitative (*See also* qt, quant)
quantity (*See also* qty)
quartile (*See also* q)
quaternary
Q (Queensland) (query) [fever]
question[able] (*See also* quest.)
quinacrine [chromosome detection fluorescent method]
quotient
radiant energy [electromagnetic wave]
reaction energy [nuclear]
reactive power [AC power system]

⚠ **Q°, q°**
every hour ⚠

⚠ **Q1°**
every hour around the clock ⚠

⚠ **Q2°**
every two hours around the clock ⚠

q
four [L. *quattuor*]
frequency of rarer allele of a gene pair
long arm of chromosome
quartile (*See also* Q)
quintal

q.
each (every) [L. *quodque*]

QA
quality assessment (assurance)
Quatrefages angle [parietal angle] (*See also* Q angle)
quinaldic acid
quisqualic acid

QAC
before every meal [L. *quodque ante cibum*]
quaternary ammonium compound (*See also* quat)

QAFT
quantitative autonomic functioning testing

QALE
quality-adjusted life expectancy

QALY
quality-adjusted life-year

⚠ **QAM**
quality assurance monitor
every morning [L. *quaque ante meridiem*] ⚠

Q angle
Quatrefages angle [parietal angle] (*See also* QA)

Q-angle
quadriceps angle

QAP
quality assurance program

QAR
quality assurance reagent
quantitative autoradiograph(y) (autoradiogram)

QA/RM
quality assurance/risk management

QAS
quality-adjusted survival
quality assurance standard

QAT
quality assurance technical [material]

QAUR
quality assurance and utilization review

QB
quantitative (electrophysiological) battery
whole blood (*See also* B, WB, W Bld)

Q_B
blood flow (*See also* BF, Q)

QBC
quantitative buffy coat

QBCA
quantitative buffy-coat analysis

QBV
whole blood volume (*See also* WBV)

QC
quad cane
quality control
Quick catheter

Qc
capillary blood flow [perfusion]

QCA
quantitative coronary angiography (arteriography)

QCD
quantum chromodynamics

QCL
quadrigeminal cistern lipoma

Q_{CO2}
quantity of carbon dioxide [mL per mg tissue dry weight per hour]

QC-PCR
quantitative competitive polymerase chain reaction

Q_{CSF}
rate of cerebrospinal fluid [uptake from cerebrospinal space by arachnoid villi]

QCSI
quantitative chemical shift imaging

QCT
quantified computed tomography
quantitative computed tomography

QCU
qualitative coronary ultrasound

⚠ **QD**
dialysate flow
every day [L. *quaque die*] (*See also* q.d.) ⚠

⚠ **q.d.**
every day [L. *quaque die*] (*See also* QD) ⚠

QDA
quadratic discriminant analysis [statistics]

⚠ **QDAM, q.d.a.m.**
once daily in the morning ⚠

QDE
quantum detection efficiency

QDN
quantum dot nanocrystals

⚠ **QDPM, q.d.p.m.**
once daily in the evening ⚠

QDR
quantitative digital radiography

QDS
qigong deviation syndrome

QE
Queyrat erythroplasia
quinidine effect

QECT
quantitative contrast-enhanced computed tomography

⚠ **QED**
every even day (*See also* q.e.d.) ⚠
quantum electrodynamics
quick and early diagnosis

⚠ **q.e.d.**
that which is to be demonstrated [L. *quod erat demonstrandum*]
every even day (*See also* QED) ⚠

QEE
quadriceps extension exercise

QEEG
quantitative electroencephalograph(y) (electroencephalogram)

QEMG
quantitative electromyography

QET
Quality Extinction Test

QEW
quick early warning

QF
quadratus femoris
quality factor [relative biologic effectiveness]
quick freeze

Qf
rate of fluid filtration

QFD
quartz fiber dosimeter

Q-FISH
quantitative fluorescence in situ hybridization

QF-PCR
quantitative fluorescence polymerase chain reaction

Q fract
quick fraction

QFV
Q fever vaccine

QGS
quantitative gated single-photon emission compared tomography (SPECT)

⚠ **q.h.**
every hour [L. *quaque hora*] ⚠

⚠ **q.2h.**
every two hours [L. *quaque secunda hora*] ⚠

⚠ **q.3h.**
every three hours [L. *quaque tertia hora*] ⚠

⚠ **q.4h.**
every four hours [L. *quaque quarta hora*] (*See also* QQH, q.q.h.) ⚠

⚠ **QHS**
at bedtime [L. *hora somni hour of sleep*] (*See also* q.h.s.) ⚠
quantitative hepatobiliary scintigraphy

⚠ **q.h.s.**
at bedtime [L. *hora somni hour of sleep*] (*See also* QHS)
every night ⚠

QI
quality improvement
Quetelet Index [body mass index]

QIAD
Quantitative Inventory of Alcohol Disorders

QID
four times daily [L. *quater in die*] (*See also* q.i.d.)

⚠ **q.i.d.**
four times daily [L. *quater in die*] (*See also* QID) ⚠

QIE
quantitative immunoelectrophoresis

QIF
Quadriplegia Index of Function

QIg
quantitative immunoglobulin

QIMT
quantitative intima media thickness

QJ
quadriceps jerk

QKD
time between QRS wave and last Korotkoff sound on blood pressure measurement

QL
quadratus lumborum
quality of life

⚠ **q.l.**
as much as desired (quantum libet) ⚠

QLF
quantitative light induced fluorescence

QLI
Quality of Life Index

QLQ
Quality of Life Questionnaire

QLQ-C30
Quality of Life Questionnaire-C30

QLS
Quality of Life Scale
quasielastic laser light-scattering spectroscope

qlty
quality (*See also* qual)

QLV
quasilinear viscoelastic [model]

QM
quantization matrix [imaging]
Quénu-Muret [sign]
quinacrine mustard

Qmax
maximal flow rate

QMB
qualified Medicare beneficiary

QMI
Q-wave myocardial infarct[ion]

QMM
qigong meridian massage

QMRI, qMRI
quantitative magnetic resonance imaging

QMT
quantitative muscle testing

QMV
quadricusp mitral valve
quantified mechanical vibration

QMWS
quasimorphine withdrawal syndrome

⚠ **q.n.**
every nighttime or bedtime ⚠

QNA
quadriceps neutral angle

QNB
quinuclidinyl benzilate [chemical weapon]

⚠ **QNS, q.n.s.**
quantity not sufficient ⚠

QNST
Quick Neurological Screening Test

QO$_2$, Q$_{O2}$
oxygen consumption
oxygen quotient
oxygen utilization

QOC
Quality of Contact

⚠ **QOD, q.o.d.**
every other day [L. *quaque aler die*] ⚠

QOL
quality of life

QOLI
Quality of Life Interview
Quality of Life Inventory

QOLIE-31
Quality of Life in Epilepsy [short form]

QOLRD
Quality of Life in Reflux and Dyspepsia [questionnaire]

QOM
quality of motion
quality of movement

QP
quadrant pain
quanti-Pirquet [reaction]

Qp
pulmonary blood flow (*See also* PBF)

⚠ **q.p.**
at will [quantum placeat] ⚠

QPC
quadrigeminal plate cistern
quality of patient care

Qpc
pulmonary capillary blood flow

QPCR, Q-PCR
quantitative polymerase chain reaction

QPD
quadrature phase detector
qualitative platelet defect

QPEEG
quantitative pharmacoelectroencephalography

⚠ **QPM, q.p.m.**
each evening [L. *quaque post meridiem*] ⚠

QPOS
Quality Point of Service

Qp:Qs
left-to-right shunt ratio [electrocardiography]
pulmonary to systemic flow ratio
pulmonary to systemic circulation ratio

QPT
Quick prothrombin time (*See also* QT)

QPVT
Quick Picture Vocabulary Test

⚠ **q.q.**
each ⚠

⚠ **QQH, q.q.h.**
every four hours [L. *quaque quarta hora*] (*See also* q.4h.) ⚠

QR
quadriradial
quality review
quieting reflex (response)
quiet room
quinaldine red

q.r.
quantity is correct [L. *quantum rectum*]

QRB
Quality Review Bulletin

Q-RB
electrocardiographic time-wave interval

QRC
qualitative radiocardiography

QRDR
quinolone resistance-determining region [gene locus]

QRE
quality-related event

QRN
quasiresonant nucleus

QRNG
quinolone-resistant *Neisseria gonorrhoeae*

QRS
electrocardiographic wave [complex or interval]

QRS-ST
electrocardiographic junction between QRS complex and ST segment

QRS-T
electrocardiographic angle between QRS and T vectors

QRZ
wheal reaction time [Ger. *Quaddel Reaktion Zeit*]

QS
every shift
Q-switched [laser]

quadriceps set
quadrilateral socket
quantitation standard
quantity sufficient (*See also* q.s.)
quiet sleep

QS2
total electromechanical systole

Qs
systemic blood flow

q.s.
quantity sufficient (*See also* QS)

QSAC
quadrant sparing acetabular component

QSAR
quantitative structure-activity relationship

QSART
quantitative sudomotor axon reflex test

QSC
quasistatic compliance

QS$_2$I
shortened electrochemical systole

Q sign
Quant sign [rickets]

Qsp
physiologic shunt flow

QSPV
quasistatic pressure volume

Qs:Qt
intrapulmonary shunt ratio
right-to-left shunt ratio

Qsrel
relative shunt flow

QSRL
Q-switched ruby laser

QSS
quantitative sacroiliac scintigraphy

QST
quantitative sensory testing

Q-S
Queckenstedt-Stookey [test for subarachnoid channel blockage]

QSYAG
Q-switched neodymium: YAG laser

QT
Quick test [eponymous test for amount of prothrombin and clotting time] (*See also* QPT)

Q-T
electrocardiographic interval from the beginning of QRS complex to end of the T wave
quick test [any rapid laboratory or psychology test]

Qt
quiet (*See also* qt, QU)

qt
quantitative (*See also* Q, quant)
quart (*See also* Q, qt)
quiet (*See also* Qt, QU)

QTB
quadriceps tendon bearing
QTC
quantitative tip culture
QTc, QT$_c$
QT corrected for heart rate
QTd
QT dispersion
qter
end of long arm of chromosome
QTL
quantitative trait locus
Q-TWIST, Q-TWiST
quality-adjusted time without symptoms
or toxicity
qty
quantity (*See also* quant)
QU
quiet (*See also* Qt, qt)
quad
quadrant
quadriceps (*See also* Q)
quadrilateral
quadriplegia (quadriplegic)
quad ex
quadriceps exercise
quadrupl.
four times as much [L. *quadruplicato*]
qual
qualitative
quality (*See also* qlty)
qual anal
qualitative analysis
QUALY
quality-adjusted life-year
QUALYS
quality-adjusted life-year saved
quant
quantitative (*See also* Q, qt)
quantity (*See also* Q, qty)
quar
quarantine
QUART
quadrantectomy, axillary dissection,
radiation therapy
quart.
fourth [L. *quartus*]
quarterly
quasi-CW
quasi-continuous wave
quat
quaternary ammonium compound
(*See also* QAC)
quer
querulous
QUEST
Quality of Upper Extremities Test

Quality, Utilization, Effectiveness,
Statistically Tabulated
quick estimation by sequential testing
quest.
question(able) (*See also* Q)
QuICCC
Questionnaire for Identifying Children
with Chronic Conditions
QUICHA
quantitative inhalation challenge
apparatus
QUICKI
quantitative insulin sensitivity check
index
quint.
fifth [L. *quintus*]
QUIPS
quantitative image processing system
QuMA
quantitative microsatellite analysis
[polymerase chain reaction]
quotid.
daily [L. *quotide*]
QuPID
Qualitative Platform Immunoassay
Device
QUS
quantitative ultrasound
q.v.
which see [literature citation] [L. *quod
vide*]
QW
every week
quality of working [life] (*See also*
QWL)
QWB
Quality of Well-Being (scale)
QWB-SA
Quality of Well-Being Scale
Self-Administered
QWE
every weekend
⚠ **q. 4 wk.**
every four weeks ⚠
⚠ **q. wk**
once a week ⚠
QWL
quality of working life (*See also* QW)
QWMI
Q-wave myocardial infarct(ion)
QWMS
quantitative wall motion
score
QYBV
Qalyub virus
QYD
Qi (and) Yin deficiency

R

arginine (*See also* Arg)
roentgen-ray exposure unit [Behnken, obsolete]
[Broadbent] registration point [craniometric]
electrocardiographic wave [in QRS complex]
gas constant [8.315 joules]
race (*See also* RC)
racemic (*See also* r, rac)
ramus
range
rare
rate
ratio
rationale
raw
react(ing) (reaction) (*See also* Rxn)
recessive
rectified average
rectum (rectal) (*See also* rect)
red [indicator color]
reference (*See also* ref)
regimen
regression coefficient [statistics]
regular (*See also* reg)
regulator [gene]
rejection [factor]
relapse
relation (*See also* REL)
relaxation
release [factor] (*See also* RF)
remission (*See also* REM, Rm)
repressor
resazurin
residuum
resistance determinant [plasmid] (*See also* RD)
resistance [electrical] (*See also* RES)
respiration (*See also* resp)
response (*See also* resp, Rs)
rest [cell cycle]
resting
restricted
reticulocyte (*See also* RET, RETIC, retic)
retinoscopy
review (*See also* REV, rev)
rhythm
rib
ribose (*See also* Rib)
Rickettsia
right (*See also* (R), RT, Rt)

Rinne [hearing test]
roentgen (*See also* r, ROE, roent)
root (*See also* rad)
rough [bacterial colony]
routine (*See also* rout., RTN)
rub
side chain in amino acid formula
stimulus [G. *Reiz*] (*See also* S, ST)
take [L. *recipe*] (*See also* Rx)
total response (*See also* TR)

R0
no residual tumor [TNM classification]

R1
longitudinal relaxivity
microscopic residual tumor [TNM classification]

R2
macroscopic residual tumor [TNM classification]
transverse relaxivity

R#1
good risk [for anesthesia]

R#2
fairly good risk [for anesthesia]

R#3
poor risk [for anesthesia]

R#4
very poor risk [for anesthesia]

R$_0$
resting radium

°R
[degree] Rankine [obsolete temperature scale]
[degree] Réaumur [obsolete temperature scale]

+R
Rinne [hearing] test positive

(R)
rectal
right (*See also* R, RT, Rt)

−R
Rinne [hearing] test negative

r
product moment [statistics]
racemic (*See also* R, rac)
radius
recombinant
reproductive potential
ring chromosome [1–22]
roentgen (*See also* R, ROE, roent)
round

r.
far [point] [L. *remotum*]

r^2
coefficient of determination

R1, RI
    type I regulatory dimer
R2, RII
    type II regulatory dimer
RA
    radial artery
    radioactive
    radiographic absorptiometry
    radionuclide angiograph(y) (angiogram)
      (*See also* RNA, RNG)
    ragocyte [rheumatic arthritis cell]
    ragweed antigen
    rales
    reactive arthritis (*See also* ReA)
    reading age
    readmission (*See also* RDM, RE,
      readm)
    reciprocal asymmetrical
    refractory anemia
    refractory ascites
    regional anesthesia
    remittance advice
    renal artery
    renin activity
    renin-angiotensin
    repeat action [drugs]
    residual air
    retinoic acid
    rheumatoid agglutinin (*See also* RhA,
      Rh agglut)
    rheumatoid arthritis
    rhinocerebral aspergillosis
    right angle
    right arm
    right atrial
    right atrium
    right auricle [obsolete for heart]
    Rokitansky-Aschoff [sinus] (*See also*
      RAS)
    room air
    rotational angiography
    rotational atherectomy
5α-RA
    5-alpha-reductase activity
R_A
    airways resistance (*See also* AR, RAW,
      R_{AW}, R_{AW}, R (AW))
Ra
    radium
    Rayleigh number [fluid mechanics]
Ra-A, B, C, C1, C2, D, E, F
    decay products of radium
^{226}Ra
    radium-226
rA
    riboadenylate
RAA
    renin-angiotensin-aldosterone [system]
      (*See also* RAAS)

    right aortic arch
    right atrial abnormality
    right atrial appendage
RAAA
    ruptured abdominal aortic aneurysm
RA-ABG
    room air arterial blood gas
RAAGG
    rheumatoid arthritis agglutinin
RAAPI
    resting ankle-arm pressure index
RAAS
    renin-angiotensin-aldosterone system
      (*See also* RAA)
rAAT
    recombinant alpha-1 antitrypsin
RAB
    rabies vaccine, not otherwise
      specified
    remote afterload (afterloading)
      brachytherapy
    rice, applesauce, and banana [diet]
Rab
    rabbit
RABA
    rabbit antibladder antibody
    radioantigen-binding assay
RABDEV
    rabies vaccine, duck embryo
      culture
RABFRhl-2
    rabies vaccine, diploid
      fetal-rhesus-lung-2 cell line
RABG
    room air blood gas
RABHDCV
    rabies vaccine, human diploid cell
      culture
RABig
    rabies immune globulin
      immunoglobulin
RAbody
    right atrium body
RABP
    retinoic acid-binding protein
RABPCEC
    rabies vaccine, purified chick embryo
      cell culture
RAC
    radial artery catheter
    retinal artery collapse
    right antecubital
    right arterial catheter
    right atrial contraction
RAC3
    receptor-associated coactivator 3
rac
    racemate
    racemic (*See also* R, r)

RACAT
rapid acquisition computed axial tomography

RACCO
right anterior caudocranial oblique

RACE
rapid antigen uptake into cytosol enterocytes

RACT
recalcified (whole-blood) activated clotting time

RAD
ionizing radiation unit [obsolete]
radical
radiology (*See also* Rad, Radiol)
reactive airways disease
reactive attachment disorder
regional alveolar damage
restricted activity day
right anterior descending
right atrial diameter
right axis deviation
roentgen administered dose

Rad
radiology (*See also* RAD, Radiol)
radiotherapy (*See also* RADIO, Rad Ther, RATx, RoRx, RT, RTx, RXT)

rad
radial
radian [measure of angle]
radiation (roentgen) absorbed dose [symbol rd]
radiculitis
root [L. *radix*] (*See also* R)

RADA
right acromion dorsoanterior (acromiodorsoanterior) [fetal position]

RADAR
Rapid Assessment of Disease Activity in Rheumatology [questionnaire]

RADCA
right anterior descending coronary artery

rad imp
radium implant

RADIO
radiotherapy (*See also* Rad, Rad Ther, RATx, RoRx, RT, RTx, RXT)

Radiol
radiology (*See also* RAD, Rad)

RADISH
rheumatoid arthritis, diffuse idiopathic skeletal hyperostosis

RAD ISO VENO BILAT
radioactive isotopic venogram, bilateral

RADIUS
routine antenatal diagnostic imaging with ultrasound

RADIV
Radi virus

RadLV
radiation leukemia virus

RADP
right acromion dorsoposterior (acromiodorsoposterior) [fetal position]

RADS
rapid assay delivery system
reactive airways disease (dysfunction) syndrome
retrospective assessment of drug safety
Reynolds Adolescent Depression Scale

rad/s
radian per second

RADT
rapid antigen-detection test

Rad Ther
radiotherapy (*See also* Rad, RADIO, RATx, RoRx, RT, RTx, RXT)

RADTS
rabbit antidog-thymus serum

Rad Ul
radius-ulna

RADWASTE
radioactive waste

RAE
retinol activity equivalent
right atrial enlargement
Ring-Adair-Elwyn [orofacial surgery ET tube]

RaE
rabbit erythrocyte

RAEB
refractory anemia with excess blasts

RAEBT, RAEB-t
refractory anemia with excess blasts in transformation

RAEM
refractory anemia with excess myeloblasts

RAF
rapid atrial fibrillation
rheumatoid arthritis factor

RAFF
rectus abdominis free flap

RAFT
Rehabilitative Addicted Family Treatment

RAG
ragweed (*See also* RW)
recombination activation gene
room air gas

Rd
rutherford [unit of radioactivity]
rd
rad [metric unit radiation dose]
(*See also* rad)
RDA
recommended daily (dietary) allowance
representational difference analysis
right dorsum anterior (dorsoanterior)
[fetal position]
right ductus arteriosus
rubidium dihydrogenarsenate
RdA
reading age
RDB
randomized double-blind [trial]
research and development board
RDC
research diagnostic criteria
RDD
radiation dispersal device
random digital dialing
renal dose dopamine
RDDA
recommended daily dietary allowance
RDDP
RNA-dependent DNA polymerase
(*See also* RDPase)
RDE
receptor-destroying enzyme
remote data entry
RDEA
right deviation of electrical axis
RDEB
recessive dystrophic epidermolysis
bullosa
RDES
remote data entry system
RDF
rapid dissolution formula
rotary door flap
RDFC
recurring digital fibroma of childhood
RDFS
ratio of decayed and filled surfaces
RDFT
ratio of decayed and filled teeth
RDG
retrograde duodenogastroscopy
right dorsogluteal
RDHBF
regional distribution of hepatic blood
flow
RDI
recommended daily (dietary) intake
relative dose intensity
respiratory distress (disturbance) index
Retirement Descriptive Index
rupture-delivery interval

RDIH
right direct inguinal hernia
RDLBBB
rate-dependent left bundle branch
block
RDLS
Reynell Development Language Scales
[psychologic test]
RDM
reactive drug metabolite
readmission (*See also* RA, RE, readm)
right deltoid muscle
rod disc membrane
rDNA
recombinant deoxyribonucleic acid
(DNA)
ribosomal deoxyribonucleic acid (DNA)
⚠ **RDOD**
retinal detachment, oculus dexter (right
eye) ⚠
⚠ **RDOS**
retinal detachment, oculus sinister (left
eye) ⚠
RDP
radiopharmaceutical drug product
random-donor platelet
right dorsum posterior (dorsoposterior)
[fetal position]
RDPA
right descending pulmonary artery
RDPase
RNA-dependent DNA polymerase
(*See also* RDDP)
RDPE
reticular degeneration of pigment
epithelium
RDQ
respiratory disease questionnaire
RdQ
reading quotient (*See also* RQ)
RDR
rate-drop response
RDRC
radioactive drug research committee
RDRV
rhesus diploid [cell strain] rabies
vaccine
RDS
radioisotope delivery system
random-dot stereogram
Raskin Depression Scale
respiratory distress syndrome
reticuloendothelial depressing substance
rDsg
recombinant desmoglein
RDT
regular [hemo]dialysis treatment
retinal damage threshold
routine dialysis therapy

RDTD
referral, diagnosis, treatment, discharge
RDU
recreational drug use
RDVT
recurrent deep vein thrombosis
RDW
red [blood cell] distribution width
[index]
RDWr
reticulocyte distribution width
RE
regarding [concerning]
racemic epinephrine
radiodermatitis emulsion
radium emanation
Rasmussen encephalitis
readmission (*See also* RA, RDM,
readm)
rectal examination
reflux esophagitis
regional enteritis
regular education
renal and electrolyte
renal excretion
resistive exercise
resting energy
reticuloendothelial
retinol equivalent
right ear (*See also* AD, a.d.)
right extremity
right eye (*See also* OD, o.d.)
ring enhancement
rostral end
rowing ergometer
R&E
research and education
rest and exercise
round and equal
R↑E
right upper extremity (*See also* RUE,
RUX)
RE√
recheck
R$_E$
respiratory exchange ratio (*See also*
RER)
R$_e$
Reynolds number [fluid mechanics]
Re
rhenium
^{186}Re
rhenium-186
^{188}Re
rhenium-188
REA
radiation emergency area

radioenzymatic assay
renal anastomosis
restriction endonuclease analysis
restriction enzyme analysis
right ear advantage
ReA
reactive arthritis (*See also* RA)
REAB
reactive anemia with excess blasts
READ
restriction endonuclease analysis
readm
readmission (*See also* R, RA, RDM,
RE)
REAL
Revised European-American
[Classification of] Lymphoid
[Neoplasms]
REALM
Rapid Estimation of Adult Literacy in
Medicine
REAS
reasonably expected as safe
REB
roentgen-equivalent biologic
rubber-reinforced bandage
R-EBD-HS
recessive epidermolysis bullosa
dystrophica–Hallopeau-Siemens
[syndrome]
REC
radioelectrocomplexing
rearend collision
receptor
recommend(ation)
record
recovery
recreation
recur (recurrence) (recurrent)
right external carotid
rec
reactive
recent
recombinant chromosome
RECA
right external carotid artery
recd, rec'd
received
RE CEL
reticulum cell
RECG
radioelectrocardiograph(y)
(radioelectrocardiogram) (*See also*
RCG)
recip
recipient
reciprocal

recom
  smallest unit of DNA capable of
    recombination
recond
  recondition(ed)
  reconditioning
reconstr
  reconstruction
RecOS
  reconstruction occlusal surface
recryst
  recrystallization
rect
  rectal (*See also* R)
  rectification (rectified)
  rectum (*See also* R)
  rectus [muscle]
recur.
  recurrence (recurrent)
RED
  radiation experience data
  rapid erythrocyte degeneration
  rectal evacuatory disorder
  reproductive endocrine disorder
  rigid external distraction
Re-D
  reevaluation deadline
red.
  reduce
  reducing
  reduction (*See also* redn)
redn
  reduction (*See also* red.)
redox
  oxidation-reduction
REDS
  receptors for endogenous danger
    signals
  remote endoscopic digital spectroscopy
RED SUBS
  reducing substances
REE
  rapid extinction effect
  rare earth element
  resting energy expenditure
re-ed
  reeducation
REEDS
  retention [of tears], ectrodactyly,
    ectodermal dysplasia, and strange
    [hair, skin, teeth syndrome]
REEG
  radioelectroencephalograph(y)
    (radioelelectroencephalogram)
R-EEG
  resting electroencephalogram
REEL
  Receptive-Expressive Emergent
    Language (Scale)

REEL-2
  Receptive-Expressive Emergent
    Language [Scale], Second Edition
ReEND
  reproductive endocrinology
REEP
  right end-expiratory pressure
  role exchange/education-practice
REF
  ejection fraction at rest
  referred
  refused
  renal erythropoietic factor
  right ventricular ejection fraction
ref
  reference (*See also* R)
  reflex (*See also* Refl)
Ref Doc
  referring doctor
REFI
  regional ejection fraction image
    (imaging)
ref ind
  refractive index (*See also* RI, RI)
Refl
  reflect(ion)
  reflex (*See also* ref)
Ref Phys
  referring physician
REFRAD
  released from active duty
REG
  radiation exposure guide
  radioencephalograph(y)
    (radioencephalogram)
  random event generator
  regenerating gene I
  regression analysis
  rheoencephalograph(y)
reg
  regarding
  region
  regular
  regulation
Reg block
  regional block anesthesia
regen
  regenerate
  regeneration
reg rhy
  regular rhythm
reg R&R
  regular rate and rhythm (*See also* RRR)
reg. umb.
  umbilical region [L. *regio umbilici*]
regurg
  regurgitation
REH
  renin essential hypertension

REHAB, rehab
rehabilitate(d) (rehabilitation)
REL
rate of energy loss
recommended exposure level (limit)
relative (related) (relation)
religion
resting expiratory level
RELE
resistive exercise of lower extremities
REM
rapid eye movement [sleep] (*See also* REMS)
recent event memory
remarried
remission
reticular erythematous mucinosis
return electrode monitor
rem
radiation (roentgen) equivalent in man
removal
REMA
repetitive excess mixed anhydride [method]
REMAB
radiation-equivalent-manikin absorption
REMBL
retroflexed endoscopic multiple band ligation
REMCAL
radiation-equivalent-manikin calibration
REMP
roentgen-equivalent-man period
REMS
rapid eye movement sleep (*See also* REM)
REN, ren
renal (*See also* RN)
ren mai channel [acupuncture]
reproductive endocrinology
REO
Receptive-Expressive Observation [Scale]
respiratory enteric orphan [virus]
REON
renal epithelioid oxyphilic neoplasm
ReoV
reovirus
REP
rapid electrophoresis
reactive eosinophilic pleuritis
repair
repeat (*See also* rep., rept)
report (*See also* rept)
resistive exercise products
rest-exercise program
retrograde pyelograph(y) (pyelogram) (*See also* retro pyelo, RGP, RP, RPG)

Rochester Epidemiology Project
roentgen equivalent-physical
[surgical] repair
rep.
let it be repeated [L. *repetatur*]
rep B&S
repetitive bending and stooping
REPC
reticuloendothelial phagocytic capacity
REP CK
rapid electrophoresis creatine kinase
REPE
reexpansion pulmonary edema
REPL
recurrent early pregnancy loss
r-EPO
recombinant human erythropoietin
repol
repolarization
REP-PCR, Rep-PCR
repetitive extragenic palindromic polymerase chain reaction
reprep
re-preparation
REPS
reactive extensor postural synergy
repetitions
rept
repeat (*See also* REP)
report (*See also* REP)
Re-PUVA
combination retinoid and PUVA therapy
RE-Q
recuperation [period]
req
request(ed)
requir(ed)
REQF
wrong test requested-floor error
RER
peak respiratory ratio
renal excretion rate
respiratory exchange ratio (*See also* R_E)
rough endoplasmic reticulum
RER−
replication error negative
RER+
replication error positive
RES
resistance [electrical] (*See also* R)
radionuclide esophageal scintigraphy
recurrent erosion syndrome
resection
research
reserve
residence

RES *(continued)*
residue
reticuloendothelial system
RESC, resc
resuscitation (*See also* resus)
resist. ex.
resistive exercise
resp
respective(ly)
respiration (*See also* R)
respiratory
response (*See also* R, RS)
responsible
RESP-A
respiratory battery, acute
REST
Raynaud [phenomenon], esophageal
[motor dysfunction], sclerodactyly, and
telangiectasia [syndrome]
regressive electric shock (electroshock)
therapy
restoration
Restricted Environment Stimulation
Therapy
reticulospinal tract
resus
resuscitation (*See also* RESC, resc)
RESV
Restan virus
RET
retarded (*See also* rtd)
rational-emotive therapy
rearranged during transfection
retention
reticulocyte (*See also* R, RETIC,
retic)
retina
retired (*See also* ret, rtd)
return (*See also* rtn)
right esotropia
ret
rad equivalent therapeutic
retired (*See also* RET)
RETA
rete testis aspiration
RETC
rat embryo tissue culture
ret cath
retention catheter (*See also* RC)
ret detach
retinal detachment
RE-TEM
rectal expander-assisted transanal
endoscopic microsurgery
RETHINK
recognize, empathize, think, hear,
integrate, notice, keep
RETIC, retic
reticulocyte (*See also* R, RET)

retic ct
reticulocyte count
retro pyelo
retrograde pyelogram (*See also* REP,
RGP, RP, RPG)
RETRX
retraction
RETUL
reticulum cell
RetV
retrovirus
Re-Tx
retransplant(ation)
REU
rectal endoscopic ultrasonography
reu
radiation effect unit
REUE
resistive exercises to upper extremities
REUS
rectal endoscopic ultrasonography
REV, rev
reticuloendotheliosis virus
reversal
review (*See also* R)
revision
revolution
room's eye view
Rev
ribonucleic acid (RNA) encoding viral
[sequence-specific RNA-binding
protein]
REVL
to be reviewed by laboratory
[pathologist]
rev/min
revolution per minute
Rev of Sys
review of systems
REx
resistive exercise
re-x
reexamination
REZ
root exit zone
RF
radial fiber [of cochlea]
radiofrequency
rapid filling
rate of flow [chromatography]
receptive field [of visual cortex]
recognition factor
reduction fixation
reflecting [platelet]
regurgitant fraction
relative flow
relative fluorescence
release factor (*See also* R)
releasing factor

R

renal failure
replicative form
resistance factor
resorcinol-formaldehyde [resin]
respiratory failure
respiratory frequency
restricted fluids
retardation factor
reticular formation
retroflexed
retroperitoneal fibromatosis
rheumatic fever
rheumatoid factor
riboflavin
right foot
ring finger
risk factor
root [canal] filling
rosette formation

RF6
rejection-free survival at 6 months
[posttransplantation]

R&F
radiographic and fluoroscopic

Rf
rutherfordium

rFVIIa
recombinant factor VIIA [7a]

RFXAP
regulatory factor X (RFX)-associated
protein

RFA
radiofluorescent antibody
radiofrequency ablation
right femoral artery
right forearm
right frontoanterior [fetal position]
(See also FDA)

RFB
radial flow chromatography
residual functional capacity
retained foreign body
rheumatoid factor binding

RFb
respiratory feedback

RFC
radiofrequency coil
radiofrequency current
reduced folate carrier
retrograde femoral catheter
right frontal craniotomy
rosette-forming cell

RFCA
radiofrequency catheter ablation

RFD
reference dose
residue-free diet
rice-fruit diet

RFDT
Reach in Four Directions Test

RFE
relative fluorescence efficiency
return flow enema

RF-FAST
radiofrequency spoiled Fourier-acquired
steady state

RFFF
radial forearm free flap

RFFIT
rapid fluorescent focus inhibition test

RFg
visual fields by Goldmann-type
perimeter

rFGF-2
recombinant fibroblast growth factor 2

RFH
right femoral hernia

RFI
recurrence-free interval
renal failure index

RFIED
round femoral inferior epiphysis
dysplasia

RFIPC
Rating Form of IBD (inflammatory
bowel disease) Patient Concerns

RFL
radionuclide functional
lymphoscintigraphy
recurrent fetal loss
right frontolateral [fetal position]

RFLA
rheumatoid factorlike activity

RFLC
resistant Friend leukemia cell

RFLF
retained fetal lung fluid

RFLP
restriction fragment length
polymorphism (See also RLP)

RFLS
rheumatoid factorlike substance

RFOL
results to follow

RFP
rapid filling period
recurrent facial paralysis
renal function panel
request for payment
request for proposal
ret-fused protein
right frontoposterior [fetal position]
(See also FDP)

RF-PMR
radiofrequency percutaneous myocardial
revascularization

RFR
  rapid filling rate
  refraction
RFS
  rapid frozen section
  refeeding syndrome
  relapse-free survival
  renal function study
rFSH
  recombinant follicle-stimulating hormone
RFT
  respiratory function test
  right fibrous trigone
  right frontotransverse [fetal position]
    (*See also* FDT)
  rod-and-frame test
  routine fever therapy
RFTA
  radiofrequency thermal ablation
RFTB
  riboflavin tetrabutyrate
RFTC
  radiofrequency thermocoagulation
RFTSW
  right foot switch
RFTVR
  radiofrequency tissue volume
    reduction
RFUT
  radioactive fibrinogen uptake
RFV
  reason for visit
  right femoral vein
  Royal Farm virus
RFVII
  Reading-Free Vocational Interest
    Inventory
RFVTR
  radiofrequency volumetric tissue
    reduction
RFW
  rapid filling wave
RFX
  reflex
RG
  regurgitated [infant feeding]
  retrograde
  right gluteus (gluteal)
  Rodgers [antibody in Chido-Rodgers
    blood group]
R/G
  red/green
RGA
  right gastroepiploic artery
RGAS
  retained gastric antrum syndrome
RGBMT
  renal glomerular basement membrane
    thickness

RGC
  radio gas (radiogas) chromatography
  remnant gastric cancer
  respiratory glycoconjugate
  retinal ganglion cell
  right giant cell
RGD
  range-gated Doppler
RGE
  relative gas expansion
  respiratory gas equation
RGEA
  right gastroepiploic artery
RGEPS
  Rucker-Gable Educational Programming
    Scale
RGH
  rat growth hormone
  recurrent gross hematuria
RGM
  rapidly growing mycobacteria
  recurrent glioblastoma multiforme
  right gluteus maximus [muscle]
  right gluteus medius [muscle]
RGMT
  reciprocal geometric mean titer
RGO
  reciprocal gait orthotic (orthosis)
  reciprocating (reciprocation) gait orthosis
RGP
  retrograde pyelograph(y) (pyelogram)
    (*See also* REP, retro pyelo, RP, RPG)
  rigid gas-permeable [contact lens]
  rural general practitioner
RGR
  relative growth rate
RGS5
  regulator of G protein signaling protein
    5
RGT
  reversed gastric tube
RGV
  Rio Grande virus
RH
  radial hemolysis
  radiant heat
  radical hysterectomy
  radiologic health
  reactive hyperemia
  recurrent herpes
  regional heparinization
  regulatory hormone
  relative humidity
  releasing hormone
  renal hemolysis
  rest home
  retinal hemorrhage
  rheumatoid
  right hand

right hemisphere
right hyperphoria
room humidifier

Rh
rhesus [blood factor] (*See also* Rhf)
rhinion [craniometric]
rhodium

Rh+, Rh pos
rhesus positive

Rh−, Rh neg
rhesus negative

rh
rheuma (*See also* rheum)
rheumatic (*See also* rheum)
rhonchi

r/h, R/h
roentgen per hour (*See also* R/hr)

RHA
right hepatic artery

RhA
rheumatoid agglutinin (*See also* RA, Rh
agglut)

Rha
L-rhamnose

rHA
recombinant human albumin

Rh agglut
rheumatoid agglutinins (*See also* RA,
RhA)

RHAMM
receptor for hyaluronan-mediated
motility

rhAPC
recombinant human activated
protein C

RHB
raise head of bed
right heart border
right heart bypass

rHBcAg
recombinant hepatitis Bc antigen

RHBF
reactive hyperemia blood flow

rhBMP-2, rHuBMP-2
recombinant human bone morphogenetic
protein

RH/BSO
radical hysterectomy and bilateral
salpingo-oophorectomy

RHBV
right heart blood volume

RHC
resin hemoperfusion column
respiration has ceased
right heart catheterization
right hemicolectomy
right hypochondrium

routine health care
rural health clinic

RhC
rhesus antigen C [Rh blood group]

RHCT
renal helical computed tomography

RHD
radial head dislocation
radiant heat device
radiologic health data
relative hepatic dullness
renal hypertensive disease
rheumatic heart disease (*See also* rheu
ht dis)
right-hand dominant
right hemisphere [brain] damage
round heart disease

RhD
rhesus antigen D [Rh blood group]
rhesus (hemolytic) disease

RHE
respiratory heat exchange
retinohepatoendocrinologic [syndrome]

RhE
rhesus antigen E [Rh blood group]

RHEED
reflection high-energy electron
diffraction

rheo
rheostat

rh-EPO
recombinant human erythropoietin

rheu ht dis
rheumatic heart disease (*See also* RHD)

rheum
rheuma (*See also* rh)
rheumatic (*See also* rh)

RhEx
rhythmic exercise

RHF
rheumatic fever vaccine
right heart failure

Rhf
rhesus factor (*See also* Rh)

RHG
radial hemolysis in gel
relative hemoglobin
right hand grip

rhG-CSF
recombinant human granulocyte
colony-stimulating factor

rhGH
recombinant human growth hormone

rhGM-CSF
recombinant human
granulocyte-macrophage
colony-stimulating factor

RHH
  right homonymous hemianopia
Rhi, Rhin
  rhinology
RhIg
  rhesus immune globulin
    (immunoglobulin)
rhIGF
  recombinant human insulinlike growth
    factor
RhIgIV
  Rh immune globulin intravenous
rhIL, rHuIL 1–11
  recombinant human interleukin 1–11
rhin
  rhinitis
rhino
  rhinoplasty
RHINOS
  fiberoptic rhinoscopy
r-hirudin
  recombinant hirudin
RHL
  recurrent herpes labialis
  right hemisphere lesion
  right hepatic lobe
RHLB
  Right Hemisphere Language Battery
RHLN
  right hilar lymph node
RHM
  routine health management
Rhm
  roentgen per hour at one meter
rhMCAF
  recombinant human
    macrophage-monocyte chemotactic and
    activating factor
rHM-CSF
  recombinant human macrophage
    colony-stimulating factor
rHm EPO, rHuEPO
  recombinant human erythropoietin
RhMk, RhMk, RhMkK
  rhesus monkey kidney (*See also*
    RMK)
RHMV
  right heart mixing volume
RHN
  Rockwell hardness number
Rh$_{null}$
  rhesus factor null [all Rh factors are
    lacking]
ρ, rho
  electrical resistivity
  rho [17th letter of Greek alphabet
    lowercase]
RHO
  right heeloff

RHOB
  raise head of bed
RHOCS
  right-handed orthogonal coordinate
    system
rhom
  rhomboid [muscle]
RHP
  resting head pressure
  right hemiparesis
  right hemiplegia
RHPA
  reverse hemolytic plaque assay
rhPDGF, rHuPDGF
  recombinant human platelet-derived
    growth factor
RHR
  resting heart rate
R/hr
  roentgen per hour (*See also* r/h,
    R/h)
Rh-Rh
  rhodium-rhodium target filter
    combination
RHS
  radial head subluxation
  reciprocal hindlimb-scratching
    (syndrome)
  right-hand side
  right heel strike
  rough hard sphere
rhSOD
  recombinant human superoxide
    dismutase
RHT
  regional hyperthermia
  renal homotransplantation
  right hypertropia
r-hT-FPI
  recombinant human tissue factor
    pathway inhibitor
rhTSH
  recombinant human thyroid-stimulating
    hormone
RHU
  rheumatology
rhuG-CSF
  recombinant human granulocyte
    colony-stimulating factor
rhuKGF
  recombinant human keratinocyte growth
    factor
rhuMAb HER2
  recombinant anti-p185HER2 monoclonal
    antibody
rhuMAb-VEGF
  recombinant humanized monoclonal
    antibody to vascular endothelial cell
    growth factor

RHV
  right hepatic vein
  rotating hemostatic valve
RhV
  rhinovirus (*See also* RV)
rhVEGF
  recombinant human vascular endothelial
  growth factor
RHW
  radiant heat warmer
RI
  input resistor
  radiation intensity
  radioactive isotope
  radioimmunology
  radioisotope
  ramus intermedius [coronary artery]
  recession index
  recombinant inbred [strain]
  reference interval
  refractive index (*See also* ref ind, n)
  regenerative index
  regional ileitis
  relapse incidence
  relative intensity
  release inhibition
  remission induced (induction)
  renal index
  renal insufficiency
  replicative intermediate
  resistance index
  resistive index
  respiratory illness
  respiratory index
  response interval
  reticulocyte index
  retroactive inhibition
  retroactive interference
  retroillumination
  rhythmic initiation
  ribosome
  right iliac [crest] (*See also* RIC)
  Rohrer index [wt/ht^3; weight in kg,
  height in meters]
  rooming in
  rosette inhibition
R$_i$
  inhibitory receptor
R/I
  rule in
RIA
  radioimmunoassay
  relaxation-induced anxiety
  reversible ischemic attack
  right iliac artery
RIA-DA
  radioimmunoassay double antibody [test]

RIAST
  Reitan Indiana Aphasic Screening Test
RIAT
  radioimmune antiglobulin test
Rib
  ribose (*See also* R)
RIBA
  radioimmunoblot assay
  recombinant immunoblot assay
  recombinant immunosorbent assay
RIBLS
  Riley Inventory of Basic Learning
  Skills
RIBP
  radiation-induced brachial plexopathy
RIBS
  rutherford ion backscattering
RIC
  reduced intensity conditioning
  Rehabilitation Impairment Categories
  renomedullary interstitial cell
  right iliac crest (*See also* RI)
  right internal capsule
  right internal carotid
  right interventricular coronary
  [artery]
RICA
  reverse immune cytoadhesion
  right internal carotid artery
RICE
  rest, ice, compresses, (compression)
  elevation
RICM
  right intercostal margin
RICP
  recurrent intrahepatic cholestasis of
  pregnancy
RICS
  right intercostal space
RICU
  respiratory intensive care unit
RID
  radial immunodiffusion
  (radioimmunodiffusion)
  radioimmunodetection (*See also* RAID)
  remission-inducing drug
  remove intoxicated driver
  right [ventricular] internal diameter
  ruptured intervertebral disc
RIDCSF
  radial immunodiffusion cerebrospinal
  fluid
RIE, RIEP
  radiation-induced emesis
  reactive ion etching
  relative inspiratory effort
  rocket immunoelectrophoresis

R

RIES
Revised Impact of Events Scale
RIF
radiation-induced fibrosis
release-inhibiting factor
replication inhibition factor
resistance-inducing factor
right iliac fossa
right index finger
rigid internal fixation
rosette inhibitory factor
RIFA
radioiodinated fatty acid
RIFC
rat intrinsic factor concentrate
rIFN-A, rIFN-α, rIFN-a, rIFN-alpha
recombinant interferon alpha (α)
rIFN-gamma (γ)
recombinant interferon gamma (γ)
RIg
rabies immune globulin
(immunoglobulin)
RIgH
rabies immune globulin, human
RIGS
radioimmunoguided surgery
RIH
right inguinal hernia
RIHD
radiation-induced heart disease
RIHP
renal interstitial hydrostatic pressure
RIHSA
radioactive iodinated (radioiodinated)
human serum albumin
RIIE
respiratory isolation implementation
efficiency
RIIS
respiratory isolation implementation
sensitivity
RIJ
right internal jugular [vein or catheter]
rIL
recombinant interleukin
RILD
radiation-induced liver disease
RILT
rabbit ileal loop test
RIM
radioisotope medicine
rapid identification method
recurrent induced malaria
relative-intensity measure
RIMA
reversible inhibitor of monoamine
oxidase-type A
right internal mammary anastomosis
right internal mammary artery

RIMS
resonance ionization mass spectrometry
RIN
radiation-induced necrosis
radiation-induced neoplasm
rat insulinoma
RINB
Reitan-Indiana Neuropsychological
Battery
RIND
resolving ischemic neurologic deficit
reversible ischemic neurologic deficit
(disability)
RINN
recommended international
nonproprietary name
R_int
intrinsic flow resistance
RINV
radiation-induced nausea and vomiting
RIO
right inferior oblique [muscle]
RIOJ
recurrent intrahepatic obstructive
jaundice
R-IOL
remove intraocular lens
RIP
radioimmunoprecipitation (test)
radioisotopic pathology
rapid infusion pump
receptor interacting protein
reflex-inhibiting pattern
respiratory inductance (inductive)
plethysmograph(y)
respiratory inversion point
rhythmic inhibitory pattern
RIPA
radioimmunoprecipitation assay
ristocetin-induced platelet agglutination
RIPIS
Rhode Island Pupil Identification Scale
RIPP
resistive-intermittent positive pressure
[ventilation]
RIPV
right inferior pulmonary vein
RIR
right iliac region
right inferior rectus [muscle]
RIRB
radioiodinated rose bengal [dye]
RIRS
retrograde intrarenal surgery
RIS
radiographic imaging system
radioimmunoglobulin scintigraphy
rapid immunofluorescence
(immunofluorescent) staining

relative intensity score
resonance ionization spectroscopy
respiratory index score
responding to internal stimuli
RI
Rehabilitation Indicator
RISA
radioactive iodinated serum albumin
radioimmunosorbent assay
radioiodinated serum albumin
Responsibility and Independence Scale
for Adolescents
RISB
Rotter Incomplete Sentences Blank
RISCC
ratio of ingested saturated fat and
cholesterol to calories [rating]
RISHN
radiation-induced sarcoma of head and
neck
RIST
radioimmunosorbent test
RIT
radioimmunoglobulin therapy
radioimmunotherapy
radioiodinated triolein
radioiodine treatment
Rorschach Inkblot Test (*See also* Ror)
rosette inhibition titer
rush immunotherapy
RITA
radiofrequency interstitial tissue ablation
right internal thoracic artery
RITC
rhodamine isothiocyanate
rhodamine isothiocyanate conjugated
RITE
rapid intraoperative tissue expansion
RIU
radioactive iodine (radioiodine) uptake
(*See also* RAIU)
RIV
ramus interventricularis
right innominate vein
RIVC
radionuclide [imaging of] inferior vena
cava
right inferior vena cava
RIVD
ruptured intervertebral disc
RIVS
ruptured interventricular septum
RIX
radiation-induced xerostomia
RJ
radial jerk [reflex]
right jugular

RJA
regurgitant jet area
RJI
radionuclide joint imaging
RJS
reduced joint survey
RK
rabbit kidney
radial keratotomy
right kidney
RKE-R
Rabideau Kitchen Evaluation Revised
RKG
radio(electro)cardiogram
RKID
right kidney
RKS
renal kidney stone
retrograde kidney study
RKV
rabbit kidney vacuolating [virus]
RKW
renal kalium (potassium) wasting
RKY
roentgen kymography
RL
coarse rales
radiation laboratory
recidivans leishmaniasis
reduction level
renal dysplasia-limb defect [syndrome]
resistive load
reticular lamina
right lateral (*See also* R LAT, R Lat,
RT LAT, rt lat)
right leg
right lower
right lung
Ringer lactate [solution] (*See also* RLS)
rotation left
R L, R-L, R→L, R/L
right-to-left [shunt] (*See also* rl-sh)
R or L
right or left
R&L
right and left
R$_L$
resistance of lung [pulmonary
resistance]
Rl
medium rales
rl
fine rales
RL₁
few fine rales
Rl₂
moderate number of medium rales

RL₃
numerous coarse rales
RLA
radiographic lung area
right lower arm
right lung apex
R LAT, R Lat
right lateral (*See also* RL, RT LAT, rt lat)
RLB
rickettsialike bodies
right lateral bending
RLBCD
right lower border of cardiac dullness
RLC
rectus and longus capitis [muscle]
residual lung capacity
rhodopsin-lipid complex
RLD
related living donor
resistive load detection
right lateral decubitus [position]
ruptured lumbar disc
RLDP
right lateral decubitus position
RLDS
Reynell Language Developmental Scale
RLE
recent life events
remaining life expectancy
right lower extremity
RLF
retained lung fluid
retrolental fibroplasia
right lateral femoral
RLFP
Remaining Lifetime Fracture Probability
RLG
right lateral gaze
RLGS
restriction landmark genomic scanning
RLH
reactive lymphoid hyperplasia
recurrent lobar hemorrhage
RLI
Reasons for Living Inventory
RLL
right liver lobe
right lower lid
right lower limb
right lower lobe
RLM
right lower medial
RLMA
reinforced laryngeal mask airway
RLMD
rat liver mitochondria [and submitochondrial particles derived by] digitonin [treatment]

RLN
recurrent laryngeal nerve
regional lymph node
RLNC
regional lymph node cell
RLND
regional lymph node dissection
retroperitoneal lymph node dissection
RLO
residual lymphocyte output
Right-Left Orientation Test
RLP
radiation leukemia protection
rectal linitis plastica
remnantlike lipoprotein particle
restriction fragment length polymorphism (*See also* RFLP)
ribosomelike particle
RLP-C
remnantlike lipoprotein particles-cholesterol
RLPV
right lower pulmonary vein
RLQ
right lower quadrant
RLQD
right lower quadrant defect
RLR
right lateral rectus [muscle]
RLRTD
recurrent lower respiratory tract disease
RLS
person who stammers having difficulty enunciating R, L, and S
rat lung strip
Reaction Level Scale
resonance light scattering
restless legs syndrome
rheumatoid lung silicosis
right-to-left shunt
Ringer lactate solution (*See also* RL)
Roussy-Levy syndrome
RLSB
right lower scapular border
right lower sternal border
rl-sh
right-left shunt (*See also* R L, R-L, R→L, R/L)
RLT
reactive lymphoid tissue
red light therapy
reduced liver transplant(ation)
right lateral thigh
RLTCS
repeat low transverse cesarean section
RLU
relative light unit
RLV
Rauscher leukemia virus

RLWD
routine laboratory work done
RLX
right lower extremity
RLZ
right lower zone
RM
radical mastectomy
radon monitor
random migration
range of (motion) movement (*See also* ROM)
red marrow
reference material
regional myocardial
rehabilitation medicine
repetition maximum
resistive movement
respiratory metabolism
respiratory movement
respiratory muscle
rhabdomyosarcoma
Riehl melanosis
right median
risk management
risk model
room (*See also* rm)
ruptured membranes
1-RM
1 repetition maximum
R&M
routine and microscopic
Rm
relative mobility
remission
rm
room (*See also* RM)
RMA
reduction in metabolic activity
refused medical advice
relative medullary area [kidney]
right mentum anterior (mentoanterior) [fetal position] (*See also* MDA)
Rivermead motor assessment
RMB
right mainstem bronchus
RMBF
regional myocardial blood flow
RMBPC
Revised Memory and Behavior Problems Checklist
RMC
Richards maximum contact
right middle cerebral [artery]
Rozsos microcholecystectomy
RMCA, R-MCA
right main coronary artery
right middle cerebral artery

RMCAT
right middle cerebral artery thrombosis
RMCE
recombinase mediated cassette exchange
RMCL
right midclavicular line
RMCP
rat mast cell protease
RMCT
rat mast cell technique
RMD
rapid movement disorder
ratio of midsagittal diameter
recommended maintenance dose
retromanubrial dullness
right manubrial dullness
rippling muscle disease
RME
rapid maxillary expansion
reasonable maximum exposure
resting metabolic expenditure
right mediolateral episiotomy (*See also* RMLE)
RMEE
right middle ear exploration
rMETase
recombinant methioninase
r-metHuLeptin
recombinant methionyl human leptin
RMF
right middle finger
RMI
Reading Miscue Inventory
recent myocardial infarction
Rivermead Mobility Index
RMIC
renomedullary interstitial cell
RMK
rhesus monkey kidney
RMK #1
remark number 1
RML
radiation myeloid leukemia
right mediolateral
right mentum lateral (mentolateral) [fetal position]
right middle lobe [of lung]
RMLB
right middle lobe bronchus
RMLE
right mediolateral episiotomy (*See also* RME)
RMLS
right middle lobe syndrome
RMLV
Rauscher murine leukemia virus (*See also* RMuLV)

R

689

RMM
rapid micromedia method
RMMA
rhythmic masticatory muscle activity
rMOG
recombinant myelin oligodendrocyte
glycoprotein
RMP
rapidly miscible pool
rapid manual processing
resting membrane potential
right mentum posterior (mentoposterior)
[fetal position] (*See also* MDP)
risk management program
RMQ
Roland-Morris Questionnaire
RMR
resting metabolic rate
right medial rectus [muscle]
root mean square residue
rMRGlu
glucose metabolism
RMRM
right modified radical mastectomy
RMS
rectal morphine sulfate [suppository]
red-man syndrome
repetitive motion syndrome
respiratory muscle strength
rhabdomyosarcoma (*See also* RD)
rheumatic mitral stenosis
rigid-man syndrome
Rocky Mountain spotted fever vaccine
root-mean-square [statistics] (*See also*
rms)
Ruvalcaba-Myhre-Smith
rms
root-mean-square [statistics] (*See also*
RMS)
RMSB
right middle sternal border
RMSD
root-mean-square deviation [statistics]
RMSE
root-mean-square error [statistics]
RMSF
Rocky Mountain spotted fever
RMT
relative medullary thickness
retromolar trigone
right mentum transverse
(mentotransverse) [fetal position]
RMTD
rhythmical midtemporal discharge
rMTT
regional mean transit time
rMu
recombinant murine [mouse
protein]

RMUI
relief medication unit index
RMuLV
Rauscher murine leukemia virus
(*See also* RMLV)
RMV
respiratory minute volume
RN
radionuclide [scan]
red nucleus
reflex nephropathy
renal [disease] (*See also* REN, ren)
reticular nucleus
right nostril (naris)
R/N
renew
Rn
radon
^{222}Rn
radon-222
RNA
radionuclide angiograph(y) (angiogram)
(*See also* RA, RNG)
ribonucleic acid
rough, noncapsulated, avirulent [bacterial
culture]
RNAA
radiochemical neutron activation analysis
RNAi
ribonucleic acid interference
RNA-PCR
ribonucleic acid-polymerase chain
reaction
RNAse, RNase
ribonuclease
RNase D
ribonuclease D
RNAse H
ribonuclease H
RNase P
ribonuclease P
RNBA
refractory normoblastic anemia
RND
radical neck dissection
reactive neurotic depression
RNEF
resting (radio)nuclide ejection fraction
RNFL
retinal nerve fiber layer
RNG
radionuclide angiograph(y) (angiogram)
(*See also* RA, RNA)
RNI
reactive nitrogen intermediates
reference (recommended) nutrient
intake
RNL
renal laboratory profile

RNP
  restorative nursing program
  ribonuclear protein (ribonucleoprotein)
RNR
  ribonucleotide reductase
RNS
  reference normal serum
  repetitive nerve stimulation (stimulator)
  replacement normal saline [0.9%
    sodium chloride]
  responsive neurostimulator
RNSC
  radionuclide superior cavography
RNST
  reactive nonstress test
RNT
  radioassayable neurotensin
Rnt
  roentgenology (*See also* roent)
RNTC
  rat nephroma tissue culture
RNUD
  recurrent nonulcer dyspepsia
RNV
  radionuclide venography
  radionuclide ventriculograph(y)
    (ventriculogram) (*See also* RNVG)
rNV
  recombinant [capsid protein of] Norwalk
    virus
RNVG
  radionuclide ventriculograph(y)
    (ventriculogram) (*See also* RNV)
RO
  radiation oncology
  reality orientation (oriented)
  relative odds
  report of
  reverse osmosis
  Ritter-Oleson [technique]
  routine order
  rule out (*See also* R/O)
R/O
  rule out (*See also* RO)
ROA
  radiologic osteoarthritis
  regurgitant orifice area
  reversal of antagonist
  right occiput anterior (occipitoanterior)
    [fetal position] (*See also* ODA)
ROAC
  repeated oral [doses of] activated
    charcoal
ROAD
  reversible obstructive airways disease
ROAF
  reversed ophthalmic artery flow

ROAM
  roaming optical access multiscope
ROAT
  repeat open-application testing
ROATS
  rabbit ovarian antitumor serum
rob.
  robertsonian [translocation]
ROBC
  residual infiltrating breast cancer
ROC
  receiver operating characteristic
    [statistics]
  record of contact
  residual organic carbon
roc
  reciprocal ohm centimeter
ROCF, ROCFT
  Rey-Estreich Complex Figure Test
Roch-Ochs
  Rochester-Ochsner [forceps]
ROCM
  radiopaque contrast media
ROCV
  Rocio virus
ROD
  rapid opiate (opioid) detoxification
  renal osteodystrophy
RODA
  rapid opiate (opioid) detoxification
    under anesthesia
RODAC
  replicate organism detection and
    counting
RODAC-TM
  replicate organism direct agar
    contact
RODEO
  rotating delivery of excitation off
    resonance
RODS
  resolution of delusions scale
ROE
  report of event
  return on equity
  right otitis externa
  roentgen (*See also* R, r, roent)
rOEF
  regional oxygen extraction fraction
roent
  roentgen (*See also* R, r, ROE)
  roentgenology (*See also* Rnt)
ROF
  review of outside films
ROH
  rat ovarian hyperemia [test]
  rubbing alcohol

R

ROI
　reactive oxygen intermediate
　region of interest
　release of information
ROIDS
　hemorrhoids
ROIH
　right oblique inguinal hernia
ROJM
　range of joint motion
ROL
　right occiput lateral (occipitolateral)
　[fetal position]
ROLC
　roentgenographically occult lung cancer
　roentgenologically occult lung cancer
ROLS
　Reinverting Operating Lens System
ROM
　range of motion (movement) (*See also* RM)
　reactive oxygen metabolite
　removal of metal [pins or plates in orthopedic surgery]
　right otitis media
　rupture of membranes
Rom, Romb
　Romberg [sign]
rom
　reciprocal ohm meter
ROM C P
　range of motion complete and pain-free
ROMI
　rule out myocardial infarct(ion)
romied
　ruled out for myocardial infarct(ion)
ROMSA
　right otitis media, suppurative, acute
ROMSC
　right otitis media, suppurative, chronic
ROM WNL
　range of motion within normal limits
RON
　radiation optic neuropathy
ROOF
　retroorbicularis oculi fat
　retroorbicularis orbital fat
ROP
　regional organ procurement
　retinopathy of prematurity
　right occiput posterior (occipitoposterior) [fetal position] (*See also* ODP)
ROPA
　Regional Organ Procurement Agency
ROPE
　respiratory ordered phase encoding
ROQ
　Rhinitis Outcomes Questionnaire

ROR
　measles-mumps-rubella vaccine [French acronym]
　retinoic acid-related orphan receptor
Ror
　Rorschach [Inkblot Test] (*See also* RIT)
RoRx
　roentgen (radiation) therapy (radiotherapy) (*See also* Rad, RADIO, Rad Ther, RATx, RT, RTx, RXT)
ROS
　reactive oxygen species
　review of systems (*See also* Rev of Sys)
　rod outer segment
RoS
　rostral sulcus
ROSA
　rank-order stability analysis
ROSC
　restoration (return) of spontaneous circulation
ROSNI
　round spermatid nucleus injection
rOspA
　recombinant outer surface protein A
ROSS
　review of signs and symptoms
　review of (other) subjective symptoms
ROT
　real oxygen transport
　remedial occupational therapy
　right occiput transverse (occipitotransverse) [fetal position]
　rotating (*See also* Rot, rot.)
　rotation
　rotator
　rule of thumb
ROTA
　rotablator atherectomy
ROTACS
　rotational angioplasty catheter system
rot. ny
　rotatory nystagmus
ROU
　recurrent oral ulcer
ROUL
　rouleau [singular] (rouleaux [plural])
rout.
　routine (*See also* R, RTN)
ROW
　rat ovarian weight
　rest of [the] week
ROWPVT
　Receptive One-Word Picture Vocabulary Test
RP
　radial pulse
　radical prostatectomy

radiographic planimetry
radiopharmaceutical
rapid processing [of film]
Raynaud phenomenon
reaction product
reactive protein
readiness potential
rectal prolapse
red phosphorus
reduced profile
reentrant pathway
refractory period
regulatory protein
relapsing polychondritis
relative potency
respiratory to pulse rate index
responsible party
resting position
resting potential
resting pressure
restorative proctocolectomy
rest pain
retinitis pigmentosa
retinitis proliferans (*See also* R Pr)
retrograde pyelograph(y) (pyelogram)
  (*See also* REP, retro pyelo, RGP,
  RPG)
retroperitoneal
reverse phase
rheumatoid polyarthritis
ribose phosphate
root plane

R_p, Rp
  pulmonary resistance
RPA
  radial photon absorptiometry
  recurrent pleomorphic adenoma
  replication protein A
  restenosis postangioplasty
  resultant physiologic acceleration
  retroperitoneal adenitis
  retroperitoneal approach
  reverse passive anaphylaxis
  ribonuclease protection assay
  right pulmonary artery
r-PA
  recombinant plasminogen activator
RPAB
  Rivermead Perceptual Assessment
    Battery
RPAW
  right pulmonary artery withdrawal
RPBD
  rating of perceived breathing difficulty
rPBF
  regional pulmonary blood flow
RPC
  reactive perforating collagenosis

recurrent pyogenic cholangitis
recurrent pyogenic cholangiohepatitis
relapsing polychondritis
relative proliferative capacity
restorative proctocolectomy
retained products of conception
root planing and curettage
RP&C
  root planing and curettage
RPCA
  reverse passive cutaneous anaphylaxis
RPCF, RPCFT
  Reiter protein complement-fixation
    [test]
RPCGN
  rapidly progressive crescentic
    glomerulonephritis
RPCV
  retropubic cytourethropexy
RPD
  rapid
  removable partial denture
rPDGF
  recombinant platelet-derived growth
    factor
R-PDQ
  Revised Denver Prescreening
    Development Questionnaire
RPDSI
  Riley Preschool Developmental
    Screening Inventory
RPE
  rated perceived exertion
  rate of perceived exertion
  rating of perceived exertion
  recurrent pulmonary emboli
  retinal pigment epithelium (epithelial
    cell)
RPED
  retinal pigment epithelium detachment
r-PEG
  recombinant polyethylene glycol
RPEP
  rabies postexposure prophylaxis
  right pre ejection period
RPET
  rapid partial exchange transfusion
RPF
  Reiter protein fixation test
  relaxed pelvic floor
  renal plasma flow
  retroperitoneal fibrosis
rPF4
  recombinant platelet factor 4
RPF^a
  arterial renal plasma flow
RPFS
  Rosenzweig Picture-Frustration Study

RPF^v
venous renal plasma flow
RPG
radiation protection guide
research project grant
retrograde percutaneous gastrostomy
retrograde pyelograph(y) (pyelogram)
(*See also* REP, retro pyelo, RGP, RP)
rheoplethysmography
RPGG
retroplacental gamma globulin
RPGN
rapidly progressive glomerulonephritis
RPGR
retinitis pigmentosa GTPase regulator
gene
RPH
retroperitoneal hemorrhage
RPHA
reversed passive hemagglutination
[reaction]
RPHAMCFA
reversed passive hemagglutination by
miniature centrifugal fast analysis
RP-HPLC
reversed phase high-performance liquid
chromatography
RPI
Racial Perceptions Inventory
resting pressure index
reticulocyte (reticulocytic) production
index
RPICA
right posterior internal carotid artery
RPICC
regional perinatal intensive care
center
RPICCE
round pupil intracapsular cataract
extraction
RPIPP
reversed phase ion-pair partition
RPL, RPLAD
retroperitoneal lymphadenectomy
RPLA
reversed passive latex particle
agglutination
reverse passive latex agglutination
RPLC
reversed-phase liquid chromatography
RPLD
repair of potentially lethal damage
retroperitoneal [lymph node] dissection
(*See also* RPLND)
RPLE
reversible posterior leukencephalopathy
RPLND
retroperitoneal pelvic lymph node
dissection

RPLS
reversible posterior leukoencephalopathy
syndrome
RPM, rpm
radical pair mechanism
rapid processing mode
Raven Progressive Matrices
real-time position management
revolution per minute
rotation per minute
RPMD
rheumatic pain modulation disorder
RPMPR
radical posteromedial and plantar release
RPM-R
Raven progressive matrices-Revised
RPN
renal papillary necrosis
RPND
retroperitoneal [lymph] node dissection
RPNG
rapidly progressive necrotizing
glomerulonephritis
RPO
radiation protection officer
reflectance pulse oximetry
right posterior oblique [radiologic view]
RPP
radical perineal prostatectomy
rate-pressure product
retinal periphlebitis
retropubic prostatectomy
RPPC
regional pediatric pulmonary center
RPPI
role perception picture inventory
RPPR
red [blood cell] precursor production
rate
RPPS
retropatellar pain syndrome
RPR
rapid plasma reagin
Reiter protein reagin
R Pr
retinitis proliferans (*See also* RP)
RPr
rotational panoramic radiography
RPRCF
rapid plasma reagin complement
fixation
RPRCT, RPR-CT
rapid plasma reagin card test
rapid plasma reagin circle test
RPRF
rapidly progressive renal failure
RPS, rps
renal pressor substance
reverse pivot shift

review per screen [imaging]
revolution per second
RPT
rapid pull-through (pullthrough)
(technique)
refractory period of transmission
rpt
report
RPTA
renal percutaneous transluminal
angioplasty
rptd
rupture(d) (*See also* rupt)
RPTK
receptor protein tyrosine kinase
RPU
retropubic urethropexy
RPV
right portal vein
right pulmonary vein
RPVP
right posterior ventricular preexcitation
RPx
revised prognosis
Rpx
Rathke pouch homeobox transcription
factor
RQ
reading quotient (*See also* RdQ)
recovery quotient
respiratory quotient
RQLQ
Respiratory Quality of Life
Questionnaire
rhinoconjunctivitis-specific Quality of
Life Questionnaire
RQS
repeated quick stretch
RQS-E
repeated quick stretch from elongation
RQS-SEC
repeated quick stretch superimposed
upon an existing contraction
RR
radial rate
radiation reaction
radiation response
rapid radiometric
rate ratio
reading retarded
recovery room
red reflex
regular rate
regular respiration
relative response
relative risk
renin release

resistant relapse
respiratory rate
respiratory reserve
response rate
retinal reflex
rheumatoid rosette
right rotation
risk ratio
Riva-Rocci [sphygmomanometer]
(*See also* RRS)
road rash
roentgenographic pelvimetry
rotation right
ruthenium red
R/R
rales/rhonchi
R&R
rate and rhythm
recent and remote
recess(ion) and resect(ion)
rest and recuperation
rest and relaxation
RRA
radioreceptor assay (activity)
right radial artery
right renal artery
RRAM
rapid rhythmic alternating movements
relative response attributable to
maneuver
RRB
rigid rockerbottom
rrBF
relative regional blood flow
RRC
relative risk cohort
risk reduction component
routine respiratory care
RRCT no (m)
regular rate, clear tones, no
murmurs
RRD
rhegmatogenous retinal detachment
RRE
radiation-related eosinophilia
regressive resistive exercise
Rev (RNA-encoding viral protein)-
response element
round, regular, and equal [pupils]
(*See also* RR&E)
RR&E
round, regular, and equal [pupils]
(*See also* RRE)
RRED
Rapid Rare Event Detection [system]
RREF
resting radionuclide ejection fraction

RREID
  rapid rabies enzyme immunodiagnosis
RRF
  ragged red fiber
  residual renal function
  right rectus femoris
RRFC
  renal reserve filtration capacity
RR-HPO
  rapid recompression-high pressure
    oxygen
RRI
  recurrent respiratory infection
  reflex relaxation index
  relative response index
  renal resistive index
RR-IOL
  remove and replace intraocular lens
RRIS
  recurrent respiratory infection
    syndrome
RRM
  reduced renal mass
  right radial mastectomy
RRMS
  relapsing-remitting multiple sclerosis
rRNA
  ribosomal ribonucleic acid
RRND
  right radical neck dissection
RROM
  resistive range of motion
R rot
  right rotation
RRP
  radical retropubic prostatectomy
  readily releasable pool
  recurrent respiratory papilloma(tosis)
  relative refractory period
RRpm
  respiratory rate per minute
RRQG
  right rostral quarter ganglion
RRR
  recovery room routine
  regular rate and rhythm
  relative risk reduction
  renin-release rate (ratio)
  risk rescue rating
RRRN
  round, regular, react normally [pupils]
RRS
  retrorectal space
  Riva-Rocci sphygmomanometer (*See also*
    RR)
Rrs
  respiratory resistance
R$_{rs}$
  resistance respiratory system

RRSS
  race-related stressor scale
RRT
  randomized response technique
  recommended replacement time [battery]
  relative retention time
  resazurin reduction time
RRTM
  retroperitoneal residual tumor mass
RRU
  rapid reintegration unit
  respiratory resistance unit
RRV
  rhesus rotavirus vaccine
  right renal vein
  Ross River virus
RRVN
  retrolabyrinthine/retrosigmoidal vestibular
    neurectomy
RRVO
  repair relaxed vaginal outlet
RRVS
  recovery room vital signs
RRV-TV
  rhesus rotavirus-tetravalent vaccine
RRW
  rales, rhonchi, wheezes
RRx
  radiation treatment
RS
  radiosurgery
  random sample
  rapid smoking
  rating schedule
  reactive site
  reading of standard
  recipient's serum
  rectal sinus
  rectal suppository
  rectal swab
  rectosigmoid
  recurrent seizures
  Reed-Sternberg [cell] (*See also* R-S)
  rehydrating solution
  reinforcing stimulus
  relative survival
  remnant stomach
  Repression-Sensitization [Scale]
  reproductive success
  reschedule
  resolved sarcoidosis
  resorcinol-sulfur
  respiratory symptom
  respiratory syncytial [virus]
  respiratory system
  restart
  reticulated siderocyte (*See also* R-S)
  rheumatoid spondylitis
  rhythm strip

right sacrum
right septum
right side
right stellate [ganglion]
right subclavian
Ringer solution
ring sideroblast
Ritchie sedimentation
rumination syndrome

R:S

response to stimulus ratio

R-S

Reed-Sternberg [cell]
reticulated siderocyte (*See also* RS)
rough-smooth [variation]

R/S

reschedule
rest stress
rupture spontaneous

R/S I

resuscitation status one [full
resuscitative effort]

R/S II

resuscitation status two [no code,
therapeutic measures only]

R/S III

resuscitation status three [no code,
comfort measures only]

R&S

restraint and seclusion

R/s

roentgen per second

4 Rs

remove, replace, reinoculate, repair

Rs

resolution
respond
response (*See also* R, resp)
(total) systemic resistance

R$_s$

stimulatory receptor

r$_s$

rank correlation coefficient [statistics]

RSA

rabbit serum albumin (*See also* RbSA)
rapid susceptibility assay
rat serum albumin
recurrent spontaneous abortion
regular spiking activity
relative specific activity
relative standard accuracy
respiratory sinus arrhythmia
reticulum [cell] sarcoma (*See also* RCS)
right sacrum anterior (sacroanterior)
[fetal position] (*See also* SDA)
right subclavian artery
roentgen stereophotogrammetric analysis

Rsa

[total] systemic arterial resistance

RSA-BF

respiratory sinus arrhythmia biofeedback

RSAPE

remitting seronegative arthritis with
pitting edema

RSB

reticulocyte standard buffer
right sternal border

RSBA

refractory sideroblastic anemia

RSBD

rapid eye movement (REM) sleep
behavior disorder

RSBI

Rapid Shallow Breathing Index

RSBT

rhythmic sensory bombardment therapy

RSC

radioscaphocapitate
rat spleen cell
rectosigmoid neocolpopoiesis
rested state contraction
reversible sickle cell
right side colon
right subclavian [artery or vein]

RScA

right scapula anterior (scapuloanterior)
[fetal position] (*See also* ScDA)

RSCCD

Rating Scale of Communication in
Cognitive Decline

rsCD4

recombinant soluble CD4 [cells]

RSCL

Rotterdam Symptom Check List

RSCN

reactive spindle cell nodule

RScP

right scapula posterior (scapuloposterior)
[fetal position] (*See also* ScDP)

RSCS

respiratory system compliance score

RSCT

Rach Sentence Completion Test
Rotter Sentence Completion Test

rscu-PA

recombinant, single-chain, urokinase-type
plasminogen activator

RSCVP

right subclavian central venous

RSD

rad surface dose
reflex sympathetic dystrophy
relative sagittal depth
relative standard deviation

RSDP
  random single-donor platelets
RSDS
  reflex sympathetic dystrophy syndrome
RSE
  rat synaptic ending
  reactive subdural effusion
  refractory status epilepticus
  reverse sutured eye
  right sternal edge
RSEP
  right somatosensory evoked potential
RSES
  Rosenberg Self-Esteem Scale
RSF
  raw soybean flour
RSG
  Reitan Strength of Grip
RSG/IAC
  retrosigmoid/internal auditory canal
RSH
  rectus sheath hematoma
  reduced sulfhydryl group
RSI
  rapid sequence intubation (intubation)
  repetitive strain (stress) injury
RSIVP
  rapid-sequence intravenous pyelography
RSL
  renal solute load
  right sacrum lateral (sacrolateral) [fetal position]
RSLD
  repair of sublethal damage
RSLR
  reverse straight leg raise
RSLT
  reduced-size liver transplant(ation)
RSLTx
  right single lung transplant(ation)
RSM
  remote study monitoring
  risk-screening model
RSMR
  relative standardized mortality ratio
RSN
  right substantia nigra
RSNI
  round spermatid nuclear injection
RSO
  right salpingo-oophorectomy
  right superior oblique [muscle]
rSO2, rSO$_2$
  regional oxygen saturation
RSOM-31
  Rhinosinusitis Outcome Measure 31 questionnaire
RSOP
  right superior oblique palsy

RSP
  rapid steady progression
  rapid straight pacing
  rat serum protein
  recirculating single pass
  recurrent spontaneous pneumothorax
  removable silicone plug
  rhinoseptoplasty
  right sacrum posterior (sacroposterior) [fetal position] (*See also* SDP)
RS3PE
  remitting seronegative symmetric synovitis with pitting edema
RSPK
  recurrent spontaneous psychokinesis
RSPM
  Raven Standard Progressive Matrices
RSPV
  right superior pulmonary vein
RSR
  rectosphincteric reflex
  regular sinus rhythm
  relative survival rate
  response to stimulus ratio
  right superior rectus [muscle]
rSR′
  abnormal EKG rhythm of small-R wave, bigger-R wave of QRS [aberrant conduction of supraventricular beat]
RSRI
  renal to systemic renin index
RSS
  rat stomach strip
  rearfoot stability system
  recombination signal sequence
  rectosigmoidoscope (rectosigmoidoscopy)
  reduced space symbologies
  repetitive stress syndrome
  representative sample sectioned
  right subscapular skinfold [thickness, measurement]
  rotatory subluxation of scaphoid
  Russian spring-summer [encephalitis]
RSs
  relative supersaturation
RSSE
  Russian spring-summer encephalitis (*See also* RSS)
RSSEV
  Russian spring-summer encephalitis virus
RSSR
  relatively slow sinus rate
RST
  radiosensitivity test
  rapid simple test
  rapid surfactant test
  reagin screen test

repeated significance test [statistics]
right sacrum transverse (sacrotransverse)
  [fetal position] (*See also* SDT)
rubrospinal tract
RSTL
relaxed skin tension line
RSTS
retropharyngeal soft tissue space
RSTs
Rodney Smith tubes
RSV
regurgitant stroke volume
respiratory syncytial virus
right subclavian vein
Rous sarcoma virus
RSVA
ruptured sinus of Valsalva aneurysm
RSVB
respiratory syncytial virus bronchiolitis
RSVC
right superior vena cava
RSV-IgIV
respiratory syncytial virus immune
  globulin (immunoglobulin) intravenous
Rous sarcoma virus immune globulin
  (immunoglobulin) intravenous
RSVP
rapid serial visual presentation
rejuvenation with sparing of vascular
  perforators
RSW
right-sided weakness
RT
rabbit trachea
radiation therapy (radiotherapy)
  (*See also* Rad, RADIO, Rad Ther,
  RATx, RoRx, RTx, RXT)
radiologic technology
radiotelemetry
radium therapy
random transfusion
raphe transection
rational therapy
reaction time
reading task (test) (time)
receptor transforming
reciprocating tachycardia
recovery time
recreational therapy
rectal temperature (*See also* R/T)
red tetrazolium
reduction time
related to
relaxation time
renal transplant(ation) (*See also* RTx)
repetition time
Reporter's Test

reptilase time
resistance training
resistance transfer
respiratory technology
respiratory therapy
rest tremor
retransformation
reverse transcriptase
right (*See also* R, (R), Rt)
right thigh
right triceps
room temperature
running total
R/T
rectal temperature (*See also* RT)
related to (*See also* R/t)
R$_T$
total pulmonary resistance
Rt
right (*See also* R, (R), RT)
R/t
related to (*See also* R/T)
rT
ribothymidine
RT$_3$
[serum] resin triiodothyronine [uptake]
  (*See also* RT$_3$U)
rT$_3$
reverse triiodothyronine
RT$_4$
resin thyroxine [test] thyroxine
RTA
renal tubular acidosis
renal tubular antigen
retinal thickness analyzer (analysis)
road traffic accident
routine tests administered
RTA-I–RTA-IV
renal tubular acidosis I–IV
RTAD
renal tubular acidification defect
RTAH
right anterior hemiblock
RTAS
radiology telephone access system
rapid telephone access system
RTAT
right anterior thigh
RTAV
Resistencia virus
RTAVI
Risk-Taking, Attitude, Values Inventory
RTB
return to baseline
RTC
(a)round the clock
randomized trial, controlled

RTC *(continued)*
 Readiness to Change [questionnaire]
 renal tubular cell
 return to clinic
 reverse thrust catheter
RT-CT
 radiotherapy dedicated computed
  tomography
RTD
 renal tubular dysgenesis
 renal tubular dysplasia
 repetitive trauma disorder
 residual thermal damage
 resubmission turnaround document
 routine test dilution
RTD-1
 rhesus theta defensin 1
rtd
 retarded (*See also* RET)
 retired (*See also* RET)
RTE
 rabbit thymus extract
 renal tubular epithelial
RTER
 return to emergency room
RTF
 replication and transfer
 resistance transfer factor
 respiratory tract fluid
 return to flow
RTFNA
 real-time fine-needle aspiration
RTH
 resistance to thyroid hormone
RtH
 right-handed
RTI
 reproductive tract infection
 respiratory tract infection
 retrograde tracheal intubation
 reverse transcriptase inhibitor
Rti
 tissue resistance
RTK
 receptor tyrosine kinase
 rhabdoid tumor of kidney
RTKP
 radiothermokeratoplasty
RTL
 reactive to light (pupils)
rtl
 rectal
RT LAT, rt lat
 right lateral (*See also* RL, R LAT, R
  Lat)
RTLF
 respiratory tract lining fluid
RTLX
 real-time, low-intensity x-ray

RTM
 reciprocal tension membrane
 routine medical care
R$_{tmf}$
 total matrix formation rate
rTMP
 ribothymidylic acid (*See also* TMP)
rTMS
 rapid transcranial magnetic stimulation
 repetitive transcranial magnetic
  stimulation
RTN
 renal tubular necrosis
 routine (*See also* R, rout.)
 routine tests negative
rtn
 return (*See also* RET)
rTNFα, rTNF alpha
 recombinant tumor necrosis factor alpha
  (α)
rTNM
 retreatment [TNM classification]
RTO
 return to office
 right toe-off
Rtot
 total airways resistance
RTP
 radiation therapy (treatment) plan(ning)
 renal transplant(ation) patient
 return to play
 reverse transcriptase-producing [agent]
RTPA, rt PA, rtPA, rt-PA
 recombinant tissue-type plasminogen
  activator
RT-PCR
 reverse transcriptase (transcription)
  polymerase chain reaction
RTPE
 reverse transcriptase primer extension
RTPS
 radiation therapy planning system
RTR
 red [blood cell] turnover rate
 renal transplant(ation) recipient
 retention time ratio
 return to room
RTRR
 return to recovery room
RTRT
 real-time tumor tracking radiation
  therapy
RTS
 radiation therapy system
 real-time scan
 relative tumor size
 return to sender
 Revised Trauma Score
 right toe strike

rTSAB
rodent thyroid-stimulating antibody
rt scap bord
right scapular border
rTSH
recombinant thyrotropin contrast agent
RTSW
Repeated Test of Sustained Wakefulness
r_{tt}
obtained coefficient
reliability coefficient
RTU
ready to use
real-time ultrasonography (*See also* RTUS)
relative time unit
RT₃U
resin triiodothyronine uptake (*See also* RT₃)
rTU
ribosomal ribonucleic acid transcription unit
RTUS
real-time ultrasonography (*See also* RTU)
RTV
rhinotracheitis virus
room temperature vulcanize(d) (vulcanization) (vulcanizing)
RTW
return to work (*See also* R/W)
RTWD
return to work determination
RTX
real-time transmission
RTx
radiation therapy (radiotherapy)
renal transplant(ation) (*See also* Rad, RADIO, Rad Ther, RATx, RoRx, RT, RXT)
RU
radioactive uptake
radioulnar
rat unit
reading of unknown
recall urticaria
rectourethral
recurrent ulcer
residual urine
resin uptake
resistance unit
retrograde urogram
retroverted uterus
right uninjured
right uninvolved
right upper
rodent ulcer

roentgen unit
routine urinalysis
RU-1
human embryonic lung fibroblast
Ru
ruthenium
⁸²Ru
rubidium-82
RUA
right upper arm
routine urine analysis
RuBP
ribulose bisphophate
RUBV
rubella virus
RUD
recurrent ulcer of duodenal bulb
RUDS
random urine drug screen
reactive upper airways dysfunction syndrome
RUDT
respiratory and upper digestive tract
RUE
right upper extremity (*See also* R↑E, RUX)
RUFIS
rotating ultra-fast imaging sequence
RUG
resource utilization group
retrograde urethrograph(y) (urethrogram)
r-UK
recombinant urokinase
RUL
right upper (eye)lid
right upper lateral
right upper limb
right upper lobe
right upper lung
RUM
right upper medial
RUMI
Rowden uterine manipulator-injector
RUO
right ureteral orifice
RUOQ
right upper outer quadrant
RUP
rat urine protein
right upper pole
rupt
rupture(d) (*See also* rptd)
RUPV
right upper pulmonary vein
RUQ
right upper quadrant

RUR
resin uptake ratio
RURTI
recurrent upper respiratory tract
infection
RUS
radioulnar synostosis
real-time ultrasonography
recurrent ulcerative stomatitis
RUSB
right upper sternal border
RUSP, RVSP
right ventricular systolic pressure
RUSS
recurrent ulcerative scarifying stomatitis
RUT
rapid urease test
RUV
residual urine volume
RUX
right upper extremity (*See also* R↑E,
RUE)
RV
random variable
rat virus
Rauscher virus
rectal vault
rectovaginal
reference value
regurgitant [stroke] volume
reinforcement value
renal vein (venous)
reovirus
reserve volume
residual volume
respiratory volume
retinal vasculitis
retrovaginal
retroversion
retrovesical
return visit
rhabdovirus
rheumatoid vasculitis
rhinovirus (*See also* RhV)
right ventricle (ventricular)
rotavirus
rubella vaccine
rubella virus
Russell viper [time] (*See also* RVT,
RVVT)
R$_V$
radius of view
RVA
rabies vaccine adsorbed
recombinant virus assay
reduced visual acuity
reentrant ventricular arrhythmia
renal vascular resistance
right ventricular abnormality

right ventricular activation
right ventricular apex (apical)
right vertebral artery
RVAD
right ventricular assist device
RVAW
right ventricle anterior wall
RVB
red venous blood
RVBF
reversed vertebral blood flow
RVC
radioactivity of vegetative cells
respond to verbal command
RVCB
right ventricular copulsation balloon
RVD
reference vessel diameter
relative vertebral density
relative volume decrease
right ventricular dimension
right ventricular dysfunction
right ventricular dysplasia
right vertebral density
RVDO
right ventricular diastolic overload
RVDP
right ventricular diastolic pressure
RVDT
retinal venous dilation and
tortuosity
RVDV
right ventricular diastolic volume
RVE
reduced ventricular effort
right ventricular enlargement
RVECP
right ventricular endocardial potential
RVEDD
right ventricular end-diastolic diameter
RVEDP
right ventricular end-diastolic pressure
RVEDV
right ventricular end-diastolic volume
RVEDVI
right ventricular end-diastolic volume
index
RVEF
right ventricular ejection fraction
right ventricular end-flow
RVERP
right ventricular refractory period
RVESV
right ventricular end-systolic volume
RVESVI
right ventricular end-systolic volume
index
RVET
right ventricular ejection time

RVF
    renal vascular failure
    Rift Valley fever
    right ventricular failure
    right ventricular function
    right visual field
RVFP
    right ventricular filling pressure
RVFV
    Rift Valley fever virus
RVG
    radionuclide ventriculograph(y)
      (ventriculogram)
    radiovisiography
    relative value guide
    right ventral gluteus [muscle]
      [veterinary]
    right ventrogluteal
    right visceral ganglion
RVH
    renal vascular (renovascular)
      hypertension
    right ventricular hypertrophy
RVHD
    rheumatic valvular heart disease
RVI
    relative value index
    right ventricle infarct(ion)
RVID
    right ventricular internal diameter
    right ventricular internal dimension
RVIDd
    right ventricle internal dimension
      diastole
RVIDP
    right ventricular initial diastolic pressure
RVIT
    right ventricular inflow tract [view]
RVL
    right vastus lateralis
RVLG
    right ventrolateral gluteal
RVLM
    rostral ventrolateral medulla
RVM
    right ventricular mass
RVN
    radionuclide ventriculogram
    retrolabyrinthine vestibular
      neurectomy
RVO
    relaxed vaginal outlet
    retinal vein occlusion
    right ventricular outflow
    right ventricular overactivity
RVol
    regurgitant volume

RVOT
    right ventricular outflow tract
RVOTH
    right ventricular outflow tract
      hypertrophy
RVP
    red veterinary petrolatum
    renovascular pressure
    resting venous pressure
    right ventricular pressure
RVPFR
    right ventricular peak filling rate
RVP:LVP
    right ventricular to left ventricular
      pressure ratio
RVPRA
    renal vein plasma renin activity
RVR
    rapid ventricular response
    reduced vascular response
    reduced vestibular response
    relative vascular resistance
    renal vascular resistance
    renal vein renin
    renovascular resistance
    repetitive ventricular response
    resistance to venous return
    right ventricular rhythm
RVRA
    renal vein renin activity
    renal vein (venous) renin assay
RV:RA
    renal vein to renal activity
      ratio
RVRC
    renal vein renin concentration
RV/RF
    retroverted/retroflexed
RVRI
    renal vascular (renovascular) resistance
      index
RVS
    rabies vaccine, adsorbed
    recognizable viral syndrome
    relative value scale
    relative value schedule
    relative value study
    reported visual sensation
    retrovaginal space
    Rokeach Value Survey [psychologic
      test]
RVSO
    right ventricle stroke output
RVSP
    right ventricular systolic pressure
RVSV
    right ventricular stroke volume

RVSW
    right ventricular stroke work
RVSWI
    right ventricular stroke work index
RVT
    recurrent ventricular tachycardia
    renal vein thrombosis
    Russell viper [venom] time (*See also* RV, RVVT)
RVTE
    recurring venous thromboembolism
RV:TLC
    residual volume to total lung capacity ratio
RVU
    relative value unit
RVV
    rubella vaccinelike virus
    rubella virus vaccine
    Russell viper venom
RVVT
    Russell viper venom time (*See also* RV, RVT)
RVW
    right ventricular wall
RVWD
    right ventricular wall device
R-W
    Rideal-Walker [coefficient]
RW
    radiant warmer
    radiologic warfare
    ragweed (*See also* RAG)
    red welt
    respiratory work
    right [ear], warm [stimulus] [Bárány caloric test]
    rolling walker
    round window
R/W
    return to work (*See also* RTW)
RWA
    right wing authoritarianism
RWAGE
    ragweed antigen E
RWBT
    rapid whole blood test
RWECochG
    round window electrocochleography
RWG
    rye whole grain
RWIS
    restraint and water immersion stress
RWJF
    Robert Wood Johnson Foundation
RWM
    regional wall motion

RWMA
    regional wall motion abnormality
RWP
    ragweed pollen
    R-wave progression [electrocardiography]
RWS
    ragweed sensitivity
RWT
    relative wall thickness
    Roche, Wainer, and Thissen [method of height prediction]
    R-wave threshold [electrocardiography]
RX
    rapid exchange
    residual tumor not assessed [TNM classification]
Rx
    drug
    medication
    pharmacy
    prescribe
    prescription
    prescription drug
    take [L. *recipe*] (*See also* R)
    therapy
    treatment
r(X)
    right X [chromosome]
Rxd
    treatment [prescribed]
Rx'd US
    treated with ultrasound, diathermy, and traction
RXLI
    recessive X-linked ichthyosis
Rxn
    react(ing) (reaction) (*See also* R)
Rx Phys
    treating physician
RXR
    9-cis retinoic acid receptor
    retinoid X receptor
RXRE
    Rex [protein] responsive element
RXT
    radiation therapy (radiotherapy) (*See also* Rad, RADIO, Rad Ther, RATx, RoRx, RT, RTx)
    right exotropia
R-Y
    Roux-en-Y [anastomosis]
RYGB
    Roux-en-Y gastric bypass
RZ
    reserve zone
RZR
    retinoid Z receptor

S

apparent power [electrical]
entropy [in thermodynamics]
exposure time [radiology]
half [L. *semis*] (*See also* HF, hf, sem., semi, ss)
label, write [L. *sigma*] [L. *sigma* mark, write on] (*See also* /S/, SG, sig.)
left [L. *sinister*] (*See also* s)
let it be written, labeled [L. *signetur*] (*See also* /S/, SG, sig.)
mean dose per unit cumulated activity [radiopharmacy]
response to white space [Rorschach]
sacral
saline (*See also* SA, SAL)
Salmonella
same
saturate(d) (*See also* SAT, sat., sat'd, std)
saturation (*See also* SAT, sat., satn, sats)
Schistosoma
screen-containing cassette
section (*See also* s, SEC, sec, sect)
sella (turcica) [center, craniometric]
senile
senility
sensitivity (*See also* sens)
sequential
series (*See also* s, ser)
serine (*See also* Ser)
serum
Shigella
sick
siemens [SI unit of electric conductance, susceptance, admittance]
sigmoid
signature [prescription] (*See also* /S/, SG, sig.)
sign(ed) (*See also* /S/, SG, sig.)
signs (*See also* Sx, S$_x$, sx)
single [marital status]
singular (*See also* sing.)
sinus
sister (*See also* SIS)
small (*See also* Sm)
smooth [bacterial colony]
soft
soil
solid
soluble (*See also* sol.)
solute (*See also* SOL, solu)
son
sone [unit of subjective loudness]
south

space (*See also* sp)
spasm
spatial aptitude [in General Aptitude Test Battery]
spheric(al) [lens] (*See also* sph)
Spirillum
spleen
sponge
sporadic
Staphylococcus
stimulus (*See also* R, ST stim, stimn)
Streptococcus
subject
subjective [findings]
substrate
sulcus
sulfur
sum [of arithmetic series]
supravergence
surface
Svedberg [sedimentation coefficient, ultra-centrifuge]
swine
Swiss (mouse)
sympathetic
synthesis [phase in cell cycle]
systole (*See also* syst)
without (*See also* ō, sin., WO, wo)

S'

shoulder

S1–S4

first through fourth heart sounds
suicide risk classification

S1–S5

first to fifth sacral nerve
first to fifth sacral vertebra

S7

summation gallop [heart sounds]

^{35}S

sulfur-35

/S/, /s/

label, write [L. *signa*] (*See also* S, SG, sig.)
let it be written, labeled [L. *signetur*] (*See also* S, SG, sig.)
sign(ed) (*See also* S, SG, sig.)
signature [prescription] (*See also* S, SG, sig.)

s

atomic orbital with angular momentum quantum number zero
label [L. *signa*] (*See also* S, sig)
left [L. *sinister*] (*See also* S)
length of path
standard deviation (see also σ)

s *(continued)*
sample variance (*See also* s^2)
satellite [chromosome]
scruple [apothecary]
second (*See also* S)
section (*See also* S, SEC, sec, sect)
sedimentation coefficient
selection coefficient
series (*See also* S, ser)
suckling

s^2
sample variance (*See also* s)

7s
serial sevens test [mental status evaluation] (*See also* serial 7s)

SA
according to art [L. *secundum artem*]
NATO code for arsine
sacroanterior (sacrum anterior) [fetal position]
saline (*See also* S, SAL)
salt added
salvage angioplasty
sarcoma (*See also* sarc)
Schizophrenics Anonymous
second antibody
secondary amenorrhea
secondary anemia
secondary arrest
self-agglutinating
self-analysis
semen analysis
sensitizing antibody
sensory awareness
septal apical
serratus anterior
serum albumin (*See also* SAB)
serum aldolase
severe asthma
Sexaholics Anonymous
short acting
sialic acid
sialoadenectomy
siblings [raised] apart
simian adenovirus
sinuatrial (sinoatrial) (*See also* S-A, SN)
sinus arrest (arrhythmia) (*See also* S Arrh)
skeletal age
sleep apnea
slightly active
slow acetylator
social acquiescence
social age
soluble in alkaline [medium]
spatial average
specific activity
spectrum analysis

sperm abnormality
sperm agglutinin
spiking activity
spinal anesthesia
splenic artery
standard accuracy
Staphylococcus aureus
status asthmaticus
stimulus artifact
Stokes-Adams [attack, syndrome] (*See also* SAA)
subarachnoid
subcarinal angle
substance abuse
suicide alert
suicide attempt
surface antigen
surface area
sustained action
sympathetic activity
systemic artery
systemic aspergillosis

S-A
sinuatrial (sinoatrial) (*See also* SA, SN)

S/A
same as
sugar and acetone (*See also* S&A)

S&A
sickness and accident [insurance]
sugar and acetone (*See also* S/A)

SAA
same as above
serum amyloid [type] A
severe aplastic anemia
Sex Addicts Anonymous
splenic artery aneurysm
Stokes-Adams attack (*See also* SA)
synthetic amino acids

SAAG
serum ascites-albumin gradient

SAAND
selective apoptotic antineoplastic drug

SAAP
selective aortic arch perfusion

SAARD
slow-acting antirheumatic drug

SAAST
Self-Administered Alcoholism Screening test

SAAV
simultaneous acquisition of artery and vein

SAB
sequential androgen blockade
serum albumin (*See also* SA)
short-acting block
side air bags
significant asymptomatic bacteriuria
sinuatrial (sinoatrial) block

spontaneous abortion
Staphylococcus aureus bacteremia
streptavidin-biotin [peroxidase
complex]
subarachnoid bleed
subarachnoid block
SABA
short-acting beta agonist
SABOV
Sabo virus
SABP
spontaneous acute bacterial
peritonitis
SABR
screening auditory brainstem
response
SABV
Saboya virus
SAC
saccharin
screening and acute care
seasonal acute conjunctivitis
seasonal allergic conjunctivitis
segmental antigen challenge
serial autocorrelation
serum aminoglycoside concentration
short arm cast
shoulder adhesive capsulitis
sideline assessment of concussion
space available for cord
splenic adherent cell
stable access cannula
SACA
Service Assessment for Children and
Adolescents
SACC
short arm cylinder cast
sacc
cogwheel respiration [Fr. *saccades* to
jerk]
SACD
subacute combined degeneration [of
spinal cord] (*See also* SCD)
SACE
serum angiotensin-converting enzyme
SACH
small animal care hospital
soft ankle, cushioned heel [orthopedic
appliance]
solid ankle-cushion heel [articulated foot
prosthesis]
SACHT
serum antichymotrypsin
sac-il
sacroiliac (*See also* SI)
SACL
Sales Attitude Check List

SACQ
Student Adaptation to College
Questionnaire
SACS
secondary anticoagulation system
SACSF
subarachnoid cerebrospinal fluid
SACT
sinuatrial (sinoatrial) conduction time
SAD
Scale of Anxiety and Depression
schizoaffective disorder
seasonal affective disorder
Self-Assessment Depression [Scale]
separation anxiety disorder
serial-agitated dilution
severe autoimmune disease
sinoaortic denervation
small airways disease (dysfunction)
social anxiety disorder
social avoidance and distress
source-to-axis distance
specific antibody deficiency
subacromial decompression
subacute dialysis
sugar and acetone determination
sugar, acetone, diacetic acid [test]
(*See also* SADA)
superior axis deviation
suppressor-activating determinant
SADA
sugar, acetone, diacetic acid [test]
(*See also* SAD)
SADBE
squaric acid dibutylester
SADD
Standardized Assessment of Depressive
Disorders
SADDAN
severe achondroplasia with
developmental delay and acanthosis
nigricans
SADIA
small-angle double-incidence
angiogram
SADL
simulated activities of daily living
SAD PERSONS
sex, age, depression, previous attempt,
ethanol, rational thinking loss,
separated, divorced, widowed,
organized plan, no social support,
stated future intent [suicide
assessment]
SADQ
Self-Administered Dependency
Questionnaire

S

SADR
suspected adverse drug reaction
SADS
Schedule for Affective Disorders and
Schizophrenia
seasonal affective disorder syndrome
Self-Assessment Depression Scale
sudden arrhythmic death syndrome
SADS-C
Schedule for Affective Disorders and
Schizophrenia-Change
SADS-L
Schedule for Affective Disorders and
Schizophrenia-Lifetime [Version]
SADT
Stetson Auditory Discrimination
Test
SAE
serious adverse event
short above-elbow [cast]
specific action exercise
stimulated acoustic emission
subcortical arteriosclerotic
(atherosclerotic) encephalopathy
supported arm exercise
SAEB
sinuatrial (sinoatrial) entrance block
SAECG, SaECG, SAEKG
signal averaging (averaged)
electrocardiograph(y)
(electrocardiogram)
SAED
selected area electron diffusion
semiautomatic external defibrillator
SAEP
Salmonella abortus equi pyrogen
SAESU
substance abuse evaluation screen
unit
SAF
Self-Analysis Form
self-articulating femoral
[hip prosthesis]
serum accelerator factor
simultaneous auditory feedback
subcutaneous abdominal fat
SAFA
soluble antigen fluorescent antibody
[test]
SAFE
sexual assault forensic evidence
simulated aircraft fire and emergency
solid ankle flexible endoskeletal [foot
prosthesis]
stationary ankle flexible endoskeleton
[foot prosthesis]
stationary attachment flexible
endoskeletal [prosthesis]
support, autonomy, fusion, empathy

SAFER
Safety Assessment of Function and
Environment for Rehabilitation
SAFHS
sonic-accelerated fracture-healing
system
SAFK
single-axis friction knee [prosthesis]
SAFTEE
Systematic Assessment for Treatment of
Emergent Events
SAFV
Saint-Floris virus
SAG
sodium antimony gluconate
sonoangiograph(y) (sonangiogram)
Swiss(-type) agammaglobulinemia
sag
sagittal
SAGB
Swedish Adjustable Gastric Band
Sag D
sagittal diameter
SAGE
serial analysis of gene expression
SAGES-P
Screening Assessment for Gifted
Elementary Students, Primary
SAGM
sodium chloride, adenine, glucose,
mannitol [preservative]
SAGV
Sagiyama virus
SAH
S-adenosyl-L-homocysteine (*See also*
AdoHcy)
subarachnoid hemorrhage
systemic arterial hypertension
SAHA
seborrhea-hypertrichosis/hirsutism-
alopecia [syndrome]
SAHEM
self-applied health enhancement method
SAHIES
Staphylococcus aureus
hyperimmunoglobulinemia E syndrome
SAHS
sleep apnea-hypersomnolence syndrome
sleep apnea-hypopnea syndrome
SAHS-UAO
sleep apnea hypersomnolence syndrome
associated with upper airways
obstruction
SAI
Schedule for Assessment of Insight
Schema Assessment instrument
self-administered injectable
Self-Analysis Inventory
Sexual Arousability Inventory

Social Adequacy Index
sodium amytal interview
Student Adjustment Inventory
surface asymmetry index
systemic active immunotherapy

SAICAR

succinyl aminoimidazole carboxamide
ribotide

SAID

specific adaptation to imposed demand
steroidal antiinflammatory drug

SAIDS

sexually acquired immune deficiency
(immunodeficiency) syndrome
simian acquired immunodeficiency
syndrome

SAKV

Sakhalin virus

SAL

salicylate (See also sal)
salicylic and lactic acid [wart paint]
saline (See also S, SA, Sa, sal)
self-aligning [knee prosthesis]
sensorineural acuity level
sensory acuity level
specified antilymphocytic
sterility assurance level
suction-assisted lipectomy
suction-assisted lipoplasty
synchronous airway lesion

SAL 12

sequential analysis of twelve chemistry
constituents

sal

salicylate (See also SAL)
salicylic
saliva
salt

SALF

subacute liver failure

SALK

single-axis locking knee [prosthesis]
surgical arthroscopy, left knee

SALT

skin-associated lymphoid tissue

SALT-P

Slosson Articulation Language Test with
Phonology

SALV

Salehabad virus

SAM

S-adenosyl-L-methionine
scanning acoustic microscope
selective antimicrobial modulation
self-administered medication
sex arousal mechanism
short arc motion

Skills Assessment Module
sleep apnea monitor
smart anesthesia multigas
spinal analysis machine
structural aluminum malleable [splint]
subcutaneous augmentation material
sulfated acid mucopolysaccharide
surface-active material
surface adherent monocyte
synthetic, adhesive, moisture [vapor
permeable]
systolic anterior motion [of mitral
valve]

SAMA

schizoaffective mania mainly affective
[type]

SAMBA

simultaneous areolar mastopexy and
breast augmentation

SAME

syndrome of arthralgias, myalgias,
edema

SAMe, SAM-e

S-adenosylmethionine

SAMF

single antibody Millipore filtration

SAMI

socially acceptable monitoring
instrument

sAMS

adenylosuccinic acid

SAMS

Study Attitudes and Methods Survey

SAMSHA

[United States Department of Health
and Human Services] Substance Abuse
and Mental Health Administration

S-AMY

serum amylase

SAN

side-arm nebulizer
sinuatrial (sinoatrial) node (See also SN)
slept all night
solitary autonomous nodule

SANA

sinuatrial (sinoatrial) node artery

sanat

sanatorium

SANC

short arm navicular cast

SANDO

sensory ataxic neuropathy with
dysarthria and ophthalmoplegia

SANDR

sinuatrial (sinoatrial) nodal reentry

sang.

sanguineous

S

sanit
>sanitarium
>sanitary
>sanitation

SANS
>Scale for the Assessment of Negative Symptoms
>Stoller afferent nerve stimulation
>sympathetic autonomic nervous system

SANV
>Sango virus

SAO
>small airways obstruction
>Southeast Asian ovalocytosis
>splanchnic artery occlusion
>subclavian artery occlusion

SaO$_2$, S$_{AO2}$
>arterial oxygen saturation

SAOF
>Self-Assessment of Occupational Functioning

SAP
>saline-assisted polypectomy
>sensory action potential
>serum acid phosphatase
>serum alkaline phosphatase
>serum amyloid P
>severe acute pancreatitis
>shock-absorbing pylons
>situs ambiguus with polysplenia
>sporadic adenomatous polyps
>stable angina pectoris
>standard automated perimetry
>*Staphylococcus aureus* protease
>systemic arterial pressure
>systolic arterial pressure

SAP-1
>stress-activated protein 1

SAP1
>sphingolipid activator protein 1

sap.
>saponification (*See also* sapon)
>saponify (*See also* sapon)

SAPA
>spatial average-pulse average [ultrasound]

SAPASI
>Self-Administered Psoriasis Area and Severity Index

SAPD
>self-administration of psychoactive (psychotropic) drug
>signal-averaged P-wave duration

SAPF
>simultaneous anterior and posterior [spinal] fusion

SAPH
>saphenous

SAPHO
>synovitis, acne, pustulosis, hyperostosis, osteitis [syndrome]

SAPK
>stress-activated protein kinase

SAPK2
>stress-activated protein kinase 2

SAP-MS
>sodium acrylate and vinyl alcohol copolymer microsphere
>superabsorbent polymer microsphere

SAPMS
>short arm posterior-molded splint

sapon
>saponification (*See also* sap.)
>saponify (*See also* sap.)

SAPP
>sodium acid pyrophosphate

SAPS
>Scale for the Assessment of Positive Symptoms
>short arm plaster splint
>Simplified Acute Physiology Score
>single-action pumping system

SAPS II
>Simplified Acute Physiology Score version II

SAQ
>School Atmosphere Questionnaire
>Seattle angina questionnaire
>Sexual Adjustment Questionnaire
>short-arc quadriceps [test]
>Substance Abuse Questionnaire

SAQC
>statistical analysis and quality control

SAQLI
>Sleep Apnea Quality of Life Index

SAR
>scaffold-associated regions
>scatter to air ratio
>seasonal allergic rhinitis
>sexual attitude reassessment
>sexual attitude restructuring
>somatoautonomic reflex
>specific absorption rate
>structure-activity relationship
>supplied air respirator
>survival after recurrence

Sar
>sarcosine
>sulfarsphenamine

SARA
>sexually acquired reactive arthritis
>system for anesthetic and respiratory administration

SARC
>seasonal allergic rhinoconjunctivitis

sarc
>sarcoma (*See also* SA)

SARK
surgical arthroscopy, right knee
SARM
selective androgen-receptor modulator
SARME
surgically assisted rapid maxillary expansion
SARPE
surgically assisted rapid palatal expansion
S Arrh
sinus arrest (arrhythmia) (*See also* SA)
SARS
severe acute respiratory syndrome
SARS-CoV
severe acute respiratory syndrome coronavirus
SART
sinuatrial (sinoatrial) recovery time
standard acid reflux test
SARV
Santa Rosa virus
SAS
saline, agent, and saline
scalenus anticus syndrome
School Assessment Survey
School Attitude Survey
Sedation-Agitation Scale
see assessment sheet
self-rating anxiety scale
short arm splint
shoulder arm system
signs and symptoms (*See also* S&S, SS)
Simpson-Angus Scale [neuroleptic-induced parkinsonism]
simultaneous analog stimulation
Situational Attitude Scale
Sklar Aphasia Scale
sleep apnea syndrome
slide agglutination serotyping
small animal surgery
small aorta syndrome
Social Adaptation Status
Social Adjustment Scale
sodium amylosulfate
space-adaptation syndrome
Specific Activity Scale
static adjustable stretch
statistical analysis system
statistical applications software
sterile aqueous solution
sterile aqueous suspension
subaortic stenosis
subarachnoid space
subaxial subluxation
supravalvular aortic stenosis (*See also* SVAS)

surface-active substance
synthetic absorbable suture
SASD
secundum artem septal defect
SA-SD
subacromial-subdeltoid [bursa]
SaSE
saline solution enema
SASH
saline, agent, saline, heparin
SASI
Separation Anxiety Symptom Inventory
SASMAS
skin-adipose superficial musculoaponeurotic system
SASPP
syndrome of absence of septum pellucidum with porencephaly
SASQ
seasonal allergies symptoms questionnaire
SASRS
Social Adjustment Self-Report Scale
SASS
Social Adaptation Self-Evaluation Scale
SASSAD
six-area, six-sign atopic dermatitis
SASSI
Substance Abuse Subtle Screening Inventory
SAT
satellite
saturate(d) (*See also* S, sat., sat'd, std)
saturation (*See also* S, sat., satn, sats)
Scholastic Aptitude Test
School Ability Test
School Attitude Test
self-administered therapy
Senior Apperception Technique
Senior Apperception Test
serum antitrypsin
Shapes Analysis Test
single-agent therapy
slide agglutination test
specific antithymocytic [globulin]
speech awareness threshold
spermatogenic activity test
spinal attunement technique
spontaneous activity test
spontaneous autoimmune thyroiditis
Stanford Achievement Test
structural atypia
subacute thrombosis
subacute thyroiditis
subcutaneous adipose tissue
symptomless autoimmune thyroiditis

S

SAT *(continued)*
  systematized assertive therapy
  systemic assertive therapy
sat.
  satisfactory
  saturate(d) (*See also* S, SAT, sat'd, std)
  saturation (*See also* S, SAT, satn, sats)
SATA
  Scholastic Abilities Test for Adults
  spatial average-temporal average
    [ultrasound]
SATB
  Special Aptitude Test Battery
sat. cond
  satisfactory condition
sat'd
  saturated (*See also* std) (*See also* S,
    SAT, sat., std)
SATL
  surgical Achilles tendon lengthening
SATM
  sodium aurothiomalate [injectable gold]
satn
  saturation (*See also* S, SAT, sat., sats)
SATP
  spatial average-temporal peak
    [ultrasound]
  substance abuse treatment program
SATS
  streptococcus A toxic shock
sats
  [oxygen] saturation (*See also* S, SAT,
    sat., satn)
sat. sol., sat. soln.
  saturated solution
SATV
  Sathuperi virus
SAV
  San Angelo virus
  sequential atrioventricular [pacing]
  specific allergy vaccination
  streptavidin
  supraannular valve
SA:V
  surface area to volume ratio
SAVANT
  Surgical Anatomy Visualization And
    Navigation Tools
SAVD
  spontaneous assisted vaginal
    delivery
SAVED
  saphenous vein graft de novo
SAWV
  sawgrass virus
SAX
  short axis
SAXT
  slow axoplasmic transport

SB
  safety belt
  sandbag
  scleral buckle
  seat belt
  seen by
  septal basal
  serum bilirubin
  shortness of breath (*See also* SOB)
  sick bay [military]
  sick boy
  side bend
  sideroblast
  single blind
  single breath
  sinus bradycardia
  slide board
  small bowel
  sodium balance
  Southern blot
  soybean
  spike burst [electroencephalogram]
  spina bifida
  sponge bath
  spontaneous blastogenesis
  spontaneously breathing
  stand by [assistance] (*See also* ST BY)
  Stanford-Binet [Intelligence Scale]
    (*See also* SBIS)
  stereotyped behavior
  sternal border
  stillbirth
  stillborn (*See also* STB, Stb,
    stillb)
  stone basketing
  subarachnoid block [anesthesia]
  suction biopsy
  surface binding [protein]
S-B
  Sengstaken-Blakemore [tube]
+SB
  wearing seat belt
S/B
  seen by
  side bending
SB-
  not wearing seat belt
Sb
  antimony [L. *stibium*]
  strabismus (*See also* strab)
sb
  stilb [unit of luminous intensity]
SBA
  serum bactericidal activity
  serum bile acid
  sideroblastic anemia
  soybean agglutinin
  spina bifida aperta
  standby angioplasty

standby assistance
Summary Basis of Approval [FDA]
SBAC
small-bowel adenocarcinoma
SBAI
Social Behavior Assessment Inventory
SBB
simultaneous binaural bithermal
small-bowel biopsy
stereotactic breast biopsy
stimulation-bound behavior
Sudan black B [dye, stain]
SBBO
small-bowel bacterial overgrowth
SBC
sensory binocular cooperation
serum bactericidal concentration
single base cane
skull base chordoma
special back care
standard bicarbonate
strict bed confinement
sunburn cell
superficial bladder cancer
SBD
sleep-related brain disorder
straight bag drainage
suggested brain dysfunction
Supervisory Behavior Description
S-BD
seizure-brain damage
SbDH
sorbitol dehydrogenase
SBDX
scanning-beam digital x-ray
SBE
saturated base excess
self-breast examination
short below-elbow [cast]
shortness of breath on exertion
(*See also* SOBE, SOBOE)
short-segment Barrett esophagus
small-bowel enteroscopy
subacute bacterial endocarditis
SBEP
somatosensory brainstem evoked
potential
S/β, s/beta
sickle cell beta (β)
SBF
serologic-blocking factor
serum blocking factor
specific blocking factor
splanchnic blood flow
splenic blood flow
systemic blood flow
SBFE
Stanford-Binet Fourth Edition

SBFT
small-bowel follow-through
(followthrough) (*See also* SMBFT)
SBG
selenite brilliant green
standby guard
SBGM
self blood-glucose monitoring
SBH
sea-blue histiocyte
sequencing by hybridization
SBHC
school-based health center
SBI
silent brain infarct(ion)
silicone [gel-containing] breast
implant
soybean trypsin inhibitor
systemic bacterial infection
SBIAB
secondary bacterial infection acute
bronchitis
SBIS
Stanford-Binet Intelligence Scale
(*See also* SB)
SBJ
skin, bones, joints
SBK
spinnbarkeit [cervical mucus]
SBL
serum bactericidal level
soybean lecithin
sponge blood loss
sBLA
supplemental Biologics License
Application
SBLLA
sarcoma, breast and brain tumors,
leukemia, laryngeal and lung
adenomas [syndrome]
SB-LM
Stanford-Binet Intelligence Test Form
LM
SBM
selective broth medium
subbasement membrane
subepithelial basement membrane
SBMPL
simultaneous binaural midplane
localizatison
SBN$_2$, SB$_{N2}$, SBNT
single-breath nitrogen [test]
SBNW
single-breath nitrogen washout
SBO
small-bowel obstruction
specified bovine offal
spina bifida occulta

S

⚠ SBOD
scleral buckle, oculus dexter
(right eye) ⚠
SBOE
surgical blood order equation
SBOH
State Board of Health
SBOM
soybean oil meal
⚠ SBOS
scleral buckle, oculus sinister
(left eye) ⚠
SBP
school breakfast program
scleral buckling procedure
selenium-binding protein
serotonin-binding protein
small-bowel phytobezoar
solitary bone plasmacytoma
spontaneous bacterial peritonitis
spontaneous biliary perforation
steroid-binding plasma (protein)
sulfobromophthalein
systemic blood pressure
systolic blood pressure (*See also* SYS
BP)
SBPA
satellite-borne phased array
SBPN
simultaneous bilateral percutaneous
nephrolithotomy
SBQ
Smoking Behavior Questionnaire
SBQC
small-based quad cane
SBR
Scarff-Bloom-Richardson [breast cancer
grading system]
sluggish blood return
small-bowel resection
spleen to body [weight] ratio
stillbirth rate
strict bedrest
styrene-butadiene rubber
SBRN
sensory branch of radial nerve
SBRT
split beat rotation therapy
SBS
serum blood sugar
shaken baby syndrome
short bowel syndrome
sick building syndrome
side to back to side
side by side
sinobronchial syndrome
small-bowel series
social breakdown syndrome

staff burnout scale
straight back syndrome
SBSE
supine bicycle stress echocardiography
SBSM
self-blood sugar monitoring
SBSP
simultaneous bilateral spontaneous
pneumothorax
SBSRT
Spreen-Benton Sentence Repetition Test
SBSS
Seligmann balanced salt solution
SBT
sequenced-based typing
serous borderline tumor
serum bactericidal test
serum bactericidal titer
serum bacteriologic titer
single-breath test
skin bleeding time
spontaneous breathing trial
SBTB
sinus breakthrough beat
SBTI
soybean trypsin inhibitor (*See also*
STI)
SBTPE
State Boards Test Pool Examination
SBTT
small-bowel transit time
SBTx
small-bowel transplant(ation)
SBV
single binocular vision
SBW
seat belts worn
standard body weight
SBX
symphysis, buttocks, xiphoid
⚠ SC
sacrococcygeal
schedule change
schizophrenia
Schwann cell
Sciana [blood group antigen]
sciatic [nerve]
science (scientific) (*See also* Sc, Sci)
scleral cautery
sclerosing cholangitis
secondary cleavage
secretory coil
secretory component
self-care
self-control
semicircular
semiclosed
semilunar-valve closure

serum complement
serum creatinine (*See also* SCr)
service connected
sex chromatin
Sezary cell
shallow compartment
short circuit
sick call
sickle cell
sieving coefficient
sigmoid colon
silicone coated
single chemical
skin conductance (conduction)
slow component
small [blood pressure] cuff
Smeloff-Cutter [heart valve prosthesis]
Snellen chart
sodium citrate
soluble complex
special care
specific characteristic
specific conductance [water]
spinal cord
spindle (-cell) carcinoma
spleen cell (*See also* SPC)
sport cord
squamous carcinoma
statistical control
stellate cell
stem cell
stepped care
sternoclavicular
stimulus, conditioned
stratum corneum
stroke count
subcellular
subclavian
subclavian catheter
subcostal
subcorneal
subcortical
subcutaneous(ly) (*See also* sc, SQ,
  subcu, subcut, subq) △
subtotal colectomy
succinylcholine (*See also* SCH, Succ,
  sux)
sugar coated
sulfur colloid
sulfur containing
superior colliculus
superior constrictor [muscles of
  pharynx]
superior cornu
supplementary canal
supportive care
suppressor cell

supraclavicular
supracondylar
surface colony
surgical cone
surveillance cultures
systemic candidiasis
systolic click

S&C
sclera and conjunctiva [singular]
sclerae and conjunctivae [plural]
singly and consensually

Sc
scandium
scapula [singular] (scapulae [plural])
  (*See also* SCAP)
science (*See also* SC, Sci)
scientific (*See also* SC, Sci)

⁴⁷Sc
scandium-47

△ **sc**
scant
sclera
subcutaneous(ly) (*See also* SC, SQ,
  subcu, subcut, subq) △

s̄c
without correction [glasses] [L. *sine
  correctione*]

SCA
School and College Ability [test]
selective coronary angiogram
selfcare agency
severe congenital anomaly
sickle cell anemia
single-camera autostereoscopy
  [imaging]
single-chain antigen-binding
  [protein]
single-channel analyzer
sperm-coating antigen
spinocerebellar ataxia
spleen colony assay
steroidal-cell antibody
subclavian artery
subcutaneous abdominal [block]
sudden cardiac arrest
superior cerebellar artery
suppressor cell activity

SCA1
spinocerebellar ataxia, type 1

SCa, S_Ca
serum calcium

ScA
scapula anterior (scapuloanterior) [fetal
  position]

SCAA
sporadic cerebral amyloid
  angiopathy

SCAb
autoantibody to stratum corneum
SCABG
single coronary artery bypass graft
SCAD
segmental colitis associated with
diverticulosis
short-chain acyl coenzyme A
dehydrogenase [deficiency]
spontaneous coronary artery dissection
spontaneous cervical artery dissection
SCAE
subcortical arteriosclerotic
(atherosclerotic) encephalopathy
SCAG
single coronary artery graft
SCAL
Self-Concept as a Learner
SCALE
Scaled Curriculum Achievement Levels
Test
Scales of Creativity and Learning
Environment
SCAMI
Self-Concept and Motivation Inventory
SCAMP 1–5
secretory carrier membrane protein
1–5
SCAN
Screening [Test for Identifying] Central
Auditory Disorder
suspected child abuse [and/or] neglect
systolic coronary artery narrowing
SCAP
scapular
scapula [singular] scapulae [plural]
(See also SC)
stem cell apheresis
SCARED
Screen for Child Anxiety-Related
Emotional Disorders
SCARF
skeletal [abnormalities], cutis [laxa],
craniostenosis, [psychomotor]
retardation, facial [abnormalities]
SCARMD
severe childhood autosomal recessive
muscular dystrophy
SCAS
Self-Care Assessment Schedule
semicontinuous activated sludge
SCAT
School and College Ability Test
sheep cell agglutination test (titer)
short-contact treatment
sickle cell anemia test
SCATBI
Scales of Cognitive Ability for
Traumatic Brain Injury

SCAV
Sunday Canyon virus
SCB
sedative cabinet bath
strictly confined to bed
SCBA
self-contained breathing apparatus
SCBC
small-cell bronchogenic carcinoma
SCBE
single-contrast barium enema
SCBF
spinal cord blood flow
SCBG
symmetrical calcification of basal
[cerebral] ganglia
SCBH
systemic cutaneous basophil
hypersensitivity
SCBP
stratum corneum basic protein
SCBS
survival and coping beliefs scale
ScBU
screening bacteriuria
SCC
sequential combination chemotherapy
services for crippled children
short calcaneocuboid
short circuit current
short-course chemotherapy
sickle cell crisis
side-chain cleavage
small-cell cancer (carcinoma)
small cleaved cell
spinal cord compression
squamous carcinoma of cervix
squamous cell cancer (carcinoma)
(See also SCCA, SQC, SqCA,
SqCCA, sq cell ca)
subcutaneous sarcoidosis
SC4C
subcostal four-chamber [view on
echocardiogram]
SCCA
semiclosed circle absorber (system)
squamous cell cancer (carcinoma)
(See also SCC, SQC, SqCA, SqCCA,
sq cell ca)
squamous cell carcinoma antigen
(See also SCC-Ag)
SCC-Ag
squamous cell carcinoma antigen
(See also SCCA)
SCCB
small-cell cancer of bladder
small-cell carcinoma of bronchus
SCCC
squamous cell cervical carcinoma

SCCD
Schnyder crystalline corneal dystrophy
subacute cortical cerebellar
degeneration
SCCE
squamous cell carcinoma of esophagus
SCCH
sternocostoclavicular hyperostosis
SCCHN
squamous cell carcinoma of head and
neck
SCCHO
sternocostoclavicular hyperostosis
SCCI
subcutaneous continuous infusion
S-CCK-Pz
secretin, cholecystokinin, pancreozymin
SCCL
small-cell carcinoma of lung
SCCM
Sertoli cell culture medium
SCCMS
slow-channel congenital myasthenic
syndrome
SCCOT
squamous cell carcinoma of oral tongue
squamous cell carcinoma of tongue
SCCT
severe cerebrocranial trauma
SCD
sagittal canal diameter
sequential compression device
service-connected disability
sickle cell disease
spinal cord disease
spinocerebellar degeneration
subacute combined degeneration [of
spinal cord] (*See also* SACD)
subacute coronary disease
sudden cardiac death
sudden coronary death
sulfur-carbon drug
systemic carnitine deficiency
sCD4
soluble recombinant human CD4
ScDA
right scapula anterior (scapuloanterior)
[fetal position] [L. *scapulodextra
anterior*] (*See also* RScA)
S-C disease
sickle cell-hemoglobin C disease
SCDM
soybean-casein digest medium
ScDP
right scapula posterior (scapuloposterior)
[fetal position] [L. *scapulodextra
posterior*] (*See also* RScP)

SCE
saturated calomel electrode
secretory carcinoma of endometrium
serous choroidal effusion
sister chromatid exchange
soft-cooked egg
specialized columnar epithelium
spinal cord ependymoma
split hand-cleft lip/palate and ectodermal
dysplasia
subcutaneous emphysema (*See also*
SQE)
SCEMIA
self-contained enzymatic membrane
immunoassay
SCEP
sandwich counterelectrophoresis
somatosensory cortical evoked potential
SCER
sister chromatid exchange rate
SCF
somatic cell-derived growth factor
special care formula
stem cell factor
supercritical fluid
SCFA
short-chain fatty acid
SCFE
slipped capital femoral epiphysis
SCFGT
Southern California Figure Ground
Test
SCFI
specific clotting factor and inhibitor
scFv
single-chain variable fragment
SCG
seismocardiography
serum chemistry [to analyze] graft
serum chemogram
substitute caregiver
superior cervical ganglion
SCGE
single-cell gel electrophoresis
SCGYEM
serum, casein, glucose, yeast extract
medium
SCH
Schirmer [test]
schistosomiasis (*Schistosoma* spp.)
vaccine
sole community hospital
spinal cord hemangioma
subclinical hypothyroidism
subconjunctival hemorrhage
succinylcholine (*See also* SC, SUCC,
SUX)

S

SCH *(continued)*
suprachiasmatic
suprachoroidal hemorrhage
SCh
succinylcholine chloride
SCHAD
short-chain hydroxyacyl-coenzyme A
dehydrogenase
SCHC
sickle cell hemoglobin C disease
SChE
serum cholinesterase
sched
schedule
SCHISTO, SCHIZ
schistocyte (schizocyte)
schiz
schizophrenia
SCHL
subcapsular hematoma of liver
SCHLP
supracricoid hemilaryngopharyngectomy
SCHNC
squamous cell head and neck
cancer
SCHT
subcutaneous histamine test
SCI
Science Citation Index
Sertoli cell index
short crus of incus
silent cerebral infarct(ion)
spinal cord injury
structured clinical interview
subcoma insulin
Sci
science (scientific) (*See also* SC, Sc)
SCIA
superficial circumflex iliac artery
SCIBTA
stem cell indicated by transplant(ation)
assay
SCID
severe combined immunodeficiency
(immune deficiency) [disease,
disorder]
Structured Clinical Interview for
DSM-IV
SCID-II
Structured Clinical Interview (for
DSM-IV) Axis II Personality
Disorders
SCID-IV
Structured Clinical Interview for
DSM-IV Dissociative
Disorders
SCIDA
[Athabascan type] severe combined
immunodeficiency disease

SCID-CV
Structured Clinical Interview (for
DSM-IV Axis I Disorders): Clinician
Version
SCID-D
Structured Clinical Interview (for
DSM-IV) Dissociative Disorders
SCID-P
Structured Clinical Interview (for
DSM-IV) Patient Version
SCID-PD
Structured Clinical Interview (for
DSM-IV) Psychotic Disorders
SCIDS
severe combined immunodeficiency
(immune deficiency) syndrome
(*See also* SCID)
SCIDX
severe combined immunodeficiency
(immune deficiency) X-linked
⚠ **SCIG**
subcutaneous immunoglobulin ⚠
SCII
Strong-Campbell Interest Inventory
SCINT
scintigraphy
SCIP
Screening and Crisis Intervention
Program
SCIPP
sacrococcygeal to inferior pubic point
SCIS
surface carcinoma in situ
SCIT
single-chain immunotoxin
SCIU
spinal cord injury unit
⚠ **SCIV**
subclavian intravenous
subcutaneous and intravenous ⚠
SCIWORA, SCIWOA
spinal cord injury without radiographic
(radiologic) abnormality
SCJ
squamocolumnar junction
sternoclavicular joint
sCJD
sporadic Creutzfeldt-Jakob disease
SCK
serum creatine kinase
sc-kit
soluble c-kit [gene]
SCL
scaphocapitolunate arthrodesis
scleroderma (*See also* SD)
serum copper level
sinus cycle length
skin conductance level
soft contact lens

spinocervicolemniscal
symptom checklist
syndrome checklist
SCL-90
Symptoms Checklist 90 [items]
Scl, scl
sclerosis
sclerotic
ScLA
left scapula anterior (scapuloanterior)
[fetal position] [L. *scapulolaeva
anterior*] (*See also* LScA)
SCLAX
subcostal long axis
SCLBCL
secondary cutaneous large B-cell
lymphoma
SCLC
small-cell lung cancer (carcinoma)
SCLD
sickle cell lung disease
SCLE
subacute cutaneous lupus
erythematosus
subcutaneous lupus erythematosus
SCLND
selective complete lymph node
dissection
ScLP
left scapula posterior (scapuloposterior)
[fetal position] [L. *scapulolaeva
posterior*] (*See also* LScP)
SCL-90R, SCL-90-R
Symptoms Checklist 90 Revised
SCLS
systemic capillary leak syndrome
SCL
synthetic combinatorial libraries
[gene]
SCM
scalene muscle (*See also* ScM)
scanning capacitance microscope
Schwann cell membrane
sensation, circulation, motion
soluble cytotoxic medium
spinal cord malformation
spleen-cell conditioned medium
split-cord malformation
spondylotic caudal myelopathy
steatocystoma multiplex
sternocleidomastoid [muscle]
streptococcal cell membrane
structure of cytoplasmic matrix
subclavian muscle
supraclavicular muscle
surface-connecting membrane
synovial chondromatosis

ScM
scalene muscle (*See also* SCM)
SCMC
sodium carboxymethylcellulose
sperm-cervical mucus contact
spontaneous cell-mediated cytotoxicity
SCMD
senile choroidal macular degeneration
SCMI
single central maxillary incisor
SCML
small-cell malignant lymphoma
SCMV
serogroup C meningococcal vaccine
SCN
serum thiocyanate
severe chronic neutropenia
severe congenital neutropenia
sodium thiocyanate
suprachiasmatic nucleus
SC$_{Na}$
sieving coefficient for sodium
SCNB
stereotactically guided core needle
biopsy
stereotactic core-needle biopsy
SCNC
small-cell neuroendocrine carcinoma
SCNS
subcutaneous nerve stimulation
SCNT
somatic cell nuclear transfer
SCO
Sertoli cell only [tumor]
somatic crossing-over
subcommissural organ
S:CO
signal to cutoff ratio
SCOB
Schedule-Controlled Operant Behavior
SCOI
Southern California Orthopaedic
Institute
scoli
scoliosis
SCOP, scop
Structural Classification of Proteins
SCOPE
arthroscopy
Surveillance and Control of Pathogens
of Epidemiologic Importance [CDC]
systematic, complete, objective,
practical, empirical
scope
perform endoscopy
SCOR
skin conductance orienting response

S

SCORAD
  Severity Scoring of Atopic Dermatitis
SCORE
  Simple Calculated Osteoporosis Risk Estimation
SCOT
  succinyl CoA:3-ketoacid CoA transferase [enzyme, deficiency]
SCP
  secondary care provider
  single-celled protein
  sodium cellulose phosphate
  soluble cytoplasmic protein
  squamous cell papilloma
  standardized care plan
  submucous cleft palate
  superior cerebellar peduncle
  supracristal plane
SCP-2
  sterol carrier protein 2
ScP
  scapula posterior (scapuloposterior) [fetal position]
scp
  spherical candle power
SCPF
  stem cell proliferation factor
SCPK, S-CPK
  serum creatine phosphokinase
SCPL
  supracricoid partial laryngectomy
SCPL-CHEP
  supracricoid partial laryngectomy with cricohyoidoepiglottopexy
SCPN
  serum carboxypeptidase N
SCPNT
  Southern California Postrotary Nystagmus Test
SCPP
  spinal cord perfusion pressure
SCPR
  standard cardiopulmonary resuscitation
SCPUFA
  short-chain polyunsaturated fatty acid
SCQ
  situational confidence questionnaire
SCR
  silicon-controlled rectifier
  skin conductance response
  spondylotic caudal radiculopathy
  standard care regimen
  stem cell rescue
SCr
  serum creatinine (*See also* SC)
sCR
  soluble complement receptor
sCR1
  soluble complement receptor type 1

sCRAG
  serum cryptococcal antigen
SCRAM
  speech-controlled respirometer for ambulatory measurement
SCRAP
  Simple-Complex Reaction-Time Apparatus
SCREEN
  Screening Children for Related Early Educational Needs
script
  prescription (*See also* PS, Rx)
SC-RNV
  subcutaneous radionuclide venography
SC/RP
  scaling and root planing
SCRS
  Short Clinical Rating Scale
SCRT
  stereotactic conformation radiotherapy
SCS
  Self-Control Scale
  shaken child syndrome
  silicon-controlled switch
  Social Climate Scale
  spinal canal stenosis
  spinal cord stimulation (stimulator)
  splatter control shield
  stem cell support
  subacute confusional state
  suspected catheter sepsis
  synovial chondrosarcoma
  systolic click syndrome
SCSAX
  subcostal short axis
SCSIT
  Southern California Sensory Integration Tests
SCSP, SC-SP
  supracondylar-suprapatellar
SCSR
  standard cervical spine radiography
SCSVT
  Southern California Space Visualization Test
S-CT
  spiral computed tomography
SCT
  allogeneic stem-cell transplant(ation)
  salmon calcitonin
  Sentence Completion Test
  Sertoli cell tumor
  sex chromatin test
  Sexual Compatibility Test
  sickle cell trait
  solid cystic tumor
  sperm cytotoxic
  spinal computed tomography

spinocervicothalamic
spiral computed tomography
squamous cell carcinoma of thyroid
staphylococcal clumping test
star-cancellation test
stem cell transplant(ation)
sugar-coated tablet

SCTA
spiral computed tomography
arteriography (angiography)

SCTAT
sex cord tumor with annular tubule

SCTP
solid and cystic tumors of
pancreas

SCTX
static cervical traction

SCTx
spinal cervical traction

scuba
self-contained underwater breathing
apparatus

SCUCP
small-cell undifferentiated carcinoma of
prostate

SCUD
schizophrenia, chronic undifferentiated
septicemic cutaneous ulcerative
disease

SCUF
slow continuous ultrafiltration

SCUM
secondary carcinoma of upper
mediastinum

SCUNC
small-cell undifferentiated
neuroendocrine carcinoma

SCUT
schizophrenia, chronic undifferentiated
type

SCV
sensory conduction velocity
Sixgun City virus
slow-component velocity
smooth, capsulated, virulent
[bacteria]
squamous cell carcinoma [of] vulva
subclavian vein
subcutaneous vaginal [block]

SCVB
subcutaneous vaginal block

SCV-CPR
simultaneous compression
ventilation-cardiopulmonary
resuscitation

SCWT
Stroop Color Word Test

SCY
scytonemin

SCZ
schizophrenia

SCZ-PTSD
comorbid schizophrenia and
posttraumatic stress disorder

SD
sagittal depth (of cornea)
scleroderma (*See also* SCL)
seborrheic dermatitis
secretion droplet
seizure disorder
senile dementia
sensory deficit
septal defect
serologically defined (detectable)
(determined)
serum defect
severe deficit
severe disability
severely disabled
shallow distance [aquatic therapy]
shoulder disarticulation
shoulder dislocation
shoulder dystocia
single dose
skin destruction
skin dose
sleep deprived (deprivation)
social desirability
socialized delinquency
socialized dementia
solvent-detergent
somadendritic
somatic dysfunction
somatization disorder
spasmodic dysphonia
speech discrimination
spontaneous delivery
sporadic depression
Sprague-Dawley [rat]
spreading depression
stable disease
standard diet
statistical documentation
Stensen duct
sterile dressing
stimulus drive (*See also* Sd)
stone disintegration
straight drainage
succinate dehydrogenase (*See also* SDG)
sudden death
suicide-depression
superoxide dismutase
surgical drain
systolic discharge

S-D

sickle cell [hemoglobin] D [disease]
strength-duration [curve]
suicide-depression

S/D

sharp/dull
solvent/detergent [treated plasma]

S:D

systolic to diastolic ratio

S&D

seen and discussed
stomach and duodenum

S^d

stimulus, discriminative

Sd

stimulus drive (*See also* SD)

SDA

right sacrum anterior (sacroanterior)
[fetal position] [L. *sacrodextra
anterior*] (*See also* RSA)
Sabouraud dextrose agar
salt-dependent agglutinin
same day admission
serotonin/dopamine antagonist
shoulder disarticulation
sialodacryoadenitis [virus]
specific dynamic action
steroid-dependent asthmatic
strand displacement amplification
succinic dehydrogenase activity
superficial distal axillary [node]

SDAP

single-donor apheresis platelets

SDAT

senile dementia of Alzheimer
type

SDAV

sialodacryoadenitis virus

SDAVF

spinal dural arteriovenous fistula

SDB

Sabouraud dextrose broth
self-destructive behavior
sleep-disordered breathing
subdeltoid bursitis

SDBP

seated diastolic blood pressure
standing diastolic blood pressure
supine diastolic blood pressure

SDC

salivary duct carcinoma
sensitivity depth compensation
[imaging]
serum digoxin concentration
serum drug concentration
size/date consistency [fetus]
subclavian dialysis catheter

SD&C

suction, dilation, and curettage

SDCL

symptom distress check list

SD-CT

standard-dose chemotherapy

SDCT

single-detector computed tomography

SDD

selective digestive [tract]
decontamination
specific developmental disorder
sporadic depressive disease
sterile dry dressing
subantimicrobial dose doxycycline
surfactant deficiency disorder

SDDT

selective decontamination of digestive
tract

SDE

specific dynamic effect
subdural empyema

SDEEG

stereotactic depth electroencephalogram

SDES

symptomatic diffuse esophageal spasm

SDF

sexual dysfunction
slow death factor
stream dilution factor
stress distribution factor
stromal cell derived factor

SDF-1

stromal cell derived factor 1

SDFP

single-donor frozen plasma

SDG

short distance group
succinate dehydrogenase (*See also* SD)
sucrose density gradient

SDGC

sucrose density gradient centrifugation

SDGU

sucrose density gradient
ultracentrifugation

SDH

serine dehydrase
sorbitol dehydrogenase
spinal detrusor hyperreflexia
spinal dorsal horn
subdural hematoma
subdural hemorrhage
subjacent dorsal horn
succinate dehydrogenase [activity]
systolic-diastolic hypertension

SDHD

succinate dehydrogenase complex
subunit D
sudden death heart disease

SDI

Self-Description Inventory

sexual desire index
size/date inconsistency [fetus]
standard deviation interval
State Disability Insurance
Surtees Difficulties Index
SDIHD
sudden death ischemic heart disease
SDII
sudden death in infancy
SDKT
simultaneous double kidney
transplant(ation)
SDL
self-directed learning
serum digoxin level
serum drug level
speech discrimination loss
SDLE
sex difference in life expectancy
somatic dysfunction lower extremity
SDLRS
self-directed-learning readiness scale
sdly
sidelying
SDM
sensory detection method
single, divorced, married
soft drusen maculopathy
standard deviation of mean [statistics]
S/D/M
systolic, diastolic, mean [blood
pressure]
SDMT
Symbol Digit Modalities Test
SDN
sexually dimorphic nucleus
sporadic dysplastic nevus
SD:N
signal difference to noise ratio
SDNA
single-strand deoxyribonucleic acid
SDNN
standard deviation of normal-to-normal
beats
SDNV
Serra do Navio virus
SDO
sudden-dosage onset
surgical diagnostic oncology
SDP
right sacrum posterior (sacroposterior)
[fetal position] [L. *sacrodextra
posterior*] (*See also* RSP)
single-donor platelets
stomach, duodenum, pancreas
SDPC
Suicide-Depression Proneness Checklist

SDQII
Self-Description Questionnaire II
SDR
selective dorsal rhizotomy
sequential diagrammatic reformulation
short-duration response
spontaneously diabetic rat
surgical dressing room
SDRI
small, deep, recent infarct(ion)
SDRT
Stanford Diagnostic Reading Test
SDS
same day surgery
school dental service
Self-Directed Search
Self-Rating Depression Scale
sensory deprivation syndrome
sexual differentiation scale
simple descriptive scale
single-dose suppression
slow deflate system
sodium dodecyl sulfate (*See also*
NaDodSO$_4$)
somatropin deficiency syndrome
specific diagnosis service
speech discrimination score
standard deviation score
stent delivery system
Student Disability Survey
sudden death syndrome
sustained depolarizing shift
Symptom Distress Scale
syringe-driven system
Sds, sds
sounds
SDSEM
spinocerebellar degeneration [with] slow
eye movements [syndrome]
SD-SK
streptodornase-streptokinase
SDSO
same day surgery overnight
SDS-PAGE
sodium dodecyl sulfate-polyacrylamide
gel electrophoresis
SDT
right sacrum transverse (sacrotransverse)
[fetal position] [L. *sacrodextra
transversa*] (*See also* RST)
sensory decision theory
single-donor transfusion
speech detectability (detection)
threshold
SDU
short double upright
Standard Deviation Unit

SDUE
somatic dysfunction upper extremity
SDW
separated, divorced, widowed
SE
saline enema
sanitary engineering
Seeing Eye
self-examination
self-explanatory
sheep erythrocyte
side effect
Signed English
sleep efficiency
smoke exposure
smoke extract
soft exudate
solid extract
special education
sphenoethmoidal
spherical equivalent
spin-echo
spongiform encephalopathy
squamous epithelium
staff escort
standard error [statistics]
staphylococcal enterotoxin
starch equivalent
Starr-Edwards [prosthesis] (*See also* SEP)
status epilepticus
sterol ester
subendocardial
subendothelial
supernormal excitability
supportive-expressive
surgical excision
sustained engraftment
S&E
safety and efficiency
seen and examined
S/E
suicidal and eloper
Se
selenium
75Se
selenium-75
SEA
seronegativity, enthesopathy, arthropathy
sheep erythrocyte agglutination
shock-elicited aggression
side-entry access
soluble egg antigen
Southeast Asia
spinal epidural abscess
spondylitis, enthesitis, arthritis
spontaneous electrical activity
staphylococcal enterotoxin A

subdural electrode array
Survey of Employee Access
synaptic electronic activation
SEAR
Southeast Asia refugee
SEAT
sheep erythrocyte agglutination test
SEB
Scale for Emotional Blunting
seborrhea
staphylococcal enterotoxin B
surrogate end-point biomarker
SEBA
staphylococcal enterotoxin B antiserum
seb derm
seborrheic dermatitis
SEBI
stereotactic external-beam irradiation
seb ker
seborrheic keratosis (*See also* SK)
SEBL
self-emptying blind loop
SEBR
spontaneous eye blink rate
SEC
according to [L. *secundum*]
school handicap condition
secondary (*See also* sec)
secretin
secretion
section (*See also* S, s, sec, sect)
series elastic component [of muscles]
sertoliform endometrioid carcinoma
serum electrolyte concentration
Singapore epidemic conjunctivitis
sinusoidal endothelial cell
size exclusion chromatography
soft elastic capsule
spontaneous echo contrast
sporadic erythrocytosis
squamous epithelial cell (*See also* SqEP, squ epi)
steric exclusion chromatography
strong exchange capacity [resin]
subepidermal connective tissue
superficial esophageal carcinoma
sec
second (*See also* s)
secretary
section (*See also* S, s, SEC, sect)
SECG
scalp electrocardiogram [fetal]
stress electrocardiography
SECL
seclusion
SECPR
standard external cardiopulmonary resuscitation

SE-CPT
single-electrode current perception threshold

SECRET
stiffness of joints, elderly, constitutional [symptoms], arthritis, elevated erythrocyte sedimentation rate (ESR), temporal arteritis [polymyalgia rheumatica]

SECSY
spin-echo correlated spectroscopy

sect
section (*See also* S, s, SEC, sec)

SECTL
single enhancing CT lesion

SED
sedimentation [rate] (*See also* SR, sed rate, sed rt)
semielemental diet
serious emotional disturbance
skin erythema dose
socially and emotionally disturbed
spondyloepiphysial dysplasia
standard error of difference
standard erythema dose
staphylococcal enterotoxin D
strain energy density
suberythemal dose

sed.
sedate
sedative
stool [L. *sedes*]

SeDBP
seated diastolic blood pressure

SEDC
spondyloepiphysial dysplasia congenita

SEDD
Szondi Experimental Diagnostics of Drives

SEDDS
self-emulsifying drug-delivery system

SEDL
spondyloepiphysial (spondyloepiphyseal) dysplasia, late

SED NET
severely emotional disturbed network

sed rate, sed rt
sedimentation rate (*See also* SED, SR)

SeDS
sedentary death syndrome

SEDT-PA
spondyloepiphysial (spondyloepiphyseal) dysplasia tarda-progressive arthropathy

SEE
series elastic element [of muscles]
standard error of estimate
Surgical Eye Expeditions

SEE₁
Seeing Essential English

SEE₂
Signing Exact English

SEEG
stereotactic electroencephalogram

SEEP
small end-expiratory pressure

SEER
Surveillance, Epidemiology and End Results [network, program]

SEF
somatically evoked field
spectral edge frequency
staphylococcal enterotoxin F
suction effusion fluid

SEG
segment(ed) (segmental) (segmentation)
soft elastic gelatin (capsule)
sonoencephalograph(y) (sonoencephalogram)

seg
segmented neutrophil (*See also* segs)

SEGA
subependymal giant cell astrocytoma

SEG-CES
segmental cement extraction system

sEGF
salivary epidermal growth factor

segm
segment(ed)

segs
segmented neutrophils [leukocytes, white blood cells] (*See also* seg)

SEH
School Handicap Condition Scale
severe emotional handicap
spinal epidural hematoma
spinal epidural hemorrhage
subdural effusion with hydrocephalus
subependymal hemorrhage

SeHCAT
selenium-labeled homocholic acid conjugated with taurine

SEI
scaling, erythema, induration
Scar Elevation Index
Self-Esteem Index (Inventory)
subendocardial infarct
subepithelial [corneal] infiltrate
Suretee Events Index

S-EIA
stick-enzyme immunoassay

SE/IVH
subependymal/intraventricular hemorrhage

SEL
serum ethanol level
spontaneous esophageal lesion
SELCA
smooth excimer laser coronary
angioplasty
SELD
slow expressive language development
SELDI
surface enhanced laser
desorption/ionization
SELDI-MS
surface-enhanced laser
desorption/ionization mass
spectrometry
SELDI-TOF
surface-enhanced laser
desorption/ionization time-of-flight
SELDI-TOF-MS
surface-enhanced laser desorption
ionization time-of-flight mass
spectrometry
SELF
Self-Evaluation of Life Function scale
SELFVD
sterile elective low forceps vaginal
delivery
SELI
specific expressive language
impairment
SELU
seromuscular enterocystoplasty lined
with urothelium
SELV
Seletar virus
SEM
scanning electron micrograph
scanning electron microscope
(microscopy)
secondary enrichment medium
self-expanding metallic [stent]
semen (seminal)
serum methylguanidine
skin, eye, mucocutaneous
slow eye movement
smoke exposure machine
standard error of mean [statistics]
systolic ejection murmur
[verbal] sample evaluation
method
sem.
half [L. *semis*] (*See also* HF, hf, S,
semi, ss)
SEMD
spondyloepimetaphysial dysplasia
SEMDIT
spondyloepimetaphysial
(spondyloepimetaphyseal) dysplasia,
Irapa type

SEMDJL
spondyloepimetaphysial dysplasia (with)
joint laxity
SEMG, sEMG
surface electromyography
SEMI
subendocardial myocardial infarct(ion)
subendocardial myocardial injury
semi
half [L. *semis*] (*See also* HF, hf, S,
sem., ss)
semid
half a dram
SEMS
self-expanding metallic stent
self-expanding microporous stent
sem ves
seminal vesicle
SENA
sympathetic efferent nerve activity
sens
sensation
sensitivity (*See also* S)
sensorium
sensory
SENSE
sensitivity encoding
SEOC
serous epithelial ovarian carcinoma
SEOV
Seoul virus
SEP
sclerose en plaques [French for multiple
sclerosis]
sclerosing encapsulating peritonitis
sensory evoked potential
separate(ly) (separation)
separation of ghosts [biochemistry]
serum electrophoresis
somatosensory evoked potential
(*See also* SSEP)
sperm entry point
spinal evoked potential
Starr-Edwards prosthesis (*See also* SE)
Stroke Education Program
surface epithelium
syringe exchange program
systolic ejection period
SEPA
superficial external pudendal artery
separ
separatel(y) (separation)
SEPI
segmented (spiral) echo-planar imaging
SEPS
subfascial endoscopic perforator
surgery
sept
septum

sept.
seven [L. *septem*]
SEPV
Sepik virus
SEQ
side-effects questionnaire
simultaneous equation
seq
sequel
sequela (singular) (sequelae
[plural])
sequence
sequestrum
seq dev ex
sequential developmental exercises
SER
scanning equalization radiography
sebum excretion rate
sensory evoked response
service (*See also* serv)
side effects records
signal enhancement ratio
smooth endoplasmic reticulum (*See also*
sER)
somatosensory evoked response
supination external rotation [type of
fracture, I–IV]
suppressive E-receptor
systolic ejection rate
Ser
serine (*See also* S)
sER
smooth endoplasmic reticulum (*See also*
SER)
ser
serial
series (*See also* S, s)
serology
SERCA
sarcoplasmic-endoplasmic reticulum
calcium ATPase
SEREX
serological analysis of recombinant
cDNA [complementary
deoxyribonucleic acid] expression
SERF
Severity of Exacerbation and Risk
Factors
SERI
Spondee Error Index
serial 7s
serial sevens test [mental status
evaluation] (*See also* 7s)
ser ind
serum index
SERLINE
Serials on Line

SERM
selective estrogen receptor modulator
(modifier)
sero, serol
serologic
serology
SERPACWA
skin exposure reduction paste against
chemical warfare agents
SERPIN
serine protease inhibitor
ser sect
serial sections
SERT
serotonin reuptake transporter
sustained ethanol release tube
Ser/Thr
serine/threonine
serv
service (*See also* SER)
SERVHEL
service and health [records]
SES
seroepidemiological study
sexual experience survey
sick euthyroid syndrome
socioeconomic status
spatial emotional stimuli
sphenoethmoidal suture
standard electrolyte solution
subendothelial space
SESAP
Surgical Education and Self-Assessment
Program
SeSBP
seated systolic blood pressure
SESE
somatosensory evoked spike
epilepsy
sess
sessile
SEST
supine empty stress test
SET
serial end-point titration
shredding embolectomy thrombectomy
signal extraction technology
skin endpoint titration
social environmental therapy
support, empathy, truth
surrogate embryo transfer
systolic ejection time
SETTLE
spindle-cell epithelial tumor with
thymus-like differentiation
SEV
Starr-Edwards valve

S

SEV 1–18, 125, 203
 simian enterovirus 1–18, 125, 203
sev
 severe(ly) (severity) (*See also* SV)
 sever(ed)
SEW
 slice excitation wave
SEWHO
 shoulder, elbow, wrist, hand orthosis
SEXAF
 surface extended x-ray absorption fine
 [structure]
SeXO
 serum xanthine oxidase
SF
 Sabin-Feldman [dye test for
 Toxoplasma]
 safety factor
 salt free
 saturated fat
 scarlet fever
 seizure frequency
 seminal fluid
 serosal fluid
 serum factor
 serum ferritin
 serum fibrinogen
 sham feeding
 shell fragment
 shrapnel fragment
 shunt flow
 sickle [cell hemoglobin] F
 simian foam-virus
 skin fibroblast
 skin fluorescence
 skin fold
 skull fracture
 slow function
 small finger
 snack food
 sodiumazide, fecal [medium]
 soft feces
 sound field
 spinal fluid (*See also* sp fl, sp/fl)
 spontaneous fibrillation
 spontaneous fission [radioactive
 isotopes]
 spontaneous fluctuation
 spontaneous fracture
 stable factor
 starch-free
 sterile female
 stimulating factor
 stress formula
 sucrose-free
 sugar-free
 sulfation factor [of blood serum]
 superior facet
 suppressor factor

 suprasternal fossa
 survival fraction
 symptom free
 synovial fluid (*See also* syn fl)
SF-1
 steroidogenic factor 1
SF6, SF-6, SF$_6$
 sulfur hexafluoride (sulfahexafluoride)
 [gas used in eye surgery]
SF-36
 36-item short form health survey
 Short Form-36 General Health
 Survey
S&F
 soft and flat
 slip and fall
SF%
 shortening fraction percentage
S$_f$, Sf
 flotation constant [Svedberg]
Sf
 Streptococcus faecalis
SFA
 saturated fatty acid
 seminal fluid analysis (assay)
 serum folic acid
 skinfold anthropometry
 stimulated fibrinolytic activity
 subclavian flap aortoplasty
 superficial femoral angioplasty
 superficial femoral artery
sFas
 soluble Fas [gene]
sFasL
 soluble FasL [gene]
SFB
 saphenofemoral bypass
 single-frequency bioimpedance
 spinal fluid block
 surgical foreign body
SFBL
 self-filling blind loop
SFC
 serum fungicidal
 soluble fibrin-fibrinogen complex
 spinal fluid count
 subarachnoid fluid collection
SFCD
 sequential foot compression device
SFD
 scaphoid fossa depression
 sheep factor delta (δ)
 short foot drape
 skin-film distance
 skin-to-film distance
 small for dates [gestational age]
 source film distance
 soy-free diet
 spectral frequency distribution

SFE
supercritical fluid extraction
SFEMG
single-fiber electromyography
SFF
silver-fork fracture
speaking fundamental frequency
SFFA
serum-free fatty acid
SFFF
sedimentation field flow fractionation
SFFV
[Friend] spleen focus virus
SFG
spotted fever group
SFH
schizophrenia family history
serum-free hemoglobin
stroma-free hemoglobin
SFHb
pyridoxalated stroma-free hemoglobin
stroma-free hemoglobin pyridoxalated
SFI
sciatic function index
Sexual Functioning Index
sexual function score
Social Function Index
SFIQ
Sexual Function Inventory Questionnaire
SFJ
saphenofemoral junction
SFL
synovial fluid lymphocyte
SFLE
Stress From Life Experience
SFM
scanning force microscopy
serum-free medium
soluble fibrin monomer
SFMC
soluble fibrin monomer complex
SFNM
subfoveal neovascular membrane
SFNV
sandfly fever Naples virus
SFO
subfornical organ
SFo
speaking phonation
SFOM
suppurative focal osteomyelitis
SFP
scanned focal point
screen filtration pressure
simulated fluorescence process
simultaneous foveal perception
spinal fluid pressure

stopped flow pressure
synostotic frontal plagiocephaly
SFPT
standard fixation preference test
SFR
screen-filtration resistance
stenotic flow reserve
stroke with full recovery
SFRT
stereotactic fractionated
radiotherapy
SFS
serial focus seizures
serum fungistatic
small-fragment system
split function study
superficial fascial system
SFSV
sandfly fever Sicilian virus
SFT
Sabin-Feldman test [toxoplasmosis]
sensory feedback therapy
serum-free thyroxin
skinfold thickness
solitary fibrous tumor
SFTAA
Short Form Test of Academic
Aptitude
SFTP
solitary fibrous tumor of pleura
SFTR
sagittal, frontal, transverse, rotation
SFUP
surgical followup
SFV
simian foamy viruses
superficial femoral vein
SFW
sexual function of women
shell fragment wound
shrapnel fragment wound
slow-filling wave
SFWB
social/family well-being
SFWD
symptom-free walking distance
SG
Sachs-Georgi [test] (*See also* S-Gt)
salivary gland
scrotography
sebaceous gland
secretory granule
serous granule
serum globulin
serum glucose
side glide
sign(ed) (*See also* S, /S/, sig.)

S

SG *(continued)*
    signature [prescription] (*See also* S, /S/, sig.)
    skin graft
    soluble gelatin
    specific gravity (*See also* SpG, sp gr, sp. gr.)
    stent graft
    stratum granulosum
    substantia gelatinosa
    supplemental groove
    Swan-Ganz [catheter] (*See also* SGC)

S/G
    swallow/gag

SGA
    second generation antihistamine
    second generation antipsychotic
    senile genital atrophy
    small for gestational age
    subjective global assessment [dietary history and physical examination]
    substantial gainful activity [employment]

S-GAP
    superior gluteal artery perforator

SGAR
    spectral gradient acoustic reflectometry

SGAT
    salivary gland anlage tumor

SGAV
    Salanga virus

SGAW, SG$_{AW}$
    specific airways conductance

SGB
    stellate ganglion block
    strawberry gallbladder
    Swiss gym ball

SGBI
    silicone gel-filled breast implant

SGC
    salivary gland carcinoma
    spermicide-germicide compound
    Swan-Ganz catheter (*See also* SG)
    sweat gland carcinoma

sGC
    soluble guanylate cyclase

SGCA
    subependymal giant-cell astrocytoma

SGCNB
    stereotactic guided core-needle biopsy

SgCV
    saguaro cactus virus

SGD
    [neutrophil-]specific granule deficiency
    salivary gland dysfunction
    single gene disorder
    specific growth delay
    speech-generating device
    straight gravity drainage
    sweat gland density

SGE
    secondary generalized epilepsy
    significant glandular enlargement
    spoiled gradient echo

SGF
    sarcoma growth factor
    silica gel filtered
    simulated gastric fluid
    skeletal growth factor

SGF2
    smoke generator fog 2 [fog oil device]

SGFR
    single-nephron glomerular filtration rate (*See also* SNGFR)

SGGT
    serum gamma-glutamyltransferase

SGH
    sebaceous gland hyperplasia
    subgaleal hematoma

SGHL
    superior glenohumeral ligament

SGIB
    severe gastrointestinal bleeding

SGL
    salivary gland lymphocyte

s̄ gl
    without glasses

SGLPG
    sulfate-3-glucuronyl lactosaminyl paragloboside

SGLT
    sodium-dependent glucose transporter [family]
    sodium glucose cotransporter [gene]

SGLT1
    sodium glucose cotransporter 1

SGM
    serum glucose monitoring

SGMI
    silicone gel-filled mammary implant

SGO
    Surgeon General's Office
    surgery, gynecology, obstetrics

SGOT
    serum glutamic-oxaloacetic transaminase

SGP
    scaled gradient projection [radiotherapy]
    serine glycerophosphatide
    sialoglycoprotein
    soluble glycoprotein
    stress-generated potential

SGP-2
    sulfated glycoprotein 2

SGPA
    salivary gland pleomorphic adenoma
    supragenicular popliteal artery
SGPG
    sulfate-3-glucuronyl paragloboside
SGPT
    serum glutamic-pyruvic transaminase
SGR
    Sachs-Georgi reaction
    Shwartzman generalized reaction
    skin galvanic reflex
SGRQ
    St. Georges Respiratory Questionnaire
SGRQ-A
    St. Georges Respiratory Questionnaire
    translated into American English
SGS
    second generation sulfonylurea
    short gut syndrome
    silicone gel sheeting
    stroke guidance system
    subglottic stenosis
sGS
    surgical Gleason score
S-Gt
    Sachs-Georgi test (*See also* SG)
SGTCS
    secondarily generalized tonic-clonic
    seizure
SGTT
    standard glucose tolerance test
SGTX
    surugatoxin [mollusc toxin]
SGtx1
    Scodra griseipes toxin [spider]
SGV
    salivary gland virus
    selective gastric vagotomy
    small granular vesicle
SGV&P
    selective gastric vagotomy and
    pyloroplasty
SH
    Salter-Harris [fracture]
    Schönlein-Henoch [purpura] (*See also*
    SHP)
    serum hepatitis
    service hours
    sex hormone
    sexual harassment
    sham [operation]
    shared haplotype
    Sherman [rat]
    short
    short hydrophobic [protein, gene]
    shoulder (*See also* S', SHLD)
    shower

    sick (in) hospital
    sinus histiocytosis
    sitting height
    social history
    somatotrophic hormone (*See also*
    STH)
    spontaneously hypertensive [rat]
    (*See also* SHR)
    state hospital
    sulfhydryl
    suprachoroidal hemorrhage
    surgical history
    symptomatic hypoglycemia
    systemic hyperthermia
S&H
    speech and hearing
S/H
    sample and hold
    suicidal/homicidal [ideation]
SH2
    Src homology 2
sh
    sheep
SHA
    soluble human leukocyte antigen
    staphylococcal hemagglutinating
    antibody
    super-heated aerosol
SHAA
    serum hepatitis-associated antigen
SHAA-Ab
    serum hepatitis-associated antigen
    antibody
SHAART
    salvage highly active antiretroviral
    therapy
SHAFT
    sad, hostile, anxious, frustrated,
    tenacious [patient]
SHAL
    standard hyperalimentation
SHARP
    School Health Additional Referral
    Program
    shared prepulse
SHAS
    Supplement to HIV/AIDS Surveillance
    [CDC]
    supravalvular hypertrophic aortic
    stenosis
SHAV
    Shamonda virus
    superior hemiazygos vein
SHB
    scapulohumeral bursitis
    sequential hemibody [irradiation]
    subacute hepatitis with bridging

S

SHb, S-Hb
sulfhemoglobin (*See also* HbS, SULFHb)

SHBD
serum hydroxybutyrate dehydrogenase

SHBG
serum hemoglobin [and] blood glucose
sex hormone-binding globulin
steroid hormone-binding globulin

sHBO2T
systemic hyperbaric oxygen therapy

SHC
sclerosing hepatic carcinoma
sinus histiocytosis
subsequent hospital care

SHCO
sulfated hydrogenated caster oil

SHD
satellite hemodialysis [telemedicine]
scapulohumeral dystrophy
structural heart disease

SHDI
supraoptical hypophysial diabetes insipidus

SHE
subclinical hepatic encephalopathy
Syrian hamster embryo

SHEENT
skin, head, eyes, ears, nose, throat

SHF
simian hemorrhagic fever
subfulminant hepatic failure

shf
super high frequency

SHFD
split hand/foot deformity

SHFM
split hand/split foot malformation

SHFV
simian hemorrhagic fever virus

SHG
shigellosis (*Shigella* sp.) vaccine
sonohysterography
synthetic human gastrin

SHGT
somatic cell human gene therapy

SHH
sonic hedgehog [gene]
syndrome of hyporeninemic hypoaldosteronism

SHHH
Self-Help for Hard of Hearing People

SHHP
semihorizontal heart position

SHI
second harmonic imaging
Self-Harm Inventory
severe head injury
standard heparin infusion

SHIP
Sgarlato hammertoe implant

SHIV
simian-human immunodeficiency virus

SHL
sensorineural hearing loss (*See also* SNHL)
sudden hearing loss
supraglottic horizontal laryngectomy

sHLA
soluble human leukocyte antigen

SHLD
shoulder (*See also* S', SH)

SHM
simple harmonic motion

SHML
sinus histiocytosis with massive lymphadenopathy

SHMT
serine hydroxymethyltransferase

SHN
spontaneous hemorrhagic necrosis
subacute hepatic necrosis

SHO
secondary hypertrophic osteoarthropathy
shoulder holster orthosis

SHORT, S-H-O-R-T
short [stature], hyperextensibility [of joints or] hernia [or both], ocular [depression], Rieger [anomaly], teething [delayed]

short-FRAME
short stature, facial anomalies, Rieger anomaly, midline anomalies, enamel defects [syndrome]

SHOV
Shokwe virus

SHOX
short stature homeobox [gene]

SHP
Schönlein-Henoch purpura (*See also* SH)
secondary hyperparathyroidism
secondary hypertension, pulmonary
small heterodimer partner [gene]
state health plan
summer-type hypersensitivity pneumonitis
surgical hypoparathyroidism

SHP1–SHP2
Src homology domain-containing phosphatase 1–2

SHPL
sacral horizontal plane line

sHPT
secondary hyperparathyroidism

SHQ
self-healing style of qigong

SHR
scapulohumeral rhythm
sinusoidal heart rate
spontaneously hypertensive rat (*See also* SH)

ShR
shading response [Rorschach]

SHRC
shortened, held, resisted, contracted

SHS
Sayre head sling
sheep hemolysate supernatant
Shipley-Hartford Scale [psychology]
shoulder-hand syndrome
student health service
super high speed

SHSP
spontaneously hypertensive stroke-prone [rat]

SHSS
Stanford Hypnotic Susceptibility Scale

SHT
simple hypocalcemic tetany
STYCAR Hearing Test
subcutaneous histamine test
symptomatic hemorrhage

SHUR
System for Hospital Uniform Reporting

SHUV
Shuni virus

SHV
short hepatic vein
simian herpes virus
Southampton virus
sulfhydryl variant

SHVC
suprahepatic inferior vena cava

SHx
social history

SI
International System of Units [Fr. *Systéme International d'Unites*]
sacroiliac (*See also* sac-il)
sagittal index
Salience Inventory
saline infusion (injection)
saturation index
sector iridotomy
self-inflicted
sensitive index
sensory integration
serious illness
serum insulin
serum iron
service index
severity index

sex inventory
sexual intercourse
signal intensity
Singh Index [radiology]
single injection
sinus irregularity
small intestine
small-intestine channel [acupuncture] (*See also* si)
social introversion
soluble insulin
special intervention
stimulation index
stress incontinence
strict isolation
stroke index
structure of intellect
sucrase-isomaltase
suicidal ideation
sulfated insulin
superior-inferior
suppression index
syncytium-inducing
syncytium-inhibiting
Systematic Inquiry
systolic index

S&I
suction and irrigation
support and interpretation

S:I
sucrose to isomaltase ratio

S/I
superior/inferior

Si
most anterior point on lower contour of sella turcica [craniometric]
silicon [element]
[venous] sinus

si
small-intestine channel [acupuncture] (*See also* SI)

SIA
serum inhibitory activity
slide immunoenzymatic assay
small-intestine atresia
stimulation-induced analgesia
stress-induced analgesia
stress-induced anesthesia
stretch-induced arrhythmia
subacute infectious arthritis
synalbumin-insulin antagonism
syncytia induction assay

Sia
sialic acids

SIAD
syndrome of inappropriate antidiuresis

S

SIADH
syndrome of inappropriate [secretion of] antidiuretic hormone

SIAT
supervised intermittent ambulatory treatment

SIB
self-inflating bulb
self-injurious behavior

sib, sibs
sibling(s) (*See also* SS)

SIBC
serum iron-binding capacity
synchronous ipsilateral breast cancer

SIBD
silent ischemic brain damage

SIBDQ
Short Inflammatory Bowel Disease Questionnaire

SIBIS
self-injurious-behavior inhibiting system

SIBO
small-intestine bacterial overgrowth

SIC
dry [L. *siccus*]
selective intrapartum chemoprophylaxis
self-intermittent catheterization
serum inhibitory concentration
serum insulin concentration
squamous intraepithelial cell
Standard Industrial Classification

SiC
silicon carbide

sICAM
soluble intracellular adhesion molecule

SICD
Sequenced Inventory of Communication Development
serum isocitrate dehydrogenase
serum isocitric dehydrogenase
sudden infant crib death

SICH
spontaneous intracerebral hemorrhage

SICSVA
sequential impaction cascade sieve volumetric air [sampler]

SICT
selective intracoronary thrombolysis

SID
selective intestinal decontamination
sensory integration dysfunction
source-to-image [receptor] distance
sucrase-isomaltase deficiency
sudden inexplicable death
sudden infant death
suggested indication of diagnosis
systemic inflammatory disease

⚠ **s.i.d.**
once a day [L. *semel in die*] ⚠

SIDA
síndrome da imunodeficiéncia adquirida [French and Spanish abbreviation for AIDS]

SIDAM-A
structured interview for diagnosis of Alzheimer dementia, infarct dementia, and dementias of other etiology [ICD-10 and DSM-III-R]

SIDD
syndrome of isolated diastolic dysfunction

SIDER
siderocyte

SIDFF
superimposed dorsiflexion of foot

SIDS
sudden infant death syndrome
sulfoiduronate sulfatase deficiency

SIE
stroke in evolution
subacute infective endocarditis

SIEA
superficial inferior epigastric artery

SIEP
serum immunoelectrophoresis

SIER
sonication-induced epitope retrieval

SIESTA
snooze-induced excitation of sympathetic triggered activity

SIF
sacral insufficiency fracture
serum inhibitory factor
simulated intestinal fluid
small intensely fluorescent
somatotropin release-inhibiting factor (*See also* SRIF)

Sif
segment inferior

SIFE
serum immunofixation electrophoresis

SIFT
selected ion flow tube
sperm intrafallopian transfer

SIFTER
Screening Instrument for Targeting Educational Risk

SIG
sigmoidoscope (sigmoidoscopy)
special interest group

SIg, sIg
serum immune globulin (immunoglobulin)
surface immunoglobulin

sig
signal
significant

sig.
label, write [L. *signa*] (*See also* S, /S/, SG)
let it be written, labeled [L. *signetur*] (*See also* S, /S/, SG)
signature [prescription] (*See also* S, /S/, SG)

SIgA
surface immunoglobulin A

sIgA
secretory IgA

SIGI
System for Interactive Guidance Information

Siglish
Signed English

Σ, sigma
foaminess
sigma [18th letter of Greek alphabet uppercase]
summation
syphilis (*See also* SY, syph)

σ, sigma
standard deviation (*See also* S)
sigma [18th letter of Greek alphabet lowercase]
Stefan-Boltzman constant [constant of proportionality in Stefan-Boltzman law]

sigmo
sigmoidoscope (sigmoidoscopy)

Signal 99
patient in cardiac or respiratory distress

SIGSS
selective imaging and graphics for stereotactic surgery

SIH
secondary intracranial hypertension
somatotropin release-inhibiting hormone
spontaneous intracranial hypotension
stimulation-induced hypalgesia
stress-induced hyperthermia
suction-induced hypoxemia

SIHC
surgically implanted hemodialysis catheter

SIHE
spontaneous intramural hematoma of esophagus

SI/HI
suicidal ideation/homicidal ideation

SI-I
shunt index via inferior mesenteric vein

SII
self-inflicted injury

SIJ, SI jt
sacroiliac joint

SIJS
sacroiliac joint syndrome

SIL
seriously ill list
sister-in-law
specimen in lab
speech interference level
squamous intraepithelial lesion

SIL/ASCUS
squamous intraepithelial lesion/atypical squamous cell of undetermined significance

SILD
Sequenced Inventory of Language Development

SILFVD
sterile indicated low forceps vaginal delivery

SILL
subischial leg length

sIL-1R
soluble type 1 interleukin-1 receptor

SILS
Shipley Institute of Living Scale

SILV
Silverwater virus
simultaneous independent lung ventilation

SIM
selected ion monitoring
small-intestine mesentery
specialized intestinal metaplasia
sucrose-isomaltose
sulfide, indole, motility [medium]
surface-induced mineralization

sim 1–27
simian adenovirus 1–27

SIMA
single internal mammary artery

simkin
simulation kinetics (analysis)

simp.
simple [L. *simplex*]

SIMS
secondary ion mass spectroscopy
surgical indication monitoring system

simul
simultaneous(ly)

SIMV
Simbu virus
spontaneous intermittent mandatory ventilation
synchronized intermittent mandatory ventilation

SIN
salpingitis isthmica nodosa

S

sin.
without [L. *sine*] (*See also* S, ō, WO, wo)
SINES
short interspersed elements
sing.
singular (*See also* S)
SINV
Sindbis virus
SIO
sacroiliac orthosis
Si-O
silicon-oxygen
SiO₂
silicon dioxide (silica)
SIOD
Schimke immune osseous (immunoosseous) dysplasia
SIP
saturation inversion projection
segment inertial properties
Sickness Impact Profile
slow inhibitory potential
spontaneous intestinal perforation
stroke in progression
summarized intensity projection [computer-assisted radiography]
surface inductive plethysmography
sympathetically independent pain
SIPI
Short Imaginal Processes Inventory
SIPS
sympathetically independent pain syndrome
SIPT
Sensory Integration and Praxis Tests
sIPTH
serum immunoreactive parathyroid hormone
SIQ
sick in quarters [military]
SIQ-JR
Suicidal Ideation Questionnaire-Junior
SIR
single isomorphous replacement
specific immune release
standardized incidence ratio
SIREF
specific immune-response-enhancing factor
SIRF
severely impaired renal function
SIRIS
sputter-initiated resonance ionization spectroscopy
SIRNA, siRNA
silencing ribonucleic acid
small (short) interfering ribonucleic acid

SIRS
soluble immune response suppressor
Structured Interview of Reported Symptoms
systemic inflammatory response syndrome
SIRT
selective internal radiation therapy
SI-S
shunt index [via] superior [mesenteric vein]
SIS
saline infusion sonography
saline infusion sonohysterography
Second International Standard
serotonin irritation syndrome
simulator-induced syndrome
sister (*See also* S)
Skin Intensity Score
small-intestine submucosa
social information system
Social Interaction Scale
spontaneous interictal spike
sterile injectable solution
sterile injectable suspension
Stress Impact Scale
Stroke Impact Scale
Surgical Infection Stratification [system]
SISA
stenting in small arteries
SISCOM
subtraction ictal single photon emission computed tomography coregistered to magnetic resonance imaging (MRI)
SISI
short increment sensitivity index
small increment sensitivity index
SISPA
sequence-independent single primer amplification
SISS
serum inhibitor of streptolysin S
severe invasion streptococcal syndrome
SIT
serum-inhibiting titer
serum inhibitory titer
silicon-intensified target
Simultaneous Interview Technique
Slosson Intelligence Test
specific immunotherapy [allergy]
sperm immobilization test
strategic intermittent therapy
stress inoculation training
structured interrupted therapy
supraspinatus, infraspinatus, teres [muscle insertions]
surgical intensive therapy

SITA
standard infertility treatment algorithm
Swedish interactive thresholding
algorithm
SIT BAL
sitting balance
SIT-F
Sperm Immobilization Test-Fjallbrant
SIT-I
Sperm Immobilization Test-Isojima
SIT TOL
sitting tolerance
SITx
small-intestine transplant(ation)
SIUD
subcortical ischemic vascular dementia
sudden intrauterine unexplained death
SIV
simian immunodeficiency virus
Sprague-Dawley-Ivanovas [rat]
Survey of Interpersonal Values
SIVP
slow intravenous push
SIW
self-inflicted wound
SIWIP
self-induced water intoxication [and]
psychosis
SJ, sj
sanjiao channel [acupuncture]
SJA
subtalar joint axis
SJAV
Sandjimba virus
SJC
swollen joint count
SJF
subtalar joint function
SJK
Scheuermann juvenile kyphosis
SJM
St. Jude Medical [prosthesis] [valve]
SjO₂, SjVO₂
jugular venous oxygen saturation
S-JRA
systemic juvenile rheumatoid
arthritis
SJV
San Juan virus
SK
seborrheic keratosis (See also seb ker)
senile keratosis
skin (See also SKI)
Sloan-Kettering [hospital]
solar keratosis
spontaneous killer [cell]
streptokinase (See also STK)

striae keratopathy
swine kidney
S&K
single and keeping [baby]
sk
skeletal (skeleton) (See also skel)
skim(med)
SKA, SKAO
skills, knowledge, abilities [ratings]
supracondylar knee-ankle [orthosis]
SKAb
skeletal antibody
SKAT
Sex Knowledge and Attitude Test
SKBM
Summit Krumeich-Barraquer
microkeratome
SKC
single knee to chest
skel
skeletal (skeleton) (See also sk)
SKI
Skill Indicators
skin (See also SK)
SKILL
Smith-Kettlewell Institute low luminance
[test, card]
SKL
serum-killing level
SKOLD
Screening Kit of Language
Development
SKPT
simultaneous kidney-pancreas
transplant(ation) (See also SPK)
SKS
syphilitic knee synovitis
SKSD, SK-SD
streptokinase-streptodornase
SKT
simple knee test
sk tr
skeletal traction
SKU
stock keeping unit [related to product
identification]
SKY
spectral karyotype (karyotyping)
SL
salt loser
saline lock
sarcolemma
satellite-like
scapholunate
Schwalbe line
sclerosing leukoencephalopathy
secondary leukemia

SL *(continued)*
    segment length
    sensation level [of hearing]
    sensory latency
    sentinel lymphadenectomy
    septal leaflet
    serious list
    serotonin level
    serum lipid
    short leg [cast] (*See also* SLC)
    Sibley-Lehninger [aldolase method/unit]
    sidelying
    signal level
    slight
    slit-lamp
    small leukocyte
    small lymphocyte
    soda lime
    sodium lactate
    solidified liquid
    sound level
    spinal length
    spin-lock
    staging laparoscopy
    standard laparoscopy
    stereolithography
    sublingual(ly) (*See also* subl, subling)

S:L
    sucrase to lactase ratio

Sl
    Steel [mouse]

sl
    slice
    slow
    slyke [unit of buffer value]

SLA
    left sacrum anterior (sacroanterior) [fetal position] [L. *sacrolaeva anterior*] (*See also* LSA)
    sandblasted, large-grit, acid-etched [surfaced implant]
    sex and love addiction
    single-cell liquid cytotoxic assay
    slide latex agglutination
    soluble liver antigen
    superficial linear array
    surfactantlike activity
    [The] Satisfaction with Life Areas [test]

SLAC
    scaphoid-lunate (scapholunate) advanced collapse
    scapholunate arthritic (arthritis) collapse

SLAM
    scanning laser acoustic microscope
    signaling lymphocytic activation molecule
    simultaneous latram and mastectomy
    Systemic Lupus Activity Measure

SLAP
    serum leucine aminopeptidase
    superior labrum anterior and posterior [lesion, fracture]

SLAS
    salt-losing adrenogenital syndrome

SLAT
    simultaneous laryngoscopy and abdominal thrusts

SLB
    short leg brace
    surgical lung biopsy

SLBB
    single living baby boy

SLBG
    single living baby girl

SLC
    secondary lymphoid tissue chemokine
    short leg cast (*See also* SL)
    Sociopolitical Locus of Control
    sodium-lithium countertransport(er)
    synovial lining cell

SLCC
    short leg cylinder cast
    sulfated lithocholic conjugate

SLCG
    sulfolithocholylglycine

SLCT
    Sertoli-Leydig cell tumor

SLD
    scapholunate dissociation
    second-line drug
    serum lactate dehydrogenase
    specific language disorder

SLDH
    serum lactate dehydrogenase

SLDR
    sublethal damage repair [genetic]

SLE
    slit-lamp examination (*See also* SLEX)
    St. Louis encephalitis (*See also* STLE)
    systemic lupus erythematosus

SLED
    slow low-efficiency dialysis
    sustained low-efficiency dialysis

SLEDAI
    Systemic Lupus Erythematosus Disease Activity Index

SLEM
    slow lateral eye movement

SLEP
    Shelf-Life Extension Program
    short latent-evoked potential

SLEV
    St. Louis encephalitis virus [serology]

SLEX
    slit-lamp examination [ophthalmology, biomicroscopy] (*See also* SLE)

SLeX
    sialyl Lewis X [blood group antigen]
SLF
    selected low frequency
SLFIA
    substrate-labeled fluorescent
      immunoassay
    substrate-linked fluorescent immunoassay
SLFVD
    sterile low forceps vaginal delivery
SL-GRE
    spin lock gradient-echo
SLGXT
    symptom-limited graded exercise test
SLHR
    sex-linked hypophosphatemic rickets
SLI
    secretin-like immunoreactivity
    selective lymphoid irradiation
    somatostatin-like immunoreactivity
      (*See also* SLIR)
    specific language impairment
    speech and language impaired
    splenic localization index
    subdermal levonorgestrel implant
SLINKY
    sliding interleaved kY [MRA technique]
SLIP
    Singer-Loomis Inventory of Personality
SLIR
    somatostatin-like immunoreactivity
      (*See also* SLI)
SLIT
    sublingual immunotherapy
SLJM
    syndrome of limited joint mobility
SLK, SLKC
    superior limbic keratoconjunctivitis
SLL
    second-look laparotomy
    serum lidocaine level
    small lymphocytic lymphoma
    spinolaminar line
SLM
    sound level meter
    spatial light modulator
SLMC
    spontaneous lymphocyte-mediated
      cytotoxicity
SLMFD, SLMFVD
    sterile low midforceps [vaginal]
      delivery
SLMMS
    slightly more marked since
SLMN
    sarcomalike mural nodule
SLMP
    since last menstrual period

SLN
    sentinel lymph node
    sublentiform nucleus
    superior laryngeal nerve
SLNB
    sentinel lymph node biopsy
SLND
    sentinel lymph node detection
SLNM
    sentinel lymph node mapping
SLNTG
    sublingual nitroglycerin
SLNWBC
    short leg nonweightbearing cast
SLNWC
    short leg nonwalking cast
SLO
    scanning laser ophthalmoscope
    second-look operation
    shark liver oil
    streptolysin O
S-LOST
    sulfur mustard, Lommel and Steinkopf
      [chemical weapon]
SLOtest
    streptolysin O test
SLP
    left sacroposterior (sacrum posterior)
      [fetal position] [L. *sacrolaeva*
      posterior] (*See also* LSP)
    scanning laser polarimeter (polarimetry)
    segmental limb [systolic] pressure
    sex-limited protein
    short luteal phase
    single-limb progression
    speech-language pathology
    subluxation of patella
    superficial lamina propria
    super long pulse [laser, hair removal]
SLPI
    secretory leukocyte protease inhibitor
      (leukoprotease)
    secretory leukocyte proteinase inhibition
      (leukoproteinase)
SLPMS
    short leg posterior-molded splint
SLPP
    serum lipophosphoprotein
SLR
    Shwartzman local reaction
    single lens reflex
    straight-leg raise (raising)
    Streptococcus lactis R
SLRS
    stereotactic LINAC radiosurgery
SLRT
    straight-leg raising tenderness
    straight-leg raising test

S

SLS
scleroderma-like syndrome
second-look sonography
segment long-spacing [collagen]
selective laser sintering
short leg splint
shrinking lung syndrome
single leg stance
single limb support
stagnate loop syndrome

SLSQ
Speech and Language Screening
Questionnaire

SLT
left sacrum transverse (sacrotransverse)
[fetal position] [L. *sacrolaeva
transversa*] (*See also* LST)
scanning laser tomography
secondary lymphatic tissue
selective laser trabeculoplasty
sex-linked thrombocytopenia
Shiga-like toxin
single-lung transplant(ation)
split-liver transplant(ation)
spontaneous labor at term
STYCAR Language Test
swing light test

SLT-1
Shiga-like toxin I

SLTA
severe life-threatening asthma
standard language test for
aphasia

SLTEC
Shigella-like toxin-producing *Escherichia
coli*

SlTr
silent treatment

sl.tr.
slight trace

SLUD
salivation, lacrimation, urination,
defecation

SLUDGE
salivation, lacrimation, urination,
defecation, gastrointestinal distress,
emesis

SLV
since last visit

SLVD
systolic left ventricular dysfunction

SLVL
splenic lymphoma with villous
lymphocyte

SLWB
severely low birth weight

SLWC
short leg walking cast

SLZ
serum lysozyme

SM
sadomasochism
segmental mastectomy
self-medication
self-monitoring
self-mutilation
semimembranous
service mark
Sexual Myths [Scale]
Shigella mutant
simple mastectomy
skim milk
small (*See also* S)
smoker
smooth muscle
somatomedin
sonomicrometry
space medicine
sphingomyelin
spinal manipulation
splenic macrophage
splenomegaly
sports medicine
stapedius muscle
staphylococcus medium
submandibular
submucosal
submucous
substituted metabolite
substitute for morphine
suckling mouse (*See also* sM)
sucrose medium
suction method
superior mesenteric
supramamillary [nucleus]
surrogate mother
sustained medication
symptom(s) (*See also* Sx, S_x, sx, sym,
symp, sympt)
synaptic membrane
synovial membrane
systolic mean [pressure]
systolic motion
systolic murmur

SM1
primary sensorimotor cortex

S&M, S/M
sadism and masochism
sadomasochism

Sm
samarium
Smith [antigen]

^{153}Sm
samarium 153

SMA
schedule of maximal allowance

sequential (simultaneous) (serial)
multiple (multichannel) autoanalyzer
(autoanalysis) (analysis) (analyzer)
(*See also* SMAC)
serum muramidase activity
shape-memory alloy
small muscle atrophy
smallpox vaccine, not otherwise
specified
smooth muscle actin
smooth muscle antibody
smooth muscle autoantibody
spinal muscular atrophy [type I–III]
spontaneous motor activity
standard method agar
superior mesenteric artery
supplemental motor area [epilepsy]

SM-A
somatomedin A

SMA-II
spinal muscular atrophy, type II

SMA-6
Sequential Multiple Analysis—six
different blood tests

SMA 6/60
Sequential Multiple Analysis—six
different blood tests in sixty minutes

SMA-12
Sequential Multiple Analysis—twelve
different blood tests [biochemical
profile]

SMA 12/60
Sequential Multiple Analysis—twelve
different blood tests in sixty minutes

SMA-20
Sequential Multiple Analysis—twenty
chemical constituents of blood

SMA-60
Sequential Multiple Analysis—sixty
chemical constituents of blood

SMABF
superior mesenteric artery blood flow

SMABV
superior mesenteric artery blood
velocity

SMAC
Sequential Multiple Analyzer Computer
(*See also* SMA)

SMAD
Sma- and Mad-related protein

SMAE
superior mesenteric artery embolus

SMAF
smooth muscle activating factor
specific macrophage-arming factor
superior mesenteric artery (blood)
flow

SMAI
superior-medial acetabular index

SMAL
serum methyl alcohol level

SMALL
same-day microsurgical arthroscopic
lateral-approach laser-assisted

sm an
small animal

SMAO
superior mesenteric artery occlusion

SMAP
systemic mean arterial pressure

SMAR
self-medication administration record

SMART
sensitive membrane antigen rapid test
shape-memory alloy recoverable
technology
simultaneous multiple-angle
reconstruction technique
sperm microaspiration retrieval
technique
surgical myomectomy as reproductive
therapy

SMAS
submucosal aponeurotic system
[flap]
superficial musculoaponeurotic
system
superior mesenteric artery syndrome

SMASH
self-massage acupressure for self-
healing
simultaneous acquisition of spatial
harmonics

SMAST
Short Michigan Alcoholism Screening
Test

SMAT
School Motivation Analysis Test

SMAvac
smallpox vaccine [vaccinia virus]
(*See also* SPX$_V$)

SMB
selected mucosal biopsy
simulated moving bed [chromatography]
standard mineral base

SMBA
spinal bulbar muscular atrophy

SMBFT
small-bowel follow-through
(followthrough) (*See also* SBFT)

SMBG
self-monitored blood glucose

SMBP
serum myelin basic protein

S

SMC
sensorimotor cortex
skeletal myxoid chondrosarcoma
smooth muscle cell
special monthly compensation
special mouth care
succinylmonocholine
supplementary motor cortex
supernumerary marker chromosome

SM-C, Sm-C
somatomedin C

SMCA
smooth muscle contracting agent
sorbitol MacConkey agar

SMCD
senile macular chorioretinal
degeneration
systemic mast cell disease
systemic meningococcal disease

SM-C/IGF
somatomedin C/insulin-like growth
factor

SMD
senile macular degeneration
standardized mean difference
[statistics]
stereotypic movement disorder
sternocleidomastoid diameter
submanubrial dullness

SMDA
Safe Medical Device Act
starch methylenedianiline

SMDS
secondary myelodysplastic syndrome

SME
severe myoclonic epilepsy
significant medical event

SMECE
sclerosing mucoepidermoid carcinoma
with eosinophilia

SMED
spondylometaphysial
(spondylometaphyseal) dysplasia

SMEDI
stillbirth, mummification, embryonic
death, infertility [syndrome]

SMEI
severe myoclonic epilepsy in infancy

SMEM
supplemented [Eagle] minimal essential
medium

SMEPP
subminiature end plate potential

SMF
static magnetic field

SMFA
Short Musculoskeletal Function
Assessment
sodium monofluoroacetate

sm-FeSV
McDonough strain of feline sarcoma
virus

SMFM
shear modulation force microscope

SMFP
state medical facilities plan

SMFVD
sterile midforceps vaginal delivery

SMG
submandibular gland
supramarginal gyrus

SMGCT
secondary malignant giant cell
tumor

SMH
state mental hospital
strongyloidiasis with massive
hyperinfection

SMI
Self-Motivation Inventory
sensory motor integration
serious mental illness
severely mentally impaired
silent myocardial infarct(ion)
small volume infusion
stress myocardial image
Style of Mind Inventory
suggested minimum increment
supplementary medical insurance
sustained maximal inspiration

SMIDS
suppertime mixed insulin and daytime
sulfonylureas

SmIg
surface membrane immunoglobulin

SMILE
safety, monitoring, intervention, length
of stay, evaluation
subperiosteal minimally invasive laser
endoscopic [facelift]
sustained maximal inspiratory lung
exercise

SMIT
standard mycological identification
technique

SML
single major locus
smoldering leukemia

SMM
scintimammography

SMMD
specimen mass measurement device

SMMI
Senoussi Multiphasic Marital
Inventory

SMMVT
sustained monomorphic ventricular
tachycardia

SMN
second malignant neoplasm
surgical microscope navigation
survival motor neuron
SMNB
submaximal neuromuscular block
SMN
survival motor neuron [gene]
SMO
Sarns membrane oxygenator
serum monoamine oxidase
site management organization(s)
slip made out
smoothened [gene]
supramalleolar orthosis (orthotic)
SMo
stainless steel and molybdenum
SMOH
smoothened [*Drosophila*] homolog
SMON
subacute myelooptic neuropathy
SMOR
standardized mortality odds ratio
SMP
self-management program
simultaneous macular perception
skeletal muscle protein
slow-moving protease
special monthly pension
standard medical practice (procedure)
submitochondrial particle
sympathetically maintained pain
SMPC
submucous palatal cleft
SMPN
sensorimotor polyneuropathy
SMPS
sympathetically mediated pain syndrome
SMPV
superior mesenteric portal vein
SM-PVC
superior mesenteric-portal vein
confluence
SMR
scatter to maximum ratio
sensorimotor rhythm
severe mental retardation
sex (sexual) maturity rating
skeletal muscle relaxant
sleeping metabolic rate
somnolent metabolic rate
standard(ized) metabolic rate
standard(ized) morbidity (mortality) ratio
stroke with minimal residuum
submucous resection
SMRR
submucous resection and rhinoplasty

SMRT
silencing mediator of retinoic acid and
thyroid hormone receptor
SMRV
squirrel monkey virus
SMS
scalded mouth syndrome
serial motor seizures
somatostatin (*See also* SOM, SST)
stiff-man syndrome
supplemental minimal sodium
SMSA
standard metropolitan statistical area
SMSV
San Miguel sea lion virus
SMT
Sertoli-cell mesenchyme tumor
smooth muscle tumor
Snider Match Test
spinal manipulative therapy
spindle microtubule
spontaneous mammary tumor
standard medical therapy
stereotactic mesencephalic tractotomy
SMTUMP
smooth muscle tumor of uncertain
malignant potential
SMV
Sena Madureira virus
slow-moving vehicle
small volume
spiral vein of modiolus
stentless mitral valve
submental vertex (submentovertical)
[orthodontic x-rays]
superior mesenteric vein
SMVR
supraannular mitral valve replacement
SMVT
sustained monomorphic ventricular
tachycardia
SMZL
splenic marginal zone lymphoma
SN
sciatic notch
sclerema neonatorum
sensorineural
sensory neuron
seronegative
serum neutralization (neutralizing)
single nephron
sinuatrial (sinoatrial) node (*See also*
SAN)
sinus node
spinal needle
spontaneous nystagmus
standard nomenclature

S

SN *(continued)*
streptonigrin
stromal nodule
subnormal
substantia nigra
superior nasal
supernatant
supernormal
suprasternal notch (*See also* SSN)

S-N
sella to nasion [craniometric]

S:N
sample to negative control ratio
signal to noise ratio (*See also* SNR)
speech to noise ratio

Sn
subnasale [craniometric]
tin [L. *stannum*]

¹¹³Sn
tin-113

SNA
sinonasal adenocarcinoma
specimen not available
superior nasal artery
sympathetic nerve activity
systems network architecture

S-N-A, SNA
sella-nasion-subspinale (point A, craniometric)

SNa
serum sodium [concentration]

SNAC
scaphoid nonunion advanced collapse

SNagg
serum normal agglutinator

SNAGS
sustained natural apophysial glides

SNAI
Standard Nomenclature of Athletic Injuries

SNAP
scheduled nursing activities program
Score for Neonatal Acute Physiology
sensory nerve action potential
soluble NSF (N-ethylmaleimide-sensitive fusion) attachment protein
Swanson, Nolan, and Pelham [psychology rating scale]

SNAP-25
synaptosome-associated protein of 25 kilodalton

SNAP-PE
Score for Neonatal Acute Physiology-Perinatal Extension

SNARE
sensory nerve action potential receptor
soluble *N*-ethylmaleimide-sensitive factor attachment protein receptor

SNaRI
serotonin noradrenergic reuptake inhibitor

SNAT
suspected nonaccidental trauma

SNB
scalene node biopsy
sentinel [lymph] node biopsy
Silverman needle biopsy

S-N-B, SNB
sella-nasion-supramentale (point B, craniometric)

SNBR
sentinel node to background ratio

SNC
skilled nursing care
small noncleaved cell (*See also* SNCC)
spontaneous neonatal chylothorax

SNc, Snc
substantia nigra pars compacta

SNCB
stereotactic needle core biopsy

SNCC
small noncleaved cell (*See also* SNC)

SNCCL
small noncleaved cell lymphoma

SNCD
sinonasal carcinoma with neuroendocrine differentiation

SNCL
sinus node cycle length

SNC, n-B/B
small noncleaved cell, non-Burkitt lymphoma

SNCS
sensory nerve conduction study

SNCV
sensory nerve conduction velocity

SND
selective neck dissection
single-needle device
sinus node disease [dysfunction]
striatonigral degeneration
sympathetic nerve discharge
systemic nodal dissection

SNDA
Supplemental New Drug Application [FDA]

SNE
sinus node electrogram
spatial nonemotional [stimuli]
subacute necrotizing encephalomyelopathy

SNEF
skilled nursing extended (care) facility

SNES
suprascapular nerve entrapment syndrome

SnET₂
  tin ethyl
SNF
  Simon nitinol filter
  sinus node formation
  skilled nursing facility
  Student-Newman-Keuls [test, statistics]
SnF2
  stannous fluoride
SNFH
  schizophrenia nonfamily history
SNF/MR
  skilled nursing facility for mentally
  retarded
SNGBF
  single-nephron glomerular blood flow
SNGFR
  single-nephron glomerular filtration rate
  (*See also* SGFR)
SNGP
  supranuclear gaze palsy
SNGPF
  single-nephron glomerular plasma flow
SNHHD
  simplified nocturnal home hemodialysis
SNHL
  sensorineural hearing loss (*See also* SHL)
SNIP
  silver nitrate immunoperoxidase
  strict no information in paper
SNIPA
  seronegative inflammatory polyarthritis
SNIPPV
  synchronized nasal intermittent
  positive-pressure ventilation
SNM
  sentinel [lymph] node mapping
  serotonergic neuroenteric modulator
SNMT
  systematic nutritional muscle testing
SN-N
  sternal notch to nipple
SNO
  substantive negative outcome
SnO₂
  tin oxide
SNODO, SNDO
  Standard Nomenclature of Diseases and
  Operations
SNOMED
  Systematized Nomenclature of Medicine
SNOMED CT
  Systematized Nomenclature of Medicine
  Clinical Terms
SNOMED RT
  Systematized Nomenclature of Medicine
  Reference Terminology

SNOOP
  Systematic Nursing Observation of
  Psychopathology
SNOP
  Systematized Nomenclature of Pathology
SNOs
  S-nitrosothiols
SNOT-16
  Sinonasal Outcome Test 16
SNP
  simple neonatal procedure
  single nucleotide polymorphism
  sinus node potential
SNP-LP
  single nucleotide polymorphism linkage
  disequilibrium
SnPP
  tin protoporphyrin
SNPV
  single nucleopolyhedrovirus
SNQ
  superior nasal quadrant
SNR
  selective nerve root [block]
  signal to noise ratio [imaging] (*See also*
  S:N)
  specific neurotic syndrome
  substantia nigra zona reticulata
  supernumerary rib
Snr
  substantia nigra pars reticulata
SNRB
  selective nerve root block
SNRI
  selective noradrenergic reuptake
  inhibitor
  serotonin-norepinephrine reuptake
  inhibitor
snRNA
  small nuclear ribonucleic acid
SNRP, snRNP
  small nuclear ribonucleoprotein
SNRPN
  small nuclear
  ribonucleoprotein-associated
  polypeptide
SNRT
  sinus node recovery time (*See also*
  SRT)
SNRTd
  sinus node recovery time, direct
  [measuring]
SNS
  sacral nerve stimulation
  sterile normal saline
  Strategic National Stockpile [drugs,
  medical supplies]

S

SNS *(continued)*
  surgical navigation system
  sympathetic nervous system
SNSA
  seronegative spondyloarthropathy
  sympathetic nervous system activity
SNT
  sinuses, nose, throat
  spectral noise threshold
  Suppan nail technique
SNTSC
  sinonasal teratocarcinosarcoma
SNUC
  sinonasal undifferentiated
    carcinoma
SNV
  Sin Nombre virus
  spleen necrosis virus
  superior nasal vein
  systemic necrotizing vasculitis
SO
  salpingo-oophorectomy
  second opinion
  sex offender
  shoulder orthosis
  significant other
  slow oxidative
  special observation
  sphenooccipital [synchondrosis]
  sphincter of Oddi
  spinal orthosis
  standing orders
  suboccipital
  suggestive of
  suicide observation
  superior oblique
  supraoptic
  supraorbital
  sutures out
  sympathetic ophthalmia
SO$_3$
  sulfite
SO$_4$
  sulfate
S&O
  salpingo-oophorectomy
⚠ **SO$_2$**
  oxygen saturation (*See also* OS, O$_2$ sat.,
    SaO$_2$, S$_{AO_2}$) ⚠
  sulfur dioxide ⚠
^{82}So
  strontium-82
SOA
  serum opsonic activity
  shortness of air
  spinal opioid analgesia
  stimulus onset asynchrony
  supraorbital artery
  swelling of ankles

SoA
  Scedosporium apiospermum [fungus]
SOAA, SOAMA
  signed out against [medical] advice
    (*See also* SOMA)
SOAE
  spontaneous otoacoustic emission
SOAM
  stitches (sutures) out in morning
SOA-MCA
  superficial occipital artery to middle
    cerebral artery
SOAP
  subjective [data], objective [data],
    assessment, plan [problem-oriented
    record]
  symptom, objective finding, assessment,
    plan
SOAPIE
  subjective [data], objective [data],
    assessment, plan, implementation,
    evaluation [problem-oriented record]
SOAPS
  suction, oxygen, apparatus,
    pharmaceuticals, saline [anesthesia
    equipment]
SOB
  see order blank
  see order book
  shortness of breath (*See also* SB)
  side of bed
  stool occult blood
  suboccipitobregmatic
SOBE, SOBOE
  shortness of breath on exertion
    (*See also* SBE)
SOBT
  solution-oriented brief therapy
SOC
  see old chart
  sequential oral contraceptive
  snap-off compression [pin]
  socialization
  stages of change
  standard of care
  start of care
  state of consciousness (*See also* SoC)
  sum of cylinder [method]
  surgical overhead canopy
  syphilitic osteochondritis
  system organ class
S&OC
  signed and on chart
SoC
  state of consciousness (*See also*
    SOC)
soc
  social
  society

SOCD
separation of circle-diamond
SOCS
sized orthotics for children
suppressor of cytokine signaling
[protein]
SocSec
Social Security
S-OCT
serum ornithine carbamoyltransferase
SOD
sinovenous occlusive disease
sphincter of Oddi dysfunction
spike occurrence density
superoxide dismutase
sod.
sodium (*See also* Na)
SODA
Severity of Dyspepsia Assessment
SODAS
spheroidal oral drug absorption
system
sod bicarb
sodium bicarbonate
SODD
silencer of death domain [gene]
SOE
source of embolism
SOF
superior orbital fissure
SOFA
sepsis-related organ failure
assessment
sequential organ failure
assessment
stromal osteoclast-forming activity
SOFAS
Social and Occupational Functioning
Assessment
SOFS
spontaneous osteoporotic fracture of
sacrum
superior orbital fissure syndrome
SOFT
Sorting of Figures Test
SOG
suggestive of good
supraorbital groove
SOGS
South Oaks gambling screen
SOH
sexually oriented hallucination
sympathetic orthostatic
hypotension
SOHN
supraoptic hypothalamic nucleus
SOHND
supraomohyoid neck dissection

SOHS
severe ovarian hyperstimulation
syndrome
SoHx
social history
SOI
severity of illness
slipped on ice
Student Opinion Inventory
sudden overwhelming infection
surgical orthotopic implantation
[implant]
syrup of ipecac
SOKV
Sokuluk virus
SOL
solute (*See also* S, solu)
solution (*See also* sol., soln)
space-occupying lesion
SOL I–III
special observations level 1–3
sol.
soluble (*See also* S)
solution (*See also* SOL, soln)
SOLER
squarely [face person], open [posture],
lean [toward person], eye [contact],
relaxed
soln.
solution (*See also* SOL, sol.)
SOLST
Stephens Oral Language Screening
Test
solu
solute (*See also* S, SOL)
SOLV
Soldado virus
solv
dissolve [L. *solve*]
solvent
SOM
secretory otitis media
sensitivity of method
serous otitis media
somatization
somatostatin (*See also* SMS, SST)
somatotropin
somnolent
sphincter of Oddi manometry
superior oblique muscle
suppurative otitis media
supraorbital margin
SOMA
signed out against medical advice
(*See also* SOAA, SOAMA)
subjective, objective, management,
analytic
System of Multicultural Assessment

somat
somatic
SOMI
sternal occipital mandibular immobilization (immobilizer)
sternooccipital-mandibular immobilization (immobilizer) [brace, orthosis]
SOMPA
System of Multicultural Pluralistic Assessment
SOMT
Spatial Orientation Memory Test
SON
supraoptic nucleus [of hypothalamus]
SONH
spontaneous osteonecrosis of hip
SONK
spontaneous osteonecrosis of knee
sono
sonograph(y) (sonogram)
SONP
soft organs not palpable
solid organs not palpable
SOOF
suborbicularis oculi fat
SOOL
spontaneous onset of labor
SOP
sphincter of Oddi pressure
spinal osteophytosis
standard operating procedure
SOPA
Survey of Pain Attitudes
syndrome of primary aldosteronism
SOPCA
sporadic olivopontocerebellar ataxia
SOPM
stitches out in afternoon
SOPP
splanchnic occluded portal pressure
SOPWA
survivor of a person with AIDS
SOQ
Suicide Opinion Questionnaire
SOR
sign own release
stimulus-organism response
strength of recommendation
SOr
supraorbitale [craniometric]
SORA
stable on room air
sorb
sorbitol
SOREMP
sleep-onset rapid eye movement period
SORT-R
Slosson Oral Reading Test-Revised

SORV
Sororoca virus
SOS
save our ship [universal call for emergency]
self-obtained smear
shortness of stature
silicone-only suspension
sinusoidal obstruction syndrome
son of sevenless [gene]
speed of sound
stimulation of senses
Student Orientations Survey
suicidal observation status
supplemental oxygen system
Surgitek One-Step
SOSF
single organ system failure
SOSOB
sit on side of bed
SOT
sacrooccipital technique
Sensory Organization Test
solid organ transplant(ation)
something other than
squamous odontogenic tumor
stream of thought
superficial ocular trauma
systemic oxygen transport
SOTO
step out, turn out
SOTP
sex offender treatment provider
SOTT
synthetic medium old tuberculin trichloroacetic acid [precipitated]
SOV
Sabin oral vaccine
SOW
scope of work
SOWS
subjective opiate withdrawal scale
SP
sacral promontory
sacroposterior (sacrum posterior) [fetal position]
sacrum to pubis
salivary progesterone
scale of psychosis
schizotypal personality
secretory piece
semiprivate
senile plaque
septal pore
septum pellucidum
sequential pulse
serine proteinase
seropositive
serum protein

shoulder press
shunt pressure
shunt procedure
silent period
skin potential
small protein
soft palate
solid phase
spastic dysphonia
spastic paraplegia
spatial peak
speech (*See also* Sp)
speech pathology
spike potential
spine
spirometry
spleen
spleen channel [acupuncture] (*See also* Sp)
spontaneous pneumothorax
spouse
standard of performance
standard practice
standard procedure
stand and pivot (*See also* S/P)
staphylococcal protease
status positive
status post (*See also* S/P)
steady potential
stool preservative
subdural peritoneal
subliminal perception
substance P
subtilopeptidase
suicide precaution
summating potential
suprapatellar
suprapatellar pouch
suprapubic
suprapubic puncture
surfactant protein
symphysis pubis
synthase phosphatase
systolic pressure

S/P
stand and pivot (*See also* SP)
status post (*See also* SP)

S&P
sharp and pink

Sp
most posterior point on posterior contour of sella turcica [craniometric]
sacropubic
speech (*See also* SP)
Streptococcus pneumoniae
summation potential

sP
senile parkinsonism

sp
space (*See also* S)
specific (*See also* spec)
spinal (*See also* spin.)
spleen channel [acupuncture] (*See also* SP)

sp.
species [singular]
spirit, alcohol [L. *spiritus*] (*See also* spir.)

SP1
stimulatory protein 1

SP 1–2
suicide precautions number 1–2

SPA
salt-poor albumin
schizophrenia with premorbid asociality
scintillation proximity assay
serum prothrombin activity
sheep pulmonary adenomatosis
single-photon absorptiometry
spastic ataxia
speech pathology and audiology
sperm penetration assay
sphenopalatine artery
spinal progressive amyotrophy
spondyloarthropathy
spontaneous platelet aggregation
stimulation-produced analgesia
subperiosteal abscess
suprapatellar amputation
suprapubic aspiration

SP-A–SP-C
surfactant protein A–C

SpA
spondyloarthropathy
staphylococcal protein A

SPAC
satisfactory postanesthesia course
sectionally processed antibody coated

SPACE
single potential analysis cavernous electrical activity
spatial and chemical-shift encoded excitation

SPAD
selective antipolysaccharide antibody deficiency
stenosing peripheral arterial disease
subcutaneous peritoneal access (administration) device

SPAG
small-particle aerosol generator

S

SPAI
steroid protein activity index
SPAIR
short scar, periareolar, inferior pedicle reduction
SPAM
scanning photoacoustic microscope (microscopy)
SPAMM
spatial modulation of magnetization
span.
spansule
sPAP
systolic pulmonary artery pressure
SPAQ
Seasonal Pattern Assessment Questionnaire
SPAR
sensitivity prediction by acoustic reflex
SPARC
secreted protein acidic and rich in cysteine [glycoprotein]
SPARS
spatially resolved spectroscopy
SPAT
slide platelet aggregation test
slow paroxysmal atrial tachycardia
SPB
solitary plasmacytoma of bone
SPBE
saw palmetto berry extract
SPBI
serum protein-bound iodine
S-PBIgG
serum-platelet bindable immunoglobulin G
SPBMD
spinal bone mineral density
SPBT
suprapubic bladder tap
SPC
saturated phosphatidylcholine
scaphopisocapitate
sclerosing pancreatocholangitis
second primary cancer
serum phenylalanine concentration
sickle-shaped particle cell
simultaneous prism [and] cover test
single palmar crease
single photoelectron counting
single-point cane
single photon counting
small pyramidal cell
spike-processed contraction
spleen cell (*See also* SC)
standard platelet count
statistical process control
Summary of Product Characteristics [Europe]

suprapatellar cuff
suprapubic catheter
synthesizing protein complex
sPC
sequential postremission chemotherapy
SPCA
coagulation factor VII (serum prothrombin conversion accelerator) [gene F7]
systemic pulmonary collateral artery
SPCD
syndrome of primary ciliary dyskinesia
sp cd, sp/cd
spinal cord
SPCG
spectral phonocardiography
SPCT
simultaneous prism and cover test
SPD
salmon-poisoning disease
schizotypal personality disorder
silicon photodiode
sociopathic personality disorder (disturbance)
somatoform pain disorder
specific paroxysmal discharge
spectral power distribution
standard peak dilution
subcorneal pustular dermatosis
suprapubic drainage
synpolydactyly
S-2PD
static two-point discrimination
Spd
spermidine
SPDC
striopallidodentate calcinosis
SPDP
N-succinimidylproprionate
SPDT
single-pole, double-throw (switch)
SPE
saw palmetto extract
Sensory Perceptual Examination
septic pulmonary edema
serum protein [and] electrolytes
serum protein electrophoresis
serum protein electrophoretogram
solid-phase extraction
soy phytoestrogen extract
streptococcal pyrogenic exotoxin
subjective paranormal experience
sucrose polyester
superficial punctate erosion
SPEA
streptococcal exotoxin A
SPEAK
spectral peak

SPEAR
    selective parenteral and enteral
        antisepsis regimen
SPEB
    streptococcal pyrogenic exotoxin B
SPEC
    streptococcal pyrogenic exotoxin C
spec
    special
    specialist
    specialty
    specific (*See also* sp)
    specimen
    speculum
Spec Ed
    special education
SPECS
    System to Plan Early Childhood
        Services
SPECT
    single-photon emission computed
        tomography
SPEEP
    spontaneous positive end expiratory
        pressure
SPEG
    serum protein electrophoretogram
SPEL
    syndactyly-polydactyly-earlobe
        [syndrome]
SPELT-P
    Structure Photographic Expressive
        Language Test-II
SPEM
    smooth pursuit eye movement
SPEP
    serum protein electrophoresis
SPERM
    spastic paraplegia-epilepsy-mental
        retardation [syndrome]
SPES
    short psychiatric evaluation
        scale
SPET
    single-photon emission tomography
SPF
    semipermeable film
    specific pathogen free
    spectrophotofluorometer
    S-phase fraction [tumors]
    split products of fibrin
    standard perfusion fluid
    streptococcal proliferative factor
    Stuart-Prower factor [human clotting
        factor X]
    sun protection factor
    systemic pulmonary fistula

SPFI
    solid-phase fluorescence (fluorescent)
        immunoassay
SPFIA
    solid phase fluorescence (fluorescent)
        immunoassay
sp fl, sp/fl
    spinal fluid (*See also* SF)
SPFT
    Sixteen Personality Factors Test
SPG
    scrotopenogram
    serine phosphoglyceride
    spastic paraplegia
    sphenopalatine ganglion
    stereophotogrammetry
    sucrose-phosphate-glutamic acid
        [buffer]
    symmetrical peripheral gangrene
SpG
    specific gravity (*See also* SG, sp gr, sp.
        gr.)
spg
    sponge
SP-GCT
    soft parts giant cell tumor
SPGR
    spoiled gradient recalled
sp gr, sp. gr.
    specific gravity (*See also* SG, SpG)
SPGX
    spastic paraplegia, X-linked
SPGY
    spermatogenesis on Y [gene]
SPH
    secondary pulmonary hemosiderosis
    severely and profoundly handicapped
    sigh per hour
    spherocyte
    spherocytosis
    sphingomyelin
    suprarenal pseudohermaphroditism
SPh
    simple phobia
Sph
    sphenoidale [craniometric]
sph
    sphere
    spheric(al) [lens] (*See also* S)
    spheroid
SPHE, SPHER
    spherocyte
SPI
    selective population inversion
    selective protein index
    Self-Perception Inventory
    sensor position indicator

S

SPI *(continued)*
serum precipitable iodine
serum protein index
Shipley Personal Inventory
somatotyping ponderal index
speech processor interface
Standards for Pediatric Immunization
structured pain interview
subclinical papillomavirus infection
surgical peripheral iridectomy
symptom problem index

SPIA
solid phase immunosorbent assay
(immunoassay)

SPIB
Social and Prevocational Information
Battery

SPICU
surgical pulmonary intensive care
unit

SPID
summed pain intensity difference

SPIDER
steady-state projection imaging with
dynamic echo-train readout
structured platform-independent data
entry and reporting

SPIF
solid-phase immunoassay fluorescence
(fluorescent)
spontaneous peak inspiratory force

SPIFE
serum protein and immunofixation
electrophoresis [system]

SPIH
superimposed pregnancy-induced
hypertension

S-PIN
Steinmann pin

spin.
spinal
spine

SPINK1
serine protease inhibitor Kazal type 1
[gene]

SPIO
superparamagnetic iron oxide [imaging
agent]

SPIR
selective partial inversion-recovery [MRI
technique]
spectral presaturation with inversion
recovery

spir
spiral

spir.
spirit, alcohol [L. *spiritus*] (*See also*
sp.)

spiss.
dried [L. *spiritus*]
inspissated, [thickened by evaporation]
[L. *spiritus*]

SPK
serum pyruvate kinase
simultaneous pancreas-kidney
[transplantation] (*See also* SKPT)
single parent keeping [baby]
superficial punctate keratitis

spkr
speaker

SPKT
superficial punctate keratitis of
Thygeson

SPL
short plantar ligament
skin potential level
sound pressure level
spontaneous lesion
staphylococcal phage lysate
superior parietal lobule

SPLATT, SPLATTT
split anterior tibial tendon [transfer]

sPLM
sleep-related periodic leg movement

SPLV
serum parvo viruslike virus

Splx
splenectomy

SPM
scanning probe microscope
(microscopy)
second primary malignancy
self-phase modulation
shock per minute
significance probability mapping
[statistics]
spermine
subhuman primate model
suspended particulate matter
syllable per minute
synaptic plasma membrane

SPM96
statistical parametric mapping 96
[statistics, neuroimaging data]

SpM
spiriformis medialis [avian brain]

spm
suppression and mutation

SPMA
spinal progressive muscular atrophy

SPMB
strong partial maternal behavior

SPMD
scapuloperoneal muscular dystrophy
semipermeable membrane device [lab
testing]

SPME
solid-phase microextraction
SPMI
severely and persistently mentally ill
status post myocardial infarct(ion)
SPMR
standardized proportionate mortality
SPMS, SP-MS
secondary progressive multiple sclerosis
SPMSQ
Short Portable Mental Status
Questionnaire
S-PMVT
sustained polymorphic ventricular
fibrillation
SPN
pneumolysin
Streptococcus pneumoniae
solitary pulmonary nodule
superficial peroneal nerve
supplementary parenteral nutrition
support parenteral nutrition
sympathetic preganglionic neuron
sp. n.
new species [L. *species novum*]
SPNK
single parent not keeping (baby)
SPO
sphincter-preserving operation
status postoperative
SpO$_2$
arterial oxyhemoglobin saturation
oxygen saturation as measured using
pulse oximetry
SPOA
subperiosteal orbital abscess
SPOCS
Surgical Planning and Orientation
Computer System
SpoCS
space of cavernous sinus
SPOD
spouse's perception of disease
spon, spont
spontaneous
SPONASTRIME
spondylar changes, nasal anomaly,
striated metaphyses
SponVe
spontaneous ventilation
SPOOL
simultaneous peripheral operation
on-line
SPOP
sequential paired opposed plaques
SPORO
sporotrichosis

Sport Px
sport physical
SPOT
salpingitis after previous tubal occlusion
salpingitis in previously occluded tubes
sonographic planning of oncology
treatment
SPOV
Spondweni virus
SPP
Sexuality Preference Profile
single presentation phenotype
skin perfusion pressure
small-plaque parapsoriasis
standard pseudoisochromatic plate
stannous pyrophosphate
super packed platelets
suprapubic prostatectomy
spp.
species [plural]
SPPA
spatial peak-pulse average [ultrasound]
SPPARM
selective peroxisome
proliferator-activated receptor gamma
modulator
SPPK
striate palmoplantar keratoderma
SPPS
single-photon planar scintigraphy
solid phase peptide synthesis
stable plasma protein solution
SPPT
superprecipitation
SP-PVC
superior mesenteric-portal vein
confluence
SPPX
X-linked spastic paraplegia
SPQ
Sales Personality Questionnaire
schizotypal personality questionnaire
SPR
scanned projection radiography
scan projection radiography
selective posterior rhizotomy
serial probe recognition
simultaneous pancreatic-renal
[transplant(ation)]
skin potential reflex
solid phase radioimmunoassay (*See also*
SPRIA)
solid phase receptacle
superior peroneal retinaculum
surface plasmon resonance
SPRAS
Sheehan Patient Rated Anxiety Scale

S

SPRCA
solid phase red-cell adherence assay

SPRIA
solid phase radioimmunoassay (*See also* SPR)

SPR-MS
surface plasmon resonance mass spectrometry

SPROM
spontaneous premature rupture of membranes

SPRT
sequential probability ratio test

SPS
scapuloperoneal syndrome
sestamibi parathyroid scintigraphy
shoulder pain and stiffness
simple partial seizure
single patient system
slow-progressive schizophrenia
sodium polyanethol sulfonate [lab test tube additive]
sodium polyethylene sulfonate [heparinlike drug]
sound production sample
spastic pseudosclerosis
special Pap smear
status post surgery
stiff person syndrome
stimulated protein synthesis
sulfite polymyxin sulfadiazine [agar]
superior petrous sinus
Symonds Picture-Story [Test] (*See also* SPST)
systematic problem solving
systemic progressive sclerosis

SpS
sphenoid sinus

spSHR
stroke-prone spontaneous hypertensive

SPSI
School Problem Screening Inventory

SPSS
spontaneous portal-systemic (portosystemic) shunt
Statistical Package for Social Sciences

SPST
single-pole, single-throw [switch]
Symonds Picture-Story Test (*See also* SPS)

SPSU
straight partial sit-up

SPT
second primary tumor
selective population transfer
septic pelvic thrombophlebitis
single patch technique
single-patient trial
skin prick test
sleep period time
slow pull-through (pullthrough)
sound production task
spinal tap
Spondee Picture Test
standard psychometric test
standing pivotal transfer
station pull-through (pullthrough)
superficial papillary tumor
Supervisory Practices Test
supportive periodontal therapy
suprapubic tenderness
suprapubic tube (*See also* SP TUBE)
Symbolic Play Test

SPTA
spatial peak-temporal average [ultrasound]

Sp tap
spinal tap

SPTB
spontaneous preterm birth

SPTI
systolic pressure time index

SPTL
spontaneous preterm labor
subcutaneous panniculitis-like T-cell lymphoma

SPTP
spatial peak-temporal peak [ultrasound]

SPTS
subjective posttraumatic syndrome

SP TUBE
suprapubic tube (*See also* SPT)

SPTURP
status post transurethral resection of prostate

SPTx
static pelvic traction

SPUT
sputum

SPV
San Perlita virus
selective proximal vagotomy
Shope papillomavirus
slow-phase velocity
stentless porcine valve
sulfophosphovanillin
systolic pressure variation

SPVR
systemic peripheral vascular resistance

SPW
subxiphoid pericardial window

SPX
smallpox vaccine [not otherwise specified]

SPXv
  smallpox vaccine [vaccinia virus]
    (*See also* SMAvac)
SPZ
  secretin pancreozymin
⚠ **SQ**
  social quotient
  squalene
  square
  status quo
  subcutaneous (*See also* SC, sc, subcu,
    subcut, subq) ⚠
  survey question
  symptom questionnaire
sq
  squamous
SQC
  semiquantitative culture
  squamous cell cancer (carcinoma)
    (*See also* SCC, SCCA, SqCA, SqCCA,
    sq cell ca)
SqCa, SqCCA, sq cell ca
  squamous cell cancer (carcinoma)
    (*See also* SCC, SCCA, SQC)
sq cm
  square centimeter (*See also* cm^2)
SQE
  subcutaneous emphysema (*See also*
    SCE)
SqEp
  squamous epithelium (*See also* SEC,
    squ epi)
SQFT
  subcutaneous quadriceps fat
    thickness
sq m
  square meter (*See also* m^2)
sq mm
  square millimeter (*See also* mm^2)
SQMP
  subcutaneous morphine pump
SQ3R
  survey, question, read, review, recite
    [study system]
squ epi
  squamous epithelial [cell] (*See also*
    SEC, SqEP)
SQUID
  superconducting quantum interference
    device [array for reproductive
    assessment]
SQUIDS
  superconducting quantum interference
    device susceptometer
SR
  sarcoplasmic reticulum
  saturation recovery

  scanning radiometer
  schizophrenic reaction
  screen
  secretion rate
  sedimentation rate (*See also* SED, sed
    rate, sed rt)
  see report
  seizure resistant
  self-recording
  senior
  sensitivity response
  sensitization response [cell]
  sentence repetition
  seroreversion
  service record
  sex ratio
  short hair [guinea pig]
  side rails
  sigma reaction
  silicone rubber
  sinus rhythm
  skin resistance
  sleep and rest
  slew rate
  slow release
  smooth-rough [bacterial colony]
  social recreation
  soluble repository
  spatial resolution [imaging]
  specific release
  specific resistance
  specific response
  speech reception
  spontaneous remission
  stabilizing reversal
  stage of resistance
  steroid resistance
  stimulation ratio
  stimulus response (*See also* S-R)
  stress related
  stress relaxation
  stretch reflex
  structured reporting
  sulfonamide-resistant
  superior rectus
  sustained release [drug]
  sustained response
  suture removal
  synchronization ratio
  systemic reaction
  systemic resistance
  systems research
  systems review
S-R
  smooth-rough [bacterial colony]
    (*See also* SR)
  stimulus-response (*See also* SR)

S

S&R
seclusion and restraints
S/R
schizophrenic reaction
strong/regular (pulse)
3SR
self-sustained sequence replication
self-sustaining sequence replication
Sr
strontium
85Sr
strontium-85
87mSr
strontium-87m
89Sr
strontium-89
90Sr
strontium-90
sr
steradian [solid angle measurement]
SRA
segmented renal artery
serotonin release assay
sewing ring area
spleen repopulating activity
steroid resistant asthma
SRAM
static random access memory
SR/AP
schizophrenic reaction, acute,
paranoid
SR/AU
schizophrenic reaction, acute
undifferentiated
SRAV
Saraca virus
SR_AW
specific airways resistance
SRBC
sheep red blood cell (*See also* SRC)
sickle red blood cell
SRBOW
spontaneous rupture of bag of waters
SRC
protooncogene tyrosine-protein kinase
scleroderma renal crisis
sedimented red [blood] cell
sheep red [blood] cell (*See also*
SRBC)
Student Reactions to College
SRCA
specific red cell adherence
SRCBC
serum reserve cholesterol binding
capacity
SRCC
sarcomatoid renal cell carcinoma
SRCP
superficial renal cortical perfusion

SR/CP
schizophrenic reaction, chronic,
paranoid
SRCS
[FDA Division of] Surveillance,
Research, and Communication Support
SRCT
small round-cell tumor
SR/CU
schizophrenic reaction, chronic,
undifferentiated
SRD
service-related disability
smallest real difference [statistics]
sodium-restricted diet
specific reading difficulty (disability)
SRDS
Self-Rating Depression Scale
severe respiratory distress syndrome
SRDT
single radial diffusion test
SRE
Schedule of Recent Events
Schedule of Recent Experiences
sex and relationships education
skeletal related event
SREBP
sterol regulatory element binding
protein
SREDA
subclinical rhythmic epileptiform
discharge of adult
S-REM
simulated real ear measurement
sREM
stage rapid eye movement
SREV
Saumarez Reef virus
SRF
semirigid fiberglass cast
severe renal failure
skin-reactive factor
slow-reacting factor
somatotropin-releasing factor
split renal function
subretinal fluid
SRF-A, SRFOA
slow-reacting factor of anaphylaxis
SRFC
sheep [red blood cell] rosette-forming
cell
SRFS
split renal function study
SRGVHD
steroid resistant graft-versus-host
disease
SRH
signs of recent hemorrhage
single radial hemolysis [test]

somatotropin-releasing hormone
spontaneously resolving (responding)
  hyperthyroidism
stigmata of recent hemorrhage
SRI
serotonin reuptake inhibitor
severe renal insufficiency
social relationships index
surface regularity index
SRID
single radial immunodiffusion
SRIF
somatotropin release-inhibiting factor
  (*See also* SIF)
SRIH
somatotropin release-inhibiting hormone
SRIV
Sripur virus
SRK
Sanders-Retzlaff-Kraff formula
  [ophthalmology]
smooth-rod Kaneda [thoracolumbar
  implant]
SRL
short radiolunate
SRM
spontaneous rupture of membranes
standardized response mean [statistics]
Standard Reference Material
subretinal membrane
superior rectus muscle
SRMD
stress-related mucosal damage (disease)
SRMs
specified risk materials
SRN
subretinal neovascularization (*See also*
  SRNV)
superficial radial nerve
SRNA, sRNA
small ribonucleic acid
soluble ribonucleic acid
SR/NE
sinus rhythm, no ectopy
SRNP
soluble ribonuclear protein
SRNS
steroid-responsive nephrotic syndrome
SRNV
subretinal neovascularization (*See also*
  SRN)
SRNVM
senile retinal neovascular membrane
subretinal neovascular membrane
SRO
sagittal ramus osteotomy
single room occupancy

smallest region of overlap
sustained-release oral
SROA
sports-related osteoarthritis
SROCPI
Self-Rating Obsessive-Compulsive
  Personality Inventory
SROM
spinal range of motion
spontaneous rupture of membranes
SRP
scaling and root planing [dental]
septorhinoplasty
short rib-polydactyly (syndrome)
  (*See also* SRPS)
signal recognition particle (protein)
simple response paradigm
single reference point
spinal rehabilitation program
stapes replacement prosthesis
surgical reversal of presbyopia
synchronized retroperfusion
SR-PLLA
self-reinforced poly-L-lactide
self-reinforcing polylevolactic acid
SRPS
short rib-polydactyly syndrome (*See also*
  SRP)
SRR
short R-R interval [on
  electrocardiogram]
slow rotation room
specific reading retarded
stabilized relative response
standardized rate ratio
systematic rational restructuring
SRRS
Social Readjustment Rating Scale
SR-RSV
Schmidt-Ruppin [strain] Rous sarcoma
  virus
SRS
schizophrenic residual state
sex reassignment surgery
skeletal repair system
slow-reacting substance
social and rehabilitation service
somatostatin receptor scintigraphy
splenorenal shunt
stereotactic radiosurgery
suicide risk screen
Symptom Rating Scale
sRS
without redness or swelling
SRSA, SRS-A
slow-reacting substance of
  anaphylaxis

SRSH
    self-reported self-harm
SRSV
    small round structured virus
SRT
    Seashore Rhythm Test
    sedimentation rate test
    segmented ring tripolar
    sick role tendency
    simple reaction time
    sinus [node] recovery time (*See also*
        SNRT)
    sleep-related tumescence
    smoke removal tube
    Social Relations Test
    speech reception test
    speech reception (recognition) threshold
    spontaneously resolving thyrotoxicosis
    stereotactic radiation therapy
        (radiotherapy)
    surfactant replacement therapy
    Symptom Rating Test
SRU
    side rails up
    solitary rectal ulcer
    structural repeating unit
SrU
    strontium unit
SRUS
    solitary rectal ulcer syndrome
SRV
    Schmidt-Ruppin virus
    Shark River virus
    small round virus
    superior radicular vein
SRVC
    subcutaneous reservoir and ventricular
        catheter
SRVG
    silicone elastomer ring vertical
        gastroplasty
SRVGB
    Silastic ring vertical-banded gastric
        bypass
SRVT
    sustained reentrant ventricular
        tachyarrhythmia
SRW
    short ragweed [test]
SRX
    sex-determining region X [chromosome]
SRY
    sex-determining region Y [chromosome]
SS
    sacral sulcus
    sacrosciatic
    saline soak
    saline solution
    saliva sample

saliva substitute
Salmonella-Shigella [agar] (*See also*
    SSA)
salt sensitivity
salt substitute
saturated solution (*See also* sat. soln)
schizophrenia (schizophrenic)
    spectrum
Schizophrenia Subscale
scleral spur
seizure sensitive
septic shock
serotonin syndrome
serum sickness
short stature
short stay
siblings (*See also* sib, sibs)
sickle cell [anemia] (*See also* SSA)
side-to-side
signs and symptoms (*See also* SAS,
    S&S, S/SX)
single session [treatment]
single stranded (*See also* ss)
single strength
skull series [radiographs]
slice select [gradient]
sliding scale
slip sent
slow-wave sleep
smoking status
soapsuds
Social Security
social services
sorbitan sesquioleate
sparingly soluble
special service
sport sheath
stable sarcoidosis
staccato syndrome
stainless steel
standard score
statistically significant
steady state (*See also* ss)
sterile solution
steroid sensitivity
steroid sulfurylation
stromal sarcoma
subaortic stenosis
subscapularis
subsegmental
subsequent sibling
substernal
suction socket
sum [of] squares [statistics]
supersaturated
support (and) stimulation
susceptible
suture system
symmetrical strength

synovial sarcoma (*See also* SYS)
syringosubarachnoid shunting
systemic sclerosis (*See also* SSc)

S/S
Saturday and Sunday
sprain/strain

S&S
shower and shampoo
signs and symptoms (*See also* SAS, SS, S/SX)
sitting and supine
sling and swathe
soft and smooth [prostate]
support and stimulation
swish and spit
swish and swallow

Ss
serum soluble [antigen]
subjects [piural]

ss
half [L. *semis*] (*See also* HF, hf, S, sem., semi)
single stranded (*See also* SS)
subspinale

SSA
sagittal split advancement
salicylsalicylic acid
Salmonella-Shigella agar (*See also* SS)
sickle cell anemia
Sjögren syndrome [antigen] A
skin-sensitizing antibody
skin sympathetic activity
Social Security Administration
special somatic afferent
specific surface area
sperm-specific antigen (antiserum)
standard sedative agent
streptococcal superantigen
Subjective Symptoms Assessment
subsegmental airway
subsegmental atelectasis
sulfosalicylic acid

SSADH
succinic semialdehyde dehydrogenase [deficiency]

SSAER
steady-state auditory evoked response

SSAV
simian sarcoma-associated virus

SSB
short small-bowel
short spike burst
stereospecific binding

SS B
Sjögren syndrome [antigen] B

SSBE
short-segment Barrett esophagus

SSBG
sex steroid-binding globulin

SSBP
sitting systolic blood pressure

SSBR
see separate bacteriology report

SSC
saline sodium citrate
sign-symptom complex
silver sulfadiazine and chlorhexidine [impregnated central catheter]
single-stripe colitis
sodium chloride-sodium citrate solution
somatic stem cell
somatosensory cortex
Special Services for Children
stainless steel crown
standard saline citrate
standard straight care
Stein Sentence Completion [test]
subcutaneous sarcoidosis
superior semicircular canal
suprascapular nerve compression
syngeneic spleen cell

SSc
systemic sclerosis (*See also* SS)

SSCA
sensitized sheep cell agglutination
single shoulder contrast arthrography
spontaneous suppressor cell activity

SSCCS
slow spinal cord compression syndrome

SSCD
superior semicircular canal deficiency

SSCF
sleep-stage change frequency

SSCIF
squamous cell carcinoma inhibitory factor

SSCM
split spinal cord malformation

SSCP
single-stranded conformational polymorphism
substernal chest pain

SSCr
stainless steel crown

SSCS
segmental spinal correction system

SSCT
Sacks Sentence Completion Test
stereotactic subcaudate tractotomy

SSCVD
sterile spontaneous controlled vaginal delivery

S

SSD
segmental spinal dysgenesis
serosanguineous drainage
shaded-surface display [imaging]
shock(-induced) suppression of drinking
sickle cell disease
single saturating dose
Social Security Disability
source to surface distance
source-to-skin distance
speech-sound discrimination
succinate semialdehyde dehydrogenase
sudden sniffing death
sum of square deviations [statistics]
surface shaded display
syndrome of sudden death

SSDBS
symptom schedule for diagnosis of
borderline schizophrenia

SSDI
Social Security Disability Insurance
striatal (striatocapsular) small deep
infarction

SSDLP
subthreshold subfoveal diode laser
photocoagulation

SS-DNA, ssDNA
single-stranded deoxyribonucleic acid

SSDP
sequence-specific deoxyribonucleic acid
(DNA) primer

SSE
saline solution enema
skin self-examination
soapsuds enema
steady-state exercise
subacute spongiform encephalopathy
systemic side effects

SSEA
stage-specific embryonic antigen

SSEEG
scalp-sphenoidal electroencephalography

SSEH
spontaneous spinal epidural
hematoma

SSEP
short-latency somatosensory-evoked
potential
somatosensory-evoked potential (*See also*
SEP)
steady state evoked potential

SSER
somatosensory evoked response
(*See also* SER)

SSF
septic scarlet fever
soluble suppressor factor
subscapular skinfold [thickness]
supplementary sensory feedback

SSFI
social stress and functionability
(functionality) inventory [for psychotic
disorders]

SSFP
steady-state free precession
steady-state free progression

SSFSE
single shot fast spin echo

SSG
sublabial salivary gland

SSGS
State Shame and Guilt Scale

SSH
spinal subdural hemorrhage

SSHA
Survey of Study Habits and Attitudes

SSHb
homozygous for sickle cell hemoglobin

SSHL
severe sensorineural hearing loss
sudden sensorineural hearing loss

SSHR
steady state heart rate

SShTSE
sensitivity encoding (SENSE) [with
half-Fourier] single-shot turbo spin
echo

SSHV
snowshoe hare virus

SSI
School Setting Interview
segmental sequential irradiation
segmental spinal instrumentation
semistructured psychiatric interview
severity score index
shoulder subluxation inhibitor
sliding scale insulin
small-scale integration
Social Skills Inventory
somatic symptom index
stuttering severity instrument
subshock insulin
superior sector iridectomy
Supplemental Security Income
surgical site infection
symptom severity index
synthetic sentence identification
System Sign Inventory

SSIAM
Structured and Scaled Interview to
Assess Maladjustment

SSIDS
sibling of sudden infant death syndrome
[victim]

SSII
Safran Student's Interest Inventory

SSIS
side-to-side isoperistaltic strictureplasty

SSIT
subscapularis, supraspinatus, infraspinatus, teres minor [muscles]

SSKI
saturated solution of potassium iodide
supersaturated potassium iodide

SSL
second stage of labor
skin surface lipid
subtotal supraglottic laryngectomy
synthetic sentence list

SSLE
subacute sclerosing leukoencephalitis

S-sleep
synchronized sleep

SSLF
sacrospinous ligament fixation

SSLI
serum sicknesslike illness

SSLND
selective sentinel lymph node dissection

SSLR
seated straight leg raise

SSM
scaphoid shift maneuver
skin-sparing mastectomy
skin surface microscopy
solid state microscopy
subsynaptic membrane
superficial spreading melanoma
suprasellar meningioma

S-SMase
secretory sphingomyelinase

SSMP
spastic spinal monoplegia

SSN
[computer-assisted] surgical segment navigator
severely subnormal
Social Security number
subacute sensory neuropathy
superior salivary nucleus
suprasternal notch (See also SN)

SSNB
suprascapular nerve block

SSNHL
sudden sensorineural hearing loss

SSNS
steroid-sensitive nephrotic syndrome

SSO
sagittal split osteotomy
second surgical opinion
sequence specific oligonucleotide
Spanish-speaking only
special sense organs [of animals]

SSOC
site-specific ovarian cancer

SSOP
sequence-specific oligonucleotide probe [hybridization]
Standard System of Psychiatry

SSP
Sanarelli-Shwartzman phenomenon
sequence-specific primer
short-stay procedure
simultaneously stapled pneumonectomy
slice sensitivity profile
small spherical particle
stereotactic surface projection
subacute sclerosing panencephalitis (See also SSPE)
superior spermatic plexus
supersensitivity perception
supragingival scaling and prophylaxis

ssp.
subspecies [singular]

SSPA
staphylococcal-slime polysaccharide antigen

SSPCS
side-to-side portacaval shunt

SSPD
schizoid-schizotypal personality disorder

SSPE
subacute sclerosing panencephalitis (See also SSP)

SSPG
steady-state plasma glucose

SSPI
steady-state plasma insulin

SSPL
saturation sound pressure level

SSPP
subsynaptic plate perforation

sspp.
subspecies [plural]

SSPS
side-to-side portacaval shunt

SS-PSE
Schizophrenic Subscale of Present State Examination

SSPT
Speech-Sound Perception Test

SSQ
sequential scalar quantization
Social Support Questionnaire
Staring Spell Questionnaire

SS-QOL
stroke-specific quality of life

SSR
shaded-surface rendering [imaging]
simple sequence repeats

S

SSR *(continued)*
sleep self-reporting
solar stimulated radiation
somatosensory response
somatostatin receptor
steady-state rest
steroid-resistant rejection
substernal retraction
sympathetic skin response

SSRFC
surrounding subretinal fluid cuff

SSRI
selective serotonin reuptake inhibitor

SSRO
sagittal split ramus osteotomy

SSRP
subgingival scaling and root planing

SSRS
Social Skills Rating System

SSS
scalded skin syndrome
Scandinavian Stroke Scale
School Situation Survey
secondary Sjögren syndrome
sensation-seeking scale
Sepsis Severity Score
sick sinus syndrome
Simple Scoring System
skin and skin structures
small sharp spike
soluble specific substance
specific soluble substance
sphincter-saving surgery
Stanford Sleepiness Scale
sterile saline soak
strong soap solution
structured sensory stimulation
subclavian steal syndrome
superior sagittal sinus
systemic sicca syndrome

SSS-58
58-point Scandinavian Stroke Scale

SSSA
skin sympathetic sudomotor activity

SSSB
sagittal split setback [procedure]

SSSC
Social Support Scale for Children [test]

SSSDW
significant sharp, spike, or delta waves [EEG]

SSSE
self-sustained status epilepticus

SSSI
skin and skin structure infection

SSSS
staphylococcal scalded skin syndrome

ssSSc
systemic sclerosis sine scleroderma

SSSS-M
Sexual Self-Schema Scale-Male Version

SSST
superior sagittal sinus thrombosis

SSSV
superior sagittal sinus velocity

SST
sagittal sinus thrombosis
sclerosing stromal tumor
serum separator tube
simple shoulder test
Slingerland Screening Tests
social skills training
sodium sulfite titration
somatosensory thalamus
somatostatin (*See also* SMS, SOM)
stainless steel rod

SSTE
skin-soft tissue envelope

SSTI
skin and soft tissue infection

SSU
Saybolt seconds universal [kinematic viscosity]
sterile supply unit

SSV
sheep seminal vesicle
simian sarcoma virus

SSVC
systemic venous collateral

SSVD
sterile, spontaneous vaginal delivery

SSVEP
steady-state visual evoked potential

SSW
slow spike wave [electroencephalogram]
spike and sharp wave [electroencephalogram]
Staggered Spondaic Word Test

S/SX
signs [and] symptoms (*See also* SAS, SS, S&S)

SSYM
sign or symptom

ST
electrocardiographic wave segment
esotropia (*See also* ESO, eso, ET)
(heat-)stable (entero)toxin
sacrum transverse (sacrotransverse) [fetal position]
scala tympani
scapulothoracic
Schiotz tonometry [ophthalmology]
Schirmer test [dry eyes]
sclerotherapy
sedimentation time
semitendinosus [muscle]

septal thickness
serotonin
serum transferrin
sharp transients [EEG]
shock therapy
siblings [raised] together
similarly tested
sinus tachycardia
sinus tympani [part of temporal bone]
skin tag
skin tear
skin temperature
skin test
skin thickness
slight trace
slow twitch
smokeless tobacco
soft tissue treatment
sore throat
spasmodic torticollis
spastic torticollis
sphincter tone
split thickness
spondee threshold [speech/hearing test]
standard(ized) test
starting time
stent thrombosis
sternothyroid [muscle]
stimulus (*See also* R, S)
stomach (*See also* stom)
stomach channel [acupuncture]
store (*See also* STO)
straight
strength training
stress test
stretcher
striatum (*See also* Str)
sublingual tablet
subtalar
subtotal
surface tension
surgical therapy
surrogate tolerogenesis
survival time
symptomatic treatment
synapse time
systolic time

S-T

sickle cell thalassemia

St

stoke [CGS unit of kinematic viscosity]
stomion [median point of oral slit when
  lips are closed]

St.

saint

sT

tumor surgery [TNM classification]

sT0

tumor surgery not done [TNM
  classification]

sT1

tumor complete resection [TNM
  classification]

sT2

tumor resection, 50%–90% [TNM
  classification]

sT3

tumor resection 5% to 50% [TNM
  classification]

sT4

tumor biopsy [TNM classification]

sT5

tumor shunting [TNM classification]

st

stage (of disease)
stere [metric unit of volume]
stone [British measure of human or
  animal weight]
subtype

STA

second trimester abortion
serum thrombotic accelerator
serum tobramycin assay
spike-triggered averaging [testing]
spinothalamic ataxia
standard tube agglutination test
Staphylococcus vaccine, not otherwise
  specified
superficial temporal artery
superior temporal artery

Sta

staphylion [craniometric]
station

STAaur

Staphylococcus aureus vaccine

stab

polymorphonuclear leukocyte
stabkernige (band neutrophil)

STABS

Suinn Test Anxiety Behavior
  Scale

STACL

Screening Test for Auditory
  Comprehension of Language

STAE

subsegmental transcatheter arterial
  embolization

St AE

standard above-elbow [cast]

STAG

split-thickness autogenous graft
striped tag myocardial tagging system

S-TAG

slow-binding target-attaching globulin

S

STAI
Spielberger State-Trait Anxiety Inventory
State-Trait Anxiety Inventory

STAIC
State-Trait Anxiety Inventory for
Children

STAI-I
State Trait Anxiety Index I

STALD
Sheffield Screening Test for Acquired
Language Disorders

STA-MCA
superficial temporal artery-middle
cerebral artery

STAMP
Solid Tumor Autologous Marrow
Transplant Program

StanPsych
standard psychiatric [nomenclature]

STA-PCA
superficial temporal artery-posterior
cerebral artery

STA-peg
[Smith] subtalar joint arthroereisis
peg

staph
staphylococcus

STAPP
short-term anxiety-provoking
psychotherapy

STAR
Scandinavian total ankle replacement
Simultaneous Technique for Acuity and
Readiness Testing
specialized tissue aspirating
resectoscope
staged abdominal repair
steroidogenic acute regulatory
suture tension adjustment reel

StAR
steroidogenic acute regulatory
protein

STARD
Standards for Reporting of Diagnostic
Accuracy

STARR
stapled transanal rectal resection
procedure

STARRT
selective tubal assessment to refine
reproductive therapy

STARS
Short-Term Auditory Retrieval and
Storage [Test]

START, StaRT
stereotactic-assisted radiation therapy

STAS
sporadic testicular agenesis syndrome
State-Trait Anger Scale

STA-SCA
superficial temporal artery-superior
cerebellar artery

STAspl
staphylococcus vaccine, bacteriophage
lysate

STAT
at once [L. *statim*] (*See also* stat.)
Suprathreshold Adaptation Test

Stat
signal transducer and activator of
transcription [protein]

Stat4
signal transducer and activator of
transcription 4 [protein]

Stat5
signal transducer and activator of
transcription 5 [protein]

stat.
at once [L. *statim*] (*See also* STAT)

statA, ampere-esu
statampere

statC
statcoulomb

STAXI
State-Trait Anger Expression Inventory

STB, Stb
silicotuberculosis
stillborn (*See also* SB, stillb)

STBAL
standing balance

ST BY
stand by (*See also* SB)

STC
sarcomatoid thymic carcinoma
serum theophylline concentration
sexually transmitted condition
slow transit constipation
soft tissue calcification
stimulate to cry
subtotal colectomy
sugar-tong cast

sTCC
superficial transitional cell carcinoma

STCL
Standardized Test of Computer
Literacy

STD
selective T-cell defect
sexually transmitted disease
short-term disability
skin test done
skin test dose
skin-to-tumor distance
sodium tetradecyl (sulfate)
source-to-tray distance
standard density (reference)
standard test dose
ST-segment depression

std
> saturated (*See also* S, SAT, sat., sat'd)
> standard(ized)

STDH
> skin test for delayed-type
> hypersensitivity

STDS
> stone-tissue detection system

STDT
> standard tone-decay test

STD TF
> standard tube feeding (*See also* STF)

STE
> stimulated echo
> ST-segment elevation
> subperiosteal tissue expander

STEAM
> stimulated echo acquisition mode

STEC
> Shiga toxin (Stx 2) producing
> *Escherichia coli*

STEL
> short-term exposure limit

STEM
> scanning transmission electron
> microscope (microscopy)

STEMI
> ST-segment elevation myocardial
> infarction

STEN
> staphylococcal toxic epidermal
> necrolysis

sten
> stenose(d) (stenosis) (stenosing)

STEP
> Sequential Tests of Educational
> Study

S.T.E.P.
> Short Transitional Edge Protection

STEP-III
> Sequential Tests of Educational
> Progress, Series III

STEPS
> Screening Test for Educational
> Prerequisite Skills
> sequential treatment employing
> pharmacologic support
> [The] System for Thalidomide
> Educating and Prescribing Safety

stereo
> stereogram
> stereophonic

STET
> single-photon emission tomography
> submaximal treadmill exercise test

stet
> let it stand

STETH
> stethoscope

STEV
> short-term exposure value

STF
> serum thymic factor
> slow twitch fiber
> small third-trimester fetus
> specialized treatment facility
> special tube feeding
> standard tube feeding (*See also* STD
> TF)
> sudden transient freezing
> superficial temporal fascia

STF1
> somatostatin transcription
> factor 1

sTf-R, sTfR
> soluble transferrin receptor

STG
> short-term goal
> split-thickness graft
> superior temporal gyrus

STGC
> syncytiotrophoblastic giant cell

STH
> soft tissue hematoma
> soft tissue hemorrhage
> somatotrophic hormone (*See also* SH)
> subtotal hysterectomy
> supplemental thyroid hormone

STh, S-Thal
> sickle cell thalassemia

STHB
> said to have been

ST:HR
> ST-segment to heart rate [slope or
> ratio]

STI
> scientific and technical information
> serum trypsin inhibitor
> sexually transmitted infection
> short-term immunotherapy
> signal transduction inhibitor
> soft tissue injury
> soybean trypsin inhibitor (*See also*
> SBTI)
> sum total impression
> systolic time interval

STIC
> serum trypsin inhibition capacity
> solid-state transducer intracompartment
> [catheter]

STIF
> spinopelvic transiliac fixation

stillb
> stillborn (*See also* SB, STB, Stb)

S

stim, stimn
stimulation
stimulus (*See also* R, S, ST)

STING
subureteric Teflon injection

STIP
(basophilic) stippling

STIR
short inversion time inversion recovery [imaging]
short tau (time) (T1) inversion recovery

STJ
scapulothoracic joint
subtalar joint

STK
streptokinase (*See also* SK)

STK11
serine threonine kinase gene 11

STL
sent to laboratory
serum theophylline level
status thymicolymphaticus
swelling, tenderness, limited [motion]

STLE
St. Louis encephalitis (*See also* SLE)

STLI
subtotal lymphoid irradiation

STLOM
swelling, tenderness, limitation of motion

STLS
subacute thyroiditis-like syndrome
surface tension-lowering substance

STLV
simian T-cell lymphotropic virus

STM
scanning tunneling microscope (microscopy)
short-term memory
soft tissue mobilization

STML
short-term memory loss

StMPM
syncytiotrophoblast microvillar plasma membrane

STMS
Short Test of Mental Status

STMV
Santarem virus

STN
[computer assisted] surgical tool navigator
subtalar neutral [position]
subthalamic nucleus
supratrochlear nucleus

sTNFR
soluble tumor necrosis factor receptor

sTNF-RI
soluble tumor necrosis factor receptor type I

STNI
subtotal nodal irradiation

STNM
surgical component of TNM staging

STNP
subtalar joint neutral position

STNR
symmetric tonic neck reflex

STNS
sham transcutaneous nerve stimulation

STNV
satellite tobacco necrosis virus

STO
store (*See also* ST)
surgical treatment objective

stom
stomach (*See also* ST)

STOP
selective tubal occlusion procedure
sensitive, timely, organized program [battered spouses]
surgical termination of pregnancy

STORCH
syphilis, toxoplasmosis, other agents, rubella, cytomegalovirus, herpes simplex [virus]

STP
scientifically treated petroleum
serenity, tranquility, peace [user's term for dimethoxymethylamphetamine]
short-term plan
Sibling Training Program
standard temperature and pressure
standard temperature and pulse
step training progression

S-TPA
serum tissue polypeptide antigen

STPD
standard temperature and pressure, dry

STPI
State-Trait Personality Inventory

STPP
sodium tripolyphosphate

STPS
Short-Term Performance Status
specific thalamic projection system

STPT
second-trimester pregnancy termination

STPTIMF
soft tissue pinch thickness at inframammary fold

STPTUP
soft tissue pinch thickness upper pole

STQ
superior temporal quadrant

STR

scotopic threshold response [electroretinogram]
short tandem repeat
skeletal targeted radiotherapy
skin test reactivity
slide thin slab
small tandem repeat [marker, chromosome]
soft-tissue rheumatism
special treatment room
standard threshold shift
stone tissue recognition (system)
stretcher
subtotal resection

Str

striatum (See also ST)

strab

strabismus (See also Sb)

StrAbs

striated muscle

strep

streptococcus

strep TSS

streptococcal toxic shock syndrome

STRESS

subject's treatment-emergent symptom scale

STRP

short tandem repeat polymorphism
simple tandem repeat polymorphism

STRR

Slosson Test of Reading Readiness

STRT

simultaneous thermoradiotherapy
skin temperature recovery time

struct

sructural
structure (See also STX)

STRV

Stratford virus

STS

serology (serologic) test for syphilis
sexual tubal sterilization
short-term storage
short-term survivor
silicone thermoplastic splinting
soft tissue sarcoma
soft tissue swelling
standard test for syphilis
steroid sulfatase [deficiency]
steroid sulfate [transporter]
subtrapezial space
sugar-tong splint

STSD

secondary traumatic stress disorder

STSE

split-thickness skin excision

STSG

split-thickness skin graft

STS-MIP

sliding thin-slab maximum intensity projection

STSS

staphylococcal toxic shock syndrome
streptococcal toxic shock syndrome

STSs

sequence-tagged sites

STS-SPT

simple two-step swallowing provocation test

STT

scaphoid, trapezium, trapezoid [joint]
scaphotrapeziotrapezoid [joint]
scaphotrapezoid-trapezial [joint]
sensitization test
serial thrombin time
skin temperature test
soft tissue tumor
spinothalamic tract
standard triple therapy
subtotal thyroidectomy
superficial tibiotalar

STT #1–#2

Schirmer tear test #1–#2

STTOL

standing tolerance

STUMP

stromal tumor of unknown malignant potential

STV

short-term variability
soft tissue view
spontaneous tidal volume
superior temporal vein

STVA

subtotal villous atrophy (See also SVA)

STVS

short-term visual storage

STX

saxitoxin [neurotoxin chemical weapon TZ]
stricture
structure (See also struct)

Stx

Shiga toxin

STYCAR

Sheridan Tests for Young Children and Retardates

SU

salicyluric [acid]
sensation unit

S

SU *(continued)*
  sensory urgency
  solar urticaria
  Somogyi unit [amylase activity in
    blood]
  sorbent unit
  spectrophotometric unit
  stasis ulcer
  status uncertain
  stress ulcer
  subunit
  supine
S/U
  shoulder/umbilicus
S&U
  supine and upright [x-rays]
SUA
  serum uric acid
  single umbilical artery
  single unit activity
SUB
  Skene, urethral Bartholin [glands]
subac
  subacute
subconj
  subconjunctival
subcrep
  subcrepitant
⚠ **subcu**
  subcutaneous(ly) (*See also* SC, sc, SQ,
    subcut, subq) ⚠
subcut
  subcutaneous(ly) (*See also* SC, sc, SQ,
    subcu, subq)
subl, subling
  sublingual(ly) (*See also* SL)
submand
  submandibular
SubN
  subthalamic nucleus
⚠ **subq**
  subcutaneous(ly) (*See also* SC, sc, SQ,
    subcu, subcut) ⚠
substd
  substandard
SUCC
  succinylcholine (*See also* SC, SCH,
    SUX)
Succ
  succinate
  succinic
SUD
  skin unit dose
  subjective unit of distress
  substance use disorder
  sudden unexpected (unexplained)
    death
SuDBP
  supine diastolic blood pressure

SUDEP
  sudden unexpected (unexplained) death
    in epilepsy
SUDI
  sudden unexpected (unexplained) death
    in infancy (infants)
SUDS
  single-unit delivery system
  single-use diagnostic system
  Subjective Units of Distress Scale
  sudden unexpected (unexplained) death
    syndrome
SUE
  single-use electrode
SUF
  sequential ultrafiltration
  symptomatic uterine fibroids
SUFE
  slipped upper femoral epiphysis
suff
  sufficient
SUHT
  subject's height
SUI
  stress urinary incontinence
  suicide
SUID
  sudden unexpected (unexplained) infant
    death
SUIOS
  Simplified Urinary Incontinence
    Outcome Scale
SUKA
  subungual keratoacanthoma
sulf
  sulfate
SULFHb
  sulfhemoglobin (*See also* HbS, SHb,
    S-Hb)
sum.
  summation
SUMA
  sporadic ulcerating and mutilating
    acropathy
SUMD
  Scale for Assessment of Unawareness
    of Mental Disorder
SUN
  serum urea nitrogen
  Standard Units and Nomenclature
SUNCT
  short lasting unilateral neuralgiform
    [headache with] conjunctival injection
    [and] tearing
SUND
  sudden unexplained death
SUNDS
  sudden unexplained nocturnal death
    syndrome

SUO
  syncope of unknown origin
SUP
  stress ulcer prophylaxis
  superficial
  superior
  supination (*See also* supin)
  supinator [muscle]
  symptomatic uterine prolapse
sup
  supervision
  supervisor
SupHypArt
  superior hypophysial artery
supin
  supination (*See also* SUP)
supp
  support
suppl
  supplement(ary)
suppos
  suppository
SUR
  standardized uptake ratio
  sulfonylurea receptor
SUR1–SUR2
  sulfonylurea receptor 1, 2
SURF
  Service Utilization and Risk Factors
surf
  surfactant
SURG, surg
  surgery (*See also* Sx, S$_x$, sx)
  surgical
SURS
  solitary ulcer of rectum syndrome
SURT
  sarcoidosis of upper respiratory tract
SUS
  solitary ulcer syndrome
  strained urinary sediment
  suppressor sensitive
  sustained urinary sediment
susp
  suspend(ed)
  suspension
SUTI
  sperm-ubiquitin tag immunoassay
  symptomatic urinary tract infection
SUUD
  sudden unexpected, unexplained death
SUV
  standardized uptake value [imaging
    contrast]
SUVAG
  system universal verbotonol audition
    Guberina [hearing]

S-UVT
  sustained uniform ventricular tachycardia
SUX
  succinylcholine (*See also* SC, SCH,
    SUCC)
  suction (*See also* sx, SZ)
SUZI
  subzonal injection
  subzonal insemination
  subzonal insertion
SV
  saphenous vein
  Sapporo virus
  sarcoma virus
  satellite virus
  scimitar vein [anomalous right lung
    vein draining to inferior vena cava]
  selective vagotomy
  semilunar valve
  seminal vesicle
  Sendai virus
  severe(ly) (severity) (*See also* sev)
  sigmoid volvulus
  simian virus
  single ventricle
  sinus venosus
  snake venom
  splenic vein
  spoken voice
  spontaneous ventilation
  stroke volume
  Study of Values
  subclavian vein
  subventricular
  supravital
  systolic velocity
SV40
  simian vacuolating virus 40
S:V
  surface to volume ratio
Sv
  sievert [SI equivalent dose of radiation
    in living organisms]
sv
  single vibration
sv.
  serovar
SVA
  selective vagotomy with antrectomy
  selective visceral angiography
  sequential ventriculoatrial [pacing]
  small volume admixture
  spatial voltage [at maximal] anterior
    [force]
  special visceral afferent
  subtotal villous atrophy (*See also*
    STVA)

S

SVAB
    stereotactic vacuum-assisted biopsy
SVABB
    stereotactic vacuum-assisted breast
      biopsy
SVAS
    supravalvular aortic stenosis (*See also*
      SAS)
SVB
    saphenous vein bypass
SVBG
    saphenous vein bypass graft
SVC
    saphenous vein cutdown
    segmental venous capacitance
    selective vascular clamping
    selective venous catheterization
    slow vital capacity
    subclavian vein catheter(ization)
    subclavian vein compression
    superior vena cava
    suprahepatic vena cava
    supraventricular crest
SV-CAH
    simple virilizing congenital adrenal
      hyperplasia
SVCCS
    superior vena cava compression
      syndrome
SVCG
    spatial vectorcardiogram
SVCO
    superior vena cava obstruction
SVC-PA
    superior vena cava-pulmonary artery
      [shunt]
SVCPMS
    segmental vertebral
      cellulotenoperiosteomyalgic syndrome
SVCR
    segmented venous capacitance ratio
SVC-RPA
    superior vena cava and right pulmonary
      artery [shunt]
SVCS
    superior vena cava syndrome
SVD
    single-vessel disease
    singular value decomposition
    small-vessel disease
    spontaneous vaginal delivery
    spontaneous vertex delivery
    structural valve deterioration
    swine vesicular disease
SVDV
    swine vesicular disease virus
SVE
    slow volume encephalography
    soluble viral extract

    special visceral efferent
    spontaneous ventricular event
    sterile vaginal examination
    Streptococcus viridans endocarditis
    subcortical vascular encephalopathy
    supraventricular ectopic [beat]
    supraventricular ectopy
    supraventricular extrasystole
SV&E
    suicidal, violent, and eloper
SVG
    saphenous vein graft
    scatter and veiling glare
    seminal vesiculography
SVH
    saphenous vein harvesting
    subjective visual horizontal [test]
SVI
    seminal vesicle invasion
    small-vessel infarct(ion)
    small volume infusion
    stroke volume index
    systolic velocity integral [Doppler]
SVIB
    Strong Vocational Interest Blank
SVI/BL
    severe visual impairment and
      blindness
S VISC
    serum viscosity
SVL
    severe visual loss
    superficial vastus lateralis
SVM
    seminal vesicle microsome
    spatial voltage at maximal [posterior
      force]
    syncytiovascular membrane
SVN
    small-volume nebulizer
SVO
    small-vessel occlusion
    splenic vein obstruction
SvO_2, S_{vo2}
    systemic vascular resistance index
    venous oxygen saturation
SVOM
    sequential volitional oral movement
SVOO
    systemic vascular outflow obstruction
SVP
    selective vagotomy with pyloroplasty
    small-volume parenteral [infusion]
    spatial voltage [at maximal] posterior
      [force]
    spontaneous venous pulse (pulsation)
    standing venous pressure
    static volume pressure
    superficial vascular plexus

SVPB
supraventricular premature beat
SVPC
supraventricular premature contraction
SV:PP
stroke volume to pulse pressure ratio
SVPT
supraventricular paroxysmal
tachycardia
SVR
sequential vascular response
slow vertex response
supervoltage radiation
supraventricular rhythm
sustained viral (virologic) response
systemic vascular resistance
SVRI
systemic vascular resistance index
SVS
slit ventricle syndrome
SVSe
supravaginal septum
SVT
sinoventricular tachyarrhythmia
sinus-vein thrombosis
STYCAR Vision Test
subclavian vein thrombosis
superficial vein thrombosis
supraventricular tachyarrhythmia
(tachycardia)
sustained ventricular tachycardia
symptom validity test
SVV
Sal Vieja virus
SVVD
spontaneous vertex vaginal delivery
SW
seriously wounded
shallow walk [aquatic therapy]
shock wave
short wave
slow wave
social worker
spherule wall
spike wave
spiral wound
stab wound
sterile water
stroke work
Swiss Webster [mouse]
S&W
soap and water
S/W
spike wave [electroencephalogram]
Sw
swine
sw
switch

SWA
seriously wounded in action
slow-wave activity
[electroencephalogram]
SWAMI
Speech with Alternating Masking Index
SWAMP
swine-associated mucoprotein
SWAP
short wavelength automated perimetry
SWAT
skin wound assessment and treatment
stationary wavelet transform [imaging]
SWBS
Spiritual Well-Being Scale
SWC
submaximal working capacity
S&WC
spike and wave complex [EEG]
SW-CAH
salt-wasting congenital adrenal
hyperplasia
SWD
shortwave diathermy
SWE
slow-wave encephalography
SWEL
sleep-awake experience list
SWFI
sterile water for injection (*See also*
SWI)
SWG
standard wire gauge
SWGD
sterile water gastric drip
SWI
skin and wound isolation (*See also*
S&WI)
sterile water for injection (*See also*
SWFI)
stroke-work index
surgical wound infection
S&WI
skin and wound isolation (*See also*
SWI)
SWIM
sperm-washing insemination method
SWIORA
spinal cord injury without radiologic
abnormality
SWL
shock wave lithotripsy
SWM
segmental wall motion
SWMA
segmental wall motion abnormality
SWMF
Semmes-Weinstein monofilament

SWO
superficial white onychomycosis
SWORD
Surveillance of Work-related and
Occupational Respiratory Disease
[CDC]
SWOT
strengths, weaknesses, opportunities,
threats [analysis]
SWP
small whirlpool
SWR
serum Wassermann reaction
surface wrinkling retinopathy
SWS
sheltered workshop
slow-wave sleep
spike-wave stupor
steroid-wasting syndrome
SWSD
shift-work sleep disorder
SWT
shock-wave therapy
shuttle-walk test [endurance capacity in
COPD and CHF]
sine-wave threshold
Speech Weber Test
stab wound of throat
SWU
septic workup
SWW
static wall walk [aquatic therapy]
Sx, S$_x$, sx
signs (*See also* S)
surgery (*See also* SURG, surg)
symptom(s) (*See also* SM, sym, symp,
sympt)
sx
suction (*See also* SUX, SZ)
SXA
single-energy x-ray absorptiometer
SXCT
spiral x-ray computed tomography
SXPL
strictureplasty
SXR
skull x-ray
SY
syphilis (*See also* Σ, syph)
syphilitic (*See also* syph)
SYA
subacute yellow atrophy
SYC
small, yellow, constipated [stool]
sym
symmetric(al)
symptom(s) (*See also* SM, Sx, S$_x$, sx,
symp, sympt)

symb
symbol(ic)
symp, sympt
sympathetic (*See also* sympath)
symptom(s) (*See also* SM, Sx, S$_x$, sx,
sym)
sympath
sympathetic (*See also* symp, sympt)
symph
symphysis
SYN
synaptophysin
syn, synd
syndrome
synonym
synovial
synovitis
sync
synchronous (synchronize)
syndet
synthetic detergent
syn fl
synovial fluid (*See also* SF)
Synip
syntaxin 4 interacting protein
synth
synthetic
syph
syphilis (*See also* Σ, SY)
syphilitic (*See also* SY)
SYR
Syrian [hamster]
syr
syringe
syrup
syrupus [apothecary]
SYS
stretching-yawning syndrome
synovial sarcoma (*See also* SS)
sys
system (*See also* syst)
systemic (*See also* syst)
SYS BP
systolic blood pressure (*See also*
SBP)
syst
system (*See also* sys)
systemic (*See also* sys)
systole (*See also* S)
systolic
SZ
schizophrenic
seizure
suction (*See also* SUX, sx)
Sz
skin impedance
SZD
streptozocin diabetes

T

electrocardiographic wave corresponding
  to repolarization of ventricles
obtained under test conditions
period [time]
ribothymidine (*See also* Thd)
tablespoon(ful) (*See also* tbs, TBS, tbsp)
tanycyte [type of ependymal cell]
tau [19th letter of Greek alphabet
  uppercase]
telomere [chromosome]
temperature (*See also* temp, TPR)
temporal [electrode placement in
  electroencephalography] (*See also*
  temp)
temporary (*See also* temp)
tender
tension (*See also* TEN, TN)
tera- [trillion]
term
terminal [banding region in
  chromosomes]
tertiary (*See also* ter, tert)
tesla [SI derived unit of magnetic flux
  density]
testicle
testosterone (*See also* testos)
tetra
thoracic (*See also* Th, thor)
thoracoabdominal (*See also* TA)
thorax (*See also* Th, thor, TX)
threatened [animal]
threonine (*See also* Thr)
thrombus (*See also* throm, thromb)
thymidine (*See also* TdR)
thymine (*See also* Thy)
thymus [cell] (*See also* thy.)
thymus-derived [lymphocyte] (*See also* T
  cell)
thyroid (*See also* Th, thr)
tidal
time (*See also* t)
tincture (*See also* TCT, tinc, tinct,
  TR, Tr)
tocopherol
tone
tonometer [vitamin E]
torque
total (*See also* ttl)
Toxoplasma
trace (*See also* t, TR, Tr)
transformation [zone] (*See also* TMZ)
transition [point] (*See also* TP)
tray
Treponema (*See also* Trep)

triangulation
trigger(ed)
tritium [hydrogen isotope H3] (*See also*
  ^{3}H)
tuberculin (*See also* TB)
tuberculum
tuberosity
tumor (*See also* TM)
type (*See also* Ty)

⚠ Ṫ, ṪṪ, ṪṪṪ

quantity of drug to be used (*See also* i,
  ii, iii) ⚠

T 1/2, T$^1\!/_2$

[mitral] pressure half-time [Doppler]
terminal half-life [of isotopes]

T0

tumor cannot be assessed [TNM
  classification]

T$_1$

monoiodotyronine
tricuspid first heart sound

T1

first twitch height
spin-lattice or longitudinal relaxation
  time [MRI scan]

T−1, T−2, T−3
decreased intraocular pressure 1–3
T+1−T+3
increased intraocular pressure 1–3
T1−T4
tumors progressing in size, number,
  penetration [TNM classification]
T1−T12
thoracic nerves 1–12
thoracic vertebrae 1–12 (*See also*
  D1–D12)

T$_2$

diiodothyronine
tricuspid second heart sound

T2

spin-spin or transverse relaxation time
  [MRI scan]

T$_3$

3,5,3′-triiodothyronine (*See also* TIT,
  TITh, TRIT)

⚠ T3

transurethral thermoablation
  therapy
Tylenol with codeine [30 mg] ⚠

T$_4$

tetraiodothyronine (thyroxine)

T$_7$

free thyroxine (T4)
T28

Trapezoidal-28 [hip prosthesis]

T-1824
 Evans blue [dye]
2,4,5-T
 (2,4,5-trichlorophenoxy)acetic acid
T+
 increased intraocular tension
 increased tension (pressure)
T−
 decreased tension (pressure)
t¹/₂
 reaction half-time
 time taken for half of initial
  concentration of deoxyribonucleic acid
  to renature
t
 duration
 life (time) (*See also* T)
 teaspoon(ful) (*See also* teasp, ts, tsp)
 terminal (*See also* term., TRML, trml)
 time (*See also* T)
 ton [2000 pounds]
 tonne [metric, 1000 mg]
 trace (*See also* T, TR, Tr)
 transformer
 translocation
t.
 three [times] [L. *ter*] (*See also* ter)
TA
 tactile afferent
 Takayasu arteritis
 T-amplifier
 technical assistance
 teichoic acid
 temperature, axillary (*See also* T(A))
 temporal arteritis
 temporal artery
 temporal average
 temporary abstinence
 tendon of Achilles [tendo Achillis]
 tension applanation (*See also* TAP)
 tension, arterial
 terminal antrum
 terminal arteriole
 Terminologia Anatomica
 test age
 therapeutic abortion (*See also* TAB,
  TAb)
 thermophilic *Actinomyces*
 thoracoabdominal (*See also* T)
 thymocytotoxic autoantibody
 thyroarytenoid
 thyroglobulin autoprecipitation
 thyroglobulin autoprecipitin
 thyroid antibody
 thyroid autoantibody
 tibialis anterior
 titratable acid
 toothache
 total alkaloids

toxic adenoma
toxin-antitoxin (*See also* TAT)
tracheal aspirate
traffic accident
transactional analysis
transaldolase (*See also* TRA)
transantral
transplant(ation) antigen
trapped air
treatment adherence
treatment assignment
tricholomic acid
tricuspid anuloplasty (annuloplasty)
tricuspid atresia (*See also* TCA, TriA)
trophoblast antigen
true anomaly
true apex
truncus arteriosus
tryptamine
tryptose agar
tube agglutination
tuberculin, alkaline
tumor antigen
tumor associated
T&A
 tonsillectomy and adenoidectomy
 tonsils and adenoids
T/A
 time and amount
T(A)
 temperature, axillary (*See also* TA)
Tα₁, TA1
 thymosin alpha (α) 1
Ta
 tantalum
¹⁷⁸Ta
 tantalum-178
¹⁸²Ta
 tantalum-182
TAA
 thoracic aortic aneurysm
 total ankle arthroplasty
 transcoronary alcohol ablation
 transverse aortic arch
 tumor-associated antigen
TAAA
 thoracoabdominal aortic aneurysm
TAAF
 thromblastic activity of amniotic fluid
TA-AIDS
 transfusion-associated AIDS
TAB
 tablet (*See also* tab.)
 temporal artery biopsy
 therapeutic abortion (*See also* TA, TAb)
 total androgen blockade
 total atrial blanking
 triple antibiotic
 tumescent absorbent bandage

typhoid, paratyphoid A, and paratyphoid B [vaccine]

TAb
therapeutic abortion (*See also* TA, TAB)

tab.
tablet (*See also* TAB)

TABC
total aerobic bacteria count
typhoid, paratyphoid A, paratyphoid B, and paratyphoid C [vaccine]

TABTD
typhoid, paratyphoid A, paratyphoid B, tetanus toxoid, and diphtheria toxoid [vaccine]

TAC
terminal antrum contraction
terminal atrial contraction
tibial artery catheter
time-activity curve
timed average concentration
total abdominal colectomy
total aganglionosis coli
total allergen content
total arterial compliance
transient aplastic crisis
transiently amplifying cell

TACC
thoracic aortic cross-clamping

TACE
teichoic acid crude extract
transarterial catheter embolization
transarterial chemoembolization
transcatheter arterial chemoembolization
trianisylchloroethylene

tach, tachy
tachycardia

TACI
total anterior circulation infarct

TACK
Translating and Congruent Mobile-Bearing Knee [prosthesis]

TACL
Tests for Auditory Comprehension of Language

TACL-R
Tests for Auditory Comprehension of Language Revised

tac-MRA
timed arterial compression magnetic resonance

tachy-brady
tachycardia-bradycardia syndrome (*See also* TBS)

TACS
total anterior circulation syndrome

TACT
thermoacoustic computed tomography
tuned aperture computed tomography

TACurea
timed average concentration, urea

TAD
Test of Auditory Discrimination
thoracic asphyxiant dystrophy (*See also* ATD)
thrombin activation device
total administered dose
trans-activation domain
transient acantholytic dermatosis
transverse abdominal diameter
tricyclic antidepressant drug

TADAC
therapeutic abortion, dilation, aspiration, curettage

TADC
tumor-associated dendritic cell

TADG15
tumor-associated differentially expressed gene 15

TAE
right atrial enlargement
total abdominal evisceration
transcatheter arterial embolization

TAER
transient auditory-evoked response

TAES
transcutaneous acupoint electrical stimulation

TAF
tissue angiogenesis factor
total abdominal fat
toxoid-antitoxin floccule
tracheobronchial aspirate fluid
transactivation factor
traumatic aortocaval fistula
tuberculin, albumose-free [Ger. *Tuberculin Albumose frei*]
tumor angiogenesis (angiogenic) factor

TAFI
thrombin-activatable fibrinolysis inhibitor

TAG
target-attaching globulin
thymine, adenine, guanine
tissue anchor guide
total available glucose
triacylglycerol (*See also* TG)
tumor-associated glycoprotein

TAG-72
tumor-associated glycoprotein 72

TAGA
term, appropriate for gestational age

TAGH
triiodothyronine, amino acids, glucagon, heparin

T

TAGM
trisacryl gelatin microsphere
TAGV
Taggert virus
TA-GVHD
transfusion-associated graft-versus-host disease
TAH
total abdominal hysterectomy
total artificial heart
TAHBSO
total abdominal hysterectomy and bilateral salpingo-oophorectomy
TAHIV
transfusion-acquired human immunodeficiency virus
transfusion-associated human immunodeficiency virus
TAHV
Tahyna virus
TAI
thoracoabdominal irradiation
tissue antagonist of interferon
traumatic aortic injury
T Air
air puff tonometry [ophthalmology]
TAIV
Tai virus
TAKE
Targeting Abnormal Kinetic Effects [scale]
TAL
Achilles tendon (tendo Achillis) lengthening (*See also* ATL)
thick ascending limb
thymic alymphoplasia
total arm length
total autogenous latissimus
tumor-associated lymphocyte
TALC
transairway laryngeal control
talc
talcum
TALH
thick ascending limb of Henle
TALL, T-ALL
T-cell acute lymphoblastic leukemia
TALLA
T-cell acute lymphoblastic leukemia antigen
TALP
total alkaline phosphatase
tumor-assisted lymphoid proliferation
TALPS
Transactional Analysis Life Position Survey
TALT
testicular adrenal-like tissue

TALTFR
tendo Achillis lengthening and toe flexor release
TAM
Technology Assessment Methods Project
teenage mother
thermoacidurans agar modified
total active motion
toxin-antitoxin mixture
toxoid-antitoxoid mixture
transient abnormal myelopoiesis
transtelephonic ambulatory monitoring [system]
tricuspid annular motion
tumor-associated macrophage
TAMBA
talar axis–first metatarsal base angle
TAME
tosylarginine methyl ester
TAMe
toxoid-antitoxoid mixture esterase
TAMIS
Telemetric Automated Microbial Identification System
TAML, t-AML
therapy-related acute myelogenous (myeloid) leukemia
TAMMAS
temporary articulating methylmethacrylate antibiotic spacer
TAMV
Tamiami virus
temporal average maximal velocity [Doppler]
TAN
total adenine nucleotide
total ammonia nitrogen
treatment as needed
Treatment Authorization Number
tropical ataxic neuropathy
tan.
tandem translocation
tangent
TANI
total axial [lymph] node irradiation
TANIS
T and N integer score [staging system]
TANV
Tanga virus
TAO
thromboangiitis obliterans
thyroid-associated ophthalmopathy
turning against object
TAP
tension applanation (*See also* TA)
Thornton anterior positioner
tone and positioning
tonometry applanation (*See also* AT, T APPL)

Trainer's Assessment of Proficiency
transabdominal preperitoneal
  [laparoscopic hernia repair]
transesophageal atrial pacing (*See also*
  TEAP)
transport-associated protein
transvaginal amniotic puncture
trypsin activation peptide
trypsinogen-activating peptide
tumor-activated prodrug

TAPC
total anomalous pulmonary circulation

TAP-D
Test of Articulation
  Performance-Diagnostic

TAPE
temporary atrial pacemaker electrode

TAPET
tumor amplified protein expression
  therapy

TAPP
transabdominal preperitoneal
  polypropylene [hernioplasty,
  meshplasty]

T APPL
tonometry applanation (*See also* AT,
  TAP)

TAPS
training and placement service
trial assessment procedure scale

TAP-S
Test of Articulation Performance-Screen

TAPVC
total anomalous pulmonary venous
  connection

TAPVD
total anomalous pulmonary venous
  drainage

TAPVR
total anomalous pulmonary venous
  return

TAQW
transient abnormal Q wave

TAR
thoracic aortic rupture
thrombocytopenia and absent radius
tissue-air ratio
total abortion rate
total ankle replacement
total anorectal reconstruction
transactivator
treatment administration record
treatment authorization request

TARA
total articular replacement (resurfacing)
  arthroplasty
tumor-associated rejection antigen

TARC
thymus and activation-regulated
  chemokine

TARP
total atrial refractory period

TART
tissue [texture changes], asymmetry,
  restriction [of motion,] tenderness
tumorectomy, axillary [dissection],
  radiotherapy

TARTI
total apexcardiographic relaxation time
  index

TARU
technical advisory response unit

TAS
test for ascendance-submission
Test of Attitude Toward School
tetanus antitoxin serum
thoracoabdominal staples
thoracoabdominal syndrome
thrombolytic assessment system
Toronto Alexithymia Scale
transabdominal suture
turning against self
typical absence seizure

TASA
tumor-associated surface antigen

TASB
Teacher Assessment of Social Behavior

T'ase, Tase
tryptophan synthetase

TASH
transcoronary ablation of septal
  hypertrophy

T-ASI
Teen Addiction Severity Index

TASI
transperitoneal anterior subcostal
  incision

TASS
thyroiditis, Addison disease, Sjögren
  syndrome, sarcoidosis [syndrome]

TAS/TVS
transabdominal/transvaginal ultrasound

TAT
tandem autotransplants (transplants)
Tell a Tale [psychiatry]
tetanus antitoxin
thematic apperception test
thematic aptitude test
thrombin-antithrombin
thromboplastin activation test
till all taken
total adipose tissue
total antitryptic activity
toxin-antitoxin (*See also* TA)

T

TAT *(continued)*
    transactivator of transcription [protein]
    transaxial tomogram
    transplant-associated thrombocytopenia
    transverse axial tomography
    tray agglutination test
    treponemal antibody test
    triple advancement transposition
    tumor activity test
    turnaround time
    tyrosine aminotransferase
TATA
    tumor-associated transplantation antigen
TATD
    tyrosine aminotransferase deficiency
TATE
    tumor-associated tissue eosinophilia
TATR
    tyrosine aminotransferase regulator
TATST
    tetanus antitoxin skin test
TATT
    tired all the time
TATV
    Tataguine virus
τ, tau
    life [of radioisotope]
    relaxation time
    shear stress
    spectral transmittance
    tau [19th letter of Greek alphabet
      lowercase]
    transmission coefficient
TAU
    tumescence activity unit
TAUC
    target area under curve
    time-averaged urea concentration
TAUS
    transabdominal ultrasound
TAUSA
    thrombolysis and angioplasty in unstable
      angina
TAV
    transcutaneous [transvenous]
      aortovelography
    trapped air volume
TAWF
    Test of Adolescent/Adult Word
      Finding
TB
    Tapes for the Blind
    term birth
    terminal bronchiole
    terrible burning
    thought broadcasting
    thromboxane B
    thymol blue
    toluidine blue

    toothbrush
    total base
    total body
    total bound
    tracheal bronchial [region]
    tracheobronchitis
    trapezoid body
    tub bath
    tubercle bacillus
    tuberculin (*See also* T)
    tuberculosis
    tumor bearing
T_b
    buildup time
    temperature, body
Tb
    terbium
Tb_4
    thymosin beta (β)4
tb
    biologic half-life
TBA
    to be absorbed
    to be added
    to be administered
    to be admitted
    to be announced
    to be arranged
    to be assessed
    tertiary butyl acetate
    testosterone-binding affinity
    thiobarbituric acid
    thyroxine-binding albumin
    total bile acid
    total body [surface] area
    traditional birth attendant
    transaxillary breast augmentation
    trypsin-binding activity
    tumor-bearing animal
TBAB
    thyroid-blocking antibody
    tryptose/blood/agar base
TBAGA
    term birth appropriate for gestational
      age
T-bar
    tracheotomy bar [respiratory therapy]
TBARS
    thiobarbituric acid-reactive substance
TBB
    transbronchial biopsy (*See also* TBBx)
TBBC
    total [vitamin] B_{12} binding capacity
TBBM
    total body bone mineral
TBBMC
    total body bone mineral content
TBBMD
    total body bone mineral density

TBBx
    transbronchial biopsy (*See also* TBB)
TBC
    to be canceled
    thyroxine-binding coagulin
    total-blood cholesterol
    total body calcium
    total body clearance (*See also* Q$_B$)
    total body counting
    traumatic bone cyst
    tubercidin
    tuberculous
TBD
    to be determined
    total body density
    Toxicology Data Base
TBE
    to be evaluated
    tick-borne encephalitis
    tris-boric acid-EDTA
        (ethylenediaminetetraacetic acid)
    tuberculin bacillary emulsion
TBE$_e$
    tick-borne encephalitis, Eastern subtype
TBE$_w$
    tick-borne encephalitis, Western subtype
T-berg
    Trendelenburg [position]
TBEV
    tick-borne encephalitis virus
TBF
    temporal bone fracture
    total body fat
    tracheal blood flow
TBFB
    tracheobronchial foreign body
TBFM
    total body fat mass
TBFV
    tidal breathing flow-volume
TBFVL
    tidal breathing flow-volume loop
TBG
    testosterone-binding globulin
    thyroxine-binding globulin
    tracheobronchogram
    tris-buffered Grey [solution]
TBGE
    thyroxine-binding globulin, estimated
TBGI
    thyroxine-binding globulin index
TBGP
    total blood granulocyte pool
TBH
    total body hematocrit
TBHT
    total body hyperthermia

TBI
    thrombotic brain infarction
    thyroxine-binding index
    tick-borne illness
    tooth-brushing instruction
    total body irradiation (*See also*
        TBX)
    tracheobronchial injury
    traumatic brain injury
    tumor burden index
TBIAb
    TSH (thyroid-stimulating hormone)
        binding inhibitor antibody
TBII
    thyrotropin-binding inhibitory
        immunoglobulin
    TSH (thyroid stimulating hormone)
        binding inhibitory immunoglobulin
TBILI
    total bilirubin
TBK
    total body kalium [potassium]
TBL
    toluidine blue O [dye, stain]
TBLB
    transbronchial lung biopsy
TBLC
    term birth, living child
TBLF
    term birth, living female
TBLI
    term birth, living infant
TBLM
    term birth, living male
TBLR
    transconjunctival blepharoplasty laser
        resurfacing
TBM
    therapeutic back massage
    thin basement membrane
    total body mass
    total bone matrix
    tracheobronchomalacia
    tuberculous meningitis
    tubular basement membrane
TBMD
    thin basement membrane disease
TBMg
    total-body magnesium
TBN
    total body nitrogen
    tributyrin agar
TBNA
    total body neutron activation
    total body sodium
    transbronchial needle aspiration
    treated but not admitted

T

TBNa
    total body natrium [sodium]
TBNAA
    total body neutron activation
        analysis
t-BOC, tBoc
    tert-butyloxycarbonyl
TBP
    TATA-binding protein
    testosterone-binding protein
    thiobisdichlorophenol (bithionol)
    thyroxine-binding protein
    toe blood pressure
    total body phosphorus
    total body photograph
    total body protein
    total bypass
    tributyl phosphate
    tuberculous peritonitis
TBPA
    thyronine-binding prealbumin
    thyroxine-binding prealbumin
TBPT
    total body protein turnover
TBR
    total bed rest
    tumor-bearing rabbit
TB-RD
    tuberculosis-respiratory disease
TBRF
    tick-borne relapsing fever
TBRS
    Timed Behavioral Rating Sheet
TBS
    tablespoon(ful) (*See also* T, tbs, tbsp)
    tachycardia-bradycardia syndrome
        (*See also* tachy-brady)
    The Bethesda System
    total body scan
    total body solids
    total body solute
    total body surface
    total burn size
    tracheobronchial submucosa
    tracheobronchoscopy
    Transition Behavior Scale
    tribromsalan (tribromosalicylanilide)
    triethanolamine-buffered saline
    tris-buffered saline [solution]
    tubular bone stenosis
tbs, tbsp
    tablespoon(ful) (*See also* T, TBS)
TBSA
    temporal bone subperiosteal abscess
    total body surface area
    total burn surface area
TBSAH
    traumatic basal subarachnoid
        hemorrhage

TBT, TbT
    tolbutamide test
    tracheal bronchial (tracheobronchial)
        toilet
    tracheobronchial tree
    transbronchoscopic balloon tipped
        [catheter]
    transcervical balloon tuboplasty
TBTNR
    Toronto Biculture Test of Nonverbal
        Reasoning
TBTT
    tuberculin tine test
TBTV
    Timboteua virus
TBUT
    tear breakup time (test)
TBV
    total blood volume
    total brain volume
    trabecular bone volume
    transluminal balloon valvuloplasty
TBV$_p$
    total blood volume predicted
TBW
    total body washout
    total body water (*See also* TBWA)
    total body weight
TBWA
    total body water (*See also* TBW)
TBX
    thromboxane (*See also* Thx)
    total body irradiation (*See also*
        TBI)
TC
    to contain
    tai chi
    talocalcaneal
    tandem colonoscopy
    target cell
    taurocholate
    taurocholic [acid]
    telephone call (*See also* T/C)
    temperature compensation
    teratocarcinoma
    terminal cancer
    tertiary cleavage
    testicular cancer
    to [the] chest
    therapeutic community
    therapeutic concentrate
    thermal conductivity (detector) (*See also*
        λ, TCD)
    thermocouple
    thoracic cage
    thoracic circumference
    throat culture (*See also* TH-CULT)
    thyrocalcitonin (*See also* TCA,
        TCT)

tissue culture
tonic-clonic
tonsillar coblation
total calcium
total capacity
total cholesterol
total colectomy
total colonoscopy
total correction
tracheal collar
traffic collision
transcobalamin
transcutaneous
transhepatic cholangiograph(y)
  (cholangiogram) (*See also* THC)
transverse colon
trauma center
treatment completed
true conjugate
tuberculosis, contagious
tumor cell
tungsten carbide
type [and] crossmatch (*See also* T&C,
  T&CM, T&M, T&X, TXM)
typical carcinoid
TC I
transcobalamin I
TC II
transcobalamin II
T$_4$(C)
serum thyroxine measured by column
  chromatography
TC$_{50}$
median toxic concentration
T/C
to consider
telephone call (*See also* TC)
T:C
tumor to cerebellum ratio
T&C
test and crossmatch
turn and cough
type and crossmatch (*See also* TC,
  T&CM, T&M, T&X, TXM)
Tc
core temperature
cytotoxic T-cell
generation time of cell cycle
technetium
temporal complex
^{99}Tc
technetium-99
^{99m}Tc
technetium-99m
^{99m}Tc-DISIDA
technetium-99m diisopropyliminodiacetic
  acid

^{99m}Tc-DMSA
technetium-99m dimercaptosuccinic acid
^{99m}Tc-DPTA, ^{99m}TC-DTPA
technetium-99m diethylenetriamine
  pentaacetic acid
^{99m}Tc-ECD
technetium-99m ethyl cysteinate dimer
^{99m}Tc-GHA
technetium-99m gluceptate
  (glucoheptonate)
^{99m}Tc-GSA
technetium-99m galactosyl-human serum
  albumin
^{99m}Tc-HIDA
technetium hepatoiminodiacetic acid
  [scan]
^{99m}Tc-HMPAO
technetium-99m
  hexamethylpropyleneamine oxime
^{99m}Tc-HSA
technetium-99m labeled human serum
  albumin
^{99m}Tc-IDA
technetium iminodiacetic acid
^{99m}Tc-labeled
technetium-99m-labeled
^{99m}Tc-MAA
technetium-99m macroaggregated
  albumin
^{99m}Tc-MAG3
technetium-99m
  mercapto-acetyl-glycyl-glycyl-glycine
^{99m}Tc-MDP
technetium-99m-methylene-
  bisphosphonate
^{99m}Tc-MIBI
technetium-99m methoxyisobutylisonitrile
^{99m}Tc-MMAA
technetium-99m minimicroaggregated
  albumin
^{99m}Tc-PYP
technetium-99m pyrophosphate
^{99m}Tc-RBC
technetium-99m [tagged] red blood cell
^{99m}Tc-SC
technetium-99m sulfur colloid
tc
translational control
TCA
talocalcaneal angle
tentorium cerebelli attachment
terminal cancer (carcinoma)
tetracyclic antidepressant
thymic carcinoma
thyrocalcitonin (*See also* TC, TCT)
tissue concentrations of antibiotic(s)
tissue culture assay

TCA *(continued)*
    total cholic acid
    total circulating albumin
    total circulatory arrest
    total colonic aganglionosis
    transcondylar axis
    transluminal coronary angioplasty
    tricalcium aluminate
    tricarboxylic acid
    trichloroacetate
    trichloroacetic acid
    tricuspid atresia *(See also* TA, TriA)
    tricyclic amine
    tricyclic antidepressant *(See also* TCAD)
    tricyclic antipsychotic
    trihydrocoprostanic acid
    tumor chemosensitivity assay
    tumor clonogenic assays

TCABG, TCAG
    triple coronary artery bypass graft

TCAD
    transplant(ation) coronary artery disease
    tricyclic antidepressant *(See also* TCA)

TCAP
    targeted cryoablation of prostate

TCAT
    Toglia Category Assessment Test
    transmission computer-assisted
      tomography

TCB
    to call back
    tetrachlorobiphenyl
    total cardiopulmonary bypass
    total counts bound
    transabdominal chorionic biopsy
    transcatheter biopsy
    transconjunctival blepharoplasty
    tumor cell burden

TcB
    transcutaneous bilirubin

TCBF
    total cerebral blood flow

TCBS
    thiosulfate-citrate-bile salts-sucrose [agar]

TCC
    thromboplastic cell component
    toroidal coil chromatography
    total contact casting
    transcatheter closure
    transitional cell carcinoma
    trichlorocarbanilide

TCCA
    tissue culture cytotoxin assay
    transitional cell cancer-associated
      [virus]

TCCB
    transitional cell carcinoma of bladder

TCCD
    transcranial color-coded Doppler

TC CO$_2$
    transcutaneous carbon dioxide [monitor]

TCCS
    transcranial color-coded sonography

TCD
    thermal conductivity detector
    tissue culture dose
    transcerebellar diameter
    transcranial Doppler [sonography,
      ultrasound]
    transcystic duct
    transverse cardiac diameter
    transverse cerebellar diameter

TCD$_{50}$
    median tissue culture dose
    tissue culture infectious dose *(See also*
      TCID$_{50}$)

TC&DB
    turn, cough, deep breath

TCDC
    taurochenodeoxycholate

TCD/CBDE
    transcystic duct/common bile duct
      exploration

TCDD
    2,3,7,8-tetrachlorodibenzo-*p*-dioxin
    tetrachlorodibenzo-p-dioxin (dioxin)

TCE
    T-cell enriched
    tetrachlorodiphenyl ethane
    total colon examination
    toxicity composite endpoint
    transcatheter embolotherapy
    trichloroethanol
    trichloroethylene

T cell
    small lymphocyte *(See also* T)
    thymus-derived lymphocyte
      (See also T)

TCES
    transcutaneous cranial electrical
      stimulation

TCESOM
    trichloroethylene-extracted soybean-oil
      meal

TCET
    transcerebral electrotherapy

TCF
    time correlation function
    tissue-coding factor *(See also* TSF)
    total conjunctival flap
    total coronary flow

TCFO
    Therapy Carrot finger contracture
      orthosis

TCFU
    tumor colony-forming unit

TCG
    time compensation gain

TCGF
 T-cell growth factor
TCH
 tanned cell hemagglutination
 temporary contralateral hemiplegia
 thiophen-2-carboxylic acid hydrazide
 total circulating hemoglobin
 traumatic cephalohydrocele
 turn, cough, and hyperventilate
TC:HDL
 total cholesterol to high density
  lipoprotein ratio
TChE
 total cholinesterase
TCHR
 traditional Chinese herbal remedy
TCHT
 traditional Chinese herbal therapy
TCI
 to come in [to hospital]
 target-controlled infusion
 temperament and character
  inventory
 total cerebral ischemia
 Totman Change Index
 transient cerebral ischemia
 transitory cognitive impairment
 tricuspid insufficiency
TCi
 teracurie
TCID
 tissue culture infective dose
 tissue culture inoculated dose
TCID$_{50}$
 median tissue culture infective dose
 tissue culture infectious dose (*See also*
  TCD$_{50}$)
TCIE
 transient cerebral ischemic episode
TCIFTT
 transcervical intrafallopian tube transfer
TCIPA
 tumor-cell-induced platelet aggregation
TCIS
 T-cell immunodeficiency syndrome
 total corrected incremental score
 transitional carcinoma in situ
TCL
 tachycardia cycle length
 thermochemiluminescence
 thyroid T-cell line
 tibial collateral ligament
 total capacity of lung
 transverse carpal ligament
 triazine chlorguanide
T-CLL
 T-cell chronic lymphocytic leukemia

TCM
 thick cutaneous melanoma
 tissue culture medium
 traditional Chinese medicine
 transcutaneous monitor
T&CM
 type and crossmatch (*See also* TC,
  T&C, T&M, T&X, TXM)
TCMA
 transcortical motor aphasia
tc-MER
 motor-evoked response to transcranial
  [stimulation]
TCMH
 tumor-direct cell-mediated
  hypersensitivity
TCMI
 T-cell-mediated immunity
TCMM
 traditional Chinese materia medica
TCMP
 thematic content modification program
TCMS
 transcranial cortical magnetic stimulation
 transcranial magnetic stimulation
TCMV
 Tacaiuma virus
TCN
 talocalcaneonavicular [joint]
 terminal capillary network
TCNB
 Tru-Cut needle biopsy
TcNM
 tumor with lymph node metastases
TCNS
 transcutaneous nerve stimulator (*See also*
  TNS)
TCO
 total contact orthosis
 transcutaneous oximetry
TCO$_2$
 transcutaneous oxygen (*See also* TCPO$_2$,
  tcPO$_2$)
TcO^{4-}, TcO4-
 pertechnetate
TcO$_2$
 transcutaneous oxygen pressure (*See also*
  TCPO$_2$, tcPO$_2$)
TCOM
 transcutaneous oxygen monitor (*See also*
  TOM)
T Con
 temporary conservatorship
TCP
 teacher-child-parent
 therapeutic class profile
 therapeutic continuous penicillin

T

TCP *(continued)*
 thrombocytopenia (*See also* T-penia)
 tibial hole coronal positioning
 total circulating protein
 transcutaneous pacing
 tricalcium phosphate
 trichlorophenol
 tricresyl phosphate
 tropical calcific pancreatitis
 tumor control probability
TCPA
 tetrachlorophthalic anhydride
TCPC
 total cavopulmonary connection
TCPCO$_2$, tcPCO$_2$
 transcutaneous carbon dioxide pressure
TCPE
 trichlorophenoxyethanol
TCP III
 total condylar prosthesis III
TCPO$_2$, tcPO$_2$
 transcutaneous oxygen pressure (*See also* TCO$_2$)
TCPS
 total cavopulmonary shunt
TCPTP
 T-cell protein tyrosine phosphatase
TCR
 T-cell antigen receptor
 T-cell reactivity
 T-cell receptor
 T-cell rosette
 thalamocortical relay
 total cytoplasmic ribosome
 tricuspid regurgitation
TCRBCL
 T-cell-rich B-cell lymphoma
TCRE
 transcervical resection of endometrium
TCRF
 temperature-controlled radiofrequency
TCRFTA
 temperature-controlled radiofrequency tissue ablation
tcRNA
 translational control ribonucleic acid
TCRP
 total cellular receptor pool
TCRT
 thoracic conformal radiation therapy
TCRV
 Tacaribe virus
 total red cell volume
TCR Vb
 T cell antigen receptor Vb
TCS
 T-cell supernatant
 tethered-cord syndrome
 tonic-clonic seizure

 total calcium score
 total cellular score
 total coronary score
 transcranial stimulation
 Treacher Collins syndrome
 Tricomponent Coaxial System
 turnstile casting stand
Tcs
 T-cell-mediating contact sensitivity
TCSA
 tetrachlorosalicylanilide
TCSM
 Test of Cognitive Style in Mathematics
TCSW
 thinking creatively with sounds and words
TCT
 taurine cotransporter
 thoracic computed tomography
 thrombin clotting time
 thymic carcinoid tumor
 thyrocalcitonin (*See also* TC, TCA)
 tincture (*See also* T, tinc, tinct, TR, Tr)
 tracheal cytotoxin
 transcatheter therapy
 triple combination tablet [abacavir, lamivudine, and zidovudine]
 Trunk Control Test
 tubocurarine test
TCU
 Test of Concept Utilization
 transitional care unit
tcu-PA
 two-chain urokinase plasminogen activator
TCV
 tall cell variant
 thoracic cage volume
 three concept view
TCVA
 thromboembolic cerebral vascular accident
TD
 to deliver
 tabes dorsalis
 tardive dyskinesia (*See also* TDK)
 targeted dose
 T-cell dependent
 temperature differential
 temporary disability
 teratoma differentiated
 terminal device
 test dose
 tetanus-diphtheria (toxoid) (*See also* Td)
 tetrodotoxin (*See also* TTX)
 therapy discontinued
 thermal dilution
 thermal dysregulation
 thermodilution

thoracic duct
three [times per] day
threshold of detectability
threshold of discomfort
threshold dose
thymus-dependent
thyroid dysgenesis
tic douloureux
tidal volume (*See also* TV, VT, V_T)
timed disintegration
tocopherol deficient
tolerance dose
tone decay
torsion dystonia
total disability
total dose
totally disabled
toxic dose
tracheal diameter
tracking dye
transdermal
transition [trigger] delay
transverse diameter (*See also* Trans D, transD)
traveler's diarrhea
treatment discontinued
trichodiscoma
tuberoinfundibular dopaminergic (*See also* TIDA)
tumor dose
typhoid dysentery

T1D
type 1 diabetes [cf. IDDM] (*See also* T1DM)

T2D
type 2 diabetes [cf. NIDDM] (*See also* T2DM)

$T_4(D)$
serum thyroxine measured by displacement analysis

TD_{50}
median toxic dose

T_D
time required to double number of cells in given population

T_d
diffusion time

Td
tetanus-diphtheria [toxoid; adult type] (*See also* TD)

tD
tetanus and diphtheria

TDA
testis-determining antigen
therapeutic drug assay
tryptophan deaminase agar

TSH (thyroid stimulating hormone) displacing antibody

TDAC
tumor-derived activated cell

TDAP
thoracodorsal artery perforator flap

Tdap
combined tetanus, diphtheria, and pertussis vaccine

TDB
Toxicology Data Bank

T&D bili
total and direct bilirubin

TDC
taurodeoxycholic [acid]
thermal dilution catheter
total dietary calories

TDCO
thermodilution cardiac output

TDD
teardrop distance
Telecommunication Device [for the] Deaf
tetradecadiene
thoracic duct drainage
total daily dose
total digitalizing dose
transpulmonary thermal-dye dilution

TDDA
tetradecadiene acetate

TDE
2-dimensional echocardiography
tetrachlorodiphenylethane
thiamine deficiency encephalopathy
time-delayed exponential
tissue Doppler echocardiography
total daily energy [requirement]
total digestible energy
transthoracic Doppler echocardiography
triethylene [glycol] diglycidyl ether

TDEC
test declined [no longer offered]

TDEE
total daily energy expenditure

TDF
testis-determining factor
Thinking Disturbance Factor
thoracic duct fistula
thoracic duct flow
thoracodorsal flap
time-dose fractionation (factor)
tissue-damaging factor (*See also* TF)
total-dietary fiber
tumor dose fractionation

TDH
thermostable direct hemolysin
thoracic disc herniation

T

TDH *(continued)*
threonine dehydrogenase
total decreased histamine
toxic dose, high

T:DHT
testosterone to dihydrotestosterone
ratio

TDI
temperature difference integrator
therapeutic donor insemination
three-dimensional interlocking [hip]
tissue Doppler imaging
tolerable daily intake
toluene diisocyanate
total-dose infusion

TDK
tardive dyskinesia (*See also* TD)

TDL
temporal difference limen
thoracic duct lymphocyte
thymus-dependent lymphocyte
toxic dose, low

TDLN
tumor-draining lymph node

TDLNC
tumor-draining lymph node cell

TDLU
terminal ductal (duct) lobular unit

TDM
tartaric dimalonate
therapeutic drug monitoring
thermodeltameter
trehalose dimycolate

T1DM
type 1 diabetes mellitus [cf. IDDM]
(*See also* T1D)

T2DM
type 2 diabetes mellitus [cf. NIDDM]
(*See also* T2D)

TDMAC
tridodecylmethylammonium chloride
[graft coating material]

TD-MCT
time-domain microwave computed
tomography

TDME
tractional diabetic macular edema

TDMS
tropical diarrhea-malabsorption
syndrome

TDMV
Tindholmur virus

TDN
total digestible nutrients
totally digestible nutrients
transdermal nitroglycerin (*See also*
TDNTG)

tDNA
transfer deoxyribonucleic acid

TDNTG
transdermal nitroglycerin (*See also*
TDN)

TDNWB
touchdown nonweightbearing

TDO
trichodentoosseous [syndrome]

TDP
tenderness to digital palpation
therapist-driven protocol
thermal death point
thiamine diphosphate
thoracic duct pressure
thymidine diphosphate
time-dependent potentiation
torsade de pointes (*See also* TdP, TP)
transdermal patch

TdP
torsade de pointes (*See also* TDP, TP)

TDPDS
temporomandibular disorder pain
dysfunction syndrome

TdPVT
torsade de pointes ventricular
tachycardia

TDPWB
touchdown partial weightbearing

TDR
thymidine deoxyriboside

TdR
thymidine (*See also* T)

TDS
Teacher Drool Scale
temperature, depth, salinity
tilted disc syndrome
transduodenal sphincteroplasty
travelers diarrhea syndrome

TDSD
transient digestive system disorder

TDSNV
Trager duck spleen necrosis virus

TDSP
time domain signal processor

TDT
tentative discharge tomorrow
thermal death time
tone decay test
transmission disequilibrium test(ing)
Trieger Dot Test
tumor doubling time

TdT
terminal deoxynucleotide transferase
terminal deoxynucleotidyltransferase

TDU
time domain ultrasound

TDW
target dry weight

TDWB
touchdown weightbearing

TDYV
  Tamdy virus
TDZ
  thymus-dependent zone (of lymph node)
TE
  echo time
  tennis elbow
  terminal extension
  test ear
  tetanic contraction [electrodiagnosis]
  tetanus (*See also* TET, tet)
  threshold energy
  thromboembolic event
  thromboembolism
  thymus epithelium
  thyrotoxic exophthalmos
  tick-borne encephalitis
  time [delay] between excitation and
    echo [maximum]
  time estimation
  tissue engineering
  tissue equivalent
  tonsillectomy
  tooth extracted
  total estrogen (excretion)
  Toxoplasma encephalitis
  trace element
  tracheoesophageal
  transepithelial elimination
  transesophgeal echocardiography
  transrectal electroejaculation
  treadmill exercise
  trial [and] error (*See also* T&E)
  trichoepithelioma
T&E
  testing and evaluation
  training and experience
  trial and error (*See also* TE)
T:E
  testosterone to epitestosterone ratio
T$_E$
  expiratory time
TE$_{mic}$
  tonsillectomy with operating microscope
Te
  tellurium
te
  effective half-life [radioactivity]
    (*See also* teff)
TEA
  temporal external artery
  Test of Everyday Attention
  tetraethylammonium
  thermal energy analyzer
  thromboendarterectomy
  total elbow arthroplasty
  total endarterectomy

  transient emboligenic aortoarteritis
  transluminal extraction atherectomy
  transversely excited atmospheric
    [pressure]
  triethanolamine
TEAB
  tetraethylammonium bromide
TEAC
  tetraethylammonium chloride
TEACCH
  treatment and education of autistic and
    related communications handicapped
    children
TEA-Ch
  Test of Everyday Attention for Children
TEAE
  treatment-emergent adverse event
  triethylaminoethyl
TEAP
  transesophageal atrial pacing (*See also*
    TAP)
TEAS
  transcutaneous electrical acustimulation
teasp
  teaspoon(ful) (*See also* t, ts, tsp)
TEB
  thoracic electrical bioimpedance
  transcutaneous endomyocardial biopsy
  tris-ethylenediaminetetraacetate borate
TEBG
  testosterone-estradiol-binding globulin
TeBG
  testosterone binding globulin
TEBP
  thyroid-specific enhancer-binding protein
T4/ebp-1
  thyroid-specific enhancer binding protein
    1
TEBS
  transurethral electrical bladder
    stimulation
TEBV
  tissue-engineered blood vessel
TEC
  thromboembolic complication
  tissue-engineered construct
  Total Environment Control [system]
  total eosinophil count
  total exchange capacity
  toxic *Escherichia coli*
  transient erythroblastopenia of childhood
  transluminal endarterectomy catheter
  transluminal extraction catheter
  transluminal extraction-endarterectomy
    catheter
  transpapillary endoscopic cholecystotomy
  triethyl citrate

T&EC
trauma and emergency center
TECA
titrated extract of *Centella asiatica*
TECAB
totally endoscopic coronary artery
bypass
tech
technical
technique
TECS
transcranial electrical stimulation
TECV
traumatic epiphyseal coxa vara
TED
Tasks of Emotional Development
threshold erythema dose
thromboembolic disease [hose,
stockings]
thyroid eye disease
tracheoesophageal dysraphism
tris-ethylenediaminetetraacetate
dithiothreitol
TEDD
total end-diastolic diameter
TEDE
total effective dose equivalent
TEDP
tetraethyl dithionopyrophosphate
TEDS
thromboembolic disease stockings
transesophageal echo-Doppler
system
treatment episode data set
TEE
thermal (thermic) effect of exercise
total energy expended (expenditure)
transesophageal echocardiograph(y)
(echocardiogram)
transnasal endoscopic ethmoidectomy
tyrosine ethyl ester
TEE-DSE
transesophageal
echocardiography-dobutamine stress
echocardiography
TEEM
tanned erythrocyte electrophoretic
mobility
Test for Examining Expressive
Morphology
TEEP
tetraethylpyrophosphate
transesophageal echocardiography with
pacing
TEF
thermal (thermic) effect of food
(feeding)
thoracoepigastric flap
thyrotroph embryonic factor

tracheoesophageal fistula
trunk extension-flexion [unit]
TEF_{25}
tidal expiratory flow at 25% of tidal
volume
TEF_{50}
tidal expiratory flow at 50% of tidal
volume
TEF_{75}
tidal expiratory flow at 75% of tidal
volume
teff
effective half-life [radioactivity]
$TEF_{25}/PTEF$
ratio of tidal expiratory flow at 25% of
tidal volume and peak tidal expiratory
flow
TEFS
transmural electrical field stimulation
TEF_{50}/TIF_{50}
ratio of tidal expiratory and inspiratory
flow at 50% of tidal volume
TEG
thromboelastograph(y)
(thromboelastogram) [hemostasis
analyzer]
TEGDMA
tetraethylene glycol dimethacrylate
TEHV
Tehran virus
TEI
therapeutic equivalence interchange
total episode of illness
transesophageal imaging
TEK
total exchangeable kalium
[potassium]
TEL
telemetry (*See also* tele)
telephone
Test of Economic Literacy
tetraethyl lead
T1EL
type 1 endoleak
T2EL
type 2 endoleak
TELD
Test of Early Language Development
TELD-2
Test of Early Language Development,
Second Edition
tele
telemetry (*See also* TEL)
$t^{1}\!/_{2}$elim
elimination half-life
TEM
terminal extensor mechanism
therapeutic electromembrane
transanal endoscopic microsurgery

transmission electron microscope
(microscopy)
transtelephonic exercise monitor
transverse electromagnetic
transverse electromagnetic mode
triethylenemelamine
TEMAC
tetramethyl ammonium chloride
TEMAS
Tell-Me-A-Story
TEMI
transient episodes of myocardial
ischemia
temp
temperature (*See also* T)
temple
temporal (*See also* T)
temporary (*See also* T)
TEMT
tubular epithelial-myofibroblast
transdifferentiation
TEN
tension (*See also* T)
titanium elastic nailing
total enteral nutrition
total epidermal necrolysis
total excretory nitrogen
toxic epidermal necrolysis
(necrosis)
transepidermal neurostimulation
TENa
total exchangeable sodium
tenac
tenaculum
TENS
transcutaneous electrical neuromuscular
(nerve) stimulator (stimulation)
TENV
Tensaw virus
TENVAD
Test of Nonverbal Auditory
Discrimination
TEOAE
transient evoked otoacoustic emission
TEP
thromboendophlebectomy
total endoprosthesis
total extraperitoneal [laparoscopic hernia
repair]
totally extraperitoneal
tracheoesophageal prosthesis
tracheoesophageal puncture
transesophageal puncture
trigeminal evoked potential
tubal ectopic pregnancy
TeP
tender point (*See also* TP)

TEPA
thermic effect of physical activity
triethylenephosphoramide
triethylenethiophosphoramide
TEPG
triethylphosphine gold
TEPH
thromboembolic pulmonary hypertension
total endoprosthetic hip
TEPP
tetraethylpyrophosphate
tetraethyl pyrophosphate
TEQ
toxic equivalents
TEQU
test equivocal
TER
therapeutic external radiation
thermal enhancement ratio
total elbow replacement
total endoplasmic reticulum
total energy requirement
transcapillary escape rate
transitional endoplasmic reticulum
transurethral electroresection
ter
terminase
ternary [three compounds]
tertiary (*See also* T, tert)
threefold
three [times] (*See also* t.)
TERC
Test of Early Reading Comprehension
TERIS
Teratogen Information System
TERM
temporary endodontic restorative
material
term.
terminate
full term [infant]
terminal (*See also* t, TRML, trml)
TERT
telomerase reverse transcriptase
total end-range time
tert
tertiary (*See also* T, ter)
TERV
Termeil virus
TES
Teacher Evaluation Scale
Team Effectiveness Survey
tetradecyl sulfate, ethanol, saline
therapeutic electrical stimulation
therapeutic error signal
thoracic endometriosis syndrome
thoracic endoscopic sympathectomy

TES *(continued)*
thymic epithelial supernatant
toxic epidemic syndrome
transcutaneous electric stimulation
transmural electric stimulation
treatment of emergent symptom
tridimensional evaluation scale
TESA
testicular sperm aspiration
TESD
total end-systolic diameter
TESE
testicular sperm extraction
TESI
thoracic epidural steroid injection
TESS
Toronto Extremity Salvage Score
Toxic Exposure Surveillance System
Treatment Emergent Symptoms Scale
TEST
tubal embryo stage transfer
testos
testosterone
TET
tetanus (*See also* TE, tet)
tetralogy (of Fallot) (*See also* TF, TOF)
thymic epithelial tumor
total exchangeable thyroxine
transcranial electrostimulation therapy
treadmill exercise test
triethyltryptamine
tubal embryo transfer
tet
tetanus (*See also* TE, TET)
TETA
test-estrin timed action
triethylenetetramine
TETE
too early to evaluate
TETEV
Tete virus
TETIg
tetanus immune globulin
TETRAC
tetraiodothyroacetic acid
tE:tTOT
expiration time to total time ratio
[breathing cycle]
tet tox
tetanus toxoid (*See also* TT)
TEU
token economy unit
TEV
talipes equinovarus
TEVAP
transurethral electrovaporization of
prostate
TEVG
tissue engineered vascular graft

TEVP
transesophageal ventricular pacing
TEWL
transepidermal water loss (*See also*
TWL)
TEZ
transthoracic electric impedance
respirogram
TF
to follow
tactile fremitus
tail flick [reflex]
temperature factor
testicular feminization
tetralogy of Fallot (*See also* TET,
TOF)
Thomsen-Friedenreich [antigen]
thymol flocculation
thymus (tolerance) factor
thymus (transfer) factor
tibiofemoral
tissue-damaging factor (*See also* TDF)
tissue factor
total flow
transfer factor
transformation frequency
transfrontal
transvestic fetishism
tube feeding
tuberculin filtrate
tubular fluid
tuning fork
typhoid fever
TF5
thymosin fraction 5
T$_f$
temperature, freezing
Tf
transferrin (*See also* TFN)
TFA
thigh-foot angle
tibiofemoral angle
topical fluoride application
total fatty acids
trans fatty acids
transverse fascicular area
trifluoroacetic acid
TFAA
trifluoroacetic anhydride
TFAV
Thiafora virus
TFB
trifascicular block
TFB-PS
tibial fracture brace proximal support
TFC
thoracic fluid content
threaded fusion cage
time to following commands

total food consumption
triangular fibrocartilage
TFCC
transjugular fibrocartilage complex
triangular fibrocartilage
(fibrocartilaginous) complex
TFCI
transient focal cerebral ischemia
TFCQ
Toronto Functional Capacity
Questionnaire
TFD
target film distance
thin film dressing
transdermal fentanyl device
TFd
transfer factor, dialyzable
TFEV
timed forced expiratory volume
TFF
tangential flow filtration
trefoil family factor [peptide]
tube-fed food
TFF1
trefoil family factor peptide 1
Tf–Fe
transferrin-bound iron
TFI
transient forebrain ischemia
treatment-free interval
tubular-fertility index
tumor of follicular infundibulum
TFJ
tibiofemoral joint
TFL
tensor fasciae latae
transnasal fiberoptic laryngoplasty
trunk-forward lean
tumefactive fibroinflammatory
lesion
TFM
testicular feminization mutation
total fat mass
total fluid movement
transverse friction massage
trifluoromethylnitrophenol
Tfm
testicular feminization (syndrome)
(*See also* TFS)
TFN
total fecal nitrogen
totally functional neutrophil
transferrin (*See also* Tf)
TFNE
transient focal neurologic event
TFO
triplex-forming oligonucleotide

TFP
temporalis fascia proper
treponemal false positive
trifunctional protein deficiency
tubular fluid plasma
TF:P
tubular fluid to plasma ratio
TFPI
tissue factor pathway inhibitor
TF:PI$_r$
tubular fluid to plasma insulin ratio
TFR
total fertility rate
total flow resistance
TfR
transferrin receptor
TFRT
Tactile Form (Finger) Recognition Test
TFS
testicular feminization syndrome
(*See also* Tfm)
thyroid function study
tube-fed saline
T1FS
T1-weighted fat-suppressed [image]
TFT
thin-film transistor
Thought Field Therapy
thrombus formation time
thumb-finding test
thyroid function test
tight filum terminale
transfer factor test
trifluorothymidine
TF:UF
tubular fluid to ultrafiltrate ratio
TFV
target vessel failure
Telok Forest virus
TFVL
tidal flow-volume loop
TG
tendon graft
testosterone glucuronide
tetraglycine
thioglucose
thioglycolate [broth] (*See also* THIO)
thyroglobulin (*See also* Tg, Tgb, thg)
total gastrectomy
total gym
toxic goiter
Toxoplasma gondii
transglutaminase (*See also* TGase)
transmissible gastroenteritis (*See also*
TGE)
treated group
triacylglycerol (*See also* TAG)

TG *(continued)*
    trigeminal [neuralgia] (*See also* TGNg, TN)
    triglyceride (*See also* TGL, TRIG, trig)
    tumor growth
    type genus

6-TG
    6-thioguanine

T$_g$
    expiratory phase time
    glass transition temperature

Tg
    generation time (*See also* GT)
    thyroglobulin (*See also* TG, Tgb, thg)

tG$_2$
    time required to complete G$_2$ phase of cell cycle

tG$_1$
    time required to complete G$_1$ phase of cell cycle

TGA
    taurocholate gelatin agar
    third-generation antidepressant
    thyroglobulin antibody (*See also* TgAb)
    total glycoalkaloids
    transient global amnesia
    transposition of the great arteries
    tumor glycoprotein assay

TgAb
    thyroglobulin antibody (*See also* TGA)

TGAR
    total graft area rejected

TGase
    transglutaminase (*See also* TG)

TGB
    thyroid-binding globulin

Tgb
    thyroglobulin (*See also* TG, Tg, thg)

TGBI
    thyroid growth-blocking immunoglobulin

TGC
    tailgut cyst
    time-gain compensation (compensator)
    time-gain control
    time-varied gain control (*See also* TVGC)

TGCC
    testicular germ cell carcinoma

TGCE
    temperature gradient capillary electrophoresis

TGCT
    testicular germ cell tumor(s)

TGD
    thermal green dye
    thyroglossal duct
    tumor growth delay

TGDC
    thyroglossal duct cyst

TGE
    theoretical growth evaluation
    transgastrostomic enteroscopy
    transmissible gastroenteritis [virus] (*See also* TG)
    tryptone glucose extract

TGEF
    transabdominal thin-gauge embryofetoscopy

TG ELISA
    tissue transglutaminase ELISA

TGF
    T-cell growth factor
    therapeutic gain factor
    transforming growth factor
    trypanosome growth factor
    tubuloglomerular feedback
    tumor growth factor

TGF1
    transforming growth factor 1

TGFA
    triglyceride fatty acid

TGF-alpha, TGF-α
    transforming growth factor-alpha (α)

TGF-B, TGF-β
    transforming growth factor beta (β)

TGF-B1, TGF-β1
    transforming growth factor beta1 (β1)

TGF-B2, TGF-β2
    transforming growth factor beta2 (β2)

TGF-B3, TGF-β3
    transforming growth factor beta3 (β3)

T1GFR
    type 1 growth factor receptor

TGG
    turkey gamma globulin

TGGE
    temperature-gradient gel electrophoresis

TGI
    thyroid growth immunoglobulin
    tracheal gas insufflation
    tumor gene index

TGL
    triglyceride (*See also* TG, TRIG, trig)
    triglyceride level

TGN
    trans-Golgi network
    trigeminal neuralgia (*See also* TG, TN)

TGOR
    transverse groove of oblique ridge

TGP
    tobacco glycoprotein

TGR
    tenderness, guarding, rigidity [abdominal exam]

T group, T-group
    training group

TGS
tincture of green soap
triglycine sulfate
TGT
thromboplastin generation test
thromboplastin generation time
tolbutamide-glucagon test
transdermal glyceryl trinitrate
TGTL
total glottic transverse laryngectomy
TGV
thoracic gas volume
transposition of the great vessels
(*See also* TOGV)
trapped gas volume
TGXT
thallium-graded exercise test
TGY, TGYA
tryptone glucose yeast (agar)
TH
Tamm-Horsfall [protein] (*See also* TNP)
tentorial herniation
T helper [cell]
thermite [reaction]
thrill
thyrohyoid
thyroid hormone
thyrotropic hormone (*See also* TTH)
topical hypothermia
torcular herophili [archaic]
total hydroperoxide
total hysterectomy
triple heater channel [acupuncture]
tube holder
tyrosine hydroxylase
T&H
type and hold
Th
thenar
thoracic (*See also* T, thor)
thorax (*See also* T, thor)
thorium
throat
thyroid (*See also* T, thr)
TH1–TH3
T-helper [cell] 1–3
THA
tetrahydroacridine
tetrahydroaminoacridine
total hip arthroplasty
total hydroxyapatite
transient hemispheric attack
Treponema hemagglutination
ThA
thoracic aorta
THAA
thyroid hormone autoantibodies
tubular hypoplasia of aortic arch

THABEST
Third Heir Avidin Biotin Enzyme
System Test
THAD
transient hepatic attenuation difference
THAL, Thal
thalassemia
THAM
Tris(hydroxymethyl)-aminomethane
(*See also* TRIS)
THAN
transient hyperammonemia of newborn
THARIES
total hip articular replacement by
internal eccentric shells
THAT
Toronto Hospital Alertness Test
THb
total hemoglobin
THBG
thyroid hormone binding globulin
THBI
thyroid hormone binding index
THBO$_2$
total hyperbaric oxygen
THbO$_2$
total oxyhemoglobin
THBR
thyroid hormone-binding ratio
THC
tetrahydrocannabinol (*See also*
Δ-9-THC)
tetrahydrocortisol
tetrahydrocortisone
thigh circumference
thiocarbanidin
transhepatic cholangiograph(y)
(cholangiogram) (*See also* TC)
transplantable hepatocellular carcinoma
Δ-9-THC
delta-9-tetrahydrocannabinol (*See also*
THC)
THCA
trihydroxycoprostanoic acid
THCCRC
tetrahydrocannabinol cross-reacting
cannabinoids
THCT
triple-phase helical computer
tomography
TH-CULT
throat culture (*See also* TC)
tHcy
total homocysteine (level)
THC: YAG
thulium-holmium-chromium: YAG [laser]
THD
transverse heart diameter

Thd
ribothymidine (*See also* T)
THDA
tuberohypophysial dopaminergic neuron
THE
tetrahydrocortisone E
tonic hind (limb) extension
total head excursion
transhepatic embolization
transhiatal esophagectomy
tropical hypereosinophilia
theor
theoretical
theory
ther
therapeutic (*See also* therap)
therapy (*See also* therap, TX, T_x, tx)
thermometer (*See also* therm)
therap
therapeutic (*See also* ther)
therapy (*See also* ther, TX, T_x, tx)
ther ex
therapeutic exercise
therm
thermal
thermometer (*See also* ther)
Θ, theta
thermodynamic temperature
theta [eighth letter of Greek alphabet uppercase]
θ, theta
angular coordinate variable
customary temperature
latent trait [statistics]
temperature interval
theta [eighth letter of Greek alphabet lowercase]
THF
humoral thymic factor
tetrahydrocortisone F
tetrahydrofluorenone
tetrahydrofolate
tetrahydrofuran
thymic humoral factor
THFA
tetrahydrofolic acid
tetrahydrofurfuryl alcohol
THg
total mercury
thg
thyroglobulin (*See also* TG, Tg, Tgb)
THH
targetoid hemosiderotic hemangioma
telangiectasia hereditaria haemorrhagica
THI
Texas Heart Institute
therapeutic husband-insemination
tissue harmonic imaging
transient hypogammaglobulinemia of infancy
trihydroxyindole
THIO
thioglycolate (*See also* TG)
thio-T, thio-TEPA
thiotriethylene phosphoramide
THIP
tetrahydroisoxazolopyridinol
THIQ
tetrahydraisoquinolone (*See also* TIQ)
THIV
Thimiri virus
THKAFO
trunk-hip-knee-ankle-foot orthosis
THL
transvaginal hydrolaparoscopy
true histiocytic lymphoma
THLAA
tubular hypoplasia of left aortic arch
THM
Tamm-Horsfall mucoprotein
total heme mass
TH_2O
titrated water
THOR
thoracentesis [fluid]
thor
thoracic (*See also* T, Th)
thorax (*See also* T, Th, TX)
THORP
titanium hollow-screw osseointegrating reconstruction plate
thou.
thousand (*See also* K)
THOV
Thogoto virus
THOX
thyroid oxidase
THP
take home pack
Tamm-Horsfall protein (*See also* TH)
tetrahydropapaveroline
tissue hydrostatic pressure
total hip precautions
total hip prosthesis
total hydroxyproline
transhepatic portography
trihexyphenidyl
THPA
tetrahydropteric acid
THPC
tetrabis (hydroxymethyl) phosphonium chloride
tHPT
tertiary hyperparathyroidism
THPV
transhepatic portal vein

THQ
  tetroquinone
THR
  target heart rate
  thrombin receptor
  thyroid hormone receptor
  total hip replacement
  training heart rate
  transhepatic resistance
Thr
  threonine (*See also* T)
thr
  thyroid (*See also* T, Th)
  thyroidectomy
THR-CT
  thrombin control
THRF
  thyrotropic hormone-releasing factor
ThRIA
  thyroid radioisotope assay
THRL
  total hip replacement, left
throm, thromb
  thrombosis
  thrombus (*See also* T)
THRR
  total hip replacement, right
  transient hyperemic response ratio
THS
  tetrahydro-compound S
  tetrahydrodeoxycortisol
THSC
  totipotent hematopoietic stem cell
THSP
  titanium hollow screw plate [system]
THTV
  therapeutic home trial visit
THU
  tetrahydrouridine
THUG
  thyroid uptake gradient
THV
  therapeutic home visit
THVO
  terminal hepatic vein obliteration
Thx
  thromboxane (*See also* TBX)
Thy
  thymine (*See also* T)
thy.
  thymectomy
  thymus (*See also* T)
THz
  terahertz
TI
  inversion time
  temporal integration

terminal ileum
thalassemia intermedia
therapeutic index
thoracic index
thought insertion
threshold of intelligibility
thymic irradiation
thymus independent
thyroxine iodine
time information
time interval
tonic immobility
total iron
transischial
translational inhibition
transverse [diameter between] ischia
transverse [diameter of obstetric] inlet
tricuspid incompetence (insufficiency)
trunk index
tubulointerstitial
tumor inducing
tumor induction
T$_I$
  duration of inspiration
  inspiratory time
Ti
  titanium
TIA
  T-cell-restricted intracellular antigen
  Test Anxiety Inventory
  transient ischemic attack
  tumor-induced angiogenesis
TIAH
  total implantation of artificial heart
TIA-IR
  transient ischemic attack, incomplete
    recovery
TIAP
  totally implantable access port
TIB
  This I Believe [test]
  tumor immunology bank
Tib, tib
  tibia
TIBC
  total iron-binding capacity
tib-fib
  tibia and fibula
TIBV
  Tibrogargan virus
TIC
  time intensity curve
  Toxicology Information Center
  trypsin-inhibitory capability (capacity)
  tumor-inducing complex
tic
  diverticulum [singular]

T

TICA
terminal internal carotid artery
traumatic intracranial aneurysm
TICCC
time interval between cessation of
contraception and conception
TICH
thrombolysis-related intracranial
hemorrhage
TI-CMV
tissue-invasive cytomegalovirus
TICS
diverticulosis
diverticular [plural]
TID
three times daily
three times a day [L. *ter in die*]
time interval difference
titrated initial dose
transient ischemic dilatation (dilation)
tubal inflammatory damage
t.i.d.
three times daily
three times a day [L. *ter in die*]
TIDA
tuberoinfundibular dopaminergic [neuron,
system] (*See also* TD)
TIDM
three times daily with meals
TIE
transient ischemic episode (event)
TIES
The Instructional Environment Scale
TIF
testicular interstitial fluid
tracheal intubation fiberscope
tropic immersion foot
tumor-inducing factor
tumor-inhibiting factor
TIF2
transcriptional intermediary factor 2
TIF$_{50}$
tidal inspiratory flow at 50% of tidal
volume
TIFB
thrombin-increasing fibrinopeptide B
TIg
tetanus immune globulin
(immunoglobulin)
TIGR
trabecular meshwork-inducible
glucocorticoid response
TIH
time interval histogram
tumor-inducing hypercalcemia
TII
terminal ileum intubation
TIL
tumor-infiltrating lymphocyte

TILV
Tilligerry virus
TIM
tissue-infiltrating macrophage
topical immunomodulator
transthoracic intracardiac monitoring
triose isomerase
TIMC
tumor-induced marrow cytotoxicity
TIME
Toddler and Infant Motor Evaluation
TiMesh
titanium mesh
TIMP
Test of Infant Motor Performance
tissue inhibitor of metalloproteinase
TIMP-1–TIMP-3
tissue inhibitor of metalloproteinase 1–3
TIMV
Timbo virus
TIN
testicular intraepithelial neoplasia
three (times) in night [L. *ter in nocte*]
Tone in Noise [test]
tubulointerstitial nephritis (nephropathy)
tinc, tinct
tincture (*See also* T, TCT, TR, Tr)
TIND
Treatment Investigational New Drug
[FDA]
TINEM
there is no evidence of malignancy
TINU
tubulointerstitial nephritis and uveitis
[syndrome]
TINV
Tinaroo virus
TIP
terbutaline infusion pump
terminal interphalangeal
thermal inactivation point
time to pregnancy
toxic interstitial pneumonitis
Toxicology Information Program
translation-inhibiting protein
tubularized incised plate [urethroplasty]
tumor-inhibiting principle
TIPJ
terminal interphalangeal joint
TIPP
The Injury Prevention Program
TIPPB
transperineal interstitial permanent
prostate brachytherapy
TIPPS
tetraiodophenolphthalein sodium
TIPS
transjugular intrahepatic portosystemic
shunt

transvenous intrahepatic portosystemic
shunt
TIPSS
transjugular intrahepatic portosystemic
stent shunt
TIQ
tetrahydroisoquinoline (*See also* THIQ)
TIR
terminal innervation ratio
toll-interleukin 1 receptor
total immunoreactive
trophoblast in regression
TIRAP
toll-interleukin 1 receptor
domain-containing adapter protein
TIRES
transient infrared emission spectroscopy
TIRFM
total internal reflection microscopy
TIRI
total immunoreactive insulin
TIRP
transcatheter intravascular ring platform
TIS
telemedicine information system
tetracycline-induced stenosis
titanium interbody spacer
trabecular insular solid
transdermal infusion system
trypsin-insoluble segment
tumor, immune, systemic
Tis
tumor in situ [TNM classification]
TISP
total immunoreactive serum pepsinogen
TISS
Therapeutic Intervention Scoring System
TIT
Treponema [*pallidum*] immobilization
test (*See also* TPI)
triiodothyronine (*See also* T_3, TITh,
TRIT)
triple intrathecal therapy
TITh
triiodothyronine (*See also* T_3, TIT,
TRIT)
3,5,3'-triiodothyronine (*See also* T_3)
titr
titrate
T_I:T_{TOT}
inspiratory time to total cycle time ratio
tI:tTOT
inspiration time and total time of
breathing cycle ratio
TIU
trypsin-inhibiting unit
TIUP
term intrauterine pregnancy

TIUV
total intrauterine volume
TIV
total intracranial volume
TIVA
total intravenous anesthesia
TIVC
thoracic inferior vena cava
⚠ **TIW, tiw, tiwk**
three times a week ⚠
three times weekly ⚠
TJ
tendon jerk
tetrajoule
tight junction
triceps jerk
TJA
total joint arthroplasty
TJC
tender joint count
TJLB
transjugular liver biopsy
TJN
tongue, jaw, neck [dissection]
twin jet nebulizer
TJP
tracheojejunal puncture
TJR
total joint replacement
T-JTA
Taylor-Johnson Temperament Analysis
TK
through the knee
thymidine kinase
tourniquet (*See also* TQ)
toxicokinetics
transketolase
triose-kinase
TKA
total knee arthroplasty (arthroscopy)
transketolase activity
trochanter-knee-ankle [line]
tyrosine kinase activity
TKC
torticollis-keloids-cryptorchidism
[syndrome]
TKCR
torticollis, keloids, cryptorchidism, renal
dysplasia [syndrome]
TKD
thymidine kinase deficiency
tokodynamometer (*See also* TOCO)
TKE
terminal knee extension
TKG
tocodynagraph (tokodynagraph)
TKIC
true knot in cord

T

TKLI
tachykinin-like immunoreactivity
TKM
thymidine kinase, mitochondrial
TKNO
to keep needle open
TKO
to keep open [vein for I.V.]
TKP
temporary keratoprosthesis
thermal keratoplasty
thermokeratoplasty
total knee prosthesis
TKR
total knee (a)rthroscopy
total knee replacement
TKRL
total knee replacement, left
TKRR
total knee replacement, right
TKS
thermokinetic selectivity
thymidine kinase, soluble
TKVO
to keep vein open
TL
taper-lock
temporal lobe
terminal limen [end point]
thermolabile
thermoluminescence
thoracolumbar
Thorndike-Lorge written frequency
threat to life
thymic lymphocyte antigen
thymus(-dependent) lymphocyte
thymus leukemia [antigen]
thymus lymphoma
time lapse
time limited
tolerance level
total laryngectomy
total lipids
total lung [capacity]
transverse line
trial leave
true lumen
tubal ligation
T/L
terminal latency [electromyography]
Tl
thallium
201Tl
thallium-201
TLA
thigh-leg angle
tissue lactase activity
total laboratory automation
translaryngeal aspiration

translumbar aortograph(y) (aortogram)
transluminal angioplasty
transperitoneal laparoscopic
adrenalectomy
trypsinlike amidase
TLAA
T-lymphocyte-associated antigen
TLAC
Test of Learning (Listening) Accuracy
in Children
triple lumen Arrow catheter
Tlam
thoracic laminectomy
TLB
transjugular liver biopsy
TL BLT
tubal ligation, bilateral
TLC
telephone-linked care
tender loving care
Test of Language Competence
therapeutic lifestyle change
thin-layer chromatography
titanium linear cutter
T-lymphocyte choriocarcinoma
total L-chain concentration
total lung capacity
total lung compliance
total lymphocyte count
transitional living center
transverse loop colostomy
triple-lumen catheter
TLC-C
Test of Language Competence for
Children
201TlCl
thallium-201 chloride
TLCO
carbon monoxide transfer factor of the
lungs
TLD
thermoluminescence detector
thermoluminescent dosimeter [rod]
thoracic lymphatic duct
transluminescent dosimeter
tumor lethal dose
T/LD$_{100}$
minimal (minimum) tumor dose causing
100% death or malformation
TLE
temporal lobe epilepsy
thin-layer electrophoresis
total life expectancy
total lipid extract
TLESR
transient lower esophageal
relaxation
TLFB
timeline follow-back [interview]

TLH
  total laparoscopic hysterectomy
TLI
  thymidine labeling index
  tonic labyrinthine inverted
  total lymphatic (lymphoid)
    irradiation
  Totman Loss Index
  translaryngeal intubation
  tritiated thymidine labeling index
  trypsin-like immunoactivity
  Tucker-Lewis index [statistics]
TLIF
  thoracolumbar interbody fusion
  thoracolumbar intervertebral fusion
  translumbar interbody fusion
TLK
  thermal laser keratoplasty
TLM
  torn lateral meniscus
TlmA
  translumbar arteriogram
TLN
  transperitoneal laparoscopic
    nephrectomy
TLNB
  term living newborn
TLND
  therapeutic lymph node dissection
TLNV
  Tlacotalpan virus
TLP
  time-limited psychotherapy
  total laryngopharyngectomy
  transitional living program
  tumor-liberated particle
TLQ
  total living quotient
TLR
  target lesion reintervention
    (revascularization)
  toll-like receptor
  tonic labyrinthine reflex
TLR4
  toll-like receptor 4 [gene]
TLS
  thoracolumbosacral
  thoracolumbosacral strain
  tight lens syndrome
  tumor lysis syndrome
TLSO
  thoracolumbar spinal orthosis
  thoracolumbosacral orthosis
TLSO-FELR
  thoracolumbosacral orthosis—flexion,
    extension, lateral [bending], and
    [transverse] rotation

TLSSO
  thoracolumbosacral spinal orthosis
TLT
  tonsillectomy
  tryptophan load test
TLV
  threshold limit value
  tidal liquid ventilation
  total liquid ventilation
  total lung volume
TLW
  total lung water
TLX
  trophoblast-lymphocyte cross-reactive
    (reactivity)
TM
  tectorial membrane
  telangiectatic matting
  temperature by mouth
  temporalis muscle
  temporomandibular [joint]
  teres major [muscle]
  term milk
  thalassemia major
  Thayer-Martin [medium]
  thrombomodulin
  Tibetan medicine
  time and modifying
  time motion
  trabecular meshwork
  trademark
  Transcendental Meditation
  transitional mucosa
  transmediastinal
  transmetatarsal
  transport maximum
  transport mechanism
  transport medium
  transverse myelitis
  treadmill
  trimester (*See also* TRI)
  tropical medicine
  tuberculosis meningitis
  tubular myelin
  tumor
  tympanic membrane (*See also* MT)
  tympanometric
T&M
  type and crossmatch (*See also* TC,
    T&C, T&CM, T&X, T&M, TXM)
Tm, T$_m$
  melting temperature
  temperature, muscle
  thulium
  tubular maximal (maximum) [excretory
    capacity of kidneys]
  tumor-bearing mice

T

tM
time required to complete M phase of cell cycle

t$_m$, t_m
temperature midpoint

TMA
tetramethylammonium
thrombotic microangiopathy
thyroid microsomal antibody (*See also* TMAb)
tissue microarray
transcortical mixed aphasia
transcription-mediated amplification
transmalleolar axis
transmetatarsal amputation
trimethoxyamphetamine
trimethoxyphenyl aminopropane
trimethylamine [hallucinogen]
trimethylxanthine [caffeine]
true metatarsus adductus

TMA-2
2,4,5-trimethoxyamphetamine [designer drug]

T/MA
tracheostomy mask [anesthesia]

TMAb
thyroid microsomal antibody (*See also* TMA)

TMAF
temporary master apical file

TMAH
trimethylphenylammonium (anilinium) hydroxide

TMAI
trimethylphenylammonium (anilinium) iodide

TMAO
trimethylamine oxide

TMAS
Taylor Manifest Anxiety Scale

TMA-uria
trimethylaminuria

T-MAX, T-max, T$_{max}$
maximum temperature
time of maximal (concentration)

TMB
tetramethyl benzidine (tetramethylbenzidine)
total (transient) monocular blindness
trimethoxybenzoate
tris-maleate buffer

TMBA
trimethoxybenzaldehyde
trimethylbenzanthracene

TMC
transmural colitis
Transtheoretical Model of Change [psychology]
trapeziometacarpal [joint]

TMCA
trimethylcolchicinic acid

TMD
temporomandibular dysfunction (disorder)
transmural drainage
treating physician

T-MDS, TMDS, t-MDS
therapy-related myelodysplasia
therapy-related myelodysplastic syndrome

TME
thermolysin-like metalloendopeptidase
total mesorectal excision
total metabolizable energy
transmissible mink encephalopathy
transmural enteritis
trapezium-metacarpal eburnation

TMEP
telangiectasia macularis eruptiva perstans

TMET
treadmill exercise test

TMEV
Tembe virus
Theiler murine encephalomyelitis virus

TMF
transformed mink fibroblast
transmitral flow

TMG
toxic multinodular goiter (*See also* TMNG)

TmG, TM$_G$
maximal tubular reabsorption rate for glucose

TMH
tetramethylammonium hydroxide
trainable mentally handicapped

TMI
threatened myocardial infarct(ion)
transmandibular implant
transmural infarct(ion)

⚠ T>MIC
time above minimum inhibitory concentration ⚠

TMIF
tumor cell migration-inhibition factor

TMIS
Technicon Medical Information System

TMJ
temporomandibular joint

TMJD
temporomandibular joint dysfunction

TMJ-OA
temporomandibular joint osteoarthritis

TMJ-PDS
temporomandibular joint pain-dysfunction syndrome (*See also* TMPDS)

TMJS
temporomandibular joint syndrome
TMJ-SF
temporomandibular joint synovial fluid
TML
terminal motor latency
tetramethyl lead
tongue midline
treadmill
TMLR
transmyocardial laser revascularization
TMM
tissue mimicking material
torn medial meniscus
total muscle mass
Tmm
McKay-Marg tension
TMNG
toxic multinodular goiter (*See also* TMG)
TMNST
tethered median nerve stress test
TMO
transcaruncular medial orbitotomy
[frontoethmoid mucocele surgery]
TMP
ribothymidylic acid (*See also* rTMP)
taste-modifying protein
thallium myocardial perfusion
thymidine monophosphate
thymolphthalein
transmembrane [hydrostatic] pressure
transmembrane potential
trimandibular plate
trimethyl psoralen
TMPD
temporomandibular pain dysfunction
tetramethyl-para-phenylenediamine
transmucosal potential difference
TMPDS
temporomandibular [joint] pain
dysfunction syndrome (*See also*
TMJ-PDS)
TMPRSS3
transmembrane protease serine 3
[gene]
TMR
temporomesial region
tetramethylrhodamine
tissue-maximum ratio
topical magnetic resonance
trainable mentally retarded
transmyocardial revascularization
TMRE
tetra-methylrhodamine ethyl ester
TmrHisto
tumor histology

TMRI
tetramethylrhodamine isothiocyanate
tetramethylrhodamine isothionate
TMS
telematic monitoring service
[telemedicine]
tetramethylsilane
thallium myocardial scintigraphy
thread mate system
total morbidity score
transcranial magnetic stimulation
trapezoidocephaly-multiple synostosis
[syndrome]
trimethylsilane
trimethylsilyl (*See also* TMSi)
trimodal spectroscopy
TMS-1
Topographic Modeling System 1
TMSI
trimethylsilylimidazole
TMSi
trimethylsilyl (*See also* TMS)
TMST
Task Management Strategy Index
treadmill stress test (*See also* TST)
TMT
tarsometatarsal
temporalis muscle temperature
teratoma with malignant transformation
Trail-Making Test [psychiatry]
treadmill test (*See also* TT)
tympanic membrane thermometer
TMTC
too many to count
TMU
tetramethylurea
TMUGS
Tumor Marker Utility Grading Scale
TMUV
Tembusu virus
TMV
tobacco mosaic virus
tracheal mucous velocity
TMZ
transformation zone (*See also* T)
TN
[intraocular] tension, normal (*See also*
Tn)
talonavicular [joint]
tarsonavicular [joint]
temperature normal
tension
tension, normal
total negatives
tree nut [allergy]
trigeminal neuralgia
trigeminal nucleus

T

TN *(continued)*
trochlear nucleus
true negative

T₄N
normal serum thyroxine

T&N
tar and nicotine
tension and nervousness
tingling and numbness

Tn
[intraocular] tension, normal (*See also* TN)
thoron
transposon
troponin

TNA
total nutrient admixture

TNAB
transthoracic needle aspiration biopsy

TNAP
tissue-nonspecific alkaline phosphatase

TNB
term newborn
transnasal butorphanol
transrectal needle biopsy [of prostate] (*See also* TNBP)
transthoracic needle biopsy
Tru-Cut needle biopsy

TNBP
transurethral needle biopsy of prostate (*See also* TNB)

TNC
turbid, no creamy [layer]

TnC
troponin C

TNCB
trinitrochlorobenzene

TND
term normal delivery
transient neonatal diabetes
twenty-nail dystrophy

TNDM
transient neonatal diabetes mellitus

TNE
transnasal esophagoscopy

TNEE
titrated norepinephrine excretion

TNF
tissue necrosis factor
trinitrofluorenone
true negative fraction
tumor necrosis factor

TNF-alpha, TNF-α
tumor necrosis factor alpha (α)

TNF-beta, TNF-β
tumor necrosis factor beta (β)

TNF-bp
tumor necrosis factor-binding protein

TNFR
tumor necrosis factor receptor

TNFSF
tumor necrosis factor superfamily

TNG
toxic nodular goiter
trinitroglycerol (nitroglycerin)

tng
tongue
training

TNH
transient neonatal hyperammonemia

TNI
total nodal irradiation

TnI
troponin I [cardiac marker]

T/NK
T/natural killer [cell]

TNM
[primary] tumor, [regional lymph] node, [remote] metastases [classification, staging]
tumor, node, metastasis

T/NM
tumor with node metastasis

TNMR
tritium nuclear magnetic resonance

TNNSS
total nonnasal symptom score

t-NNT
threshold number needed to treat [epidemiology]

TNP
total net positive
trinitrophenyl

TNPM
transient neonatal pustular melanosis

TNR
tonic neck reflex
true negative rate

TNS
tension night splint
total nuclear score
transcutaneous nerve stimulator
transient neurologic symptom
tumor necrosis serum

TnSNPV
Trichoplusia ni single capsid nuclear polyhedrosis (SNPV) [virus]

TNSS
total nasal symptom score

TNT
trinitrotoluene

TnT
troponin T [cardiac marker]

TNTC
too numerous to count

TNU
tobacco nonuser

TNV
tobacco necrosis virus
TNVAD
Test of Nonverbal Auditory Discrimination
TNY
trichomonas and yeast (*See also* T&Y)
TO
original (old) tuberculin
target organ
telephone order
temperature, oral (*See also* T(O))
Theiler original [strain of mouse encephalomyelitis virus]
thoracic orthosis
thromboangiitis obliterans
thrombotic occlusion
time off
time out
tincture of opium (*See also* t.o.)
total obstruction
tracheo-oesophageal [British]
transfer out
tuboovarian
turned on
turnover
T&O
tandem and ovoid [applicator]
tubes and ovaries
T/O
time out
T(O)
oral temperature (*See also* TO)
TO₂
oxygen transport [rate]
t.o.
tincture of opium (*See also* TO)
TOA
time of arrival
tuboovarian abscess
TOAA
to affected areas
TOAL
Test of Adolescent Language
TOAPOT
tuboovarian abscess after previous tubal occlusion
TOB
tobacco
TOBE
tests of basic experience
TOBEC
total body electrical conductivity
TOBI
tobramycin solution for inhalation (*See also* TSI)

TobRV
tobacco ringspot virus (*See also* TRSV)
TOC
table of contents
test of cure
total occlusal convergence
total organic carbon
tuboovarian complex
TOCE
transcatheter oily chemoembolization
TOCO
tocodynamometer (*See also* TKD)
TOCP
triorthocresyl phosphate
TOCSY
total correlation spectroscopy
TOCU
transoral carotid ultrasonography
⚠ **TOD**
tail-on detector [gene]
target organ damage (disease)
tension oculus dexter [tension of right eye] ⚠
time of death
time of departure
Time-Oriented Data [Bank]
tubal occlusion device
TOD/CCD
target organ disease/clinical cardiovascular disease
TODE
total organ dose equivalent
TODS
toxic organic dust syndrome
TOE
tender on examination
tracheoesophageal
trans-oesophageal echography [British]
TOES
toxic oil epidemic syndrome
TOF
tetralogy of Fallot (*See also* TET, TF)
time of flight [radiology]
tracheo-oesophageal fistula [British]
train of four [neuromuscular blockade]
T of A
transposition of aorta
TOFA
time-of-flight and absorbance
TOF MRA
time-of-flight magnetic resonance angiography
TOFMS
time-of-flight mass spectometry
TOGV
transposition of the great vessels (*See also* TGV)

TOH
throughout hospitalization
Tower of Hanoi [mathematics]
transient osteoporosis of hip

TOL
trial of labor

tol
tolerance
tolerated

TOLA
temporary leave of absence
Test of Oral and Limb Apraxia

TOLD
Test of Language Development

TOLD-I
Test of Language
Development-Intermediate

TOLD-I:2
Test of Language Development-
Intermediate, Second Edition

TOLD-P
Test of Language Development-Primary

TOLD-P:2
Test of Language Development-
Primary, Second Edition

TOM
therapeutic outcomes monitoring
tomorrow
transcutaneous oxygen monitor (*See also*
TCOM)
tube observation model

ToM
theory-of-mind

TOMAL
Test of Memory and Learning

TOMM
Test of Memory Malingering

tomo
tomogram

TON
tonight
traumatic optic neuropathy

TONAR
the oral to nasal acoustic ratio

TONE
tilted optimized nonsaturating
excitation

TONI
Test of Nonverbal Intelligence

TOP
temporal, occipital, parietal
tendency-oriented perimetry
termination of pregnancy
test orientation procedure
tissue oncotic pressure
Topografov [virus]
total ossicular prosthesis

TOP-8
Treatment Outcome PTSD [scale]

ToP
Test of Playfulness

top.
topical (*See also* T)

TOPA
topical oropharyngeal anesthesia

TOPL
Test of Pragmatic Language

TOPO
topographic simulated keratometric
power

TOPO I–II
topoisomerase I–II

TOPO-II-alpha (α)
topoisomerase II-alpha (α)

TOPOSS
Tests of Perception of Scientists and
Self

TOPS
Take Off Pounds Sensibly
Taxonomy of Problematic Social
Situations
total ozone portable spectrometer

TopSS
Topographic Scanning System

TopSS/ICG
Topographic Scanning
System/indocyanine green

TOPV
trivalent oral polio (poliomyelitis)
(poliovirus) vaccine

TOR
target of rapamycin [protein]

TORB
telephone order readback

TORC
Test of Reading Comprehension

TORCH
toxoplasmosis, other agents, rubella,
cytomegalovirus, herpes simplex
toxoplasmosis, other infections, rubella,
cytomegalovirus, and herpes simplex

TOR-I
target of rapamycin inhibitor

TORP
Test of Orientation for Rehabilitation
Patients
reconstruction (replacement) procedure
(prosthesis)

⚠ **TOS**
tension oculus sinister [tension of left
eye] ⚠
thoracic outlet stenosis
(syndrome)
toxic oil syndrome

TOSS
total suppression of sideband

TOSV
Toscana virus

TOT
tincture of time
tip-of-the-tongue
total operating time
tubal ovum transfer
TOTAL-C
total cholesterol
TOT BILI
total bilirubin (*See also* TB, TBIL, T Bili)
TOTM
trioctyltrimellitate
TOTP
triorthotolyl phosphate
TOTPAR
total pain relief
tot prot
total protein (*See also* TP, T PROT)
TOV
thrombosed oral varix [singular] (varices [plural])
trial of void
TOVA
Test of Variables of Attention
TOVF
testing of visual fields
TOWER
testing, orientation, work, evaluation, rehabilitation
TOWL
Test of Written Language
tox
toxic
toxicity
toxicology
toxin
toxoid
TOXGR
toxic granulation
TOXICON
Toxicology Information Conversational On-Line Network
TOXLINE
Toxicology Information On-Line
TOXO, toxo
toxoplasmosis
TP
tail pinch
temperature and pressure
temperature probe
temporal peak
temporoparietal
tender point (*See also* TeP)
tension pneumothorax
terminal phalanx
tetanus-pertussis
therapeutic pass

therapeutic profile
thickly padded
ThinPrep Pap [test]
thought process
threshold potential
thrombocytopenic purpura
thrombophlebitis
thymic polypeptide
thymidine phosphorylase
thymus protein
time to progression (*See also* TTP)
tissue pressure
Todd paralysis
toe pressure
toilet paper
torsade de pointes (*See also* TDP, TdP)
total population
total positives
total protein (*See also* tot prot, T PROT)
T piece
trailing pole
transforming principle
transition point (*See also* T)
transpyloric
transverse polarization
treating physician
treatment period
Treponema pallidum
triphosphate
true positive
tryptophan pyrrolase
tube precipitin
tuberculin precipitation (precipitate)
tumor protein
TP1
telomerase-associated protein
TP-1
thymostimuline
TP5
thymopoietin pentapeptide
T&P, T+P
temperature and pulse
turn and position
T:P
trough to peak ratio
Tp
tampon
tp
physical half-life
TPA
12-O-tetradecanoylphorbol 13-acetate
tannic acid, polyphosphomolybdic acid, and amido acid [staining technique]
temporary portacaval anastomosis
temporopolar artery
third-party administrator

T

TPA *(continued)*
thrombotic pulmonary artery
tissue plasminogen activator (*See also*
tPA)
tissue polypeptide antigen
total parenteral alimentation
total phobic anxiety
Treponema pallidum agglutination
tumor polypeptide antigen
tPA
tissue plasminogen activator (*See also*
TPA)
TPAC
torso phased-array coil
TPAI
tissue plasminogen activator inhibitor
TPAL
term [infants], premature [infants],
abortions, living [children] [obstetric
history]
TPB
Theory of Planned Behavior
transient posttraumatic blindness
transpalatal bar
tryptone phosphate broth
TPBA
thermal/perfusion balloon angioplasty
TPBF
total pulmonary blood flow
TPBS
three-phase [radionuclide] bone scanning
(scintigraphy)
triphasic bone scintigraphy
TPC
target plasma concentration
telescoping plugged catheter
telopeptide-poor collagen
tender point count
thenar palmar crease
thromboplastic plasma component
thyroid papillary carcinoma
time to peak contrast
time-to-pulse-height converter
total patient care
total plasma catecholamines
total plasma cholesterol
touch preparation cytology
transverse palmar crease
treatment planning conference
Treponema pallidum complement
tympanocentesis
TPCC
Treponema pallidum cryolysis
complement
TPCF
Treponema pallidum complement
fixation
TPCV
total packed cell volume

TPD
temporary partial disability
thiamine propyldisulfide
tidal peritoneal dialysis
title peritoneal dialysis
tropical pancreatic diabetes
tumor-producing dose
typhoid vaccine, not otherwise specified
TPDa
typhoid vaccine, attenuated live [oral
Ty21a strain]
TPDAKD
typhoid vaccine, acetone-killed and
dried [U.S. military]
TPDHP
typhoid vaccine, heat and phenol
inactivated, dried
TPDS
tropical pancreatic diabetes syndrome
TPDVI
typhoid vaccine, Vi capsular
polysaccharide
TPE
2-photon excitation
therapeutic plasma exchange
thermoplastic elastomer
tissue-protective, end-cutting
total pelvic exenteration
total placental estrogens
total protective environment
Tpe
expiratory pause time
T-penia
thrombocytopenia (*See also* TCP)
TPERM
time of peak emptying rate of mouth
TPERP
time of peak emptying rate of pharynx
TPEY
tellurite polymyxin egg yolk [agar]
TPF
temporoparietal fascial flap
thymus permeability factor
trained participating father [at birth]
true positive fraction
TPFR
time to peak filling rate
TPFRE
time of peak filling rate of esophagus
TPG
therapeutic play group
transmembrane potential gradient
transplacental gradient
transpulmonary gradient
transvalvular pressure gradient
tryptophan peptone glucose [broth]
TPGYT
trypticase-peptone-glucose-yeast
extract-trypsin [medium]

TPH

thromboembolic pulmonary hypertension
trained participating husband [at birth]
transient postictal hemianopia
(hemianopsia)
transplacental hemorrhage
transrectal prostatic hyperthermia
treponemal hemagglutination
Treponema pallidum hemagglutination
(*See also* TPHA)
tryptophan hydroxylase

TPHA

Treponema pallidum hemagglutination
assay [test] (*See also* TPH)

TPHOS

triple phosphate [crystal]

TPI

tender point index
Treatment Priority Index
Treponema pallidum immobilization
[test] (*See also* TIT)
trigger point injection
triose phosphate isomerase

Tpi

inspiratory pause time

TPIA

Treponema pallidum immobilization
(immune) adherence

TPIT

trigger point injection therapy

tpk

time to peak (*See also* TTP)

TPL

triphosphate of lime
tyrosine phenol-lyase

T plasty

tympanoplasty

T-PLL

T-cell prolymphocytic leukemia

TPLS

The Primary Language Screen

TPLSM

two-photon laser-scanning microscope

TPLV

transient pulmonary vascular lability

TPM

temporary pacemaker
thrombophlebitis migrans
total particulate matter
total passive motion
triphenylmethane

tPME

time to peak of maximum enhancement

TPMT

thiopurine methyltransferase

TPMV

Thottapalayam virus

TPN

thalamic projection neuron
total parenteral nutrition
triphosphopyridine nucleotide

TPNH

triphosphopyridine nucleotide,
[reduced]

TPO

temporoparietooccipital
thrombopoietin
thyroid peroxidase (thyroperoxidase)
trial prescription order
tryptophan peroxidase

TPO Ab

thyroid-peroxidase autoantibody
thyroperoxidase antibody

TPP

tetraphenylporphyrin
thiamin pyrophosphate
thrust plate prosthesis
transpulmonary pressure
tubal perfusion pressure

TP&P

time, place, and person

TPPase

thiamine pyrophosphatase

TPPD

thoracic-pelvic-phalangeal dystrophy

TPPI

time-proportional phase incrementation

TPPMMC

trapezoidal paddle pectoralis major
myocutaneous [flap]

TPPN

total peripheral parenteral nutrition

TPPS

Toddler-Preschooler Postoperative Pain
Scale

TPPT

thrombus precursor protein

TPPV

trans pars plana vitrectomy

TPQ

tridimensional personality questionnaire

TPR

temperature
temperature, pulse, respiration
testosterone production rate
Thompson-Parkridge-Richards [ankle
orthosis]
tissue-phantom ratio
total peripheral resistance
total pulmonary resistance
transsphenoidal pituitary resection
true positive rate

T2 PRE

T2 proton relaxation enhancement

T

TPRI
total peripheral resistance index
T-PRK
tracker-assisted photorefractive
keratectomy
T PROT
total protein (*See also* tot prot, TP)
TPS
telescopic plate spacer
tender point score
titanium plasma sprayed
trypsin (*See also* Tr)
tumor polysaccharide substance
typhus [*Rickettsiae* spp.] vaccine
tPSA
total prostate specific antigen
TPST
true positive stress test
TPSV
tumor peak systolic velocity
TPT
Tactile Performance Test
tetraphenyl tetrazolium
time to peak tension
total protein tuberculin
transpyloric tube
treadmill performance test
trigger point therapy
typhoid-paratyphoid [vaccine]
tPTEF
time to peak expiratory flow
tPTEF/tE
time to peak expiratory flow and total
expiration time
TPTHS
total parathyroid hormone secretion
tPTIF
time to peak inspiratory flow
TPTX
thyroid-parathyroidectomy
thyroparathyroidectomy
TPTZ
tripyridyltriazine
TPU
tropical phagedenic ulcer
TPUR
transperineal urethral resection
T-putty
Theraputty
TPV
tetanus-pertussis vaccine
TPVA
tibioperoneal vessel angioplasty
TPVR
total peripheral vascular resistance
total pulmonary vascular resistance
TPWBBI
triphasic whole-body bone imaging

TPWM
temporoparietal white matter
tympanoplasty with mastoidectomy
TPWOM
tympanoplasty without mastoidectomy
TQ
time questionnaire
tocopherolquinone
tourniquet (*See also* TK)
TQM
total quality management
T-R
test-retest
TR
recovery time
rectal temperature (*See also* T(R))
repetition time
residual tuberculin
terminal repeat
tetrazolium reduction
therapeutic radiology
therapeutic reaction
therapeutic recreation
thioredoxin reductase
thyroid hormone receptor
timed release
time to repeat
time to repetition
tincture (*See also* T, TCT, tinc, tinct,
TR, Tr)
to return
total repair
total resistance
total response (*See also* R)
trace (*See also* T, t, Tr)
trachea
transfusion reaction (*See also* TRANS
Rx)
transplant recipient
transrectal
transverse relaxation
treatment (*See also* treat., trt, trx, TX,
T_x, tx)
tremor
tricuspid regurgitation
triiodothyronine receptor
triradial
true reading
tuberculin residue
tuberculin Ruckland [new tuberculin]
tubular resorption (reabsorption)
tumor registry
turbidity reducing
turnover rate
T&R
tenderness and rebound
treated and released
turn and reposition

T:R
thickness to radius ratio
T(R)
rectal temperature (*See also* TR)
T(°R)
absolute temperature on Rankine scale
T$_r$
radiologic half-life
retention time
Tr
tincture (*See also* T, TCT, tinc, tinct, TR)
trace (*See also* T, t, TR)
tragion [craniometric]
trypsin (*See also* TPS)
TRA
[I.V.] to run at [rate]
total renin activity
transaldolase (*See also* TA)
trans-retinoic acid
traumatic rupture of thoracic aorta
tumor regression antigen
tumor rejection antigen
tumor-resistant antigen
tra
transfer (*See also* trf)
TRAb
thyrotropin receptor autoantibody
TSH (thyroid stimulating hormone) receptor antibody
TRAC
traction (*See also* Tx, T$_x$, tx)
TRACE
time-resolved amplified cryptate emission [lab method]
trach
trachea(l)
tracheostomy (*See also* trake)
tracheotomy (*See also* trake)
trach asp
tracheal aspiration
TR-ACP, TRAcP
tartrate resistant acid phosphatase
TRADD
TNF (tumor necrosis factor) receptor-associated death domain
TRAF
TNF (tumor necrosis factor) receptor-associated factor
TRAFO
tone-reducing ankle-foot orthosis
TRAIDS
transfusion-related AIDS
TRAIL
TNF (tumor necrosis factor) related apoptosis-inducing ligand

TRAJ
timed repetitive ankle jerk
TRAK
total reference air kerma
trake
tracheostomy (*See also* trach)
trachotomy (*See also* trach)
TRALD
transfusion-related acute lung disease
TRALI
transfusion-related acute lung injury
TRAM
transverse rectus abdominis muscle
transverse rectus abdominis musculocutaneous (myocutaneous) [flap for breast reconstruction]
Treatment Rating Assessment Matrix
Treatment Response Assessment Method
TRAMP
transverse rectus abdominis musculoperitoneal [flap, breast reconstruction]
TRAMPE
tricho-rhino-auriculo-phalangeal multiple exostoses
TRAN
transfusion (*See also* TX, Tx, T$_x$, tx)
TRANCE
TNF (tumor necrosis factor) related activation-induced cytokine
trans
transference
transverse (*See also* TV)
Trans D, trans D
transverse diameter (*See also* TD)
transm
transmission
transmit(ted)
transpl
transplant(ation) (*See also* TX, Tx, T$_x$, tx, Txn)
transplant(ed)
TRANS Rx
transfusion reaction (*See also* TR)
trans sect
transverse section (*See also* TS, T sect)
transsex
transsexual (*See also* TS)
TRAP
tartrate-resistant acid phosphatase
telomere (telomeric) repeat amplification protocol
thrombin receptor-activating peptide
thrombospondin-related anonymous protein
total radical-trapping antioxidant parameter (potential) [assay]

T

TRAP *(continued)*
total reactive antioxidant potential
trapezius [muscle]
twin reversed arterial perfusion

TRAP-6
thrombin receptor-activating peptide 6

TRAPS
TNF (tumor necrosis factor) receptor-associated periodic syndrome
twin reversed arterial perfusion sequence

TRAS
transesophageal atrial stimulation
transplant(ation) renal artery stenosis

TRASHES
tuberculosis, radiotherapy, ankylosing spondylitis, histoplasmosis, extrinsic allergic alveolitis, silicosis [chest x-ray findings]

trau, traum
trauma
traumatic

TRB
return to baseline

TRb
trilateral retinoblastoma

TRBC
total red blood cells

TRBF
total renal blood flow

TRBV
Tribec virus

TRC
tanned red [blood] cell
total renin concentration
total respiratory conductance
total ridge count

TRCA
tanned red [blood] cell agglutination

TRCH
tanned red [blood] cell hemagglutination

Trch
Trichophyton

TRCHI
tanned red [blood] cell hemagglutination inhibition

TRCV
total red [blood] cell volume

TRD
tinnitus relief device
tongue-retaining device
total retinal detachment
traction (tractional) retinal detachment
traumatic rupture of diaphragm
treatment-related death
treatment-resistant depression

TRDN
transient respiratory distress of newborn

TRDS
transient respiratory distress syndrome

TRE
negative triiodothyronine response element
thyroid response element
traumatic retinal edema
true radiation emission

T$_3$RE
triiodothyronine responsive element

TREA
thoroughness, reliability, efficiency, analytic [ability]
triethanolamine

treat.
treatment (*See also* TR, trt, trx, T$_x$, tx)

TREC
T-cell receptor-rearrangement excision circles

Tren, TREND
Trendelenburg [position] (*See also* TRND)

Trep
Treponema (*See also* T)

TRF
T-cell replacing factor
Teacher Rating (Report) Form
telomeric restriction fragment
terminal restriction fragment
thyrotropin releasing factor
time-resolved (fluorometry) fluorescence

trf
transfer (*See also* tra)

TRFC
total rosette-forming cell

TRG
tumor regression grade

trg, trng
training

TRGI
Teacher's Reading Global Improvement (scale, test)
triglycerides incalculable

TRH
tension-reducing hypothesis
thyroid-releasing hormone
thyrotropin-releasing hormone

TRH-DE
thyrotropin-releasing hormone degrading ectoenzyme

TRH-R
thyrotropin-releasing hormone receptor

TRH-ST
thyrotropin-releasing hormone stimulation test

TRI
tetrazolium reduction inhibition
total response index
transient radicular irritation

transient response imaging
trifocal
trimester *(See also* TM)
tubuloreticular inclusion
tri
tricentric
TriA
tricuspid atresia
TRIAC, triac
triiodothyroacetic acid
(3,5,3′-triiodothyroacetic acid)
T₃RIA, T₃(RIA)
triiodothyronine radioimmunoassay
(See also T₄RIA)
T₄RIA, T₄(RIA)
tetraiodothyronine (thyroxine)
radioimmunoassay [radioisotope assay]
TRIADS
time-resolved imaging by automatic data
segmentation
TRIC
trachoma (and) inclusion conjunctivitis
TRICB
trichlorobiphenyl
TRICH, Trich
trichinosis
Trichomonas
TRICKS
time-resolved imaging contrast kinetics
TRIG, trig
triglyceride *(See also* TG)
TRIMIS
Tri-Service Medical Information
System
TRINS
totally reversible ischemic neurological
symptoms
TRIS, tris
tris (hydroxymethyl)aminomethane
(See also THAM)
TRISS
Trauma and Injury Severity Scores
TRIT
triiodothyronine *(See also* T3, TIT,
TITh)
Trit, trit
triturate
TRITC
tetramethylrhodamine isothiocyanate
tetrarhodamine isothiocyanate
TRK
total rotating knee
transketolase
TRK-A–TRK-B
tyrosine receptor kinase A–B
TRL
triglyceride-rich lipoprotein

TRLI
transfusion-related lung injury
TR-LSC
time-resolved liquid scintillation
counting
TRM
transplant(ation)-related mortality
treatment-related mortality
TRMA
thiamine-responsive megaloblastic
anemia
TRML, trml
terminal *(See also* t, term.)
tRNA
transfer ribonucleic acid
TRNBP
transrectal needle biopsy of
prostate
TRND
Trendelenburg [position] *(See also* Tren,
TREND)
TRNG
tetracycline-resistant *Neisseria
gonorrhoeae*
TRO
to return to office
thyroid-related ophthalmopathy
tissue reflectance oximeter
TROCA
tangible reinforcement of operant
conditioned audiometry
TROCH, Troch, troch
troche (trochiscus) [lozenge]
TROM
torque range of motion
total range of motion
trop
tropical
TROPCAB
total revascularization off-pump by
coronary artery bypass
TRP
Tactile Reproduction Pegboard
total refractory period
trichorhinophalangeal [syndrome]
tubular reabsorption of phosphate
TRP-1
tyrosine-related protein 1
Trp
tryptophan *(See also* W)
TRPA
tryptophan-rich prealbumin
TRPL, TrPl
treatment plan
TRPM-2
testosterone-repressed prostate message
2 [gene]

TRPS
  trichorhinophalangeal syndrome
TrP
  trigger point
TRPT
  theoretical renal phosphorus threshold
TRR
  total respiratory resistance
TRRP
  Thackray Reading Readiness Profile
TR-RXR
  thyroid hormone receptor-retinoid X
  receptor
TRS
  testicular regression syndrome
  Therapeutic Recreation Specialist
  total reducing sugars
  tubuloreticular structure
TrS
  traumatic surgery
TRST
  triage risk screening tool
TRSV
  tobacco ringspot virus (*See also*
  TobRV)
TRT
  tangential radiation therapy
  testosterone replacement
  thermoradiotherapy
  thoracic radiation therapy
  tinnitus-retraining therapy
  total reading time
  treatment-related toxicity
trt
  treatment (*See also* TR, treat., trt, trx,
  Tx, T$_x$, tx)
TR:TE
  repetition time to echo time ratio
TrTr
  transfer training
T-RTS
  triage-revised trauma score
TRU
  turbidity-reducing unit
T$_3$RU
  triiodothyronine (T$_3$) resin uptake
TrueFISP
  true fast imaging with steady-state
  precession
TRUS
  transrectal ultrasonography
  transrectal ultrasound-guided sextant
  [biopsy]
  transrectal ultrasound scan(ning)
  transurethral ultrasound
TRUSP
  transrectal ultrasound of prostate
TRUST
  toluidine red unheated serum test

TRUV
  Trubanaman virus
TRV
  Tanjong Rabok virus
  tobacco rattle virus
TRVV
  total right ventricular volume
TRW
  teboroxime resting washout
TRX
  thioredoxin
trx
  treatment [prescription] (*See also* TR,
  treat., trt, Tx, T$_x$, tx)
TrxR
  thioredoxin reductase
Tryp
  Trypanosoma
TRZ
  tartrazine
TS
  (2′-deoxy)thymidylate synthase
  telomerase
  temperature sensitive (sensitivity)
  temporal stem
  terminal sedation
  terminal sensation
  test solution
  thermostable
  thiosporin
  thoracic spine
  thoracic surgery
  throat swab
  thymidylate synthase
  tissue space
  tocopherol supplemented
  toe sign
  total solids
  toxic shock
  toxic substance
  toxic syndrome
  trabecular separation
  tracheal sound
  tracheal spiral
  transitional sleep
  transsexual (*See also* transsex)
  transverse section (*See also* trans sect, T
  sect)
  transverse sinus
  Trauma Score
  treadmill score
  trichostasis spinulosa
  tricuspid stenosis
  triple strength
  tropical sprue
  trypticase soy [plate]
  T suppressor [cell]
  tuberous sclerosis
  tubular sound

tumor specific
type specific

T-S

type and screen (*See also* TXS)

T:S

thyroid to serum iodide ratio

Ts

skin temperature
tension by Schiotz [tonometer]
T helper suppressor cell
tosylate

tS

time required to complete S phase of
cell cycle

ts, tsp

teaspoon(ful) (*See also* t, teasp)

TSA

technical surgical assistance
Test of Syntactic Ability
tissue-specific antigens
toluene sulfonic acid
total severity assessment
total shoulder arthroplasty
total solute absorption
toxic shock antigen
transcortical sensory aphasia
trypticase soy agar
tryptone soy agar
tumor-specific antigen
tumor surface antigen
tumor-susceptible antigen
type-specific antibody
tyramide signal amplification

T$_4$SA

thyroxine-specific activity

TSAb

thyroid-stimulating antibody

TSAE

transcatheter splenic arterial
embolization

TSAH

traumatic subarachnoid hemorrhage

TSAP

toxic shock-associated protein

Tsaph

temperature in saphenous [vein]

TSAR

tape-surrounded Appli-ruler

TSAS

total severity assessment score

TSAT

tube slide agglutination test

TSB

total serum bilirubin
trypticase soy broth
tryptone soy broth

TSBA

total serum bile acids

TSBB

transtracheal selective bronchial
brushing

TSBC

Time-Sample Behavioral Checklist

TSBP

testis-specific binding protein

TSC

theophylline serum concentration
thiosemicarbazide [stain]
total static compliance
total symptom complex
total symptom count
transient spontaneous circulation
transverse spinal sclerosis
tuberous sclerosis complex

TSCA

Toxic Substance Control Act

TSCC

Trauma Symptom Checklist for
Children

TSCS

Tennessee Self-Concept Scale

TSC1–TSC2

tuberous sclerosis complex 1–2

TSD

target-skin distance
theory of signal detectability
total sleep deprivation
transfer summary dictated
tumor stage downstaging

TSDP

tapered steroid dosing package

TSE

targeted systemic exposure
testicular self-examination
time since exposure
total skin examination
transcutaneous spinal electroanesthesia
transmissible spongiform encephalopathy
trisodium edetate
turbo spin echo

TSEB

total skin electron beam

TSEBT

total skin electron beam therapy

T sect

transverse section (*See also* trans, sect,
TS)

TSEM

transmission scanning electron
microscopy (microscope)

TSENSE

time-adaptive sensitivity encoding
(SENSE)

T set, T-set

tracheotomy set
tracheostomy set

TSF
thickness of skin fold
thrombopoiesis-stimulating factor
tissue-(coding) factor (*See also* TCF)
total systemic flow
triceps skinfold (thickness)
T-suppressor factor

TSFS
transseptal frontal sinusotomy

TSG
tumor-specific glycoprotein
tumor-suppressor gene

TSGA
term, small for gestational age

TSGE
temperature sweep gel electrophoresis

TSH
thyroid-stimulating hormone

TSHBAb
TSH (thyroid stimulating hormone)
blocking antibody

TSH-oma
TSH (thyroid stimulating hormone)
secreting pituitary adenoma

TSH-R
thyroid-stimulating hormone receptor
thyrotropin receptor

TSHR
thyroid-stimulating hormone receptor
thyrotropin-receptor antibody

TSH-RAb
thyroid-stimulating hormone receptor
antibody
thyroid-stimulating hormone receptor
autoantibody
thyrotropin receptor-stimulating
antibody

TSH-RF
thyroid-stimulating hormone-releasing
factor

TSH-RH
thyroid-stimulating hormone-releasing
hormone

TSI
Test of Social Inferences
thyroid-stimulating immunoglobulin
tobramycin solution for inhalation
(*See also* TOBI)
triple sugar iron (agar) (*See also* TSIA)

TSIA
total small-intestine allotransplantation
triple sugar iron agar (*See also* TSI)

tSIDS
totally unexplained sudden infant death
syndrome

TSIF
Tooth Surface Index of Fluorosis

T-SKULL
trauma skull

TSL
terminal sensory latency

TSLS
toxic shocklike syndrome

TSM
two-spotted spider mite
type-specific M protein

TSN
tryptophan peptone sulfide neomycin
(agar)

TSNA
tobacco-specific nitrosamine

TSNP
two-step nested polymerase chain
reaction

TSOP
time from symptom onset to
presentation

TSP
testis-specific protein
thrombospondin
tibial hole sagittal positioning
tibial sesamoid position
topical skin protection
total serum protein
total sleep period
total suspended particulate
tribasic sodium phosphate
trisodium phosphate
tropical spastic paraparesis

TSP-1
thrombospondin 1

TSPA
thiophosphoramide (Thiotepa)

TSPAP
total serum prostatic acid
phosphatase

TSP/HAM
tropical spastic paraparesis/HTLV-I
associated myelopathy

T-spica
thumb spica [bandage]

T-spine, T/spine
thoracic spine

TSPP
tetrasodium pyrophosphate

TSR
testosterone-sterilized [female] rat
thyroid-serum ratio
tissue scatter ratio [radiotherapy]
tissue standard ratio [radiotherapy]
total saturation recovery
total shoulder replacement
total systemic resistance
transient situational reaction

TSRBC
trypsinized sheep red blood cell

TSRH
Texas Scottish Rite Hospital

TSRI
Teacher School Readiness Inventory
TS III ROP
threshold stage III of retinopathy of prematurity
TSRPC
totally stapled restorative proctocolectomy
TSRS
tissue-stone recognition system
TSS
total serum solids
total symptom score
toxic shock syndrome
transsphenoidal surgery
transverse spinal sclerosis
tropical splenomegaly syndrome
tumor score system
TSSA
tumor-specific [cell] surface antigen
TSSE
toxic shock syndrome exoprotein
toxic shock syndrome exotoxin
TS-SPCL
transsclerally sutured posterior chamber lens
TS/SS
transverse/sigmoid sinus
TSST
toxic shock syndrome toxin
Trier social stress test
TSST-1
toxic shock syndrome toxin 1
TSSU
theatre sterile supply unit [British for operating room supply]
TST
thromboplastin screening test
Titmus stereoacuity test
total sleep time
transition state theory
transscrotal testosterone
treadmill stress test (*See also* TMST)
triceps (tricipital) skinfold thickness
tuberculin skin test
tumor skin test
Twenty Statements Test
TSTA
toxoplasmin skin test antigen
tumor-specific tissue antigen
tumor-specific transplant(ation) antigen
TSTI
tumor-specific transplant(ation) immunity
TSTM
too small to measure
TSU
triple sugar urea (agar)

T₃SU
triiodothyronine serum uptake
TSUV
Tsuruse virus
TSV
total stomach volume
total stroke volume
total systemic vascular resistance
TSY
trypticase soy yeast
TT
tablet triturate
tactile tension
talar tilt
talking task
telescopic and torsional
tendon transfer
terminal transferase
testicular torsion
Test Tape
tetanus toxin
tetanus toxoid (*See also* tet tox)
tetrathionate [broth]
tetrazol
Text Telephone
therapeutic touch
thoracotomy tube
thrombin time
thrombolytic therapy (*See also* TTx)
thromboplastin time
thymol turbidity
tibial torsion
tibial tubercle
tibial tuberosity
tilt table
tine test
token test
tolerance test
tonometry
tooth treatment
total thyroidectomy
total time
total transfer
trabecular thickness
transferred to
transfusion transmitted [virus]
transient tachypnea
transit time
transpupillary thermotherapy
transthoracic
transtracheal
treadmill test (*See also* TMT)
treponemal test
triple therapy
tuberculin test
tube thoracostomy
tumor thrombus

T

TT (*continued*)
 turnover time
 twitch tension
 tympanic temperature
 tympanostomy tube
 tyrosine transaminase
T-T
 time-to-time
T/T
 trace of/trace of [substances]
T&T
 time and temperature
 touch and tone
 tympanotomy and tube [insertion]
TT₃
 total triiodothyronine
TT₄
 total thyroxine
TTA
 tetanus toxoid antibody
 timed therapeutic absence
 tissue texture abnormality
 total toe arthroplasty
 transtracheal aspiration
T-TAC
 transcervical tubal access catheter
TTAP
 threaded titanium acetabular
  prosthesis
TTAT
 toe touch as tolerated
TTB
 third trimester bleeding
TTBS
 Tween-TRIS-buffered saline solution
TTBV
 total trabecular bone volume
TTC
 transtracheal catheter
 triphenyl tetrazolium chloride
 T-tube cholangiogram
TTCT
 Torrance Tests of Creative thinking
TTD
 tarsal tunnel decompression
 temporary total disability
 tissue tolerance dose
 total temporary disability
 total tumor dose
 transfusion-transmitted disease
 transient tic disorder
 transverse thoracic diameter
TTD 2
 trichothiodystrophy 2
TTDE
 touch tone data entry
 transthoracic Doppler echocardiography
TTDF
 time to distant failure

TTDP
 time-to-disease progression
TTE
 total thoracic esophagectomy
 transthoracic echocardiograph(y)
  (echocardiogram)
 trial terminated early
 two-dimensional transthoracic
  echocardiography
TTF
 thyroid transcription factor
 time-to-treatment failure
TTF-1–TTF-2
 thyroid transcription factor 1–2
TTFD
 thiamine tetrahydrofurfuryl disulfide
TTG, TTGA
 tellurite, taurocholate, gelatin [agar]
Ttg, tTG
 tissue transglutaminase
TTGE
 temporal temperature gradient gel
  electrophoresis
 timed-temperature gradient
  electrophoresis
TTH
 tension-type headache
 thyrotropic hormone (*See also* TH)
TTI
 Teflon tube insertion
 tension-time index
 time-temperature indicator
 time-tension index
 time-to-intubation
 tissue thromboplastin inhibition (test)
 total time to intubation
 transfer to intermediate
 transtracheal insufflation
TTIB
 tension-time index per beat
TTII
 thyrotropin-binding inhibitory
  immunoglobulins
TTIT
 tissue thromboplastin inhibition test
TTJV
 transtracheal jet ventilation
TTKG
 transtubular potassium concentration
  gradient
TTL
 total lymphocyte
 training and test lung
ttl
 total (*See also* T)
TTLC
 true total lung capacity
TTLF
 time to local failure

TTM
    total tumor mass
    transtelephonic monitoring
    trichotillomania
TTMAD
    Testing-Teaching Module of Auditory
    Discrimination
TTN
    time to normalization
    toxic thyroid nodule
    transient tachypnea of newborn
      (*See also* TTNB)
TTNA
    transthoracic needle aspiration
TTNAB
    transthoracic needle aspiration biopsy
      (*See also* TTNB)
TTNB
    transient tachypnea of newborn
      (*See also* TTN)
    transthoracic needle [aspiration] biopsy
      (*See also* TTNAB)
TTND
    time to nondetectable
TTO
    to take out
    tea tree oil
    time trade-off
    transfer to open
    transtracheal oxygen (*See also* TTO$_2$)
TTO$_2$
    transtracheal oxygen (*See also* TTO)
TTOD
    tetanus toxoid outdated
TTOT
    transtracheal oxygen therapy
Ttot
    total respiratory time
T$_3$-toxicosis
    triiodothyronine toxicosis
TTP
    temporary transvenous pacemaker
    tender to palpation
    tender to pressure
    Testicular Tumor Panel
    thrombotic thrombocytopenic
     purpura
    thymidine triphosphate
    thyrotoxic paralysis
    time to peak (*See also* tpk)
    time to pregnancy
    time to progression (*See also* TP)
    time to tumor progression
    transtrabecular plane
    transtubercular plane
TTPA
    triethylene thiophosphoramide

TTPD
    thoracic-pelvic-phalangeal dystrophy
TTP-HUS
    thrombocytopenic purpura/hemolytic
     uremic syndrome
    thrombotic thrombocytopenic purpura
     and hemolytic uremic syndrome
TTR
    tarsal tunnel release
    time in therapeutic range
    transthoracic resistance
    transthyretin
    Trauma Triage Rule
    triceps tendon reflex
    type to token ratio
T-tropic
    T-cell trophic
TTS
    tarsal tunnel syndrome
    temporary threshold shift
    testosterone transdermal system
    through the skin
    through-the-scope
    tight-to-shaft
    tilt table standing
    transdermal therapeutic system
    transfusion therapy service
    trigeminal trophic syndrome
    twin-to-twin transfusion syndrome
     (*See also* TTTS)
TTT
    thymol turbidity test
    tibial talar [tibiotalar] tilt
    tilt-table test
    tolbutamide tolerance test
    total tourniquet time
    total twitch time
    transpupillary thermal therapy
    tuberculin tine test
    twin-to-twin transfusion [syndrome]
     (*See also* TTS, TTTS)
TTTS
    twin-to-twin transfusion syndrome
     (*See also* TTS, TTT)
TTTT
    test tube turbidity test
T-TURP
    total transurethral resection of
     prostate
TTUTD
    tetanus toxoid up-to-date
TTV
    therapeutic trial visit
    total tumor volume
    tracheal transport velocity
    transfusion-transmitted virus
    TT virus

T

TTVP
  temporary transvenous pacemaker
TTWB
  touch-toe weightbearing
TTX
  tetrodotoxin (*See also* TD)
TTx
  thrombolytic therapy (*See also* TT)
TU
  thiourea
  thyroidal uptake
  Todd unit
  toxic unit
  toxin unit
  transmission unit
  transrectal ultrasound
  transurethral
  tuberculin unit
  turbidity unit
1-TU
  1 tuberculin unit
T₃U
  triiodothyronine uptake (*See also* T₃UP)
5-TU
  5 tuberculin unit
250-TU
  250 tuberculin unit
TUAV
  Turuna virus
TUB
  tuberculosis vaccine, not BCG
  tubouterine [junction]
TUBA
  transumbilical breast augmentation
TUBS
  traumatic unidirectional Bankart lesion
  surgery
TUD
  total urethral discharge
TUDC, TUDCA
  tauroursodeoxycholate
  tauroursodeoxycholic acid
TUDOR
  transvaginal ultrasound-directed oocyte
  retrieval
TUDS
  temporary ureteral drainage system
TUE
  transurethral extraction
TUEP, TUEVP
  transurethral electrovaporization
  (evaporation) of prostate (*See also*
  TUVP)
TUF
  tissue ultrafiltration
  total ultrafiltration
TUG
  timed up and go (*See also* TUGT)
  total urinary gonadotropin

TUGSE
  traumatic ulcerative granuloma with
  stromal eosinophilia
TUGT
  timed up-and-go test (*See also* TUG)
TUI
  transurethral incision
TUIBN
  transurethral incision of bladder neck
TUIP
  transurethral incision of prostate
TUL
  transurethral ureterolithotripsy
  tularemia (*Francisella tularensis*)
  vaccine
  tumescent ultrasound liposculpture
TULIP
  transurethral ultrasound-guided
  laser-induced prostatectomy [system]
TULIPS
  touch-up and loop incorporated primers
  [PCR method]
TUMT
  transurethral microwave thermotherapy
TUN
  total urinary nitrogen
TUNA
  transurethral needle ablation
TUNEL
  TdT (terminal deoxynucleotidyltransferase)-mediated d(UTP)
  2′-deoxyuridine 5′-triphosphate)-biotin
  nick-end labeling [method]
TUP
  transumbilical plane
T₃UP
  triiodothyronine uptake (*See also* T₃U)
TUPR
  transurethral prostatic resection
TUR
  transurethral resection
T₃UR
  triiodothyronine uptake ratio
TURB, TURBT
  transurethral resection of bladder
turb
  turbid(ity)
TURBN
  transurethral resection of bladder neck
turboFLASH
  turbo fast low-angle shot
turboGRE
  turbo gradient-refocused echo
TURM
  transurethral microwave
TURP
  transurethral resection of prostate
TURS
  transurethral resection syndrome

TURV
transurethral resection of valve
Turlock virus

TURVN
transurethral resection of vesical neck

TUS
trauma ultrasound

TUSSI
Temple University Short Syntax
Inventory

T₄U
thyroxine uptake

TUTL
transuterine tubal lavage

TUU
transureteroureterostomy

TUV
transurethral valve

TUVP, TUVRP
transurethral electrovaporization
(vaporization) of prostate
transurethral vaporization-resection of
prostate (*See also* TUEP, TUEVP)

TV
talipes varus
target volume
television
Tellina virus
temporary visit
tetrazolium violet
Thermoactinomyces vulgaris
thoracic vertebra
thyroid volume
tick-borne virus
tidal volume (*See also* TD, VT, V$_T$)
tonic vergence
total volume
toxic vertigo
transfer vesicle
transvaginal
transvenous
transverse (*See also* trans)
trial visit
Trichomonas vaginalis
tricuspid valve
trivalent
true vertebra
truncal vagotomy
tuberculin volutin
tubulovesicular
tumor virus
typhoid vaccine

T/V
touch/verbal

TVA
true visual acuity
truncal vagotomy [plus] antrectomy

TVC
third ventricle cyst
timed ventilatory capacity
timed vital capacity
total viable cells
total volume capacity
transvaginal cone
triple voiding cystogram
true vocal cord

TVc
tricuspid valve closure

TV-CDS
transvaginal color Doppler sonography

TVCS
transverse vertical cross section

TVCV
transvenous cardioversion

TVD
transmissible virus dementia
triple vessel disease

TVDALV
triple vessel disease with abnormal left
ventricle

TV$_E$
tidal expiratory volume

TVF
tactile vocal fremitus
Thiry-Vella fistula
true vocal fold

TVG
time-varied gain
transvalvular gradient

TVGC
time-varied gain control (*See also*
TGC)

TVH
total vaginal hysterectomy
turkey virus hepatitis

TVHS
transvaginal hysterosonography

TVI
Temperament and Values Inventory
time velocity integral
total vascular isolation

TV$_I$
tidal inspiratory volume

T3:T4ind
triiodothyronine to thyroxine index

TVL
tenth value layer [radiation]

TVMS
Test of Visual-Motor Skills

TVMS:UL
Test of Visual-Motor Skills: Upper
Level Adolescents and Adults

TVN
tonic vibration response

TVO
transtrochanteric valgus osteotomy
TVOR
transvaginal oocyte retrieval
TVP
tensor veli palati
textured vegetable protein
transurethral vaporization of prostate
transvenous pacemaker
transvesical prostatectomy
tricuspid valve prolapse
truncal vagotomy [plus] pyloroplasty
TVPS
Test of Visual-Perception Skills
TVPS:UL
Test of Visual-Perceptual Skills: Upper
Level Adolescents and Adults
TVR
target vessel revascularization
tonic vibration reflex
total vascular resistance
total vibration reflex
tricuspid valve replacement
triple valve replacement
TVRE
transvaginal resection of endometrium
TVRSS
total vasomotor rhinitis symptom score
TVS
transvaginal sonography
transvaginal suturing
transvenous system
transvesical sonography
trigeminovascular system
TVSC
transvaginal scan
TVT
tension-free vaginal tape
transmissible venereal tumor
transvaginal taping
transvaginal tension-free
tunica vaginalis testis
TVTV
trivittatus virus
TVU
total volume of urine
transvaginal ultrasonography (ultrasound)
(*See also* TVUS, TV-UST)
TVUS, TV-UST
transvaginal ultrasonography (ultrasound)
(*See also* TVU)
TVV
Trichomonas vaginalis virus
TVX
tumor virus X
TW
talked with
tap water
terminal web

test weight
thin wall(ed)
thought withdrawal
thymic weight
total water
traveling wave
Trophermyma whippleii
T-wave
TW2
Tanner-Whitehouse mark 2 [method for
bone-age assessment]
5TW
five times a week
TWA
time-weighted average
total wrist arthroplasty
T-wave alternans
TWAR
Taiwan acute respiratory [virus]
T wave
electrocardiographic wave corresponding
to repolarization of ventricles
TWB
total weight bearing
Twb
wet bulb temperature
TWBC
total white blood cells
TWCS
Test of Work Competency and Stability
TWD
total white and differential [cell count]
TWE
tap water enema
tepid water enema
TWEAK
TNF (tumor necrosis factor) inducer of
apoptosis weak
TWETC
tap water enema til clear
TWF
Test of Word Finding
TWFD
Test of Word Finding in Discourse
TWG
total water gradient
total weight gain
TWH
transitional wall hyperplasia
TWHW
toe walking and heel walking
TWHW ok
toe walking and heel walking all right
TWI
tooth wear index
T-wave inversion
T1WI
T1 weighted image [magnetic
resonance]

T2WI
T2 weighted image [magnetic resonance]
TWIST
time without symptoms of disease and subjective toxic effects of treatment
TWL
transepidermal water loss (*See also* TEWL)
TWN
twin
TWOC
trial without catheter
TWR
total wrist replacement
TWSTRS
Toronto Western Spasmodic Torticollis Rating Scale
TWT
timed walking test
TWWD
tap water wet dressing
TX
derivative of contagious tuberculin
no evidence of primary tumor [TNM classification]
thorax
thyroidectomized
transplant(ation) (*See also* transpl)
T&X
type and crossmatch (*See also* T&C, T&CM, T&M, TXM)
Tx, T$_x$, tx
therapist
therapy (*See also* ther, therap)
traction (*See also* TRAC)
transcription
transfuse
transfusion (*See also* TRAN)
transplant(ation) (*See also* transpl., Txn)
treatment (*See also* TR, treat., trt, trx)
tympanostomy (*See also* tymp)
TXA, TxA
thromboxane A
TXA2, TXA$_2$
thromboxane A2

TXB2, TXB$_2$
thromboxane B2
TxCAD
transplant(ation) coronary artery disease
TXM
T-cell crossmatch
type and crossmatch (*See also* T&C, T&CM, T&M, T&X)
Txn
transplant(ation) (*See also* Tx, T$_x$, tx)
TXS
type and screen (*See also* T-S)
TXT
treadmill exercise test
T&Y
trichomonas and yeast (*See also* TNY)
Ty
type (*See also* T)
typhoid
Tyk-2
tyrosine kinase 2
Tyl
tyloma
TYMP
tympanogram
tymp
tympanic
tympanicity [auscultation of chest]
tympanum
tympanostomy (*See also* Tx, T$_x$, tx)
typ
typical
TYR
tyramine
Tyrode [solution]
Tyr
tyrosine (*See also* Y)
TyRIA
thyroid radioimmunoassay (*See also* T$_3$ RIA)
TYUV
Tyuleniy virus
TZ
transition zone
TZD
thiazolidinedione [class of drug]

T

U

internal energy
Mann-Whitney U test [rank sum statistic]
ulcer
ulna (*See also* uln)
umbilicus (*See also* UMB, umb)
uncertain
unerupted
unit ⚠
unknown (*See also* UK, UNK, unk, unkn)
upper
uracil (*See also* URA, Ura)
uranium
urea
urethra (*See also* UA, ureth)
uridine (*See also* Urd)
uridylic acid (*See also* UMP)
urinary
urine (*See also* UR)
uvula
wave on electrocardiogram

U

internal energy

U/

at umbilicus

1/U

one fingerbreadth above umbilicus

U/1

one fingerbreadth below umbilicus

U/2

upper half

U/3

upper third [of long bone]

24U

24 hour urine [collection]

u

unified atomic mass unit

UA

Ulex agglutinin
ultraaudible [sound]
ultrasonic arteriograph(y) (arteriogram)
umbilical artery
unaggregated
unauthorized absence
uncertain about
unicystic ameloblastoma
unit of analysis
unrelated [children raised] apart
unstable angina
upper airways
upper arm (*See also* U-ARM)
urethra (*See also* U, ureth)

uric acid (*See also* UR AC, URIC A, URC-A)
urinalysis
urinary aldosterone
urine aliquot
urocanic acid
uterine artery
uterine aspiration

UABD

upper airways bronchodilation

UAC

umbilical artery catheter
underactive
unusual-appearing child
upper airways congestion

UA:C

uric acid to creatinine ratio
urinary albumin to creatinine ratio

UACE

unplanned acute care encounter

UACL

ulcer-associated cell lineage

UACP

upper airways closing pressure

UAD

upper aerodigestive [tract] (*See also* UADT)
upper airways disease (disorder)
uric acid dysmetabolism

UADT

upper aerodigestive tract (*See also* UAD)

UAE

unilateral absence of excretion
unsupported arm exercise
urinary albumin excretion
uterine artery embolization

UAER

urinary albumin excretion rate

UAG

uracil-adenine-guanine

UAGA

Uniform Anatomical Gift Act

UAI

uterine activity integral

UAI-C

unprotected anal intercourse with casual partners

UAL

ultrasonic-assisted lipoplasty (liposuction) (lipectomy)
umbilical artery line (*See also* umb A line)
up [out of bed] as desired [up + L. *ad libitum*] (*See also* U/P)

U

UALTE
　　unexplained apparent life-threatening
　　event
UA&M
　　urinalysis and microscopy
U-AMY
　　urinary amylase
UAN
　　uric acid nitrogen
UA/NQMI
　　unstable angina/non-Q-wave myocardial
　　infarction
UA/NSEMI
　　unstable angina and non-ST-segment
　　elevation myocardial infarction
UAO
　　upper airways obstruction
　　urine acid output
UAOP
　　upper airways opening pressure
UAP
　　unstable angina pectoris (*See also*
　　USAP)
　　upper abdominal pain
　　upper airways patency
　　urinary acid phosphatase
　　urinary alkaline phosphatase
UAPA
　　unilateral absence of pulmonary
　　artery
UAPF
　　upon arrival patient found
UAPs
　　unlicensed assistive personnel
UAR
　　upper airways resistance
U-ARM
　　upper arm (*See also* UA)
UARS
　　upper airways resistance (respiratory)
　　syndrome
UAS
　　undifferentiated autoimmune
　　syndrome
　　upper abdominal surgery
　　upstream activating sequence
　　uterine arteriosclerosis
UASA
　　upper airways sleep apnea
UAT
　　up [out of bed] as tolerated
UAU
　　uterine activity unit
UAVC
　　univentricular atrioventricular
　　connection
UB
　　ultimobranchial body [embryology]
　　Unna boot

　　upper back
　　urinary bladder
ub
　　urinary bladder channel [acupuncture]
UBA
　　undenatured bacterial antigen
　　urethral bulking agent
UBB
　　unconjugated benign bilirubinemia
UBBC
　　unsaturated [vitamin] B_{12}-binding
　　capacity
UBC
　　University of British Columbia [brace]
　　unsaturated binding capacity
UBD
　　universal blood donor
UBE
　　uniaxial balance evaluation
　　upper body ergometer
UbetaCF
　　urinary beta-core fragment
UBF
　　unknown black female
　　uterine blood flow
U-BFP
　　urinary basic fetoprotein
UBG
　　ultimobranchial gland [embryology,
　　fish]
　　urobilinogen
UBI
　　ultraviolet blood irradiation
ubiq
　　ubiquitin
UBIS
　　ultrasound bone imaging sonometer
UBL
　　undifferentiated B-cell lymphoma
UBM
　　ultrasound backscatter microscopy
　　ultrasound biomicroscopy
　　unknown black male
　　urothelial basement membrane
UBO
　　undetermined brain opacity
　　unidentified bright object
UBP
　　universal bone plate
　　ureteral back pressure
UBPS
　　ultrasound bone profile score
UBS
　　unidentified bright signal [MRI]
UBT
　　urea breath test
　　uterine balloon therapy
UBW
　　usual body weight

UC
ulcerative colitis
Uldall [vasuclar access] catheter
ultracentrifugal
umbilical cholesterol
umbilical cord
unchanged
unclassifiable
unconscious (*See also* UCS)
undifferentiated carcinoma
undifferentiated cells
unfixed cryostat
unsatisfactory condition
untreated cell
urea clearance (*See also* UCL)
urethral (urinary) catheter(ization)
urine concentrate
urine culture (*See also* UCX)
usual care
uterine contraction

U:C
umbilical artery to middle cerebral
artery [pulsatility index ratio]

U&C
urethral and cervical [cultures]
usual and customary

UCA
ultrasound contrast agent
unicystic ameloblastoma

UcA
urothelial carcinoma

UCAC
uterine cornual access catheter

UCAD
unstable coronary artery disease

U$_{Ca}$V
urinary calcium volume [excretion rate]

UCB
umbilical cord blood
unconjugated bilirubin (*See also* UCBR)
Unicorn Campbell Boy [orthotics]
unilateral calcaneal brace

UCBC
umbilical cord blood culture

UCBL
University of California, Berkeley
Laboratory

UCBR
unconjugated bilirubin (*See also* UCB)

UCBT
unrelated cord-blood transplant(ation)

UCC
urgent care center

UCD
urine collection device
usual childhood diseases (*See also*
UCHD, UDC)

UCE
upper completely edentulous
urea cycle enzymopathy

U-cell
undefined cell

UCF
unexplained chronic fatigue

UCG
ultrasonic cardiograph(y) (cardiogram)
urine (urinary) chorionic gonadotropin

UCHD
usual childhood diseases (*See also*
UCD, UDC)

UCHI
usual childhood illnesses (*See also*
UCI)

UCHS
uncontrolled hemorrhagic shock

UCI
umbilical coiling index
University of California, Irvine
urethral (urinary) catheter in
usual childhood illnesses (*See also*
UCHI)

UCL
ulnar collateral ligament
uncomfortable listening (loudness) level
(*See also* UCLL, ULL)
upper collateral ligament
upper confidence limit
urea clearance (*See also* UC)

UCLA
University of California, Los Angeles

UCLC
ulnar collateral ligament complex

UCLL
uncomfortable listening (loudness) level
(*See also* UCL, ULL)

UCLP
unilateral cleft of lip and palate

UCN
undifferentiated carcinoma of
nasopharynx

UCO
ultrasonic cardiac output
urethral catheter out
urinary catheter out

UCOD
underlying cause of death

UCP
ultrasound catheter probe
umbilical cord prolapse
uncoupling protein
urethral closure pressure
urinary coproporphyrin
urinary C-peptide
urine collection pad

U

UCP1–UCP3
uncoupling protein 1–3
UCPP
urethral closure pressure profile
UCPT
urinary coproporphyrin test
UCR
unconditioned reflex (response) (*See also* UR)
usual, customary, and reasonable [fees]
Ucr
urine creatinine (*See also* UCRE)
UCRE
urine creatinine (*See also* Ucr)
UCRP
Universal Control Reference Plasma
UCS
unconditioned stimulus (*See also* UnCS, unCS, UnS, US)
unconscious (*See also* UC)
unicoronal synostosis
uterine compression syndrome
UC&S
urine culture and sensitivity
UCT
ultrasound computed tomography
unchanged conventional treatment
UCTD
unclassifiable connective tissue disease
undifferentiated connective tissue disease
UCTS
undifferentiated connective tissue syndrome
UCV
uncontrolled variable
unconventional viral [disease, infection]
UCVA
uncorrected visual acuity
UCX
urine culture (*See also* UC)
UD
ulcerative dermatosis
ulnar deviation
underdeveloped
undesirable discharge [military]
undetermined
unipolar depression
unit dose
urethral dilatation
urethral discharge
urodynamics
uroporphyrinogen decarboxylase
uterine delivery
uterine distention
uterus delivery
UDA
under direct vision

UD-BMT
unrelated donor bone marrow transplant(ation)
UDC
uninhibited detrusor [muscle] capacity
ursodeoxycholate
usual diseases of childhood (*See also* UCD, UCHD)
UDCA
ursodeoxycholic acid (*See also* URSO)
UDE
undetermined etiology
user defined edge [aortic tomography]
UDG
uracil deoxyribonucleic acid (DNA) glycosylase
UDI
urinary diagnostic index
Urogenital Distress Inventory
UDIR
underdose [to] isodose range [radiation]
UDMA
urethane dimethacrylate
UDN
ulcerative dermal necrosis
updraft nebulizer
UDO
undetermined origin
UDP
unassisted diastolic pressure
uridine diphosphate (uridine 5'-diphosphate)
urine drug panel
UDPG, UDPGlc
uridine diphosphoglucose
UDPGA, UDP-GlcUA
uridine diphosphoglucuronic acid
UDPGal
uridine diphosphogalactose
UDPGT
uridine diphosphate glucuronosyltransferase
uridine diphosphoglucuronyl transferase
UdR
uracil deoxyriboside (deoxyuridine)
UDR-BMD
ultradistal radius bone mineral density
UDRP
urine diribose phosphate
UDS
ultra–Doppler sonography
ultrasound Doppler sonography
unscheduled deoxyribonucleic acid synthesis
urine drug screen
UDSTSS
ultradelicate split-thickness scalp skin [graft]

UDT
　undescended testicle
UE
　Ulex europaeus
　uncertain etiology
　under elbow
　undetermined etiology
　uninvolved epidermis
　upper esophagus
　upper extremity
U&E
　urea and electrolytes [test]
uE3
　unconjugated estriol [test]
UEA
　upper extremity arterial
UEA-1
　Ulex europaeus agglutinin 1
UEBW
　ultrasound-estimated bladder weight
UEC
　uterine endometrial carcinoma
UED
　unilateral epileptiform discharge
UEG
　ultrasonic encephalography
　unifocal eosinophilic granuloma
UEM
　universal electron microscope
UEMC
　unidentified endosteal marrow cell
UEP
　urinary excretion of protein
UER
　unaided equalization reference
UES
　undifferentiated embryonal sarcoma
　Unpleasant Events Schedule
　upper esophageal sphincter
UESEP
　upper extremity somatosensory evoked
　　potential
UESL
　undifferentiated embryonal sarcoma of
　　liver
UESP
　upper esophageal sphincter pressure
UESR
　upper esophageal sphincter relaxation
UEVT
　upper extremity venous thrombosis
u/ext
　upper extremity
UF
　ulcerating form
　ultrafiltrable (ultrafiltrate) (ultrafiltration)
　ultrafine

　ultrasonic frequency
　unaffected female
　uncertainty factor
　unflexed
　universal feeder
　unknown factor
　until finished
　urea formaldehyde
UFA
　unesterified fatty acid
UFB
　urinary fat bodies
UFC
　urinary (urine) free cortisol
UFCT
　ultrafast computed tomography
UFD
　ultrasonic flow detector
　unilateral facet dislocation
UFE
　uniform food encoding
　uterine fibroid embolization
UFF
　unusual facial features
UFFI
　urea formaldehyde foam insulation
UFH
　unfractionated heparin
UFISH
　ultrasensitive fluorescence in situ
　　hybridization
UFN
　until further notice
UFO
　unflagged order
　unidentified flying (foreign) object
　universal plantar fasciitis orthotic
UFOS
　universal frame outer socket
UFOV
　useful field of view
UFR
　ultrafiltration rate
　urine filtration rate
　uroflowmetry
UFS
　unilateral facial spasm
uFSH
　urinary follicle-stimulating hormone
UFT
　unified field theory
UFV
　ultrafiltration volume
　unclassified fecal virus
UG
　until gone
　urinary glucose

U

UG *(continued)*
urogastrone
urogenital *(See also* URO-GEN)
uteroglobulin

UGA
under general anesthesia
urogenital atrophy

UGCR
ultrasound-guided compression repair

UGD
urogenital diaphragm

UGF
unidentified growth factor
urinary gonadotropin fragment

UGH
uveitis, glaucoma, hyphema [syndrome]

UGH+
uveitis, glaucoma, hyphema plus
[vitreous hemorrhage]

UGI
upper gastrointestinal [tract, series]
(See also UGIT, UGIS)

UGIB
upper gastrointestinal bleeding

UGIE
upper gastrointestinal endoscopy

UGIH
upper gastrointestinal [tract]
hemorrhage

UGIS
upper gastrointestinal series *(See also*
UGI)

UGIT
upper gastrointestinal tract *(See also*
UGI)

UGI w/SBFT
upper gastrointestinal [series] with
small-bowel follow-through

UGK
urine glucose [and] ketone

UGNB
ultrasonically guided needle biopsy

UGP
urinary gonadotropin peptide

UGPP
uridyl diphosphate glucose
pyrophosphorylase

UGS
urogenital sinus

UGSV
Uganda S virus

UGTI
ultrasound-guided thrombin
injection

UGVA
ultrasound-guided vascular access

UH
umbilical hernia
unaffected hemisphere

uncontrolled hemorrhage
unfavorable history
upper half

U24H
24 hour urine

UHBI
upper hemibody irradiation

UHC
ultrahigh carbon

UHD
ulcer-healing drug
unstable hemoglobin disease

UHDDS
Uniform Hospital Discharge Data
Set

UHDRS
Unified Huntington Disease Rating
Scale

UHF
ultrahigh frequency

u-hFSH
urinary-derived human
follicle-stimulating hormone

UHFV
ultrahigh-frequency ventilation

UHL
universal hypertrichosis lanuginosa

UHMM
ultrahigh magnification mammography

UHMW
ultrahigh molecular weight

UHMWPE, UHMWPe
ultrahigh molecular weight
polyethylene

UHP
University Health Plan

UHR
underlying heart rhythm
universal head replacement

UHS
uncontrolled hemorrhagic shock

UHT
ultrahigh temperature

UHV
ultrahigh vacuum
ultrahigh voltage

UI
Ulcer Index
urethral inclination
urinary incontinence
uroporphyrin isomerase
uteroplacental insufficiency

U/I
unidentified

UIB
Unemployment Insurance Benefits

UIBC
unbound iron-binding capacity
unsaturated iron-binding capacity

UICC
Union Internationale Contre le Cancer
[International Union Against Cancer]
UID
unilateral interfacetal dislocation
UID/S
unilateral interfacetal dislocation or
subluxation
UIEP
urine immunoelectrophoresis
UIF
undegraded insulin factor
UIFE
urine immunofixation electrophoresis
UIP
unintended pregnancy
usual interstitial pneumonia
[of Liebow]
UIQ
upper inner quadrant
UIS
Utilization Information Service
UJ
uncovertebral joint
universal joint [syndrome]
UJT
unijunction transistor
UK
United Kingdom
unknown (See also U)
urine potassium
urokinase
UKA
unicompartmental knee arthroplasty
UKa
urinary kallikrein
UKE
unknown etiology
UK IC
urokinase intracoronary
UKM
urea kinetic modeling
UKNDS
United Kingdom Neurological Disability
Score
UKO
unknown origin
UKT
urine ketone testing
UKTSSA
United Kingdom Transplant Support
Service Authority
U$_k$V
urinary potassium volume [excretion
rate]
UL
unauthorized leave
undifferentiated lymphoma

upper left
upper lid
upper limb
upper limit
upper lobe
urethral length
utterance length
⚠ **U/L**
unit per liter ⚠
upper and lower (See also U&L)
U&L
upper and lower (See also U/L)
U:L
upper [body segment] to lower [body
segment] ratio
ULA
undedicated logic array
ULBW
ultralow birth weight
ULDH
urinary lactate dehydrogenase
ULDR
ultralow dose rate
ULE
unilateral laterothoracic
exanthem
ULF
ultralow frequency
uLH
urinary luteinizing hormone
ULL
ultra-lipo-lift
uncomfortable listening (loudness) level
(See also UCL, UCLC)
ULLE
upper lid left eye
ULM
unprotected left main
ULMS
uterine leiomyosarcoma
ULN
upper limits of normal
uln
ulna(r) (See also U)
ULO
upper limb orthosis
ULP
ultralow profile
upper lid ptosis
upper limb prosthesis
ULPA
ultralow particulate air
ULPE
upper lobe pulmonary edema
ULQ
upper left quadrant
ULRE
upper lid right eye

U

ULSB
upper left sternal border
ULT
ultralow temperature
ult
ultimate(ly)
ULTT
upper limb tension test
ULTT1
upper limb tension test 1 [median nerve]
ULTT2a
upper limb tension test 2a [medial nerve]
ULTT2b
upper limb tension test 2b [radial nerve]
ULTT3
upper limb tension test 3 [ulnar nerve]
ULV
ultralow volume
ULYTES
urine electrolytes
UM
unmarried
upper motor [neuron]
uterine monitor
Utilization Management
UMA
upright membrane assay
urinary muramidase activity
UMAV
Umatilla virus
Umax
maximal urinary osmolality
UMB, umb
umbilical
umbilicus
umb A line
umbilical artery line (See also UV)
UMBV
Umbre virus
umb ven
umbilical vein (See also UV)
umb V line
umbilical vein (venous) line (See also UVL)
UMCD
uremic medullary cystic disease
UMCL
upper midclavicular line
UMCV-TO
ulnar motor conduction velocity [across] thoracic outlet
$U_{Mg}V$
urinary magnesium volume [excretion rate]

UMI
urinary meconium index
uterine manipulator/injector
UMLS
Unified Medical Language System
UMN
upper motor neuron
UMNB
upper motor neurogenic bladder
UMNL
upper motor neuron lesion
UMNS
upper motor neuron syndrome
UMP
undetermined malignant potential
uridine monophosphate (uridine 5′-monophosphate) [uridylic acid]
UMPK
uridine monophosphate kinase
UMRI
ultrafast magnetic resonance imaging
UMS
upper [fossa active], medial [knee pain], and short [leg on side ipsilateral to weak fossa]
urethral manipulation syndrome
UMT
unit of medical time
UN
ulnar nerve
undernourished
unilateral neglect
updraft nebulizer
urea nitrogen
urinary nitrogen
UNA
urinary nitrogen appearance
U_{Na}, **UNa**
urinary sodium
unacc, unaccomp
unaccompanied
unaff
unaffected
UNAIDS
Joint United Nations Programme on HIV/AIDS
UNAV
Una virus
UNaV
urinary sodium voided [excretion]
UNC
uncrossed
urine net charge
UNCB
ultrasound-guided needle core biopsy
uncomp
uncompensated
uncomplicated

uncond
  unconditioned
uncor
  uncorrected
UnCS, unCS
  unconditioned stimulus (*See also* UCS, UnS, US)
UNCV
  ulnar nerve conduction velocity
UNCVA
  uncorrected visual acuity
UNDEL
  undelivered
undet
  undetermined
undiff
  undifferentiated
UNE
  ulnar neuropathy [at the] elbow
  unopposed estrogen
  urinary norepinephrine
UNG
  uracil-N-glycosylase
ung
  ointment [apothecary]
U$_{NH4}$-
  urinary ammonia
UNHS, UNHSP
  Universal Neonatal (Newborn) Hearing Screening
UNID
  unidentified
unilat
  unilateral
univ
  universal
UNK, unk, unkn
  unknown
UNL
  upper normal limit
unoff
  unofficial
UNOS
  United Network for Organ Sharing
UN/P
  unpatched [eye]
UNPC
  undifferentiated nasopharyngeal carcinoma
⚠ **UN/P OD**
  unpatched right eye ⚠
⚠ **UN/P OS**
  unpatched left eye ⚠
UNS, uns
  unsatisfactory (*See also* unsat)
  unsymmetrical (*See also* unsym)

UnS
  unconditioned stimulus (*See also* UCS, UnCS, unCS, US)
unsat
  unsatisfactory (*See also* UNS, uns)
  unsaturated
unsym
  unsymmetrical (*See also* UNS)
UNTS
  unilateral nevoid telangiectasia syndrome
UNX
  uninephrectomy
UO
  under observation
  undetermined origin
  ureteral orifice
  urinary output (*See also* UOP)
UOAC
  uterine ostial access catheter
UONP
  unilateral oculomotor nerve paralysis
UONx
  unilateral optic nerve transection
UOP
  urinary output (*See also* UO)
UOQ
  upper outer quadrant
UOR
  unusual occurrence report
UOS
  undifferentiated osteosarcoma
UOsm, Uosm
  urinary osmolality
UOV
  unit of variance
UOZ
  upper outer zone [quadrant]
UP
  ulcerative proctitis
  ultrahigh purity
  uniformly positive
  unipolar
  Unna-Pappenheim [stain]
  upright posture
  ureteropelvic
  uridine phosphorylase
  uroporphyrin
  uteroplacental
UPI
  uroplakin I
UPII
  uroplakin II
UPIII
  uroplakin III

U

U/P
up [out of bed] as desired [up + L. *ad libitum*] (*See also* UAL)

U:P
urine to plasma ratio

UPA
unpressurized aerosol
uteroplacental apoplexy

uPA, u-PA
urokinase plasminogen activator

uPAR
urokinase plasminogen activator receptor (response)

UPC
unknown primary carcinoma
usual provider continuity

UPD
uniparental disomy
upper partial denture
urinary production [rate]

UPDRS
Unified Parkinson Disease Rating Scale

UPE
upper partially edentulous

UPEC
uropathogenic *Escherichia coli*

UPEP
urinary (urine) protein electrophoresis

UPF
universal proximal femur [prosthesis]

UPG
uroporphyrinogen

UPI
uteroplacental insufficiency
uteroplacental ischemia

UPIN
unique physician (provider) identification number

UPJ
ureteropelvic junction

UPJO
ureteropelvic junction obstruction

UPL
unusual position of limbs

UPLIF
unilateral posterior lumbar interbody fusion

UPLIFT
uterine positioning via ligament investment fixation and truncation

UPN
unique patient number

UPO
[metastatic carcinoma of] unknown primary origin

UPOC
Ultramatic Project-O-Chart projector

UPOR
usual place of residence

UPOV
Upolu virus

UPP
urethral pressure profile (profilometry)
uteroplacental profilometry
uvulopalatoplasty

UPPP
uvulopalatopharyngoplasty

UPPRA
upright peripheral plasma renin activity

UPRBC
unit of packed red blood cells

UPS
ubiquitin-dependent proteosomal system
ultraviolet photoelectron spectroscopy
uroporphyrinogen synthase
uterine progesterone system

UPSC
uterine papillary serous carcinoma

Y
upsilon [20th letter of Greek alphabet uppercase]

υ
kinematic viscosity (*See also* v)
upsilon [20th letter of Greek alphabet lowercase]

UPSIT
University of Pennsylvania Smell Identification Test

UPT
Up-Converting Phosphor technology [immunoassay]
uptake
urine pregnancy test
uveoparotitis

UQ
ubiquinone
upper quadrant

UQS
upper quadrant syndrome

UR
unconditioned reflex (response) (*See also* UCR)
unrelated
upper respiratory
upper right
uptake ratio
urinal
urinary retention
urine (*See also* U)
urology
utilization review

URA, Ura
unilateral renal agenesis
uracil (*See also* U)
urethral resistance factor

UR AC, URC-A
uric acid (*See also* UA, URIC A)

ur anal
urine analysis (urinalysis) (*See also* UA)
URAS
unilateral renal artery stenosis
URC
upper respiratory condition
upper rib cage
utilization review committee
URC SP
uric acid spot [test]
URD
undifferentiated respiratory disease
unrelated donor
unspecified respiratory disease
upper respiratory disease
Urd
uridine (*See also* U)
UREA-S
urea nitrogen spot [test]
URED
unable to read (lab result)
URES
University Residence Environment
Scale
ureth
urethra (*See also* U, UA)
URF
unidentified reading frame
uterine-relaxing factor
UR-FST
urine-fasting
urg
urgent
UR HR
urine [number of] hours [glucose
tolerance]
URI
upper respiratory [tract] infection
(illness)
URIC A
uric acid (*See also* UA, UR AC,
URC-A)
URIN
random urine
URL
upper rate limit [pacemaker]
url
unrelated
UR&M
urinalysis, routine and microscopic
URO
upper respiratory obstruction
urology (*See also* Urol)
uroporphyrin
uroporphyrinogen
UROB, UROBIL
urobilinogen

UROD
ultra-rapid opiate detoxification [under
anesthesia]
uroporphyrinogen decarboxylase
URO-GEN
urogenital (*See also* UG)
URO-2H
urobilinogen—2 hours
Urol
urology (*See also* URO)
UROS
uroporphyrinogen synthetase
U-RPFA
Ultegra rapid platelet function assay
URQ
upper right quadrant (of abdomen)
URR
upstream regulatory region
urea reduction ratio
URS
transurethral ureterorenoscopy
ultrasonic renal scan(ning)
urologic surgery
URSB
upper right sternal border
URSO
ursodeoxycholic (acid) (*See also* UDCA)
UR2SV
avian sarcoma virus UR2
URSx
upper respiratory [tract] symptom
URT
upper respiratory tract
uterine resting tone
URTI
upper respiratory tract illness (infection)
UR-TIM
urine-time
URUV
Urucuri virus
URVD
unilateral renovascular disease
UR VOL
urine volume
US
ultrasonic
ultrasonograph(y)
ultrasound
unconditioned stimulus (*See also* UCS,
UnCS, unCS)
upper segment
urinary sugar
urine specimen
U.S.
United States
USA
unilateral spatial agnosia
unstable angina

U

USAMRIID
United States Army Medical Research Institute of Infectious Diseases

USAN
United States Adopted Names [generic drugs, USP]

USAP
unstable angina pectoris (*See also* UAP)

USAS
uncomplicated supraclavicular aortic stenosis

USB
upper sternal border

USC
uterine serous carcinoma

US-CNB, USCNB
ultrasound-guided (ultrasonographically guided) core-needle biopsy

U-SCOPE
ureteroscopy

USCT
ultrasound computed tomography

USCVD
unsterile controlled vaginal delivery

USE
ultrasonic echography

US-FNAB
ultrasound-guided fine-needle aspiration biopsy

USG
ultrasonograph(y) (ultrasonogram)
urine specific gravity

USH
United Services for Handicapped
usual state of health (*See also* USOH)

USI
universal salt iodization
urinary stress incontinence

USL
ultrasound lithotripsy

US:LS
upper strength to lower strength ratio

USM
ultrasonic mist

USN
ultrasonic nebulizer
unilateral spatial neglect

USO
unilateral salpingo-oophorectomy

USOGH
usual state of good health

USOH
usual state of health (*See also* USH)

USP
unassisted systolic pressure
United States Pharmacopeia
uterine-stimulating potency

USPDI
United States Pharmacopeia Drug Information

USPHS
United States Public Health Service

USPI
ulnar styloid process index

USPIO
ultrasmall-particle superparamagnetic iron oxide

USR
unheated serum reagin

USRDS
United States Renal Data System

USS
ultrasound scan(ning)
Universal Spine System

UST
upper single tooth

USUCVD
unsterile uncontrolled vaginal delivery

USUV
Usutu virus

USVMD
urine specimen volume measuring device

USVMS
urine specimen volume measuring system

USW
ultrashort wave

UT
unrelated [children raised] together
untested
untreated
upper thoracic
upper trapezius [muscle]
urea transporter
urethral thickness
urinary tract
urticaria

uT
unbound testosterone

ut
uterus

UTA
urinary tract anomaly

U$_{TA}$
urinary titrable acidity

UTBG
unbound thyroxine-binding globulin

UTC
urinary tract calculus

UTD
unable to determine
up to date

UTE
ultrashort echo time

UTF
　usual throat flora
UTI
　urinary tract infection
　urinary trypsin inhibitor
UTIV
　Utinga virus
UTJ
　uterotubal junction
UTL
　unable to locate
UTLD
　Utah Test of Language
　　Development
UTM
　urinary tract malformation
UTO
　unable to obtain
　upper tibial osteotomy
　urinary tract obstruction
UTP
　unilateral tension pneumothorax
　uridine triphosphate (uridine
　　5′-triphosphate)
UTPC
　usual type papillary carcinoma
UTR
　untranslated region
UTROSCT
　uterine tumor resembling an ovarian
　　sex-cord tumor
UTS
　ulnar tunnel syndrome
　ultimate tensile strength
　ultrasound (*See also* US, UTZ)
UTTS
　ultrathin-walled two-stage [catheter]
UTY
　ubiquitously transcribed
　　tetratricopeptide
UTZ
　ultrasound (*See also* US, UTS)
UU
　urinary urea (*See also* UREA)
　urine urobilinogen
U/U
　uterine fundus at umbilicus
U/U+
　uterine fundus above umbilicus [number
　　of fingerbreadths]
U/U−
　uterine fundus below umbilicus [number
　　of fingerbreadths]
UUD
　uncontrolled unsterile delivery
UUKV
　Uukuniemi virus

UUN
　urinary urea nitrogen excretion
　urine urea nitrogen
UUO
　unilateral ureteral obstruction
　　(occlusion)
UUP
　urine uroporphyrin
U UREA
　urinary [concentration of] urea (*See also*
　　UU)
UUT
　unsustained ventricular tachycardia
UUTI
　uncomplicated urinary tract
　　infection
UV
　ultraviolet [light] (*See also* UVL)
　umbilical vein (*See also* umb ven)
　ureterovesical
　urine volume
UVA
　ultraviolet A [long wavelength]
　ureterovesical angle
　urethrovesical angle
UVAC
　uterine vacuum aspirating curette
UVB
　ultraviolet B [midrange
　　wavelength]
UVC
　ultraviolet C [short wavelength]
　umbilical vein (venous) catheter
UVCP
　unilateral vocal cord paralysis
UVEB
　unifocal ventricular ectopic beat
UVER
　ultraviolet-enhanced reactivation
UVGI
　ultraviolet germicidal irradiation
UVH
　univentricular heart
UVI
　ultraviolet irradiation
uVIB
　ultraviolet irradiation of blood
UVJ
　ureterovesical junction
UVL
　ultraviolet light (*See also* UV)
　umbilical vein (venous) line (*See also*
　　umb V line)
UVM
　universal ventilation meter
UV/MV
　umbilical vein to maternal vein

U

UVP
ultraviolet photometry
UVPP
uvulopalatopharyngoplasty
UVR
ultraviolet radiation
UV-VIS
ultraviolet-visible [spectrometer]
UW
unilateral weakness
University of Wisconsin [solution]
UWB
unit of whole blood
UWCDot
University of Waterloo Colored Dot
Test
UWF
unknown white female

UWL
unstirred water layer
UWM
unknown white male
unwed mother
UWS
underwater seal [drainage]
UWSC
unstimulated whole saliva
collection
UWW
underwater weight
UX
uranium X (proactinium)
UXO
unexploded ordnance
UYP
upper yield point

V

 unipolar chest lead
 vaccinate(d) (vaccination) (*See also*
  VAcc)
 vaccine (*See also* vac)
 vagina (*See also* VAG, Vag, vag)
 valine (*See also* Val)
 valve (*See also* val)
 vanadium [element]
 variable (*See also* var)
 variation (*See also* var)
 varnish
 vector (*See also* vect)
 vegetarian
 vegetation (*See also* VEG)
 velocity (*See also* vel, veloc)
 venous [blood] (*See also* VB)
 venous tumor invasion [TNM
  classification]
 ventilation (*See also* V̇, VE, vent)
 ventral (*See also* vent)
 ventricle (*See also* vent, ventric)
 ventricular [fibrillation or wave]
  (*See also* vent, ventric)
 venule
 verb
 verbal [comprehension factor] (*See also*
  V factor)
 vertebra(l) (*See also* vert)
 vertex (*See also* VE, VTX, Vx)
 vertex sharp transient
  [electroencephalography]
 Viagra [as in vitamin V]
 Vibrio (*See also* Vib)
 violet
 viral (*See also* VIR)
 virulence (*See also* VI)
 vision (*See also* VIS, vsn)
 visual acuity (*See also* VA)
 visual capacity (*See also* VC)
 voice
 volt(age) (*See also* V)
 volume (*See also* vol)
 vomit(ing) (*See also* vom)

V

 voltage [electrical potential difference]
  (*See also* V)

V0

 no evidence of venous invasion [TNM
  classification]

V1

 primary visual area
 venous [tumor] invasion [TNM
  classification]

V₁-V₆

 precordial chest leads

V4

 fourth ventricle

V̇

 gas volume per unit of time [gas flow]
 ventilation

+V

 positive vertical divergence (*See also*
  +VD)

v

 rate of reaction catalyzed by an
  enzyme
 specific volume
 vena (vein) [singular]

v̄

 mixed venous [blood]

v-

 vicinal isomer

VA

 alveolar ventilation (*See also* V$_A$)
 alveolar volume (*See also* V$_A$)
 vacuum aspiration
 valeric acid
 variant angina
 vasodilator agent
 venoarterial
 ventricular aneurysm
 ventricular arrhythmia
 ventriculoatrial
 ventroanterior
 vertebral artery
 Veterans Administration [U.S.
  Department of Veterans Affairs]
 Veterans Administration [hospital]
 viral antigen
 virtual angioscopy
 visual activity
 visual acuity (*See also* V)
 visual aid
 visual axis
 volcanic ash
 volt-ampere
 volume, alveolar [gas] (*See also* V$_A$)
 volume averaging

V&A

 vagotomy and antrectomy

V$_A$

 alveolar ventilation (*See also* VA)
 volume of alveolar gas (*See also* VA)

Va

 volume arterial gas

VAA

 verbal-auditory agnosia

VAAESS
Vaccine-Associated Adverse Events Surveillance Systems [Canada] [obsolete, see CAEFISS]

VAB
vacuum-assisted [breast] biopsy
variable atrial blockage
violent antisocial behavior

VABES
vasoablative endothelial sarcoma

VABP
venoarterial bypass pumping

VABS
Vineland Adaptive Behavior Scales [Revised]

VAC
vacuum-assisted closure [dressing]
ventriculoarterial connection
ventriculoatrial condition
ventriculoatrial conduction

V-AC
volume-assist control

vac
vaccine (*See also* V)
vacuum

VACA
valvuloplasty and angioplasty of congenital anomalies

VacA
vacuolating toxin gene A

VACB
vacuum-assisted core biopsy

VA cc, Va_cc, VA ccl
[distance] visual acuity with correction

vacc
vaccinate(d) (vaccination)

VAC EXT
vacuum extractor

VACIg
vaccinia immune globulin

VACTERL
vertebral, anal, cardiac, tracheal, esophageal, renal, limb [abnormalities, anomalies]

VACV
vaccinia virus

VAD
vascular (venous) access device
vascular access dressing
ventricular assist device
vertebral artery dissection
virus-adjusting diluent
vitamin A deficiency

VaD
vascular dementia

VADCS
ventricular atrial distal coronary sinus

VADD
vitamin A deficiency disorder

VADS
Visual Aural Digit Span Test

VAE
venous air embolism

V_Aeff
effective alveolar ventilation

VA-EMCO
venoarterial extracorporeal membrane oxygenation

VAER
visual auditory evoked response

VAERS
Vaccine Adverse Events Reporting System [CDC and FDA]

VAF
visceral abdominal fat

VAFD
vascular access flush device

VAG, Vag, vag
vagina (*See also* V)
vaginal (*See also* V)
vascular access graft

VAg
visual agnosia

VAG HYST
vaginal hysterectomy (*See also* VH)

VAH
vertebral ankylosing hyperostosis
virilizing adrenal hyperplasia

VAHBE
ventricular atrial His bundle electrocardiogram

VAHRA
ventricular atrial height right atrium

VAHS
virus-associated hemophagocytic syndrome

VAI
vertebral artery injury

VAIN
vaginal intraepithelial neoplasia (neoplasm)

VAK
vestibuloauditory keratitis

VAKT
visual, association, kinesthetic, tactile (reading)

Val
valine (*See also* V)

val
valve (*See also* V)

VALE
visual acuity, left eye (*See also* VAOS)

VALI
ventilator-associated lung injury

VAM
ventricular arrhythmia monitor

VAMP
 venous/arterial [blood] management
  protection
 vesicle-associated membrane protein
VAMS
 Visual Analogue Mood Scale
VAN
 vein, artery, nerve
 ventricular aneurysmectomy
⚠ **VAOD**
 visual acuity, right eye ⚠
⚠ **VAOS**
 visual acuity, left eye (*See also*
  VALE) ⚠
⚠ **VA OS LP with P**
 visual acuity, left eye, left perception
  with projection ⚠
VAP
 average path velocity
 vaginal acid phosphatase
 variant angina pectoris
 vascular (venous) access port
 ventilator-associated pneumonia
vap
 vapor
VAPC
 Veterans Administration Prosthetic
  Center
VAPCS
 ventricular atrial proximal coronary
  sinus
VAPP
 vaccine-associated paralytic
  polio(myelitis)
VAPS
 visual analog pain score
 volume-assured pressure support
VAR
 varicella [chickenpox, varicella zoster
  virus] vaccine
 visual auditory range
var
 variable (*See also* V)
 variant
 variation (*See also* V)
 variety
 various
VARE
 visual acuity, right eye
VARIg
 varicella-zoster immune globulin
VARPRO
 variable projection [method]
VARV
 variola virus
VAS
 vagus nerve stimulation

 variable-angle spinning
 vascular (*See also* vasc)
 vasculotropin
 vasectomy (*See also* vas)
 ventriculoatrial shunt
 vesicle attachment site
 vestibular aqueduct syndrome
 vibratory acoustic stimulation
 vibroacoustic stimulation
 viral arthritis syndrome
 visual analog scale
vas
 vasectomy (*See also* VAS)
VASC
 Verbal Auditory Screen for Children
 Visual Auditory Screen for Children
VA sc, VA scl
 [distance] visual acuity without
  correction
vasc
 vascular (*See also* VAS)
VASER
 Vibration of Amplification of Sound
  Energy at Resonance
vasodil
 vasodilation (*See also* VD)
 vasodilator (*See also* VD)
VASPI
 Visual Analogue Self Assessment Scales
  For Pain Intensity
VAS RAD
 vascular radiology
VAT
 variable antigen type
 vasoocclusive angiotherapy
 ventilatory anaerobic threshold
 ventricular accommodation test
 ventricular activation time
 ventricular [pacing], atrial [sensing],
  triggered [mode, pacemaker]
 vertebral artery test
 vestibular autorotational (autorotation)
  testing
 video-assisted thoracoscopy (*See also*
  VATS)
 visceral adipose tissue
 visual action time
 visual apperception test
 Vocational Apperception Test
VATER
 vertebral [abnormality], anal
  [imperforation], tracheoesophageal
  [fistula], and radial, ray, or renal
  [anomalies or dysplasia]
VATS
 video-assisted thoracic surgery
 video-assisted thoracoscopic surgery

V

VATS *(continued)*
video-assisted thoracoscopy *(See also VAT)*
video-assisted transthoracic surgery
VATs
variable antigen, surface
VAF:TAF
visceral abdominal fat to total abdominal fat ratio
VAT:TAT
visceral adipose tissue to total adipose tissue ratio
VAV
variable air volume
VAVD
vacuum-assisted vaginal delivery
vacuum-assisted venous drainage
VAX-D
vertebral axial decompression
VB
vagina bulbi
vaginal bleeding
valence bond
Van Buren [catheter]
venous blood *(See also V)*
ventrobasal
Veronal buffer
vertebrobasilar
viable birth
virtual bronchoscopy
voided bladder
VB1–VB3
first, second, and third midstream voided [bladder specimen]
VBAC
vaginal birth after cesarean [section]
VBAC-TOL
vaginal birth after cesarean—trial of labor
VBAI, VBAIN
vertebrobasilar artery insufficiency
VBD
vanishing bile duct [syndrome] *(See also VBDS)*
Veronal-buffered diluent
VBDS
vanishing bile duct syndrome *(See also VBD)*
VBEF
vanB phenotype *Enterococcus faecium*
VBG
vagotomy and Billroth gastroenterostomy
vascularized bone graft
venoaortocoronary artery bypass graft
venous blood gas
venous bypass graft
Veronal-buffered [serum with] gelatin

vertical banded gastroplasty *(See also VBGP)*
VBGP
vertical-banded gastroplasty *(See also VBG)*
VBH
Vogele-Bale-Hohner [mouthpiece]
VBI
vertebrobasilar insufficiency
vertebrobasilar ischemia
VBIO
Video Binocular indirect ophthalmoscope
VBM
vertebral bone mass
vBMD
volumetric bone mineral density
VBMT
vascularized bone marrow transplant(ation)
VBOS
Veronal-buffered oxalated saline
VBP
venous blood pressure
VBR
ventricle to brain ratio
VBS
venous blood sample
Veronal-buffered saline
vertebrobasilar [artery] system
videofluoroscopic barium swallow [evaluation]
VBS:FBS
Veronal-buffered saline to fetal bovine serum ratio
VBT
vertebral body tenderness
VC
color vision
vaginal candidiasis
variance cardiography
vascular catheterization
vascular change
vasoconstriction
vena cava
venous capacitance
venous capillary
ventilatory capacity
ventral column
ventricular contraction
verbal comprehension
verbal cues
vertebral canal
videocassette
vinyl chloride
virtual colonoscopy
vision, color
visual capacity
visual communication

visual cortex
vital capacity
vocal cord
volume, capillary
volume control
voluntary closing
voluntary control
voluntary cough
vomiting center
vowel-consonant

V:C
ventilation to circulation ratio

V&C
vertical and centric [bite]

Vc, V$_c$
pulmonary capillary [gas] volume
ventrocaudal [nucleus]

VCA
vasoconstrictor assay
vertical-center-anterior [angle]
viral capsid antigen

VCA-EB
viral capsid antigen, Epstein-Barr

VCAM
vascular cell adhesion molecule

VCAM-1
vascular cell adhesion molecule 1

VCB
ventricular capture beat

VCC
vasoconstrictor center
ventral cell column

Vcc
vision with correction

VCCA
velocity, common carotid artery

VC-CFMV
volume-controlled constant flow
mechanical ventilation

VCD
vacuum constriction device
vibrational circular dichroism
vocal cord dysfunction

VCDF
volume-cycled decelerating-flow
ventilation

VCDQ
verbal comprehension deviation
quotient

VCDR
vertical cup to disc ratio

VCE
vagina, ectocervix, endocervix (*See also* VEE)
vaginal, cervical, endocervical [smear]
vein contrast enhancer

V$_{CE}$
velocity of contractile element

VCF
vaginal contraceptive film
velocity of circumferential fiber [shortening] (*See also* V$_{CF}$)
ventricular contractility function
vertebral compression fracture

V$_{CF}$
velocity of circumferential fiber [shortening] (*See also* VCF)

VCFS
velocardiofacial syndrome

VCG
vectorcardiograph(y) (vectorcardiogram)
voiding cystogram
volumetric cardiogram

VCI
volatile corrosion inhibitor

VCIU
voluntary control (of) involuntary
utterances

vCJD
variant Creutzfeldt-Jakob disease

VCL
curvilinear velocity
volar carpal ligament

VCM
vinyl chloride monomer

VCMG
videocystometrography

VCN
vancomycin (hydrochloride),
colistimethate (sodium), nysatatin
[medium]
vestibulocochlear nerve
Vibrio cholerae neuraminidase

VCO, V$_{CO}$
carbon monoxide [endogenous
production]
ventilator-CPAP-oxyhood

VCO$_2$, V$_{CO2}$
venous carbon dioxide [production]
volume, carbon dioxide [elimination]
(*See also* V$_E$CO$_2$)

VCP
vocal cord paralysis

VCR
vasoconstriction rate
video cassette recorder
volume clearance rate

VCS
vaginal cuff smear
vasoconstrictor substance
ventricular conduction system
vesicocervical space
Vocabulary Comprehension Scale

V

VCSA
viral cell surface antigen
VCSF
ventricular cerebrospinal fluid
VCSPS
variable circumference suprapatellar
socket
VCT
venous clotting time
voluntary counseling and testing
VCTS
vitreal corneal touch syndrome
VCU, VCUG
vesicoureterogram
videocystourethrograph(y)
(videocystourethrogram)
voiding cystourethrograph(y)
(cystourethrogram)
VCu
verbal cue
VCV
ventricular conduction velocity
volume-control(led) ventilation
vowel-consonant-vowel
VD
valvular disease
vapor density
vascular disease
vasodilation (*See also* vasodil)
vasodilator (*See also* vasodil)
venereal disease
ventricular dilator
vertical deviation
vessel disease
video densitometry
viral diarrhea
voided
voiding diary
volume of distribution
V&D
vertigo and deafness
vomiting and diarrhea
+VD
positive vertical divergence
V_D
ventilation per minute of dead space
volume of dead space (*See also*
VDS)
V_d
apparent volume of distribution
VDA
vascular-disrupting agent
venous digital angiogram
vertigo, diplopia, ataxia
video dimensional analysis
visual discriminatory acuity
V_DA
ventilation of alveolar dead space
volume of alveolar dead space

VDAC
vaginal delivery after cesarean
voltage-dependent anion channel
V_Dan
ventilation of anatomic dead space
volume of anatomic dead space
VD-auto-SMASH
variable density simultaneous acquisition
of spatial harmonics
VDBR
volume of distribution of bilirubin
VDC
vasodilator center
VDCC
voltage-dependent calcium channel
VDD
atrial synchronous ventricular inhibited
pacing
vitamin D-dependent
VDDR
pseudovitamin D deficiency rickets
vitamin D-dependent rickets
VDDR-I–VDDR-II
vitamin D dependent rickets type I, II
VDE
vasodilatory edema
VDEL
Venereal Disease Experimental
Laboratory
VDEM
vasodepressor material
VDEPT
virus-directed enzyme prodrug therapy
VDF
ventricular diastolic fragmentation
VDG, VD-G
venereal disease, gonorrhea
vdg
voiding
VDH
valvular (vascular) disease of heart
VDI
venous distensibility index
VDJ
variable diversity joining
VDL
vasodepressor lipid
visual detection level
VD or M
venous distention or mass
VDM
vasodepressor material
V_{DM}
volume of mechanical dead space
VDO
varus derotational osteotomy
VDPCA
variable-dose patient-controlled
anesthesia

VDR
venous diameter ratio
vitamin D receptor
volumetric diffusive respirator

V$_D$rb
rebreathing ventilation

VDRE
vitamin D-response element

VDRF
ventilator-dependent respiratory failure

VDRL
Venereal Disease Research Laboratory [test]

VDRR
vitamin D-resistant rickets

VDRS
Verdun Depression Rating Scale

VDRT
venereal disease reference test

VDS, VD-S
variable distance stereoacuity
vasodepressor syncope
vasodilator substance
venereal disease, syphilis
venous duplex scanning
ventral derotating spinal [implant]
ventral derotation spondylodesis
volume of dead space (*See also* V$_D$)

VDT
video display terminal
visual display terminal
visual distortion test

VDTS
video display terminal simulator

VDU
video (visual) display unit

VDV
ventricular (end-)diastolic volume

VD:VT
volume dead-space gas to volume tidal gas ratio

VE
expired volume
NATO code for nerve agent O-ethyl S-[2-(diethylamino)ethyl] ethylphosphonothioate
vacuum extraction
vaginal examination
vasoepididymostomy
Venezuelan encephalitis [virus]
venous emptying
venous extension
ventilation
ventilatory effect
ventricular elasticity
ventricular escape
ventricular extrasystole

vertex
vesicular exanthema
Vietnam era
viral encephalitis
virtual endoscopy
virtual environment
visual efficiency
visual examination
vitamin E
vocational evaluation
volume ejection
voluntary effort

V&E
Vinethine and ether [anesthesia]

V/E
violent [and] eloper

V$_E$
environmental variance
minute ventilation
peak exercise ventilation
respiratory minute volume
[volume] airflow per unit of time
volume of expired gas

VEA
vasopermeation enhancement agent
ventricular ectopic activity
ventricular ectopic arrhythmia
viral envelope antigen
viscoelastic agent

VEB
ventricular ectopic beat
ventricular extra beat

VEC
velocity-encoded cine

VE-cadherin
vascular endothelial cadherin

VECG
vector electrocardiogram

VEC-MR
velocity-encoded cine magnetic resonance

VEC-MRI
velocity-encoded cine magnetic resonance imaging

V$_E$CO$_2$
expired volume of carbon dioxide (*See also* VCO$_2$, V$_{CO_2}$)

VECP
visual-evoked cortical potential
visually evoked cortical potential

vect
vector (*See also* V)

VED
vacuum erection device
vacuum extraction delivery
ventricular ectopic depolarization
vital exhaustion and depression

V

VEDP
ventricular end-diastolic pressure
VEE
vagina, ectocervix, endocervix (*See also* VCE)
Venezuelan equine encephalomyelitis (encephalitis) [virus]
VEEa
Venezuelan equine encephalitis vaccine, attenuated live
V-EEG
vigilance-controlled electroencephalogram
VEEI
Venezuelan equine encephalitis vaccine, inactivated
VEF
ventricular ejection fraction
visually evoked field
VEFR
visually evoked flow response
VEG
vegetations [bacterial]
VEGAS
ventricular enlargement with gait apraxia syndrome
VEGF
vascular endothelial growth factor
VEGF2
vascular endothelial growth factor 2
VEGF-C
vascular endothelial growth factor C
VEGFR3
vascular endothelial growth factor receptor 3
VEGF/VPF
vascular endothelial growth factor/vascular permeability factor
VEGI
vascular endothelial cell growth inhibitor
VEGP
von Ebner gland protein
V$_{EH}$
extrahepatic distribution
vehic
vehicle
VEI
volume [lung] at end of inspiration
vel, veloc
velocity (*See also* V)
VELS
Vane Evaluation of Language Scale
VELV
Vellore virus
VEM
vasoexcitor material
vergence eye movements
V$_{E\,max}$
maximal flow per unit of time

VEMP
vestibular-evoked myogenic potential
VENC
velocity encoding value
venostasis
visual evoked potential
vent
ventilation (*See also* V, V̇, VE)
ventilator (respirator)
ventral
ventricle (ventricular) (*See also* V, ventric)
vent fib
ventricular fibrillation (*See also* VF, v fib)
ventric
ventricle (ventricular) (*See also* V, vent)
VEOS
very early onset schizophrenia
VEP
visual evoked potential
voluntary eye propulsion
VER
ventricular escape rhythm
veratridine
visual evoked response
VERIS
visual evoked response imaging system
VERP
ventricular effective refractory period
VERT
velocity-enhanced resistance training
vert
vertebra(l) (*See also* V)
vertical
VES
ventricular extrasystole
video-endoscopic surgery
ves.
bladder [L. *vesica*]
vesicle (vesicular) (*See also* vesic)
vessel
vesic
vesicle (vesicular) (*See also* ves.)
VESS
videoendoscopic swallowing study
VEST
virtual endoscopic surgery trainer
vest
vestibule (vestibular)
VESV
vesicular exanthema of swine virus
VET
vacuum erection technology
ventricular ejection time
vestigial testis

vet
veteran
veterinarian
veterinary
VETS
Veterans (Adjustment) Scale
VE/VCO$_2$
ventilation/carbon dioxide production
VEWA
Vocational Evaluation and Work Adjustment
VF
left leg electrode [electrocardiogram]
ventricular fibrillation (*See also* vent fib, v fib)
ventricular fluid
ventricular flutter
ventricular function
ventricular fusion
vertical float [aquatic therapy]
videofluorography
video frequency
vigil, fatiguing
visual field (*See also* VFD)
vitreous fluorophotometry
vocal fremitus
V$_f$
variant frequency
VFA
volatile fatty acid
Vfactor
verbal [comprehension] factor (*See also* V)
VFC
Vaccines for Children [program]
venous flow controller
ventricular function curve
viscous fluid controller
VFCB
vertical flow clean bench
VFD
visual feedback display
visual field (*See also* VF)
visual field defect
vocal fold dysfunction
VFDF
very fast death factor
VFDT
Visual Form Discrimination Test
VFES
videofluorographic evaluation of swallowing
VFFC
visual fields full to confrontation
VFI
visual field intact (*See also* VFIT)
Visual Functioning index
vocal fold injection

v fib
ventricular fibrillation (*See also* vent fib, VF)
VFIT
visual field intact (*See also* VFI)
VFL
ventricular flutter
VFMI
vocal fold motion impairment
VFO
variable flexion overhinge
VFP
ventricular filling pressure
ventricular fluid pressure
vertical float progression [aquatic therapy]
vitreous fluorophotometry
vocal fold paralysis
VFQ
Visual Function Questionnaire
VFQ-25
25-Item Visual Function Questionnaire
VFR
voiding flow rate
VFS
vascular fragility syndrome
VFSS
videofluoroscopic swallowing study
VFT
venous filling time
ventricular fibrillation threshold
Verbal Fluency Test
VF/VT
ventricular fibrillation [and/or] ventricular tachycardia
VG
NATO code for nerve agent O,O-diethyl S-[2-(diethylamino)ethyl] phosphonothioate
vein graft
ventilated group
ventricular gallop
ventrogluteal
very good
V&G
vagotomy and gastroenterotomy
V$_G$
genetic variance
VGA
villoglandular adenocarcinoma
VGAD
vein of Galen aneurysmal dilatation
VGAM
vein of Galen aneurysmal malformation
VGCC
voltage-gated calcium channel
VGE
viral gastroenteritis

V

VGFI
vented gas forced infusion
VGH
very good health
veterinary general hospital
VGKC
voltage-gated potassium channel
VGM
vein (venous) graft myringoplasty
ventriculogram
VGP
viral glycoprotein
VGPO
volume-guaranteed pressure option
VGS
video game-induced seizure
VGTT
video graphic tool technology
VH
vaginal hysterectomy (*See also* VAG
HYST)
venous hematocrit
ventricular hypertrophy
vestibular hyperreactivity
Veterans Hospital
viral hepatitis
visual hallucination
vitreous hemorrhage
von Herrick [optometry, anterior
chamber grade system]
V$_H$
hepatic distribution volume
variable domain of heavy chain
immunoglobulin
VH I
von Herrick I [very narrow anterior
chamber angles]
VH II
von Herrick II [moderately narrow
anterior chamber angles]
VH III
von Herrick III [moderately wide open
anterior chamber angles]
VH IV
von Herrick IV [wide open anterior
chamber angles]
VHA
Veterans Health Administration
VHAI
van Hees [Crohn disease] Activity
Index
VHC
valved holding chamber
VHD
valvular heart disease
vascular hemostatic device
ventricular heart disease
viral hematodepressive
disease

VHDL
very-high-density lipoprotein
VHDPB
very high dose phenobarbital
VHF
very high frequency
viral hemorrhagic fever
visual half-field
VHI
voice handicap index
Vhigh
high regional wall motion velocity
VHL
von Hippel-Lindau [gene]
VHN
Vickers hardness number
VHP
vaporized hydrogen peroxide
VHR
ventricular heart rate
VHSV
viral hemorrhagic septicemia virus
VI
inspired ventilation
virgin [untouched girl] [L. *virgo
intacta*]
vaginal irrigation
variable interval
vascular invasion
vastus intermedius
velocity index
ventilation index
ventricular index
virulence (virulent)
viscosity index
visual imagery
visual impairment
visual inspection
visually impaired
vitality index
volume index
V$_I$
volume of inspired gas [per minute]
VIA
virus-inactivating agent
virus infection-associated antigen
VIB
viral inclusion body
Vocational Interest Blank
Vib
Vibrio (*See also* V)
vib
vibration
VIBE
volumetric interpolated breath-hold
examination
VIBRANT
volume imaging for breast
assessment

VIBS
Victim's Information Bureau Service
vocabulary, information, block [design], and similarities [psychology]

VIC
Values Inventory for Children
vasoinhibitory center
vehicle for initial crawling
visual communication [therapy]
voice intensity controller

VICA
velocity internal carotid artery

V-ICD
ventricular implantable cardioverter-defibrillator

VICP
Vaccine Injury Compensation Program

VI-CTS
vibration-induced carpal tunnel syndrome

VID
vaginal intraepithelial dysplasia
videodensitometry
visible iris diameter
vitellointestinal duct

VIDA
vitiligo disease activity

VIED
vehicular improvised explosive device

VIESA
Vocational Interest, Experience, and Skill Assessment

VIF
virus-induced interferon

VIg
vaccinia immunoglobulin (immune globulin)

vig
vigorous

VIGRE
velocity imaging with gradient-recalled echo

VIH
human immunodeficiency virus [Spanish and French abbreviation]
violence-induced handicap

VILI
ventilator-induced lung injury

VIM
ventralis intermedius
video-intensification microscopy

VIN
vaginal (vulvar) intraepithelial neoplasia

VINV
Vinces virus

VIP
Validity Indicator Profile
vasoactive intestinal peptide (polypeptide)
vasoactive intracorporeal pharmacotherapy
vasoinhibitory peptide
Vattikuti Institute prostatectomy [laparoscopic robotic]
venous impedance plethysmography
very important patient
very important person
voluntary interruption of pregnancy

VIP-CT
vascularized interpositional periosteal-connective tissue [flap]

VIP-DAC
vaginal interruption of pregnancy with dilatation and curettage

VIP-IR
vasoactive intestinal polypeptide immunoreactivity

VIPoma
vasoactive intestinal peptide-secreting tumor

VIQ
Verbal Intelligence Quotient
Vocational Interest Questionnaire

VIR
virology (viral) (virus) (*See also* V)

vir
green [L. *viridis*]

VIS
Vaccine Information Statement
vaginal irrigation smear
venous insufficiency syndrome
vertebral irritation syndrome
video imaging system
visceral [manipulative treatment]
visible
vision (*See also* V)
(visitor) visit(ed) (visiting) (*See also* VIS)
visual
Visual Impairment Service
visual information storage
vocational interest schedule

VISA
vancomycin-insensitive *Staphylococcus aureus*
vancomycin-intermediate-resistant *Staphylococcus aureus*
Vocational Interest and Sophistication Assessment

VISC
vitreous infusion suction cutter

visc
viscera(l)
viscosity (viscous)

V

VISI
Vaccine Identification Standards Initiative
volar [flexed] intercalated segment instability

Viso
volume of isoflow

VISTA
Vermont Interdependent Services Team Approach [educational support services]

VIT
venom immunotherapy
vital
vitamin
vitrectomy (*See also* Vx)
vitreous

vit cap
vital capacity
vitamin capsule

vitel.
yolk [L. *vitellus*]

vitr, vitr.
glass [L. *vitrum*]
vitreous

vits
vitamins

VIU
visual internal urethrotomy

viz
visualized

viz.
that is, namely [L. *videlicet*]

VJ
ventriculojugular [shunt]
Vogel-Johnson [agar]

VK
vervet [African green monkey] kidney [cell]

VKA
vitamin K antagonist

VKC
vernal keratoconjunctivitis

VKDB
vitamin K deficiency bleeding

VL
left arm electrode [electrocardiogram]
Valuation of Life
vastus lateralis
[nucleus] ventralis lateralis
ventrolateral
vial
viral load
visceral leishmaniasis
vision, left [eye]

V_L
[actual] volume of lung
variable domain of light chain immunoglobulin

VLA
vanillacetic acid
very late activation
very late antigen
viruslike action
viruslike agent

VLA-1–VLA-5
very late antigen 1–5

VLAD
variable life-adjusted display

VLAP
vaporization laser ablation of prostate
visual laser ablation of prostate
visual laser-assisted prostatectomy

VLBR
very low birth rate

VLBW
very low birth weight

VLBWPN
very low birth weight preterm neonate

VLCAD
very long chain acyl coenzyme A dehydrogenase

VLCD
very low calorie diet

VLCFA
very long chain fatty acid

VLD
very low density

VLDL, VLDLP
very low density lipoprotein

VLDL-C
very low density lipoprotein C

VLDL-TG
very low density lipoprotein-triglyceride

VLDS
Verbal Language Development Scale

VLE
vision left eye (*See also* VOS)

VLF
very low frequency

VLG
ventral [nucleus of] lateral geniculate [body]

VLH
ventrolateral [nucleus of] hypothalamus

VLIA
viruslike infectious agent

VLM
ventrolateral medulla
virtual labor monitor
visceral larva migrans

VLO
vastus lateralis obliquus [muscle]

VLP
ventricular late potential
ventriculolumbar perfusion
viruslike particle

VLPP
Valsalva leak point pressure
VLR
vastus lateralis release
VLS
vanishing lung syndrome
vascular leak syndrome
VLSI
very large scale integration
VLT
video lottery terminal
VM
NATO code for nerve agent O-ethyl
S-[2-(diethylamino)ethyl]
methylphosphonothioate
Valsalva maneuver
vasomotor
vastus medialis
vector magnitude
venous malformation
ventilated mask (Ventimask)
ventricular mass
ventriculomegaly
ventriculometry
ventromedial
Venturi mask
vestibular membrane
viral myocarditis
voltmeter
V/m
volt per meter [electric field strength]
VMA
vanillylmandelic acid
vastus medialis advancement
V-mask
Venturi mask
VMAT
vesicular monoamine transporter
V$_{max}$
maximal (maximum) velocity
peak flow velocity [Doppler]
VMC
vasomotor center
void metal composite
von Meyenburg complex
VMCG
vector magnetocardiogram
VMD
vertical maxillary deficiency
VME
vertical maxillary excess
VMETH
volumetric multiple exposure
transmission holography
VMF
vasomotor flushing
VMGT
Visual-Motor Gestalt Test

VMH
ventromedial hypothalamic [neuron,
nucleus]
VMHL
ventromedial hypothalamic lesion
V-MI
Volpe-Manhold Index [dental calculus
score]
VMI
visual-motor integration
VMIT
visual-motor integration test
VMN
ventromedial nucleus [of hypothalamus]
VMO
[musculus] vastus medialis obliquus
vaccinia melanoma oncolysate
[immunotherapy vaccine]
vastus medialis oblique [muscle]
VMO:VL
vastus medialis obliquus to vastus
lateralis ratio
VMO:VL EMG
vastus medialis obliquus to vastus
lateralis ratio electromyographic
VMR
vasomotor response
vasomotor rhinitis
VMS
vanilla milkshake
Visual Memory Score
visual memory span
VMSC
Vineland Measurement of Social
Competence
VMST
Visual-Motor Sequencing Test
VMT
vasomotor tone
ventilatory muscle training
ventromedial tegmentum
visceral malignant tumor
VMU
vertebral motion unit
VN
vesical neck
vestibular neurectomy
vestibular nucleus
virus neutralization (neutralizing)
visceral nucleus
visual naming
vomeronasal
VNA
virus-neutralizing antibody
VNC
vesical neck contracture
VNDPT
Visual Numerical Discrimination Pretest

V

VNE
verbal nonemotional stimuli
video nasendoscopy
VNO
vomeronasal organ
VNR
ventral nerve root
verbal, numerical, and
reasoning
VNS
vagus nerve stimulation
villonodular synovitis
VNS-fMRI
vagus nerve stimulated functional
magnetic resonance imaging
VNSSL
video-assisted thoracic surgical
nonrib-spreading lobectomy
VNTR
variable numbers of tandem
repeats
VO
verbal order
visual observation
volume overload
voluntary opening
VO₂
volume of oxygen consumption per unit
of time [aerobic capacity]
V_O
oral airflow [liters per second]
Voa
[nucleus] ventralis oralis anterior
VOC
volatile organic compound
voc
vocational
vocab
vocabulary
VOCOR
vasoocclusive crisis
void on-call to operating room
(*See also* VOCTOR)
VOCTOR
void on-call to operating room
(*See also* VOCOR)
⚠ **VOD**
venoocclusive disease
visio oculus dextra [vision of
right eye] (*See also* VR, VRE) ⚠
VOE
vascular occlusive episode
VO₂ HR
volume of oxygen intake-heart rate
VOI
Vocational Opinion Index
volume of interest
VO2I
oxygen consumption index

vol
volar
volatile
volume (*See also* V)
volumetric
voluntary
volunteer
vol%
volume percent
vol adm
voluntary admission
vol:vol
volume per volume ratio
VOM
volt-ohm-millimeter
vom
vomit(ing) (*See also* V)
VO₂ max, VO₂max
maximum (maximal) oxygen
consumption
maximal oxygen uptake
VOO
continuous ventricular asynchronous
pacing
ventricular pacing, no sensing, no other
function [pacemaker]
VOOD
vesical-outlet occlusive disease
VOP
venous occlusion plethysmography
ventralis oralis posterior
VOR
vestibular ocular (vestibuloocular) reflex
vestibuloocular response
VORP
vibrating ossicular prosthesis
⚠ **VOS**
visio oculus sinister [vision of left eye]
(*See also* VLE) ⚠
voice outcome survey
VOSS
visual observation shivering score
VOT
Visual Organization Test
voice onset time
VOTC
ventral occipitotemporal [visual] cortex
⚠ **VOU**
visio oculus uterque [vision of both
eyes, each eye] ⚠
voxel
volume element
VP
vagal paraganglioma
vapor pressure (*See also* vp)
variably positive
variegate porphyria
vascular permeability
vasopressin

velopharyngeal
venipuncture
venous pressure (*See also* Pv)
venous (volume) plethysmograph
ventricle to peritoneal cavity [shunt]
ventricular pacing
ventricular pericardium
ventricular peritoneal
  (ventriculoperitoneal) [shunt]
ventricular premature [beat] (*See also*
  VPB)
ventroposterior
vertex potential
viral protein
virus protein
visual perception
Voges-Proskauer [medium, test]
voiding pressure
volume-pressure
vulnerable period

V&P
vagotomy and pyloroplasty
ventilation and perfusion

Vp
plasma volume (*See also* PV)
volumetric lung depth

vp
vapor pressure (*See also* VP)

VPA
ventricular premature activation
ventricular pseudoaneurysm
vigorous physical activity
Vocal Profiles Analysis

v-PA
vascular plasminogen activator

V-Pad
sanitary napkin

VPAP
variable positive airway pressure

VPB
ventricular premature beat (*See also* VP)

VPC
vapor-phase chromatography
velopharyngeal competence
ventricular premature complex
ventricular premature contraction
volume of packed cells
volume percentage

VPCM
vulnerable populations conceptual model

VPCT
ventricular premature contraction
  threshold

VPD
vaccine-preventable disease
velopharyngeal dysfunction
ventricular premature depolarization

VPd
venous dialysis pressure

VPDC
ventricular premature depolarization
  contraction

VPDF
vegetable protein diet [plus] fiber

V$_{pe}$
peak ejection velocity

VPF
vascular permeability factor

VPF/VEGF
vascular permeability factor/vascular
  endothelial cell growth factor

VPG
velopharyngeal gap
venting percutaneous gastrostomy

VPGSS
venous pressure gradient support
  stockings

VPI
vasopeptidase inhibitor
velopharyngeal incompetence
velopharyngeal insufficiency
ventral posterior inferior
  (ventroposteroinferior)
Vocational Planning Inventory
Vocational Preference Inventory

VPL
ventral posterolateral
  (ventroposterolateral)

VPLN
vaccine-primed lymph node [cells]

VPLS
ventilation-perfusion lung scan

VPM
Vantage Performance monitor
venous pressure module
ventilator pressure manometer
[nucleus] ventralis posteromedialis
ventroposteromedial

vpm
vibration per minute

7VPnC
7-valent pneumococcal conjugate

VPO
velopharyngeal opening

VPP
viral porcine pneumonia

VPR
virtual patient record
Voges-Proskauer reaction
volume-pressure response

vpr
viral protein R

VPRC, VPRBC
volume of packed red [blood] cells

V

VPS
  valvular pulmonic stenosis
  vascular pulmonic stenosis
  ventriculoperitoneal shunt
  verbal pain scale
  view per segment
  visual pleural space
vps
  vibration per second
VPT
  vascularized patellar tendon
  vibration perception threshold
VPTEF:VT
  volume to peak expiratory flow and
    total expiratory volume ratio
VQ
  voice quality
V̇:Q̇, V:Q
  ventilation to perfusion ratio
V$_A$:Qc
  alveolar ventilation to pulmonary
    capillary perfusion ratio
VQR
  ventilation/perfusion ratio
VR
  right arm electrode
    [electrocardiogram]
  valve replacement
  valvular regurgitation
  variable rate
  variable ratio
  vascular resistance
  velocity ratio
  venous reflux
  venous resistance
  venous return
  ventilation rate
  ventilation ratio
  ventral root
  ventricular rate
  ventricular response
  ventricular rhythm
  verbal reprimand
  vesicular rosette
  vision, right [eye] (*See also* VRE,
    VOD)
  visual reproduction
  vital record
  vitreoretinal
  vocal resonance
  vocational rehabilitation
  volume rendering
V2R
  vasopressin receptor
Vr
  volume of relaxation
VRA
  visual reinforcement audiometry
  visual response audiometry

VRBC
  volume of red blood cells
VRC
  venous renin concentration
  vocational rehabilitation counselor
VRCP
  vitreoretinochoroidopathy
VRD
  ventricular radial dysplasia
  Virtual Retinal Display
VRE
  vancomycin-resistant *Enterococcus*
  vision right eye (*See also* VR, VOD)
VR&E
  vocational rehabilitation and education
VREF
  vancomycin-resistant *Enterococcus
    faecium*
VRG
  vertical ring gastroplasty
VRI
  viral respiratory infection
VRL
  ventral root, lumbar
VRNA
  viral ribonucleic acid
VRO
  varus rotational osteotomy
VROM
  voluntary range of motion
VRP
  very reliable product
  vocational rehabilitation program
VRR
  ventral root reflex
VRS
  viral rhinosinusitis
  volume reduction surgery
VRSA
  vancomycin-resistant *Staphylococcus
    aureus*
VRT
  variance of resident time
  venous refill time
  venous return time
  ventral root, thoracic
  vertical radiation topography
  Visual Retention Test
  vocational rehabilitation therapy
  volume replacement therapy
VRU
  ventilator rehabilitation unit
VRV
  ventricular rate variability
  ventricular residual volume
  Virgin River virus
VS
  vaccination scar
  vaccine serotype

vagal stimulation
valve system
variable softness
vascular surgery
vasospasm (vascular spasm)
vegetative state
venesection
ventral subiculum
ventricular sense
ventricular septum
ventriculosubarachnoid
verbal scale
vertical shear
very sensitive
vesicular sound
vesicular stomatitis
vestibular schwannoma
veterinary surgeon
videostroboscopy
villonodular synovitis
virilization syndrome
(visitor) visit(ed) (visiting) (*See also* VIS)
visual storage
vital signs
volume support
volumetric solution
voluntary sterilization

V · s
volt-second

vs
single vibration
vibration-second
voids [urine]

Vs.
against [L. *versus*]

VSA
variant-specific surface antigen
vasospastic angina

VSADP
vocational skills assessment and development program

VSAT
Visual Search and Attention Test

VSAV
vesicular stomatitis Alagoas virus

VSBE
very short below elbow [cast]

VSC
vertebral subluxation complex
volatile sulfur compound
voluntary surgical contraception

VSCC
voltage-sensitive calcium channel

VSCS
ventricular specialized conduction system

VSD
Vaccine Safety Datalink
ventricular septal (ventriculoseptal) defect
vesical external sphincter dyssynergia
vesicular stomatitis virus
virtually safe dose

VSED
voluntarily stopping eating and drinking

VSF
Vermont spinal fixator

VSFP
venous stop flow pressure

VSG
variant surface glycoprotein

VSGP
vertical supranuclear gaze palsy

VSHD
ventricular septal heart defect

VSI
vascular status intact

VSIV
vesicular stomatitis Indiana virus

VSL
straight line velocity

VSM
vascular smooth muscle

VSMC
vascular smooth muscle cell

VSMS
Vineland Social Maturity Scale

VSN
vital signs normal

vsn
vision

VSNJV
vesicular stomatitis New Jersey virus

VSO
vertical sagittal split osteotomy
vertical subcondylar oblique [fracture]
vertical supranuclear ophthalmoplegia

VSOK
vital signs okay [normal]

VSP
variable screw placement
variable screw plate
variable spinal plating
vertical stabilization program

VSQOL
Vital Signs Quality of Life

VSR
venereal spirochetosis of rabbits
venous stasis retinopathy
ventriculoseptal rupture
visceral to subcutaneous [adipose tissue] ratio

V

VSRA
variable speech rate audiometry
VSS
[apparent] volume [of distribution] steady state
variable spot scanning
videofluoroscopic swallowing study
visual sexual stimulation
vital signs stable
VSSAF
vital signs stable, afebrile
VST
visual search task
VSULA
vaccination scar upper left arm
VSV
vesicular stomatitis virus
VSW
ventricular stroke work
V SYNC
vertical synchronization pulse
Vsys
systolic wall motion velocity
VT
tetrazolium violet [stain]
tidal volume (*See also* TD, TV, V_T)
total ventilation
unsustained ventricular tachycardia
vacuum tube
vacuum tuberculin
validation therapy
variable temperature
vasotocin
venous thrombosis
ventricular tachyarrhythmia
ventricular tachycardia
verocytotoxin
verotoxin
video telemetry
V&T
volume and tension
V_T
tidal volume (*See also* TD, TV, VT)
total ventilation
V_t
volume of pulmonary parenchymal tissue
VTA
ventral tegmental area
ventricular tachyarrhythmia
V_TA
alveolar tidal volume
V-TACH, V tach
ventricular tachycardia
VTB
virtual tracheobronchoscopy
VTBI
volume to be infused

VTCL
ventricular tachycardia cycle length
VTE
venous thromboembolism
ventricular tachycardia event
vicarious trial and error
VTEC
verocytotoxin-producing *Escherichia coli*
verotoxin-producing *Escherichia coli*
VTED
venous thromboembolic disease
V-test
Voluter test [radiology]
VTG, V_{TG}
volume thoracic gas
VTI
volume thickness index
VTL
viscerotropic leishmaniasis
VTM
mechanical tidal volume
variegated translocation mosaicism
virus transport medium
VT-NS
ventricular tachycardia nonsustained
VTO
visualized treatment objective
VTOP, VTP
vaginal termination of pregnancy
voluntary termination of pregnancy
VTQS
Voc-Tech Quick Screener
VTS
vesicular transport system
VT-S
ventricular tachycardia sustained
VTSRS
Verdun Target Symptom Rating Scale
VTT
voice termination time
VT/VF
ventricular tachycardia/ventricular fibrillation
VTVM
vacuum tube voltmeter
VTX
vertex [presentation] (*See also* V, VE, V_X)
VU
varicose ulcer
venous ulcer
very urgent
vesicoureteral [reflux]
vesicoureterogram
volume unit [meter]
V/U
verbalize understanding

VUC
vacuum uterine cannula
voiding urine cytology
VUD
voluntary unrelated donor
VUD-BMT
volunteer unrelated-donor bone marrow
transplant(ation)
VUDS
video urodynamics
VUE
villitis of unknown etiology
VUJ
vesicoureteral junction
VUO
vesicoureteral orifice
VUPM
voiding urethral pressure measurement
VUPP
voiding urethral pressure profile
VUR
vesicoureteral reflux [grade I–V]
VURD
valves, unilateral reflux, dysplasia
vesicoureteral reflux and renal dysplasia
V-US
volumetric ultrasonography
VUSE
variable-angle uniform signal excitation
VUV
vacuum ultraviolet
VV
vaccinia virus
varicose vein
venovenous
vesicovaginal [fistula] (*See also* VVF)
viper venom
vulva and vagina (*See also* V&V)
V-V
venovenous [bypass]
ventriculovenous [shunt]
V:V
volume to volume ratio
V&V
vulva and vagina (*See also* VV)
vv
venae (veins) [plural]
v/v
vice versa
VVA
venous-to-venous anastomosis
VVB
venovenous bypass
VVC
vulvovaginal candidiasis
VVD
vaginal vertex delivery
vascular volume of distribution

VVETP
Vietnam Veterans Evaluation and
Treatment Program
VVF
vesicovaginal fistula (*See also* VV)
VVFR
vesicovaginal fistula repair
VVG
Verhoeff-Van Gieson [stain]
VVI
venous valvular insufficiency
ventricular pacing, ventricular sensing,
inhibited mode [pacemaker]
vvi
vocal velocity index
VVIR
ventricular demand inhibited
[pacemaker]
VVL
varicose veins ligation
verruca vulgaris of larynx
VVLBW
very very low birth weight
VVM
vertical vesicomyotomy
VVOR
visually enhanced vestibuloocular reflex
visual vestibuloocular reflex
VVQ
verbalizer-visualization questionnaire
VVR
ventricular response rate [pacemaker]
ventricle-ventricle repolarization
vvRI
venae rectales inferiores (*See also* PRI)
VVS
vasovagal syncope
vesicovaginal space
vulvar vestibulitis syndrome
VVT
ventricular pacing, ventricular sensing,
triggered mode [pacemaker]
VW
vascular wall
vessel wall
v/w
volume per weight
VWD
ventral wall defect
VWF
velocity waveform
vibration-induced white finger
vWF
von Willebrand factor
VWFA
visual word form area
VWFT
variable-width forms tractor

VWM

ventricular wall motion

VX

NATO code for an extremely toxic persistent nerve agent [no common chemical name]

no evidence of venous invasion [TNM classification]

Vx

vaccination (*See also* vacc)

vertex (*See also* V, VE, VTX)

vitrectomy (*See also* VIT)

V-XT

V-pattern exotropia

V-Y

shape of incisions in V-Y plasty

VZ, V-Z

varicella-zoster [virus] [chickenpox] (*See also* VZV)

VZIg

varicella-zoster immunoglobin (immune globulin)

VZV

varicella-zoster virus [chickenpox] (*See also* VZ)

VZVV

varicella-zoster virus vaccine

W
shape of incisions in W-plasty
tryptophan (*See also* Trp)
tungsten [Ger. *wolfram,*]
wash
water
watt
wearing glasses
Weber [hearing test]
week (*See also* WK, wk)
Wehnelt [cylinder electrode in electrode gun]
weight (*See also* wgt, wt)
well
west
wetting
white (*See also* Wh, wt)
white [blood] cell (*See also* WC)
whole [response] (*See also* WR, Wr, wr)
width
wife
Wilcoxon rank sum test [statistics] (*See also* WRST)
Wistar [rat]
with (*See also* c̄, w̄, w/)
wolframium [tungsten]
word fluency (*See also* WF)
work [energy] (*See also* WK, wk)

W-1
wheal 1 [insignificant allergies]

W-3
wheal 2 [minimal allergies]

W3
World Wide Web

W-5
wheal 5 [moderate allergies]

W-7
wheal 7 [moderate-severe allergies]

W-9
wheal 9 [severe allergies]

W-22
22 word list [Central Institute for the Deaf]

188W
tungsten-188

W+
weakly positive

w/, w̄
with (*See also* W, c̄)

WA
when awake
while awake
wide awake
with assistance

W&A
weakness and atrophy

W/A
watt/ampere

W or A
weakness or atrophy

WAB
Western Aphasia Battery

WACH
wedge adjustable cushioned heel [shoe]

WADAO
weak and dizzy all over

WADIC
Wing Autistic Disorder Interview Checklist

WAF
weakness, atrophy, fasciculation

WAGR
Wilms [tumor], aniridia, genitourinary [abnormalities], and [mental] retardation

WAI
Weinberger Adjustment Inventory
wheat amylase inhibitor

WAIHA
warm autoimmune hemolytic anemia

WAIS
Wechsler Adult Intelligence Scale

WAIS-III
Wechsler Adult Intelligence Scale Third Edition

WAIS-R
Wechsler Adult Intelligence Scale, Revised

WAK
wearable artificial kidney

WakiTrak
wide aperture kinematic table with isotropic resolution

WALK
weight-activated locking knee [prosthesis]

WALV
Wallal virus

WAMBA
Wise areola mastopexy breast augmentation

WANV
Wanowrie virus

WAP
wandering atrial pacemaker
whole abdominopelvic [irradiation]

WAPRT
whole abdominopelvic radiation therapy

W

WAPT
Weidel Auditory Processing Test
WAQ
Work Attitudes Questionnaire
WAR
whole abdominal radiation
WARI
wheezing associated respiratory infection
WARV
Warrego virus
WAS
Ward Atmosphere Scale [psychology]
weekly activity summary
whiplash-associated disorder
WASO
wake after sleep onset
WASP
Weber Advanced Spatial Perception
[test]
Wiskott-Aldrich syndrome protein
Wass
Wasserman [reaction, test]
WAT
white adipose tissue
Word Association Test
WB
waist belt
washable base
washed bladder
water baby
water bottle
Wechsler-Bellevue [Scale]
weightbearing
well baby
Western blot
wet bulb
wheezy bronchitis
whole blood (*See also* B, QB, W Bld)
whole body
Wb
weber SI [unit of magnetic flux]
WBA
wax bean agglutinin
Western blot assay
whole-body activity
Wb/A
weber per ampere
WBACT
whole-blood activated clotting time
WBAPT
whole-blood activated partial
thromboplastin [time, test] (*See also*
WBAPTT)
WBAPTT
whole-blood activated partial
thromboplastin time (*See also*
WBAPT)
WBAT
weightbearing as tolerated

WBC
weightbearing with crutches
well-baby clinic
white blood cell (corpuscle)
WBC/hpf
white blood cell per high-power field
WBCT
whole-blood clotting time
WBD
weeks by dates [gestational age]
WBDS
whole-body digital scanner
WBE
weeks by examination [gestational
age]
whole-body extract
WBF
whole-blood folate
WBGD
whole-body glucose disposal
WBGT
wet bulb globe temperature
WBH
weight-based heparin [dosing]
whole-blood hematocrit
whole-body hyperthermia
WBI
whole-body irradiation
whole-bowel irrigation
will be in
W Bld
whole blood (*See also* B, QB, WB)
WBM
whole boiled milk
Wb/m²
weber per square meter
WBN
well-baby nursery
well-born nursery
wide band noise
WBNAA
whole-brain N-acetylaspartate
WBOS
wide base of support
WBP
whole body protein
WBPT
whole-blood partial thromboplastin [test,
time] (*See also* WBPTT)
WBPTT
whole-blood partial thromboplastin time
(*See also* WBPT)
WBQC
wide-base quad cane
WBR
whole-body radiation
whole-body retention
WBRS
Ward Behavior Rating Scale

WBRT
whole-blood recalcification time
whole-brain radiation therapy
(radiotherapy)
whole-breast radiation therapy
WBS
Wechsler-Bellevue Scale
weeks by size [gestational age]
whole-body scan
whole-body shower
withdrawal body shakes
wound-breaking strength
WBT
wet bulb temperature
WBTF
Waring Blender tube feeding
WBTT
weightbearing to tolerance
WBUS
weeks by ultrasound [gestational age]
WBV
whole-blood volume (*See also* QBV)
WC
ward confinement
warm compress
water closet [British]
wet compress
wheelchair (*See also* wh ch)
when called
white [blood] cell (*See also* W, WBC)
white [cell] cast
white [cell] count (*See also* WCC)
whole complement
whooping cough
will call
work capacity
workers' compensation
writer's cramp
WCA
work capacity assessment
WCB
will call back
WCC
well-child care
white [blood] cell count (*See also* WC)
WCCD
white cell count with differential
WCD
wearable cardioverter-defibrillator
WCE
white coat effect
wireless capsule endoscopy
work capacity evaluation
WCH
white coat hypertension
WCHE
well-child health examination

WCL
Wenckebach cycle length
whole-cell lysate
WC/LS
warm compresses and lid scrubs
WCM
whole cow's milk
WCOT
wall coated open tubular
[chromatography]
wcp
whole chromosome paint
WCR
Walthard cell rest
WCS
white coat syndrome
Wisconsin Compression System
WCST
Wisconsin Card Sorting Test
WCT
wide-complex tachycardia
WD
wallerian degeneration
ward
warm and dry (*See also* W/D)
well-developed
well-differentiated
wet dressing
Whitney Damon [dextrose]
with disease
withdrawal dyskinesia
without dyskinesia
word
working distance
wound(ed) (*See also* WND, wnd)
wrist disarticulation
W4D
Worth four-dot [eye test for fusion,
depth perception]
W/D
warm [and] dry (*See also* WD)
withdrawal
withdrawn
W→D
wet-to-dry (*See also* WTD)
WDA
wrist disarticulation
WDCA
well-differentiated carcinoma
WDCC
well-developed collateral
circulation
WDE
wound dressing emulsion
WDEIA
wheat-dependent, exercise-induced
anaphylaxis

W

WDF
white divorced female

WDFA
well-differentiated fetal adenocarcinoma

WDHA
watery diarrhea, hypokalemia, and achlorhydria [syndrome]
watery diarrhea with hypokalemic alkalosis

WDHH
watery diarrhea, hypokalemia, hypochlorhydria
watery diarrhea, hypokalemia, hypovolemia

WDI
warfarin dose index

WDL
well-differentiated lymphocyte
within defined limits
Wood-Downes-Lecks [clinical asthma score]

WDLL
well-differentiated lymphocytic lymphoma

WDPM
well-differentiated papillary mesothelioma

WDRC
wide dynamic range compression

WDS
watery diarrhea syndrome
wet dog shakes [syndrome]
word discrimination score
wounds

WDSCC
well-differentiated squamous-cell carcinoma

WDSCL
well-differentiated small-cell lymphoma

WDTC
well-differentiated thyroid cancer

WDWG
well-dressed, well-groomed

WDWN, WD,WN
well-developed, well-nourished

WDXRF
wavelength-dispersive x-ray fluorescence

WE
wage earner
wandering edema
wax ester
weekend
Wernicke encephalopathy
Western encephalitis (encephalomyelitis)
whiskey equivalent
wide excision

WEBINO
wall-eyed bilateral internuclear ophthalmoplegia

WE-D
withdrawal-emergent dyskinesia

WEE
Western equine encephalomyelitis [virus]

WeeFIM
Functional Independence Measure for Children

WEFT
water eliminated Fourier transform

WEG
water-ethylene glycol

WEH/CHOP
Wills Eye Hospital/Children's Hospital of Philadelphia

WEIS
Work Environment Impact Scale

WEMINO
wall-eyed monocular internuclear ophthalmoplegia

W3-EMRS
World Wide Web electronic medical records system

WEP
weekend pass

WES
wall-echo shadow [sign]

WESR
Westergren erythrocyte sedimentation rate
Wintrobe erythrocyte sedimentation rate

WESSV
Wesselsbron virus

WEST
Weinstein enhanced sensory test
work evaluation systems technology

WEUP
willful exposure to unwanted pregnancy

WE
wound of entry

WF
Weil-Felix [*Proteus* agglutination test]
well-flexed
wet film
white female
wide field
Wistar-Furth [rat]
word fluency
Working Formulation for Clinical Usage

W&F
weakness and fatigue

WFB
wooden foreign body

WFE, WFEx
Williams flexion exercises [lower back pain]

W FEEDS
with feedings

WFH
white-faced hornet

WFI
water for injection

WFL
within full limits [within functional limits]

WFLC
white female living child

WFNS
World Federation of Neurological Societies [grade, scale]

WF-O
will follow in office

WFR
Weil-Felix reaction
wheal-and-flare reaction

WFRT
wide-field radiation therapy

WFSS
Wolpe Fear Survey Schedule

WG
water gauge
Wegener granulomatosis
Wright-Giemsa [stain]

WGA
wheat germ agglutinin
whole genome amplification

WGRV
Wongorr virus

wgt
weight (See also W, wt)

WGTS
whole-gut transit scintigraphy

WH
walking heel [cast]
well-healed
well-hydrated
whole homogenate
work hardening
wound healing

W/H
weight/height

Wh
watt-hour
white (See also W, wt)

wh
whisper(ed)

WHA
warmed humidified air

WHAS
Women's Health Assessment Scale

WHAV
Whataroa virus

wh ch
wheelchair (See also WC)
white child

WHCR
Wolf-Hirschhorn chromosome region

WHECS
wrist hand extension compression support

WHI
Women's Health Initiative

WHIM
warts, hypogammaglobulinemia, infections, myelokathexis [syndrome]

WHIS
War Head Injury Score

WHMS
well-healed midline scar

WHNR
well-healed, no residuals

WHNS
well-healed, nonsymptomatic
well-healed, no sequelae

WHO
World Health Organization
wrist-hand orthosis

WHOART
World Health Organization Adverse Reaction Terms [Terminology]

WHO/LAR
World Health Organization/International League Against Rheumatism

WHOQOL-100
World Health Organization Quality of Life 100-Item (instrument)

WHP, Whp, whp
whirlpool (See also WP)

WHPB
whirlpool bath (See also WPB)

WHR
waist to hip ratio

WHS
Women's Health Study

WHV
woodchuck hepatic virus

WHVP
wedge(d) hepatic venous pressure

WH/WD
withholding/withdrawal [of life support]

WHYMPI
Westhaven Yale Multidimensional Pain Inventory

WHZ
wheeze(s)

WI
ventricular demand pacing
walk-in [patient]
wash-in
water ingestion
waviness index
weaning index

W/I
within (See also w/in)

W

W&I
work and interest
WIA
wounded in action
WIC
women, infants, children [federal program]
wid
widow(ed)
widower
WIED
walk-in emergency department
WIF
WNT [protein, gene] inhibitory factor
WIFC
widely invasive follicular carcinoma
w/in
within (*See also* W/I)
win.
wound-induced
WIP
work in progress
WIPI
Word Intelligibility by Picture Identification
WIQ
Walking Impairment Questionnaire
Waring Intimacy Questionnaire
WIS
Ward Incapacity Scale (Wechsler Intelligence Scale)
WISC
Wechsler Intelligence Scale for Children
WISC-III
Wechsler Intelligence Scale for Children III
WISC-R
Wechsler Intelligence Scale for Children Revised
WISH
wearable information system for human healthcare
Wistar Institute Susan Hayflick [cell]
WISP1
WNT1 inducible signaling pathway protein
WIST
Whitaker Index of Schizophrenic Thinking
WIT
water-induced thermotherapy
WITT
Wittenborn [Psychiatric Rating Scale]
WITV
Witwatersrand virus
W-J
Whitmore-Jewett [prostate cancer staging]

WJPB
Woodcock-Johnson Psychoeducational Battery
WK, wk
week (*See also* W)
work
WKF
well-known fact
W/kg
watt per kilogram
WKI
Wakefield Inventory [psychology]
WKS
Wernicke-Korsakoff syndrome
WKY
Wistar-Kyoto [rat]
WL
waiting list
waterload [test]
wavelength (*See also* λ)
weight loss
workload
WLB
Western ligand blot
WLE
wide local excision
WLF
whole lymphocyte fraction
WLI
weight-length index
WLM
work-level month
WLQ
Work Limitation Questionnaire
WLR
within-list recognition
WLS
weight-loss surgery
wet lung syndrome
WLT
waterload test
whole-lung tomography
WLU
workload unit
WM
Waldenström macroglobulinemia
wall motion
warm, moist
wet mount
white matter
whole milk
whole mount (microscopy)
woman's milk
working memory
W/m$_2$
watt per square meter
WMA
wall motion abnormality
white matter [signal] abnormality

Wmax
    peak work rate
WMBT
    weighted moving beam
    therapy
WMC
    weight-matched control
WMD
    warm moist dressing [sterile]
    weapons of mass destruction
    weighted mean difference
    white matter damage
WMFT
    Wolf Motor Function Test
WMHI
    white matter hyperintensity
WMI
    wall motion index
    weighted mean index
WML
    white matter lesion [cerebral]
WMLC
    white male living child
WMP
    warm moist pack [unsterile]
    weight management program
WMR
    wedge matrix resection
    work metabolic rate
WMS
    wall motion study
    Wechsler Memory Scale
WMSI
    wall motion score index
WMT
    Word Memory Test
WMV
    Wad Medani virus
WMX
    whirlpool, massage, exercise
WN, W/N, w/n, wn
    well-nourished
WN$_t$^{50}
    Wagner-Nelson time [drug absorption]
    50 hours
WND, wnd
    wound(ed) (*See also* WD)
WNE
    West Nile encephalitis
WNF
    well-nourished female
    West Nile fever
WNL
    within normal limits
WNLS
    weighted nonlinear least squares
    [statistics]

WNL x 4
    upper and lower extremities within
    normal limits
WNM
    well-nourished male (man)
WNR
    within normal range
WNV
    West Nile virus
WO, wo
    wash-out
    weeks old
    wide open
    without (*See also* ō, S, s̄, sin. wo)
    written order
W/O
    water [in] oil [emulsion]
WOB
    work of breathing
WOC
    ways of coping [checklist]
WOC-CA
    Ways of Coping, Cancer Version
WOCF
    worst observation carried forward
    [statistics]
WOL
    weakness of limbs
WOMAC
    Western Ontario and McMaster
    Universities Osteoarthritis Index
WOMAC-PF
    Western Ontario and McMaster
    Universities Osteoarthritis Index
    Physical Functioning subscale and
    chair performance
WONV
    Wongal virus
WOP
    whole organ pancreas [transplantation]
    without pain
WORC
    Western Ontario Rotator Cuff [index]
WORD
    Wechsler Objective Reading Dimension
WOSI
    Western Ontario Instability Index
W/O/W
    water-in-oil-in-water
WOWS
    weak opiate withdrawal scale
WP
    water packed
    wavelet packet [Fourier transform]
    weakly positive
    wet pack (*See also* WPk)
    wettable powder

W

WP *(continued)*
whirlpool (*See also* WHP, Whp, whp)
white phosphorus
white pulp
working point
wrong position

W:P
water to powder ratio

WPAI
Work Productivity and Activity
Impairment [questionnaire]

WPB
whirlpool bath (*See also* WHPB)

WPBT
whirlpool, body temperature

WPC
washed packed cells

WPCU
weighted patient care unit

WPFM
Wright peak flowmeter

WPH
whole person healing

WPk
ward pack
wet pack (*See also* WP)

WPM
wandering pacemaker

WPOA
wearing patch on arrival

WPP
wide pulse pressure

WPPSI, WPP
Wechsler Preschool and Primary Scale
of Intelligence

WPPSI-R
Wechsler Preschool and Primary Scale
of Intelligence Revised

WPR
written progress report

WPRS
Wittenborn Psychiatric Rating Scale

WPSI
Wittenborn Psychiatric Symptoms
Inventory

WPT
warbled pure tone

WPV
within-person variability

WPW
Wolff-Parkinson-White [syndrome]

WR, Wr, wr
Waldeyer ring
washroom
Wassermann reaction
water retention
weakly reactive
whole response (*See also* W)
wide range

wiping reaction
work rate
wrist

W/R
with respect [to]

Wr^a
Wright antigens

WRA
with-the-rule astigmatism

WRAIR
Walter Reed Army Institute of
Research

WRAMC
Walter Reed Army Medical Center

WRAML
Wide Range Assessment of Memory
and Learning

WRAT
Wide Range Achievement Test

WRAT-R
Wide Range Achievement Test
Revised

WRBC
washed red blood cell (*See also* WRC)

WRC
washed red [blood] cell (*See also*
WRBC)
water-retention coefficient

WRE
whole ragweed extract

WRI
Worker Role Interview

WRISS
Weapons Related Injury Surveillance
System

WRK
Woodward reagent K

WRL
World Reference Laboratory [for
foot-and-mouth disease, UK]

WRMD
work-related musculoskeletal disorder

WRMT
Woodcock Reading Mastery Test

WRN
Werner syndrome protein [mutation]

WRST
Wilcoxon rank sum test [statistics]
(*See also* W)

WRT
weekly radiation therapy

WRUED
work-related upper extremity disorder

WRVP
wedged renal vein pressure

WS
walking speed
Warthin-Starry [stain]
watermelon stomach

water soluble
water swallow
wet swallow
whole [response plus white] space
Wiener spectrum [x-ray]
Wilder silver [stain]
work simplification
work simulation
work status

W&S
wound and skin

W·s
watt-second

WSA
water-soluble antibiotic

WSB
wheat-soy blend

WSCM
water-soluble contrast medium

WSCP
Williams Syndrome Cognitive Profile

WSD
water seal drainage
weak syllable deletion

WSEP
Williams syndrome, early puberty

WSI
Weekly Stress Inventory

WSI-E
Weekly Stress Inventory, Event

WSI-I
Weekly Stress Inventory, Impact

WSLP
Williams syndrome, late puberty

WSO
white superficial onychomycosis

WSOC
water-soluble organic compounds

WSP
wearable speech processor

WSQ
wavelet scalar quantization

WSR
Westergren [erythrocyte] sedimentation
rate (See also WESR)
whole system research

W/sr
watt per steradian

WSS
wrinkly skin syndrome

WSU
weak stream urination

WSW
women [who have] sex [with] women

WT
walking tank
walking training

wall thickness
water temperature
wild type [strain]
Wilms tumor
wisdom teeth
work therapy

0WT
zero work tolerance

wt
weight (See also W, wgt)
white (See also W, Wh)

WTD
wet tail disease [veterinary]
wet to dry (See also W→D)

WTE
whole time equivalent

WTF
weight transferral frequency

WTI
Wilms tumor 1 [gene]

WTP
willingness to pay

WTS
whole tomography slice

WTV
wound tumor virus

WTW
wet to wet (See also W→W)

W/U, w/u
workup

WUP
Waldenstrom uveoparotitis

WURS
Wender Utah Rating Scale

WUSPI
Wheelchair User's Shoulder Pain
Index

WV
walking ventilation
whispered voice

W/V, w/v
weight [of solute] per volume [of
solution]

W$_v$
variable dominant spotting [mouse]

WV:MBC
walking ventilation to maximal
breathing capacity ratio

WVTR
water vapor transmission rate

WWI
World War I

WWII
World War II

W/W
wet weight
wheeled walker

W

W/W, w/w
  weight [of solute] per weight [of solvent]

W→W
  wet to wet (*See also* WTW)

[188]W
  tungsten-188

WWAC
  walk with aid of cane

WW Brd
  whole wheat bread

WWIF
  warm water immersion foot

WWTP
  wastewater treatment plant

WWW
  World Wide Web

WX
  wound of exit

WxB
  wax bite

WxP
  wax pattern

WY
  women years

WY/NRT
  Weidel Yes/No Reliability Test

WYOU
  women years of usage

WYOV
  Wyeomyia virus

WZa
  wide zone alpha [hemolysis]

χ
chi [22nd letter of Greek alphabet lowercase]

X
androgenic [zone]
break
chi [22nd letter of Greek alphabet uppercase]
cross
cross-bite (crossbite)
crossed with
crossmatch (*See also* XM, X-mat., X-match, XMT)
cross-section
decimal scale of potency or dilution
Ecstasy [methylenedioxymethamphetamine]
except
exophoria distance (*See also* x)
exposure
extra
female sex chromosome
homeopathic symbol for decimal scale of potencies
ionization exposure rate
Kienböck unit [of x-ray exposure]
removal of
respirations [anesthesia chart]
sample mean (*See also* χ)
start of anesthesia
ten [Roman numeral]
transverse
unknown quantity
xanthine
xanthosine (*See also* Xao)
xerophthalmia
X unit (*See also* xu)

χ$_v$
magnetic susceptibility

χ^2
chi-square [statistics]

X3
[orientation as to] time, place and person

X′, x′
exophoria, near viewing

X+
xiphoid plus [number of fingerbreadths]

x
axis of cylindric lens
exophoria distance (*See also* X)
horizontal axis of rectangular coordinate system
mole fraction
multiplied by [sign]

roentgen [rays]
sample mean (*See also* X)

x̄
mean

X-A
xylene-alcohol [mixture]

XA
xanthurenic acid

X:A
X chromosome to autosome ratio

Xa
chiasma [singular]

Xaa
unknown amino acid

XAb
xenoantibody

X-ALD
X-linked adrenoleukodystrophy

Xan
xanthine

XANT
xanthochromic

Xanth
xanthomatosis

Xao
xanthosine (*See also* X)

XAT
xylose absorption test

XBSN
X-linked bulbospinal neuropathy

XBT
xylose breath test

XC
excretory cystograph(y) (cystogram)

Xc
reactance [electricity, in ohms]

XCCE
extracapsular cataract extraction (*See also* ECCE)

XCCL
exaggerated craniocaudal lateral [angle, view]

XCF
aortic cross clamp off

X-CGD
X-linked chronic granulomatous disease

XCO
aortic cross clamp on

XCT
x-ray computed tomography

⚠ **XD**
times daily ⚠
xanthoma disseminatum
X-linked dominant

X

X&D
examination and diagnosis
⚠ **X2d**
times two days ⚠
⚠ **5xD**
five times a day ⚠
XDH
xanthine dehydrogenase
XDP
xanthine diphosphate
xeroderma pigmentosum (*See also* XP)
XDR
transducer
XDT
defibrillation threshold (*See also* DFT)
diversional therapy
Xe
xenon
¹²⁷Xe
xenon-127
¹²⁹Xe
xenon-129
¹³³Xe
xenon-133
Xe-CBF
xenon [enhanced] cerebral blood flow
XeCl
xenon chloride
XECT, XeCT, Xe-CT
xenon-enhanced computed tomography
X-ed
crossed
XEF
excess ejection fraction
xero
xeromammography (*See also* XMM)
XES
x-ray energy spectrometry
XF
xerophthalmic fundus
XFER
transfer
Xfmr
transformer
XFS
exfoliation syndrome
XG
xanthogranuloma
XGP
xanthogranulomatous pyelonephritis
(*See also* XPN)
XH
extra high
ξ
xi [14th letter of Greek alphabet lowercase]
Ξ
xi [14th letter of Greek alphabet uppercase]

XIBV
Xiburema virus
XIC
X inactivation center
x-ray in cast
XIH
idiopathic hypercalcuria
XIP
x-ray in plaster
XIST, Xist
X inactive, specific transcript
XKO
not knocked out
XL
excess lactate
extra large
extra long [extended release drug]
inductive reactance
xylose-lysine [agar base]
X-LA, XLA
X-linked agammaglobulinemia
XLAS
X-linked Alport syndrome
X-linked aqueductal stenosis
XLCM
X-linked cardiomyopathy
XLD
X-linked dominant [genetic, inheritance]
xylose-lysine-deoxycholate [agar]
X-leg
crossleg
XLFDP
crosslinked fibrin degradation product
XLH
X-linked hydrocephalus
X-linked hypophosphatemia
XLHN
X-linked hypercalciuric nephrolithiasis
XLHR
X-linked hypophosphatemic rickets
XLI
X-linked ichthyosis
XLJR
X-linked juvenile retinoschisis
XLMR
X-linked mental retardation
XLMR/MCA
X-linked mental retardation/multiple
congenital anomalies
XLMTM
X-linked myotubular myopathy
XLOS
X-linked Opitz syndrome
XLP, XLP1
X-linked lymphoproliferative [disease]
XLR
X-linked recessive [genetic, inheritance]
XLRP
X-linked retinitis pigmentosa

XLRS
X-linked retinoschisis

XLT
X-linked thrombocytopenia

XM, X-mat., X-match
crossmatch (*See also* X, XMT)

XMG
x-ray mammogram

XMM
xeromammography (*See also* xero)

XMP
xanthine monophosphate
xanthosine 5′-monophosphate

XMR
x-ray and magnetic resonance

XMT
crossmatch (*See also* X, XM, X-mat., X-match)

XN
night blindness

XNA
xenoreactive natural antibody

XO
gonadal dysgenesis of Turner type [Turner syndrome]
presence of only one sex chromosome [Turner syndrome]
xanthine oxidase

XOAN
X-linked ocular albinism

XOC
x-ray out of cast

XOM
extraocular movement

XOP
x-ray out of plaster

XOR
exclusive operating room

XP
xeroderma pigmentosum (*See also* XDP)

Xp
short arm of chromosome X

Xp-
deletion of short arm of chromosome X

XPA
xeroderma pigmentosum [group] A

XPC
xeroderma pigmentosum [group] C

XPID
X-linked polyendocrinopathy immune dysfunction and diarrhea

XPN
xanthogranulomatous pyelonephritis (*See also* XGP)

XPS
xiphoid process syndrome
x-ray photoemission spectroscopy

XPTB
extrapulmonary tuberculosis

Xq
long arm of chromosome X

Xq-
deletion of long arm of chromosome X

XR
extended release [drug designation]
x-linked recessive
x-ray

X/R
reactance and resistance [electricity, in ohms]

XRA
x-ray arteriography

XRD
x-ray diffraction

XRE
xenobiotic-response element

XRF
x-ray fluorescence

XRITC
rhodamine X isothiocyanate

XRN
X-linked recessive nephrolithiasis

XRT
external radiation therapy (radiotherapy)
x-ray therapy (radiotherapy) (*See also* RT)

XS
corneal scar
cross-section
excess
excessive
xiphisternum

XSA
cross-sectional area
xenograph surface area

X-SCID, XSCID
X-linked severe combined immunodeficiency

XS-LIM
exceeds limits [of procedure]

XSLR
crossed straight leg raising [sign]

XSP
xanthoma striatum palmare

XT, xT
exercise test
exotropia
extract
extracted

X(T), x(T)
intermittent exotropia

X(T′)
intermittent exotropia at 33 cm

X

Xta

chiasmata [plural of chiasma]

Xtab

crosstabulating

XTC

Ecstasy
[methylenedioxymethamphetamine]

XTLE

extratemporal-lobe epilepsy

XTM

xanthoma tuberosum multiplex
x-ray tomographic microscope

XTP

xanthosine triphosphate (xanthosine
5′-triphosphate)

XU

excretory urograph(y) (urogram)

xu

X unit (*See also* X)

XULN

times upper limit of normal

XUV

extreme ultraviolet

xvse

transverse

XX

double strength
normal female sex chromosome type

XX/XY

sex karyotypes

XY

normal male sex chromosome type

Xy, Xyl

xylose

Y
coordinate axis in plane
male sex chromosome
ordinate
tyrosine (*See also* Tyr)
vertical axis of rectangular coordinate system
year (*See also* yr)
yellow (*See also* Yel, yel)
yes
Yersinia (*See also* Yer)
young
yttrium

^{50}Y
yttrium-50

^{90}Y
yttrium-90

y
wave on phlebogram
yield

YA
Yersinia arthritis

YAC
yeast artificial chromosome

YACP
young adult chronic patient

YACV
Yacaaba virus

YADH
yeast alcohol dehydrogenase

YAG
yttrium argon garnet [laser]

YAPA
young adult psychiatric assessment

YATAV
Yata virus

YB1
Y-box binding protein

Y/B
yellow/blue

Yb
ytterbium

YBOCS
Yale-Brown Obsessive-Compulsive Scale

YBR
yellow brick road [drug dependence]

YBT
Yerkes-Bridges Test (psychology)

YBV
Yug Bogdanovac virus

YCB
yeast carbon base

yd
yard

YDES
yin deficiency-yang excess syndrome

YE
yeast extract
yellow enzyme

YEH$_2$
reduced yellow enzyme

YEI
Yersinia enterocolitica infection

Yel, yel
yellow (*See also* Y)

YEPQ
Yale Eating Patterns Questionnaire

Yer
Yersinia (*See also* Y)

YES
Youth Enjoying Sobriety

YET
Youth Effectiveness Training

YF
yellow fever

YFH
yellow-faced hornet

YFI
yellow fever immunization

YFV
yellow fever virus

YF-VAX
yellow fever vaccine

Y-Fx
Y fracture

YGTSS
Yale Global Tic Severity Scale

YHL
years of healthy life

YHMD
yellow hyaline membrane disease

YHT
Young-Helmholtz theory [trichromatic color vision]

YHV
Yaquina Head virus

YJV
yellow jacket venom

Y2K
year 2000 [obsolete]

Yk
York [antibody]

YLC
youngest living child

YLD
years of life with disability

YLF
yttrium lithium fluoride [laser]

YLL
years of life lost
YLS
years of life saved
YM
yeast and mannitol
YMA
yeast morphology agar
yellow mutant albinism
YMRS
Young Mania Rating Scale
YMTV
Yaba monkey tumor virus
YMV
yam mosaic virus
Y/N
yes/no
YNB
yeast nitrogen base
YNS
yellow nail syndrome
YNSA
Yamamoto new scalp acupuncture
YO, yo
years old
year-old
YOB
year of birth
YOD
year of death
YOGV
Yogue virus
YORA
younger-onset rheumatoid arthritis
YP
yeast phase
yield point
yield pressure
Y-P
Y plasty
YPA
yeast, peptone, adenine [sulfate]

YPC
YAG (yttrium aluminum garnet laser) posterior capsulotomy
YPLL
years of potential life lost [before age 65]
YR
Young rule [to calculate pediatric dose]
yr
year (*See also* Y)
YRBS
youth risk behavioral survey
YRD
Yangtze River disease
YRRM
Y chromosome RNA recognition motif
YS
yellow spot
yolk sac
Yoshida sarcoma
Y-S
Y set [peritoneal dialysis equipment]
YSC
yolk sac carcinoma
YSP
Yergason sign positive [biceps tendon injury]
YSR
youth self-report
YST
yeast [cells]
yolk sac tumor
YTD
year to date
YTDY
yesterday
YV
yellow vernix
YVS
yellow vernix syndrome

Z

atomic number [proton]
carbobenzoxy-group
contraction [Ger. *Zuckung*]
disc [band, line] that separates
  sacromeres [Ger. *Zwischenscheibe*
  intermediate disc]
glutamic acid (glutamate) (*See also* E,
  Glu, Glx)
glutamine (*See also* Glx)
glutaminyl and/or glutamyl [indicates
  uncertainly between Glu and Gln]
  (*See also* Glx)
impedance
ionic charge number
no effect
point of line perpendicular to
  nasion-menton line through anterior
  nasal spine [craniometric]
section modulus
shape of surgical incision in
  Z-plasty
standardized deviate (*See also* z)
standard score
zero
zeta [sixth letter of Greek alphabet
  uppercase]
zone
zusammen

Z

proton [atomic number]

z

algebraic unknown or space
  coordinate
axis of three-dimensional rectangular
  coordinate system
catalytic amount
standard normal deviate (*See also* Z)
zepto-

ZAP

Zaldivar anterior [chamber] procedure
zoster-associated pain

ZAP-70

zeta-associated protein 70

ZAS

zymosan-activated autologous serum

ZAT

Zondek-Aschheim test [pregnancy]

ZB

zebra body

ZC

zona compacta

ZCP

zinc chloride poisoning

ZD

zero defect
zero discharge
zinc deficient
zona drilling

ZDDP

zinc dialkyldithiophosphate

Z-DNA

zig-zag [left handed helical]
  deoxyribonucleic acid

ZDO

zero differential overlap

ZDS

zinc depletion syndrome
Zung [self-rating] Depression
  Scale

zDVH

z-dependent dose-volume histogram [3D
  treatment planning tool]

ZEBRA

Epstein-Barr virus transactivator protein
  antibody

ZEEP

zero end-expiratory pressure

ZEGV

Zegla virus

ZEPI

zonal echo planar imaging

Z-ESR

zeta erythrocyte sedimentation
  rate

ζ

zeta [sixth letter of Greek alphabet
  lowercase]

ZF

zero frequency
zona fasciculata
zygomaticofrontal

ZFP

zero-flow pressure
zinc finger protein

ZG

zona glomerulosa

Z/G

zoster [serum] immunoglobulin (*See also*
  ZIG, ZIg)

ZGG

zinc gluconate glycine

ZGM

zinc glycinate marker

ZI

zona incerta

ZIFT

zygote intrafallopian [tube] transfer

ZIg
zoster immune globulin
(immunoglobulin)
ZIKAV
Zika virus
ZIP
zero-fill interpolation
zoster immune plasma
ZIRTL
zinc-iron regulated transporterlike [gene]
ZIRV
Zirqa virus
ZLN
zosteriform lentiginous nevus
Zm
zygomaxillare [craniometric]
ZMA
zinc meta-arsenite
ZMC
zygomatic maxillary complex
[zygomaticomaxillary complex]
[zygomaxillary complex]
Z-[^{123}I]MIVE
^{123}I-labeled cis-11beta-methoxy-17alpha-
iodovinyl-estradiol [scintigraphy]
ZN
Ziehl-Neelsen [method, stain] (*See also*
ZNS)
Zn
zinc
^{65}Zn
zinc-65
Zn fl
zinc flocculation [test] (*See also*
ZnFT)
ZnFT
zinc flocculation test (*See also* Zn fl)
ZnO
zinc oxide
ZnPc
zinc phthalocyanine
ZNPP
zinc protoporphyrin
ZNS
Ziehl-Neelsen stain (*See also* ZN)
ZnSO$_4$
zinc sulfate
ZnSR
zinc sedimentation rate
ZO
zonula occludens
ZOE, ZnOE
zinc oxide-eugenol [base, cement,
temporary filling]
ZOG
zona glomerulosa protein
ZOI
zone of inhibition

Zool
zoology
ZOOM
Guarana [herb]
ZOT, zot
zonula occludens toxin
Z-P
Z-plasty [surgical relaxation of
contracture]
ZP
zona pellucida
ZP1–ZP3
zona pellucida 1–3
ZPA
zone of polarizing activity
ZPC
zero point of charge
zone of preparatory calcification
ZPG
zero population growth
ZPI
Z-dependent protease inhibitor
ZPLS
Zimmerman Preschool Language
Scale
ZPO
zinc peroxide
ZPP
zinc protoporphyrin
zone of partial preservation
ZPP/H
zinc protoporphyrin/heme
ZR
zona reticularis
Zr
zirconium
ZrSiO$_4$
zirconium silicate
ZSB
zero stool [since] birth
ZSC
zone of slow conduction
ZSO
zinc suboptimal
zygomatic sandwich osteotomy
ZSR
ζ (zeta) sedimentation rate
ZSRDS
Zung Self-Rating Depression Scale
ZTGN
zheng ti guan nian [holistic thinking,
Chinese medicine]
ZTS
zymosan-treated serum
ZTT
zinc turbidity test
ZTV
Zaliv Terpeniya virus

ZUMI
    Zinnanti uterine manipulator-
      injector
ZY
    zinc, yellow [plating]
Zy
    zygion [craniometric]

zz.
    ginger [L. *zingiber*]
ZZR
    zinc turbidity test
Z, Z′, Z″
    increasing degrees of contraction [Ger.
    Zuckung] (*See also* Z)

Z

Contents: The Appendices

Symbols

∧	above	>	reveals
	diastolic blood pressure		shows
	(anesthesia records)		to
	elevated		toward
	enlarged		worse than
	improved		yields
	increased		
	superior (position)	<	caused by
	upper		derived from
∨	below		less severe than ⚠
	decreased		less than ⚠
	deficiency		produced by
	deficit		proximal
	depressed	∠	angle
	deteriorated		flexion
	diminished		flexor
	down		
	inferior (position)	∠ₑ	angle of entry
	lower	∠ₓ	angle of exit
	systolic blood pressure		
	(anesthesia records)	⌋	right lower quadrant
>	causes	⌐	right upper quadrant
	demonstrates	⌐	left upper quadrant
	distal	∟	left lower quadrant
	followed by		
	derived from	Δ	anion gap
	greater than ⚠		centrad prism
	indicates		change
	leads to		delta gap
	more severe than		heat
	produces		increment
	radiates (radiating) to		occipital triangle
	results in		prism diopter
			temperature (anesthesia
			records)

Δ+	time interval	Ⓘⱽ		intravenous intravenously
Δ *A*	change in absorbance	Ⓛ		left
Δ dB	difference in decibels	Ⓜ		murmur
Δ P	change in intraocular pressure	ⓜ		by mouth mouth (temperature) murmur
Δ pH	change in pH			
Δ t	time interval	√ⓜ		factitial murmur
Δ H, H Δ	Hesselbach triangle	Ⓞ		by mouth oral orally
○	respiration (anesthesia records)			
♀	female female sex	Ⓡ		rectal rectally rectum (temperature) right
♂	male male sex			
Ⓐ, ⓐₓ	axilla (temperature)	Ⓧ		end of anesthesia (anesthesia records) end of operation
Ⓗ, ⓗ	hypodermic hypodermically			
Ⓘᴹ	intramuscular intramuscularly			

Arrows

↑	above elevated (elevation) enlarged gas greater than improved increase(d) more than rising superior (position) up(per)	↑g	increasing rising
		↑v	increase due to in vivo effect (laboratory)
		↓	below decrease(d) deficiency deficit depressed depression deteriorated, deteriorating

↓
diminished
diminution
down
falling
inferior (position)
less than
low
normal plantar reflex
precipitate(s)
slower

↓g
decreasing
diminishing
falling
lowering

↓V
decrease due to in vivo
  effect (laboratory)

↗
deviated
displaced
increasing

↘
decreasing

→
approaches limit of
causes
demonstrates direction
  of flow or reaction
distal
due to
followed by
indicates
leads to
produces

→
radiating to
results in
reveals
shows
to
to right
toward
yields

←
caused by
derived from
direction of flow or
  reaction
due to
produced by
proximal
resulting from
secondary to
to left

⇈
extensor response (up
  bilaterally, positive
  Babinski sign)
testes undescended

⇊
plantar response (down
  bilaterally, normal)
testes descended

⇅
reversible reaction
up and down

⇌
reversible (chemical)
  reaction

Genetic Symbols

□	male	⊟⊘	adopted individuals
○	female	♂ ♀	individual died without leaving offspring
◇	sex unspecified	□⊤○	no issue
□ ○	normal people	■ ●	affected individuals
■ ● ◆	affected person (with ≥ 2 conditions, the symbol is partitioned and shaded with a different fill defined in a key or legend)	■ ●	proband or propositus (first affected family member coming to medical attention)
⑤ ⑤ ◇	multiple individuals, number known (number of siblings written inside symbol)	⊞	examined professionally normal for trait
		⊡	not examined dubiously reported to have trait
ⓝ ⓝ ◇	multiple individuals, number unknown ("n" used in place of specific number)	◫	not examined reliably reported to have trait
□○	mating	◧ ◐	heterozygotes for autosomal recessive
□○	consanguinity	⊙	carrier of sex-linked recessive
(+)	uncommon or uncertain mode of inheritance	⊘ ∅	death
I II	parents and offspring, in generations	⊘ ∅ ⊘ SB SB SB 28wk 30wk 34wk	stillbirth (SB)
	dizygotic twins	P Ⓟ ◇P LMP 20wk 7/1/94	pregnancy (P); gestational age and karotype (if known) below symbol
	monozygotic twins		
④ ③	number of children of sex indicated		

consultand (individual seeking genetic counseling/testing)

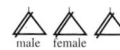 termination of pregnancy (TOP)

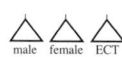 spontaneous abortion (SAB); ECT below symbol indicates ectopic pregnancy

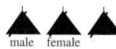 affected TOP (key or legend used to define shading)

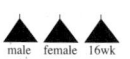 affected SAB (gestational age, if known, below symbol, and key or legend used to define shading)

Source: Genetic symbols are public domain. We credit and gratefully acknowledge the *American Journal of Human Genetics* (56:746–747, 1995) as our source for these symbols.

Numbers

0	completely absent (pulse) no response (reflexes)	+4, 4+	normal (pulse)
+1, 1+	markedly impaired (pulse)	4+	hyperactive (reflexes) large amount, pronounced reaction (laboratory tests)
1+	low normal or somewhat diminished (reflexes) slight reaction or trace (laboratory tests)	•	very brisk (reflexes)
+2, 2+	moderately impaired (pulse)	$\overline{1}$	bowel movement (numeral indicates number of stools in a given period)
2+	average or normal (reflexes) noticeable reaction or trace (laboratory tests)	1×	once one time
+3, 3+	slightly impaired (pulse)	2×, ×2	twice two times
3+	moderate reaction (laboratory tests) brisker than average (reflexes)	3×, ×3	three times, etc.

Arabic	Roman	Arabic	Roman
0		17	XVII
1	I, i	18	XVIII
2	II, ii	19	XIX
3	III, iii	20	XX
4	IV, iv	30	XXX
5	V, v	40	XL
6	VI, vi	50	L
7	VII, vii	60	LX
8	VIII, viii	70	LXX
9	IX, ix	80	LXXX
10	X, x	90	XC
11	XI, xi	100	C
12	XII, xii	1,000	M
13	XIII, xiii	5,000	$\overline{V}$
14	XIV, xiv	10,000	$\overline{X}$
15	XV	100,000	$\overline{C}$
16	XVI	1,000,000	$\overline{M}$

Pluses, Minuses, and Equivalencies

+	acid (reaction) added to△ convex lens decreased or diminished (reflexes) excess less than 50% inhibition of hemolysis (Wassermann) low normal (reflexes) markedly impaired (pulse) mild (pain or severity) plus△ positive (laboratory tests) present slight reaction or trace (laboratory tests) sluggish (reflexes) somewhat diminished (reflexes)	(+)	significant
		(+)ive	positive
		+ to ++	slight pain
		++	average (reflexes) 50% inhibition of hemolysis (Wassermann) moderate (pain or severity) moderately impaired (pulse) normally active (reflexes) noticeable reaction or trace (laboratory tests)
		+++	increased reflexes 75% inhibition of hemolysis (Wassermann) moderate amount

+++	moderate reaction (laboratory tests) moderately hyperative (reflexes) moderately severe (pain or severity) brisker than average (reflexes) slightly impaired (pulse)	±	possibly significant questionable suggestive variable very slight (reaction, severity, trace) with or without
		(±)	possibly significant
++++	complete inhibition of hemolysis (Wassermann) large amount (laboratory tests) markedly hyperactive (reflexes) markedly severe (pain or severity) normal (pulse) pronounced reaction (laboratory tests) very brisk (reflexes)	± to +	minimal pain
		∓	minus or plus
		⧺	moderate (severity) normally active (reflexes)
		#	fracture gauge number pound(s) weight
−	absent alkaline (reaction) concave lens deficiency, deficient minus negative (laboratory test) none subtract without	∼	about approximate(ly) proportionate to
		≈	approximately equal to
		=	equal to
		≠	not equal to
(−)	insignificant	◯	combined with
±	doubtful either positive or negative equivocal (reflexes, qualitative tests) flicker (reflexes) indefinite more or less plus or minus	⇌	equivalent
		⇋	not equivalent to
		≡	identical with
		≢	not identical with
		≑	nearly equal to
		≒	approximately equal

≅	approximately	>	greater than △
	approximately equal to	≯	not greater than
	congruent to	<	less than △
≐	approaches	≮	not less than
=	equilateral	≥, ⩾	greater than or equal to
≙	equiangular	≤, ⩽	less than or equal to

Primes, Checks, Dots, Roots, and Other Symbols

?	doubtful	"	bivalent
	equivocal (reflexes)		ditto
	flicker (reflexes)		inch
	not tested (severity)		minute
			second (1/60 degree)
	possible	'''	line (1/12 inch)
	questionable		trivalent
	question of		
	suggested	√	check
	suggestive (severity)		observe for
			urine
	unknown		voided (urine)
!	factorial product	⩒̇	urine and defecation
†	death		voided and bowels moved
	deceased		
		√c̄	check with
/	divided by	√d	checked
	either meaning		observed
	extension		
	extensors fraction of	√g, √ing	checking
	per△	√qs	voided quantity sufficient
	to	√‾	radical root
'	foot	²√‾	square root
	hour	³√‾	cube root
	univalent		

*	birth	:	is to, ratio
	multiplication sign (genetics)	...	no data (in given category)
	not verified		
	presumed	∴	therefore
	supposed	∵	because
°	degree, measurement (1/360 of circle)	::	as
	severity (burns, wounds)		equality between ratios
	temperature		proportion
	time (hour)$^{\triangle}$		proportionate to

Statistical Symbols

α	probability of Type I error	N	population size
	significance level	n	sample size
β	probability of Type II error	$n!$	n factorial
		O	observed frequency in a contingency table
1-β	power of statistical test		
		ϕ	ability continuum
$nCk; \left(\frac{n}{k}\right)$	binomial coefficient		phi coefficient
	number of combination of n things taken k at a time	P	probability
		p	probability of success in independent trials
χ^2	chi-squared statistic		
E	expected frequency in cell of contingency table	$P(A)$	probability that event A occurs
		$P(A\backslash B)$	conditional probability that A occurs given that B has occurred
$E(X)$	expected value of random variable X		
F	F statistic (variance ratio)	r	sample correlation coefficient, usually the Pearson product-moment correlation
f	frequency		
H_0	null hypothesis	r^2	coefficient of determination
H_1	alternative hypothesis		
μ ⚠	population mean	r_s	Spearman rank correlation coefficient

Appendix 1

ρ	population correlation coefficient	t	Student t statistic (test variable)
s	sample standard deviation	θ	latent trait
s^2	sample variance	U	Mann-Whitney rank sum statistic
SE	standard error of estimate		
σ	population standard deviation	W	Wilcoxon rank sum statistic
σ^2	population variance	$\overline{X}$	sample mean
σdiff.	standard error of difference between scores	$|x|$	absolute value of x
		$\sqrt{x}$	square root of x
σest.	standard error of estimate	z	standard score
σmeas.	standard error of measurement	∞	infinity

Greek Name	English Equivalent	Greek Upper Case	Greek Lower Case
alpha	a	A	α classifier in nomenclature of many sciences alpha particle angle of optic rotation aromatic substituent on an aliphatic chain Bunsen solubility coefficient degree of dissociation direction of chemical bond away from viewers first in a series (general) first of a series of closely related compounds (chemistry) position immediately adjacent to a carboxyl group (chemistry)
beta	b	B	β anomer of carbohydrate buffer capacity constituent of plasma protein fraction direction of chemical bond toward viewer second in a series (general) second carbon from a functional group (chemistry)
gamma	g	Γ	γ activity coefficient fourth carbon in an aliphatic acid position 2 removed from the α position in heavy chain of IgG

Greek Name	English Equivalent	Greek Upper Case	Greek Lower Case
gamma	g	Γ	γ photon (gamma ray) plasma protein (globulin) symbol for 10^{-4} gauss surface tension third in a series (general)
delta	d	Δ absence of heat treatment (chemistry) application of heat in reaction (chemistry) change double bond (chemistry) triangular surface (anatomy)	δ chemical shift in NMR distance between two atoms in a molecule position of a substituent located on the 4th atom from the carboxyl or other functional group (chemistry) thickness
epsilon	e	E	ε fifth in a series (general) heavy chain of IgE molar absorption coefficient or extinction coefficient position of a substituent located on the 5th atom from the carboxyl or other functional group (chemistry)
zeta	z	Z atomic number symbol	ζ electrokinetic potential position of a substituent located on the 6th atom from the carboxyl or other functional group (chemistry) sixth in a series (general)

Greek Name	English Equivalent	Greek Upper Case	Greek Lower Case

eta	h	H	η
			position of a substituent
			  located on the 7th atom
			  from the carboxyl or other
			  functional group (chemistry)
			viscosity

theta	th	Θ	θ angle

iota	i	I	ι
			ninth in a series (general)
			position of a substituent
			  located on the 9th atom
			  from the carboxyl or other
			  functional group (chemistry)

kappa	k	K	κ
			position of a substituent
			  located on the 10th atom
			  from the carboxyl or other
			  functional group (chemistry)
			tenth in a series (general)

lambda	l	Λ
		Avogadro number
		Ostwald solubility
		  coefficient
		radioactive constant
		wavelength
			λ
			craniometric point at
			  junction of sagittal and
			  lambdoid suture

mu	m	M	μ ⚠ chemical potential dynamic viscosity magnetic or electric dipole moment of molecule micro- ⚠

Appendix 2

Greek Name	English Equivalent	Greek Upper Case	Greek Lower Case
mu	m	M	μ ⚠ micron ⚠ position of a substituent located on the 12th atom from the carboxyl or other functional group (chemistry)
nu	n	N	ν frequency kinematic viscosity position of a susbstituent located on the 13th atom from the carboxyl or other functional group (chemistry) stoichiometric number
xi	x	Ξ	ξ
omicron	o	O	o
pi	p	Π osmotic pressure	π ratio of circumference of a circle to its diameter, 3.14159
rho	r	P	ρ density population correlation coefficient
sigma	s	Σ summation of a series	σ factor in prokaryotic RNA initiation reflection coefficient standard deviation surface tension wavenumber (frequency)

Greek Name	English Equivalent	Greek Upper Case	Greek Lower Case
tau	t	T	τ protein associated with plaque in Alzheimer disease relaxation time tele
upsilon	u	Y	υ
phi	ph	Φ magnetic flux phenyl potential energy	φ plane angle quantum yield volume fraction
chi	ch	X	χ twenty-second in a series (general) dihedral angle between α-carbon and side chains of amino acids in peptides and proteins
psi	ps	Ψ psychology	ψ
omega	o	Ω ohm	ω

Dangerous use of Greeks: Abbreviations starting with the Greek μ should not ever be used. The correct expansions are shown here. Terms containing the Greek μ in the middle or at the end can also be dangerous, and it is best to substitute "micro" within the expansion.

μ	micron	μin	microinch
μμ	micromicron, micromicro-	μIU	one-millionth International Unit
μΩ	microhm	μkat	microkatal (micromole per second)
μA	microampere	μL	microliter
μB	microbar	μL	microliter
μC	microcoloumb	μmm	micromilli
μCi	microcurie	μm³	cubic micrometerμm
μCi/hr	microcurie per hour	μmHg	micrometer of mercury
μEq	microequivalent	μmol	micromole
μF	microfarad	μN	micronewton
μμg	micromicrogram	μOsm	microsmolar
μg	microgram	μR	microroentgen
μγ	microgamma	μs, μsec	microsecond
μg/kg	microgram per kilogram	μV	microvolt
μg/L	microgram per liter	μW	microwatt
μGy	microgray	μU	microunit
μH	microhenry		

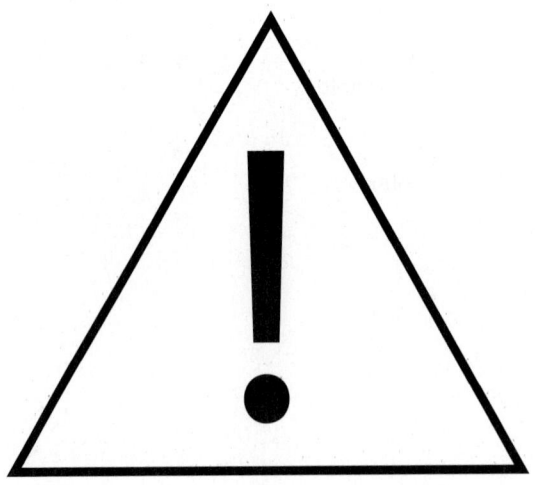

Appendix 3
Elements and Their Symbols

Element	Symbol		Element	Symbol
Actinium	Ac		Francium	Fr
Silver	Ag		Gallium	Ga
Aluminum	Al		Gadolinium	Gd
Argon	Ar		Germanium	Ge
Arsenic	As		Hydrogen	H
Astatine	At		Helium	He
Gold	Au		Hafnium	Hf
Boron	B		Mercury	Hg
Barium	Ba		Holmium	Ho
Beryllium	Be		Iodine	I
Bismuth	Bi		Indium	In
Bromine	Br		Iridium	Ir
Carbon	C		Potassium	K
Calcium	Ca		Krypton	Kr
Cadmium	Cd		Lanthanum	La
Cerium	Ce		Lithium	Li
Chlorine	Cl		Lutetium	Lu
Cobalt	Co		Magnesium	Mg
Chromium	Cr		Manganese	Mn
Cesium	Cs		Molybdenum	Mo
Copper	Cu		Nitrogen	N
Dysprosium	Dy		Sodium	Na
Erbium	Er		Niobium	Nb
Europium	Eu		Neodymium	Nd
Fluorine	F		Neon	Ne
Iron	Fe		Nickel	Ni

Element	Symbol	Element	Symbol
Oxygen	O	Silicon	Si
Osmium	Os	Samarium	Sm
Phosphorus	P	Tin	Sn
Protactinium	Pa	Strontium	Sr
Lead	Pb	Tantalum	Ta
Palladium	Pd	Terbium	Tb
Promethium	Pm	Technetium	Tc
Polonium	Po	Tellurium	Te
Praseodymium	Pr	Thorium	Th
Platinum	Pt	Titanium	Ti
Radium	Ra	Thallium	Tl
Rubidium	Rb	Thulium	Tm
Rhenium	Re	Uranium	U
Rhodium	Rh	Vanadium	V
Radon	Rn	Tungsten	W
Ruthenium	Ru	Xenon	Xe
Sulfur	S	Yttrium	Y
Antimony	Sb	Ytterbium	Yb
Scandium	Sc	Zinc	Zn
Selenium	Se	Zirconium	Zr

ISMP's List of Error-Prone Abbreviations, Symbols, and Dose Designations

Intended Abbreviation	Meaning	Misinterpretation	Correction
μ	Microgram	Mistaken as **mg**	Use **mcg** or **microgram**
AD, AS, AU	Right ear, left ear, each ear	Mistaken as OD, OS, OU (right eye, left eye, each eye)	Use **right ear**, **left ear**, or **each ear**
OD, OS, OU	Right eye, left eye, each eye	Mistaken as AD, AS, AU (right ear, left ear, each ear)	Use **right eye**, **left eye**, or or **each eye**
BT	Bedtime	Mistaken as **BID** (twice daily)	Use **bedtime**
cc	Cubic centimeters	Mistaken as **u** (units)	Use **mL**
D/C	Discharge or discontinue	Premature discontinuation of medications if D/C (intended to mean **discharge**) has been misinterpreted as **discontinued** when followed by a list of discharge medications	Use **discharge** and **discontinue**
IJ	Injection	Mistaken as **IV** or **intrajugular**	Use **injection**
IN	Intranasal	Mistaken as **IM** or **IV**	Use **intranasal** or **NAS**
HS	Half-strength	Mistaken as bedtime	Use **half-strength** or **bedtime**

Abbreviation	Intended Meaning	Misinterpretation	Correction
hs	At bedtime, hours of sleep	Mistaken as half-strength	Use **at bedtime**
IU△	International unit	Mistaken as IV (intravenous) or 10 (ten)	Use **units**
o.d. or OD	Once daily	Mistaken as **right eye** (OD-oculus dexter), leading to oral liquid medications administered in the eye	Use **daily**
OJ	Orange juice	Mistaken as OD or OS (right or left eye); drugs meant to be diluted in orange juice may be given in the eye	Use **orange juice**
Per os	By mouth, orally	The **os** can be mistaken as **left eye** (OS—oculus sinister)	Use **PO**, **by mouth**, or **orally**
q.d. or QD△	Every day	Mistaken as q.i.d., especially if the period after the **q** or the tail of the **q** is misunderstood as an **i**	Use **daily**
qhs	At bedtime	Mistaken as **qhr** or every hour	Use **at bedtime**

Abbreviation	Intended Meaning	Misinterpretation	Correction
qn	Nightly	Mistaken as **qh** (every hour)	Use **nightly**
q.o.d. or QOD△	Every other day	Mistaken as **q.d.** (daily) or **q.i.d.** (four times daily) if the **o** is poorly written	Use **every other day**
q1d	Daily	Mistaken as q.i.d. (four times daily)	Use **daily**
q6PM, etc.	Every evening at 6 PM	Mistaken as every 6 hours	Use **6 PM nightly** or **6 PM daily**
SC, SQ, sub q	Subcutaneous	SC mistaken as SL (sublingual); SQ mistaken as **5 every**; the **q** in **sub q** has been mistaken as **every** (e.g., a heparin dose ordered **sub q 2 hours before surgery** misunderstood as every 2 hours before surgery)	Use **subcut** or **subcutaneously**
ss	Sliding scale (insulin) or 1/2 (apothecary)	Mistaken as **55**	Spell out **sliding scale**; use **one-half** or **1/2**
SSRI	Sliding scale regular insulin	Mistaken as selective-serotonin reuptake inhibitor	Spell out **sliding scale (insulin)**
SSI	Sliding scale insulin	Mistaken as Strong Solution of Iodine (Lugol's)	Spell out **sliding scale (insulin)**
i̅/d	One daily	Mistaken as **tid**	Use **1 daily**

Abbreviation	Intended Meaning	Misinterpretation	Correction
TIW or tiw	3 times a week	Mistaken as **3 times a day** or **twice in a week**	Use **3 times weekly**
U or u△	Unit	Mistaken as the number O or 4, causing a tenfold overdose or greater (e.g., 4U seen as **40** or 4u seen as **44**); mistaken as **cc** so dose given in volume instead of units (e.g., 4u seen as 4cc)	Use **unit**

△ Identified abbreviations above are also included on the JCAHO's "minimum list" of Error-Prone Abbreviations, acronyms, and symbols that must be included on an organization's "Do Not Use" list, effective January 1, 2004. Visit www.jcaho.org for more information about this JCAHO requirement.
© ISMP 2006
Reprinted with permission from the Institute for Safe Medication Practices.

Dose Designations and Other Information	Intended Meaning	Misinterpretation	Correction
Trailing zero after decimal point (e.g., 1.0 mg)△	1 mg	Mistaken as 10 mg if the decimal point is not seen	Do not use trailing zeros for doses expressed in whole numbers
No leading zero before a decimal dose (e.g., .5 mg)△	0.5 mg	Mistaken as 5 mg if the decimal point is not seen	Use zero before a decimal point when the dose is less than a whole unit
Drug name and dose run together (especially problematic for drug names that end in "L" such as Inderal40 mg; Tegretol300 mg)	Inderal 40 mg Tegretol 300 mg	Mistaken as Inderal 140 mg Mistaken as Tegretol 1300 mg	Place adequate space between the drug name, dose, and unit of measure
Numeric dose and unit of measure run together (e.g., 10mg, 100mL)	10 mg 100 mL	The **m** is sometimes mistaken for a zero or two zeros, risking a 10- to 100-foldover dose	Place adequate space between the dose and unit of measure
Abbreviations such as mg. or mL. with a period following the abbreviation	mg mL	The period is unnecessary and could be mistaken as the number 1 if written poorly	Use mg, mL, and such abbreviations without a terminal period
Large doses without properly placed commas (e.g., 100000 units; 1000000 units)	100,000 units 1,000,000 units	100000 has been mistaken as 10,000 or 1,000,000; 1000000 has been mistaken as 100,000	Use commas for dosing units at or above 1,000, or use words such as **100 thousand** or **1 million** to improve readability

Drug Name Abbreviation	Intended Meaning	Misinterpretation	Correction
ARA A	vidarabine	Mistaken as cytarabine (ARA C)	Use complete drug name
AZT	zidovudine (Retrovir)	Mistaken as azathioprine or aztreonam	Use complete drug name
CPZ	Compazine (prochlorperazine)	Mistaken as chlorpromazine	Use complete drug name
DPT	Demerol-Phenergan-Thorazine	Mistaken as diphtheria-pertussis-tetanus (vaccine)	Use complete drug name
DTO	Diluted tincture of opium, or deodorized tincture of opium (Paregoric)	Mistaken as tincture of opium	Use complete drug name
HCl	hydrochloric acid or hydrochloride	Mistaken as potassium chloride (The **H** is misinterpreted as **K**)	Use complete drug name unless expressed as a salt of a drug
HCT	hydrocortisone	Mistaken as hydrochlorothiazide	Use complete drug name
HCTZ	hydrochlorothiazide	Mistaken as hydrocortisone (seen as HCT250 mg)	Use complete drug name
MgSO4$^{\triangle}$	magnesium sulfate	Mistaken as morphine sulfate	Use complete drug name
MS, MSO4$^{\triangle}$	morphine sulfate	Mistaken as magnesium sulfate	Use complete drug name
MTX	methotrexate	Mistaken as mitoxantrone	Use complete drug name

Drug Name Abbreviation	Intended Meaning	Misinterpretation	Correction
PCA	procainamide	Mistaken as **Patient Controlled Analgesia**	Use complete drug name
PTU	propylthiouracil	Mistaken as **mercaptopurine**	Use complete drug name
T3	Tylenol with codeine No. 3	Mistaken as **liothyronine**	Use complete drug name
TAC	triamcinolone	Mistaken as **tetracaine, Adrenalin, cocaine**	Use complete drug name
TNK	TNKase	Mistaken as **TPA**	Use complete drug name
ZnSO4	zinc sulfate	Mistaken as **morphine sulfate**	Use complete drug name

Stemmed Drug Name	Intended Meaning	Misinterpretation	Correction
Nitro drip	nitroglycerin infusion	Mistaken as sodium nitroprusside infusion	Use complete drug name
Norflox	norfloxacin	Mistaken as Norflex	Use complete drug name
IV Vanc	intravenous vancomycine	Mistaken as Invanz	Use complete drug nam

Symbols Abbreviations	Intended Meaning	Misinterpretation	Correction
℥ ♍	Dram	Symbol for dram mistaken as **3**	Use the metric system
	Minim	Symbol for minim mistaken as **mL**	Use the metric system
x3d	For 3 days	Mistaken as **3 doses**	Use **for three days**
> and <	Greater than and less than	Mistaken as opposite of intended; mistakenly use incorrect symbol; **< 10** mistaken as **40**	Use **greater than** or **less than**
/ (slash mark)	Separates two doses or indicates **per**	Mistaken as the number 1 (**e.g., 25 units/10 units** misread as **25 units and 110** units)	Use **per** rather than a slash mark to separate doses
@	At	Mistaken as **2**	Use **at**
&	And	Mistaken as **2**	Use **and**
+	Plus or and	Mistaken as **4**	Use **and**
°	Hour	Mistaken as a zero (e.g., q2° seen as q 20)	Use **hr, h,** or **hour**

⚠ Identified abbreviations above are also included on the JCAHO's "minimum list" of Error-Prone Abbreviations, acronyms, and symbols that must be included on an organization's "Do Not Use" list, effective January 1, 2004. Visit www.jcaho.org for more information about this JCAHO requirement.
© ISMP 2006
Reprinted with permission from the Institute for Safe Medication Practices.

Appendix 5
Weights and Measures

Scale of the Metric System and SI

Prefix	Symbol	Power
yotta-	Y	10^{24}
zetta-	Z	10^{21}
exa-	E	10^{18}
peta-	P	10^{15}
tera-	T	10^{12}
giga-	G	10^9
mega-	M	10^6
kilo-	k	10^3
hecto-	h	10^2
deca-	da	10^1
UNIT		
deci-	d	10^{-1}
centi-	c	10^{-2}
milli-	m	10^{-3}
micro-	mc	10^{-6}
nano-	n	10^{-9}
pico-	p	10^{-12}
femto-	f	10^{-15}

SI Base Units

Quantity	Name	Symbol
length	meter	m
mass*	kilogram†	kg
time	second	s
electric current	ampere	A
thermodynamic temperature	kelvin‡	K
luminous intensity	candela	cd
amount of substance	mole	mol

* In commercial and everyday use, "weight" usually means mass; e.g.,when speaking of a person's weight, the quantity referred to is mass.

† For historic reasons, kilogram is the only base unit with a prefix. Multiples and submultiples of the kilogram are formed by attaching the appropriate prefix to the stem word "gram" (e.g.,milligram) and the appropriate prefix symbol to the symbol "g" (e.g.,mg.).

‡ The degree Celsius (°C) is still widely accepted usage for expressing temperature and temperature intervals. Celsius (formerly centigrade) temperature is converted to kelvin (K) thermodynamic temperature by adding 273.16 to the Celsius scale. For temperature interval,1°C equals K.

Some SI Derived Units Expressed in Terms of Base Units

Quantity	Name	SI Derived Unit
area	square meter	m^2
volume*	cubic meter	m^3
specific volume	cubic meter per kilogram	m^3/kg
speed, velocity	meter per second	m/s
acceleration	meter per second squared	m/s^2
mass density	kilogram per cubic meter	kg/m^3
concentration	mole per cubic meter	mol/m^3
luminance	candela per square meter	cd/m^2

* Liter (L, l). 1023 m3, is regarded as a special name for the cubic decimeter.

Some SI Derived Units with Special Names

Quantity	Name	Symbol	SI Derived Name	Expression
frequency	hertz	Hz	—	s^{-1}
force	newton	N	—	$m{\cdot}kg{\cdot}s^{-2}$
pressure, stress	pascal	Pa	N/m^2	$m^{-1}{\cdot}kg{\cdot}s^{-2}$
energy, work, quantity of heat	joule	J	$N{\cdot}m$	$m^2{\cdot}kg{\cdot}s^{-2}$
power, radiant flux	watt	W	J/s	$m^2{\cdot}kg{\cdot}s^{-3}$
electric charge, quantity of electricity	coulomb	C	—	$s{\cdot}A$
electric potential difference, electromotive force	volt	V	W/A	$m^2{\cdot}kg{\cdot}s^{-3}{\cdot}A^{-1}$
capacitance	farad	F	C/V	$m^{-2}{\cdot}kg^{-1}{\cdot}s^4{\cdot}A^2$
electrical resistance	ohm	Ω	V/A	$m^2{\cdot}kg{\cdot}s^{-3}{\cdot}A^{-2}$
electrical conductance	siemens	S	A/V	$m^2{\cdot}kg^{-1}{\cdot}s^{-3}{\cdot}A^2$
magnetic flux	weber	Wb	$V{\cdot}s$	$m^2{\cdot}kg{\cdot}s^{-2}{\cdot}A^{-1}$
magnetic flux density	tesla	T	Wb/m^2	$kg{\cdot}s^{-2}{\cdot}A^{-1}$
activity of radionuclide	becquerel*	Bq	—	$-s^{-1}$
absorbed dose of radiation, specific energy (imparted), kerma	gray†	Gy	J/kg	$m^2{\cdot}s^{-2}$
exposure (x and γ radiation)	coulomb per kilogram‡	—	C/kg	$kg{\cdot}1{\cdot}s{\cdot}A$

* Replacing the curie (Ci), 3.7 3 1010 s21.

† Replacing the rad (rad), 1022 J kg21.

‡ Replacing the roentgen (R), 2.58 3 1024 C kg21.

Measures of Length

Micro-meters	Milli-meters	Centi-meters	Meters	Kilometers	Miles	Yards	Feet	Inches
1	0.001	10^{-4}						0.000039
10^3	1	10^{-1}					0.00328	0.03937
10^4	10	1	0.01			0.0109	0.03281	.3937
25,400	25.4	2.54	0.0254			0.0278	0.0833	1
	304.8	30.48	0.3048			0.333	1	12
10^6	10^3	10^2	1	0.001	0.0006213	1.0936	3.2808	39.37
914,400	914.40	91.44	0.9144	0.009	0.0005681	1	3	36
10^9	10^6	10^5	10^3	1	0.6215	1093.6121	3280.8	
			1609.0	1.609	1	1760.0	5280.0	

To convert:
Millimeters to inches: divide by 25.4
Inches to millimeters: multiply by 25.4
Centimeters to feet: divide by 30.7
Feet to centimeters: multiply by 30.7
Meters to yards: multiply by 1.09375
Yards to meters: multiply by 0.9143
Kilometers to miles: multiply by 0.625
Miles to kilometers: multiply by 1.6

Measures of Mass (Weight)

Avoirdupois

| Grains | Drams | Ounces | Pounds | Metric Equivalents | | |
				Milligrams	Grams	Kilograms
1	0.0366	0.0023	0.00014	64.8	0.0648	0.000065
27.34	1	0.0625	0.0039		1.772	0.001772
437.5	16	1	0.0625		28.350	0.028350
7,000	256	16	1		453.5924	0.453592
0.0154				1	0.001	
15.4324	0.5648	0.0353	0.002205	1000	1	0.001
15,432.358	564.32	35.27	2.2046		1000	1

To convert (approximately):
Kilograms to pounds: multiply by 2.2
Pounds to kilograms: multiply by 0.454
Grams to ounces: multiply by 0.03527
Ounces to grams: multiply by 28.35

Measures of Mass (Weight)
Apothecaries' Measures

Grains	Scruples	Drams	Ounces	Pounds	Metric Equivalents		
					Milligrams	Grams	Kilograms
1	0.05	0.0167	0.0021	0.00017	64.8	0.0648	0.000065
20	1	0.0333	0.042	0.0035		1.296	0.001296
60	3	1	0.125	0.0104		3.888	0.000389
480	24	8	1	0.0833		31.103	0.031103
5,760	288	96	12	1		373.2418	0.373242
0.0154				1	1	0.001	
15.4324		0.2572	0.0322	0.0024	1000	1	0.001
15,432.358		257.2	32.15	2.6792		1000	1

Measures of Capacity
Apothecaries' Measures

Minims	Fluid Drams	Fluid Ounces	Pints	Quarts	Gallons	Metric Equivalents	
						Liters	Milliliters
1	0.0166	0.002	0.00013			0.0006	0.06161
60	1	0.125	0.0078	0.0039		0.0037	3.6967
480	8	1	0.0625	0.0312	0.0078	0.0296	29.5737
7,680	128	16	1	0.5	0.125	0.4732	473.166
15,360	256	32	2	1	0.25	0.9464	946.358
61,440	1024	128	8	4	1	3.7854	3785.434
16,230	270.52	33.8418	2.1134	1.0567	0.2642	1	1000
16.23	0.2705	0.0338	0.00212	0.00106	0.000265	0.001	1

To convert (approximately):
1 British imperial gallon = 1.201 U.
1 U.S. gallon = 0.8327 British imperial
Liters to gallons: multiply by 0.264
Gallons to liters: multiply by 3.788
Liters to pints: multiply by 2.1
Pints to liters: multiply by 0.4762

Approximate Household Measures and Weights*
Avoirdupois

Teaspoons	Tablespoons	Cups or Glasses	Drams	Fluid Ounces	Milliliters	Grams
1			1	0.125	5	5
3	1		4	0.50	15	15
48	16***	1	64	8	237	240

* A drop is a measure of uncertain quantity, depending on the liquid as well as the shape of the container and of the opening from which the liquid falls. One drop of water is roughly equivalent to 1 mimin.
** Tumbler or glass is generally intended to mean 8 fl. oz.
*** For dry measure, 12 tablespoons equals 1 cup.

Professional Titles and Degrees

AA
Anesthesiologist Assistant

AARCF
American Association for Respiratory
Care Fellow

AAS
Associate in Applied Science

ABD
All But Dissertation

ACHRN
Advanced Certified Hyperbaric Nurse

ACP
Advanced Clinical Practitioner

ACRN
AIDS Certified Hyperbaric Nurse

AD
Associate Degree

ADN
Associate Degree in Nursing

AHI
Allied Health Instructor (American
Medical Technologists)

AHN
Army Head Nurse
Assistant Head Nurse

AHP
Assistant House Physician

AHS
Assistant House Surgeon

AMO
Assistant Medical Officer

ANP
Adult Nurse Practitioner
Advanced Nurse Practitioner

AOCN
Advanced Oncology Certified Nurse

AOCNP
Advanced Oncology Certified Nurse
Practitioner

AOCNS
Advanced Oncology Certified Nurse
Specialist

APRN
Advance Practice Registered Nurse

APRN, BC
Advanced Practice Registered Nurse,
Board Certified

APRN, BC-PCM
Advanced Practice Registered Nurse,
Board Certified-Palliative Care
Management

ARNP
Advanced Registered Nurse Practitioner

ART
Accredited Records Technologist

AT(ASCP)
Apheresis Technician (American
Society for Clinical Pathology)

ATC
Athletic Trainer, Certified

AuD
Doctorate of Audiology

BA
Bachelor of Arts

BAMS
Bachelor of Ayurvedic Medicine and
Surgery

BAO
Bachelor of Arts of Obstetrics

BB(ASCP)
Technologist in Blood Banking certified
by the American Society for Clinical
Pathology

BCCS
Board Certified in Clinical Social Work

BChD
Bachelor of Dentistry

BCNP
Board Certified Nuclear Pharmacist

BCNSP
Board Certified Nutrition Support
Pharmacist

BCPS
Board Certified Pharmacotherapy
Specialist

BDSc
Bachelor of Dental Science

BDS
Bachelor of Dental Surgery

BHS
Bachelor of Health Science

BHyg
Bachelor of Hygiene

BM, BMed
Bachelor of Medicine

BM BCH
Bachelor of Medicine and Chirurgiae
Baccalaureus (Bachelor of Surgery)

BMedBiol
Bachelor of Medical Biology

BMedSci, BMS
Bachelor of Medical Science

BMic
Bachelor of Microbiology

BMT
Bachelor of Medical Technology

BN
Bachelor of Nursing

BNEd
Bachelor of Nursing Education

BNSc
Bachelor of Nursing Science

BO
Bachelor of Osteopathy

BP, BPharm
Bachelor of Pharmacy

BPH
Bachelor of Public Health

BPHEng
Bachelor of Public Health Engineering

BPHN
Bachelor of Public Health Nursing

BS, BSc
Bachelor of Science

BSM, BScM
Bachelor of Science in Medicine

BSN, BScN
Bachelor of Science in Nursing

BSOT
Bachelor of Science in Occupational Therapy

BSPh, BScPh
Bachelor of Science in Pharmacy

BSS
Bachelor of Sanitary Science

BSW
Bachelor of Social Work

BVMS
Bachelor of Veterinary Medicine and Surgery

BVSc
Bachelor of Veterinary Science

CA
Certified Acupuncturist

CADC
Certified Alcohol and Drug Counselor

CALN
Clinical Administrative Liaison Nurse

C(ASCP)
Technologist in Chemistry certified by the American Society for Clinical Pathology

CAPA
Certified Ambulatory Perianesthesia Nurse

CAT(C)
Certified Athletic Therapist (Canada)

CBI
Certificate in Breast Imaging

CCC-A
Certificate of Clinical Competence in Audiology

CCCP
Board Certified in Child and Adolescent Psychology

CCC-SLP
Certificate in Clinical Competence in Speech-Language Pathology

CCEMT-P
Critical Care Emergency Medical Technician–Paramedic

CCHP
Certified Correctional Health
  Professional

CCM
Certified Case Manager

CCMHC
Certified Clinical Mental Health
  Counselor

CCNS
Critical Care Nurse Specialist

CCP
Certified Clinical Perfusionist

CCRN
Critical Care Registered Nurse

CCS
Cardiopulmonary Certified Specialist
Certified Coding Specialist

CDA
Certified Dental Assistant

CDE
Certified Diabetes Educator

CDMS
Certified Disability Management
  Specialist

CDN
Certified Dialysis Nurse

CDT
Certified Dental Technician

CEN
Certified Emergency Nurse

CEO
Chief Executive Officer

CFNP
Certified Family Nurse Practitioner

CFO
Chief Financial Officer

CFP
Clinical Fellowship Program

CFRN
Certified Emergency Flight Nurse

CGC
Certified Gastrointestinal Clinician

CGRN
Certified Gastroenterology Registered
  Nurse

CGT
Certified Gastroenterology Technician

ChB, CB
Chirurgiae Baccalaureus (Bachelor of
  Surgery)

ChD, Chir.Doct.
Chirurgiae Doctor (Doctor of Surgery)

CHE
Certified Healthcare Executive

ChM, CM
Chirurgiae Magister (Master of
  Surgery)

CHN
Certified Hemodialysis Nurse
Community Health Nurse

Professional Titles
and Degrees

CHP
Coordinating Hospital Physician

CHPN
Certified Hospice and Palliative Nurse

CHRN
Certified Hyperbaric Nurse

CIC
Certified Infection Control

CIH
Certificate in Industrial Health

CISW
Certified Independent Social Worker

CLA
Certified Laboratory Assistant

CLA(ASCP)
Clinical Laboratory Assistant certified by the American Society for Clinical Pathology

CLDir(NCA)
Clinical Laboratory Director certified by National Credentialing Agency for Laboratory Personnel

CLPlb(NCA)
Clinical Laboratory Phlebotomist certified by National Credentialing Agency for Laboratory Personnel

CLS
Clinical Laboratory Scientist

CLS(NCA)
Clinical Laboratory Scientist certified by National Credentialing Agency for Laboratory Personnel

CLSP
Clinical Laboratory Specialist

CLSp(CG)(NCA)
Clinical Laboratory Specialist in Cytogenetics certified by National Credentialing Agency for Laboratory Personnel

CLSp(MB)(NCA)
Clinical Laboratory Specialist in Molecular Biology certified by National Credentialing Agency for Laboratory Personnel

CLSup(NCA)
Clinical Laboratory Supervisor certified by National Credentialing Agency for Laboratory Personnel

CLT
Certified Laboratory Technician
Clinical Laboratory Technician
Clinical Laboratory Technologist

CLT(NCA)
Clinical Laboratory Technician certified by National Credentialing Agency for Laboratory Personnel

CM
Certified Midwife

CMA
Certified Medical Assistant

CMA-A
Certified Medical Assistant, Administrative

CMA-C
Certified Medical Assistant, Clinical

CMAS
Certified Medical Administrative Specialist (American Medical Technologists)

CMFT
Certified Marriage and Family Therapist

CMHN
Community Mental Health Nurse

CMO
Chief Medical Officer

CMS
Certificate in Management Studies

CMSRN
Certified Medical-Surgical Registered Nurse

CMT
Certified Medical Transcriptionist (American Association for Medical Transcription)

CNA
Certified Nursing Assistant

CNIM
Certification in Neurophysiologic Intraoperative Monitoring (American Board of Registration of Electroencephalographic and Evoked Potential Technologists)

CNM
Certified Nurse-Midwife

CNMT
Certified Nuclear Medicine Technologist

CNN
Certified Nephrology Nurse

CNOR
Certified Nurse Operating Room

CNP
Community Nurse Practitioner

CNRN
Certified Neuroscience Registered Nurse

CNS
Clinical Nurse Specialist

CNSD
Certified Nutrition Support Dietician

CNSN
Certified Nutrition Support Nurse

CNSP
Certified Nutrition Support Physician

CO
Certified Orthotist

COCN
Certified Continence Care Nurse

COLT
Certified Office Laboratory Technician (American Medical Technologists)

COMA
Certified Ophthalmic Medical Assistant

COMT
Certified Ophthalmic Medical Technologist

CORD
Commissioned Officer Residency
  Deferment

CORN
Certified Operating Room Nurse

CORT
Certified Operating Room Technician

COS, CS
Chief of Staff

COTA
Certified Occupational Therapy
  Assistant (National Board for
  Certification in Occupational
  Therapy)

CP
Certified Prosthetist
Certified Psychologist
Clinical Psychologist

CPAN
Certified Post-Anesthesia Nurse

CPed
Certified Pedorthist

CPFT
Certified Pulmonary Function
  Technologist (National Board of
  Respiratory Care)

CPH
Certificate in Public Health

CPN
Certified Pediatric Nurse

CPNP
Certified Pediatric Nurse Practitioner

CPO
Certified Prosthetist and Orthotist

CPON
Certified Pediatric Oncology Nurse

CPNP
Certified Pediatric Nurse Practitioner

CR
Chief Resident

CRCS
Canadian Registered Cardiac
  Sonographer

CRGS
Canadian Registered General
  Sonographer

CRL
Certified Record Librarian

CRNA
Certified Registered Nurse Anesthetist

CRNI
Certified Registered Nurse Intravenous

CRNP
Certified Registered Nurse Practitioner

CRRN
Certified Rehabilitation Registered
  Nurse

CRRN-A
Certified Rehabilitation Registered
  Nurse-Advanced

CRT
Certified Respiratory Therapist

CRTT
Certified Respiratory Therapy Technician

CRVS
Canadian Registered Vascular Sonographer

CSCS
Certified Strength and Conditioning Specialist

CST
Certified Surgical Technologist

CSW
Certified Social Worker
Clinical Social Worker

CT
Cardiovascular Technologist
Cytotechnologist

CT(ASCP)
Cytotechnologist certified by the American Society for Clinical Pathology

CTIC
Computed Tomography Imaging Certificate

CTR
Certified Tumor Reistrar

CUCNS
Certified Urologic Clinical Nurse Specialist

CUNP
Certified Urologic Nurse Practitioner

CURN
Certified Urological Registered Nurse

CVO
Chief Veterinary Officer

CVT
Certified Veterinary Technician

CWCN
Certified Wound Care Nurse

CWOCN
Certified Wound, Ostomy, and Continence Nurse

D, Dip
diplomate

DA
Dental Assistant
Diploma in Anesthetics

D&E
Diploma of Applied Parasitology and Entomology

DBIR
Director of Biotechnology Information Resources

DC
Doctor of Chiropractic

DCH
Diploma in Child Health

DCh
Doctor Chirurgiae (Doctor of Surgery)

DchO
Doctor of Ophthalmic Surgery

DCM
Doctor of Comparative Medicine

DCO
Diploma of the College of Optics

DCP
Diploma in Clinical Pathology
Diploma in Clinical Psychology
District Community Physician

DD
Doctor of Divinity

DDH
Diploma in Dental Health

DDM
Diploma in Dermatological Medicine
Doctor of Dental Medicine

DDO
Diploma in Dental Orthopaedics

DDR
Diploma in Diagnostic Radiology

DDS
Doctor of Dental Surgery

DDSc
Doctor of Dental Science

DFHom
Diplomat Faculty of Homeopathy

DGO
Diploma in Gynaecology and Obstetrics

DH
Dental Hygienist

DHg, Dhyg, DHy, DHyg, DrHyg
Doctor of Hygiene

DHMSA
Diploma of History of Medicine,
Society of Apothecaries

Diet. Tech.
Dietetic Technician

DipBact
Diploma in Bacteriology

DipChem
Diploma in Chemistry

DipClinPath
Diploma in Clinical Pathology

DipMicrobiol
Diploma in Microbiology

DipSocMed
Diploma in Social Medicine

DLO
Diploma in Laryngology and Otology

DLM(ASCP)
Diplomat in Laboratory Management
certified by the American Society for
Clinical Pathology

DM
Doctor Medicinae (Doctor of Medicine)

DMA
Director of Medical Affairs

DMD
Doctor of Dental Medicine

DME
Director of Medical Education

DMJ
Diploma in Medical Jurisprudence

DMR
Diploma in Medical Radiology
Directorate of Medical Research

DMRE
Diploma in Medical Radiology and
Electrology

DMS, DMSc
Doctor of Medical Science

DMT
Doctor of Medical Technology

DMV
Doctor of Veterinary Medicine

DN
Diploma in Nursing
Diploma in Nutrition
District Nurse
Doctor of Nursing

DNB
Diplomate of the National Board (of
Medical Examiners)

DNC
Dermatology Nurse Certified

DNE
Director of Nursing Education
Doctor of Nursing Education

DNO
District Nursing Officer

DNP
Doctor of Nursing Practice

DNS
Doctor of Nursing Services

DO
Diploma in Ophthalmology
Diploma in Osteopathy
Doctor of Ophthalmology
Doctor of Osteopathy

DOHyg
Diploma in Occupational Hygiene

DOM
Doctor of Oriental Medicine

DOMS
Diploma in Ophthalmic Medicine and
Surgery
Doctor of Orthopedic Medicine and
Surgery

DON
Director of Nursing

Doph
Doctor of Ophthalmology

DOPS
Director of Pharmacy Services

Dorth
Diploma in Orthodontics
Diploma in Orthoptics

DOS, DOSc
Doctor of Ocular Science
Doctor of Optical Science

DP
Doctor of Podiatry
Doctor of Pharmacy

DPD
Diploma in Public Dentistry

DPH
Doctor of Public Health
Doctor of Public Hygiene

DPharm
Doctor of Pharmacy

DPhC
Doctor of Pharmaceutical Chemistry

DPhc
Doctor of Pharmacology

DPHN
Doctor of Public Health Nursing

Dphys
Diploma in Physiotherapy

DphysMed
Diploma in Physical Medicine

DPM
Diploma in Psychological Medicine
Doctor of Physical Medicine
Doctor of Podiatric Medicine
Doctor of Preventive Medicine
Doctor of Psychiatric Medicine

DPR
Department of Professional Regulation

DPsy
Doctor of Psychology

DPT
Doctor of Physical Therapy

Dr, DR
doctor

DrHyg
Doctor of Hygiene

Dr Med
Doctor of Medicine

DrMT
Doctor of Mechanotherapy

DrPH
Doctor of Public Health/Hygiene

DS, DSc
Doctor of Science

DSC
Doctor of Surgical Chiropody

DSE
Doctor of Sanitary Engineering

DSIM
Doctor of Science in Industrial
 Medicine

DSM
Diploma in Social Medicine

DSSc
Diploma in Sanitary Science

DSur
Doctor of Surgery

DSW
Doctor of Social Work

DTCD
Diploma in Tuberculosis and Chest
Diseases

D&D
Diploma in Venereology and
Dermatology

DVM
Doctor of Veterinary Medicine

DVMS
Doctor of Veterinary Medicine and
Surgery

DVR
Diploma in Vocational Rehabilitation
Doctor of Veterinary Radiology

DVS
Doctor of Veterinary Science
Doctor of Veterinary Surgery

DVSc
Doctor of Veterinary Science

ECS
(Clinical) Electrophysiologic Certified
Specialist (American Physical
Therapists Association)

EdD
Doctor of Education

EEG T
Electroencephalographic Technologist

EFDA
Expanded Function Dental Auxiliary

EMT
Emergency Medical Technician

EMT-A
Emergency Medical Technician–
Advanced
Emergency Medical Technician–
Ambulance

EMT-B
Emergency Medical Technician–Basic
(DOT classification; locales may
vary)

EMT-D
Emergency Medical Technician–
Defibrillation

EMT-I
Emergency Medical Technician–
Intermediate (DOT classification;
locales may vary)

EMT-I/85
Emergency Medical Technician–
Intermediate (DOT classification;
locales may vary)

EMT-I/99
Emergency Medical Technician–
Intermediate (DOT classification;
locales may vary)

EMT-M
Emergency Medical Technician–
Military

EMT-P
Emergency Medical Technician–
Paramedic (DOT classification;
locales may vary)

EN
Enrolled Nurse

ENP
Emergency Nurse Practitioner

ENPC
Emergency Nursing Pediatric Course

ET
Enterostomal Therapist

FAAN
Fellow of the American Academy of
Nursing
Fellow of the American Academy of
Neurology

FAAFP
Fellow of the American Academy of
Family Physicians

FAAP
Fellow of the American Academy of
Pediatrics

FAAMT
Fellow, American Association for
Medical Transcription

FAARC
Fellow of the American Association for
Respiratory Care

FACA
Fellow of the American College of
Anesthesiology

FACAAI
Fellow of the American College of
Allergy, Asthma and Immunology

FACAG
Fellow of the American College of
Angiology

FACAI
Fellow of the American College of
Allergy and Immunology

FACAL
Fellow of the American College of
Allergy

FACAN
Fellow of the American College of
Anesthesiologists

FACAS
Fellow of the American College of
Abdominal Surgeons

FACC
Fellow of the American College of
Cardiologists

FACCP
Fellow of the American College of
Chest Physicians

FACCPC
Fellow of the American College of
Pharmacology and Chemotherapy

FACD
Fellow of the American College of
Dentists

FACEM
Fellow of the American College of
Emergency Medicine

FACEP
Fellow of the American College of
Emergency Physicians

FACFP
Fellow of the American College of
Family Physicians

FACFS
Fellow of the American College of Foot
    Surgeons

FACG
Fellow of the American College of
    Gastroenterology

FACHA
Fellow of the American College of
    Hospital Administrators

FACHE
Fellow of the American College of
    Healthcare Executives

FACLM
Fellow of the American College of
    Legal Medicine

FACN
Fellow of the American College of
    Nutrition

FACNM
Fellow of the American College of
    Nuclear Medicine

FACNP
Fellow of the American College of
    Neuropsychopharmacology
Fellow of the American College of
    Nuclear Physicians

FACO
Fellow of the American College of
    Otolaryngology

FACOG
Fellow of the American College of
    Obstetricians and Gynecologists

FACOS
Fellow of the American College of
    Osteopathic Surgeons

FACP
Fellow of the American College of
    Physicians
Fellow of the American College of
    Prosthodontists

FACPM
Fellow of the American College of
    Preventive Medicine

FACR
Fellow of the American College of
    Radiology

FACS
Fellow of the American College of
    Surgeons

FACSM
Fellow of the American College of
    Sports Medicine

FADA
Fellow of the American Dietetic
    Association

FAMA
Fellow of the American Medical
    Association

FAOTA
Fellow of the American Occupational
    Therapy Association

FAPA
Fellow of the American Psychiatric
    Association

FAPHA
Fellow of the American Public Health
Association

FAPTA
Fellow of the American Physical
Therapy Association

FASHP
Fellow of the American Society of
Health-System Pharmacists

FCAP
Fellow of the College of American
Pathologists

FCCP
Fellow of the American College of
Chest Physicians

FCGP
Fellow of the College of General
Practitioners

FChS
Fellow of the Society of Chiropodists

FCMS
Fellow of the College of Medicine and
Surgery

FCO
Fellow of the College of Osteopathy

FCPS, FCS
Fellow of the College of Physicians and
Surgeons

FCSP
Fellow of the Chartered Society of
Physiotherapy

FCST
Fellow of the College of Speech
Therapists

FDS
Fellow in Dental Surgery

FDSRCSEng
Fellow in Dental Surgery of the Royal
College of Surgeons of England

FFA
Fellow of the Faculty of Anaesthetists
(UK)

FFARCS
Fellow of the Faculty of Anaesthetists
of the Royal College of Surgeons
(UK)

FFCM
Fellow of the Faculty of Community
Medicine

FFD
Fellow in the Faculty of Dentistry

FFHom
Fellow of the Faculty of Homeopathy

FFOM
Fellow of the Faculty of Occupational
Medicine

FFR
Fellow of the Faculty of Radiologists

FHA
Fellow of the Institute of Hospital
Administrators

FIAC
Fellow of the International Academy of
Cytology

FIB
Fellow of the Institute of Biology

FIC
Fellow of the Institute of Chemistry

FICC
Fellow of the International College of
  Chiropractors

FICD
Fellow of the International College of
  Dentists

FICS
Fellow of the International College of
  Surgeons

FIMLT
Fellow of the Institute of Medical
  Laboratory Technology

FMCA
Forensic Medicine Consultant Advisor

FMS
Fellow of the Medical Society

FNAAOM
Fellow of the National Academy of
  Acupuncture and Oriental Medicine

FNP
Family Nurse Practitioner

FPS
Fellow of the Pathological Society
Fellow of the Pharmaceutical Society

FRCD
Fellow of the Royal College of Dentists
  (UK)

FRCD(C)
Fellow of the Royal College of Dentists
  of Canada

FRCGP
Fellow of the Royal College of General
  Practitioners

FRCOG
Fellow of the Royal College of
  Obstetricians and Gynaecologists
  (UK)

FRCP
Fellow of the Royal College of
  Physicians (England)

FRCPA
Fellow of the Royal College of
  Physicians of Australia

FRCPath
Fellow of the Royal College of
  Pathologists

FRCPC
Fellow of the Royal College of
  Physicians of Canada

FRCPE
Fellow of the Royal College of
  Physicians of Edinburgh

FRCP(I)
Fellow of the Royal College of
  Physicians (Ireland)

FRCPSC
Fellow of the Royal College of
  Physicians and Surgeons of Canada

FRCR
Fellow of the Royal College of
Radiologists

FRCS
Fellow of the Royal College of
Surgeons (England)

FRCSC
Fellow of the Royal College of
Surgeons of Canada

FRS
Fellow of the Royal Society (Australia,
Canada, Scotland, Ireland, UK)

FRSC
Fellow of the Royal Society, Canada

FRSM
Fellow of the Royal Society of
Medicine of England

FSCAI
Fellow of the Society for
Cardiovascular Angiography and
Interventions

FSR
Fellow of the Society of Radiographers

GCS
Geriatric Certified Specialist

GDMO
General Duties Medical Officer

GMO
General Medical Officer

GN
Graduate Nurse

GNP
Gerontological Nurse Practitioner

GNS
Gerontological Nurse Specialist

GNT
Graduate Nurse Technician

GNTP
Graduate Nurse Transition Program

GP
General Practitioner

GPN
Graduate Practical Nurse

GRT
Graduate Respiratory Therapist

GRTT
Graduate Respiratory Therapist
Technician

H(ASCP)
Technologist in Hematology certified by
the American Society for Clinical
Pathology

HAD
Hospital Administrator

HHA
Home Health Aid

HHD
Doctor of Holistic Health

HNC
Holistic Nurse Certified

HOC
Health Officer Certificate

HP
House Physician

HP(ASCP)
Hemapheresis Practitioner certified by the American Society for Clinical Pathology

HT
Histologic Technician

HT(ASCP)
Histotechnician certified by the American Society for Clinical Pathology

HTL(ASCP)
Histotechnologist certified by the American Society for Clinical Pathology

I(ASCP)
Technologist in Immunology certified by the American Society for Clinical Pathology

IBCLC
International Board Certified Lactation Consultant

ICN
Infection Control Nurse

ICP
Infection Control Practitioner

IEMT
Intermediate Emergency Medical Technician

IG
Inspector General

IME
Independent Medical Examiner

IMP
Individual Medical Practitioner

IMS
Indian Medical Service

JAR
Junior Assistant Resident

JD
Doctor of Jurisprudence

JHMO
Junior Hospital Medical Officer

JMS
Junior Medical Student

Lac
Licensed Acupuncturist

LAT
Licensed Athletic Trainer

LATC
Licensed Athletic Trainer, Certified

LCSW
Licensed Clinical Social Worker

LD
Licensed Dietician

LDS
Licentiate in Dental Surgery

LISW
Licensed Independent Social Worker

LM
Licentiate in Midwifery

LMCC
Licentiate of the Medical Council of Canada

LMFCC
Licensed Marriage, Family, and Child Counselor

LMFT
Licensed Marriage and Family Therapist

LMP
Licensed Massage Practitioner

LMT
Licensed Massage Therapist
Licensed Massage Technician

LNCC
Legal Nurse Consultant Certified

LOT
Licensed Occupational Therapist

LPC
Licensed Professional Counselor

LPCC
Licensed Professional Certified Counselor

LPN
Licensed Practical Nurse

LPN, CLTC
Licensed Practical Nurse, Certified Long-Term Care

LPN, NCP
Licensed Practical Nurse, Certified Pharmacology

LPT
Licensed Physical Therapist

LPTN
Licensed Psychiatric Technical Nurse

LRCP
Licentiate of the Royal College of Physicians (England)

LRCP(E)
Licentiate of the Royal College of Physicians (Edinburgh)

LRCP(I)
Licentiate of the Royal College of Physicians (Ireland)

LRCS
Licentiate of the Royal College of Surgeons

LSW
Licensed Social Worker

LT
Laboratory Technician

LVN
Licensed Vocational Nurse

LVN, CLTC
Licensed Vocational Nurse, Certified Long-Term Care

LVN, NCP
Licensed Vocational Nurse, Certified
  Pharmacology

LVT
Licensed Veterinary Technician

MA
Master of Arts
Medical Assistant

M(ASCP)
Technologist in Microbiology certified
  by the American Society for Clinical
  Pathology

MACCC
Master of Arts Certified Clinical
  Competence

MASc
Master of Ayurvedic Science

MB
Bachelor of Medicine

MBA
Master of Business Administration

MBBS
Bachelor of Medicine, Bachelor of
  Surgery

MBChB
Bachelor of Medicine, Bachelor of
  Surgery

MC
Master of Chirurgiae (Master of
  Surgery)
Master of Counseling

MCE
Medicare Code Editor

MCh
Master of Surgery

MChD
Master of Dental Surgery

MChOrth
Master of Orthopaedic Surgery

MChOtol
Master of Otology

MClSci
Master of Clinical Science

MCommH
Master of Community Health

MCPS
Member of the College of Physicians
  and Surgeons

MD
Doctor of Medicine

MDD
Doctor of Dental Medicine

MDentSc
Master of Dental Science

MDS
Master of Dental Surgery

MDT
Mechanical Diagnostic Therapist

ME
Medical Examiner

MEd
Master of Education

MEDEX
extension of physician (physician
assistant program using former
medical corpsman)

MEDIHC
Military Experience Directed into
Health Careers

MEDScD
Doctor of Medical Science

Med Tech
Medical Technician
Medical Technologist

MFC
Marriage and Family Counselor

MFCC
Marriage, Family, and Child Counselor

MFCT
Marriage, Family, and Child Therapist

MFST
Medical Field Service Technician

MHT
Mental Health Technician

ML
Licentiate in Midwifery

MLDT
Manual Lymph Drainage Therapist

MLPN
Medical Licensed Practical Nurse

MLT
Medical Laboratory Technician

MLT(AMT)
Medical Laboratory Technician certified
by the American Medical
Technologists

MLT(ASCP)
Medical Laboratory Technician certified
by American Society for Clinical
Pathology

MLT(ASCPi)
International Medical Laboratory
Technician (American Society for
Clinical Pathology)

MMed
Master of Medicine

MMS, MMSc
Master of Medical Science

MMSA
Master of Midwifery, Society of
Apothecaries

MMSc
Master of Medical Science

MN
Master of Nursing

MNSc
Master of Nursing Science

MO
Master of Obstetrics
Master of Osteopathy

MOC
Medical Officer on Call

MOD
Medical Officer of the Day

MOH
Medical Officer of Health

MOOW
Medical Officer of the Watch

MP(ASCP)
Technologist in Molecular Pathology certified by the American Society for Clinical Pathology

MPH
Master of Public Health

MPharm
Master in Pharmacy (Australia, New Zealand, UK, Ireland)

MPM
Master of Psychological Medicine

MPT
Master of Physical Therapy

MRad
Master of Radiology

MRC
Master of Rehabilitation Counseling

MRCP
Member of the Royal College of Physicians (England)

MRCP(E)
Member of the Royal College of Physicians (Edinburgh)

MRCP(I)
Member of the Royal College of Physicians (Ireland)

MRCS
Member of the Royal College of Surgeons (England)

MRL
Medical Records Librarian

MRT
Medical Records Technician

MS, MSc
Master of Science

MS I, II, III, IV
medical student: first, second, third, and fourth year

MSCCC
Master of Science Certified Clinical Competence

MScD
Doctor of Medical Science
Master of Dental Science

MScMed
Master of Science in Medicine

MScN
Master of Science in Nursing

MSD
Master of Science in Dentistry

MSHyg
Master of Science in Hygiene

MSM
Master of Medical Science

MSN
Master of Science in Nursing

MSPH
Master of Science in Public Health

MSPhar
Master of Science in Pharmacy

MS Rad
Master of Science in Radiology

MSS
Master of Social Science

MSSc
Master of Sanitary Science

MSSE
Master of Science in Sanitary
   Engineering

MSSW
Master of Science in Social Work

MSurg
Master of Surgery

MSW
Master of Social Welfare
Master of Social Work
Medical Social Worker

MT
Medical Technologist
Medical Transcriptionist
Monitor Technician

MTA
Medical Technical Assistant

MT(AMT)
Medical Technologist certified by the
   American Medical Technologists

MT(ASCP)
Medical Technologist certified by the
   American Society for Clinical
   Pathology

MT(ASCPi)
International Medical Technologist
   (American Society for Clinical
   Pathology)

MT(ASCP)SBB
Medical Technologist Specialist in
   Blood Banking certified by the
   American Society for Clinical
   Pathology

MTBC
Music Therapist-Board Certified

MTO
Medical Transport Officer

MTR
Music Therapist, Registered

MTRS
Licensed Master Therapeutic
   Recreation Specialist

MV
Medicus Veterinarius (Veterinary
   Doctor)

MVD
Doctor of Veterinary Medicine

NA
Network Administrator
Nurse Anesthetist

NCC
National Certified Counselor

NCS
Neurologic Certified Specialist
  (American Physical Therapists
  Association)

NCSN
National Certified School Nurse

NCT
Nursing Care Technician

NCTM
Nationally Certified in Therapeutic
  Massage (National Certification
  Board for Therapeutic Massage and
  Bodywork)

NCTMB
Nationally Certified Therapeutic
  Massage and Bodywork (National
  Certification Board for Therapeutic
  Massage and Bodywork)

ND
Doctor of Naturopathy (Naturopathic
  Doctor)
Naturopathic Doctor
Nursing Doctorate

NDP
Nurse Discharge Planner

NIRMP
National Intern and Resident Matching
  Program

NMD
Doctor of Naturopathic Medicine

NMT
Nuclear Medicine Technologist
Nurse Massage Therapist

NMT(R)
Nuclear Medicine Technologist
  Registered

NOA
Nurse Obstetric Assistant

NOSTA
Naval Ophthalmic Support and Training
  Activity

NNP
Neonatal Nurse Practitioner

NP
Nurse Practitioner

NP-C
Nurse Practitioner Certified

NPOD
Neuropsychiatric Officer of the Day

NREMT
National Registry Emergency Medical
  Technician—Basic or Candidate

NREMT-1
National Registry Emergency Medical
  Technician Basic–Intermediate

NREMT-P
National Registry Emergency Medical
  Technician–Paramedic

OA
Orthopedic Assistant

Professional Titles
and Degrees

OccTh
Occupational Therapist

OCN
Oncology Certified Nurse

OCS
Orthopedic Certified Specialist
(American Physical Therapists
Association)

OD
Doctor of Optometry

OHN
Occupational Health Nurse

OHT
Occupational Health Technician

ON
Office Nurse
Orthopedic Nurse

ONC
Orthopedic Nursing Certificate
Orthopedic Nurse Certified

OphD
Doctor of Ophthalmology

ORN
Orthopedic Nurse

ORT
Operating Room Technician
Registered Occupational Therapist

Osteo
Osteopathologist

OT
Occupational Therapist

OT-C
Orthopedic Technician, Certified

OTD
Doctor of Occupational Therapy

OT/L
Occupational Therapist, Licensed

OTR
Occupational Therapist, Registered
(National Board for Certification in
Occupational Therapy)

OTRL
Occupational Therapist, Registered
Licensed

PA
Physician Assistant
Psychological Associate

PA(ASCP)
Pathologists Assistant (American
Society for Clinical Pathology)

PA-C, PAC
Physician Assistant, Certified

PA-S
Physician Assistant, Student

PBM
Pharmacy Benefit Manager

PBT(ASCP)
Phlebotomy Technician certified by the
American Society for Clinical
Pathology

PC
Psychiatric Counselor

PCLN
Psychiatric Consultation Liaison Nurse

PCMO
Principal Clinical Medical Officer

PCP
Primary Care Physician

PCS
Pediatric Certified Specialist (American Physical Therapists Association)

PD
Doctor of Pharmacy

Phar G
Graduate in Pharmacy

Pharm D
Pharmaciae Doctor (Doctor of Pharmacy)

PhC
Pharmaceutical Chemist

PhD
Pharmaciae Doctor (Doctor of Pharmacy)
Philosophiae Doctor (Doctor of Philosophy)

PhG
Graduate in Pharmacy (historic)

PHN
Public Health Nurse

PHNC
Public Health Nurse Coordinator

PhTD
Doctor of Physical Therapy

PMO
Principal Medical Officer

PN
Practical Nurse

PNA
Pediatric Nurse Associate

PNC
Psychiatric Nurse Clinician

PNNP
Perinatal Nurse Practitioner

PNO
Principal Nursing Officer

PNP
Pediatric Nurse Practitioner

PNS
Practical Nursing Student

Pod D
Doctor of Podiatry

PSMT
Psychiatric Services Management Team

PST
Patient Service Technician

PsyD
Doctor of Psychology

PT
Physical Therapist

PTA
Physical Therapy Assistant

QMRP
Qualified Mental Retardation
   Professional

RACP
Royal Australasian College of
   Physicians

RCGP
Royal College of General Practitioners

RCP
Respiratory Care Practitioner

RCPT
Royal College of Physicians of
   Thailand

RCT
Registered Care Technologist

RD
Registered Dietician

RDA
Registered Dental Assistant (American
   Medical Technologists)

RDCS
Registered Diagnostic Cardiac
   Sonographer (American Registry for
   Diagnostic Medical Sonography)

RDH
Registered Dental Hygienist

RDMS
Registered Diagnostic Medical
   Sonographer (American Registry for
   Diagnostic Medical Sonography)

RDN
Registered Dietician/Nutritionist

REEGT
Registered Electroencephalographic
   Technician (American Board of
   Registration of
   Electroencephalographic and Evoked
   Potential Technologists)

REPT
Registered Evoked Potential
   Technologist (American Board of
   Registration of
   Electroencephalographic and Evoked
   Potential Technologists)

RGN
Registered General Nurse

RHCP
Registered Health Care Provider

RHIA
Registered Health Information
   Administrator (American Health
   Information Management
   Association)

RHIT
Registered Health Information
   Technologist (American Health
   Information Management
   Association)

RHU
Registered Health Underwriter

RISW
Registered Independent Social Worker

RKT
Registered Kinesiotherapist

RMA
Registered Medical Assistant (American Medical Technologists)

RMO
Resident Medical Officer
Responsible Medical Officer

RMT
Registered Music Therapist
Registered Massage Therapist (Canada)

RN
Registered Nurse

RNA
Registered Nurse Anesthetist

RN, BC
Registered Nurse, Board Certified

RNC
Registered Nurse, Certified

RNCD
Registered Nurse, Chemical Dependency

RNCNA
Registered Nurse, Certified in Nursing Administration

RNCNAA
Registered Nurse, Certified in Nursing Administration Advanced

RNCS
Registered Nurse, Certified Specialist

RNLP
Registered Nurse, license pending

RNMT
Registered Nuclear Medicine Technologist

RNP
Registered Nurse Practitioner

ROUB
Registered Ophthalmic Ultrasound Biometrist

RP
Registered Pharmacist

RPAC
Registered Physician Assistant Certified

RPFT
Registered Pulmonary Function Therapist (National Board of Respiratory Care)

RPh
Registered Pharmacist

RPSGT
Registered Polysomnographic Technologist (American Association of Sleep Technologists)

RPT
Registered Phlebotomy Technician (American Medical Technologists)
Registered Physical Therapist

RPTA
Registered Physical Therapist Assistant

RPVT
Registered Physician in Vascular Interpretation (American Registry for Diagnostic Medical Sonography)

Professional Titles and Degrees

RRA
Registered Records Administrator

RRNA
Resident Registered Nurse Anesthetist

RRT
Registered Respiratory Therapist

RSCN
Registered Sick Children's Nurse
(Ireland)

RSO
Resident Surgical Officer

RT
Radiologic Technologist
Registered Technologist
Respiratory Therapist

RT(ARRT)
Registered Technologist American
Registry of Radiologic Technologists

RT(BD)(ARRT)
Registered Technologist–Bone
Densitometry (American Registry of
Radiologic Technologists)

RT(BS) (AART)
Registered Technologist–Breast
Sonography (American Registry of
Radiologic Technologists)

RT(CI) (AART)
Registered Technologist–Cardiac-
Interventional Radiography
(American Registry of Radiologic
Technologists)

RT(CT)(AART)
Registered Technologist–Computed
Tomography (American Registry of
Radiologic Technologists)

RT(CV)(AART)
Registered
Technologist–Cardiovascular
Interventional Technology (American
Registry of Radiologic
Technologists)

RT(M)(AART)
Registered
Technologist–Mammography
(American Registry of Radiologic
Technologists)

RT(MR)(AART)
Registered Technologist–Magnetic
Resonance Imaging (American
Registry of Radiologic
Technologists)

RT(N)(AART)
Registered Technologist–Nuclear
Medicine(American Registry of
Radiologic Technologists)

RT(QM))(AART)
Registered TechnologistQuality
Management (American Registry of
Radiologic Technologists)

RT(R)
Recreational Therapist, Registered
Registered Technologist in Radiography

RTR(ARRT)
Registered Technologist in Radiography
American Registry of Radiologic
Technologists

RT(S)(AART)
Registered Technologist–Sonography
(Ultrasound) (American Registry of
Radiologic Technologists)

RT(T)(AART)
Registered Technologist in Radiation
Therapy (American Registry of
Radiologic Technologists)

RTT
Respiratory Therapy Technician

RTT(AART)
Radiologic Technologist in Radiation
Therapy American Registry of
Radiologic Technologists

RT(VI)(AART)
Registered Technologist–Vacular
Interventional Radiography
(American Registry of Radiologic
Technologists)

RVS
Registered Vascular Specialist

RVT
Registered Vascular Technologist
Registered Veterinary Technician

SA
Surgeon Assistant
Surgical Assistant

SAC
Substance Abuse Counselor

SAMO
Senior Administrative Medical Officer

SAR
Senior Assistant Resident

SAT
Supervisory Athletic Therapist (Canada)

SBB(ASCP)
Specialist in Blood Banking Technology
certified by the American Society for
Clinical Pathology

SC(ASCP)
Specialist in Chemistry certified by the
American Society for Clinical
Pathology

ScD
Doctor of Science

SCM
State Certified Midwife

SCMO
Senior Clerical Medical Officer

SCS
Sports Certified Specialist

SCT(ASCP)
Specialist in Cytotechnology certified
by the American Society for Clinical
Pathology

SED
Surgeon, Emergency Department

SEN
State Enrolled Nurse

SEO
Surgical Emergency Officer

SG
Surgeon General

SGO
Society of Gynecologic Oncologists

SH(ASCP)
Specialist in Hematology certified by the American Society for Clinical Pathology

SHMO
Senior Hospital Medical Officer

SHO
Senior House Officer

SI(ASCP)
Specialist in Immunology certified by the American Society for Clinical Pathology

SL (ASCP)
Laboratory Safety Specialist (American Society for Clinical Pathology)

SLP
Speech-Language Pathologist

SLS(ASCP)
Specialist in Laboratory Safety certified by the American Society for Clinical Pathology

SM
Master of Science
Master of Surgery

SM(ASCP)
Specialist in Microbiology certified by the American Society for Clinical Pathology

SMI
Senior Medical Investigator

SMO
Senior Medical Officer

SMOH
Senior Medical Officer of Health

SN
Student Nurse

SNA
Student Nursing Assistant

SNM
Student Nurse Midwife

SNP
School Nurse Practitioner

SP
Speech Pathologist

SPA
Student Physician Assistant

SPN
Student Practical Nurse

SR
Senior Resident

SRP
State Registered Physiotherapist

SRT
Stroke Rehabilitation Technician

SV(ASCP)
Specialist in Virology certified by the American Society for Clinical Pathology

SW
Social Worker

TAS
Therapeutic Activities Specialist

TMA
Trained Medication Aide

TNCC
Trauma Nursing Core Course

UC
Unit Coordinator

UL
Unit Leader

USFMG
United States Foreign Medical Graduate

USMG
United States Medical Graduate

Vet Med
Veterinary Medicine

Vet Sci
Veterinary Science

VMC
Village Malaria Communicator

VMD
Veterinariae Medicinae Doctor (Doctor of Veterinary Medicine)

VN
Visiting Nurse
Vocational Nurse

VRTA
Vocational Rehabilitation Therapy Assistant

VTS
Veterinary Technician Specialist

WC
Ward Clerk

WOC
Wound, Ostomy, and Continence Nurse (previously called Enterostomal Therapy nurse, United Kingdom)

WS
Ward Secretary

XRT
X-Ray Technician

Professional Associations and Organizations including Government and Regulatory Agencies

AABB
American Association of Blood Banks

AACAP
American Academy of Child and Adolescent Psychiatry

AACC
American Association for Clinical Chemistry

AACD
American Academy of Cosmetic Dentistry

AACN
American Association of Critical-Care Nurses

AACOM
American Association of Colleges of Osteopathic Medicine

AACR
American Association for Cancer Research

AACVPR
American Association of Cardiovascular and Pulmonary Rehabilitation

AAD
American Academy of Dermatology

AAE
American Association of Endodontists

AAFP
American Academy of Family Physicians

AAGP
American Association for Geriatric Psychiatry

AAHP
American Association of Homeopathic Pharmacists

AAHSA
American Association of Homes and Services for the Aging

AAI
American Association of Immunologists

AAM
American Academy of Microbiologists

AAMA
American Academy of Medical Acupuncture

AAMC
Association of American Medical Colleges

AAMFT
American Association for Marriage and Family Therapy

AAMI
Association for the Advancement of Medical Instrumentation

AAMR
American Association on Mental Retardation

AAMT
American Association for Medical Transcription

AAN
American Academy of Neurology
American Association of Neuropathologists
American Academy of Nursing

AANA
American Association of Nurse Anesthetists

AANP
American Association of Naturopathic Physicians
American Association of Nurse Practitioners

AAO
American Academy of Ophthalmology
American Academy of Optometry
American Association of Orthodontists

AAOA
Advocates for the American Osteopathic Association
American Academy of Otolaryngic Allergy

AAO-HNS
American Academy of Otolaryngology Head and Neck Surgery

AAOS
American Academy of Orthopaedic Surgeons

AAP
American Academy of Pediatrics
American Academy of Periodontology

AAPA
American Association of Pathologist Assistants
American Academy of Physician Assistants

AAPB
Association for Applied Psychophysiology and Biofeedback

AAPCC
American Association of Poison Control Centers

AAPMR
American Academy of Physical Medicine and Rehabilitation

AARP
American Association of Retired Persons

AASLD
American Association for the Study of Liver Diseases

AAST
American Association for the Surgery of Trauma

AAWC
Association for the Advancement of Wound Care

ABA
American Bar Association
American Board of Anesthesiology
Association for Behavior Analysis

ABC
American Botanical Council

ABIM
American Board of Internal Medicine

ABPH
American Board of Psychological Hypnosis

ABPN
American Board of Psychiatry and Neurology
American Board of Professional Neuropsychology

ABR
American Board of Radiology

ABS
American Board of Surgery

ABTA
American Brain Tumor Association

ACA
American Chiropractic Association
American Counseling Association
American Council on Alcoholism

ACB
American Council of the Blind

ACC
American College of Cardiology

ACC/AHA
American College of Cardiology/American Heart Association

ACG
American College of Gastroenterology

ACGME
Accreditation Council for Graduate Medical Education
American College of Graduate Medical Education

AHAF
American Health Assistance Foundation

AHCA
American Health Care Association

AHF
AIDS Healthcare Foundation
American Health Foundation

AHFS-DI
American Hospital Formulary Service-Drug Information

AHHA
American Holistic Health Association

AHRA
American Healthcare Radiology Administrators

AHRQ
Agency for Healthcare Research and Quality

AHTA
American Horticultural Therapy Association

AIP
American Institute of Physics

AIUM
American Institute of Ultrasound in Medicine

AJCC
American Joint Committee on Cancer

AJCC/UICC
American Joint Committee on Cancer/International Union Against Cancer

ALA
American Lung Association

ALF
American Liver Foundation

ALFA
Assisted Living Federation of America
AMA
American Medical Association

AMDA
American Medical Directors Association

AMF
American Menopause Foundation

AMPAC
Alternative Medicine Program Advisory Council

AMT
American Medical Technologists

AMTA
American Massage Therapy Association
American Music Therapy Association

AMVET
American Veterans of World War II

ANA
American Nurses Association
American Neurological Association

ANRC
American National Red Cross

ANSCII
American National Standard Code for Information Interchange

ANSI
American National Standards Institute

AO
Academy of Osseointegration

AoA
Administration on Aging

AOA
American Optometric Association
American Orthopaedic Association
American Osteopathic Association
American Obesity Association

AOFAS
American Orthopaedic Foot and Ankle Society

AONE
American Organization of Nurse Executives

AORN
Association of Perioperative Registered Nurses

AOTA
American Occupational Therapy Association, Inc.

APA
American Psychiatric Association
American Psychological Association

APDA
American Parkinson's Disease Association

APhA
American Pharmaceutical Association

APHA
American Public Health Association

APMA
American Podiatric Medical Association

APNA
American Psychiatric Nurses Association

APRL
Army Prosthetics Research Laboratory

APSA
American Pediatric Surgical Association

APTA
American Physical Therapy Association
American Polarity Therapy Association

ARA
American Rheumatism Association

ARC
American Red Cross
Association for Retarded Citizens

ARCBS
American Red Cross Blood Services

ARDMS
American Registry of Diagnostic Medical Sonographers

ARN
Association of Rehabilitation Nurses

ARSAC
Administration of Radioactive Substances Advisory Committee

ASA
American Society of Anesthesiologists
American Society on Aging
American Standards Association
American Stroke Association

ASAPS
American Society for Aesthetic Plastic Surgery

ASCCP
American Society for Colposcopy and Cervical Pathology

ASCI
American Society for Clinical Investigation

ASCLT
American Society of Clinical Laboratory Technicians

ASCP
American Society for Clinical Pathology

ASCRS
American Society for Colon and Rectal Surgeons

ASDA
American Sleep Disorders Association

ASGE
American Society for Gastrointestinal Endoscopy

ASH
American Society of Hematology

ASHA
American Speech-Language-Hearing Association

ASIA
American Spinal Injury Association

ASIF
Association for the Study of Internal Fixation

ASIM
American Society of Internal Medicine

ASM
American Society for Microbiology

ASPO
American Society of Preventive Oncology

ASPS
American Society of Plastic Surgeons

ASRT
American Society of Radiologic Technologists

ASSH
American Society for Surgery of the Hand

ASTM
American Society for Testing and Materials

ASTRO
American Society for Therapeutic Radiology and Oncology

ASTS
American Society of Transplant Surgeons

ATA
American Tinnitus Association

ATPO
Association of Technical Personnel in Ophthalmology

ATS
American Thoracic Society

AUA
American Urological Association

AUR
Association of University Radiologists

BCA
Blue Cross Association

BCCG
British Cooperative Clinical Group

BCDSP
Boston Collaborative Drug Surveillance Program

BCHS
Bureau of Community Health Services

BCIA
Biofeedback Certification Institute of America

BDA
British Dental Association

BDAC
Bureau of Drug Abuse Control

BEAR
Biological Effects of Atomic Radiation (Committee)

BHP, BHPr
Bureau of Health Professions

BIPM
Bureau International des Poids et Mesures; International Bureau of Weights and Measures

BMD
Bureau of Medical Devices

BNDD
Bureau of Narcotics and Dangerous Drugs

BOD
Bureau of Drugs

BQA
Bureau of Quality Assurance

BSI
British Standards Institution

BTTP
British Testicular Tumour Panel

BVI
Better Vision Institute

BVM
Bureau of Veterinary Medicine

CAFMHS
Child, Adolescent, and Family Mental Health Service

CANE
Clearinghouse on Abuse and Neglect of the Elderly

CAP
College of American Pathologists

CARF
Commission on Accreditation of Rehabilitation Facilities

CAS
Center for Alcohol Studies

CASCSP
Center for the Advancement of State Community Services Programs

CBBB
Council of Better Business Bureaus

CBER
Center for Biologics Evaluation and Research (FDA)

CBIRF
Chemical Biological Incident Response Force (of the U.S. Marine Corps)

CBN
Commission on Biological Nomenclature

CBTC
Childhood Brain Tumor Consortium

CCAC
Continuing Care Accreditation Commission

CCE
Council on Chiropractic Education

CCFA
Crohn's and Colitis Foundation of America

CCNSC
Cancer Chemotherapy National Service Center

CCS
Canadian Cardiovascular Society

CCUSA
Catholic Charities USA

CDC
Centers for Disease Control and Prevention

CDHNF
Children's Digestive Health and Nutrition Foundation

CDS
Christian Dental Society

CEQ
Council on Environmental Quality

CERAD
Consortium to Establish a Registry for Alzheimer's Disease

CFF
Cystic Fibrosis Foundation

CFH
Council on Family Health

CFSTI
Clearinghouse for Federal Scientific and Technical Information

CGA
Catholic Golden Age

CHAS
Center for Health Administration Studies

CHC
Community Health Council

CHEP
Cuban/Haitian Entrant Program

CHIP
Children's Health Insurance Program

CHT
Center for Health Technology

CID
Central Institute for the Deaf

CLMA
Clinical Laboratory Management Association

CMB
Central Midwives Board

CMHS
Center for Mental Health Services

CMS
Centers for Medicare Services (formerly HCFA)

CNME
Council on Naturopathic Medical Education

CODATA
Committee on Data for Science and Technology

COHSE
Confederation of Health Service Employees

COLA
Commission on Office Laboratory Accreditation

COTH
Council of Teaching Hospitals

CPEHS
Consumer Protection and Environmental Health Service

CPHA
Commission on Professional and Hospital Activities

CPSC
Consumer Product Safety Commission

CREOG
Council on Resident Education in Obstetrics and Gynecology

CRHL
Collaborative Radiological Health Laboratory

CSCD
Center for Sickle Cell Disease

CSIN
Chemical Substances Information Network

CSM
Committee on Safety of Medicines

CSTI
Clearinghouse for Scientific and Technical Information

CTAA
Community Transportation Association of America

DAIDS
Division of AIDS (of the National Institute of Allergy and Infectious Diseases, National Institutes of Health)

DAV
Disabled American Veterans

DAWN
Drug Abuse Warning Network

DBS
Division of Biological Standards

DCC
Disaster Control Center

DCFS
Department of Children and Family Services

DCS
Department of Children's Services

DCYS
Department of Children and Youth Services

DDD
Division of Developmental Disabilities

DDNC
Digestive Disease National Coalition

DDPA
Delta Dental Plans Association

DEBRA
Dystrophic Epidermolysis Bullosa Research Association of America

DEHS
Division of Emergency Health Services

DEM
Department of Emergency Medicine

DFS
Division of Family Services

DHES
Division of Health Examination Statistics

DHEW
Department of Health, Education, and Welfare (now Department of Health and Human Services)

DHS
Department of Human Services

DMH
Department of Mental Health
Department of Mental Hygiene

DMS
Department of Medicine and Surgery

DOD
Department of Defense

DOH
Department of Health

DOJ
Department of Justice

DOL
Department of Labor

DOSS
Department of Social Services

DOT
Department of Transportation

DPA
Department of Public Assistance

DPSS
Department of Public Social Services

DRME
Division of Research in Medical Education

DSHS
Department of Social and Health Services

DSMB
Data and Safety Monitoring Board

DSS
Department of Social Services

DTBE
Division of Tuberculosis Elimination

DTEG
Dermatology Teachers Exchange Group

DVA
Department of Veterans Affairs

DVH
Division for the Visually Handicapped

DVR
Division of Vocational Rehabilitation

EBAA
Eye Bank Association of America

EC
Enzyme Commission (of International Union of Biochemistry)

ECaP
Exceptional Cancer Patients

ECFMG
Educational Commission on Foreign Medical Graduates

ECLM
European Confederation for Laboratory Medicine

EEOC
Equal Employment Opportunity Commission

EHA
Environmental Health Agency

EIS
Epidemic Intelligence Service

ELS
European Laryngological Societies

ELSO
Extracorporeal Life Support Organization

EMCRO
Experimental Medical Care Review Organization

EMEA
European Medicines Evaluation Agency

ENTIS
European Network of Teratology Information Services

EORTC
European Organization for Research and Treatment of Cancer

EOS
European Orthodontic Society

EPA
Environmental Protection Agency

EPA/RCRA
Environmental Protection Agency Resource Conservation and Recovery Act

ERDA
Energy Research and Development Administration

ESCOP
European Scientific Cooperative on Phytotherapy

ESPGHAN
European Society of Paediatric Gastroenterology, Hepatology, and Nutrition

EU
European Union

EULAR
European League Against Rheumatism

FACCT
Foundation for Accountability

FACMTA
Federal Advisory Council on Medical Training Aids

FACOSH
Federal Advisory Committee on Occupational Safety and Health

FAH
Federation of American Hospitals

FAO
Food and Agriculture Organization

FBR
Foundation for Biomedical Research

FCER
Foundation for Chiropractic Education and Research

FCIC
Federal Consumer Information Center

FDA
Food and Drug Administration

FDCPA
Food, Drug, and Consumer Product Agency

FDD
Food and Drug Directorate

FEHBP
Federal Employee Health Benefits Program

FEMA
Federal Emergency Management Agency

FFS
Fight For Sight

FHC
Faith and Health Consortium

FIA
Family Independence Agency (formerly Department of Social Services)

FICA
Federal Insurance Contributions Act

FIGO
Federation International de Gynecologie et Obstetrique
International Federation of Gynecology and Obstetrics

FPO
Federation of Prosthodontic Organizations

FSA
Family Services Association

FWPCA
Federal Water Pollution Control Administration

GAO
General Accounting Office

GDB
Guide Dogs for the Blind

GDC
General Dental Council

GMENAC
Graduate Medical Education National Advisory Committee

GMS
General Medical Service

GNC
General Nursing Council

GOG
Gynecologic Oncology Group (of National Cancer Institute)

GPA
Global Program on AIDS

GRF
Glaucoma Research Foundation

GSA
Gerontological Society of America

GT
Generations Together

HAIC
Hearing Aid Industry Conference

HASP
Hospital Admissions and Surveillance Program

HC
Hospital Corps

HCIS
Health Care Information System

HCSD
Health Care Studies Division

HDSA
Huntington's Disease Society of America

HEC
Health Education Council

HER
HIV Epidemiology Research

HERS
Hysterectomy Educational Resources and Services Foundation

HEW
(Department of) Health, Education, and Welfare

HHCA
Home Health Care Agency

HHS
(Department of) Health and Human Services

HIAA
Health Insurance Association of America

HIBAC
Health Insurance Benefits Advisory Council

HIC
Heart Information Center

HICPAC
Hospital Infection Control Practices Advisory Committee

HII
Health Insurance Institute

HIVNET
Human Immunodeficiency Virus Project Network

HMAC
Health Manpower Advisory Council

HMSS
Hospital Management Systems Society

HRA
Human Resources Administration

HRRC
Human Research Review Committee

HRSA
Health Resources and Services Administration

HSA
Health Services Administration
Health Systems Agency

HSMHA
Health Services and Mental Health Administration

HSQB
Health Standards and Quality Bureau

HSRC
Health Services Research Center
Human Subjects Review Committee

HSRI
Health Systems Research Institute

HTA
Herb Trade Association

IAB
Industrial Accident Board

IADR
International Association for Dental Research

IAEA
International Atomic Energy Agency

IAET
International Association for Enterostomal Therapy

IAG
International Academy of Gnathology

IAM
Institute of Aviation Medicine

IAO
International Association for Orthodontics

IAP
International Academy of Pathology

IAPAAS
International Association of Physical Activity, Aging, and Sports

IARC
International Agency for Research on Cancer

IASHS
Institute for Advanced Study in Human Sexuality

IASP
International Association for the Study of Pain

IAVI
International AIDS Vaccine Initiative

IBC
Institutional Biosafety Committee

ICA
International Chiropractic Association

ICAAC
Interscience Conference on Antimicrobial Agents and Chemotherapy

ICAO
International Civil Aviation Organization

ICCIDD
International Council for Control of Iodine Deficiency Disorder

ICCR
International Committee for Contraceptive Research

ICDRG
International Contact Dermatitis Research Group

ICH
International Council on Harmonization

ICHPPC
International Classification of Health Problems in Primary Care

ICIC
International Cancer Information Center

ICLH
Imperial College, London Hospital

ICOPER
International Cooperative Pulmonary Embolism Registry

ICRC
International Committee of the Red Cross

ICRETT
International Cancer Research Technology Transfer

ICRP
International Commission on Radiological Protection

ICRS
Index Chemicus Registry System

ICRU
International Commission on Radiological Units

ICS
International Continence Society

ICSH
International Committee for Standardization in Hematology

IDSA
Infectious Disease Society of America

IEPS
International Education Program Service (US Department of Education)

IFCC
International Federation of Clinical Chemistry

IHS
Indian Health Service
International Headache Society

IIME
Institute of International Medical Education

IKDC
International Knee Documentation Committee

ILAE
International League Against Epilepsy

ILAR
International League of Associations for Rheumatology

ILO
International Labor Organization

ILSI
International Life Science Institute

IMA
Interchurch Medical Assistance, Inc

IMIC
International Medical Information Center

IMR
Institute for Medical Research
Institution for the Mentally Retarded

INCC
Institut National du Cancer du Canada

IOA
International Ostomy Association

IOM
Institute of Medicine

IP
L'Institut Pasteur

IRC
International Red Cross

IRH
Institute for Religion and Health

IRIS
International Research Information Service (IEPS, US Department of Education

ISA
Incest Survivors Anonymous

ISCLT
International Society for Clinical Laboratory Technology

ISCP
International Society of Comparative Pathology

ISGYP
International Society of Gynecologic Pathologists

ISH
International Society of Hematology

ISHLT
International Society for Heart and Lung Transplantation

ISHT
International Society for Heart Transplantation

ISM
International Society of Microbiologists

ISMP
Institute for Safe Medication Practices

ISO
International Standards Organization

ISR
Institute for Sex Research
Institute of Surgical Research

ISSVD
International Society for the Study of Vulvar Diseases

ISUP
International Society for Urological Pathology

ITC
Interagency Testing Committee (US Environmental Protection Agency)

ITF
International Tremor Foundation

IUPAC
International Union of Pure and Applied Chemistry

JACL
Japanese American Citizens League

JCAH
Joint Commission on Accreditation of Hospitals

JCAHO
Joint Commission on Accreditation of Healthcare Organizations

JCAHPO
Joint Commission on Allied Health Personnel in Ophthalmology

JCMHC
Joint Commission on Mental Health of Children

JFS
Jewish Family Services

JOA
Japanese Orthopaedic Association

JTF-CS
Joint Task Force for Civil Support (of the Defense Department)

LC
Library of Congress

LCDC
Laboratory Centre for Disease Control (Canada)

LCE
Legal Counsel for the Elderly

LFA
Lupus Foundation of America

LHI
Labor Health Institute

LIA
Laser Institute of America

LLS
Leukemia and Lymphoma Society, Inc.

LNCVA
Lighthouse National Center for Vision and Aging

LRN
Laboratory Response Network

LSE
Legal Services for the Elderly

LSUMC
Louisiana State University Medical Center

MAOP
Mid-Atlantic Oncology Program

MCA
Medicines Control Agency (United Kingdom)

MCB
Medicines Control Board

MDA
Medical Devices Agency (United Kingdom)

MDPH
Michigan Department of Public Health

MEDICO
Medical International Cooperation

MFCU
Medicaid Fraud Control Unit

MFSS
Medical Field Service School (US Army)

MGMA
Medical Group Management Association

MHA
Mental Health Association

MHCS
Mental Hygiene Consultation Service

MHHP
Minnesota Heart Health Program

MHI
Mental Health Institute

MHRI
Mental Health Research Institute

MLA
Medical Library Association

MMAP
Maine Medical Assessment Program

MMIS
Medicaid Management Information System

MMRS
Metropolitan Medical Response Systems

MOH
Ministry of Health

MORC
Medical Officers Reserve Corps

MOWAA
Meals on Wheels Association of America

MPA
Medical Products Agency (Sweden)

MPU
Medical Practitioners Union

MRI
Medical Research Institute

MSA
Medical Services Administration

MSC
Medical Service Corps

MSKCC
Memorial Sloan-Kettering Cancer Center

MSSP
Maternal Support Services Program

MSTS
Musculoskeletal Tumor Society

MTF
Musculoskeletal Transplant Foundation

MTSO
Medical Transcription Service Organization

N4A
National Association of Area Agencies on Aging

NAACLS
National Accrediting Agency for Clinical Laboratory Sciences

NACHC
National Association of Community Health Centers

NACI
National Advisory Committee on Immunization

NAD
National Association of the Deaf

NADL
National Association of Dental Laboratories

NAELA
National Academy of Elder Law Attorneys, Inc.

NAEPP
National Asthma Education and Prevention Program

NAFC
National Association for Continence

NAHC
National Association for Home Care

NAHD
National Association for Human Development

NAHF
National Association for Health & Fitness

NAHOF
National Association on HIV Over Fifty

NAMCS
National Ambulatory Medical Care Survey

NAMI
National Alliance for the Mentally Ill

NAMS
North American Menopause Society

NANASP
National Association of Nutrition and Aging Service Programs

NANDA
North American Nursing Diagnosis Association

NAPCA
National Asian Pacific Center on Aging

NAPGCM
National Association of Professional Geriatric Care Managers

NAPNAP
National Association of Pediatric Nurse Associates and Practitioners

NAPNES
National Association for Practical Nurse Education and Services

NARIC
National Rehabilitation Information Center

NASDAD
National Association of Seventh-Day Adventist Dentists

NAS-NRC
National Academy of Science-National Research Council

NASPGHAN
North American Society for Pediatric Gastroenterology, Hepatology and Nutrition

NASPGN
North American Society for Pediatric Gastroenterology and Nutrition

NASUA
National Association of State Units on Aging

NASW
National Association of Social Workers

NBA
National Bar Association

NBCE
National Board of Chiropractic Examiners

NBME
National Board of Medical Examiners

NBTS
National Blood Transfusion Service

NC
Nurse Corps

NCADD
National Council on Alcoholism and Drug Dependence

NCAHF
National Council Against Health Fraud

NCAI
National Coalition for Adult Immunization

NCBA
National Caucus and Center on Black Aged, Inc.

NCCAM
National Center for Complementary and Alternative Medicine

NCCAN
National Center for Child Abuse and Neglect

NCCAOM
National Certification Committee for Acupuncture and Oriental Medicine

NCCDS
National Cooperative Collaborative Crohn's Disease Study

NCCLS
National Committee for Clinical Laboratory Standards

NCCN
National Comprehensive Cancer Network

NCCNHR
National Citizen's Coalition for Nursing Home Reform

NCCS
National Coalition for Cancer Survivorship

NCDB
National Cancer Data Base

NCEA
National Center on Elder Abuse

NCHS
National Center for Health Statistics

NCI
National Cancer Institute

NCIC
National Cancer Institute of Canada

NCL
National Consumer's League

NCLR
National Council of La Raza

NCME
Network for Continuing Medical Education

NCMHD
National Center on Minority Health and Health Disparities (National Institutes of Health)

NCOA
National Council on Aging, Inc.

NCPIE
National Council on Patient Information and Education

NCPSSM
National Committee to Preserve Social Security and Medicare

NCQA
National Commission for Quality Assurance

NCRA
National Cancer Registrars Association

NCRP
National Council on Radiation Protection and Measurements

NCRR
National Center for Research Resources (National Institutes of Health)

NCTC
National Collection of Type Cultures

NCYC
National Collection of Yeast Cultures

NDA
National Dental Association

NDC
National Drug Code

NDDIC
National Digestive Diseases Information Clearinghouse

NDIC
National Diabetes Information Clearinghouse

NDS
Naval Dental School

NDTI
National Disease and Therapeutic Index

NECHI
Northeastern Consortium for Health Information

NEHCRC
Native Elder Health Care Resource Center

NEHEP
National Eye Health Education Program

NEI
National Eye Institute

NEISS
National Electronic Injury Surveillance System

NEOB
New England Organ Bank

NEOPO
Northeast Organ Procurement Organization

NERICP
New England Regional Infant Cardiac Program

NESO
Northeastern Society of Orthodontists

NFB
National Foundation for the Blind

NFCA
National Family Caregivers Association

NGNA
National Gerontological Nursing Association

NGTF
National Gay Task Force

NHCOA
National Hispanic Council on Aging

NHF
National Hospital Foundation

NHGRI
National Human Genome Research Institute (National Institutes of Health)

NHIC
National Health Information Center

NHLBI
National Heart, Lung, and Blood Institute

NHPCO
National Hospice and Palliative Care Organization

NHPF
National Health Policy Forum

NHS
National Health Service (United Kingdom)

NHSR
National Hospital Service Reserve

NIA
National Institute on Aging (National Institutes of Health)

NIA-RI
National Institute on Aging-Reagan Institute

NIAAA
National Institute on Alcohol Abuse and Alcoholism (National Institutes of Health)

NIAID
National Institute of Allergy and Infectious Diseases (National Institutes of Health)

NIAMD
National Institute of Arthritis and Metabolic Diseases (National Institutes of Health)

NIAMS
National Institute of Arthritis and Musculoskeletal and Skin Diseases (National Institutes of Health)

NIBIB
National Institute of Biomedical Imaging and Bioengineering

NICA
National Interfaith Coalition on Aging

NICE
National Institute for Clinical Excellence (United Kingdom)

NICHD
National Institute of Child Health and Human Development

NICOA
National Indian Council on Aging

NIDA
National Institute on Drug Abuse (National Institutes of Health)

NIDCD
National Institute on Deafness and Other Communication Disorders

NIDCR
National Institute of Dental and Craniofacial Research

NIDDK
National Institute of Diabetes and Digestive and Kidney Disease

NIEHS
National Institute of Environmental Health Sciences (National Institutes of Health)

NIGMS
National Institute of General Medical Sciences (NIH)

NIH
National Institutes of Health

NIH-ORBD-NRC
NIH (National Institutes of Health) Osteoporosis and Related Bone Diseases National Resource Center

NIHR
National Institute for Healthcare Research

NIIC
National Injury Information Clearinghouse

NIMH
National Institute of Mental Health (National Institutes of Health)

NINDS
National Institute of Neurological Disorders and Stroke (National Institutes of Health)

NINR
National Institute for Nursing Research (National Institutes of Health)

NIOSH
National Institute of Occupational Safety and Health (National Institutes of Health)

NIST
National Institute of Standards and Technology

NJCLD
National Joint Committee on Learning Disabilities

NKF
National Kidney Foundation

NKUDIC
National Kidney and Urological Diseases Information Clearinghouse

NLHEP
National Lung Health Education Program

NLM
National Library of Medicine (National Institutes of Health)

NLSBPH
National Library Service for the Blind and Physically Handicapped

NMA
National Medical Association

NMAC
National Medical Audiovisual Center

NMDP
National Marrow Donor Program

NMFI
National Master Facility Inventory

NMHA
National Mental Health Association

NML
National Medical Library

NMRDC
Naval Medical Research and Development Command

NMRT
National Medical Response Team

NMRU
Naval Medical Research Unit

NMSS
National Multiple Sclerosis Society

NMTCB
Nuclear Medicine Technology Certification Board

NNDC
National Naval Dental Center

NNFA
National Nutritional Foods Association

NNIS
National Nosocomial Infections Surveillance

NOCSAE
National Operating Committee on Standards for Athletic Equipment

NOCTI
National Occupation Competency Testing Institute

NOF
National Osteoporosis Foundation

NORD
National Organization for Rare Disorders

NOVA
National Organization of Victim Assistance

NOVS
National Office of Vital Statistics

NPCTG
National Prostatic Cancer Treatment Group

NPF
National Psoriasis Foundation

NPIN
National Prevention Information Network

NPRCWA
National Policy and Resource Center on Women and Aging

NPSF
National Patient Safety Foundation

NPTR
National Pediatric Trauma Registry

NRC
National Research Council
Nuclear Regulatory Commission

NRCC
National Registry in Clinical Chemistry

NRCDLTC
National Resource Center: Diversity and Long-Term Care

NRCNAA
National Resource Center on Native American Aging

NREMT
National Registry of Emergency Medical Technicians

NRHA
National Rural Health Association

NRIC
National Resource and Information Center

NRM
National Registry of Microbiologists

NRMP
National Residency Matching Plan

NRPB
National Radiological Protection Board

NRSFPS
National Reporting System for Family Planning Services
NSA
National Stroke Association

NSCERC
National Senior Citizens Education and Research Center

NSCIDRC
National Spinal Cord Injury Data Research Center

NSCLC
National Senior Citizens Law Center

NSF
National Sleep Foundation

NSGA
National Senior Games Association

NSHC
National Self-Help Clearinghouse

NTIS
National Technical Information Service

NTL
National Training Laboratories

NTP
National Toxicology Program

NVAC
National Vaccine Advisory Committee

NWHIC
National Women's Health Information Center

NWHN
National Women's Health Network

OAA
Opticians Association of America

OAM
Office of Alternative Medicine

OASDHI
Old Age, Survivors, Disability, and Health Insurance

OCA
Organization of Chinese Americans

OCCAM
Office of Cancer Complementary and Alternative Medicine

OCD
Office of Child Development
Office of Civil Defense

OCIS
Oncology Center Information System

ODAC
Oncologic Drugs Advisory Committee (of the US Food and Drug Administration)

ODSS
Office of Disability Support Services

OGD
Office of Generic Drugs (of the Food and Drug Administration)

OHTA
Office of Health Technology Assessment

OIF
Osteogenesis Imperfecta Foundation

OIG
Office of the Inspector General

OME
Office of the Medical Examiner

ONS
Office for National Statistics (United Kingdom)
Oncology Nursing Society

OPD
Office of Orphan Products Development

OPO
Organ Procurement Organization

OPS
Ophthalmic Photographers Society

OPTN
Organ Procurement and Transplantation Network

ORLAU
Orthotic Research and Locomotor Assessment Unit

ORNL
Oak Ridge National Laboratory

OSEP
Office of Special Education Programs

OSH
Office on Smoking and Health

OSHA
Occupational Safety and Health Administration

OTIS
Organization of Teratology Information Services

OTOD
Organization of Teachers of Oral Diagnosis

OTSG
Office of the Surgeon General

OVR
Office of Vocational Rehabilitation

OWL
Older Women's League

PACE
Program of All-Inclusive Care for the Elderly

PAHO
Pan American Health Organization

PBA
Prevent Blindness America

PCC
Poison Control Center

PCPFS
President's Council on Physical Fitness and Sports

PDF
Parkinson's Disease Foundation

PFC
Partnership for Caring

PFF
Pulmonary Fibrosis Foundation

PFS
Patient and Family Services

PHLS
Public Health Laboratory Service

PHO
Physician/Hospital Organization

PhRMA
Pharmaceutical Research and Manufacturers of America (formerly the
Pharmaceutical Manufacturers Association)

PHS
Public Health Service

PMIS
PSRO (Professional Standards Review Organization) Management Information
System

POCAAN
People of Color Against AIDS Network

PPFA
Planned Parenthood Federation of America

PPRC
Physician Payment Review Commission

PQRI
Product Quality Research Initiative

PRC
Pension Rights Center

PRO
Peer Review Organization
Professional Review Organization

ProPAC
Prospective Payment Assessment Commission

PSEF
Plastic Surgery Educational Foundation

PSR
Physicians for Social Responsibility

PSRC
Plastic Surgery Research Council

PSRO
Professional Standards Review Organization

PWBA
Pension and Welfare Benefits Administration

PWP
Parents Without Partners

RC
Red Cross

RCOG
Royal College of Obstetricians and Gynaecologists

RCP
Royal College of Physicians (of England)

RCPE
Royal College of Physicians of Edinburgh

RCPI
Royal College of Physicians of Ireland

RCS
Royal College of Surgeons of England

RCSED
Royal College of Surgeons of Edinburgh

RCSI
Royal College of Surgeons of Ireland

RDG
Research Discussion Group

REACH
Reassurance to Each (assistance to families of mentally ill)

ROPA
Regional Organ Procurement Agency

RTECS
Registry of Toxic Effects of Chemical Substances

SADD
Students Against Drunk Driving

SAGES
Society of American Gastrointestinal Endoscopic Surgeons

SAMHSA
Substance Abuse and Mental Health Services Administration

SART
Society for Assisted Reproductive Technology

SASA
Sex Abuse Survivors Anonymous

SBH, SBOH
State Board of Health

SCHIP
State Children's Health Insurance Program

SCOI
Southern California Orthopedic Institute

SERHOLD
Serials Holding database (National Library of Medicine, National Institutes of Health)

SESAP
Surgical Education and Self-Assessment Program

SHEA
Society for Healthcare Epidemiology of America

SHHH
Self-Help for Hard of Hearing People, Inc.

SHPDA
State Health Planning and Development Agency

SIECUS
Sex Information and Educational Council of the United States

SIOP
International Society of Pediatric Oncology

SJCRH
St. Jude Children's Research Hospital

SJM
St. Jude Medical

SKI
Sloan-Kettering Institute

SLAA
Sex and Love Addicts Anonymous

SNDA
Student National Dental Association

SPP
Society for Pediatric Pathology

SPRY
Setting Priorities for Retirement Years (Foundation)

SSA
Social Security Administration

SSIE
Smithsonian Science Information Exchange

SSO
Society of Surgical Oncology

SSOP
Second Surgical Opinion Program

SWOG
Southwest Oncology Group

TCDB
Traumatic Coma Data Bank

TCSG
The Center for Social Gerontology

TDB
Toxicology Data Bank

TERIS
Teratogen Information System

TGA
Therapeutic Goods Administration (Australia)

TIRR
The Institute for Rehabilitation Research

TMIC
Toxic Materials Information Center

TSRH
Texas Scottish Rite Hospital

UAPD
Union of American Physicians and Dentists

UCB
University of California, Berkeley

UCBL
University of California, Berkeley, Laboratory

UCI
University of California, Irvine

UCLA
University of California, Los Angeles

UH
University Hospital

UHSC
University Health Services Clinic

UICC
International Union Against Cancer

UKTSSA
United Kingdom Transplant Support Service Authority

UNAIDS
Joint United Nations Programme on HIV/AIDS

UNOS
United Network for Organ Sharing

UOA
United Ostomy Association

URAC
Utilization Review Accreditation Commission

USAFSAM
United States Air Force School of Aerospace Medicine

USAIDR
United States Army Institute of Dental Research

USAMEDS
United States Army Medical Service

USAMRIID
United States Army Medical Research Institute of Infectious Disease

USAMRMC
United States Army Medical Research and Material Command

USAN
United States Adopted Names (Council)

USASI
United States of America Standards Institute

USBS
United States Bureau of Standards

USD
United States Dispensary

USDA
United States Department of Agriculture

USDHHS
United States Department of Health and Human Services

USFDA
United States Food and Drug Administration

USH
United Services for Handicapped

USHC
United Seniors Health Council

USPHS
United States Public Health Service

USRDS
United States Renal Data System

VA
Department of Veterans Affairs
Veterans Administration

VAAESS
Vaccine-Associated Adverse Events Surveillance System (Canada)

VACO
Veterans Administration Central Office

VAERS
Vaccine Adverse Events Reporting System

VC
Veterinary Corps

VEDA
Vestibular Disorders Association

VHA
Veterans Health Administration

VIBS
Victims Information Bureau Service

VICP
Vaccine Injury Compensation Program

VNA
Visiting Nurse Association

VNAA
Visiting Nurse Association of America

VNS
Visiting Nursing Service

VRS
Vocational Rehabilitation Services

WARDS
Working for Animals Used in Research Drugs and Surgery

WASP
World Association of Societies of Pathology

WFC
World Federation of Chiropractic

WHO
World Health Organization

WHO/ILAR
World Health Organization/International League of Associations for Rheumatology

WMR
World Medical Relief

WOCN
Wound, Ostomy, and Continence Nurses (Society)

WRAIR
Walter Reed Army Institute of Research

WRAMC
Walter Reed Army Medical Center

WW
Weight Watchers

YMCA
Young Men's Christian Association

YWCA
Young Women's Christian Association

Chemotherapy and Other Drug Regimens

AA
ara-C and Adriamycin

AAF
2-acetylaminofluorene

AAG
17-(allylamino)-17-demethoxygeldanamycin

ABC
Adriamycin, BCNU, cyclophosphamide

ABCD
Adriamycin, bleomycin, CCNU, dacarbazine

ABCM
Adriamycin, bleomycin, cyclophosphamide, mitomycin C

ABCVEP-I
Adriamycin, bleomycin, cyclophosphamide, vincristine, etoposide, prednisolone I

ABCVEP-II
Adriamycin, bleomycin, cyclophosphamide, vincristine, etoposide, prednisolone II

ABDIC
Adriamycin, bleomycin, DTIC, CCNU, prednisone
Adriamycin, bleomycin, dacarbazine, CCNU, prednisone

ABDV
Adriamycin, bleomycin, DTIC, vinblastine

ABOS
Adriamycin, bleomycin sulfate, vincristine, streptozocin

ABP
Adriamycin, bleomycin, prednisone

ABPP
bropirimine

ABV
actinomycin D, bleomycin, vincristine
Adriamycin, bleomycin, vinblastine

ABVD
Adriamycin, bleomycin, vinblastine, dacarbazine
Adriamycin, bleomycin, vincristine, dacarbazine

ABVD-MP
Adriamycin, bleomycin, vinblastine, dacarbazine, methylprednisolone

ABVE
Adriamycin, bleomycin, vincristine, etoposide

ABVP
Adriamycin, bleomycin sulfate, vinblastine, prednisone
Adriamycin, bleomycin sulfate, vincristine, prednisone

5-AC
5-azacytidine

AC
Adriamycin and carmustine
Adriamycin and CCNU
Adriamycin/cyclophosphamide
Adriamycin and cisplatin

Ac-D-Ac
Adriamycin, daunorubicin, Adriamycin

AcD
actinomycin D (dactinomycin)

ACE
Adriamycin, cyclophosphamide, etoposide

ACFUCY
actinomycin D, 5-fluorouracil, cyclophosphamide

ACID
Adriamycin, cyclophosphamide, imidazole, dactinomycin

ACM
Adriamycin, cyclophosphamide, methotrexate

ACNU
nimustine

ACOAP
Adriamycin, cyclophosphamide, Oncovin, cytosine arabinoside, prednisone

ACOP
Adriamycin, cyclophosphamide, Oncovin, prednisone

ACOPP
Adriamycin, cyclophosphamide, Oncovin, prednisone, procarbazine

ACR
aclarubicin

ACT-C, Act-C
actinomycin C

ACT-D, Act-D
actinomycin D
dactinomycin

ACV
amifostine, cisplatin, vinblastine

ACVBP
Adriamycin, cyclophosphamide, vindesine, bleomycin, prednisone

ADBC
Adriamycin, DTIC, bleomycin, CCNU

ADCONFU
Adriamycin, cyclophosphamide, Oncovin, fluorouracil

ADE
ara-C, daunorubicin, etoposide

ADIC
Adriamycin, DTIC
Adriamycin and dacarbazine

ADM
Adriamycin

ADOAP
Adriamycin, Oncovin, arabinosylcytosine, prednisone

ADOC
Adriamycin, docetaxel, Oncovin, cyclophosphamide

ADOP
Adriamycin, Oncovin, prednisone

ADR
Adriamycin

AFM
Adriamycin, 5-fluorouracil, methotrexate

AIM
asparaginase, ifosfamide, methotrexate

ALOMAD
Adriamycin, Leukeran, Oncovin, methotrexate, actinomycin D, dacarbazine

AMD
actinomycin D

AMP
adenosine monophosphate

AOPA
ara-C, Oncovin, prednisone, asparaginase

AOPE
Adriamycin, Oncovin, prednisone, etoposide

AP
Adriamycin and Platinol

APC
AMSA, prednisone, chlorambucil

APD
aminohydroxypropylidene diphosphate

APE
ara-C, Platinol, etoposide
Adriamycin, Platinol, etoposide

APO
Adriamycin, prednisone, Oncovin

ara-A, araA
arabinosyladenine

ara-AMP
adenine arabinoside monophosphate

ara-AC
azacytosine arabinoside

ara-C
cytarabine
arabinosylcytosine
cytosine arabinoside

ara-C/HU
ara-C plus hydroxyurea

ara-G
arabinosyl guanosine

ASAP
Adriamycin, Solu-Medrol, ara-C, Platinol

ASHAP
Adriamycin, Solu-Medrol, high-dose ara-C, Platinol

ASP
asparaginase

ATAC
Arimidex, Tamoxifen, Alone or in Combination

AV
Adriamycin, vincristine

AVAD
Adriamycin, vincristine, cytarabine, dexamethasone

AVCF
Adriamycin, vincristine, cyclophosphamide, 5-fluorouracil

AVDP
asparaginase, vincristine, daunorubicin, prednisone

AVM
Adriamycin, vinblastine, methotrexate
Adriamycin, vincristine, mitomycin C

AVP
Adriamycin, vincristine, procarbazine

AVP
Actinomycin D, vincristine, Platinol

5-AZA
5-azacytidine

5-AZC
5-azacytidine

AZQ
aziridinylbenzoquinone

AZUR, AzUr
azauridine

BAC
BCNU, ara-C, cyclophosphamide

BAC
BCNU, cytarabine, cyclophosphamide

BACO
bleomycin, Adriamycin, CCNU, Oncovin

BACOD
bleomycin, Adriamycin, CCNU, Oncovin, dexamethasone

BACON
bleomycin, Adriamycin, CCNU, Oncovin, nitrogen mustard

BACOP
bleomycin, Adriamycin, cyclophosphamide, Oncovin, prednisone
bleomycin, Adriamycin, Cytoxan, Oncovin, prednisone

BACT
BCNU, ara-C, cyclophosphamide, 6-thioguanine
BCNU, ara-C, Cytoxan, 6-thioguanine
bleomycin, Adriamycin, Cytoxan, tamoxifen
bleomycin, Adriamycin, cyclophosphamide, tamoxifen

BAMON
bleomycin, Adriamycin, methotrexate, Oncovin, nitrogen mustard.

BAP
bleomycin, Adriamycin, prednisone

BAVIP
bleomycin, Adriamycin, vinblastine, imidazole carboxamide, prednisone

BBVP-M
BCNU, bleomycin, VePesid, prednisone, methotrexate

BCAP
BCNU, cyclophosphamide, Adriamycin, prednisone

B-CAV
bleomycin, CCNU, Adriamycin, Velban

BCD
bleomycin, cyclophosphamide, dactinomycin

B-CHOP
bleomycin, Cytoxan, hydroxydaunomycin, Oncovin, prednisone

BCMF
bleomycin, cyclophosphamide, methotrexate, 5-fluorouracil

BCNU
carmustine
bischloroethylnitrosourea
bischloronitrosourea

BCOP
BCNU, cyclophosphamide, Oncovin, prednisone

BCP
BCNU, cyclophosphamide, prednisone

BCVP
BCNU, cyclophosphamide, vincristine, prednisone

BCVPP
BCNU, cyclophosphamide, vinblastine, procarbazine, prednisone

B-DOPA
bleomycin, dacarbazine, Oncovin, prednisone, Adriamycin
bleomycin, DTIC, Oncovin, prednisone, Adriamycin

BEAC
BCNU, etoposide, ara-C, cyclophosphamide

BEACOPP
bleomycin, etoposide, Adriamycin, cyclophosphamide, vincristine, procarbazine,
  prednisone

BEAM
BCNU, etoposide, ara-C, melphalan

BELD
bleomycin, Eldisine, lomustine, dacarbazine

BEMP
bleomycin, Eldisine, mitomycin, Platinol

BEP
bleomycin, etoposide, Platinol

BHD
BCNU, hydroxyurea, dacarbazine

BHD-V
BCNU, hydroxyurea, dacarbazine, vincristine

BiCNU
carmustine

BIP
bleomycin, ifosfamide, Platinol
bleomycin, ifosfamide with mensa rescue, Platinol

BLEO
bleomycin

BLEO-COMF
bleomycin, cyclophosphamide, Oncovin, methotrexate, 5-fluorouracil

BLEO-MOPP, B-MOPP
bleomycin, mechlorethamine, Oncovin, procarbazine, prednisone

BMP
BCNU, methotrexate, procarbazine

BOAP
bleomycin, Oncovin, Adriamycin, prednisone

BOLD
bleomycin, Oncovin, lomustine, dacarbazine

BOMP
bleomycin, Oncovin, Matulane, prednisone
bleomycin, Oncovin, mitomycin, Platinol

BOP
bleomycin, Oncovin, Platinol
bleomycin, Oncovin, prednisone

BOPAM
bleomycin, Oncovin, prednisone, Adriamycin, mechlorethamine, methotrexate

BOPP
BCNU, Oncovin, procarbazine, prednisone

BU-CY, BU/CY
busulfan and cyclophosphamide

BVAP
BCNU, vincristine, Adriamycin, prednisone

BVCPP
BCNU, vinblastine, cyclophosphamide, procarbazine, prednisone

BVD
BCNU, vincristine, dacarbazine

BVDS
bleomycin, Velban, doxorubicin, streptozocin

BVPP
BCNU, vincristine, procarbazine, prednisone

C
carboplatin
chloramphenicol

CA
cytosine arabinoside

CA
cyclophosphamide and Adriamycin

CABOP, CA-BOP
cyclophosphamide, Adriamycin, bleomycin, Oncovin, prednisone

CABS
CCNU, Adriamycin, bleomycin, streptozocin

CAC
cisplatin, ara-C, caffeine

CA/CAF
cyclophosphamide, doxorubicin with or without 5-fluorouracil

CACP
cisplatin

CAD

cyclophosphamide, Adriamycin, dacarbazine
cytosine arabinoside and daunorubicin

CADIC

cyclophosphamide, Adriamycin, dacarbazine

CAE

cyclophosphamide, Adriamycin, etoposide

CAF

cyclophosphamide, Adriamycin, 5-fluorouracil
Cytoxan, Adriamycin, 5-fluorouracil

CAFFI

cyclophosphamide, Adriamycin, 5-fluorouracil by continuous infusion

CAFP

cyclophosphamide, Adriamycin, 5-fluorouracil, prednisone

CAFTH

Cytoxan, Adriamycin, 5-fluorouracil, tamoxifen, Halotestin
cyclophosphamide, Adriamycin, 5-fluorouracil, tamoxifen, Halotestin

CAFVP

cyclophosphamide, Adriamycin, 5-fluorouracil, vincristine, prednisone

CAI

carboxyamidotriazole

CALF

Cytoxan, Adriamycin, leucovorin calcium, 5-fluorouracil
cyclophosphamide, Adriamycin, leucovorin calcium, 5-fluorouracil

CALF-E

Cytoxan, Adriamycin, leucovorin calcium, 5-fluorouracil, ethinyl estradiol
cyclophosphamide, Adriamycin, leucovorin calcium, 5-fluorouracil, ethinyl
  estradiol

CAM

Cytoxan, Adriamycin, methotrexate
cyclophosphamide, Adriamycin, methotrexate

CAMB
Cytoxan, Adriamycin, methotrexate, bleomycin
cyclophosphamide, Adriamycin, methotrexate, bleomycin

CAMELEON
cytosine arabinoside, high-dose methotrexate, leucovorin, Oncovin

CAMEO
cyclophosphamide, Adriamycin, methotrexate, etoposide, Oncovin

CAMF
cyclophosphamide, Adriamycin, methotrexate, 5-fluorouracil

CAMLO
cytosine arabinoside, methotrexate, leucovorin, Oncovin

CAMP
cyclophosphamide, Adriamycin, methotrexate, procarbazine

CAO
cyclophosphamide, Adriamycin, Oncovin

CAP
cyclophosphamide, Adriamycin, Platinol
cyclophosphamide, Adriamycin, prednisone

CA4P
Combretastatin A4 prodrug

CAP-BOP
cyclophosphamide, Adriamycin, procarbazine, bleomycin, Oncovin, prednisone

CAP-I
cyclophosphamide, Adriamycin, Platinol

CAP-II
cyclophosphamide, Adriamycin, high-dose Platinol

CAPPR
Cytoxan, Adriamycin, Platinol, prednisone

CAPPr
cyclophosphamide, Adriamycin Platinol, prednisone

CarboPEC
carboplatin, etoposide, cyclophosphamide

CAT
cyclophosphamide, cytosine, arabinoside, topotecan
cytosine arabinoside, Adriamycin, 6-thioguanine
cytarabine, Adriamycin, 6-thioguanine
cytosine arabinoside, 6-thioguanine

CAV
cyclophosphamide, Adriamycin, vincristine
cyclophosphamide, Adriamycin, vinblastine
cyclophosphamide, Adriamycin, Velban

CAVe
CCNU, Adriamycin, vinblastine
CCNU, Adriamycin, Velban

CAVP
cyclophosphamide, Adriamycin, vincristine, prednisone

CAVP16
Cytoxan, Adriamycin, VP-16
cyclophosphamide, Adriamycin, VP-16

CAVP-I
cyclophosphamide, Adriamycin, vincristine, prednisone

CAVPM
cyclophosphamide, Adriamycin, VP-16, prednisone, methotrexate

Cb
carboplatin

CBDT
Cisplastin, BCNU, dacarbazine, tamoxifen

CBV
cyclophosphamide, BCNU, VP-16
Cytoxan, BCNU, VP-16

CBVD
CCNU, bleomycin, vinblastine, dexamethasone

CCAVV
CCNU, cyclophosphamide, Adriamycin, vincristine, VP-16

CCFE
cyclophosphamide, cisplatin, 5-fluorouracil, estramustine

CCM
cyclophosphamide, CCNU, methotrexate

CCMA
CCNU, cyclophosphamide, methotrexate, Adriamycin

CCNU
chloroethylcyclohexylnitrosourea
cyclohexylchloroethylnitrosurea

CCOB
CCNU, cyclophosphamide, Oncovin, bleomycin

CCV
CCNU, cyclophosphamide, vincristine

CCVB
CCNU, cyclophosphamide, vincristine, bleomycin

CCVPP
CCNU, cyclophosphamide, Velban, procarbazine, prednisone

CD
cytarabine, daunorubicin

CDC
carboplatin, doxorubicin, cyclophosphamide

CDDP
cis-diamminedichloroplatinum
cisplatin

CDE
Cytoxan, doxorubicin, etoposide
cyclophosphamide, doxorubicin, etoposide

CE
carboplatin, etoposide

CEB
carboplatin, etoposide, bleomycin

CECA
cisplatin, etoposide, Cytoxan, Adriamycin
cisplatin, etoposide, cyclophosphamide, Adriamycin

CEF
Cytoxan, epirubicin, 5-fluorouracil
cyclophosphamide, epirubicin, 5-fluorouracil

CEM
cytosine arabinoside, etoposide, methotrexate

CEOP
cyclophosphamide, epirubicin, Oncovin, prednisone

CEOP
cyclophosphamide, epirubicin, Oncovin, prednisolone
cyclophosphamide, epirubicin, vincristine (Oncovin), prednisone
cyclophosphamide, epirubicin, vincristine (Oncovin), prednisolone

CEOP-B
cyclophosphamide, epirubicin, Oncovin, prednisone, bleomycin

CEP
cyclophosphamide, etoposide, Platinol
CCNU, etoposide, prednimustine

CEV
cyclophosphamide, etoposide, vincristine

CEVAIE
Carboplatin, epirubicin, vincristine, actinomycin D, ifosfamide, etoposide

CEVD
cyclophosphamide, etoposide, vincristine, dexamethasone

CFEV
cyclophosphamide, 5-fluorouracil, epirubicin, vincristine

CFL
cisplatin, 5-fluorouracil, leucovorin

CFP
cyclophosphamide, 5-fluorouracil, prednisone

CFPT
cyclophosphamide, fluorouracil, prednisone, tamoxifen

CFR
citrovorum-factor rescue

CHAD
cyclophosphamide, hexamethylmelamine, Adriamycin, DDP

CHAMOCA
Cytoxan, hydroxyurea, actinomycin D, methotrexate, Oncovin, calcium folinate, Adriamycin
cyclophosphamide, hydroxyurea, actinomycin D, methotrexate, Oncovin, citrovorum factor, Adriamycin

CHAP
cyclophosphamide, hexamethylmelamine, Adriamycin, Platinol
cyclophosphamide, Hexalen, Adriamycin, Platinol

CHF
cyclophosphamide, hexamethylmelamine, 5-fluorouracil

CHIP
cis-dichlorotranshydroxy-bis-isopropylamine platinum IV
Iproplatin

CHL
chlorambucil
chloramphenicol

ChlVPP
chlorambucil, vinblastine, procarbazine, prednisone

ChlVPP/EVA
chlorambucil, vinblastine, procarbazine, prednisone, etoposide, vincristine, Adriamycin

CHO
cyclophosphamide, hydroxydaunorubicin, Oncovin

CHOB
cyclophosphamide, hydroxydaunomycin, Oncovin, bleomycin

CHOD
Cytoxan, hydroxydaunomycin, Oncovin, dexamethasone
cyclophosphamide, hydroxydaunomycin, Oncovin, dexamethasone

CHOP
cyclophosphamide, hydroxydaunomycin, Oncovin, prednisone
cyclophosphamide, Halotestin, Oncovin, prednisone

CHOP-BLEO
cyclophosphamide, hydroxydaunorubicin, Oncovin, prednisone, bleomycin

CHOPE
Cytoxan, Halotestin, Oncovin, prednisone, etoposide
cyclophosphamide, hydroxydaunomycin, Oncovin, prednisone, etoposide
cyclophosphamide, Halotestin, Oncovin, prednisone, etoposide

CHOR
cyclophosphamide, hydroxydaunorubicin, Oncovin, radiotherapy

CHVP
cyclophosphamide, hydroxydaunomycin, VM-26, prednisone

CH1-VPP
chlorambucil, vinblastine, procarbazine, prednisone

CIA
CCNU, ifosfamide, Adriamycin

CisCA
cisplatin, cyclophosphamide, Adriamycin

cis-DDP
cis-diamminedichloroplatinum
cisplatin

CLB
chlorambucil

CMC
cyclophosphamide, methotrexate, CCNU

CMC-VAP
cyclophosphamide, methotrexate, CCNU, vincristine, Adriamycin, procarbazine

CMED
cyclophosphamide, methotrexate, etoposide, dexamethasone

CMEV
cyclophosphamide, methotrexate, epirubicin, vincristine

CMF
cyclophosphamide, methotrexate, 5-fluorouracil
Cytoxan, methotrexate, 5-fluorouracil

CMF-AV
cyclophosphamide, methotrexate, 5-fluorouracil, Adriamycin, vincristine

CMFAVP
cyclophosphamide, methotrexate, 5-fluorouracil, Adriamycin, vincristine,
   prednisone

CMF-BLEO
cyclophosphamide, methotrexate, 5-fluorouracil, bleomycin

CMF-FLU
cyclophosphamide, methotrexate, 5-fluorouracil, fluoxymesterone

CMFH
cyclophosphamide, methotrexate, 5-fluorouracil, hydroxyurea

CMFP
cyclophosphamide, methotrexate, 5-fluorouracil, prednisone
Cytoxan, methotrexate, 5-fluorouracil, prednisone

CMFPT
Cytoxan, methotrexate, 5-fluorouracil, prednisone, tamoxifen
cyclophosphamide, methotrexate, 5-fluorouracil, prednisone, tamoxifen

CMFPTH
cyclophosphamide, methotrexate, 5-fluorouracil, prednisone, tamoxifen, Halotestin

CMFP-VA
cyclophosphamide, methotrexate, 5-fluorouracil, prednisone, vincristine, Adriamycin

CMFT
cyclophosphamide, methotrexate, 5-fluorouracil, tamoxifen

CMF-TAM
cyclophosphamide, methotrexate, 5-fluorouracil, tamoxifen

CM-5-FU
cyclophosphamide, methotrexate, 5-fluorouracil

CMFV
cyclophosphamide, methotrexate, 5-fluorouracil, vincristine

CMFVAT
cyclophosphamide, methotrexate, 5-fluorouracil, vincristine, Adriamycin, testosterone

CMFVP
cyclophosphamide, methotrexate, 5-fluorouracil, vincristine, prednisone
Cytoxan, methotrexate, fluorouracil, vincristine, prednisone

CMH
Cytoxan, m-AMSA, hydroxyurea
cyclophosphamide, m-AMSA, hydroxyurea

CMOPP
cyclophosphamide, mechlorethamine, Oncovin, procarbazine, prednisone

CMP
CCNU, methotrexate, procarbazine

CMPF
cyclophosphamide, methotrexate, prednisone, 5-fluorouracil

CMV
cisplatin, methotrexate, Velban
cisplatin, methotrexate, vinblastine

CNF
cyclophosphamide, Novantrone, 5-fluorouracil

CNOP

Cytoxan, Novantrone, Oncovin, prednisone
cyclophosphamide, Novantrone, Oncovin, prednisone

COAP

cyclophosphamide, Oncovin, arabinosylcytosine, prednisone
Cytoxan, Oncovin, ara-C, prednisone

COAP-BLEO

cyclophosphamide, Oncovin, ara-C, prednisone, bleomycin

COB

cisplatin, Oncovin, bleomycin

CODE

cisplatin, Oncovin, doxorubicin, etoposide

CODOX-M/IVAC

cyclophosphamide, doxorubicin, high-dose methotrexate/ifosfamide, etoposide, high-dose cytarabine

COM

cyclophosphamide, Oncovin, methotrexate
cyclophosphamide, Oncovin, methyl-CCNU
cyclophosphamide, Oncovin, meCCNU

COMA-A

cyclophosphamide, Oncovin, methotrexate, Adriamycin, ara-C

COMB

Cytoxan, Oncovin, methotrexate, bleomycin
cyclophosphamide, Oncovin, methotrexate, bleomycin
cyclophosphamide, Oncovin, meCCNU, bleomycin

COMBAP

cyclophosphamide, Oncovin, methotrexate, bleomycin, Adriamycin, prednisone

COMe

cyclophosphamide, Oncovin, methotrexate

COMET-A

cyclophosphamide, Oncovin, methotrexate, leucovorin, etoposide, ara-C

COMF
cyclophosphamide, Oncovin, methotrexate, 5-fluorouracil

COMLA
cyclophosphamide, Oncovin, methotrexate, leucovorin, arabinosylcytosine
cyclophosphamide, Oncovin, methotrexate, leucovorin, ara-C

COMP
CCNU, Oncovin, methotrexate, procarbazine
cyclophosphamide, Oncovin, methotrexate, prednisone

CONPADRI I
cyclophosphamide, Oncovin, L-phenylalanine mustard, Adriamycin

CONPADRI II
CONPADRI I plus high dose methotrexate

CONPADRI III
CONPADRI II plus intensified doxorubicin

COP
cyclophosphamide, Oncovin, prednisone

COPA
cyclophosphamide, Oncovin, prednisone, Adriamycin

COPA-BLEO
cyclophosphamide, Oncovin, prednisone, Adriamycin, bleomycin

COPAC
CCNU, Oncovin, prednisone, Adriamycin, cyclophosphamide

COPB
cyclophosphamide, Oncovin, prednisone, bleomycin

COP-BLAM
cyclophosphamide, Oncovin, prednisone, bleomycin, Adriamycin, Matulane

COP-BLEO
cyclophosphamide, Oncovin, prednisone, bleomycin

COPE
Cytoxan, Oncovin, Platinol, etoposide
cyclophosphamide, Oncovin, Platinol, etoposide

COPP
cyclophosphamide, Oncovin, procarbazine, prednisone
CCNU, Oncovin, procarbazine, prednisone

COPPA
cyclophosphamide, Oncovin, procarbazine, prednisone, Adriamycin

COPP/ABVD
cyclophosphamide, Oncovin, procarbazine, prednisone, Adriamycin, bleomycin,
    vinblastine, dacarbazine

CP
chlorambucil and prednisone

COP
cyclophosphamide and prednisone
Cytoxan and Platinol

CPA
cyclophosphamide

CPB
cyclophosphamide, Platinol, BCNU

CPC
Cytoxan, Platinol, carboplatin
cyclophosphamide, Platinol, carboplatin

CPDD
cis-platinum diammine dichloride

CPM
CCNU, procarbazine, methotrexate

CPOB
cyclophosphamide, prednisone, Oncovin, bleomycin

CPT
cisplatin

CPV
cyclophosphamide, Platinol, VP-16

CROP
cyclophosphamide, rubidazone, Oncovin, prednisone

CSA, CsA
cyclosporin A

CTCb
cyclophosphamide, thiotepa, carboplatin
Cytoxan, thiotepa, carboplatin

CTX
Cytoxan
Cyclophosphamide

CTX-Plat
cyclophosphamide and Platinol

CV
cisplatin, VePesid
Cisplatin and VP-16

CVA
cyclophosphamide, vincristine, Adriamycin

CVA-BMP
cyclophosphamide, vincristine, Adriamycin, BCNU, methotrexate, procarbazine

CVAD
Cytoxan, vincristine, Adriamycin, dexamethasone
cyclophosphamide, vincristine, Adriamycin, dexamethasone

CVB
CCNU, vinblastine, bleomycin

CVBD
CCNU, vinblastine, bleomycin, dexamethasone

CVD
cisplatin, vinblastine, dacarbazine

CVEB
cisplatin, vinblastine, etoposide, bleomycin
cisplatin, Velban, etoposide, bleomycin

CVFVP
cyclophosphamide, methotrexate, 5-fluorouracil, vincristine, prednisone

CVI
carboplatin, VePesid, ifosfamide

CVM
cyclophosphamide, vincristine, methotrexate

CVP
cyclophosphamide, vincristine, prednisone

CVP-BLEO
cyclophosphamide, vincristine, prednisone, bleomycin

CVPP
cyclophosphamide, vincristine, prednisone, procarbazine
cyclophosphamide, Velban, prednisone, procarbazine
Cytoxan, vinblastine, procarbazine, prednisone
CCNU, vinblastine, prednisone, procarbazine

CVPP-CCNU
cyclophosphamide, vinblastine, procarbazine, prednisone plus CCNU

CVXD
cyclophosphamide, vincristine, DaunoXome, Decadron

CY, Cy
cyclophosphamide
cytarabine
Cytoxan

CyADIC
cyclophosphamide, Adriamycin, DIC

CYC
cyclophosphamide

CYCLO, CyClo
cyclophosphamide

CyHOP
cyclophosphamide, Halotestin, Oncovin, prednisone

CYP, CyP
cyclophosphamide

CytaBOM
cytarabine, bleomycin, Oncovin, mechlorethamine

CY/TBI
Cytoxan/total body irradiation

CyVADACT
cyclophosphamide, vincristine, Adriamycin, dactinomycin

CyVADIC
cyclophosphamide, vincristine, Adriamycin, DTIC

CyVMAD
cyclophosphamide, vincristine, Adriamycin, DTIC

DA
daunorubicin and ara-C

DAC
deoxyazacytidine

DACE
dexamethasone, ara-C, carboplatin, etoposide

DACT
dactinomycin

DADAG
diacetyldianhydrogalactitol

DAIP
dexamethasone, ifosfamide, cisplatin, cytarabine

DAP
dianhydrogalactitol, Adriamycin, Platinol

DAPD
diaminopurine dioxolane

DAP/TMP
dapsone and trimethoprim

DAT
daunorubicin, ara-C, 6-thioguanine

DATVP
daunomycin, ara-C, 6-thioguanine, vincristine, prednisone

DAUNO
daunorubicin

DAV
dibromodulcitol, Adriamycin, vincristine

DAVA
desacetyl vinblastine amide

DAVH
dibromodulcitol, Adriamycin, vincristine, Halotestin

DAVTH
dibromodulcitol, Adriamycin, vincristine, tamoxifen, Halotestin

DBD
dibromodulcitol

DBPT
dacarbazine, carmustine, cisplatin, tamoxifen
DTIC, BCNU, Platinol, tamoxifen
dimethyltriazenoimidazole carboxamide, bischloroethylnitrosourea, Platinol, tamoxifen

DBV
dacarbazine, BCNU, vincristine

DC
daunorubicin and cytarabine

DCCMP
daunorubicin, cyclocytidine, 6-metacaptopurine, prednisone

DCEP
dexamethasone, cyclophosphamide, etoposide, cisplatin

DCF
2-deoxycoformycin

DCMP
daunorubicin, cytarabine, 6-mercaptopurine, prednisone

DCNU
chlorozotocin

DCPM
daunorubicin, cytarabine, prednisolone, mercaptopurine

DCT
daunorubicin, cytarabine, 6-thioguanine

DCV
dacarbazine, CCNU, vincristine
DTIC, CCNU, vincristine

ddC
zalcitabine

ddCMP
2´, 3´-dideoxycytidine 5´-monophosphate

DDL
dideoxyinosine

ddIno
2´, 3´-dideoxyininosine

ddN
2´, 3´-dideoxynucleoside

DDP
cis-diamminedichloroplatinum

DDS
diaminodiphenylsulfone

DEAE
diethylaminoethyl

DECAL
dexamethasone, etoposide, cisplatin, ara-C, L-asparaginase

DEM
diethyl maleate

DFDC
gemcitabine

DFV
DDP, 5-fluorouracil, VePesid

DHAC
dihydro-5-azacitidine

DHAD
dihydroxyanthracenedione

DHAP
dexamethasone, high-dose cytarabine, cisplatin

DHPG
dihydroxypropoxymethylguanine

DIC
dimethyltriazenoimidazole carboxamide

DICE
dexamethasone, ifosfamide, cisplatin, etoposide

DICEP
dose-interactive cyclophosphamide, etoposide, Platinol

DIF
DPD-inhibitory fluoropyrimidine

DL
doxorubicin and lomustine

DMC
dactinomycin, methotrexate, cyclophosphamide

DMRIE/DOPE
1,2-dimyristyloxypropyl-3-dimethylhydroxyethyl ammonium
bromide/dioleoylphosphatidylethanolamine formulation

DNJ
deoxynojirimycin

DNM
daunomycin

DNR
daunorubicin

DOAP
daunorubicin, Oncovin, ara-C, prednisone

DPPE
N, N-diethyl-2-[4-(phenylmethyl)phenoxy]ethanamine.HCl

DRB
daunorubicin

DSF
doxorubicin, streptozocin, 5-fluorouracil

d4T
didehydrodeoxythymidine
didehydrodideoxythymidine, stavudine, Zerit

DTC-101
cytarabine

DTC
diethyldithiocarbamate

DTIC
dacarbazine
dimethyltriazenoimidazole carboxamide

DTIC-ACTD
DTIC and actinomycin D

DTIC-Dome
Dacarbazine

dTK
2´-deoxythymidine kinase

DT-PACE
dexamethasone, thalidomide plus Adriamycin, cyclophosphamide, etoposide

DVB
cis-diamminedichloroplatinum, vindesine, bleomycin

DVB
DDP, vindesine, bleomycin

DVP
daunorubicin, vincristine, prednisone

DVPL-ASP
daunorubicin, vincristine, prednisone, L-asparaginase

DXR
doxorubicin

DZAPO
daunorubicin, azacytidine, ara-C, prednisone, Oncovin

EAP
etoposide, Adriamycin, Platinol

EBAP
etoposide, Adriamycin, Platinol

EBV
epirubicin, bleomycin, vinblastine

ECF
epirubicin, cisplatin, 5-fluorouracil

ECHO
etoposide, cyclophosphamide, hydroxydaunomycin, Oncovin

ECMV
etoposide, Cytoxan, methotrexate, vincristine

EDAP
etoposide, dexamethasone, ara-C, Platinol

EFP
etoposide, 5-fluorouracil, Platinol

ELF
etoposide, leucovorin, 5-fluorouracil

EMACO, EMA-CO
etoposide, methotrexate, actinomycin D, cyclophosphamide, Oncovin

EMP
estramustine phosphate

E-MVAC
escalated methotrexate, vinblastine, Adriamycin, cisplatin

EP
etoposide and Platinol

epi-ADR
epinephrine and Adriamycin

EPIC
early postoperative intraperitoneal chemotherapy
etoposide, prednisolone, ifosfamide, cisplatin

EPIDX
epidoxorubicin

EPOCH
etoposide, prednisone, Oncovin, Cytoxan, Halotestin
etoposide, prednisone, Oncovin, cyclophosphamide, Halotestin

ESAP
etoposide, Solu-Medrol, ara-C, Platino

ESHAP
etoposide, Solu-Medrol, high-dose ara-C, Platinol

ETO, ETP
etoposide

EV
etoposide and vincristine

EVA
etoposide, vinblastine, Adriamycin

EVAP
etoposide, vinblastine, Adriamycin, prednisone

FAC
5-fluorouracil, Adriamycin, cyclophosphamide

FAC-BCG
ftorafur, Adriamycin, cyclophosphamide, BCG

FAC-M
5-fluorouracil, Adriamycin, Cytoxan, methotrexate
5-fluorouracil, Adriamycin, cyclophosphamide, methotrexate

FACP
ftorafur, Adriamycin, cyclophosphamide, Platinol

FACS
5-fluorouracil, Adriamycin, cyclophosphamide, streptozocin

FACVP
5-fluorouracil Adriamycin, cyclophosphamide, VP-16

FAM
5-fluorouracil, Adriamycin, mitomycin
fludarabine, ara-C, mitoxantrone

FAM-C
5-fluorouracil, Adriamycin, methyl-CCNU

FAM-CF
5-fluorouracil, Adriamycin, mitomycin, citrovorum factor

FAMe
5-fluorouracil, Adriamycin, methyl-CCNU

FAMMe
5-fluorouracil, Adriamycin, mitomycin C, methyl-CCNU

FAMP
fludarabine monophosphate

FAM-Se
5-fluorouracil, Adriamycin, mitomycin C, streptozotocin

FAMTX
sequential high-dose methotrexate followed by 5-FU in combination with
  Adriamycin
5-fluorouracil, Adriamycin, methotrexate

FAP
5-fluorouracil, Adriamycin, Platinol

FCAP
5-fluorouracil, Cytoxan, Adriamycin, Platinol
5-fluorouracil, cyclophosphamide, Adriamycin, Platinol

FCP
5-fluorouracil, cyclophosphamide, prednisone

FEC
5-fluorouracil, epirubicin, cyclophosphamide
5-fluorouracil, epirubicin, Cytoxan

FED
5-fluorouracil, etoposide, DDP

F-FU
F-labeled 5-fluorouracil

FHX
fluorouracil, hydroxyurea, radiotherapy

FIVB
5-fluorouracil, imidazole, vincristine, BCNU

FL
flutamide and Lupron Depot

FLAC
5-fluorouracil, leucovorin calcium, Adriamycin, Cytoxan

FLAG
fludarabine, ara-C, G-CSF

FLAG-ida
fludarabine, ara-C, G-CSF, idarubicin

FLAM
fludarabine, cytarabine, mitoxantrone

FLAP
5-fluorouracil, leucovorin calcium, Adriamycin, Platinol

FLEP
5-fluorouracil, leucovorin, etoposide, Platinol

F-MACHOP
5-fluorouracil, methotrexate, ara-C, cyclophosphamide, Adriamycin, oncovin,
   prednisone

FMD
fludarabine, mitoxantrone, dexamethasone

FMV
fluorouracil, methyl-CCNU, vincristine

FND
fludarabine, mitoxantrone, dexamethasone

FMdC
fluoromethylene deoxycytidine

FMS
5-fluorouracil, mitomycin C, streptozocin

FMV
5-fluorouracil, methyl-CCNU, vincristine

FNC
5-fluorouracil, Novantrone, cyclophosphamide

FND
fludarabine, Novantrone, dexamethasone

FNM
5-fluorouracil, Novantrone, methotrexate

FOAM
5-fluorouracil, Oncovin, Adriamycin, mitomycin C

FOLFIRI
irinotecan, folinic acid, 5-fluorouracil

FOLFOX
oxaliplatin with leucovorin and 5-fluorouracil
5-fluorouracil, folinic acid, oxaliplatin

FOLFUGEM
folinic acid, leucovorin, 5-fluorouracil, gemcitabine

FOLFUGEM-OX
folinic acid, leucovorin, 5-fluorouracil, gemcitabine, oxaliplatin

FOM
5-fluorouracil, Oncovin, mitomycin C

FRACON
framycetin, colistin, nystatin

FT, Ft
ftorafur

FU
fluorouracil

5-FU
5-fluorouracil

FUDR
floxuridine
fluorodeoxyuridine

FUFA
5-fluorouracil and folinic acid

FUFOL
5-fluorouracil and folinic acid

5-FU/LV
5-fluorouracil/leucovorin

FUM
5-fluorouracil and methotrexate

FUMIR
fluorouracil, mitomycin C, radiation

FUra
fluorouracil

FURAM
ftorafur, Adriamycin, mitomycin C

FUVAC
5-fluorouracil, vinblastine, Adriamycin, Cytoxan

FZ
flutamide and Zoladex

GEM
gemcitabine

GEMOX
gemcitabine plus oxaliplatin

GEPARDO
German preoperative Adriamycin, docetaxel

GO
gemtuzumab ozogamicin

HAC
hexamethylmelamine, Adriamycin, cyclophosphamide

HAD
hexamethylmelamine, Adriamycin, DDP

HAM
hexamethylmelamine, Adriamycin, melphalan
hexamethylmelamine, Adriamycin, methotrexate

HAMP
hexamethylenamine, Adriamycin, methotrexate, Platinol

H-CAP
hexamethylmelamine, cyclophosphamide, Adriamycin, Platinol
hexamethylmelamine, Cytoxan, Adriamycin, Platinol

HDAC, HDARA-C
high-dose ara-C

HDC-ABMT
high-dose chemotherapy with autologous bone marrow transplantation

HDC/ASCR
high-dose chemotherapy with autologous bone marrow or stem cell rescue

HDC-ASCS
high-dose chemotherapy with autologous stem cell support

HDCh
high-dose chemotherapy

HD-CNVp
high-dose cyclophosphamide, mitoxantrone, VP-16

HDC-SCR
high-dose chemotherapy with stem-cell rescue

HDMTX
high-dose methotrexate

HDMTX-CF
high-dose methotrexate, citrovorum factor

HDMTX-LV
high-dose methotrexate, leucovorin

HDPEB
high-dose Platinol, etoposide, bleomycin

HD-VAC
high-dose methotrexate, vinblastine, Adriamycin, cisplatin

HEX, Hex
hexamethylmelamine

Hexa-CAF
hexamethylmelamine, cyclophosphamide, amphotericin B, fluorouracil
hexamethylmelamine, cyclophosphamide, Adriamycin, fluorouracil

HI-DAC, HiDAC
high-dose cytosine arabinoside

HMAF
hydroxymethylacylfulvene

HMM
hexamethylmelamine

HMTX
high-dose methotrexate

HN2
mechlorethamine
nitrogen mustard

HOAP-BLEO
hydroxydaunomycin, Oncovin, ara-C, prednisone, bleomycin

HOM
hexamethylmelamine, Oncovin, methotrexate

HOP
hydroxydaunomycin, Oncovin, prednisone

HPMPC
3-hydroxy-2-phosphono-methoxypropyl cytosine

4-HPR
N-(4-hydroxyphenyl)retinamide

HXM
hexamethylmelamine

hyper-CVAD
hyperfractionated cyclophosphamide, vincristine, doxorubicin, dexamethasone

ICE
ifosfamide, carboplatin, etoposide

IDA
idarubicin

IDR
idarubicin

IF, IFEX, IFM, IFO, IFOS, IFX
ifosfamide

IMP
inosine monophosphate

IMVP-16
ifosfamide, mesna uroprotection, methotrexate, etoposide

IPA
ifosfamide, Platinol, Adriamycin

IPP
isopropyl pyrrolizine

IROX
irinotecan and oxaliplatin

ITM, ITMTX
intrathecal methotrexate

IU
iodouracil

IUDR
idoxuridine

IVA
ifosfamide, vincristine, actinomycin

LAM
L-asparaginase, methotrexate

LAPOCA
L-asparaginase, prednisone, Oncovin, cytarabine, Adriamycin

L-ASP
L-asparaginase

L-CF
leucovorin-citrovorum factor

LCR
leurocristine

LED
liposomal encapsulated doxorubicin

LEU, LCV, LV,
leucovorin

Leu-Dox
N-1-leucyldoxorubicin

LMF
Leukeran, methotrexate, 5-fluorouracil

LOHP
oxaliplatin

LOMAC
leucovorin, Oncovin, methotrexate, Adriamycin, cyclophosphamide

LOPP
chlorambucil, vincristine, procarbazine, prednisone

LPAM
L-phenylalanine mustard

L-Spar
asparaginase

LV
leucovorin

L-VAM
leuprolide acetate, vinblastine, Adriamycin, mitomycin

LV5FU2
leucovorin and 5-fluorouracil

LVVP
Leukeran, vinblastine, vincristine, prednisone

M
methotrexate

M2
vincristine, carmustine, cyclophosphamide, melphalan, prednisone

3M
mitomycin, mitoxantrone, methotrexate

MABOP
Mustargen, Adriamycin, bleomycin, Oncovin, prednisone

MAC
methotrexate, actinomycin D, chlorambucil
methotrexate, Adriamycin, cyclophosphamide
Mitomycin C, Adriamycin, cyclophosphamide

MACC
methotrexate, Adriamycin, cyclophosphamide, CCNU
methotrexate, ara-C, cyclophosphamide, CCNU

MACHO
methotrexate, asparaginase, Cytoxan, hydroxydaunomycin, Oncovin
methotrexate, asparaginase, cyclophosphamide, hydroxydaunomycin, Oncovin

MACOB
methotrexate, Adriamycin, cyclophosphamide, Oncovin, bleomycin

MACOP-B
methotrexate, Adriamycin, cyclophosphamide, Oncovin, prednisone, bleomycin

MADDOC
mechlorethamine, Adriamycin, dacarbazine, DDP, Oncovin, cyclophosphamide

MAID
mesna, Adriamycin, ifosfamide, dacarbazine
mesna, Adriamycin, interleukin-3, dacarbazine
Mesnex, Adriamycin, Ifex, dacarbazine

MAP
melphalan, Adriamycin, prednisone
mitomycin C, Adriamycin, Platinol

MAZE
mAMSA, azacitidine, etoposide

M-BACOD
methotrexate, bleomycin, Adriamycin, cyclophosphamide, Oncovin,
   dexamethasone

m-BACOD
moderate-dose methotrexate, bleomycin, Adriamycin, cyclophosphamide, Oncovin,
   dexamethasone

M-BACOS
methotrexate, bleomycin, Adriamycin, cyclophosphamide, Oncovin, Solu-Medrol

MBC
methotrexate, bleomycin, cisplatin

MBD
methotrexate, bleomycin, cisplatin

MC
mitomycin C

MCBP
melphalan, cyclophosphamide, BCNU, prednisone

MCCNU
methyl-CCNU

MCP
melphalan, cyclophosphamide, prednisone

MCV
methotrexate, cisplatin, vinblastine

MDLO
metoclopramide, dexamethasone, lorazepam, ondansetron

MeCCNU
methyl-CCNU
semustine

MeCP
methyl-CCNU, cyclophosphamide, prednisone

MeCy
methotrexate, cyclophosphamide

MeFA
methyl-CCNU, 5-fluorouracil, Adriamycin

MEL
melphalan

MEP
mitomycin C, etoposide, Platinol

MF
mitomycin, 5-fluorouracil

MFEV
methotrexate, 5-fluorouracil, epirubicin, vincristine

MFL
mitoxantrone, 5-fluorouracil, leucovorin

MFP
melphalan, 5-fluorouracil, medroxyprogesterone acetate
melphalan, 5-fluorouracil, Provera

MGI-114
hydroxymethylacylfulvene

MICE
mesna rescue, ifosfamide, carboplatin, etoposide

MIFA
mitomycin, 5-fluorouracil, Adriamycin

MIME
mesna, ifosfamide, mitoxantrone, etoposide

MINE
mesna, ifosfamide, Novantrone, etoposide

MINE/ESHAP
mesna, ifosfamide, Novantrone, etoposide plus etoposide, methylprednisolone, high-dose ara-C, *cis*-platinum

mini-BEAM
BCNU, etoposide, ara-C, melphalan

mini-COAP
Cytoxan, Oncovin, ara-C, prednisone

MINT
mesna, ifosfamide, Novantrone, Taxol

MIT-C
mitomycin C

MIV
mitoxantrone, ifosfamide, VePesid

MMC
mitomycin C

MMM
mitoxantrone, methotrexate, mitomycin

MMOPP
methotrexate, mechlorethamine, Oncovin, procarbazine, prednisone

MOAD
methotrexate, Oncovin, L-asparaginase, dexamethasone

MOAP
methotrexate, Oncovin, PEG-asparaginase, prednisone

MOB
mechlorethamine, Oncovin, bleomycin
Mustargen, Oncovin, bleomycin

MOB-III
mitomycin C, Oncovin, bleomycin, cisplatin

MOCA
methotrexate, Oncovin, Cytoxan, Adriamycin

MOF
MeCCNU, Oncovin, 5-fluorouracil
methotrexate, Oncovin, fluorouracil

MOF-STREP
MeCCNU, Oncovin, 5-fluorouracil plus streptozocin

MOMP
mechlorethamine, Oncovin, methotrexate, prednisone

MOP
methylprednisolone, Oncovin, procarbazine
mechlorethamine, Oncovin, prednisone

MOP-BAP
nitrogen mustard, Oncovin, procarbazine, bleomycin, Adriamycin, prednisone
mechlorethamine, Oncovin, prednisone, bleomycin, Adriamycin, procarbazine

MOPP
mustine HCl, Oncovin, procarbazine, prednisone
methotrexate, Oncovin, procarbazine, prednisone

MOPP/ABV
mechlorethamine, Oncovin, procarbazine, prednisone, Adriamycin, bleomycin, vinblastine

MOPP/ABVD
mechlorethamine, Oncovin, procarbazine, prednisone plus Adriamycin, bleomycin, vinblastine, dacarbazine

MOPP-BLEO
mechlorethamine, Oncovin, procarbazine, prednisone, bleomycin

MOPr
mechlorethamine, Oncovin, procarbazine

MP
melphalan, prednisolone

6-MP
6-mercaptopurine

MPC
meperidine, promethazine, chlorpromazine

MPFL
methotrexate, Platinol, 5-fluorouracil, and leucovorin, calcium

MPL
Melphalan

MPL+PRED
melphalan plus prednisone

MTC
mitomycin C

MTX
methotrexate

MTX/ara-C
methotrexate and arabinoside C

MTX+MP
methotrexate plus mercaptopurine

MV
mitomycin and vinblastine
mitoxantrone, VP-16

MVAC
methotrexate, vinblastine, Adriamycin, cisplatin

MVC
mitoxantrone, vinblastine, cyclophosphamide

M-VEC
methotrexate, vinblastine, epirubicin, cisplatin

MVF
mitoxantrone, vincristine, 5-fluorouracil

MVP
mitomycin, vinblastine, Platinol

MVPP
mechlorethamine, vinblastine, procarbazine, prednisone

MVVPP
mechlorethamine, vincristine, vinblastine, procarbazine, prednisone

NAC
nitrogen mustard, Adriamycin, CCNU

9-NC
rubitecan
9-nitrocamptothecin
9-nitro-20-(S)-camptothecin

NCS
neocarzinostatin
zinostatin

NFL
Novantrone, 5-fluorouracil, leucovorin

NH2
topical nitrogen mustard

NOPP
Novantrone, Oncovin, procarbazine, prednisone

NOVP
mitoxantrone, Oncovin, vinblastine, prednisone

NVB
Navelbine

OAP
Oncovin, ara-C, prednisone

OAP-BLEO
Oncovin, ara-C, prednisone, bleomycin

O-DAP
Oncovin, dianhydrogalactitol, Adriamycin, Platinol

OEPA
Oncovin, etoposide, prednisone, Adriamycin

OM
oncostatin M

OMAD
Oncovin, methotrexate, Adriamycin, dactinomycin

7-OMEN
menogaril

OPAL
Oncovin, prednisone, L-asparaginase

OPEN
Oncovin, prednisone, etoposide, Novantrone

OPP
Oncovin, procarbazine, prednisone

OPPA
Oncovin, procarbazine, prednisone, Adriamycin

OPPA/COPP
Oncovin, procarbazine, prednisone, Adriamycin, cyclophosphamide, Oncovin, procarbazine, prednisone

OSM
oncostatin M

PAB-Esc-C
Platinol, Adriamycin, bleomycin, escalating doses of Cytoxan

PAC, PAC-1,
Platinol, Adriamycin, cyclophosphamide

PACE
Platinol, Adriamycin, cyclophosphamide, etoposide
5-fluorouracil, cisplatin, cytarabine, caffeine

PATCO
prednisone, ara-C, 6-thioguanine, cyclophosphamide, Oncovin

PAVe
procarbazine, Alkeran, Velban

PBV
Platinol, bleomycin, vinblastine

PCB
procarbazine

PCE
Platinol, Cytoxan, etoposide
Platinol, cyclophosphamide, Eldisine

P-CHOP
cisplatin, cyclophosphamide, doxorubicin, vincristine, prednisone

PCV
procarbazine, CCNU, vincristine
procarbazine, lomustine, vincristine

PCZ
procarbazine

PEB
Platinol, etoposide, bleomycin

PEC
Platinol, etoposide, cyclophosphamide

PEG-DOXO
pegylated liposomal doxorubicin

PEI
Platinol (cisplatin), etoposide, ifosfamide

PELF
cisplatin, epirubicin, folinic acid, 5-fluorouracil

PEP
Procytox, epipodophyllotoxin-derivative, prednisolone

PFE
Platinol, 5-fluorouracil, etoposide

PFL
Platinol, 5-fluorouracil, leucovorin

PFL-IFN
Platinol, 5-fluorouracil, leucovorin, interferon alfa-2b

PFM
Platinol, 5-fluorouracil, methotrexate

PFT
prednisone, 5-fluorouracil, tamoxifen
phenylalanine, 5-fluorouracil, tamoxifen

PG-TXL
polyglutamate paclitaxel

PHRT
procarbazine, hydroxyurea, radiotherapy

PIA
Platinol, ifosfamide, Adriamycin

PIAF
Platinol, interferon alfa, Adriamycin, 5-fluorouracil

PM
prednimustine

PMB
Platinol, methotrexate, bleomycin

PMF
phenylalanine mustard, methotrexate, 5-fluorouracil

P-MVAC
Platinol, methotrexate, vinblastine, Adriamycin, carboplatin

POACH
prednisone, Oncovin, ara-C, cyclophosphamide, hydroxydaunomycin

POC
procarbazine, Oncovin, CCNU

POC
procarbazine, Oncovin, lomustine

POCA
prednisone, Oncovin, cytarabine, Adriamycin

POCC
procarbazine, Oncovin, CCNU, Cytoxan
procarbazine, Oncovin, cyclophosphamide, CCNU

POMP
prednisone, Oncovin, methotrexate, Purinethol
prednisone, Oncovin, methotrexate, 6-mercaptopurine

PRIME
procarbazine, ifosfamide, methotrexate

ProMACE
prednisone, methotrexate-leucovorin, Adriamycin, cyclophosphamide, etoposide

ProMACE-CytaBOM
prednisone, methotrexate-leucovorin, Adriamycin, cyclophosphamide, etoposide
plus cytarabine, bleomycin, Oncovin, methotrexate

ProMACE-MOPP
prednisone, methotrexate, Adriamycin, cyclophosphamide, etoposide plus
mustargen, Oncovin, procarbazine, prednisone

PTX
paclitaxel

PVA
prednisone, vincristine, l-asparaginase

PVB
Platinol, vinblastine, bleomycin

PVC
paclitaxel, vinblastine, cisplatin

PVDA
prednisone, vincristine, daunorubicin, l-asparaginase

PVP
Platinol, VP-16

PXL
paclitaxel

RIDD
recombinant interleukin-2, dacarbazine, cisplatin

ROAP
rubidazone, Oncovin, ara-C, prednisone

SAM
streptozocin, Adriamycin, methyl-CCNU

SCAB
streptozocin, CCNU, Adriamycin, bleomycin

SMF
streptozotocin, mitomycin, 5-fluorouracil

Stanford V
mechlorethamine, doxorubicin, vinblastine, vincristine, bleomycin, etoposide,
prednisone

STEAM
streptonigrin, 6-thioguanine, cyclophosphamide, actinomycin, mitomycin

TAD
6-thioguanine, ara-C, daunomycin

TAM
tamoxifen

TC
6-thioguanine and cytarabine

TCG
Taxol, cisplatin, gemcitabine

TEC
thiotepa, etoposide, carboplatin

TEM
Temodal

TEMP
tamoxifen, etoposide, mitoxantrone, Platinol

6-TG
6-thioguanine

TG
thioguanine

T-MOP
6-thioguanine, methotrexate, Oncovin, prednisone

TMQ
trimetrexate

TMX
tamoxifen

TMZ
temozolomide

TOAP
6-thioguanine, Oncovin, ara-C, prednisone

TPCH
6-thioguanine, procarbazine, CCNU, hydroxyurea

TPDCV
6-thioguanine, procarbazine, dibromodulcitol, CCNU, vincristine

TPF
Taxotere, Platinol, 5-fluorouracil

TPT
topotecan

TRAP
6-thioguanine, rubidomycin, ara-C, prednisone

TT
Thiotepa

TVCa
high-dose etoposide, thiotepa, dose-adjusted carboplatin

TVD
topotecan, vincristine, doxorubicin

TZ, Tz, TZM
temozolomide

UFT
uracil, 5-fluorouracil, tegafur
uracil plus Ftorafur
uracil-tegafur

VA
vincristine and actinomycin D

VAAP
vincristine, L-asparaginase, Adriamycin, prednisone

VAB

Velban, actinomycin D, bleomycin
vincristine, actinomycin D, bleomycin

VAB 2

vinblastine, actinomycin D, bleomycin, cisplatin

VAB 3

vinblastine, actinomycin D, bleomycin, cisplatin, cyclophosphamide, chlorambucil

VAB 4

vinblastine, actinomycin D, bleomycin, cisplatin, cyclophosphamide

VAB 5

vinblastine, actinomycin D, bleomycin, cyclophosphamide, cisplatin

VAB 6

vinblastine, actinomycin D, bleomycin, cisplatin, cyclophosphamide

VABCD

vinblastine, Adriamycin, bleomycin, CCNU, DTIC

VAC

vincristine, actinomycin D, cyclophosphamide
vincristine, Adriamycin, cisplatin
vincristine, Adriamycin, cyclophosphamide

VACA

vincristine, actinomycin A, cyclophosphamide, Adriamycin
vincristine, actinomycin D, cyclophosphamide, Adriamycin

VACAD

vinblastine, Adriamycin, Cytoxan, actinomycin D, dacarbazine
vincristine, actinomycin D, cyclophosphamide, Adriamycin, dacarbazine

VACP

VePesid, Adriamycin, Cytoxan, Platinol
VePesid, Adriamycin, cyclophosphamide, Platinol

VAD

vincristine, doxorubicin, Decadron
vincristine, Adriamycin, dexamethasone

VAdCA + 1 I/E

vincristine, doxorubicin, cyclophosphamide, dactinomycin plus ifosfamide with
  mesna

VADRIAC

vincristine, doxorubicin, cyclophosphamide

VAD/V

vinblastine, Adriamycin, dexamethasone, verapamil

VAFAC

vincristine, amethopterin, 5-fluorouracil, Adriamycin, cyclophosphamide

VAI

vinblastine, actinomycin D, ifosfamide

VAIA

vincristine, actinomycin D, ifosfamide, Adriamycin

VALOP-B

etoposide, doxorubicin, cyclophosphamide, vincristine, prednisone, bleomycin

VAM

vinblastine, Adriamycin, mitomycin C
VP-16-213, Adriamycin, methotrexate

VAMP

vincristine, actinomycin, methotrexate, prednisone
vincristine, Adriamycin, methylprednisolone
vincristine, Adriamycin, methotrexate, prednisone

VAP

vinblastine, actinomycin D, Platinol
vincristine, Adriamycin, prednisone,
vincristine, Adriamycin, procarbazine

VAPA

vincristine, Adriamycin, prednisone, ara-C

VAPE

vincristine, Adriamycin, prednisone, ara-C

VAP-II
vinblastine, actinomycin D, Platinol

VAT
vinblastine, Adriamycin, thiotepa
vincristine, ara-C, 6-thioguanine

VATD
vincristine, ara-C, 6-thioguanine, daunorubicin
VATH
vinblastine, Adriamycin, thiotepa, Halotestin

VAV
VP-16-213, Adriamycin, vincristine

VB
vinblastine, bleomycin
vinblastine

VBA
vincristine, BCNU, Adriamycin

VBAP
vincristine, BCNU, Adriamycin, prednisone

VBC
vincristine, bleomycin, cisplatin
VePesid, BCNU, cyclophosphamide

VBD
vinblastine, bleomycin, DDP

VBL
vinblastine

VBM
vincristine, bleomycin, methotrexate

VBMCP
vincristine, BCNU, melphalan, cyclophosphamide, prednisone

VBMF
vinblastine, bleomycin, methotrexate, 5-fluorouracil
vincristine, bleomycin, methotrexate, 5-fluorouracil

VBMPC
vinblastine, BCNU, melphalan, prednisone, Cytoxan

VBP
vinblastine, bleomycin, Platinol

VC
vincristine
VePesid and carboplatin
vinorelbine and cisplatin

VCAP
vincristine, cyclophosphamide, Adriamycin, prednisone

VCAP-I
VP-16, cyclophosphamide, Adriamycin, Platinol

VCF
vincristine, cyclophosphamide, 5-fluorouracil

VCMP
vincristine, cyclophosphamide, melphalan, prednisone

VCP
vincristine, cyclophosphamide, prednisone

VPC-I
VP-16, cyclophosphamide, Platinol

VCR
vincristine

VDA
vincristine, daunorubicin, L-asparaginase

VDBCC
vincristine, dactinomycin, bleomycin, cisplatin, cyclophosphamide

VDC
vincristine, doxorubicin, cyclophosphamide

VDD
vincristine, doxorubicin, dexamethasone

VDP
vinblastine, dacarbazine, Platinol
vincristine, daunorubicin, prednisone

VEEP
vincristine, epirubicin, etoposide, prednisolone

VeIP
vinblastine, ifosfamide, Platinol
Velban, ifosfamide, Platinol

VEMP
vincristine, Endoxan, 6-mercaptopurine, prednisone

VEPA
vinblastine, etoposide, prednisone, Adriamycin

VEPA-B
VEPA, bleomycin

VEPA-M
vincristine, etoposide, prednisone, Adriamycin, methotrexate

VePesid
Etoposide
VP-16

VFL
vinflunine

VIC
vinblastine, ifosfamide, CCNU
VP-16, ifosfamide, carboplatin

VICE
vincristine, ifosfamide, carboplatin, etoposide

VIE

vinblastine, ifosfamide, etoposide
vincristine, ifosfamide, etoposide

VIG

vinblastine, ifosfamide, gallium (nitrate)

VIMB

VP-16, ifosfamide, mitoxantrone, bleomycin

VIP

VePesid, ifosfamide, Platinol
vinblastine, ifosfamide, Platinol
VP-16, ifosfamide, Platinol

VIP-B

VP-16, ifosfamide, Platinol, bleomycin

VLB

vincaleukoblastine

VLP

vincristine, L-asparaginase, prednisone

VM-26

teniposide

VM

vinblastine and mitomycin

VMAD

vincristine, methotrexate, Adriamycin, actinomycin D

VMC

VP-16, methotrexate, citrovorum factor

VMCP

vincristine, melphalan, cyclophosphamide, prednisone

VMP

VePesid, mitoxantrone, prednimustine

VNB
vinorelbine

VOCA
VP-16, Oncovin, cyclophosphamide, Adriamycin

VOCAP
VP-16-213, Oncovin, cyclophosphamide, Adriamycin, Platinol

VP
vincristine, prednisone

VP-16
CCNU, cyclophosphamide, Adriamycin, vincristine, VP-16

VP+A
vincristine, prednisone, L-asparaginase

VPB
vinblastine, Platinol, bleomycin

VPBCPr
vincristine, prednisone, vinblastine, chlorambucil, procarbazine

VPCA
vincristine, prednisone, cyclophosphamide, ara-C

VPCMF
vincristine, prednisone, cyclophosphamide, methotrexate, 5-fluorouracil

VPP
VP-16, Platinol
VePesid and Platinol

VPVCP
vincristine, prednisone, vinblastine, chlorambucil, procarbazine

VRB, VRL
vinorelbine

V-TAD
VePesid, 6-thioguanine, ara-C, daunorubicin

Chemotherapy Generic Drug Names

Chemotherapy abbreviations and acronyms are built on a basic group of drugs, using generic, brand, and/or chemical names to create an acronym or easily remembered word. The table below lists the generic name of the chemotherapy drug and some of the many other names that are commonly used.

GENERIC NAME	BRAND, TRADE, MISCELLANEOUS NAMES
aclarubicin	Aclacin, aclacinomycin A
aldesleukin	Proleukin, IL-2, Interleukin-2
altretamine	Hexalen
amifostine	Ethyol, Ethiofos, Gammaphos
amsacrine	mAMSA
ara-A	arabinosyladenine, Vidarabine, Anhydrous, Vira-A
ara-C	See cytarabine
asparaginase	Elspar, Oncaspar, Pegaspargase
azacytidine	5 AZC , 5-Azacytidine, 5-AC, 5-ACZR
bleomycin	Blenoxane
capecitabine	Xeloda
carboplatin	Paraplatin, CBDCA
carmustine	BCNU, BiCNU, Gliadel
chlorambucil	Leukeran
chlormethine	Mustine
chloroethylcyclohexylnitrosourea	See lomustine, CCNU
cladribine	Leustatin
citrovorum factor	See leucovorin
cisplatin	Platinol, diammine dichloroplatinum, CDDP
cyclophosphamide	Cytoxan, CytoxanIV, Neosar, CTX
cytarabine	Cytosar-U, ara-C, Cytosine arabinoside, DepoCyt, arabinosylcytosine
dacarbazine	DTIC, DTIC-Dome, dimethyltriazenoimidazolecarboxamide
dactinomycin	Cosmegen, actinomycin-D
desacetylvinblastine amide	DAVA, DVA, VDS
diaziquone	AZQ, CI-904, Diaziquone, NSC-18298
docetaxel	Taxotere
doxorubicin	Adriamycin, Rubex, hydroxydaunorubicin HCl, 14-hydroxydaunomycin
epirubicin	Ellence
etoposide	Toposar, VP-16, VePesid, EPE, Epipodophyllotoxin, VP 16–213
fludarabine	Fludara

GENERIC NAME	BRAND, TRADE, MISCELLANEOUS NAMES
fluorouracil	Adrucil, Efudex, Fluoroplex, Fluorouracil IV, 5-FU
gemcitabine	Gemzar
granisetron	Kytril
hydroxyurea	Hydrea
idarubicin	Idamycin
ifosfamide	Ifex, isophosphamide
interferon alfa	Alferon N, Intron A, Roferon-A, Wellferon
irinotecan	Camptosar, Cpt-11, HCL
levamisole	Ergamisol
leucovorin calcium	Folinic acid
leucovorin	Wellcovorin, Wellcovorin IM/IV, Leucovorin, Leucovorin IM/IV
liposomal doxorubicin	Doxil, Evacet
lomustine	CeeNU, CCNU
mechlorethamine	See nitrogen mustard
megestrol	Megace, Pallace, megestrol acet
melphalan	Alkeran
mercaptopurine	Purinethol, 6-MP
mesna	Mesnex
methotrexate	Abitrexate, amethopterin
methotrexate Injection	MTX Injection
metoclopramide	Reglan
mitomycin	Mutamycin, Mitomvcin-C
mitotane	Lysodren
mitoxantrone	Novantrone
neocarzinostatin	zinostatin
nitrogen mustard	Mustargen, mechlorethamine
oxaliplatin	Eloxatin
paclitaxel	Paxene, Taxol
pirarubicin	THP-doxorubicin
razoxane	ICRF-159
rituximab	Rituxan
streptonigrin	SN, rufochromomycin, bruneomycin
streptozoticin	STZ, Zanosar, 2-deoxy-2-methylnitro soaminocarbonylamino-d-glucopyranos
tamoxifen	Nolvadex
thioguanine	Tabloid, 6-TG, TG
topotecan hydrochloride	Hycamtin
trastuzumab	Herceptin
vinblastine	Velban, Vinblastine, vincaleukoblastine

GENERIC NAME	BRAND, TRADE, MISCELLANEOUS NAMES
vincristine	Oncovin, Vincasar
vindesine	Eldisine
vinorelbine tartrate	Navelbine

Appendix 9
Clinical Trials

AAASPS
African American Antiplatelet Stroke Prevention Study

AASK
African American Study of Kidney Disease and Hypertension

ABACAS
Adjunctive Balloon Angioplasty Following Coronary Atherectomy Study

ACAPS
Asymptomatic Carotid Artery Plaque Study

ACAS
Asymptomatic Carotid Atherosclerosis Study

ACCESS
Acute Candesartan Clinical Evaluation of Stroke Survivors

ACIT
Asymptomatic Cardiac Ischemia Trial

ACME
Angioplasty Compared to Medicine

ACOVE
Assessing Care of Vulnerable Elders

ACTG
AIDS Clinical Trials Group

ACTG 214
AIDS Clinical Treatment Group 214

ACTG 325
AIDS Clinical Treatment Group 325

ACTG 334
AIDS Clinical Treatment Group 334

ACTG 349
AIDS Clinical Treatment Group 349

ADMIT
Arterial Disease Multiple Intervention Trial

AFCAPS/TexCAPS
Air Force/Texas Coronary Atherosclerosis Prevention Study

AFFIRM
Atrial Fibrillation Followup Investigation of Rhythm Management

AIDSTRIALS
Clinical Trials of Acquired Immunodeficiency Syndrome Drugs

AIPRI
Angiotensin-Converting Enzyme Inhibition in Progressive Renal Insufficiency

AIRE
Acute Infarction Ramipril Efficacy
Acute Infarction Reperfusion Efficacy

ALLHAT
Antihypertensive and Lipid-Lowering Treatment to Prevent Heart Attack Trial

AMIS
Aspirin in Myocardial Infarction Study

AMISTAD
Acute Myocardial Infarction Study of Adenosine

APASS
Antiphospholipid Antibodies in Stroke Study

APRICOT
Antithrombotics in the Prevention of Reocclusion in Coronary Thrombolysis
Aspirin versus Coumadin Trial

APT
Atherosclerosis Prevention and Treatment

ARK
Analysis of Radial Keratotomy

ASIST
Atenolol Silent Ischemia Trial

ASPECT
Anticoagulants in Secondary Prevention of Events in Coronary Thrombosis

ASPIRE
Action on Secondary Prevention by Intervention to Reduce Events

ASS
Acute Stroke Study

ASSIST
American Stop Smoking Intervention Study (for Cancer Prevention)

ATLAS
Aspirin and Ticlid versus Anticoagulation for Stents
Assessment of Treatment with Lisinopril and Survival

AVEG
AIDS Vaccine Evaluation Group

AVEU
AIDS Vaccine Evaluation Unit

AVID
Amiodarone Versus Implantable Defibrillators
Antiarrhythmics versus Implantable Defibrillators

BARI
Bypass Angioplasty Revascularization Investigation

BCDDP
Breast Cancer Detection Demonstration Project

BCPT
Breast Cancer Prevention Trial

BECAIT
Bezafibrate Coronary Atherosclerosis Intervention Trial

BEHAVE-AD
Behavioral Pathology in Alzheimer Disease

BEST
beStent clinical trial
Beta-Blocker Evaluation of Survival Trial
Beta-Blocker Stroke Trial
Bolus Dose-Escalation Study of Tissue-Type Plasminogen Activator
Bucindolol Evaluation of Survival Trial

BEST+ICD
Beta-Blocker Strategy Plus Implantable Cardioverter-Defibrillator

beta-WRIST
Beta-Washington Radiation for In-Stent Restenosis Trial

BHAT
Beta-Blocker Heart Attack Trial

BHFS
Benazepril Heart Failure Study

BHS
Bogalusa Heart Study

BOAT
Balloon versus Optimal Atherectomy Trial

CABRI
Coronary Angioplasty versus Bypass Revascularization Investigation
Coronary Artery Bypass Revascularization Investigation

CADILLAC
Controlled Abciximab and Device Investigation to Lower Late Angioplasty
　　Complications

CADS
Captopril and Digoxin Study

CAFS
Canadian Atrial Fibrillation Study

CAMI
Canadian Assessment of Myocardial Infarction

CAMIAT
Canadian Amiodarone Myocardial Infarction Arrhythmia Trial
Canadian Myocardial Infarction Amiodarone Trial

CAPIT
Core Assessment Program for Intracerebral Transplantation

CAPPP
Captopril Prevention Project

CAPRIE
Clopidogrel versus Aspirin in Patients at Risk of Ischemic Events

CAPS
Cardiac Arrhythmia Pilot Study

CAR
Cardiac Ablation Registry

CARAT
Coronary Angioplasty and Rotablator Atherectomy Trial

CARAT II
Coronary Angioplasty and Rotablator Atherectomy Trial II

CARDIA
Coronary Artery Risk Development in Young Adults

CARE
Calcium Antagonist in Reperfusion

CARES
Cancer Rehabilitation Evaluation System

CARET
Carotene and Retinol Efficacy Trial

CASANOVA
Carotid Artery Stenosis with Asymptomatic Narrowing: Operation versus Aspirin Study

CASES
Canadian Activase for Stroke Effectiveness Study

CASS
Coronary Artery Surgery Study

CAST
Cardiac Arrhythmia Suppression Trial
Chinese Acute Stroke Trial

CAST II
Cardiac Arrhythmia Suppression Trial II

CATCH
Child and Adolescent Trial of Cardiovascular Health
Community Actions to Control High Blood Pressure

CATS
Canadian American Ticlopidine Study
Captopril and Thrombolysis Study

CAVATAS
Carotid and Vertebral Artery Transluminal Angioplasty Study

CCABOT
Cornell Coronary Artery Bypass Outcomes Trial

CCAIT
Canadian Coronary Atherosclerosis Intervention Trial

CCP
Cooperative Cardiovascular Project

CCSS
Childhood Cancer Survivor Study

CCTAT
Cooperative Clinical Trials in Adult Transplantation

CCTPT
Cooperative Clinical Trials in Pediatric Transplantation

CDP
Coronary Drug Project

CHF-STAT
Congestive Heart Failure-Survival Trial of Antiarrhythmic Therapy

CHIC
Cardiovascular Health in Children

CIBIS
Cardiac Insufficiency Bisoprolol Study

CIDS
Canadian Implantable Defibrillator Study

CIGTS
Collaborative Initial Glaucoma Treatment Study

CLAS
Cholesterol Lowering Atherosclerosis Study

CLASP
Carolinas Laparoscopic Advanced Surgery Program

CLASS
Celecoxib Long-Term Arthritis Safety Study

CLASSIC
Clopidogrel Aspirin Stent International Cooperative

CLEK
Collaborative Longitudinal Evaluation of Keratoconus

CLOUT
Clinical Outcomes with Ultrasound Trial
Core Laboratory Ultrasound Analysis

COG
Central Oncology Group

COMS
Collaborative Ocular Melanoma Study

CONSENSUS
Cooperative North Scandinavian Enalapril Survival Study

CONVINCE
Controlled Onset Verapamil Investigation for Cardiovascular Endpoints

COPERNICUS
Carvedilol Prospective Randomized Cumulative Survival

CORAMI
Cohort of Rescue Angioplasty in Myocardial Infarction

CPPT
Coronary Primary Prevention Trial

CPS
Collaborative Perinatal Study

CRC
Cancer Research Campaign

CREST
Carotid Revascularization Endarterectomy versus Stenting Trial

CRTP
Consciousness Research and Training Project

CRUISE
Can Routine Ultrasound Influence Stent Expansion

CRUSADE
Coronary Revascularization Ultrasound Angioplasty Device

CSMB
Center for Study of Multiple Births

CSSCD
Cooperative Study of Sickle Cell Disease

CTAC
Cancer Treatment Advisory Committee

CUOG
Canadian Urology Oncology Group

CURE
Clopidogrel in Unstable Angina to Prevent Recurrent Ischemic Events

CURN
Conduct and Utilization of Research in Nursing

DAIS
Diabetes Atherosclerosis Intervention Study

DART
Dilation versus Ablation Revascularization Trial

DASH
Delay in Accessing Stroke Healthcare
Dietary Approaches to Stop Hypertension

DAVID
Dual-Chamber and VVI Implantable Defibrillator (trial)

DCCT
Diabetes Control and Complications Trial

DIAD
Detection of Ischemia in Asymptomatic Diabetics

DIG
Digitalis Investigation Group

DIGAMI
Diabetes Mellitus Insulin Glucose Infusion in Acute Myocardial Infarction

DOQI
Dialysis Outcomes Quality Initiative

DPT-1
Diabetes Prevention Trial Type 1 Diabetes

DRS
Diabetes Retinopathy Study

EAST
Emory Angioplasty versus Surgery Trial

EBMT
European Group for Bone Marrow Transplantation

ECAT
European Concerted Action on Thrombosis

ECLAM
European Consensus Lupus Activity Measure

ECOG
Eastern Cooperative Oncology Group

ECST
European Carotid Surgery Trial

ELITE
Evaluation of Losartan in the Elderly

ELLDOPA
Early versus Later L-DOPA

EMIAT
European Myocardial Infarct Amiodarone Trial

EMIP
European Myocardial Infarction Project

ENDIT
European Nicotinamide Diabetes Intervention Trial

EORTC QLQ
European Organization for Research and Treatment of Cancer Quality of Life Questionnaire

EPISTENT
Evaluation of Platelet IIb-IIIa Inhibitors for Stenting

EQOL
Economics and Quality of Life Substudy of GUSTO

ERA
Enoxaparin Restenosis after Angioplasty

ERASE
Emergency Room Assessment of Sestamibi for Evaluation of Chest Pain

EROTIC
European Organization for Research and Treatment of Cancer

ESCOBAR
Emergency Stenting Compared to Conventional Balloon Angioplasty

ESPRIT
European/Australian Stroke Prevention in Reversible Ischaemia Trial

ESSENCE
Efficacy and Safety of Subcutaneous Enoxaparin in Non-Q-Wave Coronary Events

ETDRS
Early Treatment Diabetic Retinopathy Study

EUP
Experimental Use Permit

EXACTO
Excimer Laser Angioplasty in Coronary Total Occlusion

EXCEL
Expanded Clinical Evaluation of Lovastatin

FACET
Fosinopril versus Amlodipine Cardiovascular Events Randomized Trial

FASTER
Fibrinolytic and Aggrastat ST Elevation Resolution

FATS
Familial Atherosclerosis Treatment Study

FCVDS
Framingham Cardiovascular Disease Survey

FHRS
Familial Hypercholesterolemia Regression Study

FHS
Framingham Heart Study

FIR.S.T.
First Seizure Trial Group

FLUENT
Fluvastatin Long-Term Extension Trial

FOOD
Feed or Ordinary Diet

FREIR
Federal Research on Biological and Health Effects of Ionizing Radiation

FRISC
Fast Revascularization During Instability in Coronary Artery Disease
Fragmin During Instability in Coronary Artery Disease

GABI
German Angioplasty Bypass Surgery Investigation

GRAMI
Gianturco-Roubin in Acute Myocardial Infarction

GREAT
Grampian Region Early Anistreplase Trial

GUSTO
Global Utilization of Streptokinase and t-PA for Occluded Coronary Arteries

GUSTO-1
Global Utilization of Streptokinase and Tissue Plasminogen Activator for Occluded
Coronary Arteries

HALT
Heroin Antagonist and Learning Therapy

HARP
Harvard Atherosclerosis Reversibility Project

HART
Heparin Aspirin Reperfusion Trial
Hypertension Audit of Risk Factor Therapy

HEAP
Heparin in Early Patency

HEART
Healing and Early Afterload Reducing Therapy
Health Evaluation and Risk Tabulation

HeCOG
Hellenic Cooperative Oncology Group

HERO
Hirulog Early Reperfusion/Occlusion

HIPS
Heparin Infusion Prior to Stenting

HIT
Hirudin for the Improvement of Thrombolysis

HOPE
Heart Outcomes Prevention Evaluation
Hospital Outcomes Reversibility for the Elderly

HOT
Hypertensive Optimal Treatment Trial

HVTN
HIV Vaccine Trials Network

HWRS
Habits of Work and Recreation Survey

IBCSG
International Breast Cancer Study Group

ICSS
International Carotid Stenting Study

IGCCCG
International Germ Cell Cancer Colllaborative Group

IMAGE
International Multicenter Angina Exercise

IMPACT
Integrilin to Minimize Platelet Aggregation and Coronary Thrombosis

IMPACT-Stent
Integrilin to Minimize Platelet Aggregation and Coronary Thrombosis in Stenting

INRC
International Neuroblastoma Response Criteria

INTEGRITI
Integrilin and Tenecteplase in Acute Myocardial Infarction

INTIME
Intravenous t-PA for Treatment of Infarcting Myocardium Early

IONDT
Ischemic Optic Neuropathy Decompression Trial

IPSS
International Pilot Study of Schizophrenia

IPTR
International Pancreas Transplant Registry

IRAS
Insulin Resistance Atherosclerosis Study

IRSG
Intergroup Rhabdomyosarcoma Group

ISAM
Intravenous Streptokinase in Acute Myocardial Infarction

ISAR
Intracoronary Stenting and Antithrombotic Regimen

ISIS
International Study of Infarct Survival

IST
International Stroke Trial

JCOG
Japanese Clinical Oncology Group

KIGS
Kabi International Growth Study

KIHD
Kuopio Ischemia Heart Disease Risk Factor Study

LAARS
LDL Apheresis Atherosclerosis Regression Study

LACI
Laser Angioplasty for Critical Ischemia

LAPIS
Late Potential Italian Study

LARS
Laser Angioplasty for Restenosed Stents

LATE
Late Assessment of Thrombolytic Efficacy

LIFE
Longitudinal Interval Followup Evaluation

LIPID
Long-Term Intervention with Pravastatin in Ischemic Disease

LONG WRIST
Washington Radiation for In-Stent Restenosis Trial for Long Lesions

MAAS
Multicenter Antiatheroma Study
Multicenter Antiatherosclerotic Study

MACE
Mayo Asymptomatic Carotid Endarterectomy

MACS
Multicenter AIDS Cohort Study

MAPS
Multivessel Angioplasty Prognosis Study

MARS
Mevacor Atherosclerosis Regression Study
Monitored Atherosclerosis Regression Study

MASS
Medicine, Angioplasty, or Surgery Study

MAST
Multicenter Acute Stroke Trial

MDC
Metoprolol in Dilated Cardiomyopathy

MDPIT
Multicenter Diltiazem Post-Infarction Trial

MDRD
Modification of Diet in Renal Disease

MERIT-HF
Metoprolol CR/XL Controlled Release Randomized Intervention Trial in Heart
   Failure

MEXIS
Metoprolol and Xamoterol Infarction Study

MFS
Minnesota Followup Study

M-HEART
Multi-Hospital Eastern Atlantic Restenosis Trial

MIDAS
Myocardial Infarction Data Acquisition System

MILTS
Multicentre International Liver Tumor Study

MITRA
Maximal Individual Therapy in Acute Myocardial Infarction

MOS
Medical Outcomes Study

MOS-HIV
Medical Outcomes Study-Human Immunodeficiency Virus

MOS sf-20
Medical Outcomes Study, short form, 20 items

MOS sf-36
Medical Outcomes Study, short form, 36 items

MOST
Mode Selection Trial in Sinus Node Dysfunction

MPS
Macular Photocoagulation Study

MRFIT
Multiple Risk Factor Intervention Trial

MUSIC
Multicenter Ultrasound Stent in Coronary Artery Disease

MUST
Multicenter Stent Study
Multicenter Stents Ticlopidine
Medication Use Studies

MUSTT
Multicenter Unsustained Tachycardia Trial

NABTT
New Approaches to Brain Tumor Therapy

NACDG
North American Contact Dermatitis Group

NADE
New Animal Drug Evaluation

NAMIS
Nifedipine Angina Myocardial Infarction Study

NAPRTCS
North American Pediatric Renal Transplant Cooperative Study

NASCET
North American Symptomatic Carotid Endarterectomy Trial

NASTRA
North American Study of Treatment for Refractory Ascites

NBCCG
National Breast Cancer Collaborative Group

NCCTG
North Central Cancer Treatment Group

NCGS
National Cooperative Growth Study

NCIC-CTG
National Cancer Institute of Canada Clinical Trials Group

NCI-CTC
National Cancer Institute Common Toxicity Criteria

NDDG
National Diabetes Data Group

NELS
National Educational Longitudinal Study

NETT
National Emphysema Treatment Trial

NFS
National Fertility Study

NHANES
National Health and Nutrition Examination Survey

NHANES II
Second National Health and Nutrition Examination Survey

NHBPEP
National High Blood Pressure Education Program

NHDS
National Hospital Discharge Survey

NHIS
National Health Interview Survey

NIP
National Immunization Program
National Inpatient Profile

NIS-2
Second National Incidence Study

NIT
National Intelligence Test

NLTCRC
National Long-Term Care Research Center

NMCUES
National Medical Care Utilization and Expenditure Survey

NNHS
National Nursing Home Survey

NRMI
National Registry of Myocardial Infarction

NSABP
National Surgical Adjuvant Breast and Bowel Project

OARS
Optimal Atherectomy Restenosis Study

OASIS
Organization to Assess Strategies for Ischemic Syndromes

OCBAS
Optimal Coronary Balloon Angioplasty versus Stent

OMERACT
Outcome Measures in Rheumatology Clinical Trial

ONTT
Optic Neuritis Treatment Trial

OPERA
Omapatrilat in Persons with Enhanced Risk of Atherosclerotic Events

OPTIMA
Oxford Project to Investigate Memory and Aging

OPTIMAAL
Optimal Therapy in Myocardial Infarction with the Angiotensin II Antagonist Losartan
Optimal Trial in Myocardial Infarction with the Angiotensin II Antagonist Losartan

OPTIME-CHF
Outcomes of a Prospective Trial of Intravenous Milrinone for Exacerbations of Chronic Heart Failure

OPUS
Orbofiban in Patients with Unstable Coronary Syndromes

PACT
Philadelphia Association of Clinical Trials

PACTG
Pediatric AIDS Clinical Trial Group Protocol

PAMI
Primary Angioplasty in Myocardial Infarction

PARAGON
Platelet IIb/IIIa Antagonist for the Reduction of Acute Coronary Syndrome Events in a Global Organization Network

PARIS
Peripheral Artery Radiation Investigational Study

PART
Prevention of Atherosclerosis with Ramipril Therapy

PAS
Physician's Activity Study
Professional Activities Study

PASE
Physical Activity Scale for the Elderly Evaluation

PASS
Piracetam in Acute Stroke Study
Postural Assessment Scale for Stroke Patient

PATH
Partnership Approach to Health

PBTG
Philadelphia Bone Marrow Transplant Group

PCIVOT
Prostate Cancer Intervention versus Observation Trial

PEA
Pulseless Electrical Study

PEACE
Prevention of Events with ACE Inhibition

PEPI
Postmenopausal Estrogen/Progestin Intervention

PERI
Psychiatric Epidemiology Research Interview

PICS
Pacing in Cardiomyopathy Study

PICSS
Patent Foramen Ovale in Cryptogenic Stroke Study

PICTURE
Post Intracoronary Treatment Ultrasound Result Evaluation

PIOPED
Prospective Investigation of Pulmonary Embolism Diagnosis

PIVOT
Prostate Cancer Intervention versus Observation Trial

PLAC
Pravastatin Limitation of Atherosclerosis in Coronary Arteries
Pravastatin, Lipids, and Atherosclerosis in the Carotid Arteries

PLAC-2
Pravastatin, Lipids, and Atherosclerosis in the Carotid Arteries

POEM
Patency, Outcomes and Economics of MIDCAB
Patient-Oriented Evidence That Matters

PORTS
Patient Outcomes Research Team Study

POSCH
Program on the Surgical Control of Hyperlipidemias

POST
Posterior Stroke Trial

PRAISE
Prospective Randomized Amlodipine Survival Evaluation

PRCCT
Prospective Randomized Controlled Clinical Trials

PREVENT
Prevention of Recurrent Venous Thromboembolism
Proliferation Reduction with Vascular Energy Trial
Prospective Randomized Evaluation of the Vascular Effects of Norvasc Trial

PRISM
Platelet Receptor Inhibition for Ischemic Syndrome Management
Prospective Record of the Impact and Severity of Menstrual Symptoms

PRISM-PLUS
Platelet Receptor Inhibition for Ischemic Syndrome Management in Patients Limited to Very Unstable Signs and Symptoms

PROOF
Prevent Recurrence of Osteoporotic Fractures

PURSUIT
Platelet Glycoprotein IIb/IIIa in Unstable Angina; Receptor Suppression Using Integrilin Therapy

QOLHS
Quality of Life Hypertension Study

QoLITY
Quality of Life Trial Hypertension

QUIET
Quinapril Ischemic Event Trial

R3
ReoPro Readministration Registry

RACE
Ramipril Angiotensin Converting Enzyme Inhibition

RADAR
Rapid Assessment of Disease Activity in Rheumatology

RADIANCE
Randomized Assessment of Digoxin on Inhibitors of Angiotensin-Converting Enzyme

RALES
Randomized Aldactone Evaluation Study

RAPPORT
ReoPro in Acute Myocardial Infarction and Primary PTCA Organization and Randomized Trial

REGRESS
Regression Growth Evaluation Statin Study

REIN
Ramipril Efficacy in Nephropathy

REST
Restenosis Stent Trial

RESTORE
Randomized Efficacy Study of Tirofiban for Outcomes and Restenosis

RIGHT
Cerivastatin Gemfibrozil Hyperlipidemia Treatment

RISC
Research on Instability in Coronary Artery Disease

RITA
Randomized Intervention in the Treatment of Angina

ROSTER
Rotational Atherectomy versus Balloon Angioplasty for Diffuse In-Stent Restenosis

4S
Scandinavian Simvastatin Survival Study

SAVE
Survival and Ventricular Enlargement

SCAT
Simvastatin/Enalapril Coronary Atherosclerosis Regression Trial

SCD-HeFT
Sudden Cardiac Death in Heart Failure Trial

SECURE
Study to Evaluate Carotid Ultrasound Changes with Ramipril and Vitamin E

SENIC
Study on Efficacy of Nosocomial Infection Control

SEQOL
Study of Economics and Quality of Life

SHEP
Systolic Hypertension in the Elderly Program

SHS
Strong Heart Study

SICCO
Stenting in Chronic Coronary Occlusion

SLICC
Systemic Lupus International Collaborating Clinics

SMART
Second Manifestations of Arterial Disease
Serum Markers Acute Myocardial Infarction and Rapid Treatment
Study of Medicine versus Angioplasty Reperfusion Trial
Study of Microstent's Ability to Limit Restenosis Trial
Study of Monoclonal Antibody Radioimmunotherapy

SMILE
Survival of Myocardial Infarction: Long-Term Evaluation

SNAP
Study of Nitroglycerin and Chest Pain

SOLVD
Studies of Left Ventricular Dysfunction

SPAF
Stroke Prevention in Atrial Fibrillation

SPAF TEE
Stroke Prevention in Atrial Fibrillation III Transesophageal Echocardiogram

SPINAF
Stroke Prevention in Nonrheumatic Atrial Fibrillation

SPORT
Stent Implantation Post Rotational Atherectomy Trial

SPRINT
Secondary Prevention Reinfarction Israeli Nifedipine Trial

SSSS
Scandinavian Simvastatin Survival Study

STAMI
Stenting for Acute Myocardial Infarction

STAMP
Solid Tumor Autologous Marrow Transplant Program

STAR
Study of Tamoxifen and Raloxifene

STAR*ICU
Strategies to Reduce Transmission of Antimicrobial Resistant Bacteria in Intensive Care Units

STARS
Stent Antithrombotic Regimen Study

START
Selection of Thymidine Analog Regimen Therapy
Stents and Radiation Therapy
Stent versus Angioplasty Restenosis Trial
Stent versus Directional Coronary Atherectomy Randomized Trial

STENTIM
Stenting in Acute Myocardial Infarction

STENTIM-2
Stenting with Elective Wiktor Stent in Acute Myocardial Infarction

STENT PAMI
Stent Primary Angioplasty for Myocardial Infarction

STICH
Surgical Treatment for Intracerebral Hemorrhage

STOP
Stenting of Total Occlusion versus PTCA

STOP-ROP
Supplemental Therapeutic Oxygen for Prethreshold Retinopathy of Prematurity

STRATAS
Study to Determine Rotablator and Transluminal Angioplasty Strategy

STRESS
Stent Restenosis Study

SURE
Serial Ultrasound Analysis of Restenosis

SVCP
Special Virus Cancer Program

SWIFT
Should We Intervene Following Thrombolysis

SYMPHONY
Sibrafiban versus Aspirin to Yield Maximum Protection from Ischemic Heart
Events Post-Acute Coronary Syndromes

TACS
Thrombolysis and Angioplasty in Cardiogenic Shock

TACT
Ticlopidine Angioplasty Coronary Trial

TACTICS
Thrombolysis and Counterpulsation to Improve Cardiogenic Shock Survival
Treat Angina with Aggrastat and Determine Costs of Therapy with Invasive or
Conservative Strategies

TAIM
Trial of Antihypertensive Interventions and Management

TAM
Total Atherosclerosis Management

TAMI
Thrombolysis and Angioplasty in Myocardial Infarction

TASC
Trial of Angioplasty and Stents in Canada

TASS
Ticlopidine Aspirin Stroke Study

TASTE
Ticlopidine Aspirin Stent Evaluation

TAUSA
Thrombolysis and Angioplasty in Unstable Angina

TEAM
Thrombolytic Trial of Eminase in Acute Myocardial Infarction

TECBEST
Transluminal Extraction Catheter Before Stent

TIBET
Total Ischaemic Burden European Trial

TIMI
Thrombin Inhibition in Myocardial Infarction
Thrombolysis in Myocardial Infarction

TIMI-7
Thrombin Inhibition in Myocardial Ischemia

TOAST
Treatment of Acute Stroke Trial

TOHP
Trials of Hypertension Prevention

TOPIT
Transluminal Extraction Catheter or PTCA in Thrombus

TRACE
Trandolapril Cardiac Evaluation

TREAT
Tranilast Restenosis Following Angioplasty Trial

TREND
Trial Reversing Endothelial Dysfunction

TRIM
Thrombin Inhibition in Myocardial Ischemia

UGDP
University Group Diabetes Program

UKPDS
United Kingdom Prospective Diabetes Study

Val-HeFT
Valsartan Heart Failure Trial

VALIANT
Valsartan in Acute Myocardial Infarction Trial

VALUE
Valsartan Antihypertensive Long-Term Use Evaluation

VANQWISH
Veterans Affairs Non-Q-Wave Infarction Strategies in Hospital

VAS
Verapamil Angioplasty Study

VASIS
Vasovagal Syncope International Study

VEGAS
Vein Graft AngioJet Study

VeHF
Veterans Heart Failure

VEST
Vesnarinone Survival Trial

V-HeFT
Veterans Administration Heart Failure Trial

V-HeFT II
Vasodilator Heart Failure Trial II

VHS
Veterans Health Study

VIGOR
Vioxx Gastrointestinal Outcomes Research

VISP
Vitamin Intervention for Stroke Prevention

VITATOPS
Vitamins to Prevent Stroke

VOTE
Value of Transesophageal Echocardiography

VPS
Vaccine Preparedness Study

WESDR
Wisconsin Epidemiologic Study of Diabetic Retinopathy

WEST
Women's Estrogen for Stroke Trial

WIHS
Women's Interagency HIV Study

WINS
Women's Intervention Nutrition Study

WITS
Women and Infants Transmission Study

WRIST
Washington Radiation for In-Stent Restenosis Trial